THIRD EDITION

FORENSIC NEUROPATHOLOGY

THIRD EDITION

FORENSIC NEUROPATHOLOGY

Jan E. Leestma, M.D., M.B.A.

CRC Press
Taylor & Francis Group
Boca Raton London New York

CRC Press is an imprint of the
Taylor & Francis Group, an **informa** business

CRC Press
Taylor & Francis Group
6000 Broken Sound Parkway NW, Suite 300
Boca Raton, FL 33487-2742

First issued in paperback 2020

ISBN-13: 978-1-4398-8750-9 (hbk)
ISBN-13: 978-0-367-77793-7 (pbk)

Library of Congress Cataloging-in-Publication Data

Leestma, Jan E., author.
Forensic neuropathology / Jan E. Leestma. -- Third edition.
p. ; cm.
Includes bibliographical references and index.
ISBN 978-1-4398-8750-9 (hbk. : alk. paper)
I. Title.
[DNLM: 1. Forensic Pathology--methods. 2. Central Nervous System--pathology. 3. Trauma, Nervous System--pathology. W 700]

RA1147
614'.1--dc23 2013036875

Visit the Taylor & Francis Web site at
http://www.taylorandfrancis.com

and the CRC Press Web site at
http://www.crcpress.com

Contents

Foreword to the Second Edition

Over half a century ago, a medical examiner office was created for Dade County (Miami, FL) where no such facility had existed. The first chief medical examiner was Dr. Stanley H. Durlacher, 13 years my senior. I was his assistant. I lacked the experience of Dr. Durlacher and considered him my mentor for the future.

After one year in office, Dr. Durlacher experienced a fatal rupture of an aneurysm of the Circle of Willis while attending the Chicago meeting of the American Academy of Forensic Sciences. I was placed in charge and had to develop forensic experience gained from personal scene investigations while working closely with well experienced police homicide investigators, my autopsies, and courtroom cross examinations. Illustrated forensic pathology texts were useful for initial learning but lacked detail and variations demonstrated by our case material.

Neurological problems, natural and violent in origin, were common in my forensic pathology practice. Not clearly diagnosed coma cases were accepted from hospitals because CT and MRI were for the future. Ruptured aneurysms of cerebral arteries were frequent. Each case was carefully evaluated in terms of circumstances correlated with pathological findings—a constant learning experience.

Histological judgment of post event healing time based upon literature and texts failed to help us consistently judge time estimates. References were inadequate. For example, timing of skin bruises based upon published articles failed to correlate with what we had determined as correct based upon careful investigation of circumstances. Two publications appeared that taught me lessons.

In 1957, Robertson published an article on the aging of skin contusions in the *Journal of Forensic Medicine* out of South Africa. An illustration of a 5-day-old bruise appeared as fresh as a 5-minute bruise. Why? Not appreciated by his predecessors, and those since who failed to heed what he observed, was the fact that neutrophilic response was not a response to blood but was in response to escape of intracellular content from damaged tissue cells, an inconsistent component of skin bruises.

Another example concerned evidence of neuronal hypoxia prior to death. Richard Lindenberg, former Luftwaffe neuropathologist and scientist brought to the United States following World War II who served many years as a forensic neuropathologist at the Baltimore Medical Examiner's Office, produced a military publication demonstrating that structural neuronal changes of hypoxia were dependent upon the duration of the agonal period. The more rapid the death, the more changes were apparent, which reflect the fact that sudden death occurs while life functions including enzyme activities are operating to the fullest. Sudden death favored more enzymatic autolysis. Over time, many misconceptions of medical belief have come to my attention in the forensic pathology and toxicology literature.

Now is the time to address misconceptions in forensic neuropathology. The new edition of *Forensic Neuropathology* does so by including contributions from different disciplines.

Kirk Thibault, PhD, a biomechanical engineer with extensive experience in application of physical laws to the study of physical trauma adds to our understanding of craniocerebral injuries. Proper application of biomechanical principles is crucial to expert witness testimony. Conversely, improper distortion of physical laws needs recognition when such appears in literature or the court.

A pathologist is not expected to be a qualified biomechanical engineer but must accept the fact that injurious forces follow laws of physics. The pathologist must be aware of nonmedical contributions made to our understanding of trauma. Ignorant is the pathologist who denigrates the application of biomechanical disciplines to the judging of craniocerebral trauma but accepts erroneous concepts outside laws of physics. I have encountered forensic pathologists who have stated that only a medical doctor is entitled to express opinions of cause and effect of trauma—an illogical *ad hominem* argument.

Forensic in the title of the book clearly implies courts of law. Physicians must realize that the ultimate judges of their professionalism and opinions are not physicians but lawyers in courts of law and through them the public that supports legislatures. Legislators set the parameters of medical practice.

Elaine Whitfield Sharp, JD, an attorney with experience with legal issues of injury, clarifies for the reader the present legal principles that define expert witness testimony. The legal system in which we operate has developed a framework to judge the worth of expert opinion. However, that method involves the adversary system in which attorneys argue for their side of cause and effect. A forensic pathologist must understand the system and be prepared to present logical and correct justifications of opinions.

A major impetus for this creation of a totally new approach to forensic neuropathology are recent concepts associated with expansion of diagnostic criteria used by many physicians to include intent aspects of craniocerebral findings, "nonaccidental" or "abusive head trauma." Dr. Leestma has approached this subject in a logical fashion. His comments augmented by those of Drs. Thibault and Sharp, doctorates in their respective fields, develops this book into a new and refreshing approach to the interpretation of neuropathology. I regret it was not available to me over half a century ago.

Joseph H. Davis, MD

Foreword to the Third Edition

> Logical science: *I will believe it when I see it.*
> Illogical dogma: *I will see it when I believe it.*

The previous edition of *Forensic Neuropathology* appeared in late 2009. Four months later, the National Academy of Sciences' report *Strengthening Forensic Science in the United States* issued, shaking the forensic world even more than had occurred in 1993 following the U.S. Supreme Court *Daubert* decision directing trial judges to bar from the courtroom scientific testimony lacking sufficient indicia of reliability. No longer would it be sufficient that the witness offering the testimony had the proper credentials; the judge was to examine the proffered testimony itself for proper underpinnings. With the issuance of the Academy's 2009 report asserting that essentially *none* of the underpinnings of the scientific testimony used in criminal prosecution had ever been shown to be valid, the question during the post-*Daubert* years as to how knowledgeable trial judges were exercising their mandated gatekeeper role was suddenly brought into sharp relief.

As I began to write this foreword, the much loved and universally respected author of the second edition's foreword—Joseph H. ("Joe") Davis, MD—passed away in his 89th year. An outspoken advocate of fact-based medicine and scorner of medical dogma well into his ninth decade, Joe was my source for the aphorism atop this page. In his foreword, he stressed the crucial need for objectivity on the part of forensic pathologists, especially when they acted as expert witnesses in criminal trials. He ridiculed the assertion he reported encountering among some pathologists that only medical doctors were capable of addressing the causes of human trauma. As a physicist and forensic scientist, I have long been heartened by the attitude expressed by medical practitioners such as Dr. Davis, a forensic pathologist, and Dr. Norman Guthkelch, a wonderful neurosurgeon now in his 98th year, who bear witness to the scientific method by their writings and actions. For hundreds of years, scientists have known that the laws of physics determine what happens in the physical world. This being the case, it is impossible to refer to as scientists those medical practitioners who still nurture a belief in vitalism, that *something* supersedes the laws of physics where animate beings are concerned. Although they may deny this belief, they reveal it by disregarding biomechanical analyses of human injury. They reveal it by suggesting that Newton's laws may not apply to living tissue. In addition to the vitalists, it is impossible to regard as adherents to the scientific method those professors of medicine who dismiss as unhelpful the results of experiments that contradict what the professors already "know" to be true.

Then there are those medical practitioners, whether or not they are vitalists, who respond to calls from the "hard" sciences for more convincing support for their theories by pointing out the obvious, that medicine is not an exact science, and, anticipating suggestions not about to be made, that "ethics" prohibits the types of experiments that would satisfy physicists. Although this response is to a degree justified when the subject is a theory or practice aimed at improving health or extending life, it is worse than worthless when used to support a theory used to imprison persons. In 2008, Dr. Davis expressed special concern for what he perceived as the then-recent concepts used by some physicians to find criminal *intent* in certain craniocerebral findings. He was referring to the so-called shaken baby syndrome theory of murderous assault. To his disappointment, the succeeding years saw this theory spread throughout the criminal justice system and even into state legislatures, urged on by the type of advocate Eric Hofer long ago analyzed in his *True Believers.* That this theory regarding the effect of force on the human body has the support of no physical scientist or engineer and yet nevertheless continues to give rise to testimony admitted into evidence at trial is a discouraging phenomenon. Unfortunately, there is a tradition among trial judges of immunizing medical testimony for the prosecution from the reliability tests imposed on nonmedical expert testimony at least since the *Daubert* decision.

This book derives from one launched a quarter of a century ago, one that was to become a standard in its field. In 2009, Dr. Leestma, with collaborators, published the second edition, not only revising and expanding the original text, but including material on biomechanics, perhaps for the first time in a medical text written by medical people. In addition, the second edition presented a chapter on legal procedure and scientific evidence in the post-*Daubert* world. All true scientists practicing in the forensic arena should welcome this new edition in the wake of the forensic sciences report of the National Academy of Sciences, a report that was most welcome to those who already were aware of the facts that surprised so many laypersons, lawyers, and judges.

Thomas L. Bohan, PhD, JD

Preface

Forensic pathology and neuropathology have much in common. Both fields are well recognized within the medical and legal professions; both are subspecialties recognized by the American Board of Pathology, which offers certification in those fields, and both fields demand similar attributes in their practitioners. These include the basic skills of the anatomic pathologist and morbid anatomist; a broad scientific, medical, and pathological knowledge; a firm background in the basic physical and medical sciences; highly developed analytical skills; and a constant desire to confront the unusual and the unknown and to search for answers to innumerable questions that arise every day in the course of their practices. Both fields make use of all other disciplines of medicine, the physical and life sciences, and yet, traditionally, comparatively few practitioners of either discipline have developed a close working relationship with practitioners of the other to share their expertise and further their efforts toward a common goal. In part this has been due to physical separation, with comparatively few forensic pathology units being associated, administratively or physically, with hospitals or medical schools in the United States; however, this is changing.

Over the past 40+ years, as both forensic pathology and neuropathology have grown in sophistication, the two specialties have had increasing interaction, and now many forensic pathologists also have neuropathology training and often board certification in neuropathology.

A particularly seminal interaction was begun by the late Dr. Russell S. Fisher, former chief medical examiner for the state of Maryland and former member of the American Board of Pathology. Dr. Fisher, in the mid-1950s, established the first formal laboratory of neuropathology associated with a medical examiner's office in the United States and retained the full-time services of an experienced neuropathologist, Dr. Richard Lindenberg, to serve in that laboratory. Dr. Lindenberg and his faithful collaborator to the end of his life, Ms. Ella Freytag, tirelessly offered the full range of neuropathological expertise to the Maryland State Medical Examiner's Office and influenced several generations of trainees in forensic pathology, general pathology, neuropathology, neurology, and neurosurgery through their popular evening show-and-tell sessions that were held regularly for several years in the unforgettable old city morgue on the now-refurbished Baltimore waterfront and later in the modern medical examiner's buildings near the University of Maryland Medical Center. These exciting sessions drew visitors from all along the East Coast of the United States. They came to view an unparalleled array of fascinating case material, available virtually nowhere else. Those who attended these sessions and who were stimulated by the late Dr. Lindenberg have formed an ever-expanding cadre of individuals who have developed the interactions between forensic pathology and neuropathology wherever they have gone and influenced still other generations of pathologists and other specialists as to the richness of the case material to be found in the forensic neuropathological material.

It should not pass without acknowledging the passing of Dr. Joseph H. Davis, the long time Chief Medical Examiner of the Miami–Dade facility. Dr. Davis, who wrote the foreword to the second edition of this book, was a dedicated, scholarly, and knowledgeable pathologist who influenced many and made major contributions to forensic pathology over his long career.

Like any other field of science or medicine, change occurs constantly. While the autopsy rate in hospitals has declined, and with it expertise in autopsy pathology, the case load has increased for forensic pathology services all across the United States. Natural and other disasters have focused attention upon forensic pathologists and demonstrated how important this discipline is to the public welfare. DNA trace analysis technologies have changed the landscape of forensic pathology and the legal system, and many once-sacred forensic tools have been shown to be unreliable. The increasing sophistication of the legal community has increased demand for many areas of highly specialized knowledge and expertise, including neuropathology. Within forensic pathology and neuropathology, the discipline of injury biomechanics has evolved as a vital area of science to both, yet most recent forensic pathology texts make little mention or little use of the wealth of injury biomechanics information and its applications to forensics.

In the short period before the publication of this edition of *Forensic Neuropathology*, one measure of the increasing attention being paid to the forensic aspects of neuropathology has been the appearance of several new books dealing with forensic neuropathology. These include Dolinak and Matshes, *Medicolegal Neuropathology: A Color Atlas* (CRC Press); Oehmichen et al., *Forensic Neuropathology and Neurology* (Springer); Whitwell, *Forensic Neuropathology* (Hodder Arnold); and Itabashi et al., *Forensic Neuropathology: A Practical Review of the Fundamentals* (Academic Press). Each brings a different perspective to the discipline. It is hoped that this new edition of *Forensic Neuropathology* will complement the growing literature and prove as helpful to forensic pathologists as the first and second editions proved to be.

One would be remiss by not mentioning the original text with the name *Forensic Neuropathology*, by Cyril Courville (Callaghan & Co., Mundelein, IL, 1964), which is now a collector's item. In a sense this book and the numerous articles Dr. Courville published over his career pointed the way for what has become a discipline in itself—forensic neuropathology.

In the second edition of *Forensic Neuropathology*, much of the original content was nearly totally or substantially rewritten in response to the incredible increase in knowledge and scientific progress in the past 20 years. This same process applies to the third edition. A number of changes are noteworthy. The evolution of new perspectives and rules regarding expert testimony and evidence admissibility, occasioned by the landmark *Daubert* and related Supreme Court rulings on expert testimony, called for a discussion of the relevance of these decisions on how forensic pathologists, neuropathologists, and other potential experts can and must interact with the legal system. The standards for veracity and reliability of expert testimony are not the same as they were and are still evolving as courts incorporate them into their day-to-day practice. The medical profession, not necessarily driven by the legal environment but on its own, has called for so-called evidence-based medicine to underscore clinical decision making and medical education. All of these movements call for what should be and should have been the gold standard—solid science and evidence to back up the way we do things and what we purport to say we know against the basic framework of logic.

In this third edition of *Forensic Neuropathology*, much of the content of the second edition remains, but the steady march of progress in medical science and forensic medicine requires editing, additions, and in some cases deletions of material that has diminished in relevance or is in error. Regrettably, the problem of child abuse is still very much with us, and many aspects of its pathology and causality remain controversial. Injury biomechanics has continued to evolve and provide important science, which can be of enormous value to forensic pathologists. Like many relatively new additions to the body of pathology knowledge, incorporation of this information into one's armamentarium requires often painful relearning of long neglected or forgotten mathematics and physics. The expanding field of molecular genetics has more and more forensic import, and may require totally new learning to be abreast of the latest body of knowledge. It should be abundantly clear that in the field of forensics, life-long learning is no longer discretionary, it is a requirement of professionalism (and for the "Boards," which now require recertification every 10 years).

This new edition, like most new medical books, uses an all-color format for the figures. Some of the previous figures were replaced with better-quality color photographs, while many are reproduced here from the original Kodachromes. Again, modern technology has offered new opportunities not only for the authors but also for the readers. Readers will note that for this third edition of *Forensic Neuropathology*, the Taylor & Francis Group (CRC Press) continues as its publisher.

Taylor & Francis have published and continue to publish important high-quality books in forensic sciences. It is hoped that this book will complement an already strong bibliography for them. The professionalism of the staff of Taylor & Francis is appreciated by the authors.

Jan E. Leestma, MD, MBA

Acknowledgments

The authors thank the following individuals and organizations for their contributions, direct and indirect, and for making the second edition and now the third edition of *Forensic Neuropathology* possible. In the first edition, many individuals made important contributions. Their contributions are again acknowledged, even though many have retired or died. Collectively, thanks go to the pathologists at the Cook County Medical Examiner's Office during the years 1977–1986, the Department of Pathology of the District of Columbia General Hospital, Washington, DC, 1969–1971, and the many excellent pathologists at the Armed Forces Institute of Pathology, Washington, DC, with whom the lead author worked during the years 1968–1971 and who provided the opportunity to examine a wealth of forensic neuropathological material and the case material for many figures that are used in this book. Without their eager assistance, this edition and the first edition of this book would not have been possible. Specifically deserving of mention are the late Dr. Robert J. Stein, Dr. J. Douglas Balentine, Dr. Richard Lindenberg, Dr. Kenneth M. Earle, Professor Nenad Grcevic, and Dr. Joseph H. Davis. From the Cook County Medical Examiner's Office during the late 1970s and early 1980s, I acknowledge the assistance of Drs. Edmund Donoghue, Mitra Kalelkar, Shaku Teas, Eupil Choi, Ty-Lyong An, Michael Chambliss, Yuksel Konakci, Barry Lifschultz, H. Wayne Carver, Lee F. Beamer, Joann M. Richmond, and Carol Haller.

Other pathologists who have contributed in intellectual or material ways to the second edition include Drs. Joseph H. Davis (who wrote the foreword for the second edition and has recently died), John Plunkett, Janice Ophoven, Patrick Lantz, Mark Shuman, Jennian Geddes, Helen Whitwell, Waney Squier, Andreas Buettner, Edward N. Willey, Darinka Mileusnic-Polchan, David Wolfe, John Galaznik, and Willam C. Schoene, and the forensic pathologists at the Institute for Forensic Sciences, San Juan, Puerto Rico. The late professor Werner Goldsmith, of the University of California, Berkeley (Biomechanics), deserves special personal gratitude for his wisdom and kind patience even when he was desperately ill. Other biomechanicians whose advice, counsel, and contributions deserve mention are Faris Bandak, Larry Thibault (recently deceased) and his son, Kirk Thibault, and Chris Van Ee.

Others that deserve mention for contributions in the past edition and for the third edition are Drs. Edward N. Willey, Thomas L. Bohan, Steven Gabaeff, Peter J.T. Stephens, Julie Mack, Irene Scheimberg, Marta Cohen, John Lloyd, Patrick D. Barnes, and many others. I particularly wish to acknowledge the continued assistance and counsel of Becky Masterman of CRC Press/Taylor & Francis, the publishers of this book.

As often happens when one collects and shares case materials with colleagues, microscopic slides and photographs often lose identifications of origin. It is inevitable that some photographs will appear in this book, as they did in the prior ones, that do not have an attribution, simply because it has been lost or strayed. In some cases, the origin of previously published figures was discovered and attribution is now given or corrected. If a reader should happen to recognize one of his or her cases without attribution, we hope that this oversight will be understood and that satisfaction might be gained for having shared a good example of a process for the benefit of a larger audience, perhaps advancing someone else's learning. For all such anonymous individuals, I thank you for your kindness in sharing your case material with me and our readers.

Author

Jan E. Leestma, MD, MBA, is the lead author of this third edition of *Forensic Neuropathology*. He received a BA degree in chemistry and biology from Hope College in Holland, Michigan, in 1960 and an MD degree from the University of Michigan, Ann Arbor, Michigan, in 1964. He completed residency training in anatomic and neuropathology at the University of Colorado Medical Center, Denver, and a neuropathology fellowship at the Albert Einstein College of Medicine, Bronx, New York. He is certified in both anatomic and neuropathology by the American Board of Pathology (1970). He served in the U.S. Air Force Medical Corps at the Armed Forces Institute of Pathology, Washington, DC (1968–1971), and was honorably discharged with the rank of major, USAF MC. He was granted a masters degree in management (MBA) by the J. L. Kellogg Graduate School of Management of Northwestern University, Evanston, Illinois in 1986. Dr. Leestma was an assistant and associate professor of pathology and neurology at Northwestern University School of Medicine (1971–1986) and served as chief of neuropathology at both Northwestern Memorial Hospital and the Children's Memorial Hospitals, Chicago. He was professor of pathology and neurology and dean of students for the Division of the Biological Sciences and the Pritzker School of Medicine at the University of Chicago, Chicago, Illinois (1986–1987). He was an assistant medical examiner and neuropathology consultant to the Office of the Medical Examiner, Cook County, Illinois (1977–1987). Dr. Leestma was a guest researcher at the Karolinska Institutet, Huddinge University Hospital, Pathology Institute, Stockholm, Sweden (1981–1982). He was associate medical director and chief of neuropathology at the Chicago Institute of Neurosurgery and Neuroresearch in Chicago (1987–2003). He has had a private consulting practice in forensic neuropathology since the early 1970s that continues to the present time, and he has given expert testimony in more than 40 states, Canada, and the United Kingdom. Dr. Leestma is the author of more than 100 professional publications, including numerous book chapters in texts. He was the author of *Forensic Neuropathology*, first edition, Raven Press, New York, 1988, and the second edition published by CRC Press/Taylor & Francis, Boca Raton, in 2009. He is a member of the American Association of Neuropathologists and a fellow of the American Academy of Forensic Sciences. He resides in Chicago, Illinois.

Contributors

Thomas Lynch Bohan, PhD, JD, received his SB degree in physics from the University of Chicago and PhD also in physics from the University of Illinois at Urbana–Champaign. After a career in physics research and education with the U.S. Army, the semiconductor industry, and universities in the United States and abroad, he enrolled in law school in the late 1970s, receiving his JD from the Franklin Pierce Law Center in Concord, New Hampshire in 1980. Since then, he has practiced law and forensic science, a dual career leading to a special interest in scientific-evidence admissibility, an interest that deepened following the 1993 U.S. Supreme Court *Daubert* decision. He has written and spoken extensively on the subject, being perhaps the first to speak formally regarding *Daubert* and its potential consequences. Because of his advocacy for scientific-evidence reliability, he has been especially concerned with what he perceives to be the admission into evidence of *ipse dixit* medical testimony and the slowness with which the judiciary has applied to expert medical testimony the reliability tests routinely used with other forensic testimony. In 2002, he joined the other physical scientists and engineers who support those physicians seeking to ensure that medical testimony in criminal cases is evidence-based. Dr. Bohan has served as president of the American Academy of Forensic Sciences and as an officer in other professional forensic organizations, including the Forensic Specialties Accreditation Board. He is certified by the International Board of Forensic Engineering Sciences. Over his 40-year career, he has published papers in the refereed literature of physics and forensic science as well as articles in the popular press. In 2009, he published *Crashes and Collapses*, an exposition of forensic science for the general public; from 1995 until 2006, he was the contributing editor of the two-volume set *Forensic Accident Investigation* and its annual supplements. He is a member of the bars of several state and federal jurisdictions including that of the Supreme Court of the United States. His honors and awards include being named in 2010 "Profesor Honorario" of Peru's University of San Marcos, where he served as a Fulbright Visiting Professor of Physics in the early 1970s. Dr. Bohan resides at Peaks Island, Maine.

Joseph H. Davis, MD, was a graduate of Long Island College of Medicine (1949). He served an internship and residency in pathology at the University of California School of Medicine, the University of Washington in Seattle, and the Public Health Service Hospital in New Orleans, serving also with the Public Health Service in the Department of Indian Affairs. He served on the faculty and was a coroner's pathologist at Louisiana State University and Charity Hospital in New Orleans. He is certified by the American Board of Pathology in anatomic pathology and forensic pathology. Dr. Davis became an assistant medical examiner and, later, chief medical examiner for Miami–Dade County, Florida, serving there from 1956 until his first retirement in 1996 but resuming temporary duties there again until he retired for good in 2000. He was also professor of legal medicine and professor of pathology at the University of Miami School of Medicine. In his long and distinguished career, he has served in numerous consultative positions and has been the recipient of numerous honors and awards. He has served as president of the National Association of

Medical Examiners as well as president of the American Academy of Forensic Sciences. Dr. Davis is the author of a long list of professional publications in the forensic sciences and forensic pathology, including several book chapters. Sadly, Dr. Davis died in March of 2013 at the age of 89 years.

Joel B. Kirkpatrick, MD, is a graduate of Washington University School of Medicine, St. Louis, Missouri (1962). His residency training in anatomic and neuropathology was done at Washington University and Barnes Hospital in St. Louis (1962–1967). He is certified by the American Board of Pathology in both anatomic and neuropathology. He is the author of numerous publications in neuropathology and experimental neurology. Dr. Kirkpatrick held academic positions at the University of Texas and Southwestern in Dallas, Texas, and was a consultant to the Institute of Forensic Sciences (Dr. Charles Petty), also in Dallas. He was a professor of pathology at Baylor College of Medicine and the Methodist Hospital in Houston, Texas until his retirement in 1999. He currently has an appointment as visiting assistant professor of neurology, University of Texas Southwestern Medical School, Dallas. He resides in Waxahatchie, Texas, and Baden, Austria.

Elaine Whitfield Sharp, JD, is an attorney who has focused her private practice on forensic issues and scientific evidence for more than a decade. Ms. Sharp began practicing law in 1987, when she worked on criminal appeals for both defense and prosecution agencies, after which she was sworn in as an assistant attorney general for the State of Michigan and served in the Transportation Division, the Special Litigation Division, and the Corrections Division. Ms. Sharp opened her private practice in Michigan in late 1989. Ms. Sharp was admitted to practice in Massachusetts in 1993. Ms. Sharp has handled several high-profile criminal cases in the past decade; she was the architect with the experts of the forensic defense in *Commonwealth of Massachusetts v. Louise Woodward*, and in 2000 she represented the family members of Albert DeSalvo in their bid to clear his name as the Boston Strangler and family members of Mary Sullivan, the last victim of the so-called strangler, who joined forces with them because they did not believe DeSalvo was her killer. Ms. Sharp also handles a variety of civil cases involving allegations of federal constitutional violations. As a graduate of the Wyoming-based Gerry Spence Trial Lawyers College (TLC), Ms. Sharp has written about science and the law for the TLC's journal, *The Warrior*. She was selected by her TLC peers as Warrior of the Year in 2004 for the northeastern region for her *pro bono* services in assisting other lawyers with forensic questions. Ms. Sharp has presented at the American Bar Association on several cold cases and has spoken to defense organizations and the American Academy of Forensic Sciences on scientific issues in the law. Ms. Sharp has appeared in numerous states to assist counsel in cases involving forensic issues and has consulted with lawyers in every state on such issues, frequently authoring briefs for *Daubert* or *Frye* hearings in criminal and civil cases. Ms. Sharp earned her bachelor's degree in journalism and political science from the University of Michigan at Ann Arbor in 1980, after which she wrote a variety of news articles and investigative features for numerous state and national newspapers and was a contributor to Michigan Public Radio. Ms. Sharp earned her law degree from the University of Detroit Mercy School of Law, a Jesuit law school, in 1987. Ms. Sharp has been a frequent commentator on CNN, Fox News, and other national and local news channels on cases of forensic interest. She lives and practices in Marblehead, Massachusetts and is currently working on books that detail forensic issues in high-profile cases. Her husband and partner, Daniel Sharp, Esq., is recently deceased.

Ms. Sharp is a member of the American Academy of Forensic Sciences, the New York Academy of Sciences, the American Association for the Advancement of Science, and the American Association of Justice, where she is an active member of the Medical Malpractice and Expert Witness sections. Ms. Sharp is admitted to practice in federal courts in Michigan and Massachusetts, the U.S. Court of Appeals for the First Circuit and the Sixth Circuit, and the U.S. Court of Federal Claims, where she litigates vaccine injury and death cases under the National Childhood Vaccine Injury Compensation Acts. She resides in Marblehead, Massachusetts. She is a board member of the National Lawyers Guild.

Kirk L. Thibault, PhD, earned his BSE in mechanical engineering (1991) and his MS (1993) and PhD (1997) in bioengineering from the University of Pennsylvania. Dr. Thibault's research activities have included studies of the biomechanics of central nervous system injury, with a particular emphasis on the age-dependent, pathophysiologic response of the infant and young child to head impact loading. He has extensive experience in mechanical testing, analysis, and modeling of biological materials/structures and their injury mechanisms. Dr. Thibault's current research interests include the application of his basic research to the development of an age-specific computational model of pediatric head injury and the design of a more biofidelic infant head form. Kirk has published and presented numerous articles in the field of injury biomechanics and has received a number of awards, including Centers for Disease Control Research Fellow, University of Pennsylvania Fellow, and the ASME Young Engineer Award. He is currently owner of Thibault Scientific, LLC, of Wayne, Pennsylvania.

Pathology and Neuropathology in the Forensic Setting

1

JAN E. LEESTMA
ELAINE WHITFIELD SHARP

Contents

The Pathologist and the Justice System

Medical professionals have had a long history of providing valued services to the legal profession as advisers, experts, and sometimes also as attorneys. The legal system has often looked to the medical profession for guidance in attempting to offer justice to the people. Many times this service is advisory to the court, as a so-called friend of the court (*amicus curiae*) regarding interpretation of complex issues of a medical–technical nature. More often, medical professionals are approved, selected, and may be engaged by the court to assist counsels for prosecution or defense in their cases and the court in its judgments. In the course of legal history, the role of the expert (medical and otherwise) has had varying influence on the judicial process and has been subject to evolving standards before the court that will be discussed in detail in Chapter 2.

Most often, a responsible government entity looks to a pathologist to certify deaths that are not otherwise certified by a practicing physician who had knowledge of the deceased. In years past, the bulk of such work was done by hospital pathologists on a contractual basis, but in recent years, forensic pathologists acting as coroner's physicians or medical examiners have assumed much of this role. The forensic pathologist generally functions within the framework of a state, county, or city governmental agency in an official, volunteer, or consulting capacity. He or she may work within a coroner's system in which an appointed or elected official, not necessarily a pathologist or even a physician, is responsible for the administration of the office. There has been a trend toward development of medical examiner systems in which administrative direction is provided not only by a physician pathologist but also by a board-certified forensic pathologist who supervises a staff of other forensic pathologists. Whatever the system, the mission of the forensic pathologist, regardless of his or her position, is essentially to generate a death certificate under circumstances specified by statute.

Certification of Death

Although any licensed physician is empowered to sign a death certification, it frequently may fall to a coroner or medical examiner to generate such a document because there are circumstances that call for a forensic analysis or there is no physician who is willing or able to generate a death certificate for a given individual. If involved, in whatever capacity, the pathologist must endeavor to determine, by whatever method he or she deems appropriate, the medical cause or causes that led to a death and also the manner of death. In most states or other governmental units, the manner of death must fall into one of five categories: homicide, suicide, accident, natural, or undetermined. This quasi-judicial assignment has been criticized by many forensic pathologists as often being arbitrary, confusing, prejudicial, and limiting. Various replacement terminologies have been suggested. Nevertheless, the judgment as to which category a given case belongs resides with the coroner/medical examiner and the forensic pathologist. These determinations are based on the best interpretation of the available facts or may be determined by a coroner's jury or coroner's inquest (in the case of a coroner's system and certain local practices). The determination of the cause and manner of death must appear on the certificate of death, which over the years has become a nearly standard document in the United States. To amplify the information provided on the certificate, contributing causes of death may also appear.

Although the types of cases and the manner in which they come to the attention of the authorities may vary slightly from place to place, according to either convention or statute, in general, the medical examiner or coroner must be notified when [1–4]

1. An individual has died and there is no one who can or will sign the death certificate (unattended by a physician) or a body is unclaimed,
2. There is evidence or suspicion of foul play, accident, criminal abortion, or suicide (violent or unnatural death),
3. An individual dies suddenly and unexpectedly while in apparent good health (found dead),

4. An individual dies within 24 hours of admission to a hospital,
5. Death occurs under anesthesia during an operation, childbirth, or therapeutic procedure,
6. Death occurs during incarceration or while in police or institutional custody,
7. Death occurs in the workplace or the possibility exists that death was due to a toxic agent,
8. Death may be due to some cause that poses a threat to public health,
9. A body is to be cremated, dissected, or buried at sea.

When notified by a hospital, nursing home, police, or other official, the medical examiner or coroner must determine whether the case falls within his or her jurisdiction. If this is found to be so, the medical examiner/coroner, or designee, must determine the cause and manner of death and generate a death certificate before any disposition of the body may take place. Information regarding the circumstances of death may be obtained from investigative staff, personal observations, and interviews at the scene, as well as observations of police or other officials or of medical personnel who may have been associated with the case. The method of collection of information and evidence in any case varies enormously from location to location and may be performed by the coroner or medical examiner, the police or other law enforcement agencies, the state or local health department, the state or local crime laboratory, etc. In special cases, federal agencies or the military may be involved, as in the cases of transportation accidents; deaths in or near military or governmental facilities, Indian reservations, or institutions; deaths on a large scale, as in natural disasters or terrorist attacks; and suspicious or violent deaths of military, diplomatic, governmental, or elected officials. In addition, in the course of investigating special crimes (civil rights violations, kidnapping, environmental disasters, sabotage, terrorist actions, espionage, etc.) or crimes involving interstate issues, federal authorities may have special authority, and responsibility that may involve but rarely supersede those of the local medical examiner/coroner. In recent years, the U.S. Military Services have established their own medical examiner system (AFMES), which descended from the Forensic Pathology Branch at the Armed Forces Institute of Pathology. It is located at Dover Air Force Base, Dover, Delaware.

Based on preliminary data, the coroner or medical examiner may elect not to examine the body in detail and may "certify" death with or without taking blood or other fluids for toxicological examination. As an alternative, it may be decided a more detailed examination is indicated that may include a complete postmortem examination. In most locations, the coroner or medical examiner is able to request a postmortem examination without the necessity of obtaining permission from the next of kin and may also have the power of subpoena to secure evidence or interview persons in connection with the death or may have other powers [3]. When there is some argument or objection to an autopsy or any other function in the death investigation on the part of the next of kin for personal or religious reasons, the issue of whether a forensic autopsy will be performed or whether the investigative method is appropriate may have to be resolved in court.

The Forensic Autopsy

When an autopsy for forensic purposes (official determination of cause and manner of death) is performed, at least in the United States, the designated pathologist generally has wide latitude in the methods to be employed. These may include nonstandard incisions or dissections (as compared to usual hospital autopsy) and retention of any body parts deemed necessary [1,3], including dissection and retention of projectile wounds to any part of the body and dissection of the head, neck, spine, and extremities, with removal and retention of bones and other tissues if needed. If necessary, the entire body may be retained for whatever period of time is required to complete the investigation. The forensic pathologist may not be officially concerned with all the medical aspects of a case, but only those that bear on the ability to identify the deceased, establish natural disease processes that might be present, establish any injuries that may have an exogenous or inflicted basis, and determine the cause and manner of death. This goal-directed approach is often criticized by hospital pathologists as being "sloppy" or unenlightened; nevertheless, it is appropriate that the forensic pathologist perform the procedure required and that the hospital pathologist should do the same. Often, the forensic autopsy is far more detailed and rigorous than any hospital autopsy, for reasons dictated by the facts surrounding the case and the fact that the autopsy rate has fallen in hospital deaths and many pathologists emerging from training programs have comparatively little autopsy experience or interest in the process.

From time to time, unanswered medical questions come back to haunt the forensic pathologist, especially in cases in which a civil suit is brought regarding the death, where the issues may involve underlying or coexistent disease in an individual whose immediate cause and manner of death are obvious, for example, in a vehicular accident in which the victim is burned. In recent years, there have been successful suits that have won huge judgments against defendants in product liability and other liability actions, and many cases are proving to be highly complex and to rely heavily upon pathological expertise not envisioned or employed previously. For example, in claims against automobile manufacturers that allege faulty design of fuel tanks, and with state laws that allow for punitive financial damages for "conscious pain and suffering" prior to death, it may become necessary to exhume and reautopsy victims who had been quite properly "signed out" by forensic authorities as having suffered accidental death due to trauma or burning after a visual inspection of the body and toxicological examination of blood. Such reexaminations may be required to gain insight into whether traumatic injuries underlying the burning or other scenarios were sufficient to render a victim unconscious and thus oblivious to the injuries that followed.

One might argue that the medical examiner/coroner pathologist should have developed this information initially and extended his or her responsibility to avoid any later questions, but strictly speaking, he or she is not compelled to perform studies to suit other parties, only to fulfill the statutory responsibility. It is in cases where complex medical, functional, or mechanistic questions arise in connection with litigation that the consultant neuropathologist or another subspecialist may be asked to become involved.

On many occasions, for one reason or another, a valid autopsy permit may have been obtained on a coroner's case if the death occurred in a hospital or other medical care institution. In such a circumstance, the coroner or medical examiner may deputize or elect to permit the hospital pathologist to perform the examination, with the stipulation that a copy of the report be sent to his or her office in due course, or he or she may preempt this examination and direct that the body be transported to an official facility. At times there may be considerable negotiation over who will perform an autopsy, especially when a given case proves interesting or important for medical reasons to the physicians who had cared for the deceased, but ultimately, the medical examiner/coroner has the last word.

There is often an issue about witnesses who wish or demand to attend an autopsy. Practices vary widely on this matter. Many pathologists do not wish to have police, or other nonmedical personnel present, whereas others allow all manner of persons with various interests to attend. Regardless of what standard is adopted, the pathologist should not permit interference or influence with the task at hand to occur. The standard is that the pathologist should be unbiased, uninfluenced by desired outcomes or opinions, and follow the facts and findings as they unfold, regardless of where they lead. Further, the autopsy is a solemn and serious affair, and the pathologist must prevent, if possible, any exploitation of the proceedings or violation of the deceased's right of privacy.

The Neuropathologist's Role in Forensic Pathology

To the public and probably the legal profession, the field of pathology, and specifically neuropathology, is not understood except in vague terms influenced by popular television and mystery novels. Pathology is a recognized medical specialty with many subspecialty divisions, most of which have their own board certifications by the American Board of Pathology [5].

Pathology is the study of disease in all its forms, how it manifests itself in the various organ systems, the mechanisms by which disease occurs, how it progresses, how the body attempts to overcome the disease process, and how it kills. The effects of treatment, pro and con, are also important in pathology. It should be remembered that disease is any internal or external alteration in normal body function caused by genetic abnormalities, toxins, physical forces, neoplasms, infectious agents, autoimmunity, electromagnetic forces, and radiation, alone or in combination. The pathologist must have knowledge of the basic physical, chemical, and biological sciences as well as a good working knowledge of all the branches of medicine to accomplish his or her mission.

As a practical matter, the pathologist, in general, is not a clinician and does not treat patients as would a surgeon, internist, pediatrician, etc., although he or she may have had training at one time in a clinical specialty. In practice, the pathologist relies on the professional literature, laboratory sciences, radiology, consultants, and performance of an autopsy or examination of various tissues to discover what disease processes might be operating in a given case and how they might have interacted. The neuropathologist does the same things, only within the more focused context of the nervous system. Pathologists may function within the context of a medical care facility, teaching facility, the military, coroner/medical examiner facility, or other settings that may include government and industry. The job requirements vary from environment to environment. In the health care environment the pathologist's work product is directed ultimately to patient care and assisting the clinicians as well as the teaching of students, residents, and fellow physicians. In the forensic environment, the work product, as noted above, is mostly directed to determining cause and manner of death and providing information to the relevant governmental agency.

In the performance of their duties, forensic pathologists (coroner/medical examiners) may enlist whomever they desire to assist with the primary mission—the determination of the cause and manner of death. This often involves the use of expert consultants such as forensic dentists (odontologists), forensic anthropologists, forensic psychiatrists, biomechanicians, and neuropathologists. With regard to the latter, until recently there were very few neuropathologists working on a regular basis with forensic pathologists in coroner/medical examiner facilities, but with the declining hospital autopsy rate and the corresponding scarcity of good neuropathological autopsy material, more and more neuropathologists have sought out forensic pathologists as a source for good teaching material and have taken on the challenge of forensic work in their disciplines. In addition, with more and more professionalism in forensic pathology, the increasing prevalence of medical examiner systems, and the well-known concentration of neuropathological problems in the forensic pathology caseload, the need for subspecialty neuropathologic information has created the demand for neuropathological consultations, and a significant number of pathologists now have training and board certification in forensic pathology as well as neuropathology and function within coroner/medical examiner systems.

The issues that may involve the consulting neuropathologist include a wide range of problems, many of which will tax his or her ingenuity and professional skills. Examples include differentiation of injuries caused by blows vs. falls, interpretation of alleged accidental craniocerebral injuries in suspected child abuse cases, their probable or possible mechanisms including differentiation between accidental injuries and inflicted ones. The determination of the functional significance of brain lesions may be required. The analysis of various diseases that manifest themselves as sudden and unexpected death, and accident reconstructions based on probable neurological deficits caused by central nervous system (CNS) lesions discovered at autopsy (a forensic clinical–pathological correlation) are common tasks. In addition, the analysis may involve the diagnosis of unsuspected intracranial disease processes that may include neoplasms, infectious diseases, malformations, degenerative diseases, neurological manifestations, and effects of drugs, toxins, and other poisonous substances. An important aspect of forensic pathology and neuropathology may involve the resolution of matters that have public health impact, such as diagnosis of various forms of encephalitis, AIDS, prion-caused spongiform encephalopathy diseases (Creutzfeldt–Jakob, bovine spongiform encephalopathy ["mad" cow diseases]), rabies, and many others. It is obvious that many of these issues are normally beyond the capability of even the most skilled forensic general pathologist, and it is indeed fortunate that there is potentially someone well versed in these complex problems that can help. Such increasing interaction between forensic pathologists and neuropathologists, out of necessity and mutual interest, has dramatically facilitated and improved the mission performance of many forensic pathologists in recent years.

Whom Does the Forensic Pathologist Serve?

In a restricted sense the forensic pathologist serves the governmental, institutional, or political system that employs him or her. In a broader sense the medical examiner/coroner and his or her pathologists are servants of the public and guardians of the public health and welfare. Consumers of the service offered by the medical examiner/coroner include many diverse and often incompatible groups, such as prosecuting attorneys and defense attorneys, the courts, special interest groups of consumers, citizens' action groups, labor and other unions, news media, commercial enterprises, politicians, insurance companies, hospital administrators, physicians, and friends and relatives of victims. Each group may expect different and specific actions from the medical examiner/coroner, which he or she may not be willing or able to satisfy. Thus, in the course of his or her duties, the forensic pathologist may come into conflict with the very people who employ him or her and must tread a careful line in not only serving the system and its administrators but also serving a greater constituency in an unbiased and ethical manner. The complexity of this task is illustrated by the dilemma that faces the medical examiner when a governmental official, or prominent personage dies, when an offender or citizen dies and there are accusations of police brutality, or when some other circumstance arises where the glare of publicity, an inflamed public, or media passions intrude into his or her professional activities. In such circumstances it is often very difficult to maintain authority, objectivity, confidentiality, and security so that a professional job can be done.

Within this anxiety-producing context, the professional consultant to the office must be keenly aware of his or her position and that of the forensic pathologist, who also must carefully examine the existing professional and ethical responsibilities and act accordingly. Discretion and confidentiality are often vital, and every consultant must realize that he or she may not be free to discuss or share any findings with friends or colleagues. This restriction represents a considerable departure from the usual academic or hospital professional environment, where interchange of case information is often unfettered and proceeds without a second thought. However, considerable embarrassment and sometimes legal liabilities or complications can result from indiscrete or nonprofessional discussion of happenings or observations in connection with official duties in the forensic setting. If a consultant cannot maintain a professional demeanor that includes an awareness of professional privilege and confidentiality, it would be best that he or she not become involved in situations that require these demands. In the end, any opinion or judgment given must be unbiased, factually correct, and based upon the scientifically supportable information and data.

The Problem of the Manner of Death

As discussed above, the determination of the manner of death is one of the key responsibilities of any official forensic pathological examination and is more complex than might be realized at first. On the one hand, the pathologist is uniquely qualified to determine the medical cause of death of an individual, but on the other hand, his or her competence or supposed omniscience may be severely taxed in determining the manner of death, for this judgment involves a synthesis of medical, circumstantial, and physical evidence and, most often, simply an application of common sense. In this task, the pathologist must rely on others for information that, if collected and recorded properly, enables a cogent analysis and determination. However, as is usually the case, ancillary nonmedical information is garbled, blurred, partial, absent, or has been lost. Judgment based on such imperfect information may involve a great deal of conscientious guesswork and thus be open to error and criticism. Generally for the consultant pathologist (neuropathologist), the most valuable information is objective, i.e., material or information that exists in pure uninterpreted form, such as autopsy photographs, tissue, microscopic slides, radiographs, and scene photographs and physical evidence. Medical records represent a valuable information source but may or may not be completely factual or complete, and thus having an element of nonobjectivity. Witness accounts and other statements may or may not be true or objective and have to be put in context with the objective evidence and form the basis for questions, not answers.

Table 1.1 Certifications by Manner of Death, Cook County Medical Examiner

Natural causes	65%
Homicide	11%
Suicide	4%
Accident (total)	~17%
Drug related	2%
Motor vehicle related	6%
Home/occupational related	6%
Other	5%
Undetermined	~5%

Source: Office of the Medical Examiner, *Annual Report, 1977–1979*, Cook Country, IL, 1979.

An example of the types of cases by manner of death that one urban medical examiner facility (Cook County, Chicago) has encountered can be seen in Table 1.1 [6].

These figures are not markedly different from similar facilities in the United States in the years since 1977. It is obvious that the largest category is the natural manner of death. These types of cases most commonly involve individuals more than 40 years of age, in whom cardiovascular and cerebrovascular disease are the leading etiologies. That is not to say that these cases are always obvious, although many are. For example, if an individual is found dead at home or in the workplace, without a careful analysis that includes an autopsy, it may not be apparent if the case is a suicide (perhaps by some nonobvious means), an accident, a homicide, or a death due to some disease process (natural manner of death). The significance of such a determination may involve a double indemnity payment on a life insurance policy for accidental death, a cancellation of insurance benefits if suicide is declared, or an accusation of murder against someone if homicide is determined. The ramifications of such a decision may mean notoriety, vindication, or ruination of an individual's public reputation, not to mention significant financial reward or loss.

In some circumstances, it may not be possible for the coroner/medical examiner, in a best good-faith judgment, to determine the exact manner of death, in which case the label of "undetermined" may be assigned the case. This is, of course, professionally and intellectually unsatisfying and may lead to considerable criticism and second-guessing by others, including the press; nevertheless, sometimes there is no other option than to admit uncertainty. The consequences of this classification on disposition of certain forensic cases are frequently hotly debated. On the one hand, it might be argued that such a label, undetermined manner of death, will prejudice a State's Attorney from pursuing an indictment, the police from pressing an investigation to search for a perpetrator, or other interested parties from pressing an issue, but it should be pointed out that this judgment by the medical examiner/coroner is not the last word. Although this opinion is certainly admissible in court, the information contained in the case, plus that developed later, may in other hands (a prosecutor, defense attorney, expert witness, etc.) be developed to yield a different opinion. In addition, should other evidence come to light, the death certificate can be amended to reflect a new determination. The basic concept of this category of determination still stands—that at the time and place of the determination, the best judgment of the pathologist was that he or she could not be sure enough to be more specific. Similarly, any other manner of death may be subject to interpretation, argument, and change at some later date as well.

Issues for the Neuropathologist in the Forensic Setting

There are a number of issues and phenomena that are part of the special forensic environment of which any consultant, including the forensic neuropathologist, must be aware. These include the special mission requirements of the forensic pathologist as outlined above and the issue of preservation of evidence and the chain of custody [3,7], the requirements and elements of the forensic report, the nature of the interaction with the forensic pathologist, and the nature of the interaction of the consultant with the courts, defense, plaintiffs, and prosecuting attorneys. There are many issues that center around the consultant's function as an expert medical/scientific witness [8,9] that appear to be growing more complex with each passing year. Many of these will be covered in Chapter 2.

Preservation of Evidence and the Chain of Custody

In the course of the practice of forensic pathology (including forensic neuropathology), physical or other tangible evidence may be discovered or developed that have subsequent importance in whatever legal proceeding may occur. This may take the form of physical objects or personal effects of the deceased, including objects such as a bullet or projectile fragment or other objects discovered in a specimen recovered from the body or brain at the time of autopsy or brain cutting, or it may be the actual neuropathological specimen itself. It may also take the form of a tissue block, paraffin block, or microscopic slide derived from a given autopsy or surgical examination; notes or drawings of a body, body part, or organ; photographs of specimens or body parts; or medical or other records pertaining to the case. It is essential that such evidence or information be precisely identified by case, adequately marked, and preserved by the expert in a logical and secure manner until the case is concluded, sometimes for a considerable period thereafter. Some medical examiner's offices dispose of specimens, even slides, after only a few years, and sometimes, it appears, to frustrate anyone who might wish to reexamine the case, to destroy specimens sooner. This practice is unfortunate and possibly unethical. Preservation of evidence should be one of the earliest actions of attorneys when they become involved in a case either for the defense or for the prosecution. This is especially true of objective (physical) evidence such as a bullet or an important specimen that the neuropathologist might come to possess [1,7,9].

Not only is it important to keep such items secure and marked with sufficient information so as to provide unambiguous and certain identification of their source, but it may also be important to keep a record of where such items were kept, whether their place of storage was secure, who had access to these items, and also to whom any item was given by whom and when, and when and what was returned. Such a written record documents the chain of custody [7]. Although this sort of obsessional record might seem more than is necessary, there are times when just such a record is required, and its absence might prove not only embarrassing but also damaging personally and to the administration of justice [9,10]. Such a situation may arise when a bullet has been discovered in a specimen. It is necessary that the object be marked so as not to damage rifling grooves (an appropriate place to mark would be the base of the bullet); that it be unambiguously retained in a sealed envelope with the case identification plainly on its face with date, time, and place of its acquisition; and that a receipt record be kept of who had possession or access to the object. It may be necessary to produce this record at the time of trial or hearing. If this record does not exist or is flawed, it might be possible to cast enough doubt concerning the identity of the projectile and its connection with the case or with the defendant that the evidence becomes worthless, and an otherwise persuasive case may be terminated for lack of evidence.

As a matter of procedure, when any forensic evidence, especially of a physical nature, is collected by anyone, it should be sealed in some manner, labeled clearly, and securely stored. This may apply to a neuropathologist in the hospital setting who may have occasion to examine a specimen containing a projectile such as a bullet. Under some circumstances local law enforcement officials should be notified of its existence. In any case, if the possessor of this evidence is required or requested to give up custody of this evidence to someone else, a signed receipt should be retained that indicates what was given to whom, when, how, and why. When or if the evidence is returned, its identity should be reestablished along with its condition, and another signed receipt should be obtained (and copy given) that indicates when, how, where, and by whom the evidence was returned. Often a record of these transactions should accompany the physical evidence so as to provide a written chain that establishes the movement of the evidence and its integrity. Such an effort, which need not be in any special form, will obviate difficulties later. A more complete discussion of this issue and techniques commonly employed can be found in many standard texts and monographs.

One of the most frequent forms of evidence the neuropathologist will examine are microscopic slides. A practical procedure for documenting this evidence and all its identifying marks is to place the slides on a copy machine or scanner, and produce an image for later reference. The pathologist may also use this copy to makes notes of what is on the slides, and if photos were taken, and perhaps other information to which he/she may later refer if need be.

The Forensic Neuropathological Report

In many instances, when a consultant is called upon to examine case material and render a diagnosis, a written report may be requested, but not always. It is within the prerogative of the retaining counsel or person seeking consultation to request that no report be prepared and that findings be communicated verbally or informally. That such a request is made is in no way unethical or improper. Each jurisdiction mandates the rules concerning this matter. There are a number of appropriate reasons for this request. In a civil litigation case, a report may be "discoverable" by opposing counsel prior to trial, and various uses may be made of this report that retaining counsels, for their own reasons, may not wish to have happen. One instance of this may be that the report of the expert may not benefit the client of the attorney and might not be introduced in evidence at a trial (or the expert may not be asked to render testimony). In such a situation, one must remember that the consultant may have the burden of work product confidentiality to legal counsel and cannot take it upon himself or herself to go beyond the consulting relationship. There could, however, be circumstances in which the consultant may have a greater burden of responsibility of disclosure, in which case it would behoove one in such a situation to seek independent legal advice for a proper course of action.

The consultant's report may or may not be subject to examination by opposing attorneys, other experts and consultants, and a variety of laypersons, depending upon local practices and statutes. Occasionally, reports are wittingly or unwittingly released to the media. It is important, therefore, that any report be prepared with care. Adherence to general guidelines on the preparation of reports that have forensic import can save much explanation later and sometimes prevent embarrassment.

The consultant neuropathologist's report should identify what was examined. In the case of tissues, a simple listing of what organs were examined may suffice. In the case of microscopic slides or photographs, these should be identified in some fashion. If records or documents were examined, they should be identified and also listed. In general, a consultative report should consist of a descriptive portion dealing with the observations made on the material at hand and a separate portion dealing with conclusions based on the observations and the reasons for them, sometimes listing references. The consultant should inquire of whoever retained him or her as to the form and content desired in his or her report before preparing it. The expert report may be limited to the expert's observations and opinions only or may deal also with an evaluation of the analysis or opinions of others. The length and depth of the report can be highly variable but, as a practical matter, cannot be expected to cover every conceivable detail of the case in anticipation of every possible question an opposing counsel or anyone might have. There are some circumstances, especially in civil litigation cases in many jurisdictions, that mandate that everything the expert might wish to or be called upon to testify upon at a trial must, in some fashion, be in the report; otherwise, such possible testimony might not be permitted. Thus, it is important to have a firm knowledge of what is required before writing a report. In Canada and the United Kingdom, and in some federal jurisdictions, very specific formats for expert opinions may be required employing special verbiage.

The report need not be versed in lay terminology unless requested, but descriptions should be thorough and precise. If conclusions are to be included, they should be to the point and as clearcut as possible, avoiding conjecture, speculation, overinterpretation, and moral or personal judgments. Diagnoses, similarly, should be as precise as possible. When difficult or complex issues arise, these should be discussed clearly and concisely. The consultant should avoid wordiness or rambling interjections of personal opinion and should confine himself or herself to the medical issues at hand that are supportable scientifically. When appropriate, mechanistic conclusions may be included unless specifically requested to the contrary by counsel. Diagrams, photographs, and figures quite properly can be part of a report and may form an invaluable part of it, especially when the report contains descriptions of external lesions, wounds, or injuries. A list of references in support of relevant interpretations is often appropriate. Care should be taken that these references are correctly quoted from and cited. The pages of the report should be consecutively numbered and the last one signed and dated, usually with a statement to the effect that the foregoing is true to a reasonable degree of medical and scientific certainty. A digital, photocopy, or other copy should always be maintained. Some examples of typical forensic pathology reports and consultant's reports can be found in several current forensic pathology texts and articles [11,12].

It should be borne in mind that very often, notes and other materials relating to a report or consultation and the "working file" can be requested of the consultant by opposing counsel and might be subpoenaed (discoverable) for use in depositions, hearings, or trial. For this reason, care should be exercised in maintaining the working file. When such materials are requested, retaining counsel may request or demand that privileged attorney–client materials be removed. When there are concerns about this, they should be discussed with retaining counsel, who may need to seek a judicial ruling on the matter. At times, subpoenas will be issued to an expert to turn over an unreasonable volume of materials or personal documents that have no bearing on the case. Such requests in practical terms may not reasonably or easily be complied with. In most instances of this type, retaining counsel should be informed and can deal with the subpoena, perhaps seeking relief for the expert by a ruling of the court. In any case, a subpoena cannot be ignored and must be obeyed or formally dealt with.

Interactions of the Neuropathologist with Attorneys

The neuropathologist, in the course of normal duties, may come into contact with attorneys who desire information from him or her. There are many circumstances in which this can occur, and it is appropriate for the neuropathologist to be aware of them. In some instances, the involvement may be as an informal consultant, but quite often, the interaction may eventually involve the neuropathologist as a witness requiring an appearance in some form of legal proceeding. The parameters of this special form of interaction are discussed in detail below. One must be aware of issues of patient confidentiality in all secondary consultations.

Interactions in an Official Capacity

If the neuropathologist is involved as a consultant with the forensic pathologists of a coroner's or medical examiner's office, it is likely that he or she will be approached from time to time by attorneys interested in forensic cases in which a report was generated or in which the neuropathologist was involved. These attorneys may be from the State's Attorney's office, the public defender, or a private law firm representing a plaintiff or defendant. Because the coroner or medical examiner in most cases does not, and should not, represent any particular legal interest, and as such is, or should be, an impartial observer (a friend of the court), the consultant should also assume this position. In general, a good rule of thumb when approached about a coroner's case on which one has worked is to inform the coroner or medical examiner that information has been requested and to secure permission before consenting to an interview or responding to a request for information. In most cases, such a request is appropriate and permission given, but occasionally, this may not be so, in which case, it is important to remember that, as a consultant, the neuropathologist does not have primary responsibility for the case and that the person who engaged his or her services has the privilege to restrict access on a formal or informal basis. However, one may be compelled to respond with information or to appear at a hearing, deposition, or trial as a witness if a lawful subpoena is executed, regardless of the wishes of the other parties [13,14].

The Neuropathologist as a Witness

When a neuropathologist is asked to testify either in court, at a deposition, or before some administrative or quasi-judicial body, in most circumstances, this participation has been agreed to in advance and is a matter of choice. However, there are circumstances when the pathologist may not always be appearing voluntarily—that is, one may have been served with a subpoena requiring a mandated appearance. Such instances are rarely without warning and should not be the subject of concern. The command of a subpoena is limited: the person named must appear on the date, time, and place specified (*subpoena ad testificandum*) or may be requested to bring along certain documents or things described in the subpoena, such as reports, microscopic slides, photographs, notes, or physical evidence (*subpoena duces tecum*). In many instances, the issuance of a subpoena is a common practice or formality to ensure that a person, documents, or other evidence are present when required at a hearing, deposition, or trial to allow the orderly functioning of the judicial process and does not have any pejorative connotation for the recipient. At times, the arrival of a subpoena is inconvenient or impossible to comply with; in such cases, upon proper notification of the issuing authority, other arrangements can usually be made. Nevertheless, a subpoena must be taken seriously, for failure to honor it may result in punishment for contempt of court that may include imprisonment, fine, or both. When summoned by subpoena, the recipient is required only to comply with the specific terms of the document and is not required to perform an additional service, research or preparation, or other special activity as might be the case when a neuropathologist is participating voluntarily as a testifying expert.

In most instances in which a neuropathologist or other professional has been served with a subpoena, it is because the pathologist either has personal knowledge of the facts relevant to the particular judicial inquiry or has physical possession of relevant materials such as slides, tissues, photographs, or reports. For example, the pathologist may have performed an autopsy or neuropathological examination on a surgical specimen in connection with regular employment, only to learn years later that one's personal observations and reported findings are now material evidence in a civil or criminal case where that evidence may be important in proving or disproving a crucial material fact. In this circumstance, the pathologist is considered to be the same as any other *fact* witness in the case called to give evidence and is not an expert as such. When testifying in this capacity, one usually only receives stipulated witness and mileage fees, which vary from jurisdiction to jurisdiction. These fees are often nominal and not adequate reimbursement for the time expended. It is therefore appropriate, when served with a subpoena compelling appearance at a deposition or trial, to inquire of the party at whose insistence the subpoena was issued whether it is possible to be paid for time spent at the neuropathologist's usual hourly rate. In the State of Illinois, for example, the Illinois Supreme Court promulgated a rule that now permits a party to pay a reasonable professional fee to a physician or surgeon for the time he or she will spend testifying at any deposition, as long as the fee is paid only after testimony has been given and is only a reimbursement for time actually spent in testimony [15]. However, some jurisdictions may not permit this practice, so it is important to inquire in every instance and not expect a fee as a matter of right. In any case, no fee for professional services may be contingent on the outcome of the case. If contingency payment is involved, the expert may risk loss of his/her medical license and be subject to other penalties.

The Neuropathologist as a Retained Expert

Expert witnesses are regularly used in both criminal and civil litigation to perform an important function in the adjudication of disputes, which in most people's experience occurs at a trial. Trials may be either criminal or civil, and although there are substantive differences between them, both involve the adjudication of contested facts. Every trial involves someone to act as the trier of fact. This may involve trial before a judge only (a bench trial) or may involve a jury trial, in which, customarily, twelve or more people hear the evidence and decide on the facts. When a jury is not used, the judge is the sole determiner of fact. Regardless of the type of trial, it is the function of the expert witness to assist the trier of fact (judge or jury) in understanding the evidence and the facts at issue by testifying as to his or her opinion. The expert is qualified to perform this function by reason of his or her special scientific, technical, or other knowledge gained by experience or training. This function is fully described in the *Federal Rules of Evidence* 702 [16]. This and other rules of evidence are provided in Chapter 2.

When a neuropathologist or other professional is approached by an attorney and asked to provide assistance or to function as an expert witness, there are a number of issues that should be addressed. Not only must the prospective expert interact with the attorney to define what one's role will be in a future action, but he or she must also make other inquiries to ensure that one's participation in the case is possible, is appropriate, and will proceed smoothly and in an orderly manner. Most misunderstandings between experts and retaining attorneys can be avoided by candidly and simply discussing what each party to the arrangement expects from the other, and sometimes a letter of retention is in order.

Whom Do You Represent and Who Are the Parties Involved in the Case?

One of the first questions a prospective expert witness will want to ask of a retaining attorney is the identity of his or her client, whether the case is criminal or civil, and if the client is the plaintiff or defendant in the legal action. It is important to know this information because it is possible that the expert may be unable to represent a certain client by virtue of a conflict of interest. For the same reason, it is important also to know all the other parties involved in the case, for it is common for the expert to have many personal and professional associations, any one of which might create a conflict situation. An example would be if the expert learns that the chairman of his or her department may have been retained by opposing counsel or that his or her own institution, or one with which he or she is or was involved, is one of the parties in the action. Other examples might be having a relative, associate, or friend as one of the interested parties or some other connection that is or might be construed as having vested interest in the case. Sometimes it will happen that an expert may have been contacted by an attorney and may have been given information or materials about the case and may perform some work on a case, or decline to be involved, only to be contacted later by the attorney for the opposing side. In general, this should mean that the expert has a conflict, and prior involvement should be divulged. Failure to do so may cause serious problems later. Conflicts of interest cut both ways. Whereas the retaining attorney may not want a neuropathologist or other expert as a witness if a real or potential conflict exists, the expert himself or herself may have reasons for declining to participate in a particular case, which must be respected.

The potential conflict situation is important, because whenever a witness takes the stand during the course of a trial or other formal proceeding as a retained expert, credibility is always at issue. Any time a witness has a demonstrable bias, prejudice, or personal interest in the outcome of a case, it is reasonable to expect opposing counsel to elicit facts relating to the alleged bias in the hope of discrediting the witness's testimony in the eyes of the trier of fact. Disregarding the actual substance of the testimony and the fact that everyone likes to think that one can put aside biases and "do the right thing" when called upon to do so, opposing counsel may argue that the witness, by reason of personal bias, prejudice, or vested interest is not to be believed.

At the outset of an interaction between expert and retaining attorney, care should be taken by both parties to ensure that no disabling conflicts exist, for failure to do so can result in disqualification or impeachment, not to mention embarrassment of the witness and attorney should these facts come to light once the case is underway and considerable time and money have been expended. It is not uncommon that expert witnesses may have had prior lawsuits against them; these may be subject to examination. Credentials and their veracity, including institutional affiliations or appointments, must be factual and not embellished. If the witness has ever been prevented from testifying as an expert, this event may come to light. Any difficulty with the legal system, including arrests or substance abuse issues, must be brought to the attention of the retaining counsel. Time taken to explore these uncomfortable issues is always time well spent [13].

There may be circumstances in which an expert, once it becomes known that he or she is involved in a notorious or highly publicized case, may be subject to political pressure either to not testify or to provide certain desired testimony. Once the legal proceedings have commenced and a potential witness has been divulged to the court, such meddling is not only inappropriate but also unlawful and can expose the "meddler" to severe punishment under the general mantle of witness tampering. If one has become the target of such attempts, the court and certainly retaining counsel should be informed. In some circumstances it may be necessary to inform the State's Attorney General or U.S. Attorney's office of attempts made to coerce or influence testimony. These occasions are often taken very seriously.

What Do You Expect Me to Do?

When a pathologist is approached by an attorney and asked to act as an expert witness in his or her case, the pathologist should determine exactly what the attorney expects one to do. Not all experts perform in the same capacity in every case, and the involvement may be major and crucial or relatively minor. The expert may be asked to serve as a consultant only in the preparation of the case with no requirement for testimony, or he or she may be asked to not only consult but also be prepared to offer evidence at a deposition or trial.

Many jurisdictions have different procedures for experts, depending upon whether they will be acting as a consultant or testifying expert. For example, in some states, the identity of a consulting expert need only be disclosed to opposing counsel and the court if the attorney expects to call the expert as a witness at trial. However, disclosure may be ordered if opposing counsel demonstrates exceptional circumstances under which it is impractical for a party seeking discovery to obtain facts or opinions on the same subject by other means [17]. When testimony is anticipated, the expert's identity must be disclosed well in advance of trial so that opposing counsel can undertake a pretrial discovery regarding the expert's opinions and the bases for any opinions. Whether discovery depositions may be taken is often a local jurisdictional matter, although in civil litigation, it is generally expected. In some states, criminal cases may allow depositions of experts as well.

If a pathologist would like to do forensic work but lacks the enthusiasm for the adversarial aspects of litigation, such as being examined and cross-examined in open court, acting only as a consulting expert is a viable and appropriate option. It is not uncommon for an attorney to retain a consulting expert to assist in trial preparation and to coordinate the preparation of testifying experts, as well as to educate the retaining attorney on complex medical or technical issues involved in the case, so that he or she may more effectively examine opposing experts and present the case in court. It is certainly within the professional prerogative of an expert to choose to limit his or her participation. A consulting expert may also be asked to assist in retention of an expert who is prepared to testify, because an expert is certainly more prepared to know who are the experts in a given field than is the typical attorney. Once a prospective testifying expert has been identified, it may be appropriate and desirable for the consulting expert to make the initial contact to determine whether the individual is even interested in becoming involved. This is to the advantage of the attorney because it is more likely that a desired expert will respond favorably to an inquiry from a colleague, who can vouch for the attorney and provide initial information, than to an unsolicited call from an unknown attorney about an unfamiliar case.

A consulting expert may also be of considerable help to retaining counsel by developing a strategy to counter opposing counsel's expert witnesses, if the expert finds issues with their proposed testimony, and their testimony as it becomes known. This information usually emerges after opposing counsel identifies those experts whom he or she intends to call at trial. The attorney will then probably want to take discovery (depositions or interrogatories) of those witnesses to learn the subject matter on which the experts will testify as well as the substance of the facts and opinions and the bases for those opinions that will be presented at trial. In preparation for taking oral depositions, a consulting expert might be asked to research the publications listed in the opposing expert's *curriculum vitae* for the purpose of identifying areas of expertise, probable lines of reasoning or support for opinion, as well as exploitable weaknesses or inconsistencies that might exist. Similarly, the consulting expert may be asked to provide counsel with key literature references on the issue in question so that he or she might acquire sufficient background to examine the opposing witness at discovery. Sometimes, the consultant might be asked to formulate questions to be asked of the opposing expert. In most cases, an attorney cannot realistically hope to challenge or even adequately examine an expert on such a complex subject as neuropathology or other medical specialty unassisted, but the same cannot be said for a fellow expert. A testifying expert, unlike a consulting expert, will be expected to testify at discovery and also at trial and may also be asked to perform the same functions as a consulting expert, and it is the usual case that an expert fulfills both roles. It is generally inappropriate for a retained expert to approach an opposing expert on the case in question, or to attempt to influence the opposing expert in any manner. If contact with an opposing expert is sought by retaining or opposing counsel, it would be important that such a contact be fully agreed to by all parties, and possibly involve permission and oversight by the judge in the case.

Once the expert's precise role in the litigation has been defined by questioning the retaining attorney, the next step is to formalize the working arrangement between expert and retaining attorney. This may take the form of a letter of retention. The actual form of such a letter is unimportant, but it should contain certain basic items, including the issue of compensation. Most experts have developed an hourly rate for their services, usually determined by talking with peers about what they charge for given services. It is appropriate to charge different hourly rates or compensation for different services, for example, reviewing records, reading and research, preparation of a report, examination of microscopic slides, examination of a tissue specimen, performance of an autopsy or neuropathological examination, a special analysis or procedure, testimony at discovery deposition or trial, travel or extraordinary expenditures of time, and reimbursement for expenses. Some experts simply charge an hourly or daily fee regardless of what work was done. Despite the financial arrangements, there should be an unequivocal statement in the agreement as to who will be responsible for paying the professional's fee and when it will be paid. Furthermore, the retention agreement should expressly state that the expert's fee is in no way contingent upon the outcome of the litigation. Although attorneys commonly take some types of cases on a contingency fee basis, an expert must never do so. In many states, if any appearance of contingent testimony by an expert can be demonstrated, this may result in disqualification of the witness or be in violation of the state practice standards.

In What Court Is the Case Pending and What Difference Does This Make?

Whenever a neuropathologist or other expert is retained for the purpose of testifying, he or she will want to know the jurisdiction in which the case is pending. This is important to know because there are different procedures regarding expert testimony in different jurisdictions, which are governed to a large extent by the prevailing rules of evidence [16] that determine the admissibility and content of expert opinion and testimony as well as the manner in which these things are presented to the trier of fact (judge or jury). The U.S. (federal) district courts across the country all use the same rules of evidence, which have been codified and are called the *Federal Rules of Evidence* [16]. Many state and local jurisdictions have also adopted these rules, but many states have their own laws of evidence in spite of sharing the same historical lineage in English common law [18]. The practical implications of these differences to the testifying expert involve how the expert's opinion may be presented in court. There have been many changes in recent years relating to expert testimony and its basis. These issues are discussed in detail in Chapter 2. The nuances of laws of evidence for every circumstance are not the concern of the expert witness, but it is helpful to be aware of some of the issues relating to admissibility and suitability of testimony and how to accommodate these constraints. The retaining attorney will assist the expert in any issues relating to the law of evidence and prepare the witness so that his or her testimony can proceed smoothly and without conflict.

What Will I Be Required to Do during the Pretrial Phase of the Case?

Whether the expert is retained to act as a consultant or testifying expert, he or she can expect to be involved during the pretrial phase of the case, as mentioned above, by helping to prepare the attorney for what is to follow and to be prepared by the attorney for his or her part in the proceedings. As also mentioned above, it is common for opposing counsel to request the opportunity to discover, by means of written interrogatories or oral deposition of the witness, exactly what he or she plans to say, the scope of his testimony, and the nature and bases for his or her opinion. The underlying rationale for pretrial discovery is to allow both sides to be aware of each other's case and to avoid what was once typical in legal proceedings—surprise witnesses and so-called trial by ambush.

Discovery is usually the rule in civil cases, where the practice is rather broad and several tools exist to facilitate the process, but in criminal litigation, as dictated by local jurisdictional conventions, the discovery process may or may not be limited and may or may not involve depositions.

The Oral Deposition

As already alluded to, the oral deposition affords attorneys the opportunity to discover what information, if any, a witness possesses regarding the subject matter of a civil lawsuit and, occasionally, a criminal proceeding. As long as there is action pending, any attorney for a party to the action may ask the court to compel any person connected with the action, including expert witnesses and material witnesses, to appear at a specified time and place for the purpose of answering questions put to him or her under oath and subject to the penalties for perjury. The person whose deposition is to be taken, the deponent, may also be required by subpoena or otherwise to bring documents, reports, or other evidence with him or her to the deposition. As far as the expert witness is concerned, the process is straightforward.

At the deposition (which may be with all parties physically present, or via videoconferencing or some other process with only some of the participants physically present with the witness), a court reporter will transcribe the proceedings. The deponent first takes an oath, administered by a court reporter/stenographer, to swear that the evidence about to be given shall be the truth. The expert is then asked questions by opposing attorneys at whose insistence the deposition has been taken. All questions and responses are taken down verbatim by the reporter and form a permanent official record of the proceeding. The deposition may be brief or take days to complete. At times the deposition may be videotaped for later use in lieu of in-person testimony at trial. The initial questions usually involve a review of the training and education as well as institutional affiliations of the witness and also the time and circumstances under which he or she was retained by counsel. Inquiries may be made regarding the expert's testimony and case history. In federal courts, the expert may be asked to provide a list of cases in which sworn testimony was given for the previous 5 or more years. In some state jurisdictions, this may also be required. It is therefore appropriate for anyone who anticipates offering expert testimony to keep a file identifying those cases in which he or she has given testimony in the past. It is not a requirement to provide a listing of cases consulted upon but which never involved sworn testimony.

The questioning then usually proceeds to matters relating to the case. The scope of the inquiry is often very broad—much broader than is generally allowed by the rules of evidence in effect at the time of trial. For example, in federal civil actions, the issue is not whether the matter being inquired about is relevant, but whether the matter under inquiry might reasonably be calculated to lead to admissible evidence at time of trial [16]. In this context, it is proper for counsel to object to a question, the objection being noted for the record, but such objection does not relieve the deponent from the responsibility of answering it because there is no one present who can rule on the merits of the objection. Occasionally, a question may be so far afield or inappropriate that the retaining attorney will instruct the witness not to answer, but he or she may have to argue this position at a later time before a judge.

Good practice dictates that a retained expert spend time preparing for deposition with the same care that one would for an appearance at a trial, keeping in mind that the testimony to be given is being transcribed and can be introduced into evidence at trial in an attempt to discredit or impeach the witness if opposing counsel feels that a misstatement or incorrect or potentially conflicting information has been given. For this reason, inadequate preparation and errors may come back to haunt the deponent at the time of trial, and any experienced attorney will want to avoid this eventuality. The expert should listen carefully to the questions put to him or her; if any are unclear, a request should be made that they be read back, repeated, or rephrased. The witness should not answer open-ended or vague questions or presume to understand the meaning of the question if he or she does not. The expert should try not to volunteer information or anticipate the lines of questioning. A deposition is not a test, and a witness wins no awards for demonstrating breadth of expertise or erudition. The only obligation is to answer truthfully the questions asked. If questions are asked for which the expert does not have an answer or for which he or she cannot recall the answer, it is appropriate and necessary to so state. If questions relate to areas of expertise in which the expert does not consider himself or herself competent, these should be avoided and it should simply be stated that the matter is beyond the witness's area of professional competence. Occasionally, the expert, during the course of the deposition, will recall important details or additional information that should have been given in response to an earlier question. In this case it is appropriate to inform counsel that he or she wishes to amend an earlier answer and to do so. Remember that variances with later testimony may be used to impeach the credibility of the witness at trial.

Although it is usually the opposing counsel who will ask questions of the witness in a deposition, occasionally retaining counsel may wish to query the expert to enter certain information into the record or make clear potentially troublesome or ambiguous points. If there are several attorneys party to the action, all of them may wish to question the witness. In any case, when the deposition is completed, the expert will normally be given the option of reviewing the typed transcript of the deposition when it is available or to "waive signature." What this means is that the witness may choose to read his or her testimony and to make nonsubstantive corrections, such as spelling, in the transcript or may choose to rely on the expertise of the court reporter to have fairly taken down the testimony. As a general rule, it is good practice for the expert not to waive signature and to review the record before signing it, because many reporters have difficulty in understanding and spelling medical or technical terms and may simply have entered them phonetically in the record. Furthermore, if gross or troublesome errors have occurred, or an important word that changes the meaning of crucial testimony has been left out or added (such as an *is* instead of *isn't*) as a result of a stenographic error, retaining counsel can be warned promptly. Another benefit of reviewing one's own testimony is that it can provide valuable feedback on how one has responded to questions under pressure and can assist the expert in improving his or her technique for the future.

Written Interrogatories and Declarations

Another frequently used discovery tool is the written interrogatory, affidavit, or declaration. Interrogatories are written questions that are served by one party on another in a lawsuit. Interrogatories are not directed to the expert himself or herself but rather to retaining counsel, with the aim of discovering ahead of trial or deposition certain basic information about the witness. Under the *Federal Rules of Civil Procedure* [17], a party seeking discovery of the other side's testifying expert must first serve interrogatories that may ask the following: the identity of each expert counsel expects to call, the subject matter on which the expert is expected to testify, and the substance of the facts and opinions to which the expert is expected to testify, and a summary of the grounds for each opinion. Deposition of a witness may not take place until and unless there has been a response to these written interrogatories and the court allows for depositions to take place. It is not uncommon for the court to deny additional discovery in the form of deposition or to impose conditions, limit the scope of additional discovery, or assess fees and costs in connection with additional discovery. The procedures regarding this process vary considerably, but when this process directly affects the expert, he or she will be informed and prepared for this by his retaining attorney. In the court system of the United Kingdom, for example, depositions or testimony may take many forms that can include meetings between opposing experts and the relevant attorneys. If one is involved in non-U.S. judicial systems, it is wise to inquire and to be informed of what the particular convention regarding testimony is.

When the expert is asked to respond to specific interrogatories, they often include the following: areas of expertise (brain tumors, forensic pathology, degenerative diseases, wound ballistics, epilepsy, traumatology, behavioral illness, mental retardation, etc.), the publications relevant to these or other areas the expert has authored, the experience the expert has had in these or other areas, the number and nature of previous legal cases in which he or she was involved, and the number of hours devoted to the case in question. The expert may be asked to provide a *curriculum vitae* and certain information about his or her education, training, experience, licensure, board certification, appointments, memberships in professional organizations, honors received, and lists of abstracts and publications. For this reason, it is appropriate for the expert to prepare a complete *curriculum vitae* containing all these relevant facts, which can be referred to if necessary. The content of the *curriculum vitae* must be accurate and not embellished or nonfactual. The expert may choose to list only peer-reviewed publications (articles and books) and omit a listing of lectures, seminars, talks and other presentations, or abstracts; others include these items and more. If untruths are discovered, the witness may suffer irreparable professional damage and may be disqualified from testifying. Such discoveries are permanent and not easily overcome. There have been instances in which an expert's testimony has been stricken because of falsifications in a *curriculum vitae.* It is possible that perjury charges might be brought if falsifications are deemed serious enough to have violated the oath given at the beginning of the testimony.

Occasionally, an expert will be asked to provide a declaration or affidavit regarding his or her opinions on a case. These latter documents are often required in postjudgment appeals so that the court may assess whether some form of relief from a prior judgment might be warranted. Although essentially the same as a report, often a proscribed format is required that can be provided by retaining counsel. Often in proceedings that occur in Canada and the United Kingdom, the declaration/report may be very extensive and detailed and may call for specific verbiage and content.

What Must Be Done in Preparation for Trial?

In preparing for trial, any expert witness should undertake to review again all information about the case that is relevant to the expert's testimony and opinion as well as whatever literature review might be necessary. At this juncture, this review should involve close consultation with the retaining attorney regarding what the discovery process has disclosed in terms of additional evidence and opinions of other experts, probably in the form of their deposition transcripts and his or her own. The factual contours of a case seldom remain constant, and before the witness takes the witness stand, he or she should have a firm understanding of just how the proposed testimony fits into the case and the other evidence.

It often happens that a witness will want to use exhibits during his or her testimony. Such exhibits should be reviewed before use and may have to be disclosed to opposing counsel. Trial exhibits may be characterized as real or demonstrative. Real evidence is defined as evidence having some historical connection with the case on trial, such as a medical specimen, microscopic slides, a bullet or other projectile recovered from the victim, or photographs of some aspect of the case. Demonstrative evidence, on the other hand, is evidence used to demonstrate or illustrate a witness's testimony [19,20]. Examples of this are a brain model or anatomical diagrams or sketches that will facilitate the explanation of a difficult point or provide background for testimony [14]. Currently, PowerPoint® is a widely used and very powerful tool for communicating visual information and can include video clips and animations. Many court rooms have LCD projectors and other video equipment to facilitate the use of such software.

Experienced trial attorneys know the persuasive value of demonstrative evidence, and the testifying expert should not hesitate to suggest the use of it. To restate an old adage, a picture is worth a thousand words. Sometimes, opposing counsel will challenge the use of real or demonstrative evidence on the grounds that either it is prejudicial (especially gruesome or gory photographs in color, for example) or it is not relevant or factual. One cannot predict if the judge will allow the use of any given piece of evidence, demonstrative or real, and the expert should be prepared to go on without it if it is ruled inadmissible. One must remember that animations and "cartoons," although often graphic, may not represent the facts because of exaggeration or some other tampering with the data and may be misused.

How Is a Trial Conducted?

The culmination of the judicial process is the trial. As previously mentioned, this is the occasion when all the evidence is presented to the trier of fact, judge or jury, who decides the outcome. Evidence is normally presented at trial in specified stages by the parties involved. The plaintiff or the state (the party that has sought the action) has the burden of establishing the facts (the burden of proof) that will entitle that party to get the relief sought and, thus, presents its evidence first. In so doing, counsel will call on, in successive order, the witnesses who will present evidence to support his or her case or claims against the defendant. Such proof may consist of testimony by material witnesses for the purpose of authenticating exhibits and physical evidence or entering into evidence items of personal knowledge about when certain things occurred, what was said or done, and the like. Plaintiff's experts will be asked to present opinions on relevant issues. After the plaintiff rests, it is then the defendant's turn to call his or her witnesses and introduce his or her evidence, after which the defendant rests. At this juncture, the plaintiff may offer evidence in rebuttal, but only in relation to material already introduced into the proceedings. No new evidence may be introduced. The defendant also has the option of offering rebuttal evidence under the same restraints. In some jurisdictions and venues, the jury may submit written questions of a witness to the judge, who may then read the questions to the expert for responses. By the same token, some judges make a practice of also asking questions of the expert.

Following final statements by the attorneys for both parties, the trier of fact (judge or jury) retires to deliberate and eventually renders a verdict. The verdict is the final judgment on the case and must be abided by. There may be a series of appeals if one party or the other feels that there are errors in the proceedings, but these appeals are conducted at a later time before an appellate court where no witnesses or new testimony is usually permitted. In certain appeal proceedings, as mentioned above, declarations or affidavits by experts may be submitted to the court for consideration. These generally provide information that there is new evidence relevant to the case or that evidence presented originally was in error or omitted and should have been considered.

What Will I Be Asked to Do When I Testify?

When a witness testifies, it is under oath in a courtroom before the trier of fact (judge alone, or judge and jury). The party who calls the witness conducts what is known as the direct examination. This takes the form of a series of direct questions of the witness. The attorney will usually begin by asking questions that are designed to qualify the witness as an expert by means of establishing his or her professional credentials, such as his or her training, education, present employment, staff appointments, honors, and publications. The witness will generally be asked to define what his or her specialty is and where and how he or she practices that specialty. The expert may be asked to define the training necessary to attain competence in the field and what board certification means. The questioning may then move on to the substantive matters at hand. During this phase of the testimony, the attorney guides the directions of the testimony by continuing to ask a series of questions that must be nonleading, that is, questions that do not suggest an answer to the witness. The use of leading questions is described in Rule 611(c) of the *Federal Rules of Evidence* [16] as follows:

> Leading questions should not be used on the direct examination of a witness except as may be necessary to develop his testimony. Ordinarily leading questions should be permitted on cross-examination. When a party calls a hostile witness, an adverse party, or a witness identified with an adverse party, interrogation may be by leading questions, of control over a witness, and their use has generally been limited to cross- and re-cross-examinations. Although impossible to promulgate hard and fast rules regarding what is a leading question and what is not, it might be helpful to remember that questions prefaced with one of the following will usually be non-leading: Who? What? When? Where? How? On the other hand, questions that suggest the answer are usually deemed leading and will be objected to.

For the testifying expert, adequate preparation is the key to a successful direct examination. This preparation may involve spending time with the retaining attorney reviewing questions to be asked and the course of the expected examination, and even becoming familiar with the attorney's style by having him or her ask some typical questions and criticize the answers. Some attorneys will want to write out their questions ahead of time and may ask you to help them do so, so that the crucial information can be developed smoothly and completely. When in court and awaiting questioning, the conduct of the expert witness is important. The expert should take care to be punctual. The witness should appear well groomed and dressed in a manner that does not detract from the substance of the testimony and is consistent with a professional mien. The expert should bring only those things required for testimony, such as exhibits, evidence, and notes that may be used. In some venues the volume of notes and documents may be limited, but it is generally permitted that the expert be able to refer to notes to aid in remembrance of facts. The witness must speak slowly, clearly, and forthrightly and maintain eye contact with counsel, the trial judge, and members of the jury. The trial judge should be referred to as "Your Honor." Before leaving the witness box or before performing any demonstration, permission to do so must be obtained from the judge. The witness must ask permission if there is an intention to approach the jury with a piece of evidence or a demonstration, and care should be taken not to personally interact with any member of the jury verbally or physically unless specific permission by the court has been given.

When responding to questions, the expert should always consider the meaning of the question carefully before answering. If the question is unclear or ambiguous, he or she must ask for clarification. Generally, concise, short answers should be given when possible, but lengthy answers are entirely appropriate when necessary to convey meaning. Information should not be volunteered, and questions should not be anticipated. The witness should not pontificate, preach, or lecture. To the extent possible, the expert should face the jury to answer questions, because it is the jury that the witness is there to assist. In the case of a bench trial, it is to the judge that answers are directed.

Juries are as diverse as humankind itself and frequently represent a wide range of cultural and educational backgrounds. Some will be attentive, following every word of testimony, whereas others will appear bored or oblivious to the proceedings and may even sleep. Most experts, such as neuropathologists with teaching experience, however, are adept at dealing with these diverse forms of behavior because they occur in the classroom every day. But the expert must remember that it is the judge who may admonish a sleeping juror, not the witness.

Because much of the evidence a medical expert is likely to present is complex and probably inherently unknown to the jury, the expert must try to avoid the use of jargon as much as possible and explain the meaning of terms that might be unfamiliar to the jury. Illustrative materials and exhibits are especially helpful in this regard, as are photographic slides. The use of analogies can also be a powerful conveyer of meaning and is almost always appreciated by the jury over the dry, technical presentations of a stuffy expert.

While a witness is being examined in court, it is not uncommon for opposing counsel to make objections. Objections can relate to any number of matters, such as the form of a question asked of the witness or admissibility of an exhibit. Whenever an objection is made, the trial judge is obliged to rule on the objection. He or she may agree with the legal basis for the objection, sustain it, and instruct the jury to disregard the offending question or answer or may not allow some evidence or exhibit to be introduced. On the other hand, the judge may not agree and may overrule the objection, thus allowing the expert to proceed. Sometimes the judge may conduct a "side bar" conference with counsel before ruling, or it may be necessary to adjourn the trial for a time to the judge's chambers, where the issue in question is settled with the court reporter present. At such times, if the argument is lengthy, the witness and the jury are excused temporarily. Regardless of when, how, or by whom objections are made, the expert should take cues from the trial judge. The witness should remain silent until the matter is resolved. If allowed to proceed, he or she should do so, but if ordered otherwise, he or she should cease answering in accordance with the ruling. Sometimes objections may seem trivial or arbitrary to the expert witness;

nevertheless, the witness should not interpose himself or herself into the issue and should await instructions from the judge on how to proceed.

At times opposing counsel may interrupt the proceedings to request a *voir dire* examination of the expert. This usually involves exploration of the expert's qualifications regarding a given issue that opposing counsel may be concerned about or some other matter that deals with admissibility of testimony. Such exercises generally occur early in the direct examination, and generally, the jury is excluded from the courtroom. There may be objections over the qualification of the expert, which the judge will decide.

At the conclusion of direct examination, the opposing counsel has the opportunity to cross-examine the expert witness on the testimony and qualifications. Whereas direct examination usually proceeds smoothly and in an orderly manner, cross-examination may not be as easy. That is not to say that one cannot prepare for cross-examination because the witness may have seen opposing counsel in action at a discovery deposition and probably already knows the kinds of questions that will be asked and the areas of difficulty or challenge ahead. A self-critical approach following the deposition can prepare the witness in this regard.

The opposing counsel will certainly be thoroughly familiar with the deposition in the case and possibly other prior testimony on different cases, and he or she will hold the expert to prior opinions and testimony in an effort to show inconsistency if he or she can. Therefore, this testimony must be reviewed carefully by way of preparation. In addition, the cross-examining attorney should be expected to have reviewed any publications by the witness (perhaps with the aid of his or her own experts) in search of possible contradictory statements or opinions that can be used to undermine the witness's credibility. With this in mind, the expert should be familiar with his or her own publications, especially with those having some relevance to the issue at hand, and should be prepared to explain any differences, apparent inconsistencies, or changes of opinion. Similarly, if an expert relies on papers and books written by others, he or she should be prepared to respond intelligently to questions about them. During cross-examination, attorneys commonly attempt to impeach an expert by first eliciting from the witness an admission that a certain book, paper, or work is "authoritative" and then by reading a passage from the authoritative book that either contradicts or is at variance with the expert's prior testimony, casting doubt on the opinion. The expert must be prepared to explain this controversy. This can be done by pointing out that out of necessity any textbook is somewhat out of date owing to delays in writing and publication and that the contents of any chapter or any paper may represent that author's opinion and is not ironclad fact. It is helpful if the expert himself or herself has authored articles, textbooks, or chapters and can explain that no one has exclusive rights to the truth and that, owing to scientific and medical advances, opinions and views change and are not always reflected in an already published book.

Furthermore, the state of knowledge changes constantly, and yesterday's "facts" may have been supplanted or found wrong. The expert should also beware of being drawn into an examination of minute and highly technical points in obscure papers and placing himself or herself in the position of being tested. An attorney may "bone up" on a specialized area and attempt to discredit the expert by showing supposed mastery of a complex subject by exposing the expert's apparent lack of knowledge. This tactic can usually be met by pointing out the volume of medical literature that already exists and the new material that appears each year and noting that no one can possibly memorize every bit of it, which is what libraries and databases are for. If an article is proffered, it is wise for the expert to request to see the article and to take whatever time is necessary to familiarize himself or herself with the article before being drawn into answering specific questions.

During cross-examination, the expert should not engage in guesswork or speculation. If he or she does not know something or cannot remember, he or she should say so. By the same token, the expert should not agree to a generalization or vague statement of "fact" by counsel, or to an inexact, convoluted, or distorted restatement of the expert's opinion, in the interest of simplicity. The expert should never be forced to answer yes or no to a question that does not deserve such an answer. It is popular misconception on the part of physicians that one can be forced into such an answer. Should such an occasion arise in which an attorney attempts to badger an expert in this manner, the witness should state that he or she is unable to answer the question truthfully as posed.

A common issue for physician witnesses in a trial is the question that is often put to them about their certainty of some opinion or judgment as well as the issue of possible or probable alternate opinions or outcomes. In the everyday practice of medicine, physicians are accustomed to acknowledging that probabilities and possibilities exist in diagnosis and, hence, differential diagnosis is commonly used as a conceptual device. But in formal litigation an attorney must attempt to determine the certainty or confidence the expert has in his or her opinion. Often an attempt is made to get the expert to give a percentage of confidence or likelihood of his or her opinion's being correct. Most physicians are thoughtful and self-critical individuals who might be tempted to admit freely to colleagues of being unsure to some degree, or to being fallible, but such an exercise is not needed in court. Depending upon the circumstances (civil or criminal proceedings), the degree of assurance often can fall within the "more likely than not" or "to a reasonable degree of medical certainty" characterization. When faced with this type of questioning, the expert may simply repeat the opinion and state that it was arrived at after carefully considering all the facts to a reasonable degree of medical and scientific certainty and that this is the witness's best judgment. In criminal cases, it is the jury, not the expert, who must determine the degree of veracity and certainty of the purported facts, but the expert in such cases has an added ethical and moral burden, because of the consequences to justice of his or her testimony, that the opinion is sound and based upon robust science.

Cross-examination, although usually relating to the substance of the case and matters covered under direct examination, may pertain to issues that are tangential. Not surprisingly, most experienced trial attorneys are reluctant to fight an expert on his or her own turf, even with the pretrial assistance of another expert. The attorney cannot reasonably expect to acquire in a short time the knowledge and experience of the expert and may attempt to discredit the opposing expert on the basis of some nonsubstantive matter. For example, opposing counsel may directly question or insinuate that the witness's education, training, or experience is suspect or somehow insufficient to justify the opinions given. He or she may impugn the motives of the expert for testifying and may harp on the expert's fee. It may be suggested that if the expert has testified before, his or her opinions are "for sale." An appropriate response to such badgering is not to appear defensive or to over-explain or justify one's fee but to assert quite clearly that, of course, one is being paid to be present and for the time taken away from one's practice but that one's fee is not contingent on the outcome of the case and that, under no circumstances, is the opinion for sale. It is not uncommon for an opposing attorney to ask how much time the expert has spent on the case to date and what his or her bill is or will be, or if the past bills submitted have been paid. The expert may be asked how much income he or she has realized as a result of expert testimony in the past year and what percentage of his or her income is derived from this source. These are all proper questions, and one should be prepared to answer them without rancor or defensiveness.

At the conclusion of the cross-examination, the retaining attorney has the option of posing questions on redirect. These questions are designed to clarify any unresolved or unclear matters already testified to or entered in evidence or to counter points made by opposing counsel. No new evidence may be introduced at this time. At the conclusion of redirect, the opposing counsel has another opportunity at re-cross-examination for the same reasons. Occasionally, the judge may allow several interchanges of redirect and recross, but this is usually limited. In some jurisdictions and in military trials, members of the jury may submit questions to the judge that can be asked of the witness, and it is not uncommon for the judge to ask questions of the witness. These should be answered like any other question—truthfully and completely. Upon conclusion of the testimony, the witness is excused and may leave the stand. The expert will generally have little or nothing left to do with the case, unless the attorney wishes to make use of his or her services in other aspects of the case or in the unlikely instance in which a witness will be recalled or be permitted to hear the testimony of other witnesses. Depending upon the case and special local issues, the expert may be barred from discussing the case with others, including the media, for a finite period of time. Generally, however, once testimony is finished the expert's involvement is concluded.

Implications for the Expert of Having Given Testimony

Because legal trials are open to the public and are thus public records, the expert's testimony may be reported in the media and is certainly available to other interested parties for later examination in the form of the written transcript or recordings of the proceedings. The expert may be solicited for comments or further information about his or her testimony or other aspects of the case that has been tried. It would be entirely inappropriate for any comments to be made before a verdict or other disposition of the case has taken place and is a matter of personal judgment on what comments would be appropriate, if any, at the conclusion of the proceedings. The expert witness is generally not under any obligation to make comments regarding the testimony and may be well advised to refrain from any public pronouncements without first discussing the matter with the retaining attorney.

As a part of the public nature of a legal proceeding, excerpts from a given case, a digest of the issues involved, and a listing of the attorneys and expert witnesses may appear in a number of private legal publications at a later date for the benefit of other attorneys with similar cases. These listings are widely available, and it is possible for anyone to consult indexes of these publications to determine if an expert has testified before, when, where, and what he or she said. A full transcript of testimony can also be obtained for the cost of transcription or copying. This means that in any future case, opposing counsel can have access to any information given in a prior trial if he or she wishes to take the time and effort to seek it out. This information may be valuable in "prereading" a potential expert witness and planning strategy. When one participates in legal hearings and trials, one therefore has to assume that opposing counsel has complete information about a witness's prior participation in any public legal matter and, from review of this material, whether that witness was effective or ineffective. It is therefore in the interest of any expert witness to conduct himself or herself in a professional manner at all times in all public legal proceedings, because somewhere there will be a written record of everything he or she has said. If there are occasions in which the expert's testimony has been impeached because of inconsistency of opinion between that which appeared in an article or book and oral testimony, he or she must be prepared to be questioned about this in future proceedings in which the same issues occur.

As a result of having testified, as mentioned above, the neuropathologist expert may be contacted by other attorneys for his or her opinion on their cases, especially if his or her testimony was memorable in some respect. On these occasions, the neuropathologist should exercise good judgment in determining whether he or she wishes to become involved in the matter, as discussed above. If any expert has been very active in the legal arena and spends a significant portion of his or her professional time in legal activities, there is the risk that he or she will become characterized as a professional witness whose opinions are for sale to the highest bidder or that the expert is a defense or prosecution witness and thus unreliable. Regrettably, sometimes this is the case, but this cannot and should not be assumed to be true. It may happen that an expert has acquired special expertise that may lead to being called again and again in a certain type of case, for example, automobile crash analysts who are called repeatedly to testify on their narrow field of expertise all over the country. One might answer that because the issues in the case in question are so difficult technically, and because there are so few individuals qualified in the area, it stands to reason that an expert on the issue in question will be asked to testify whenever there is such a case. To fail to do so would deprive the triers of fact of the information required to do proper justice.

By participating in legal actions, the neuropathologist may attract attention in his or her medical community. This attention may be negative, but most frequently, it is surprisingly positive. In the latter circumstance, it is not uncommon to find other physicians seeking information about the in-court experience and any reflections one might have on the process. Advice is often sought as well. This and even the negative reactions that sometimes occur are outgrowths of the relative ignorance of much of the medical community about legal matters. It is indeed regrettable that there is such a lack of knowledge, but it is only through more enlightened participation of physicians with the legal system that both lawyers and physicians may come to work together out of mutual respect and more effectively interact for the benefit of society.

References

1. Spitz WU, Spitz DJ, eds. *Spitz and Fisher's Medicolegal Investigation of Death: Guidelines for the Application of Pathology to Crime Investigation*. Springfield, IL: Charles C. Thomas, 2006.
2. DiMaio VJ, DiMaio D. *Forensic Pathology*. Boca Raton, FL: CRC Press, 2001.
3. Camps FE, Robinson AE, Lucas BGB, eds. *Gradwohl's Legal Medicine*. Bristol, UK: A. John Wright, 1976.
4. Knight B. *Forensic Pathology*. London: Arnold, 1996.
5. American Board of Pathology. http://www.abpath.org/. Tampa, FL: American Board of Pathology, 2007.
6. Office of the Medical Examiner, *Annual Report, 1977–1979*. Cook County, IL. 1979.
7. Moenssens AA, Moses RE, Inbau, FE. *Scientific Evidence in Criminal Cases*. Mineola, NY: The Foundation Press, 1973.
8. Faigman DL, Kaye DH, Saks MJ, Sanders J. *Modern Scientific Evidence: The Law and Science of Expert Testimony*. Eagan, MN: Thomson West, 2005.

9. Broun KS, Dix GE, Imwinkelried EJ, Kaye DH, Mosteller RP, eds. *McCormick on Evidence*. Eagan, MN: Thomson West, 2006.
10. Moritz AR. Classical mistakes in forensic pathology: Alan R. Moritz (*American Journal of Clinical Pathology*, 1956). *Am J Foren Med Pathol* 1981;2:299–308.
11. Fatteh A. *Handbook of Forensic Pathology*. Philadelphia: Lippincott, 1973.
12. Kirkpatrick JB. Forensic considerations in examining the brain. *Semin Diagn Pathol* 1984; 1:98–113.
13. Horsley JE, Carlova J. *Testifying in Court*. Oradell, NJ: Medical Economics Books, 1983.
14. Quimby CW Jr. General considerations of medical testimony. In James AE Jr., ed., *Legal Medicine with Special Reference of Diagnostic Imaging*. Baltimore: Urban and Schwarzenberg, 1980, pp. 49–61.
15. *Illinois Revised Statutes*. 1985.
16. Rothstein PF. *Federal Rules of Evidence*. Eagan, MN: Thomson West, 2002.
17. *Federal Civil Judicial Procedure and Rules*. Eagan, MN: Thomson West, 2007.
18. Best A, ed. *Wigmore on Evidence*. New York: Aspen, 2007.
19. Maher TP. *Demonstrative Evidence for Complex Litigation: A Practical Guide*. Tucson, AZ: Lawyer's and Judges Publishing, 2005.
20. Rychiak RJ. *Real and Demonstrative Evidence—Applications and Theory*. Charlottesville, VA: Michie, 1995.

Scientific Evidence and the Courts

2

ELAINE WHITFIELD SHARP

Contents

Introduction

The most brilliant and lucid expert witness is worth little in the courtroom unless he or she passes muster with the judge (the "gatekeeper") and is able to have his or her evidence and opinions admitted into evidence for the jury.

The theory of this chapter is that the expert is more likely to achieve these goals if he or she understands, well in advance, the evidentiary standards he or she will have to satisfy. Those standards are well established in the federal courts but vary among state courts. Fortunately, an understanding of the federal standards will go a long way toward understanding the various state standards.

Since the publication of the second edition of this book in 2008, the National Academy of Sciences (NAS) issued a scathing report condemning the fragile state of forensic science in the United States (the NAS Report). The NAS Report, "Strengthening Forensic Science in the United States—A Path Forward," critiques the state of the multiple fields of forensic sciences and, of particular interests to readers here, that of forensic pathology. This updated chapter includes an account of that section of the NAS Report [27]. Also, in May 2011, the United Kingdom's Law Commission, which advises the UK Parliament on law reform, issued a Report (UK Report) that resonates with the NAS Report's recommendations for reform of the presentation of evidence proffered as scientific in criminal cases [28]. Relevant portions from the UK Report are included in this revised chapter [28]. In addition to the publication of the NAS and the UK reports, respectively, where the law of scientific evidence has been superseded by new standards of admissibility, most notably, Arizona, those developments are also included here.

Sea Changes in the History of Forensic Evidence

A revolution in scientific evidence began in 1993 in the United States with *Daubert*, a U.S. Supreme Court decision [1] articulating sample criteria for trial judges to use to evaluate whether evidence proffered as scientific is reliable enough for consideration by the jury to resolve a material issue of fact in the case. It continued in 1997 with *Joiner* [2] and culminated in 1999 with *Kumho* [3], also U.S. Supreme Court cases. These three cases—*Daubert*, *Kumho*, and *Joiner*—became known as the "*Daubert* trilogy" or "*Daubert* and its progeny" and now embody the law of scientific evidence in federal courts. This law, in either its pure or adapted form, has been adopted by many of the highest courts of the fifty states. It has also been used for guidance in the United Kingdom.

In 2005, the United Kingdom House of Commons Science and Technology Committee recommended the creation of a Forensic Science Advisory Council to regulate forensic evidence in the UK and observed:

> The absence of an agreed protocol for the validation of scientific techniques prior to their being admitted in court is entirely unsatisfactory. Judges are not well-placed to determine scientific validity without input from scientists. We recommend that one of the first tasks of the Forensic Science Advisory Council be to develop a "gate-keeping" test for expert evidence. This should be done in partnership with judges, scientists and other key players in the criminal justice system, and should build on the US *Daubert test* [4].

Daubert mandated a sea change in the way in which federal trial judges were instructed to evaluate scientific evidence. But it did not do so in a historical vacuum.

The *Frye* Standard

The growth of science and technology leading up to and beyond the industrial revolution put scientific issues in court at an exponential rate. In the past 150 years, the courtroom has become the proving ground for many new areas of science to determine issues pivotally relevant to criminal and civil liability, and sometimes both.

Over the last two centuries, trial judges have been asked to decide: are there unique human identifiers, such as, fingerprints? If so, are fingerprints reliable? Is the identification of a person through facial measurement (anthropometry) reliable? What about bite marks? Lip prints? Ear prints? Voice recognition? Handwriting? Is DNA reliable? Is there a machine that can tell if someone is lying or telling the truth? Is there a machine that enables us to see a person's bones right through the skin, the brain, or injury to the brain? Is there an objective way to tell how much pain a person suffered before death? How do we know if a particular bullet was discharged from a particular gun?

Experts became a permanent fixture in the courtroom and often as equally powerful, if not more so, in their influence with jurors as the trial judge's gavel.

Despite the widespread use of experts on every subject from antibodies to zoology, most state and federal trial court judges in the early 1900s had few standards, if any, by which to independently judge the question: is this "science" reliable enough for the trier of fact to consider in helping justly to resolve this case? It is fundamental to our system of justice that evidence purported to be scientific but not, in fact, reliable enough to warrant the label "scientific" evidence is not relevant and, as such, may be more unfairly prejudicial than probative on issues that impact a finding of guilty or not guilty, liable or not liable. A lack of standards in the early 1900s left judges adrift in uncertainty about what evidence to admit for consideration by a jury and what to exclude. In 1923, a federal appeals court announced a working rule of thumb, for which we have James Alphonzo Frye to thank. Mr. Frye was on trial for murder, and to prove his innocence, or at least raise reasonable doubt, he took a systolic blood pressure deception test, a crude precursor of the polygraph examination. His defense lawyer proffered the results of the test at trial, and when the trial judge sided with the government and refused to let the jurors hear the results, Mr. Frye's attorney offered to bring the "scientist" who ran the test to run it again on the defendant before the jurors. The scientist was William Marston, creator of "Wonder Woman" and her truth-inducing magic lasso and founder of Marston Comics. The trial judge ruled for the prosecutor and the jurors never heard that "scientific" evidence.

Deprived of his favorable "scientific" evidence, Mr. Frye was convicted of second-degree murder and, in a single-issue appeal, raised the question of whether, in excluding the evidence of the test and its results, the trial judge abused his discretion, creating reversible error that would entitle him to a new trial.

Mr. Frye's lawyer claimed that the 1923 "deception test" measured systolic blood pressure, the body's strongest blood pressure and that, by measuring changes in blood pressure triggered by a witness's changing emotional state, the test was able to detect truth or falsehood. Describing the underlying scientific theory of the test, the *Frye* court wrote [5]:

> Scientific experiments, it is claimed, have demonstrated that fear, rage and pain always produce a rise in systolic blood pressure and that conscious deception or falsehood, concealment of facts, or guilt of crime, accompanied by the fear of detection when the person is under examination, raises the systolic blood pressure curve, which corresponds exactly to the struggle going on in the subject's mind, between fear, as the examination touches the vital points in respect of which he is attempting to deceive the examiner. In other words, the theory seems to be that truth is spontaneous, and comes without conscious effort, while the utterance of a falsehood requires a conscious effort, which is reflected in the blood pressure.

Although there were no guiding standards about what scientific evidence should be admitted and excluded, a practice in some courts in 1923 was to allow an expert to testify about scientific or technical knowledge when, in the judge's discretion, the facts needed the interpretation or opinion of an expert to assist the jurors in understanding and deciding important issues in the case.

Confusion occurred when a party, like Mr. Frye, wanted jurors to hear scientific testimony about novel or cutting-edge "science." How was the trial judge to determine whether the "thing" that was being proffered should be heard or considered by the trier of fact?

The *Frye* court held that the standard was in the hands of the scientists, writing what has, perhaps, become one of the most famous—or depending on one's viewpoint, infamous—statements in the law of evidence [5]:

> Just when a scientific principle or discovery crosses the line between the experimental and demonstrable stages is difficult to define. Somewhere in this twilight zone the evidential force of the principle must be recognized, and while courts will go a long way in admitting expert testimony deduced from a well-recognized scientific principle or discovery, *the thing from which the deduction is made must be sufficiently established to have gained general acceptance in the particular field in which it belongs.* [Emphasis added.]

This is the *Frye* rule, sometimes also called the general acceptance rule. In *Frye*, the appeals court held that the systolic blood pressure test had not gained the kind of standing and recognition among physiologists and psychologists—the relevant scientific community—to warrant presenting the results of the tests to jurors. Holding that the trial judge had not abused his discretion, the appeals court affirmed Mr. Frye's murder conviction. As a side note, Mr. Frye was ultimately exonerated when exculpatory evidence came to light; however, the systolic blood pressure test, which spawned the modern-day polygraph, did not fare so well. In 2002, a report of the National Academy of Sciences concluded that the lie detector test, although a helpful investigative tool, was not reliable science [6].

Thus was born the test in the federal courts by which any evidence that a litigant claimed was novel science was to be judged: if a scientist opined that *the thing from which the deduction is made is established and has gained general acceptance in the particular field in which it belongs*, it could be admitted for the trier of fact to consider to resolve factual issues. The *Frye* rule applied in both criminal and civil cases. In 1943, silent movie star Charlie Chaplin tried to defend a paternity suit against him with the results of an ABO blood type test that ruled him out as the father of the child in question. The court held that the ABO test was inadmissible because it was not generally accepted in the relevant scientific community, then having been only recently discovered (in 1915). Whereas the *Frye* court addressed only the question of novel scientific evidence, later courts extended the general acceptance test of admissibility to all scientific evidence. For 70 years, the *Frye* test was the standard for judging all science in the federal courts. Most state courts adopted the *Frye* test, although some adopted hybrids of the test that imposed a duty on the trial judge to independently assess the reliability of proffered scientific testimony.

In an ideal world, if a scientific proposition has been generally accepted in the relevant community, one would expect it to be based on a well-reasoned hypothesis shown to be valid by reliably designed research consisting of sufficiently reliable data and subsequent tests validating initial results. Also, one would expect that any expert testimony about the proposition in a specific case would be the product of reliable methods and conclusions that would be properly applied to the facts of the case. *Frye*'s admissibility test of "general acceptance in the relevant scientific community" would have implicitly contemplated all of these expectations because reliability in hypothesis formation, study or experiment design, testing, and interpretation of results has historically been the hallmark of trustworthy science.

But that is an ideal world. In the real world, scientists are plagued by problems of ego, turf wars, the politics of scientific funding, faulty hypothesis formation, poor study design, poor data analysis, and otherwise intellectually tainted orientations and conclusions. Like any other human endeavor, the process of scientific investigation is far from pure, neutral, and unbiased. As Pulitzer Prize winner Paul Starr [7] wrote: "The dream of reason did not take power into account."

For more than 70 years, the *Frye* test held the world of law hostage to the world of science and its idiosyncrasies—until the U.S. Supreme Court laid out new rules for the admissibility of scientific evidence in three cases: *Daubert*, *Kumho*, and *Joiner*.

The *Daubert* Era: The Search for Reliability

Jason Daubert and Eric Schuller were born with serious birth defects. The mothers of Jason and Eric had taken the anti-nausea drug Bendectin during pregnancy, and they blamed their sons' birth defects on the drug. The boys and their parents sued Merrell Dow, the pharmaceutical company that manufactured the drug. But before trial by jury, the defendant-drug company filed a motion through which it convinced the trial judge that the case should be summarily dismissed because the boys had no generally accepted evidence under the *Frye* rule to take to a jury about what caused their birth defects. The U.S. District Court trial judge agreed: juries resolve factual disputes, and here there was no dispute about causation because the plaintiffs had no evidence to create such an issue.

Lawyers for the defendant, Merrell Dow, argued that the human statistical studies about Bendectin all showed that the drug did not cause birth defects. Lawyers for Jason and Eric argued that their evidence established that Bendectin did cause the boys' birth defects. They offered (1) *in vitro* (test tube) and *in vivo* (live animal) studies that found a link between Bendectin and malformations; (2) pharmacological studies that showed chemical structures similar to that of Bendectin that they claimed caused birth defects; and (3) a reanalysis of previously published human statistical, i.e., epidemiological, studies. (The third type of proof is sometimes called meta-analysis or data pooling.)

The trial court judge dismissed the case because, under the *Frye* test, "scientific evidence is admissible only if the principle upon which it is based is "sufficiently established to have general acceptance in the field to which it belongs." The trial court found that Jason and Eric had no way to challenge the accuracy of Merrell Dow's human statistical studies and that the plaintiffs' reanalysis or recalculation of those studies had not been available for review by the relevant scientific community to be generally accepted. Therefore, the trial court ruled, Jason's and Eric's animal cell (test tube) studies, live animal studies, and the chemical structure analyses did not establish, and could not be admitted to show, that Bendectin caused birth defects.

Jason and Eric appealed to the U.S. Court of Appeals for the Ninth Circuit. That court agreed with the trial judge: without *generally accepted* evidence of causation—and causation was an element of the plaintiff's claim—the trial judge was correct to dismiss their lawsuit.

Jason and Eric appealed to the U.S. Supreme Court to review their case on the question of the correct standard to apply in determining what is reliable science. By this time, some of the thirteen federal circuit courts of appeal were in conflict over how to answer this question. Should they use the general acceptance *Frye* test, or Federal Rule of Evidence 702, enacted by Congress in 1975? The 1975 version of Rule 702 stated:

> If *scientific*, technical, or other specialized knowledge will assist the trier of fact to understand the evidence or to determine a fact in issue, a witness qualified as an expert by knowledge, skill, experience, training, or education, may testify thereto in the form of an opinion or otherwise. [Emphasis added; see Table 2.1.]

How was this rule, enacted by Congress 52 years after *Frye*, to be applied? Was *Frye*'s general acceptance test part of it? Or was the rule independent of *Federal Rules of Evidence* (FRE) 702? If Rule 702 was independent of *Frye*, how were trial judges to interpret and apply the rule? *Daubert* presented not only an unusual conflict of evidence laws and a bitter battle of scientific experts but also a classic conflict of decisions among the thirteen federal circuit courts of appeal. The U.S. Supreme Court took the case.

In a nutshell, in *Daubert*, the Supreme Court held that scientific evidence did not have to pass *Frye*'s general acceptance test as a precondition for admissibility, that Rule 702 was the pertinent rule to apply, but that an interpretation of the rule requires trial judges to act as reliability gatekeepers to ensure that an expert's testimony rests on both reliable methods and conclusions and that it is actually relevant to the specific case. How the Supreme Court got there is another story. It is a story that is helpful in understanding how to prepare a forensic opinion with a view to meeting the standards of admissibility.

The main question for the court was: when Rule 702 speaks of "scientific evidence," what does that term mean and by what criteria should a trial court judge the "science" in deciding the question of admissibility?

Table 2.1 FRE Relevant to the Admissibility of Scientific or Expert Evidence with Commentary and Observations

Rule 104. Preliminary Questions. (a) **In General.** The court must decide any preliminary question about whether a witness is qualified, a privilege exists, or evidence is admissible. In so deciding, the court is not bound by evidence rules, except those on privilege. (b) **Relevance That Depends on a Fact.** When the relevance of evidence depends on whether a fact exists, proof must be introduced sufficient to support a finding that the fact does exist. The court may admit the proposed evidence on the condition that the proof be introduced later.... (d) **Cross-Examining a Defendant in a Criminal Case.** By testifying on a preliminary question, a defendant in a criminal case does not become subject to cross-examination on other issues in the case. (e) **Evidence Relevant to Weight and Credibility.** This rule does not limit a party's right to introduce before the jury evidence that is relevant to the weight or credibility of other evidence.

Rule 401. Test for Relevant Evidence. Evidence is relevant if: (a) it has any tendency to make a fact more or less probable than it would be without the evidence; and (b) the fact is of consequence in determining the action.

Rule 403. Excluding Relevant Evidence for Prejudice, Confusion, Waste of Time, or Other Reasons. The court may exclude relevant evidence if its probative value is substantially outweighed by a danger of one or more of the following: unfair prejudice, confusing the issues, misleading the jury, undue delay, wasting time, or needlessly presenting cumulative evidence.

Rule 702. Testimony by Expert Witnesses. A witness who is qualified as an expert by knowledge, skill, experience, training, or education may testify in the form of an opinion or otherwise if: (a) the expert's scientific, technical, or other specialized knowledge will help the trier of fact to understand the evidence or to determine a fact in issue; (b) **Examining.** The court may examine a witness regardless of who calls the witness. (c) **Objections.** A party may object to the court's calling or examining a witness either at that time or at the next opportunity when the jury is not present.

Rule 703. Bases of an Expert's Opinion Testimony. An expert may base an opinion on facts or data in the case that the expert has been made aware of or personally observed. If experts in the particular field would reasonably rely on those kinds of facts or data in forming an opinion on the subject, they need not be admissible for the opinion to be admitted. But if the facts or data would otherwise be inadmissible, the proponent of the opinion may disclose them to the jury only if their probative value in helping the jury evaluate the opinion substantially outweighs their prejudicial effect.

Rule 704. Opinion on an Ultimate Issue. (a) **In General—Not Automatically Objectionable.** An opinion is not objectionable just because it embraces an ultimate issue. (b) **Exception.** In a criminal case, an expert witness must not state an opinion about whether the defendant did or did not have a mental state or condition that constitutes an element of the crime charged or of a defense. Those matters are for the trier of fact alone.

[**Author Commentary**: Federal Rule of Evidence 704 touches a nerve that makes many lawyers and judges uncomfortable because, although the Seventh Amendment (U.S. Constitution Amendment VII) guarantees the right to trial by a jury—meaning that criminal defendants and civil litigants have the right to a determination of the facts by jurors—FRE 704 permits an expert's opinion to "embrace [] an ultimate issue". The same rule in subsection (b) draws the line at testimony regarding a criminal defendant's mental state and prohibits an expert from testifying that a defendant did or did not have the mental capacity to commit a crime. That is a jury question.]

Rule 705. Disclosing the Facts or Data Underlying an Expert's Opinion. Unless the Court orders otherwise, an expert may state an opinion—and give the reasons for it—without first testifying to the underlying facts or data. But the expert may be required to disclose those facts or data on cross-examination.

[**Author Commentary**: Federal Rule of Evidence 705, concerning the disclosure of facts or data underlying expert opinion, permits an expert to give his or her opinion without the necessity of the lawyer's laboriously laying the foundational facts for the opinion before he or she does so.]

(*continued*)

Table 2.1 (Continued) FRE Relevant to the Admissibility of Scientific or Expert Evidence with Commentary and Observations

Rule 706: Court-Appointed Expert Witnesses. (a) **Appointment Process.** On a party's motion or on its own, the court may order the parties to show cause why expert witnesses should not be appointed and may ask the parties to submit nominations. The court may appoint any expert that the parties agree on and any of its own choosing. But the court may only appoint someone who consents to the act. (b) **Expert's Role.** The court must inform the expert of the expert's duties. The court may do so in writing and have a copy filed with the clerk or may do so orally at a conference in which the parties have an opportunity to participate. The expert: (1) must advise the parties of any findings the expert makes; (2) may be deposed by any party; (3) may be called to testify by the court, or any party; and (4) may be cross-examined by any party, including the party that called the expert. (c) **Compensation.** The expert is entitled to a reasonable compensation, as set by the court. The compensation is payable as follows: (1) in a criminal case or a civil case involving just compensation under the Fifth Amendment, from any funds that are provided by the law; and (2) in any other civil case, by the parties in the proportion and at the time that the court directs—and the compensation is then charged like other costs. (d) **Disclosing the Appointment to the Jury.** The court may authorize to disclose to the jury that the court appointed the expert. (e) **Parties' Choice of Their Own Experts.** This rule does not limit a party in calling its own experts.

Educated with help from twenty-two *amici* briefs filed by several of the nation's scientific leaders, the Supreme Court cobbled together a definition of what it believes the term *scientific knowledge* means in Rule 702. "Scientific knowledge," said the court [1]:

- Implies a grounding in the methods and procedures of science;
- Implies a body of known facts, accepted on good grounds;
- Implies that an inference or assertion is derived by the scientific method; and
- Does not imply that the subject of scientific testimony must be "known to a certainty," for, arguably, there are no certainties in science. ("Science is not an encyclopedic body of knowledge about the universe. Instead it represents a process for proposing and refining theoretical explanations about the world that are subject to further testing and refinement.")

Under *Frye*, the scientists dictated what was reliable and what was not. But, under *Daubert*, the court directed trial judges that the determination of reliability was their duty. They alone were to be the gatekeepers of scientific reliability at the bar. If the trial judge determines that proffered scientific testimony is reliable, the gatekeeper should admit it for the trier of fact, usually the jury, to consider. Otherwise, the gatekeeper must exclude it. Federal Rule of Evidence 104(a) states in part: "Preliminary questions concerning the qualification of a person to be a witness…or the admissibility of evidence *shall* be determined by the court…." This was a mandate, not a choice.

The court explained that in acting as gatekeepers of scientific knowledge, there are some hallmarks of reliable science for which to look:

1. Is the thing that is being proffered as scientific capable of being tested, and has it been tested? Quoting nineteenth-century philosopher Karl Popper [8], the court wrote: "Scientific methodology today is based on generating hypotheses and testing them to see if they can be falsified; indeed, this methodology is what distinguishes science from other fields of human inquiry."

2. Has the theory or technique been subjected to peer review and publication? (Publication is not the *sine qua non* of admissibility and, indeed, is only one component of peer review. Sometimes what is published is not reliable, and sometimes that which is reliable is not published. But publication ensures "submission to the scrutiny of the scientific community" and is a "component of good science, in part, because it increases the likelihood that substantive flaws in methodology will be detected.")
3. Is there a known or potential rate of error? (Do standards exist, and are these maintained in the testing? This is important in relation to the validation of test results through the use of consistent standards and is part of good science.)
4. Is the thing generally accepted? (Depending on the case and type of proffered scientific testimony, it may be pertinent to identify a relevant scientific community and to determine the degree of acceptance within that community.)

The *Daubert* court realized that the trial judge's "focus, of course, must be solely on principles and the methodology, not on the conclusions they generate."

Determining whether the proffered science is reliable is only one part of the gatekeeper's job, said the court [1]. The trial judge must also ensure that the scientific testimony is, in fact, relevant to resolve a disputed issue in the case. There must be a "fit" between the science proffered and the facts of the case. Wrote the court: "Rule 702's 'helpfulness' standard requires a valid scientific connection to the pertinent inquiry as a precondition of admissibility." Under *Daubert*, reliability and relevancy (fit) are the two guiding principles in the determination of whether to admit scientific evidence.

Daubert's checklist of four factors to consider in determining if proffered scientific testimony should be admitted contemplated the specific type of science offered in that case. On the plaintiff's side were meta-analyses and *in vivo* and *in vitro* studies, whereas on the defendant's side were epidemiological studies, that is, the study of large groups of people from which statistical correlations may be shown. *Daubert*'s specific fact situation involved relatively esoteric areas of science.

Daubert did not answer the questions of whether and how it applied to other areas of expert knowledge, such as engineering and other applied sciences and technology, and it was not clear by what standard appeals courts were to review a trial judge's decision to admit or exclude scientific evidence. Was it a mere abuse of discretion standard under which reliance by the trial judge on any facts to admit or exclude expert testimony would be upheld? If so, that would mean that the decision of the trial judge, who already had the power to act as reliability gatekeeper, would be virtually untouchable on appeal. Or was the standard a more stringent one in which the appellate courts would completely review the trial judge's evidentiary ruling to see whether they disagreed with the lower court's findings?

The court answered these questions in *Joiner* and *Kumho*.

The *Joiner* Standard

Mr. Joiner claimed that while working as an electrician for General Electric, he developed small-cell lung cancer because of his exposure to polychlorinated biphenyls (PCBs) and their derivatives, furans and dioxins, found in the coolant fluid in transformers.

Joiner's experts on causation relied on studies performed on infant mice that developed tumors in their small air sacs after highly concentrated, massive doses of PCBs were injected directly into their stomachs and abdominal walls. In contrast, Joiner's human exposure was indirect and on a much lower scale. Joiner's experts also relied on two studies for which the authors themselves were unwilling to suggest a link between PCBs and lung cancer. The experts also relied on a third study in which a link between lung cancer and a specific mineral oil—to which Joiner had not been exposed—was found. The trial judge ruled that this testimony was inadmissible because it did not show that Joiner's small-cell lung cancer was caused by his exposure to PCBs, and his experts' testimony to the contrary, and their insistence that causation was shown, did not rise above subjective belief or unsupported speculation.

The Court of Appeals for the Eleventh Circuit disagreed. Rather than simply deciding whether the trial court had abused its discretion in coming to a manifestly erroneous factual conclusion, the Eleventh Circuit applied a stringent review. It held that, in light of the fact that the rules of evidence display a preference for admissibility, the trial judge had incorrectly excluded the plaintiff's proof of causation. The trial judge had improperly played "science" judge by reaching a different conclusion about the research than the plaintiff's experts reached. The jury, not the judge, should decide between competing views of science, the Eleventh Circuit stated.

General Electric appealed to the U.S. Supreme Court, arguing that the standard of review on appeal when a trial judge excludes scientific evidence is whether there was an abuse of discretion, that is, whether the decision was manifestly erroneous in that it lacked any reasonable, factual foundation. Looking at the trial judge's findings in that light would mean that it was not manifestly erroneous for him to exclude the plaintiff's proof of causation because there was a factual basis for the finding that this failed to make the link between Joiner's exposure to PCBs and his cancer.

The U.S. Supreme Court took the case and ruled that the appeals courts were to apply the abuse of discretion standard to review a trial judge's rulings to admit or exclude scientific evidence. Unless there was no factual basis for the trial court's decision, it was to be left untouched. This development meant that not only was the power to determine scientific reliability in the hands of the trial judge, but the trial judge's ruling was also to be virtually impregnable to attack on appeal [2].

The other question in *Joiner* was whether a trial judge had to take the word of an expert that scientific evidence was reliable. The court held that the trial court does not have to rely on the *ipse dixit*, which is Latin for the "say-so," i.e., the bare assertion, of an expert exerting his authority. Rather, the trial judge must be the reliability gatekeeper, scrutinizing not only conclusions but also the methods used by experts in reaching those. (Recall that the plaintiff's experts' claim of *ipse dixit* was that the plaintiff's cancer was linked to PCBs, but the literature upon which they relied for this proposition did support such a claim.) Affirming the trial judge's exclusion of the plaintiff's proofs, the *Joiner* court reminded trial judges who hold the reins of reliability and, therefore, relevancy:

> Conclusions and methodology are not entirely distinct from one another. Trained experts commonly extrapolate from existing data. But nothing in either *Daubert* or the *Federal Rules of Evidence* requires a [trial] court to admit opinion evidence that is connected to existing data only by the *ipse dixit* of the expert. A court may conclude that there is simply too great an analytical gap between the data and the opinion offered. [2]

Both *Daubert* and *Joiner* involved scientific knowledge. The question still nagging the federal trial bench was whether the trial judges had to be the reliability gatekeepers in all areas of knowledge, such as skills-oriented, applied sciences like engineering. Did the duty extend to testimony based on technical or other specialized knowledge, as included in Rule 702?

The *Kumho* Standard

In *Kumho*, the U.S. Supreme Court answered the question posed above. In this case, one plaintiff had been killed and others injured when a tire of the minivan they were traveling in blew out. The plaintiffs' tire failure analysis expert inspected the tire and opined that the blowout was consistent with a tire-manufacturing defect and not due to wear and tear. But he also conceded that the tire was old and worn and that it had twice previously been punctured and inadequately repaired.

Applying all four of the *Daubert* factors, the *Kumho* trial judge found that the testimony of the tire expert witness on the cause of the blowout was not reliable and dismissed the suit on grounds that the plaintiffs could not prove the element of causation. The plaintiffs moved for reconsideration on the grounds that the trial judge too rigidly applied the *Daubert* factors. They argued that these factors were to be used for areas of science akin to that in *Daubert*, and that the real focus was not on the four factors but on reliability. The *Kumho* trial judge reconsidered using reliability as the standard, after which he wrote that "the component of [the expert's] tire failure analysis which most concerned the Court [was] the methodology employed by the expert in analyzing the data obtained in the visual inspection, and the scientific basis, if any, for such an analysis." He did not agree that the plaintiffs' expert's tactile or hands-on inspection of the tire was reliable.

On appeal, the Eleventh Circuit held in the plaintiffs' favor on grounds that the *Daubert* factors only apply to scientific knowledge and not to technical or other areas of specialized knowledge in Rule 702. Kumho Tire appealed to the U.S. Supreme Court.

The Supreme Court took the case "in light of the uncertainty" about whether *Daubert* applies to all areas of knowledge listed in Rule 702, i.e., science, technology, and other specializations. The court held that it did, and, as for *Daubert*'s four factors, the court wrote [3]:

> In our view…we can neither rule out or rule in, for all cases and for all time the applicability of the factors mentioned in *Daubert*, nor can we now do so for subsets of cases categorized by category of expert or by kind of evidence. Too much depends upon the circumstances of the particular case at issue.…
>
> [That] list was meant to be helpful, not definitive. Indeed, those factors do not all necessarily apply even in every instance in which the reliability of scientific testimony is challenged. It might not be surprising in a particular case, for example, that a claim made by a scientific witness has never been the subject of peer review, for the particular application at issue may never previously have interested any scientist. Nor, on the other hand, does the presence of *Daubert*'s general acceptance factor help show that an expert's testimony is reliable where the discipline itself lacks reliability…."

The *Kumho* court also warned against litigation bias in tests. Expert witnesses must use the same degree of intellectual rigor in testing for a court case that they would in the laboratory or any other area of their practice. Methods and conclusions had to be *reliable* in all contexts.

The sum and the substance of expert witness testimony under the *Daubert* trilogy are as follows:

- *Daubert*: The trial judge is the mandated gatekeeper of scientific reliability and relevancy. Scientific knowledge has certain hallmarks that make it reliable. All scientific expert testimony must be reliable, that is, relevant to resolve an issue in the case (fit).
- *Joiner*: A trial judge's decision to admit or exclude scientific expert testimony will only be upset by the appeals court if it is an abuse of discretion, i.e., without facts to support it. The trial judge will usually have the last word. The trial judge does not have to take the word, i.e., the *ipse dixit*, of the expert that a conclusion is correct if the methodology is unreliable (fit).
- *Kumho*: Reliability analysis applies to all areas of expert testimony—scientific, technical, or other specialized knowledge—and also to methods used, and conclusions reached, in testing for litigation.

Daubert, *Joiner*, and *Kumho* together represent the search for reliability as part of the quest to do justice and are included in the now-modified Federal Rule of Evidence 702:

> If scientific, technical, or other specialized knowledge will assist the trier of fact to understand the evidence or to determine a fact in issue, a witness qualified as an expert by knowledge, skill, experience, training, or education, may testify thereto in the form of an opinion or otherwise, if (1) the testimony is based upon sufficient facts or data, (2) the testimony is the product of reliable principles and methods, and (3) the witness has applied the principles and methods reliably to the facts of the case.

In evaluating whether scientific or other expert testimony is admissible, most states follow some version of the principles found in either FRE 702 or a mix of the principles in FRE 702 and *Frye*. None of the cases in the *Daubert* trilogy or in any state on the admissibility of scientific evidence are shrouded in mystery because two unifying threads are woven throughout their fabric: reliability and relevance. In those states where evidence is admitted if it is "helpful to the jury in understanding a fact in issue," even this standard inherently assumes reliability, for that which is not reliable is not relevant. No matter the name of the case or the number of the rule of evidence governing the admissibility of scientific evidence in a given state, with few exceptions, the standards may be boiled down to reliability and relevance. (See Table 2.2 for state-by-state standards for admissibility of scientific evidence, cases, and rules, and related discussion.) When science or other areas of expert knowledge are in the courtroom, reliability is, on a fundamental level, about trying to find the truth. It is about proof beyond a reasonable doubt, clear and convincing evidence, or proof by a preponderance of the evidence. As numerous wrongful conviction/exoneration cases have illustrated, the integrity of our entire system of justice depends on a single quality: trust in the result [9].

The *Federal Rules of Evidence*

The FRE represent the culmination of centuries of common-law experience and were enacted by Congress as a federal code in 1973.

Table 2.2 Evidentiary Standards for the Admissibility of Scientific Evidence State by State Showing Death Penalty States

State	Death Penalty	*Daubert*	*Daubert* (Instructive)	*Frye* and Modifications	Rule 702 Based or Gatekeeper
Alaska		X			
Alabama	X			X	
Arizona	X	X			X
Arkansas	X	X			
California	X				X
Colorado	X				X
Connecticut	X				X
Delaware	X			X	
District of Columbia				X	
Florida	X			X	
Georgia	X				X
Hawaii			X		
Idaho	X				X
Illinois	X			X	
Indiana	X		X		
Iowa			X		
Kansas	X			X	
Kentucky	X	X			
Louisiana	X	X			
Maine			X		
Maryland	X			X	
Massachusetts			X		
Michigan		X			
Minnesota				X	
Mississippi	X	X			
Missouri	X				X
Montana	X	X			X
Nebraska	X	X			X
Nevada	X				X
New Hampshire	X	X			
New Jersey				X	
New Mexico	X	X			X
New York				X	
North Carolina	X	X			X
North Dakota					X
Ohio	X		X		
Oklahoma	X	X			
Oregon	X	X			X
Pennsylvania	X			X	
Rhode Island		X			
South Carolina	X				X
South Dakota	X	X			X
Tennessee	X		X		

(*continued*)

Table 2.2 (Continued) Evidentiary Standards for the Admissibility of Scientific Evidence State by State Showing Death Penalty States

State	Death Penalty	*Daubert*	*Daubert* (Instructive)	*Frye* and Modifications	Rule 702 Based or Gatekeeper
Texas	X	X			
Utah	X				X
Vermont		X			
Virginia	X				X
Washington	X			X	
West Virginia		X		X	
Wisconsin					X
Wyoming	X	X			

FRE 103 states: "The rules shall be construed to secure fairness in administration, elimination of unjustifiable expense and delay, and promotion of growth and development of the law of evidence to the end that the truth may be ascertained and proceedings justly determined."

Under FRE 104(a) the trial judge is mandated to serve as the gatekeeper. He or she must strive only to admit evidence that is relevant under FRE 401. Where the probative value of the evidence is outweighed by considerations such as its unfairly prejudicial nature, the trial judge is to exclude it under FRE 403.

The rules of evidence governing the admission of expert testimony are found in the "700 chapter" of the federal rules. The post-*Daubert* version of FRE 702, which is quoted above and included in the text box for convenience, is the rule governing the admissibility of expert testimony and evidence. FRE 703 allows an expert to base his or her opinion upon hearsay—upon "facts or data...perceived or made known to the expert at or before the hearing"—providing that the facts or data are of a type reasonably relied upon by experts in their respective fields. Even though the expert may rely on hearsay, the requirement of "reasonable reliance" is a further safeguard against the backdoor admission of unreliable material, sometimes called junk science, the very concern of *Frye* and then *Daubert*. (The reasonable reliance issue is more fully explored below on the section on medical and scientific literature.)

In adopting *Daubert* [1] as the standard for the admissibility of all scientific evidence, the Alaska Supreme Court cogently outlined the decision tree required under the Alaska rules of evidence for the admissibility of scientific evidence. Because this is the same decision tree that would apply under the FRE, which have been adopted in whole or in part by numerous states, it is included here:

> Several of our evidence rules bear on the admissibility of scientific evidence. Evidence Rule 104(a) assigns to the trial court the duty to determine preliminary questions concerning the qualification of a person to be a witness and the admissibility of evidence. Evidence Rule 401 defines what evidence is relevant. Evidence Rule 403 allows exclusion of relevant evidence for such reasons as prejudice, confusion, and waste of time. Evidence Rule 702 allows experts to offer helpful opinion testimony. Evidence Rule 703 allows experts to base opinions on facts or data of a type reasonably relied upon by experts in the field. Thus, expert opinion evidence is admissible if the trial court (exercising its authority under Rule 104[a]) determines that (1) the evidence is relevant (Rule 401); (2) the witness is qualified as an expert (Rule 702[a]); (3) the trier of fact will be assisted (Rule 702[a]); (4) the facts or data on which the opinion is based are of a type reasonably relied upon by experts in the particular field in forming

opinions upon the subject (Rule 703); and (5) the probative value of the evidence is not outweighed by its prejudicial effect (Rule 403). *Alaska v. Coon*, 974 P. 2d 386, 392–393 (1999).

Several states have adopted or used *Daubert* when determining the admissibility of an expert's opinion. Several states have adopted Rule 702, and some of those have also adopted *Daubert*.

The Ever-Changing Face of the Admissibility Standards of Scientific and Expert Witness Testimony

Law, like science, is never static. An expert witness needs to be aware of the fact that although states that have adopted *Daubert* are unlikely to change back to the *Frye* rule, the process of law, like science, is more often an evolutionary one. The expert should ask the retaining lawyer for guidance on the current standards in the jurisdiction where the evidence is to be proffered and, in his or her conversations with the lawyer, recognize that the standard of admissibility of expert witness testimony may differ depending on (1) the type of evidence being proffered (novel vs. established?) and (2) the forum in which it is being proffered (civil or criminal?). The *Daubert* trilogy, the *Frye* rule, and other evidentiary standards, such as state functional equivalents of FRE 702, represent a varied patchwork of law. Some state high courts have adopted only the *Daubert* reliability rule for novel evidence and then expanded it to all expert testimony under *Kumho*'s reasoning that all expert testimony must be reliable to be presented to the trier of fact. Some state high courts have adopted only *Daubert* and *Kumho* in criminal cases and then expanded it to civil cases. Some states apply *Daubert* only to novel scientific evidence. Other states have adopted a mixed *Frye* and *Daubert* approach, and still others have retained the *Frye* rule, only.

The Oklahoma Supreme Court's *Christian v. Gray* decision, more fully discussed below, presents a clear example of the evolutionary process of the evidentiary law of scientific and expert testimony. *Daubert* was first applied to criminal cases and then only to novel scientific evidence (see *Taylor v. State*, 889 P. 2d 319 [1995]). Then, in *Harris v. State*, 13 P. 3d 489 (2000), in a post-*Kumho* decision, *Daubert* was applied to all novel expert testimony. Relying on *Kumho*, the Oklahoma Supreme Court stated that in cases where the evidence is not novel, "a trial court may make that determination and avoid a prolonged *Daubert* inquiry…." The trial court "possesses the authority needed both to avoid unnecessary 'reliability' proceedings in ordinary cases where the reliability of an expert's methods is properly taken for granted, and to require appropriate proceedings in the less usual or more complex cases where cause for questioning the expert's reliability arises."

The patchwork of law of the various states in the area of expert testimony, as with all areas of law, will always be varied. It is the variety that stimulates thought and provides guidance for experts in thinking about their approach to testimony about forensic issues.

Many of the state high court *Daubert* opinions offer not only bright line rules—shifts from *Frye* to *Daubert* in civil or criminal cases, or both, for novel or established evidence, or both—but also often serve to inform the expert's role in delivering his or her product. Depending on the jurisdiction, the expert's opinion is an opinion to a reasonable degree of medical or scientific certainty or medical or scientific probability, given to the finder of fact either at a *Daubert* hearing or at trial itself. Forensic medical experts are also frequently called upon to testify, depending upon the state's criminal procedural law, at probable cause hearings to determine if there is probable cause to believe the accused may have committed the crime in question, at preliminary examinations to determine if there is sufficient evidence to bind a defendant over for trial to a felony trial court, and at state or federal grand juries before criminal indictments are issued.

Where a state high court's *Daubert* opinion expounds on some aspect of the *Daubert* trilogy, and where it may be helpful for expert witness practice, segments of various discussions of some of the state high courts are included below. Opinions from state courts that have adopted mixed *Daubert* and *Frye* standards or mixed *Frye* and *Rules of Evidence*, or that use a purely rules-based standard, are also included.

Whether the expert will be called to actually testify at either a *Daubert* or *Frye* hearing is generally a matter of discretion with the trial judge. Federal Rule of Evidence 104(a) and its state counterparts *require* the trial judge to make a pretrial finding whether evidence that is proffered as scientific either is generally accepted in the relevant scientific community (a so-called *Frye* hearing) or is reliable (a so-called *Daubert* hearing) or is a blend of these questions, depending on the state. (Of course, in federal courts, the hearing will be called a *Daubert* hearing.) The document that alerts the trial judge to the need for a *Frye* or *Daubert* hearing is called a motion *in limine*, that is, one that is filed at the outset, or *before* the trial begins. It may be filed months, weeks, or days before the trial begins. The decision as to whether to actually require a party to produce experts to offer live testimony at such a hearing, or to simply consider the matter based upon the affidavits (sworn statements) of the experts in combination with briefs and argument of counsel, is largely a matter of discretion with the trial judge. This decision may depend upon the gravity of the issue, the expense involved in bringing experts from out of state for a mini-trial on the science prior to trial, the timing of the hearing on the motion in relation to the trial, and other considerations of judicial time and economy. But this is where the discretion ends, for Rule 104(a) mandates the judge to be the gatekeeper of the evidence. In *Daubert*, the Supreme Court wrote [1]:

> Expert evidence can be both powerful and quite misleading because of the difficulty in evaluating it. Because of this risk, the judge in weighing possible prejudice against probative force under Rule 403 *exercises more control over experts than over lay witnesses.* [Emphasis added; internal citations omitted.]

Daubert and *Frye* hearings may occur at many different stages of the civil and criminal pretrial processes. For example, in a civil case, the trial or motion judge may be asked to exercise his or her gate-keeping role in the context of a motion for summary judgment, as occurred in *Daubert*, where a party argues that the opponent's evidence is not reliable to establish an essential element of a claim, such as the element of causation in a negligence case. For example, assume that in a medical negligence action where essential elements are (1) a breach of the standard of care and (2) causation, it is established that the physician did, in fact, breach the standard of care. Presented with a motion where the defense, via a motion for summary judgment, challenges the reliability of the plaintiff's experts' opinions on causation, a judge would be required to make a determination of whether the plaintiff's experts' opinions were reliable enough to create a genuine issue of material fact on the essential element of causation. If the breach of the standard of care did not *cause* the injury of which the plaintiff complains, then the element of causation is not established and the judge, in such a case, would have to summarily dismiss the case before trial because there is no genuine issue of material fact for a jury to decide.

The expert witness may be asked to testify at a *Daubert* and *Frye* pretrial or *in limine* evidentiary hearing, especially in a criminal case. An expert may also be asked to testify in person in a civil *Daubert* pretrial or hearing, but not usually. In a motion for summary judgment in a civil case, the opinions of experts are usually only submitted to the Court in the form of affidavits, although live testimony may be requested and required, depending on the preference of counsel or in the trial judge's discretion.

Daubert States

Alaska: *Daubert*. "Capricious" *Frye* Standard Rejected

In adopting *Daubert*, the Alaska Supreme Court stated one of the most widely held views on the problem of *Frye* in *State v. Coon*, 974 P. 2d 386, 389–395 (Alaska 1999): "Frye is potentially capricious because it excludes scientifically-reliable evidence which although generally accepted, cannot meet rigorous scientific scrutiny." *Daubert* and its progeny were adopted as the standard to be used by Alaska's trial court judges in determining the admissibility of *all* scientific evidence, and their analysis is to be consistent with Alaska Rules of Evidence (ARE) 702(a) and 703, which are substantially the same as FRE 702 and 703 (see federal rules above). Rule 703, with its requirement that an expert in forming an opinion may rely on facts or data "reasonably relied" upon in his or her field is seen by some courts to trump *Frye*'s general acceptance standard. See, e.g., *Alaska v. Coon*, 974 P. 2d 386 (1999) [FRE changed *Frye* test].

In *Coca-Cola Bottling Co. v. Gill*, 100 S.W. 3d 715 (2003), the Alaska Supreme Court adopted *Kumho*, holding that Rule 702 applies equally to all types of expert testimony and not simply to scientific expert testimony. All expert testimony must be shown to be both reliable and relevant. In later decisions the court applied *Coon-Daubert* to scientific evidence that was not novel, e.g., mass spectrometry and gas chromatography, which are generally accepted and recognized procedures for testing blood to determine a quantifiable amount. (*Hoyle v. State*, 2007 Ark. LEXIS 624; *Hoyle v. State*, 2007 Ark. LEXIS 624 [Ark. 2007], *Rhrg. den. Hoyle v. State*, 2008 Ark. LEXIS 12 [Ark., Jan. 10, 2008]).

Arkansas: *Daubert* and Novel Evidence

Farm Bureau Mut. Ins. Co. of Ark., Inc. v. Foote, 341 Ark. 105, 14 S.W. 3d 512, 519–520 (2000) ("Foote"). In the context of a proffer of novel evidence in an arson case that a canine's ability to detect fire accelerants is more sensitive than laboratory equipment used by forensic chemists, the court explicitly adopted *Daubert* for all novel evidence, consistent with a pre-*Daubert* holding of the Arkansas Supreme Court in *Prater v. State*, 307 Ark. 180, 820 S.W. 2d 429 (1991) applying Arkansas Rules of Evidence (ARE) 401, 402, and 702. Those rules require "the trial court to conduct a preliminary inquiry focusing on (1) the reliability of the novel process used to generate the evidence, (2) the possibility that admitting the evidence would overwhelm, confuse or mislead the jury, and (3) the connection between the evidence to be offered and the disputed factual issues in the particular case. Under this approach, reliability is the critical element. There are a number of factors that bear upon reliability, including the 'novelty' of the new technique, its relationship to more established modes of scientific analysis, the existence of specialized literature dealing with the technique, the qualifications and professional stature of expert witnesses, and the non-judicial uses to which scientific techniques are put" (*Foote*, at 116–117, citing *Prater v. State*, 307 Ark. 180, 820 S.W. 2d 429 [1991]).

Colorado: Rule Based: More Liberal Admissibility Standard to Be Tempered by Prejudice Analysis

In *People v. Shreck*, 22 P. 3d 68, 77 (Colo. 2001), the Supreme Court of Colorado held that Colorado Rule of Evidence (CRE) 702 and CRE 403 "represent a better standard [than the *Frye* rule], because their flexibility is consistent with a liberal approach that considers a wide range of issues." The *Shreck* court quoted *Daubert* with approval. The Colorado Supreme Court summarized the state's scientific testimony rules:

> To summarize, we conclude that CRE 702, rather than *Frye*, represents the appropriate standard for determining the admissibility of scientific evidence. We hold that under this standard, the focus of a trial court's inquiry should be on the reliability and relevance of the scientific evidence, and that such an inquiry requires a determination as to (1) the reliability of the scientific principles; (2) the qualifications of the witness; and (3) the usefulness of the testimony to the jury. We also hold that when a trial court applies CRE 702 to determine the reliability of scientific evidence, its inquiry should be broad in nature and consider the totality of the circumstances of each specific case. In doing so, trial court may consider a wide range of factors pertinent to the case at bar. The factors mentioned in *Daubert* and by other courts may or may not be pertinent, and thus are not necessary to every CRE 702 inquiry. *In light of this liberal standard a trial court should also apply its discretionary authority under CRE 403 to ensure that the probative value of the evidence is not substantially outweighed by unfair prejudice.* Finally, we hold that under CRE 702, a trial court must issue specific findings as it applies the CRE 702 and 403 analyses. *Id.*, at 78–79. [Emphasis added.]

Connecticut: Gatekeeper. Four-Point Test Does Not Apply to All Science

The leading case in Connecticut is *State v. Porter*, 241 Conn. 57, 698 A. 2d 739 (1997). Many physicians and scientists are befuddled by the four-part test of *Daubert*, wondering how it can apply to a specific case. This was the issue addressed by the *Kumho* court. Daubert's four-part test does not apply to all analyses of scientific reliability, and although the *Daubert* court and the *Kumho* court made it clear that the test was inclusive, not exclusive, the Connecticut Supreme Court provided a metaphor in *Porter* that speaks a thousand words: "Without a conceptual framework, using [mechanical] multiple-factor tests to evaluate science is like trying to light up a ball park with a few misaimed spotlights."

The inclusive, rather than exclusive, nature of the list in *Daubert* created an indefiniteness, noted the *Porter* court, that is a necessity because it is "impossible to formulate a specific clearly defined test that provides judges with a precise, complete list of factors to consider in evaluating the entire class of scientific evidence."

Depending upon the genre of expert testimony being proffered, the *Porter* court held that "when read and applied correctly, *Daubert* provides the proper approach to the threshold admissibility of scientific evidence." A proper application of the *Daubert* standard requires the gate keeping trial judge to evaluate the reliability of the science being offered within the framework of the particular expertise. "It is clear," wrote the court, "that [Connecticut has] been moving toward a validity standard for a number of years. We believe that it is time to complete that process, and that the *Daubert* [reliability] approach will provide structure and *guidance* to what has until now been a potentially confusing and sparsely defined area of legal analysis in our state jurisprudence.... Accordingly, we conclude that the *Daubert* approach should govern the admissibility of scientific evidence in Connecticut." [Internal citations omitted; emphasis added.]

Delaware: *Daubert,* but Still Some *Frye*

Although Delaware adopted *Daubert* for all expert testimony in *M.G. Bancorp., Inc. v. Le Beau*, 737 A. 2d 513, 522 (Del. 1999), the Delaware Supreme Court stated that the *Frye* rule would continue to apply to questions of admissibility of such expert testimony. The *Frye* rule, therefore, is part of the admissibility standard regardless of the type of expertise being proffered.

Kentucky: Reliable Science vs. Unfair Prejudice

In *Rogers v. Commonwealth*, 86 S.W. 3d 29, 42 (Ky. 2002), a case in which the Kentucky Supreme Court adopted *Daubert* and provided a fairly comprehensive statement of Kentucky law on the admissibility of scientific evidence, the court emphasized an aspect of expert witness testimony that many believe impacts the very integrity of the justice system: the potential to create unfair prejudice when jurors give it more weight than other testimony, such as that given by lay witnesses. This concern stems from the fact that the Seventh Amendment to the U.S. Constitution guarantees trial by jury, which means, fundamentally, that the jurors, and not experts, are the finders of fact.

The *Rogers* court noted that the application of Kentucky Rule of Evidence 403 (identical to FRE 403 in the text box) is especially important in cases involving science testimony where there is a risk that jurors may give greater deference to the testimony of experts than testimony given by lay witnesses. Under the *Rogers* ruling, if a trial judge determines that an expert's testimony meets the standard for scientific reliability under *Daubert*, then the judge must also determine "whether [a] KRE 403 relevancy inquiry warrants limitations on the scope of [the expert's] testimony," that is, whether parts of it may be more unfairly prejudicial than probative. If so, even though the expert witness testimony may be reliable and therefore, relevant, it may be excluded on the grounds that its probative value is outweighed by its unfair prejudice.

Louisiana: *Daubert*: Reliable Science vs. Unfair Prejudice—Where Diagnosis Is a Statement of Causation

In *State v. Foret*, 628 So. 2d 1116 (La. 1993), the Louisiana Supreme Court adopted the *Daubert* standard to determine whether expert testimony is admissible. Expert testimony often touches on the question of whether a crime was, in fact, committed (the "ultimate issue" problem of FRE 704). When such testimony is shaped by "syndrome" evidence, scientific reliability often comes into question as well as concerns about unfair prejudice.

The *Foret* Court held that the trial judge committed reversible error when he failed to determine whether the testimony of a psychologist in a child sex abuse case was scientifically reliable. Louisiana's Rule of Evidence 702 and Federal Rule of Evidence 702 were the same in 1993. The *Foret* Court stated: "Subsumed in the requirements of [Louisiana] Rule 702 is the premise that expert testimony must be reliable to be admissible." Allowing the testimony of an expert to bolster the credibility of an alleged victim, who was the state's main witness, in a case where the "science" of child sexual abuse accommodation syndrome (CSAAS), a theory lacking scientific reliability, was more unfairly prejudicial than probative. Further, "the reliability of an expert is...ensured by a requirement that there be a valid scientific connection to the pertinent inquiry." The reasoning or methodology underlying the testimony must be scientifically valid, and the trial court must determine whether this can be applied to the facts in issue. The CSAAS was not a diagnostic tool (to be used to bolster a claim, in the absence of physical evidence, that sexual abuse occurred). "The CSAAS acknowledges that there is no clinical method available to distinguish 'valid' claims from those that should be treated as fantasy or deception, and it gives no guidelines for discrimination." Rather, the syndrome was helpful only in explaining why some children delay reporting the abuse. Its use for diagnosing whether sexual abuse occurred does not pass the general acceptance or *Frye* portion of *Daubert*, and the scientific community has not, even after peer review, embraced it. Further, in one study investigating the reliability of children's claims that they had been sexually abused, there was a 32% margin of error. Although one researcher "might have been comfortable with a 32% margin of error, we are not so comfortable, especially remembering that 'the integrity of the criminal trial process is too important to permit it to be compromised by dynamic speculations'." [Internal citations omitted.] "This type of testimony has been labeled as so inherently unreliable that they cannot aid decision making in the criminal justice system."

Michigan: *Daubert*

In 2003, Michigan's Rule 702 was amended to mirror the teachings and guidance of *Daubert* and its progeny. As with many states, Michigan's codified evidence scheme closely resembles and is often textually identical to the *Federal Rules of Evidence*. Under the new Michigan Rule of Evidence 702 governing the testimony of experts:

> If the court determines that scientific, technical, or other specialized knowledge will assist the trier of fact to understand the evidence or to determine a fact in issue, a witness qualified as an expert by knowledge, skill, experience, training, or education may testify thereto in the form of an opinion or otherwise if (1) the testimony is based on sufficient facts or data, (2) the testimony is the product of reliable principles and methods, and (3) the witness has applied the principles and methods reliably to the facts of the case.

In adopting a rule that is almost identical to the federal rule, Michigan has become a *Daubert* state for all expert testimony.

Montana: *Daubert* Plus Cross-Examination

The Supreme Court of Montana adopted *Daubert in State v. Cline*, 909 P. 2d 1171 (1996), but limited its use to only proffers of novel scientific evidence. In a shoot-first-ask-questions-later approach, the *Cline* court stated that all other expert testimony is simply subject to cross-examination, *not pretrial exclusion*. One of the clearest statements of Montana's law of scientific evidence is found in *State v. Price*, 171 P. 3d 293 (2007). Bearing in mind that Montana still uses the pre-*Daubert–Kumho–Joiner* version of Rule of Evidence 702, the *Price* court stated: "The test for admissibility of expert testimony is whether the matter is sufficiently beyond common experience that the opinion of the expert will assist the trier of fact to understand the evidence or to determine a fact in issue.... Only where the introduction of 'novel scientific evidence' is sought do we apply the *Daubert* standard." [Internal citations omitted.] And, the *Cline* court added, "where *Daubert* is inapplicable it is better to admit relevant scientific evidence in the same manner as other expert testimony and allow its weight to be attacked by cross-examination and refutation," citing *Barmeyer v. Montana Power Co.*, 657 P. 2d 594 (1983) [Internal quotations omitted]; this was overruled on other grounds, *Martel v. Montana Power Co.*, 752 P. 2d 140, 145 (1988). "We adhere to the settled principle of admitting relevant scientific evidence in the same manner as other expert testimony and allowing its weight to be attacked by cross-examination and refutation." *Id.*

Montana departs from the Kumho Tire case in which the U.S. Supreme Court emphasized the mandate of FRE 104(a), which requires judges to serve as the gatekeeper of all expert testimony and, where it is found to be unreliable, to exclude it from the jury, regardless of the opportunity for cross-examination. Many lawyers, judges, and commentators take the position that no amount of cross-examination can unring the bell of unfair prejudice caused by unreliable and, therefore, irrelevant evidence, in a jury trial.

Nebraska: *Daubert*. Toxic Torts and Traps for the Unwary Expert

Toxic tort litigation has spawned controversy in law and science. It is an area in which forensic scientists are frequently called upon to testify about causation of disease and death. It is an area fraught with traps and pitfalls for the unwary, as was illustrated when the Supreme Court of Nebraska abandoned the *Frye* standard for *Daubert* in *Schafersman v. Agland Corp.*, 631 N.W. 2d 862 (2001).

The Schafersmans were dairy farmers who claimed the defendants' cattle feed was contaminated with excess minerals that caused their cows to either stop producing milk or die from what their trial expert called "multiple mineral toxicity" (MMT). On appeal, the Supreme Court noted that the plaintiffs' expert did not clinically examine or treat the cows and only examined the plaintiffs' records. The expert did not conduct any testing to rule out other causes of the cows' jaundice or reduced milk production and did not test the feed after it was mixed with other nutrients and added to the defendants' feed. The expert admitted that no single mineral in the feed was above accepted levels, that he had never studied or written about MMT, that there were no controlled studies or other scientific literature about MMT, and that his own theory did not establish any levels that would be toxic. The expert's only basis for his MMT theory was that others had observed it in the field. In reversing the plaintiffs' favorable jury verdict, the Nebraska Supreme Court determined the theory was novel such that it should have been scrutinized under *Frye*, but when it was, it failed that test because it was not generally accepted in any scientific field. Further, the expert had failed to engage in differential diagnosis of etiology. "Essentially," wrote the *Schafersman* court, "the only basis for [the expert's opinion] was that since the cows consumed the feed and then became ill, the feed must have caused the illness." If one relies only on Nebraska Rule of Evidence (NRE) 702, which, like its federal counterpart, requires that the court determine that the expert testimony will aid the trier of fact in understanding the evidence, the expert's opinion was superfluous because correlation does not prove causation. The *Schafersman* court held that the trial judge abused his discretion in admitting the MMT testimony.

"The concern about 'junk science,'" wrote the *Schafersman* court, "...now weighs in favor of adopting *Daubert/Kumho Tire* standards. The 'gatekeeper' functions exercised by trial courts under the *Daubert/Kumho Tire* analysis is, in fact, a more effective means of excluding unreliable expert testimony than is the *Frye* test. The experience in jurisdictions which have adopted the *Daubert* standards suggests that the admission of so-called junk science evidence is a minimal risk." The *Schafersman* court further noted, "While it may be that most science generally accepted in the relevant scientific community will be good science, it is not necessarily so." Therefore, the court continued, "placing the focus on reliability, rather than general acceptance, may have unexpected but not undesirable results." *Daubert*, wrote the court, not only allows the admissibility of new theories or techniques that are found to be reliable but also allows a court to find "that evidence that had previously been admitted with little discussion is no longer satisfactory, where reliability of that evidence has been appropriately challenged." The court opined, "once an issue is determined under *Frye*, it is closed to further *Frye* analysis because it is no longer 'novel.' *Daubert*, on the other hand, permits re-examination of the issue if the validity of the prior determination can be appropriately questioned.... *Frye* asks whether something is generally accepted. *Daubert* asks whether it is dependable." The gatekeeper-reliability function applies to all expert testimony "to assure that the specialized testimony is reliable and relevant [and] can help the jury evaluate foreign experience, whether the testimony reflects scientific, technical, or other specialized knowledge."

New Mexico: *Daubert*. Preserving the Line between Expert Witness Testimony and Lay Witness Credibility

In *State v. Alberico*, 116 N.M. 156, 861 P. 2d 192, 203 (N.M. 1993), the Supreme Court of New Mexico abandoned the *Frye* standard for the *Daubert* standard. The case involved the use of testimony about post-traumatic stress disorder (PTSD) in the context of two criminal cases where it was offered (1) as evidence that the alleged victims were, indeed, sexually abused, that is, as evidence that a crime had been committed, and (2) to bolster the victim's credibility. Although scientific evidence in the forensic setting often embraces an ultimate issue (i.e., whether a crime has been committed—see FRE 704 above), the *Alberico* court discussed the question of whether jurors who hear expert testimony "are automatically swayed by its aura of special reliability and trustworthiness." In this case the question was more pressing because the PTSD expert testimony arguably crossed the line between science and witness credibility. When offered to bolster the alleged victim's credibility, that use of the evidence invaded the province of the jury, and when offered to show that the symptoms of PTSD were caused by rape, that violated a cardinal rule of science that "arguably there are no certainties" (citing *Daubert* [1]).

The New Mexico Supreme Court wrote: "Rules 702, 703, 704, and 705 govern the admissibility of expert testimony. These rules do not characterize expert opinion testimony as a lesser or greater form of evidence, but rather accord the trier of fact the discretion to evaluate such evidence just like any other admissible evidence." Juries are the judges of the weight and credibility of the evidence, the court stated, adding, "expert testimony is given no more weight, at least in theory, than ordinary lay witness testimony." Based on this reasoning, the *Alberico* court did not agree that juries are prejudiced by expert testimony more than other evidence and therefore did not agree that the trial judge should guard against this. Rather, the court stated, "It is the duty of our courts, therefore, to determine initially whether expert testimony is competent under Rule 702, not whether juries will defer to it." However, the *Alberico* court did give a nod to reality when it noted that "after the expert opinion is deemed admissible under Rule 702, perhaps then a consideration of possible deference could be made under a Rule 403 analysis of whether the probative value of the evidence might be 'substantially' outweighed by the danger of unfair prejudice, confusion of the issues or misleading the jury" (citing New Mexico's Rule of Evidence 403, SCRA 1986, 11-403).

The court held that (1) PTSD testimony is grounded in scientific knowledge; (2) PTSD is probative, that is, it reliably and accurately proves what it purports to prove in that it has a tendency to prove sexual abuse, and therefore assists the trier of fact; and (3) its probative value is substantially outweighed by prejudicial effect, but it may be offered only to show that sexual abuse occurred and not for the purpose of bolstering the witness's credibility. The expert may not, however, testify that PTSD was caused by sexual abuse, only that the symptoms are consistent with it, for "allowing an expert to couch his or her testimony in terms of causality may also breach a cardinal rule of science for 'arguably, there are no certainties in science'" (citing *Daubert* [1]).

North Carolina: *Daubert* Plus Established Science

The critical case is *State v. Goode*, 461 S.E. 2nd 631 (1995). North Carolina applies *Daubert* but also recognizes that some scientific principles are so well established that they may be admitted into evidence through a procedure known as judicial notice. Experts may be surprised by this procedure, but it is a well-worn rule of evidentiary jurisprudence and one that is worth knowing about in preparing a report or to testify. Federal Rule of Evidence 201 contains the foundational requirements for judicial notice: "A judicially noticed fact must be one that is not subject to reasonable dispute in that it is either (1) generally known within the territorial jurisdiction of the trial court or (2) capable of accurate and ready determination by resort to sources whose accuracy cannot reasonably be questioned." In applying a reliability standard to blood stain and blood spatter evidence to determine how a murder was committed, the *Goode* court noted that there are times when "no specific precedent exists," and in those cases, "scientifically accepted reliability justifies admission of the testimony of qualified witnesses, and such reliability may be found *either by judicial notice* or from the testimony of scientists who are expert in the subject matter, or by a combination of the two."

The use of judicial notice, however, should not lead one through the back door to a "nose count" general acceptance rule. Reliability, wrote the *Goode* court, of a scientific procedure "is usually established by expert testimony, and the acceptance of experts within the field is one index, though not the exclusive index, of reliability. Thus, we do not adhere exclusively to the formula enunciated in *Frye* [5]." [Internal citations omitted.] "Believing that the inquiry underlying the *Frye* formula is one of the reliability of the scientific method rather than its popularity within a scientific community, we have focused on the following indices of reliability: the expert's use of established techniques, the expert's professional background in the field, the use of visual aids before the jury so that the jury is not asked 'to sacrifice its independence by accepting [the] scientific hypotheses on faith,' and independent research conducted by the expert." [Internal citations omitted.]

Oklahoma: *Daubert*. Toxic Torts—General vs. Specific Causation

Daubert applies to all genres of expert testimony in all proceedings in Oklahoma under the Oklahoma Supreme Court's decision in *Christian v. Gray*, 65 P. 3d 591 (2003). Medical experts are often asked (1) to opine as to whether a particular substance is capable of causing injury or death and (2) to opine as to whether, in a particular case, the substance was the specific cause of the injury or death. The *Christian* court's opinion is an example of this bifurcated analysis:

> Causation is now often divided into general causation and specific causation in some controversies involving allegations of injury resulting from a person's exposure to a harmful substance. General causation is whether a substance is capable of causing a particular injury or condition in the general population, while specific causation is whether that substance caused the particular individual's injury. General causation is a relatively new expression, but actually the same concept as Wigmore's [10] explanation of the probative value of evidence on the issue of causation when a thing possesses, under similar circumstances, a tendency or capacity to cause a similar effect elsewhere.

Oregon: *Daubert*

The Oregon Supreme Court adopted *Daubert* in *State v. O'Key*, 899 P. 2d 663 (1995) and *State v. Brown*, 687 P. 2d 751 (1984). The combination of *Brown* and *Daubert* "boil[s] down to a seven-step test, subject to the caveat that these factors are not an exclusive list of considerations to be applied mechanically." The factors are: (1) the technique's general acceptance in the field, (2) the expert's qualifications and stature, (3) the use that has been made of the technique, (4) the potential rate of error, (5) the existence of specialized literature, (6) the novelty of the invention, and (7) the extent to which the technique relies on the subjective interpretation of the expert.

Rhode Island: *Daubert*

The Rhode Island Supreme Court adopted *Daubert* in *DiPetrillo v. Dow Chemical Co.*, 729 A. 2d 677 (R.I. 1999) and *Gallucci v. Humbyrd*, 709 A. 2d 1059 (R.I. 1998). In Rhode Island, "*Daubert*'s general holding—setting forth the trial judge's general 'gate keeping' obligation—applies not only to testimony based on 'scientific' knowledge, but also to testimony based on 'technical' and 'other specialized' knowledge" (citing FRE 702, *Daubert* [1] and *Kumho* [3]).

South Dakota: *Daubert*

State v. Hofer, 512 N.W. 2d 482, 484 (S.D. 1994). The Supreme Court of South Dakota adopted *Daubert* in *Hofer*. "If scientific, technical, or other specialized knowledge will assist the trier of fact to understand the evidence or to determine a fact in issue, a witness qualified as an expert by knowledge, skill, experience, training, or education, may testify thereto in the form of an opinion or otherwise" (quoting FRE 702). According to this test, a trial judge must determine that an expert's testimony both rests on a reliable foundation and is relevant to the task at hand. The requirements of the test are satisfied if the expert testimony is relevant and has a reliable basis in the knowledge and experience of his discipline.

Texas: *Daubert*—A Necessary Rule in a Complex World

The Supreme Court of Texas adopted *Daubert* in *E.I. duPont de Nemours and Co. v. Robinson*, 923 S.W. 2d 549, 556, 38 Tex. Sup. Ct. J. 852 (Tex. 1995), a case in which the court underscored the need for reliability analysis by the trial judge because "the use of expert witnesses in litigation has become widespread." In addition, the *duPont* court noted, "the scientific theories about which these experts often testify have increased in complexity and have become more crucial to the outcome of the case.... These developments pose a difficult problem for trial judges ruling on the admissibility of an expert's testimony.... Professional expert witnesses are available to render an opinion on almost any theory.... While many of these experts undoubtedly hold reliable opinions which are of invaluable assistance to the jury, there are some experts who 'are more than willing to proffer opinions of dubious value for the proper fee.'" This state of affairs, wrote the *duPont* court, "can have an extremely prejudicial impact on the jury, in part because of the way in which the jury perceives a witness labeled as an expert.... To the jury an 'expert' is just an unbridled authority figure, and as such he or she is more believable."

The *duPont* court further expressed a view commonly held as one of the pressing reasons for adopting *Daubert*:

> Added to the potentially prejudicial influence of the term expert is the difficulty inherent in evaluating scientific evidence. Jurors are often expected to understand complex testimony regarding arcane scientific concepts and are even asked to resolve issues on which the experts cannot agree. *Expert witnesses may sway a jury even when the science is palpably wrong. In light of the increased use of expert witnesses and the likely prejudicial impact of their testimony, trial judges have a heightened responsibility to ensure that expert testimony show some indicia of reliability.... It is especially important that trial judges scrutinize proffered evidence for scientific reliability when it is based upon novel scientific theories, sometimes referred to as "junk science."* [Emphasis added.]

Vermont: *Daubert*

In *State v. Streich*, 163 Vt. 331, 558 A. 2d 38 (1995) and *State v. Brooks*, 162 Vt. 26, 643 A. 2d 226 (Nov. 1993), the Supreme Court of Vermont adopted *Daubert*.

Wyoming: *Daubert*

In *Bunting v. Jamieson*, 984 P. 2d 467 (1999), the Supreme Court of Wyoming adopted *Daubert*. Wyoming's Rule of Evidence (WRE) 702 was textually identical to FRE 702 in 1999. In adopting *Daubert* as part of the state's evidence jurisprudence, the Supreme Court of Wyoming wrote:

> Our traditional analysis is found in *Springfield v. State*, 860 P. 2d 435 (1993) where we stated: "In ruling upon the offer of such evidence in Wyoming, our trial courts need only be concerned with the requisite foundation. Because it does appear the *possibility of an erroneous result is more likely to arise from the testing techniques than from the procedure, it is important for the trial court to be satisfied about the manner in which the testing was performed, and the*

> *qualifications of the individual who accomplished the scientific technique*.... We noted that our approach parallels the United States Supreme Court's decision in *Daubert*, and reiterated several of the 'general observations' listed by that Court to be considered by the trial court. *We now expressly adopt the analysis provided by Daubert and its progeny as guidance for the Wyoming courts' determination whether to admit or exclude expert testimony.* In doing so, however, we do not abandon our own precedent regarding the admissibility of expert testimony [i.e., that it must have the requisite foundation], but as in *Springfield*,...find the case law of the several jurisdictions essentially compatible on this subject."

West Virginia: *Daubert* Plus Judicial Notice of Established Science

Wilt v. Buracker, 191 W.Va. 39, 443 S.E. 2d 196 (1993), cert. denied, 511 U.S. 1129, 114 S. Ct. 2137, 128 L. Ed. 2d 867 (1994). In adopting *Daubert*, the Supreme Court of Appeals of West Virginia wrote: "We also note that the Court in *Daubert* found that certain scientific theories could be judicially noticed. The [*Daubert*] Court stated: 'Of course, well-established propositions are less likely to be challenged than those that are novel, and they are more handily defended. Indeed, theories that are so firmly established as to have attained the status of scientific law, such as the laws of thermodynamics, properly are subject to judicial notice under Fed. Rule Evid. 201'." [Internal citations omitted.] The *Wilt* court continued: "We also are of the view that, under Rule 702, there is a category of expert testimony based on scientific methodology that is so longstanding and generally recognized that it may be judicially noticed, and, therefore, a trial court need not ascertain the basis for its reliability." [Internal citations omitted.]

Mississippi: *Daubert*

Following the amendment of Mississippi Rule of Evidence 702 in 2003, the state's supreme court adopted *Daubert* in *Miss. Transp. Comm'n. v. McLemore*, 863 So. 2d 31 (2003). Noting that the commentary to Mississippi's amended Rule 702 "makes no mention of *Frye* or the general acceptance test," the *McLemore* court wrote:

> Thus, the current version of Rule 702 recognizes that the *Daubert* rule, as modified, provides a superior analytical framework for evaluating the admissibility of expert witness testimony. We are confident that our learned trial judges can and will properly assume the role as gatekeeper on questions of admissibility of expert testimony. The modified *Daubert* test does not require trial judges to become scientists or experts. Every expert discipline has a body of knowledge and research to aid the court in establishing criteria which indicate reliability. The trial court can identify the specific indicia of reliability of evidence in a particular technical or scientific field. Every substantive decision requires immersion in the subject matter of the case. The modified *Daubert* test will not change the role of the trial judge nor will it alter the ever existing demand that the judge understand the subjects of the case, both in terms of claims and defenses. We are certain that the trial judges possess the capacity to undertake this review. [Internal citations omitted.]

New Hampshire: *Daubert*

New Hampshire adopted *Daubert* in *Baker Valley Lumber, Inc. v. Ingersoll Rand Co.*, 148 N.H. 609, 813 A. 2d 409, 2002 WL 31780239 (Dec. 12, 2002). In adopting *Daubert*, the Supreme Court of New Hampshire observed: "Although *Daubert* is binding only in federal court, the text of New Hampshire Rule of Evidence 702 is identical to the federal rule at the time of the *Daubert* decision.... Among the States that have adopted Rule 702's wording, the vast majority have accepted the *Daubert* standard as their own evidentiary rule.... [W]e [now] apply the *Daubert* standard to New Hampshire Rule of Evidence 702."

States Where *Daubert* Is Viewed as Instructive

Hawaii: *Daubert* Instructive

State v. Vliet, 19 P. 3d 42 (2001). The Supreme Court of Hawaii has neither accepted nor rejected *Daubert*, but because the Hawaii statute is patterned on the federal rule, construction of that rule by the federal courts is instructive. The *Vliet* court wrote: "What we endorse is a 'broad latitude,'...granted the trial judge in deciding in a particular case how to go about determining whether particular expert testimony is reliable." [Internal citations omitted.]

Indiana: *Daubert* Instructive

In *Hyppolite v. State*, 774 N.E. 2d 584 (Ind. App. 2002), the Supreme Court of Indiana wrote, "although not binding upon the determination of the state evidentiary law issues, the federal evidence law of *Daubert* and its progeny is helpful to the bench and bar in applying the Indiana Rule of Evidence."

Iowa: *Daubert* Instructive

Leaf v. Goodyear Tire & Rubber Co., 590 N.W. 2d 525 (1999). The Supreme Court of Iowa permits trial judges to apply Daubert's four factors for the analysis of scientific reliability but does not require them to do so.

> To be admissible in an Iowa court the evidence...must be relevant. Iowa R. Evid. 402. Second, it must be evidence in the form of "scientific, technical, or other specialized knowledge [that] will assist the trier of fact to understand the evidence or to determine a fact in issue." Iowa R. Evid. 702. Third, the witness must be "qualified as an expert by knowledge, skill, experience, training, or education." In addition, any potential for an exaggerated effect of the proffered evidence should be considered. We hold that trial courts are not required to apply the *Daubert* analysis in considering the admission of expert testimony. Nevertheless, trial courts may find it helpful, particularly in complex cases, to use one or more of the relevant *Daubert* "considerations" in assessing the reliability of expert testimony. Therefore, trial courts may, in their discretion, consider the following factors if deemed helpful in a particular case: (1) whether the theory or technique is scientific knowledge that can and has been tested, (2) whether the theory or technique has been subjected to peer review or publication, (3) the known or potential rate of error, or (4) whether it is generally accepted within the relevant scientific community. If a trial court considers these factors, the court should focus solely on the principles and methodology, not on the conclusions that they generate." (Citing *Daubert* [1]; Internal citations omitted.)

Massachusetts: *Daubert* Instructive

Commonwealth v. Lanigan, 641 N.E. 2d 1342 (1994). Massachusetts leans heavily toward *Daubert* but does not completely abandon *Frye*, according to the Massachusetts Supreme Judicial Court in *Commonwealth v. Lanigan*. Speaking of the *Frye* rule, the *Lanigan* court wrote: "The test has a practical usefulness because, if there is general acceptance in the relevant scientific community, the prospects are high, but not certain, that the theory or process is reliable. The ultimate test, however, is the reliability of the theory or process underlying the expert's testimony.... Thus, we have recognized the risk that reliable evidence might be kept from the fact finder by strict adherence to the *Frye* test."

The *Lanigan* court noted that there are times when the relevant scientific community has not yet digested and approved the foundation of the theory or process, but the theory or process is so logically reliable that evidence should be admitted even without its general acceptance by involved scientists.

"General acceptance is not the sole test," wrote the *Lanigan* court, adding that the *Daubert* court "thought relevant the question whether the theory or technique can be or has been tested.... Peer review and publication of the theory or process is pertinent but also not an indispensable predecessor of admissibility.... The *Daubert* opinion finds a requirement of reliability implicit in [R]ule 702 which on its face uses helpfulness to the trier of fact as the test of admissibility of expert testimony based on scientific knowledge." [Internal citations omitted.]

Although the *Lanigan* court opined that the "general proposition set forth in the *Daubert* opinion seems sound," the court noted that it gives "little guidance for the application of that proposition to the facts of a given case." Still, the *Lanigan* court added: "The expert's opinion must have a reliable basis in the knowledge and experience of his discipline.... The overarching issue is 'the scientific validity'—and thus the evidentiary relevance and reliability—of the principles that underlie a proposed submission." The trial judge's function is "significant" and, if "deciding on the admissibility of a scientific expert's opinion," the trial judge finds that the process or theory underlying the opinion "lacks reliability, that opinion should not reach the trier of fact," the *Lanigan* court wrote. The court summarized the trial judge's duties:

> Consequently, the judge must rule first on any challenge to the validity of any process or theory underlying a proffered opinion. This entails a preliminary assessment of whether the reasoning or methodology underlying the testimony is scientifically valid and of whether that reasoning or methodology properly can be applied to the facts in issue. The judge thus has a gatekeeper role. Of course, if the judge rules the opinion evidence admissible, that ruling is not final on the reliability of the opinion evidence, and the opponent of that evidence may challenge its validity before the trier of fact." [Internal citations omitted.]

The *Lanigan* court added a further point of clarification:

> "We accept the basic reasoning of the *Daubert* opinion because it is consistent with our test of demonstrated reliability. *We suspect that general acceptance in the relevant scientific community will continue to be the significant, and often the only, issue. We accept the idea, however, that a proponent of scientific opinion evidence may demonstrate the reliability or validity of the underlying scientific theory or process by some other means, that is, without establishing general acceptance.*" [Emphasis added.]

Tennessee: *Daubert* Instructive

McDaniel v. CSX Transportation, Inc., 955 S.W. 2d 257 (1997). The Supreme Court of Tennessee in *McDaniel* noted that Tennessee's adoption of Rules 702 and 703 in 1991 as part of the Rules of Evidence "supersede[s] the general acceptance test of *Frye*." Under these rules, wrote the *McDaniel* court:

> A trial court must determine whether the evidence will substantially assist the trier of fact to determine a fact in issue and whether the facts and data underlying the evidence indicate a lack of trustworthiness. The rules together necessarily require a determination as to the scientific validity or reliability of the evidence. Simply put, unless the scientific evidence is valid, it will not substantially assist the trier of fact, nor will its underlying facts and data appear to be trustworthy, but there is no requirement in the rule that it be generally accepted.
>
> Although we do not expressly adopt *Daubert*, the non-exclusive lists of factors to determine reliability [are] useful in applying our Rules 702 and 703. A Tennessee trial court may consider in determining reliability: (1) whether scientific evidence has been tested and the methodology with which it has been tested; (2) whether the evidence has been subjected to peer review or publication; (3) whether a potential rate of error is known; (4) whether, as formerly required by *Frye*, the evidence is generally accepted in the scientific community; and (5) whether the expert's research in the field has been conducted independent of litigation." [Internal citations omitted.]

Ohio: *Daubert* Instructive

Miller v. Bike Athletic Co., 687 N.E. 2d 735 (1998). The Supreme Court of Ohio cautioned that *Daubert*'s reliability analysis should not be employed by a trial judge to exclude evidence simply because the trial court disagrees that the expert's conclusions are correct. Ohio Evidence Rule 702 is more extensive than its counterparts in other states. The *Miller* court wrote:

> A witness may testify as an expert if all of the following apply: (A) The witness' testimony either relates to matters beyond the knowledge, or experience possessed by lay persons or dispels a misconception common among lay persons; (B) The witness is qualified as an expert by specialized knowledge, skill, experience, training, or education regarding the subject matter of the testimony; (C) The witness' testimony is based on reliable scientific, technical, or other specialized information. To the extent that the testimony reports the result of a procedure, test, or experiment, the testimony is reliable only if all of the following apply: (1) The theory upon which the procedure, test, or experiment is based is objectively verifiable or is validly derived from widely accepted knowledge, facts, or principles; (2) The design of the procedure, test, or experiment reliably implements the theory; (3) The particular procedure, test, or experiment was conducted in a way that will yield an accurate result.

The *Miller* court added:

> A trial court should not reject one expert opinion for another simply because it believes one theory over the other. As stated by one court, "In analyzing the admissibility of expert testimony, it is important for trial courts to keep in mind the separate functions of judge and jury, and the intent of *Daubert* to make it easier to present legitimate conflicting views of experts

for the jury's consideration" (citing *Joiner*). Thus, a trial court's role in determining whether an expert's testimony is admissible under Evid.R. 702(C) focuses on whether the opinion is based upon scientifically valid principles, not whether the expert's conclusions are correct or whether the testimony satisfies the proponent's burden of proof at trial.

Maine: *Daubert* Instructive

State v. MacDonald, 718 A. 2d 195 (Me. 1998). Noting that Maine Rule of Evidence 702 is textually identical to the federal rule, the Supreme Judicial Court of Maine has cited *Daubert*'s definition of "science" with approval:

> Construing the identical federal counterpart to the Maine [R]ule [of Evidence 702] the Supreme Court of the United States has stated, "The subject of an expert's testimony must be 'scientific…knowledge.' The adjective 'scientific' implies a grounding in the methods and procedures of science. Similarly, the word 'knowledge' connotes more than subjective belief or unsupported speculation ('the trial judge must make a discretionary determination that there is sufficient scientific basis to the proposed expert testimony so that hearing it would be helpful to the jury')."

One commentator has opined that Maine law lacks a definitive reliability standard for scientific evidence. "[F]or the admission of testimony that is ostensibly scientific into evidence, there *should* be a reliability requirement and the requirement should be articulated in such a way that its application can be evaluated by an independent observer.… Maine lacks such a standard." [11]

Frye and Modified-*Frye* States

Alabama: *Frye*

Turner v. State, 746 So. 2d 355 (1998). Alabama is a *Frye* state for all but DNA testing, for which a *Daubert* analysis is applied (see Goodwin [12]).

District of Columbia: *Frye*

The District of Columbia has a *separate state court system composed of the Superior Court (trial court) and the D.C. Court of Appeals.* The D.C. court system is funded by the federal government, but its jurisprudence for evidence and procedure, as with any state, is independent of the federal rules. For this reason, even though the District of Columbia is the so-called federal city, it is under the *Frye* rule and not *Daubert* and its progeny. The D.C. Court of Appeals articulated the test for the admissibility of expert witness testimony in the context of a police misconduct case, *Dyas v. United States*, 376 A. 2d 827 (1977):

> (1) [T]he subject matter must be so distinctively related to some science, profession, business or occupation as to be beyond the ken of the average layman; (2) the witness must have sufficient skill, knowledge, or experience in that field or calling as to make it appear that his opinion or inference will probably aid the trier in his search for truth; and (3) *the state of the pertinent art or scientific knowledge [must] permit a reasonable opinion to be asserted.* [Emphasis added; internal quote marks and citations omitted.]

Although the District of Columbia follows the *Frye* rule for novel evidence, the standard of review on appeal is *de novo*—meaning it is reviewed entirely again by the appeals court. (Other state courts and the federal circuits apply the abuse of discretion standard for all expert testimony.) In *Cook v. Edgewood Mgmt. Corp.*, 825 A. 2d 939 (2003), the D.C. Court of Appeals wrote:

> If an issue involves the admission of a...new scientific technique...or a...unique, controversial methodology, [then] this court reviews the matter *de novo*. Moreover, under *Frye*, the proponent of a new technology must demonstrate by a preponderance of the evidence that this technology has been generally accepted in the relevant scientific community. [Internal quote marks and citations omitted.]

Florida: *Frye*

Rickgauer v. Sarkar, 804 So. 2d 502, 504 (Fla. App. 2001). Florida courts still apply the *Frye* test in determining the admissibility of scientific evidence, as the Florida Supreme Court has declined to apply *Daubert*.

Illinois: *Frye*

Illinois remains fundamentally a *Frye* state but is referred to by commentators as a state with a *Frye*-plus-reliability standard for novel scientific evidence (see Hunter [13]). Under the *Frye*-plus-reliability standard, the trial court must determine if the scientific test of the novel evidence is reliable and, if that reliability is generally accepted, the field to which it belongs. Under Illinois Rule 702, the trial court must determine not only just what is being proffered but also whether it will be helpful to the jury in understanding a fact in issue in the case and, if so, whether it is scientific evidence. If it is, then the court is asked to determine if the evidence is novel or involves firmly established methods or techniques. If it is novel, the court must ask if it meets the *Frye* standard. In addition to this, the court must determine if the evidence is reliable. If the evidence is not scientific, the *Frye*-plus-analysis does not apply.

Hunter [13] writes of the Illinois courts' retention of the *Frye* rule:

> Imposition of the *Frye* test serves to (1) ensure that a minimal reserve of experts who can critically examine the validity of a scientific determination in a particular case, (2) promote a degree of uniformity of decision, (3) avoid the interjection of a time consuming and often misleading determination of the reliability of a scientific technique into the litigation, (4) assure that scientific evidence introduced will be reliable, *People v. Knox*, 459 N.E. 2d 1077 (1984) and thus relevant, (5) provide a preliminary screening to protect against the natural inclination of the jury to assign significant weight to the scientific techniques presented under circumstances where the trier of fact is in a poor position to place an accurate evaluation upon reliability and (6) impose a threshold standard of reliability, in light of the fact that cross examination by opposing counsel is unlikely to bring inaccuracies to the attention of the jury.

Hunter [13] adds:

> It is suggested that many theoretical and practical arguments support Illinois retaining adherence to Frye...and further suggested that "it is very likely that the federal courts will be returning to what amounts to a Frye test within the next few years."

Kansas: *Frye*

State v. Haddock, 897 P. 2d 152 (1995) 257 Kan. 964. The rule governing the standard for admissibility of expert witness testimony is found in Kansas Statutes Annotated (KSA) 60-456, which states:

> Testimony in form of opinion. (b) If the witness is testifying as an expert, testimony of the witness in the form of opinions or inferences is limited to such opinions as the judge finds are (1) based on facts or data perceived by or personally known or made known to the witness at the hearing and (2) within the scope of the special knowledge, skill, experience or training possessed by the witness.

Kansas law was well summarized by a panel of the Kansas Court of Appeals in *Armstrong v. City of Wichita*, 21 Kan. App. 2d 750, 907 P. 2d 923, 929 (1996), a workers' compensation case in which the court declined to adopt *Daubert*:

> The Daubert test applies only to the federal courts.... [In Daubert] the [United States] Supreme Court concluded that [the *Daubert* test] superseded the "general acceptance test" of Frye.... Daubert holds that federal trial judges, when determining admissibility of expert testimony, must assure that the proffered scientific evidence is both relevant and reliable. General acceptance in the scientific community is not necessarily a prerequisite to the admissibility of scientific evidence.... The [United States] Supreme Court indicated that a proffer of expert scientific testimony "entails a preliminary assessment of whether the reasoning or methodology underlying the testimony is scientifically valid and of whether that reasoning or methodology properly can be applied to the facts in issue...." There are a number of reasons why we decline to apply the Daubert test. *The most significant is that* Daubert *does not apply to Kansas's cases. In this state, the test utilized is the "general acceptance" test set forth in Frye.... We reject the invitation to adopt* Daubert *and hold that the* Frye *test is the proper standard to be applied in Kansas when that standard is applicable.* [Emphasis added; internal citations omitted.]

Maryland: *Frye*

Maryland courts apply the *Fryes-Reed* test to novel evidence, a test that includes the generally accepted approach but also requires experts to opine that the technique or test is reliable. *Reed v. State*, 391 A. 2d 364 (1978).

Where the evidence is not novel, trial judges may simply take judicial notice of the generally accepted technique or test, but this mechanism of admitting evidence is limited if there is a disagreement in the scientific community as to the reliability of the evidence. In the context of voice spectrographic evidence in a rape case, the *Reed* court wrote:

> On occasion, the validity and reliability of a scientific technique may be so broadly and generally accepted in the scientific community that a trial court may take judicial notice of its reliability. Such is commonly the case today with regard to ballistics tests, fingerprint identification, blood tests, and the like. Similarly, a trial court might take judicial notice of the invalidity or unreliability of procedures widely recognized in the scientific community as bogus or experimental. However, if the reliability of a particular technique cannot be judicially noticed, it is necessary that the reliability be demonstrated before testimony based on the technique can be introduced into evidence. Although this demonstration will normally include testimony by witnesses, a court can and should also take notice of law journal articles, articles from reliable sources that appear in scientific journals, and other publications

> which bear on the degree of acceptance by recognized experts that a particular process has achieved. [Internal citations omitted.]

Reed, decided in 1978, was a case that preceded the 1993 *Daubert* ruling. The Maryland Supreme Court continues to adhere to the *Reed-Frye* standard of admissibility. In 2007, the Maryland Supreme Court reaffirmed the state's expert evidence admissibility standard in *Montgomery Mut. Ins. Co. v. Chesson*, 923 A. 2d 939 (2007). The *Chesson* court wrote:

> Maryland adheres to the standard set forth in *Frye* for determining the admissibility of scientific evidence and expert scientific testimony (citing *Reed*, adopting the *Frye* standard). Under the *Frye-Reed* test, a party must establish first that any novel scientific method is reliable and accepted generally in the scientific community before the court will admit expert testimony based upon the application of the questioned scientific technique. A trial court may take judicial notice of the reliability of scientific techniques and methodologies that are widely accepted within the scientific community. A trial court also may take notice that certain scientific theories are viewed as unreliable, bogus, or experimental.... However, when it is unclear whether the scientific community accepts the validity of a novel scientific theory or methodology, we have noted that before testimony based on the questioned technique may be admitted into evidence, the reliability must be demonstrated. While the most common practice will include witness testimony, a court may take judicial notice of journal articles from reliable sources and other publications which may shed light on the degree of acceptance *vel non* [Latin for "or not"] by recognized experts of a particular process or view.... The opinion of an "expert" witness should be admitted only if the court finds that "the basis of the opinion is generally accepted *as reliable* within the expert's particular scientific field." [Emphasis added; internal citations omitted.]

Thus, Maryland, as with several *Frye* states, requires that specific attention be paid to a reliability analysis, even when the general acceptance rule is being applied to a case.

Pennsylvania: *Frye*

In Pennsylvania, expert testimony must have "gained general acceptance in the particular field in which it belongs" to be admissible. In *Commonwealth v. Davies*, 811 A. 2d 600, 604 n.2 (2002), the Supreme Court of Pennsylvania summarized the standard for admissibility of expert witness testimony:

> Since the *Frye* test represents an attempt to measure the quality of scientific evidence prior to admission,... [Pennsylvania] courts have considered this to be necessary *whenever* science enters the courtroom, because "there is the danger that the trial judge or jury will ascribe a degree of certainty to the testimony of the expert...which may not be deserved."

Minnesota: *Frye* Plus Reliability

The standard for admissibility of expert witness testimony on scientific issues in Minnesota is called the *Frye-Mack* standard, which is *Frye* plus a reliability analysis. In *Goeb v. Tharaldson*, 615 N.W. 2d 800, 814 (2000), the Minnesota Supreme Court declined to adopt *Daubert in lieu* of continued reliance on *Frye*'s general acceptance rule (adopted in Minnesota in 1952) and on the *Mack* rule (*State v. Mack*, 292 N.W. 2d 764, 768–769,

772 (1980)). Of this combination, the *Goeb* court wrote: "First, a novel scientific technique must be generally accepted in the relevant scientific community, and second, the particular evidence derived from that test must have a foundation that is scientifically reliable." Minnesota's Rule 702 is textually identical to FRE 702. The *Goeb* court stated that Rule 702 did not, in its opinion, offer sufficient guidance:

> We have previously considered whether to abandon *Frye-Mack* in favor of a standard for admission based solely on the Minnesota Rules of Evidence [702]. In reaffirming our adherence to *Frye-Mack*, we explained that the *Frye-Mack* standard for admission "facilitates more objective and uniform rulings" by the courts while a standard based solely on the rules of evidence introduces an "undesired element of subjectivity [into] evidentiary rulings." [Internal citations omitted.]

Frye critics, noted the *Goeb* court, argue that the general acceptance rule "may at times exclude cutting-edge but otherwise demonstrably reliable, probative evidence, and thus represents a more conservative approach to the admissibility of scientific evidence," and that the "*Frye* standard might exclude a new, but reliable, methodology or test because of the inherent time lag between the development of a new scientific technique and its general acceptance in the field." [Internal citations omitted.] Summarizing and critiquing critics of *Frye*, the *Goeb* court added:

> By comparison, because *Daubert* stresses a more liberal and flexible approach to the admission of scientific testimony, it has been viewed as relaxing the barriers to the admissibility of expert evidence (citing *Joiner* for the proposition that "the *Federal Rules of Evidence* allow district courts to admit a somewhat broader range of scientific testimony than would have been admissible under *Frye*"). However, in practice, *Daubert* does not necessarily make admissible expert evidence that was not admissible under *Frye*. One commentator has noted that "the post-*Daubert* era can fairly be described as the period of 'strict scrutiny' of science by non-scientifically trained judges (citing the argument that trial judges are raising the threshold of scientific proof needed to have expert causation testimony admitted)." [Internal citations omitted.]

The *Goeb* court further noted that *Daubert* has also been criticized on grounds that it "improperly defers to scientists the legal question of admissibility of scientific evidence," whereas others are "concerned that *Frye* 'abdicates' judicial responsibility for determining admissibility to scientists uneducated in the law" (citing the Alaska Supreme Court's decision adopting *Daubert* in *State v. Coon*). However, the *Goeb* court stated:

> In repossessing the power to determine admissibility for the courts, *Daubert* takes from scientists and confers upon judges uneducated in science the authority to determine what is scientific. This approach, which necessitates that trial judges be "amateur scientists," has also been frequently criticized. Scientists often have vigorous and sincere disagreements as to what research methodology is proper, what should be accepted as sufficient proof for the existence of a "fact," and whether information derived by a particular method can tell us anything useful about the subject under study. Under *Daubert*, it is the responsibility of the judiciary "to resolve disputes among respected, well-credentialed scientists about matters squarely within their expertise, in areas where there is no scientific consensus as to what is and what is not 'good science,' and occasionally to reject such expert testimony because it was not 'derived by the scientific method.'" [Internal citations omitted.]

The Minnesota Supreme Court rejected the "key assumption in this approach... that judges cannot only resolve disputes among qualified scientists who have spent years immersed in their field of study, but can do so without also adopting the substantive positions of some scientists but not others." [Internal citations omitted.]

New Jersey: *Frye*

In *State v. Free*, 798 A. 2d 83, (App. Div. 2002), a panel of the court of appeals of New Jersey stated that *Frye* is still the rule in New Jersey's criminal cases. New Jersey Rule of Evidence 702 governs the admissibility of evidence in civil cases.

New York: *Frye*

People v. Johnston, 273 A.D. 2d 514, 517–518 (N.Y. App. Div. 3d. Dep't 2000), 95 N.Y. 2d 935, 744 N.E. f2d 148, 721 N.Y.S. 2d 612 (2000) *lv denied*). In *Johnston*, New York's third appellate division summarized the state's standard of admissibility as follows:

> [D]eterminations of the admissibility and scope of expert testimony are committed to the sound discretion of the trial court, and the court's decision will not be disturbed absent a showing of serious mistake, error of law or abuse of discretion (see *People v. Perry*, 251 A.D.2d 895, 896, *lv denied* 94 N.Y.2d 827; *People v. Fish*, 235 A.D.2d 578, 579–580, *lv denied* 89 N.Y.2d 1092). Expert opinion is admissible if "it would help to clarify an issue calling for professional or technical knowledge, possessed by the expert and beyond the ken of the typical juror" (*People v. Taylor*, 75 N.Y.2d 277, 288, quoting *De Long v. County of Erie*, 60 N.Y.2d 296, 307). Accordingly, expert testimony may be precluded if it is within the average juror's understanding, not beyond the range of ordinary knowledge or intelligence and does not require professional or scientific knowledge (see *People v. Shepard*, 259 A.D.2d 775, 777, *supra; People v. Perry, supra,* at 896). Where expert testimony is deemed an appropriate aid to the jury's understanding and is based on scientific principles or procedures, then the trial court must also confirm that the principles or procedures upon which the expert's opinions will be based have gained general acceptance in its specified field (see *People v. Wesley*, 83 N.Y.2d 417, 422–423; *People v. Green*, 250 A.D.2d 143, 146, *lv denied* 93 N.Y.2d 873).

Washington: *Frye*

In *State v. Copeland*, 922 P. 2d 1304 (1996), the Supreme Court of Washington applied the *Frye* test to a novel question of DNA evidence and declined to adopt *Daubert*, articulating its rationale as follows:

> Expert testimony should be presented to the trier of fact only when the scientific community has accepted the reliability of the underlying principles.... In other words, scientists in the field must make the initial determination whether an experimental principle is reliable and accurate.... The *Frye* standard recognizes that...judges do not have the expertise required to decide whether a challenged scientific theory is correct...and therefore courts...defer this judgment to scientists. [Internal citations omitted.]

The *Copeland* court was careful to distinguish between those situations when a novel scientific principle has been generally accepted and those where there remains considerable dispute:

> The court does not itself assess the reliability of the evidence. "If there is a significant dispute between qualified experts as to the validity of scientific evidence, it may not be admitted." [Internal citations omitted.]

If the *Frye* test is satisfied, the trial court must then determine whether expert testimony should be admitted under the two-part test of Evidence Rule 702, i.e., whether the expert qualifies as an expert and whether the expert's testimony would be helpful to the trier of fact.

Further justifying its continued adherence to the *Frye* rule, the *Copeland* court wrote:

> Proponents of *Frye* agree that…it assures uniformity in evidentiary rulings, that it shields juries from any tendency to treat novel scientific evidence as infallible, that it avoids complex, expensive, and time-consuming courtroom dramas, and that it insulates the adversary system from novel evidence until a pool of experts is available to evaluate it in court.… The *Frye* standard allows "disputes concerning scientific validity to be resolved by the relevant scientific community."… In effect, *Frye* envisions an evolutionary process leading to the admissibility of scientific evidence. A novel technique must pass through an "experimental" stage in which it is scrutinized by the scientific community. Only after the technique has been tested successfully in…this stage will it receive judicial recognition. [Internal citations omitted.]

In *Copeland*, the state argued that the Washington Supreme Court should adopt *Daubert* because *Frye* is difficult to apply, to which the court responded:

> While *Frye* may be difficult to apply in some contexts, this is a result of the complexity of the particular science at issue, the extent to which the scientific community has made its views known, and the extent of any dispute in the scientific community. The same, or similar problems, arise under *Daubert*, including questions of testability, the extent to which the scientific technique or method is accepted by the scientific community, and drawing the line between legitimate science and "junk" science, along with other questions. Questions of admissibility of complex, controversial scientific techniques or methods, like those involving DNA evidence, are going to be difficult under either standard. Nevertheless, the *Frye* standard has endured for over 70 years, indicating that it has not been so difficult to apply as to call for its abandonment. [Internal citations omitted.]

In addition to the *Frye* rule, the trial judge must determine that evidence is helpful to the trier of fact in understanding a material issue in the case, thus, wrote the *Copeland* court, "providing in this jurisdiction the 'best of both worlds.'" The court continued:

> Where novel scientific evidence is at issue, the additional *Frye* inquiry allows the judiciary to defer to the scientists precisely where to do so recognizes both the need for admissibility of novel scientific evidence where it is sufficiently accepted, and the need to protect against novel scientific evidence which has not even gained general acceptance in the relevant field. The trial court's gatekeeper role under *Frye* involves by design a conservative approach, requiring careful assessment of the general acceptance of the theory and methodology of novel science, thus helping to ensure, among other things, that "pseudoscience" is kept out of the courtroom.… Evidence Rule 702 has independent force and effect, which we have both recognized and emphasized.

Idaho: Gatekeeper State

Idaho's Rule of Evidence 702 is textually identical to FRE 702 as it was before it was amended to incorporate the *Daubert–Joiner–Kumho* rulings, and it governs the admissibility of expert testimony. If the trial judge determines the expert evidence is reliable and helpful to the jury, then it is admissible. (See *Walker v. Am. Cyanamid Co.*, 948 P. 2d 1123 [1977]; *State v. Merwin*, 962 P. 2d 1026 [1998]; *Carnell v. Barker Management, Inc.*, 48 P. 2d 651 [2002].)

Idaho uses a mix of the pre-*Daubert* Rule of Evidence 702 and *Frye*, as explained by the Idaho Supreme Court in *Carnell v. Baker Management, Inc.*, 48 P. 3d 651 (2002):

> Idaho Rule of Evidence 104 in pertinent part states, "preliminary questions concerning the qualifications of a person to be a witness…or the admissibility of evidence shall be determined by the court…."

Idaho Rule of Evidence 702 states "if scientific, technical, or other specialized knowledge will assist the trier of fact to understand the evidence or to determine a fact in issue, a witness qualified as an expert by knowledge, skill, experience, training, or education, may testify thereto in the form of an opinion or otherwise." This Court has stated "that the appropriate test for measuring reliability of evidence in this state is I.R.E. 702." *State v. Merwin*, 131 Idaho 642, 646, 962 P. 2d 1026, 1030 (1998) (citing *Walker v. Am. Cyanamid Co.*, 130 Idaho 824, 832, 948 P. 2d 1123, 1131 [1997])…"The trial court's broad discretion in admitting evidence 'will only be disturbed on appeal when there has been a clear abuse of discretion.'" *Id.* In *Merwin*, the defendant argued that the studies relied upon by the experts did not meet the standards set forth in *Daubert*. This Court rejected the proposed application of *Daubert* to expert witness testimony in Idaho in *Merwin*.

Nevada: Gatekeeper State

Krause Inc. v. Little, 34 P. 3d 566, 569 (2001). Nevada Revised Statutes (NRS) 50.275 provides that "if scientific, technical or other specialized knowledge will assist the trier of fact to understand the evidence or to determine a fact in issue, a witness qualified as an expert by special knowledge, skill, experience, training or education may testify to matters within the scope of such knowledge." The *Krause* court declined to adopt *Daubert*, leaving the decision to admit or exclude scientific evidence to the trial judge who, in the court's opinion, is in the best position to determine if the expert testimony will be helpful to the jury.

Wisconsin: A Limited-Gatekeeper State

The Wisconsin legislature enacted in 1973 its own version of Rule 702:

> 907.02. Testimony by experts: If scientific, technical, or other specialized knowledge will assist the trier of fact to understand the evidence or to determine a fact in issue, a witness qualified as an expert by knowledge, skill, experience, training, or education, may testify thereto in the form of an opinion or otherwise. (Wis. Stat. § 907.02 [2006])

The Wisconsin Supreme Court in *State v. Walstad*, 119 Wis. 2d 483, 351 N.W. 2d 469 (1984) affirmatively decided that this rule would continue to be the state's governing law.

In *State v. Peters*, 192 Wis. 2d 674 (Wis. Ct. App. 1995), the Wisconsin Court of Appeals summarized the state's law of expert evidence as follows:

> Scientific evidence is admissible under the relevancy test regardless of the scientific principle that underlies the evidence.... The fundamental determination of admissibility comes at the time the witness is "qualified" as an expert. *In a state such as Wisconsin, where substantially unlimited cross-examination is permitted, the underlying theory or principle on which admissibility is based can be attacked by cross-examination or by other types of impeachment.* Whether a scientific witness whose testimony is relevant is believed is a question of credibility for the finder of fact, but it clearly is admissible. [Emphasis added.]

The *Peters* court continued:

> Although "Wisconsin confines itself to a determination of relevancy, we are compelled to acknowledge that *Wisconsin judges do serve a limited and indirect gate keeping role in reviewing the admissibility of scientific evidence. Unlike judges in* Frye *and* Daubert *jurisdictions, this role is much more oblique and does not involve a direct determination as to the reliability of the scientific principle on which the evidence is based.*" [Emphasis added.]

In addition to the standards of Wisconsin's Rule 702, Wisconsin judges may reject relevant evidence if they conclude that

> (1) the evidence is superfluous; (2) the evidence will involve a waste of judicial time and resources, *id.*; (3) the probative value of the evidence is outweighed by its prejudice to the defendant; (4) the jury is able to draw its own conclusions without it, *Valiga v. National Food Co.*, 206 N.W. 2d 377 (1973); (5) the evidence is inherently improbable; or (6) the area of testimony is not suitable for expert opinion. The foregoing list is not an exhaustive inventory of those grounds upon which the trial court may rely in refusing to admit relevant evidence. However, it demonstrates that *although Wisconsin judges do not evaluate the reliability of scientific evidence, they may restrict the admissibility of such evidence through their limited gate keeping functions.* [Emphasis added.]

Rules-Based-Plus-Reliability States

Arizona: Rule 702

Since the second edition of this text in 2008, Arizona adopted its own textually identical version of Federal Rule of Evidence 702, effective January 1, 2012 and, in doing so, made a notable departure from *Longerquist v. McVey*, 1 P. 3d 113 (2000), recognizing that "trial courts should serve as gatekeepers in assuring that proposed expert testimony is reliable, and thus helpful to the jury's determination of facts in issue." See e.g., *State v. Burke*, 2012 Ariz. Unpub. LEIXS 527 for helpful analysis, including a statement that Arizona will now look for federal decisions for guidance.

Missouri: Akin to Rule 702

A series of statutory rules of evidence enacted by the Missouri legislature, which contain language similar to that of FRE 702, applies in all civil proceedings according to the

Missouri Supreme Court's opinion in *Lasky v. Union Electric Co.*, 936 S.W. 2d 797 (1997) (*en banc*). However, unlike FRE 702, the Missouri rule, § 490.065, is restricted to civil actions. *Long v. Missouri Delta Medical Center*, 33 S.W. 3d 629, 643 (Mo. App. 2001). The *Frye* rule governs the admissibility of scientific hierarchy in criminal cases. See *State v. Stout*, 478 S.W. 2d 368 (Mo. 1972).

North Dakota: Rule 702 Plus Reliability

Hamilton v. Oppen, 2002 N.D. 185, P. 20, n.2, 653 N.W. 2d 678, 685. North Dakota's Rule 702 is the same as the pre-*Daubert* Rule 702 and, wrote the Hamilton court, it "envisions generous allowance of the use of expert testimony if the witnesses are shown to have some degree of expertise in the field in which they are to testify." However, the court cautioned, it is the trial court's responsibility to make certain expert testimony is reliable as well as relevant.

Utah: Rule 702 Plus Reliability

Utah's Rule 702 is textually identical to the federal rule. In *Franklin v. Stevenson*, 987 P. 2d 22 (1999), the Supreme Court of Utah stated the standard of admissibility for scientific evidence as follows:

> Rule 702 of the Utah Rules of Evidence, governing expert testimony, states: "If scientific, technical, or other specialized knowledge will assist the trier of fact to understand the evidence or to determine a fact in issue, a witness qualified as an expert by knowledge, skill, experience, training, or education, may testify thereto in the form of an opinion or otherwise." However, in order for *new* scientific evidence to be admissible, a threshold reliability test must be met. This court established that test nearly a decade ago in *State v. Rimmasch*, 775 P. 2d 388 (Utah 1989), *where we required a foundation establishing the reliability of the scientific evidence. We stated that "evidence not shown to be reliable cannot, as a matter of law, 'assist the trier of fact to understand the evidence or to determine a fact in issue' and, therefore, is inadmissible."* 775 P. 2d at 397–98 (quoting Utah R. Evid. 702). In making such an analysis, a trial court may either (1) take judicial notice of the "inherent reliability" of the evidence or (2) determine the inherent reliability after a hearing on the issue. [Emphasis added.]

South Carolina: Rule 702 Plus Reliability

South Carolina's Rule 702 is textually identical to FRE 702. South Carolina had not adopted the *Frye* rule prior to *Daubert.* In 1990, the standard for admitting scientific evidence in South Carolina was "the degree to which the trier of fact must accept, on faith, scientific hypotheses not capable of proof or disproof in court and not even generally accepted outside the courtroom." This standard is more liberal than the *Frye* standard. In *State v. Council*, 335 S.C. 1, 515 S.E. 2d 508, 517–518 (1999), cert. denied, 528 U.S. 1050, 120 S. Ct. 588, 145 L. Ed. 2d 489 (1999), the South Carolina Supreme Court held:

> While this Court does not adopt *Daubert*, we find the proper analysis for determining admissibility of scientific evidence is now under the SCRE. When admitting scientific evidence under Rule 702, SCRE, the trial judge must find the evidence will assist the trier of fact, the expert witness is qualified, and the underlying science is reliable. The trial judge should apply

> the Jones factors to determine reliability. Further, if the evidence is admissible under Rule 702, SCRE, the trial judge should determine if its probative value is outweighed by its prejudicial effect. Rule 403, SCRE. Once the evidence is admitted under these standards, the jury may give it such weight, as it deems appropriate.

Georgia: In a Class of Its Own

Georgia has one of the most liberal standards of admission for expert testimony. Georgia has not adopted the Federal Rule of Evidence 702, *Daubert*, or *Frye*. In *Norfolk S. Ry. v. Baker*, 514 S.E. 2d 448 (1999), a toxic tort case where the plaintiff-widow contended that her deceased railroad-worker husband contracted nasopharyngeal cancer from diesel fumes, the Supreme Court of Georgia articulated the standard:

> Citing *Daubert*, [Defendant-Appellant] Norfolk Southern [Railway] contends the trial court erred in denying its motion for directed verdict because Ms. Baker's medical expert did not offer a probable scientific basis for his opinion that diesel exhaust caused or contributed to the decedent's fatal nasopharyngeal cancer. We first note that *Daubert*...has not been adopted in Georgia. The applicable law in Georgia is [that] which provides: "the opinions of experts on any question of science, skill, trade or like questions shall always be admissible; and such opinions may be given on the facts as proved by other witnesses." Provided an expert witness is properly qualified in the field in which he offers testimony, and the facts relied upon are within the bounds of the evidence, whether there is sufficient knowledge upon which to base an opinion or whether it is based upon hearsay goes to the weight and credibility of the testimony, not its admissibility. *Jones v. Ray*, 159 Ga. App. 734, 736 (4) (285 S.E. 2d 42) (1981).

California: *Frye* Plus Reliability

California uses the *Kelly–Frye* test for admitting novel scientific evidence. It is called the *Kelly–Frye* rule because the Supreme Court of California reaffirmed its reliance on *Frye* in 1976 in *People v. Kelly*, 549 P. 2d 1240 (1976). Particular attention is given here to California because of its population and also because its jurisprudence of expert testimony is representative of the reasons other states have adhered to the *Frye* rule and continue to reject the *Daubert* trilogy.

In *Kelly*, the Supreme Court of California articulated the standard for the admissibility of expert testimony for evidence involving a novel, scientific technique:

> (1) the *reliability of the method* must be established, usually by expert testimony, and (2) the witness furnishing such testimony must be properly *qualified as an expert to give an opinion* on the subject. [Internal citations omitted.]

Although not textually identical to FRE 702, California Evidence Code Sections 720 and 801, respectively, permit experts to testify if they are qualified and if their testimony is helpful to the jury. Under California state law, the proponent of the evidence must demonstrate that correct scientific procedures were used in the particular case. (Thus, a showing of reliability in methodology is required.) In *Kelly*, the court further stated:

> The test for determining the underlying reliability of a new scientific technique was described in the germinal case of *Frye* involving the admissibility of polygraph tests: "Just when a scientific principle or discovery crosses the line between the experimental and demonstrable

stages is difficult to define. Somewhere in this twilight zone the evidential force of the principle must be recognized, and while courts will go a long way in admitting expert testimony deduced from a well-recognized scientific principle or discovery, the thing from which the deduction is made must be *sufficiently established to have gained general acceptance in the particular field in which it belongs.* [Emphasis added; internal citations omitted.]

Noting that California has "expressly adopted" the *Frye* rule, the *Kelly* court defended its position:

Some criticism has been directed at the *Frye* standard, primarily on the ground that the test is too conservative, often resulting in the prevention of the admission of relevant evidence... we are satisfied that there is ample justification for the exercise of considerable judicial caution in the acceptance of evidence developed by new scientific techniques.... Arguably, the admission of such evidence could be left, in the first instance, to the sound discretion of the trial court, in which event objections, if any, to the reliability of the evidence (or of the underlying scientific technique on which it is based) might lessen the weight of the evidence but would not necessarily prevent its admissibility. This has not been the direction taken by the California courts or by those of most states. *Frye*, and the decisions which have followed it, rather than turning to the trial judge have assigned the task of determining reliability of the evolving technique to members of the scientific community from which the new method emerges. As stated in a recent voiceprint case...[t]he requirement of general acceptance in the scientific community assures that *those most qualified to assess the general validity of a scientific method will have the determinative voice.* Additionally, the *Frye* test protects prosecution and defense alike by assuring that a minimal reserve of experts exists who can critically examine the validity of a scientific determination in a particular case. (Italics added; internal citations omitted.]

The *Kelly* court also noted that "a beneficial consequence of the *Frye* test is that it may well promote...a degree of uniformity of decision. Individual judges whose particular conclusions may differ regarding the reliability of particular scientific evidence, may discover substantial agreement and consensus in the scientific community."

However, wrote the *Kelly* court, "the primary advantage of the *Frye* test lies in its essentially conservative nature. For a variety of reasons, *Frye* was deliberately intended to interpose a substantial obstacle to the unrestrained admission of evidence based upon new scientific principles." The *Kelly* court noted that there is always "a considerable lag between advances and discoveries in scientific fields and their acceptance as evidence in a court proceeding." This reality convinced the *Kelly* court that "judicial caution" in admitting novel scientific evidence would avoid several problems, including cases where jurors may be misled by an "aura of certainty which often envelops a new scientific process, obscuring its currently experimental nature." The court added: "Scientific proof may in some instances assume a posture of mystic infallibility in the eyes of a jury." [Internal citations omitted.]

Judicial restraint is "especially warranted when the identification technique is offered to identify the perpetrator of a crime."

Moreover, once a trial court has admitted evidence based upon a new scientific technique, and that decision is affirmed on appeal by a published appellate decision, the precedent so established may control subsequent trials, at least until new evidence is presented reflecting a change in the attitude of the scientific community. [Internal citations omitted.]

More than 20 years after *Kelly*, and 6 years after *Daubert*, the Supreme Court of California affirmed its reliance on *Frye* in *People v. Soto*, 981 P. 2d 958 (1999). Although California is not a *Daubert* state, the *Soto* court introduced the notion of reliability into the judicial analysis, writing:

> Under the *Kelly* standard, evidence based upon application of a new scientific technique such as DNA profiling may be admitted only after the *reliability* of the method has been foundationally established, usually by the testimony of an expert witness who first has been properly qualified. *The proponent of the evidence must also demonstrate that correct scientific procedures were used.*
>
> The scientific technique on which evidence is being offered must have gained general acceptance in the particular field to which it belongs. However, *Kelly* does not demand that the court decide whether the procedure is *reliable as a matter of scientific fact: the court merely determines from the professional literature and expert testimony whether or not the new scientific technique is accepted as reliable in the relevant scientific community and whether...scientists significant either in number or expertise publicly oppose [a technique] as unreliable....* General acceptance under *Kelly* means a consensus drawn from a typical cross-section of the relevant, qualified scientific community. [Emphasis added; internal citations omitted.]

Medical testimony is not subject to *Kelly–Frye*, as was explained by a division of the Court of Appeals of California in *Wilson v. Phillips*, 73 Cal. App. 4th 250, 86 Cal. Rptr. 2d 204, 20–6 (1999). In *Wilson*, the plaintiffs claimed their memory of sexual abuse was repressed and then triggered. The California court refused to apply either *Frye* or *Daubert* to the plaintiffs' expert evidence, the testimony of a psychologist who was a specialist in dealing with patients who had been sexually abused and who suffered repressed memory. The *Wilson* court affirmed the trial judge's denial of a request for a *Frye* hearing and his admission of the expert's opinion that the circumstances and plaintiffs' behavior were "consistent with other individuals who had repressed their memories of childhood sexual abuse." The *Wilson* court explained:

> California distinguishes between expert medical opinion and scientific evidence; the former is not subject to the special admissibility rule of *Kelly–Frye. Kelly–Frye* applies to cases involving novel devices or processes, not to expert medical testimony, such as a psychiatrist's prediction of future dangerousness or a diagnosis of mental illness.

Similarly, the testimony of a psychologist who assesses whether a criminal defendant displays signs of deviance or abnormality is not subject to *Kelly–Frye*.

Virginia: Reliability (Neither *Daubert* nor *Frye*)

Noting that it had "declined to adopt the *Frye* test," the Supreme Court of Virginia explained the standard for admissibility of expert testimony in *Spencer v. Commonwealth*, 393 S.E. 2d 609 (1990) a case that predated *Daubert* by about 3 years:

> When scientific evidence is offered, the court must make a threshold finding of fact with respect to the reliability of the scientific method offered, unless it is of a kind so familiar and accepted as to require no foundation to establish the fundamental reliability of the system... or unless it is so unreliable that the considerations requiring its exclusion have ripened into

> rules of law, such as "lie-detector" tests…or unless its admission is regulated by statute, such as blood-alcohol test results. [Internal citations omitted.]

The *Spencer* court continued:

> In making the threshold finding of fact, the court must usually rely on expert testimony. If there is a conflict, and the trial court's finding is supported by credible evidence, it will not be disturbed on appeal. Even where the issue of scientific reliability is disputed, if the court determines that there is a sufficient foundation to warrant admission of the evidence, the court may, in its discretion, admit the evidence with appropriate instructions to the jury to consider the disputed reliability of the evidence in determining…its credibility and weight. [Internal citations omitted.]

The *Spencer* court included its view of the *Frye* rule:

> If admissibility were conditioned upon universal acceptance of forensic evidence, no new scientific methods could ever be brought to court. Indeed, if scientific unanimity of opinion were necessary, very little scientific evidence, old or new, could be used. Wide discretion must be vested in the trial court to determine, when unfamiliar scientific evidence is offered, whether the evidence is so inherently unreliable that a lay jury must be shielded from it, or whether it is of such character that the jury may safely be left to determine credibility for itself.

In *John v. Im*, 559 S.E. 2d 355 (2002), a post-*Daubert* case, the Supreme Court of Virginia stated that it has not yet considered the question of whether the *Daubert* analysis should be applied in Virginia trial courts to determine the scientific reliability of expert testimony. Although *Spencer* applies to both criminal and civil cases, the *John* Court wrote that in civil cases admissibility is also governed by Va. Code Ann. § 8.01-401.1 (2008):

> Not only must the expert testimony assist the trier of fact in understanding the evidence, but it is also subject to certain basic requirements, including the requirement that the evidence be based on an *adequate foundation*.… Expert testimony is inadmissible if it is speculative or founded on assumptions that have an insufficient factual basis.… Such testimony is also inadmissible when an expert has failed to consider all variables bearing on the inferences to be drawn from the facts observed. [Internal citations omitted.]

In both criminal and civil cases, only a physician, and not a biomechanician or biomedical engineer, may render a diagnostic opinion on the cause of injuries. In *Combs v. Norfolk & W. Ry.*, 507 S.E. 2d 355 (1998), the Supreme Court of Virginia stated:

> The practice of medicine includes the diagnosis and treatment of *human physical ailments*, conditions, diseases, pain, and infirmities. See Code Section 54.1-2900. The term "diagnose" is defined as "to determine the type and cause of a health condition on the basis of signs and symptoms of the patient." *Mosby's Medical Dictionary* 480 (5th ed. 1998). Thus, the question of causation of a human injury is a component part of a diagnosis, which in turn is part of the practice of medicine.

There are two exceptions to this rule in Virginia. First, a sexual assault nurse examiner (SANE) may testify about whether a victim was raped. In *Valazquez v. Commonwealth*,

643 S.E. 2d 131 (2007), the Supreme Court of Virginia permitted a sexual assault nurse examiner to testify about the cause of a physical human injury. Second, in *Conley v. Commonwealth*, 643 S.E. 2d 131 (Va. 2007), the Supreme Court of Virginia affirmed a trial court's admission of a psychologist's opinion in diagnosing post-traumatic stress disorder (PTSD) not only on the grounds that the psychologist was qualified to do so but, because psychology is not the sole province of physicians.

For a rapid comparison of the various states' evidentiary standards, see Table 2.2. It is clear that the veracity of the evidence that can be admitted at trial (civil or criminal) varies considerably from state to state. These differences, all with statutory or case precedent authority in their respective jurisdictions, provide an object of concern given the latitude the various standards permit or demand. This is an especially troubling issue when the outcome of an adjudication might be the death of the accused by execution. The potential for this outcome should impose upon experts who may be involved in the judicial process to provide testimony as robust and verifiable as possible, regardless of the statutory standard.

Judging the Reliability of Medical Literature Using the Three Rs, or the Reasonable Reliance Requirement, of Rule 703

The *Daubert* trilogy, and the cases of many states following it in whole or in part, focused to one degree or another on the issue of methodology. Evidence that is proffered as scientific must be the product of reliable methodology. In civil and criminal cases in which forensic pathologists and forensic neuropathologists are retained or called to testify as expert witnesses, these experts are frequently asked to disclose any and all medical or scientific literature upon which they rely for forming the basis of their opinions about causation.

The Alaska Supreme Court put it this way: As with the federal rule, "Alaska Rule of Evidence 703 employs a 'reasonably relied upon by experts' standard in contrast to *Frye*'s 'general acceptance' standard." It bears repeating the rule here:

Rule 703: Bases of Opinion Testimony by Experts

The facts or data in the particular case upon which an expert bases an opinion or inference may be those perceived by or made known to the expert at or before the hearing. If of a type *reasonably relied* upon by experts in the particular field in forming opinions or inferences upon the subject, the facts or data need not be admissible in evidence in order for the opinion or inference to be admitted.

An expert's reliance on facts and data must be reasonable because such facts and data, in and of themselves, may constitute inadmissible hearsay, a generally undesirable form of evidence because it is not subject to the crucible of cross-examination. To minimize the risk that this presents to doing justice in the context of an expert who relies on facts and data that are inadmissible hearsay, there needs to be some other guarantee of trustworthiness, and that index of trustworthiness is that it is *reasonable to rely* on such facts and data in the expert's field. If the expert, in forming his opinion to a reasonable degree of medical or scientific probability or certainty, has based his or her reliance on scientific and medical literature that is faulty and on which it is not reasonable in his field to rely, this goes beyond a mere credibility attack and, instead, is a problem with the expert's methods in reaching his conclusion. A forensic expert-physician who relies for the opinion on causation on faulty medical science not only sounds the death knell of the case but also invites rigorous examination at a deposition, expert interrogatories, or worse, cross-examination before a jury.

Under *Daubert* and its progeny, medical and scientific literature is under much greater scrutiny than before. Given the necessity of relying on medical literature to defend or attack the case for causation, it is imperative that the forensic professional, as well as the attorneys working with him or her, appreciates some of the major pitfalls in this body of knowledge. Much of this will be familiar, especially to those who are physicians, but not necessarily for lawyers. For physicians, it is hoped that the following discussion will serve to refresh some basic principles of evaluating the reliability of medical literature.

A Jury of Our Peers?

The *Daubert* court listed peer review as "ordinarily" one of the factors (depending on the proffered science) to consider in determining admissibility of evidence sponsored as scientific. Key here is the word *ordinarily* because the results and conclusions of research published in peer review journals are not always reliable and, indeed, in some cases may be *extraordinarily* unreliable. It is important to not take the term *peer review* too seriously and, even better, to approach it with much caution. A peer review journal is nothing more than a scientific "jury" asked to determine if the science in a report is valid. Just as juries in trials are subject to a wide range of foibles, so, too, are those who are on the editorial staff of, or are consultants for, peer review journals. Mainstream medical and forensic journals all have peer review boards, but they comprise mostly part-time or volunteer consultants to the journal who may fail to filter out poorly designed studies, unreliable results, or even falsified data. It is up to the expert to evaluate the scientific reliability of any references upon which he or she relies in forming a forensic opinion.

An extreme case helps illustrate how it can be dangerous to equate the term *peer review* with *reliability*. In 2005, a bogus paper based on a completely fake study concocted by some MIT students was accepted for presentation to a prestigious scientific meeting—the World Multi-Conference on Systemic, Cybernetics and Informatics (WMSCI)—in Florida. A chagrined conference chair claimed the bogus paper slipped through the cracks in the organization's standards by default: the paper was accepted simply because it was not rejected by the deadline. The paper was utter scientific gibberish generated by a computer program designed by the students to construct grammatically correct (albeit nonsensical) prose. It was even supported with a fake title, "Rooter: A Methodology for Typical Unification of Access Points and Redundancy," twenty-two fake references, fake charts, and fake diagrams. One illustration, "the schematic used by our methodology," was followed by a bar graph claiming to show "the 10th percentile seek time of our methodology, compared with other systems." (One of the students told the BBC that they played the prank to prove the lack of standards [14].)

Peer reviewers may have biases, such as financial or research interests, and refuse to publish papers that conflict with their research or financial interest, or the funding source—e.g., the pharmaceutical industry, the government, or a university may selectively fund research, which results in a skewed body of science for a particular area.

The bottom line is that peer review may not mean that the journal—in the case of a particular study—was an effective sieve for filtering out unreliable science.

Madness in the Methods

The soft underbelly of an expert's opinion may often be found in the shoddy methods used in the medical literature on which he or she relies. If it would not be reasonable for a physician to rely on articles using faulty methods to treat a patient, it is certainly not reasonable for a forensic pathologist or neuropathologist to do so in giving an opinion before a jury. Reliable methods are just as important to physicians outside the courtroom as they are to judges and lawyers in the courtroom. Writes medical research expert Trisha Greenhalgh [15]:

> It usually comes as a surprise…to learn that some (the purists would say up to 99% of) published articles belong in the bin and should certainly not be used to inform practice. In 1979, the editor of the *British Medical Journal*, Dr. Stephen Lock, wrote, "Few things are more dispiriting to a medical editor than having to reject a paper based on a good idea but with irremediable flaws in the methods used." Things have changed, but not enormously.

In a 1986 review of some 4235 research reports on the efficacy of drug trials and surgical, psychotherapeutic, and diagnostic procedures—information upon which doctors may rely to diagnose and treat our ills—three researchers concluded that only about 20% were valid studies, and some of these 4235 reports appeared in the *New England Journal of Medicine (NEJM)*, *Journal of the American Medical Association (JAMA)*, *British Medical Journal (BMJ)*, *Canadian Medical Association Journal*, *Lancet*, *American Journal of Psychiatry*, *Annals of Internal Medicine*, *Archives of Neurology and Psychiatry*, *Journal of Nervous and Mental Disease*, and *Psychiatric Quarterly*. In 1985, other researchers uncovered the fact that of more than 200 articles in two anesthesia journals, only 15% were without major errors in design or analysis. Some improvements in peer review journals have been made, with peer review journal boards using qualified statisticians and biostatisticians to review study design and check conclusions. But change is slow to come, the result of which is that the amount of bad medicine and science is still abundant and subject to attack.

A Few Basics

Most medical journal papers are written in the *IMRAD* format: introduction (why the authors did the study), methods (how they did it and how they interpreted the results), results (what they claim to have found), and discussion (the authors' interpretation of what the results mean). A shortcut to determining if the paper is reliable, regardless of how convincing the results may sound, is to go right to the methods section. If the methodology is wrong, then apply the principle of "junk in, junk out." As the *Daubert* court emphasized, the "focus of course, must be solely on principles and the methodology, not on the conclusions they generate." One might ask, "If the methodology of relying on peer review medical literature to form an opinion in a case is generally accepted in the relevant scientific community, then why shouldn't the testimony be admitted?" The answer is that *Daubert* made clear that general acceptance was only one of many considerations and is not the *sine qua non* of the admissibility of scientific evidence, as it once was. Ferreting out flaws in methodology means looking at every phase of the scientific process. That means starting out with a scientific frame of mind.

One major problem in methodology occurs when the researchers design a study or trial that inherently seeks to confirm, rather than falsify, the hypothesis. The *Daubert* court quoted twentieth-century philosopher Karl Popper [8] for the proposition that scientifically reliable results are those that stem from attempts to disprove them, that is, that seek to falsify the hypothesis. Much of today's medical literature is scientifically unreliable because either the study design or data analysis is flawed, creating confirmation bias. There is a story that has become a metaphor for this particular malady. Sir Paul Neal, a renowned seventeenth-century English astronomer, was peering through his telescope one night at the dimly visualized details of the moon when he spotted an elephant on the lunar surface. As a highly regarded member of the Royal Society, he felt it was his obligation to announce his finding to a world in which the possibility of men living on the moon had (even then) grown into a topic of serious debate among members of learned societies. However, Sir Paul and the Royal Society were publicly humiliated when it turned out that what he had taken for the trunk of an elephant was actually the tail of a mouse that had crept into his telescope. When a scientist sets out to prove a hypothesis, truth is the first casualty of the quest.

Getting Started

An opinion that has no support in the medical literature may be subject to attack as lacking scientific foundation. Sometimes, an opinion needs no published support, such as in a case where it is biologically plausible that an injury or a death was caused by a certain act, toxin, or disease, with such biological plausibility being grounded in principles of anatomy and physiology. However, when including references, the expert must be sure they pass muster under *Daubert*, *Frye*, or Rule 702. Also, in many cases, the retaining attorney will want the expert not only to provide his or her own opinion, but also to critically evaluate the opinion of the opposing expert for purposes of deposition preparation or cross-examination. Either way, it is important for the expert to obtain legible copies of any and all journal articles, textbooks, or other publications upon which he or she or the opposing expert claims to rely for his or her opinion.

Biostatistics and evidence-based medicine (EBM) now constitute a large segment of scientific and medical literature. For those unfamiliar with this topic, or even a bit rusty, there are a number of books, websites, and journal articles that are either low cost or free that provide a guide through the basics of how to analyze the scientific validity of a medical paper.

In EBM, there are several study designs, but they basically fall into two general categories: primary research and secondary research. Primary research includes randomized clinical trials (RCTs), experiments, and surveys. Forensic pathology and neuropathology medical articles are designed to answer questions about cause of death. As this book is not about clinical practice, clinical trials are not included in this discussion. Secondary research includes reviews of existing studies, such as meta-analysis by which data are aggregated from several studies, trials, or experiments.

In evaluating a medical study, one needs to first categorize it, as this will govern the standards by which it should be critiqued.

Mismatch between Design and Purpose

Flaws in study design are flaws in methodology. So, first, identify the type of study and ask yourself: What issue did the researchers set out to investigate? Make sure that the study on which the physician-expert relies matched the problem it was designed to investigate and that the study actually fits the client's case.

EBM is not always appropriate, especially in the context of death investigation. This is amusingly illustrated in a 2003 spoof study, "Hazardous Journey," for which the authors used EBM Internet research methods to search for randomized clinical trials testing the efficacy of parachutes as a treatment intervention to prevent major trauma in situations where a subject is gravitationally challenged when, for example, leaping from an airplane at a high altitude [16]. The problem to be studied? To date, the only evidence that parachutes work is merely anecdotal, i.e., observational data. The efficacy of parachutes as an intervention to prevent trauma has not been established; some people who fall from great heights have survived without a parachute, and some parachutes cause iatrogenic injury when they burst open at the wrong time or fail to open at all.

The two physicians who authored this study, published in the *British Medical Journal*, invited "the most radical protagonists of evidence based medicine" to organize and participate "in a double blind, randomized, placebo controlled, crossover trial of the parachute." That invitation went down like a lead balloon, and many people continue to rely on the time-tested parachute remedy, the efficacy of which is based only on observational (anecdotal) evidence.

Although there is an increasing number of studies that are in the genre of EBM, much of forensic pathology and neuropathology is still based upon observational data, such as case studies and case series studies. Much is also based on an understanding and application of basic medicine. Because there are many pitfalls in such studies, it is important to choose one's case studies and case series studies with caution.

Case Series Studies

Observational data are useful but, like any research, have to be applied correctly. An example of observational data is a case series study. This is a simple, descriptive account of interesting characteristics observed in a group of patients. It is one in which the "researchers" look at a group of cases and ask, "What happened?" Because the study looks back in time, it is often called a retrospective study. According to Guyatt et al. [17], a case series study, which involves unsystematic clinical observations, is the least scientifically significant [18]. This hierarchy scheme is depicted below, from best to least statistically robust [15]:

1. Systematic reviews and meta-analyses
2. Randomized controlled trials with definitive results (confidence intervals do not overlap, etc.)

3. Randomized controlled trials with non-uniform definitive results (confidence intervals overlap)
4. Cohort studies
5. Case control studies
6. Cross-sectional surveys
7. Case reports and case series

Case series studies do have a role, in that they help medical researchers to form hypotheses, and they are sometimes used to inform decisions about cause of death, but their usefulness is limited because they are subject to confirmation bias and selection bias. Under *Daubert*, the methodology would be characterized as flawed. Therefore, such studies and case reports are often scientifically unreliable.

Case series studies should be greeted with great skepticism if they claim to offer conclusions about any medical matter. In evaluating these, it is important to remember that case reports and studies based upon them frequently pose only hypotheses that require further investigation.

Selection Bias

Selection bias occurs when a researcher selects for the study only those examples or subjects that will support his or her hypothesis.

"Data dredging" is another form of selection bias and occurs when a researcher takes a small part of a study and uses it to "prove" a point that the study was not designed to show. Data dredging is often used to form hypotheses, but, unfortunately, these are then frequently presented as scientific fact. Another form of data dredging occurs when an author takes a series of case reports and tries to prove a hypothesis with these. It is particularly rampant in review articles that summarize the contents of case series studies.

A point of definition: a study riddled with the flaws of selection bias is said to suffer from confirmation bias. The easiest way to distinguish selection bias from confirmation bias is to appreciate that *confirmation bias is the end result of the selection bias process.* If one is asked to address such issues in a rebuttal report, deposition, or cross-examination, one might want to point out that the *Daubert* court relied on Karl Popper [8] for the modern-day approach to scientific inquiry: it should seek to "falsify" and not confirm a hypothesis [9]. If reasonable attempts at falsification fail, the theory or hypothesis may remain until again challenged. If the theory or hypothesis is damaged by falsification, it cannot remain viable or reliable.

Insufficient Data

Case series studies rarely provide enough clinical data to allow the reader to get behind the scientific conclusion and make his or her own determination about reliability. Therefore, peer review by fellow physicians is precluded. This flaw alone makes any case series study vulnerable to attack. The question is: is there enough information here that a physician would be able to agree with the factual foundation for the diagnosis and causation?

One of the biggest and most seductive traps that human beings fall into regarding their ideas about causality is the *post hoc ergo propter hoc* fallacy. Briefly stated, this fallacy is that a phenomenon is caused by whatever preceded it. This presupposes that the observer is fully cognizant of *everything* that preceded the phenomenon, not just the most apparent or satisfying. This, of course, is nearly impossible, or it is a very involved process. There are many paradigms for testing the veracity of a given hypothesis of causality [18]. In the case of establishing a cause for a disease, for example, Greenhalgh [15], adapting from the work of Haines [19], offers these guidelines:

1. Is there evidence from true experiments in humans?
2. Is the association strong?
3. Is the association consistent from study to study?
4. Is there a temporal relation?
5. Is there a dose-response gradient?
6. Does the association make epidemiological sense?
7. Does the association make biological or physical sense?
8. Is the association specific?
9. Is the association analogous to previously proven causal associations?

Statistics: Sometimes a Tool for Those with No Proof?

With increasing frequency, physicians who write up case reports as case series studies are attempting to breathe scientific life into them by applying statistical analysis. These reports may create a trap for the unwary because the sample sizes in case series studies are often too small to have any statistical power, i.e., statistical significance. Statistical significance means that a correlation between two or more factors is, allegedly, established to a high degree of certainty. Statistical significance in a study is related to odds ratios. However, these vary wildly, depending on the size of the sample. Case series studies are of small groups, and odds ratios jump all over the place, depending on whether the numbers are small or large. In small groups, the results are much more likely to be random. However, according to statisticians, the larger the study group, the more likely it is that the odds ratio is real. Epidemiological data that form the basis for statistics in medical articles depend on sample sizes that are large enough to be statistically significant. Like the concept of falsification of Popper [8], much of statistical testing rests on the so-called null hypothesis—that there is no difference between two samples or populations or results. Various methods can test this hypothesis and show either no difference (accept the null hypothesis) or a significant difference that can be measured (reject the null hypothesis) [20].

Data-Pooling to Conjure Up the "Statistics Boogeyman"

Sometimes proof is not medically solid and there are too few subjects sprinkled in a number of studies. As a way of covering their work with a scientific gloss, some physicians and scientists pool what they claim is data from several different studies. This may be labeled "meta-analysis" or "re-analysis" [21]. Although this might work in some areas of medical research for large, epidemiological studies, it does not always work in individual cases.

The simple reason for this is that, unlike some areas of epidemiological research, smaller study designs are an inconsistent alphabet soup of mostly case series studies of different specialties, all of which assign different clinical meanings to the same medical terms. These studies have different group sizes, different selection criteria, different analytical methods, different conclusions, and, of course, no controls. The expert should make sure that any reliance on meta-analysis is that which drew on studies that used reliable methods in design, were not substantially different in design, and used large-enough numbers to be significant. The strength of a particular meta-analysis depends upon the validity of each of the studies included in the meta-analysis. The faulty methodology of combining cases from several case series studies into a larger case review series still cannot lead to a reliable conclusion because case series studies, whether large or small, are designed to form hypotheses and not scientifically reliable conclusions.

If, when reading an article, the expert sees words like *statistics*, *statistical significance*, *odds ratio*, or *confidence interval* in the context of case series studies, this should quicken one's senses and alert the expert's faculty for critical evaluation, because, at least in the context of case series studies, statistics are for those who have no real proof. It is unscientific to apply statistics to unproved hypotheses, i.e., case series studies.

Statistics are also not a reliable way to determine causation in a case. Statistics do not, in fact, prove causation. All statistical conclusions do is report correlations. "Statistics," said Aaron Levinson, "are like bikinis. What they reveal is suggestive, but what they conceal is vital" [22,23]. Although correlations may be reliable enough for a toxic tort lawyer in cases where social policy creates proximate causation to boost the causation-in-fact proofs, statistical correlations should not help the parties in run-of-the-mill medical cases.

Case Control Studies

As with case series studies, case control studies are retrospective. They involve two groups: one group with the condition and one without the condition, that is, the control group. This type of study looks back in time and attempts to determine what risk factors, if any, existed that caused the condition in one group but not in the control group. Studies that claim to be case control studies should be analyzed for these types of biases.

Cross-Sectional Survey Studies

Cross-sectional studies analyze data collected on a group of subjects at one time, rather than over a longer period. They are snapshots in time as to what is happening now.

Cohort Studies

A cohort is a group of subjects who have something in common and who remain part of a group over an extended period of time. In medicine, the subjects in cohort studies are selected by some defining characteristic, such as one that is suspected of being a precursor to a disease.

Table 2.3 Expert Witness Rule 703 Checklist

Did the peer review process work for this article?
Do the authors in second, third, fourth places (etc.) have confidence in the data?
What was the purpose of the study?
Was the hypothesis actually tested?
What was the type/design of study?
Were there flaws in the design that, for example, allowed selection and confirmation bias?
Was the design of the study right for the problem?
Were the data properly analyzed?
Did the conclusion go beyond the data presented?
Was there data dredging?
Was there misuse of meta-analysis?
Did the conclusion understate or minimize the data presented?
Did the primary or secondary authors have a financial conflict or a research agenda that the conclusion contradicts?

Cohort studies ask the question: what will happen? Because they look forward, they are called prospective studies. They are still only observational studies, and they are still subject to all the same biases as the others of their genre. Those that claim to be scientifically reliable because they are prospective cohort studies torture the underlying definition to add a gloss of (pseudo) reliability to the conclusions. The interested reader is referred to the books and articles of references 19–21 and 24–26.

In evaluating professional publications that might be used under FRE 703, the expert would be well advised to screen anticipated publications and one's own work according to the filter in Table 2.3.

The NAS Report: The Sorry State of Forensic Science in the United States and the Risks and Challenges This Poses to Forensic Pathologists, Lawyers, and the System of Justice

"The forensic science system [in the United States] encompassing both research and practice, has serious problems," concluded the Committee on Identifying the Needs of the Forensic Science Community at the National Academy of Sciences [29]. The 2009 NAS Report—commissioned by Congress—outlines a shocking picture of the shortcomings of forensic science in the United States and calls into question the scientific reliability of much of the testimony given in death and injury investigation in the medicolegal setting. The reader is encouraged to become familiar with the NAS Report—for its title, "Strengthening Forensic Science in the United States—A Path Forward," belies the fact that the NAS Report is a serious challenge for the forensic pathologist giving expert testimony and provides fertile ground for attorneys in criminal and civil cases.

Hon. Harry T. Edwards, cochair and coauthor of the NAS Report, predicted in March 2009 that "courts [would] take the findings of the committee regarding the scientific foundation of particular types of forensic science evidence into account when considering the admissibility of such evidence in a particular case [30]." Judge Edwards later stated that because the NAS Report presents "findings about the current status of the scientific foundation of particular areas of forensic science," it would be "no surprise if the report is cited authoritatively," by judges as they evaluate the scientific reliability of evidence proffered as "scientific." [31] *Id.*

The NAS Report concludes that the practice of forensic pathology is severely hampered by the lack of research and EBM. As noted above, in the hierarchy of reliability in the medical literature, case studies, and case series studies are at the bottom. Yet, as the NAS Report authors observe: "Currently, little research is being conducted in the areas of death investigation and forensic pathology in the United States. Individual [Medical Examiner/Coroner] offices mainly utilize their databases for epidemiological *retrospective reviews.*" And, the Report continues, "[r]esearch is further limited because many offices operate training programs independent of universities.... There is a lack of broad and systematic research of forensic issue[s]." Moreover, the NAS Report continues, "[f]ew university pathology departments promote basic pathology research in forensic problems *such as* time of death, injury response and timing, or tissue response to poisoning.... Many [research] projects consist of epidemiological reviews that while of interest are not basic science." [Emphasis added] [32].

Recognizing Weaknesses in Preparing to Testify

The lack of research in basic areas of forensic pathology, such as time of death and the degree of force needed to cause soft tissue and other physical injury, creates risks for the forensic pathologist at the pretrial stage in the form of *Daubert* or *Frye* challenges to opinions, and during cross-examination. The NAS Report is a publicly available and widely distributed document that includes not only current conclusions about the weaknesses in forensic pathology, but also encapsulates many of the shortcomings of the field that have traditionally frustrated and confounded forensic pathologists. Diligent lawyers will keep the NAS Report as an arrow in their cross-examination quiver. Consider the comments of Kenneth E. Melson in 2003 made as then-president of the American Academy of Forensic Sciences (AAFS):

> [M]ore research is needed in the techniques and science already in use. With the importance of forensic science to truth and justice, the science employed and relied upon by judges and juries must be valid. It does not matter how well forensic scientists abide by testing protocols or how reliable the techniques are, if the underlying science does not actually reveal what the expert says it does. Method validation studies and new research must be ongoing even in the areas of traditional forensic science disciplines. Justice demands good science and we have an obligation to provide it. We can no longer expect the courts or public to accept the truth of our science merely because we say it is good. To maintain the integrity of both the science and the justice system, we must prove that it is so. Moreover, we cannot overlook the fact that scientific evidence was presented at many of the trials where innocent people were convicted and later exonerated by DNA. *The evidence in many of the trials showed associations between the defendants and the victims or crime scenes. While modern day science is exonerating the innocent, it is also showing us that some inferences drawn from scientific associations in the past were wrong. The use of DNA to exonerate wrongly convicted persons has certainly taught us lessons about forensic science in general and underscores the importance of continuing research.* [Emphasis added] [33].

Lack of funding for research plagues the field of forensic pathology—which is not surprising as the constituency of the dead and the indicted do not have a strong voice. Thus, it is up to the members of the forensic medical and legal professions, as Judge Edwards states, "to protect the integrity of the justice system." [34] Due to the absence of fundamental science in the field of forensic pathology, Judge Edwards urged forensic scientists to avoid testifying beyond what they actually know to be scientifically reliable: "The [NAS Report] Committee found that, as is too often the case, when there is no good scientific basis to support a forensic discipline and experts cannot quantify certainty and uncertainty, the testimony that they offer is not infrequently exaggerated and sometimes even fabricated." [35]

Thou Shalt Not Be under the Prosecutor's Thumb: Avoiding Prosecutorial Bias and the Appearance of Bias

The NAS Committee recommended in its Report the removal of all public forensic laboratories from the administrative control of law enforcement agencies or prosecutors' offices. Citing to the NAS Report, in its decision in *Melendez-Diaz*, the U.S. Supreme Court wrote:

> According to a recent study conducted under the auspices of the National Academy of Sciences, "[t]he majority of [laboratories producing forensic evidence] are administered by law enforcement agencies...where the laboratory administrator reports to the head of the agency."... And "[b]ecause forensic scientists often are driven in their work by a need to answer a particular question related to the issues of a particular case, they sometimes face pressure to sacrifice appropriate methodology for the sake of expediency." A forensic analyst responding to a request from a law enforcement official may feel pressure—or have an incentive—to alter the evidence in a manner favorable to the prosecution [36].

Following publication of the NAS Report, the National Association of Medical Examiners (NAME) studied the problem of independence and issued a position paper that made several critical points, which, because they echo the concerns of the NAS Report, warrant summary inclusion here [37]. The premise of the NAME position paper is that: "Forensic pathologist's play a vital role in the justice system in matters concerning questions of death." Based upon this fundamental premise, NAME stated:

- "Science as applied in the justice system should be objective and neutral."
- The goal of the medical examiner is to determine the cause and manner of death for death certificates and public health reporting purposes. *These goals are different than the goals of law enforcement.* Medicolegal death investigation must be independent of law enforcement interests and pressures. [Emphasis added.]
- "Accurate investigation, examination, reporting and testimony of forensic pathologists are important to determine the cause and manner of death of individuals who die under sudden, unexpected, or violent circumstances."
- "Such cases can become the focus of political or legal pressure by individuals or offices seeking to influence the pathologist's findings."
- "This pressure, even if seemingly unsuccessful in an individual case, can introduce error, bias and corruption into the medicolegal investigation process."
- [NAME's] position paper reinforces "the principle that medical examiners, coroners, and forensic pathologists should be allowed to perform medicolegal investigations free of these influences." [38]

The findings of NAME's position paper are based on surveys of the NAME membership regarding members' experience with, and reaction to, outside influences [39]. The paper underscores the fact that the NAS Committee's concerns were well-founded: According to NAME's paper, more than 70% of survey respondents had been subjected to pressures to influence their findings, and many had suffered negative consequences for resisting those influences. When law enforcement or prosecutors pressure or retaliate against forensic pathologists for taking neutral positions, the system suffers a blow to its image, and it can be expensive, such as when the appellate court in *State of Minnesota v. Beecroft*, overturned a conviction and ordered a new trial [40].

In *Beecroft*, a forensic pathologist served as an expert and consultant for the defense, and the appellate court agreed that the prosecutor had interfered. The Beecroft Court, in overturning the defendant's conviction, stated "while some police and prosecutors tend to view government-employed forensic pathologists…as members of the prosecutor's 'team,' "the courts" need these experts to…remain neutral and objective, and free from influence when they are generating reports; providing counsel to investigators, prosecutors, or criminal defendants; or testifying at trial." [41] Other findings of the NAME position paper include the following:

- Of 336 survey participants in NAME's study, more forensic pathologists working in coroner's offices were directed to change their findings (21.1%) than medical examiners systems (4.5%) by supervisors.
- Approximately 10% of respondents had been asked to sign documents (autopsy reports and/or death certificates) that were not consistent with findings at autopsy.
- Eighty-two percent of the forensic pathologists surveyed had experienced family or political pressure to change the reported cause or manner of death, with almost 10% stating this occurred on a monthly basis.
- Twenty-two percent of the forensic pathologists stated they had experienced political pressure to change death certificates from elected and/or appointed officials.
- Political pressure came in the form of verbal and/or written communications, threats, termination, intimidation, media exposure, and legal actions.
- Twenty-five percent (25%) of those forensic pathologists who resisted these pressures suffered consequences for their actions.
- Ten percent (10%) of individuals similarly reported pressure from outside sources on testimony provided in legal settings and about half of these individuals suffered consequences for resisting any changes in their expected testimony [42].

NAME's position paper authors made several recommendations:

- Forensic pathologists need to work independent of law enforcement. Medical examiners' and coroner's offices that do not have their own investigative team independent of law enforcement are subject to challenge for bias.
- To be independent in appearance and practice keep an open-door policy for defense lawyers to ask questions and discuss cases.
- Forensic pathologists should not be limited to testifying only in their employer's jurisdiction. To be so limited puts the forensic pathologist at risk for an attack on his credibility as part of the government-only "team." [43]

- Forensic pathologists should be free from fear of litigation for expressing their neutral opinions and should be given some level of qualified immunity.
- Forensic pathologists should be given some sort of employment security protection such as a contract clause that they may only be dismissed for good cause, or civil service status [44].

Science in the UK Criminal Courts

In 2011, the British judicial reform Law Commission presented a report to Parliament critiquing and recommending changes in the evaluation and presentation of expert evidence in criminal proceedings in England and Wales. The recommendations, included below, are a codification of common law, and American readers will recognize distinct parallels in them to the principles in the U.S. Supreme Court's *Daubert* trilogy.

The UK Report was published in the wake of several convictions later shown on appeal to be unsound due to unreliable scientific evidence such as ear print evidence, and assumed cases of pediatric abusive head trauma based on a triad of symptoms. The UK Report criticized the *laissez-faire* approach of admitting expert opinion without regard to its scientific reliability and refuted the assumption that cross exam would show jurors any flaws. Noting a concern that there exists a "culture of acceptance" by many trial judges who admit unreliable evidence in criminal cases, the Law Commission wrote:

> Cross examination, the adduction of contrary expert evidence and judicial guidance at the end of trial are currently assumed to provide sufficient safeguards in relation to expert evidence, by revealing to the jury factors adversely affecting reliability and weight. However… it is doubtful whether these are valid assumptions. A more credible assumption, at least in relation to complex scientific or technical fields, is that juries will often defer to the expert providing the opinion. If such an expert's opinion is unreliable, the dangers associated with deference are obvious, particularly if the opinion forms a critical link in the prosecution's case [45].

The UK Report noted that the *laissez faire* approach to admissibility was not cured in the crucible of cross examination if the cross-examiners were not competent to expose to the jury flaws in reliability of the claimed 'science.' The Law Commission wrote:

> Either way, juries may be provided with insufficient evidence to be able to come to a proper assessment of the reliability of such evidence…while cross examinations can be an effective forensic tool in the right hands for challenging many types of evidence, it would appear to be an insufficient safeguard, at least generally speaking, for expert opinion evidence adduced under a laissez-faire approach to admissibility [46].

In urging the adoption of special rules for expert opinions in the UK, the Law Commission noted that, "all experts owe an overriding duty to provide the court with impartial evidence within their area of expertise…experts owe a unique, elevated duty to the court, with a concomitant duty to ensure they do not mislead the court, regardless of the impact they may have on the party for whom they have been called." [47]

The UK Report recommended that legislation governing the admissibility of evidence proffered as scientific in criminal proceedings in England and Wales be enacted with the following provisions:

1. A statutory provision in primary legislation which would provide that expert opinion evidence is admissible only if it is sufficiently reliable to be admitted.
2. A provision which would provide [a] core test that expert opinion evidence is sufficiently reliable to be admitted if
   a. The opinion is soundly based, and
   b. The strength of the opinion is warranted having regard to the grounds on which it is based.
3. A provision which would set out of the following key (higher-order) examples of reasons why an expert's opinion evidence is *not* sufficiently reliable to be admitted:
   a. The opinion is based upon a hypothesis which has not been subjected to sufficient scrutiny (including, where appropriate, experimental or other testing), or which has failed to stand up to scrutiny.
   b. The opinion is based on an unjustifiable assumption.
   c. The opinion is based on flawed data.
   d. The opinion relies on an examination, technique, method or process which was not properly carried out or applied, or was not appropriate for use in the particular case.
   e. The opinion relies on an inference or conclusion which was not been properly reached.
4. A provision that would direct the trial judge to consider, where relevant, more specific (lower-order) factors in a Schedule to the Act and to any unspecified matters which appear to be relevant.

The requirements set out in clauses 1 and 4 of the draft bill would apply to criminal proceedings in England and Wales, and they would apply whether the expert evidence is to be given orally, in a written report, or in some other way [48].

At this time, Parliament has not enacted the legislation recommended by the Law Commission [49].

In the forensic setting, expert witnesses may utilize the content of the NAS and UK reports, and the NAME paper, to set boundaries beyond which they can refuse to stray. These reports are strong weapons against systemic pressures and are a springboard to a more fair and just legal system.

Conclusion

This chapter has attempted to give the reader a general overview of the case law governing the admissibility of scientific evidence and other expert testimony in state and federal courts and to provide a few theoretical pointers. In addition, sea changes in the public perception of the expert witness role in the justice system are afoot in the wake of the NAS Report. These changes are warning lights for the neutral expert. In the law, it is sometimes said, "there is nothing so practical as theory." If the reader masters the theory, that is, the standard for admissibility, and is wary of the pitfalls identified in the NAS Report, this will go a long way to effective expert witness representation in court; it is through that framework that expert testimony must be structured, measured, and presented.

References

1. U.S. Supreme Court. *Daubert v. Merrell Dow Pharmaceuticals, Inc.*, 1993, vol. 509, 579 pp.
2. U.S. Supreme Court. *General Electric Company, et al. v. Joiner*, 1997, vol. 522, 136 pp.
3. U.S. Supreme Court. *Kumho Tire Company v. Carmichael*, 1999, vol. 526, 137 pp.
4. House of Commons Science and Technology Committee. *Forensic Science on Trial*. London: House of Commons, 2005.
5. Columbia Co. *Frye v. United States*, D.C. Circuit, 1923, vol. 54, 1013 pp.
6. National Research Council. *The Polygraph and Lie Detection*. Washington, DC: National Academies Press, 2003.
7. Starr P. *The Social Transformation of American Medicine: The Rise of a Sovereign Profession and the Making of a Vast Industry*. New York: Basic Books, 1982.
8. Popper K. *The Logic of Scientific Discovery*. New York: Routledge, 1959.
9. Foster KR, Huber PW. *Judging Science. Scientific Knowledge and the Federal Courts*. Cambridge, MA: MIT Press, 1997.
10. Best A. *Wigmore on Evidence*. New York: Wolters Kluwer, 2007.
11. Bohan TL. Scientific evidence and forensic science since *Daubert*: Maine decides to sit out the dance. *Maine Law Rev* 2004;56:100–47.
12. Goodwin RJ. Fifty years of Frye in Alabama: The continuing debate over adopting the test established in *Daubert v. Merrell Dow Pharmaceuticals, Inc. Cumb Law Rev* 2004;35:231.
13. Hunter RS. *Trial Handbook for Illinois Lawyers—Civil*. Vol. 2. Thomson West, 2008.
14. BBC. *Prank Fools US Science Conference*. 2005. http://news.bbc.co.uk/2/hi/americas/444965/.stm
15. Greenhalgh T. *How to Read a Paper. The Basics of Evidence Based Medicine*. London: BMJ Publishing Group, 2000.
16. Smith GC, Pell JP. Parachute use to prevent death and major trauma related to gravitational challenge: Systematic review of randomised controlled trials. *BMJ* 2003;327:1459–61.
17. Guyatt GH, Sackett DL, Sinclair JC, et al. User's guides to the medical literature. IX. A method for grading health care recommendations. *JAMA* 1995;274:1800–04.
18. Donohoe M. Evidence-based medicine and shaken baby syndrome. Part I. *Am J Foren Med Pathol* 2003;29:239–42.
19. Haines A. Multipractice research: A cohort study. In Jones R, Kinmonth AL, eds., *Clinical Reading for Primary Care*. Oxford: Oxford University Press, 1995, p. 124.
20. Glantz SA. *Primer of Biostatistics*. New York: McGraw-Hill, 2002.
21. Leandro G. *Meta-Analysis in Medical Research. The Handbook for the Understanding and Practice of Meta-Analysis*. Oxford: Blackwell, 2005.
22. Huff D. *How to Lie with Statistics*. New York: W.W. Norton, 1954.
23. Milloy SJ. *Junk Science Judo: Self-Defense Against Health Scares and Scams*. Washington, DC: Cato Institute, 2001.
24. Lucy D. *Introduction to Statistics for Forensic Scientists*. Chichester, UK: John Wiley, 2005.
25. Sokal RR, Rohlf FJ. *Biometry*. New York: W.H. Freeman, 2003.
26. Huber PW. *Galileo's Revenge: Junk Science in the Courtroom*. New York: Basic Books, 1991.
27. "Strengthening Forensic Science in the United States: A Path Forward," [hereafter, "National Academies of Sciences Report," or "NAS Report"] published by The National Academies Press, Washington, DC, 2009, authored by National Academies 'Committee Committee on Identifying the Needs of the Forensic Science Community, Committee on Science, Technology, and Law Policy and Global Affairs, Committee on Applied and Theoretical Statistics,

Division on Engineering and Physical Sciences. ISBN-978-0-309-13135-3 (hardcover); ISBN 13:978-0-309-13131-5 (paperback). For a charge, the NAS Report may also be downloaded in portable document format (PDF) form by going to http://www.nap.edu/catalog/12589.html.

28. "Expert Evidence in Criminal Proceedings in England and Wales," The Law Commission, March 21, 2011 (the "UK Report"); The text of the UK Report is available at no charge in PDF at: http://www.lawcom.gov.uk/expert_evidence.htm. The UK Report was issued in the wake of several convictions, which were revered on the grounds that the science proffered by the Crown was unreliable and, most notably included the unreliably of ear print evidence; unreliability of statistical evidence of multiple cot deaths in same family; unreliability of the triad of symptoms of traumatic brain injury (TBI) in children to infer abusive head trauma. Id., at pp. 1–2.
29. See footnote 27, "Preface," to the NAS Report by Hon. T. Edwards, at pp. xix–xx.
30. "The Need to Strengthen Forensic Science in the United States: The National Academy of Science's Report on a Path Forward," Hearing Before the S. Judiciary Comm., 111th Cong. (2009) (statement of Hon. Harry T. Edwards, C.J., Emeritus, D.C. Circuit, and Co-Chair, Comm. on Identifying the Needs of the Forensic Science Community).
31. Edwards, Harry, T., Hon., "The National Academy of Sciences Report on Forensic Sciences: What it Means for Bench and Bar," Presentation at the Superior Court of the District of Columbia, Conference on "The Role of the Court in an Age of Developing Science & Technology," Washington, DC, May 6, 2010. For complete text of Judge Edwards' presentation, go to: http://www.cadc.uscourts.gov/internet/home.nsf/AttachmentsByTitle/NAS+Report+on+Forensic+Science/$FILE/Edwards,+The+NAS+Report+on+Forensic+Science.pdf
32. See footnote 27, The NAS Report, at pp. 261–263.
33. Kenneth E. Melson, President's Editorial: Strengthening Forensic Science: A Way Station on the Journey to Justice, 55 J. OF FORENSIC SCI. 5, 5–7 (2010), and see footnote 31, above, in which Judge Edwards cites Mr. Melson's comments in his discussion.
34. See footnote 31, Judge Edwards' Presentation, p. 8.
35. *Id.*
36. *Massachusetts v. Melendez-Diaz*, 557 U.S. 305, 129 S. Ct. 2527, at 2536, 174 L. Ed. 2d, at 109–112 (2009), quoting NAS Report Prepublication Copy at 6-1, S-17.
37. Melinek, J., MD, Thomas, L.C., MD, et al., National Association of Medical Examiners Position Paper: Medical Examiner, Coroner, and Forensic Pathologist Independence, NAME Position Paper, Acad Forensic Pathol 2013 3(1): 93–98, hereafter "NAME position paper."
38. *Id.*, at p. 93.
39. *Id.*, at p. 94.
40. *Id.*, at p. 94, citing *State of Minnesota v. Beecroft*, 813 N.W. 2d 814 (2012).
41. *Id.*, at p. 94.
42. *Id.*, at p. 94.
43. *Id.*, at pp. 94–95.
44. *Id.*, at pp. 94–95.
45. See footnote 28, UK Report, at p. 5.
46. See footnote 28, UK Report, at p. 5.
47. See footnote 28, UK Report, at p. 6.
48. *Id.*, at pp. 59–60.
49. Updates on the progress of the UK Law Commission's recommended legislation for the adoption of standards for the admissibility of evidence proffered as scientific in criminal cases in England and Wales may be found at: http://lawcommission.justice.gov.uk/areas/expert-evidence-in-criminal-trials.htm

Forensic Aspects of Adult and General Neuropathology

3

JAN E. LEESTMA

Contents

Introduction

The task for the pathologist, regardless of the subspecialty, is to understand the mechanisms and processes involved in human diseases, how the disease process evolves, how the body meets the challenge of the disease, how various therapies affect the diseased and normal tissues, and how this whole process is manifested at every level (gross, microscopic, submicroscopic, chemical, and physiological) at every stage of the process up to and including death and even after death. To accomplish this daunting task the pathologist must make use of the whole of the basic sciences (biology, physics, chemistry, mathematics, genetics, etc.) as well as all of the medical sciences (anatomy, physiology, biochemistry, microbiology, pathology, radiology, and the clinical sciences). Surely one cannot master all of these disciplines but one must have a good grasp of the basics in all of them, acknowledging and appreciating what one knows, how one knows it, and what one does not. It is also important to realize that no disease process can be or is fully understood at any given time by anyone. Diseases that were once thought to have been fully understood may suddenly be revealed to have a different etiology and character than had been previously "proven" owing to new methodologies and new science. One must be prepared to revise one's thinking when changes occur, provided that what is new is supported by robust science. This is often emotionally difficult especially when one has developed a belief system regarding a given disease or disease mechanism or clings to "what one was taught."

A useful context to the task of the pathologist within which diseases can be understood is anatomy and physiology (structure and function). If these are understood for the normal elements of the body, diseases, by contrast can be recognized and mechanisms for them may be realized. To begin, for the nonmedical reader, a brief primer of central nervous system (CNS) anatomy will follow. Later in other sections of this book, more complex expositions of CNS structure and function will be presented, usually relevant to the disease process to which they are important.

Causes of Death in the General Population

In the United States in 2009, about 2.5 million people died. The breakdown of the causes of death for all ages is displayed in Table 3.1 (by sex) and Table 3.2 (by race) [1]. By far, the most common causes of death are "natural" conditions, heart disease, and cancer accounting for about 50% of all deaths. On a global scale [2], in 2010, there were 52.8 million deaths. The breakdown for causes presents a very different picture than for the United States. In 2010, about 25% of all deaths were due to communicable diseases (diarrheal disease, pneumonia, measles, tetanus, etc.), maternal-neonatal deaths, and nutrition-related conditions. Human immunovirus (HIV)/acquired immune deficiency syndrome (AIDS) accounted for 1.5 million deaths. Malaria killed 1.17 million people as did tuberculosis. Many of these

Table 3.1 Causes of Death in American Men and Women (%), 2009

Cause of Death	Males	Females
Heart disease	25.2	24
Cancer	24.4	22.2
Accidents	8.2	3.5
Chronic lung disease	5.3	5.9
Stroke	4.3	6.3
Diabetes mellitus	2.9	2.8
Suicide	2.4	<1
Influenza and pneumonia	2.1	2.3
Kidney disease	2	2
AD	2	4.5
Septicemia	<1	1.6

Source: Centers for Disease Control, *National Vital Statistics Reports*.
Note: In 2009, death from all causes involved 2,437,163 individuals.

Table 3.2 Causes of Death by Race (%) in the United States, 2009 (2,437,163 deaths in 2009)

Cause of Death	White (2,086,355)	Black (286,623)	Native American (14,960)	Asian-Pacific (49,225)
Heart disease	24.7	24.3	18.5	23.1
Cancer	23.3	22.6	18.1	27
Chronic lung disease	6.1	3	4.1	3
Cerebrovascular disease	5.2	5.5	3.8	7.4
Accidents	4.9	4.2	11.6	4.2
AD	3.5	1.8	1.3	2.1
Diabetes mellitus	2.6	4.2	5.3	3.8
Influenza and pneumonia	2.2	1.8	2.7	3.2
Renal disease	1.9	3.1	2.1	2.2
Suicide	1.6	0.7	2.9	2
Septicemia	1.4	2.2	1.8	1.2
Liver disease	1.3	0.9	4.8	0.9
Homicide	0.4	2.7	1.7	0.7
HIV	0.2	1.9	0.4	0.1

Source: Centers for Disease Control, *National Vital Statistics Reports*.

disease categories have considerable regional preponderances. The forensic importance of causes of death in the majority of the world is statistically minimal, and the role of forensic neuropathology is smaller still, having relevance basically only in the Western countries. Nevertheless, it is useful to have a perspective from which to proceed.

Anatomy of the CNS

To fully appreciate how diseases and especially trauma affect the CNS, it is essential that one have some appreciation of the organ and its external and internal components. A full exposition of the brain's anatomy is not appropriate here but a brief review for those readers who may require it may provide a context for learning. There are many fine texts and atlases of neuroanatomy from varying perspectives (gross and sectional anatomy [3–5], clinical-correlative neuroanatomy [6–9], neuroanatomy from the imaging–radiological perspective [10], macroscopic and microscopic neuroanatomy [11], and other points of view).

Most anatomists divide the CNS into the cerebral hemispheres (cerebrum), the cerebellum, the brain stem (midbrain, pons, and medulla), and the spinal cord. The cerebrum is arbitrarily divided into the frontal lobes (frontal lobe tips to the anterior margin of the central sulcus (fissure of Rolando) and above the Sylvian fissure (see Figures 3.1 through 3.3). The temporal lobe lies below and deep to the Sylvian fissure and extends posteriorly to meet the parietal lobe. The parietal lobe extends from the posterior margin of the central sulcus to the parieto-occipital fissure and the occipital lobe lies posterior to this same fissure.

The surface of the cerebrum has a myriad of convolutions not all of which have names, rather many can be grouped. For example, the frontal and temporal lobes can conveniently be divided into the horizontal groups of superior, middle, and inferior convolutions that are more or less recognizable. If the Sylvian fissure if pried open, one can make out the

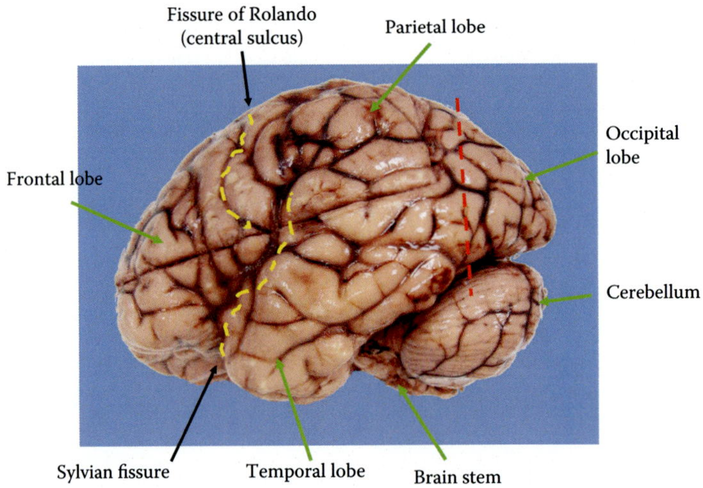

Figure 3.1 This photograph of the left side of the brain in a fixed specimen illustrates the major anatomic divisions and landmarks of the frontal, temporal, parietal, and occipital lobes as well as the cerebellum and brain stem. The central sulcus (Rolandic fissure) and Sylvian fissures are traced in yellow. Other fissures have names and define the divisions of the parietal lobe not shown here.

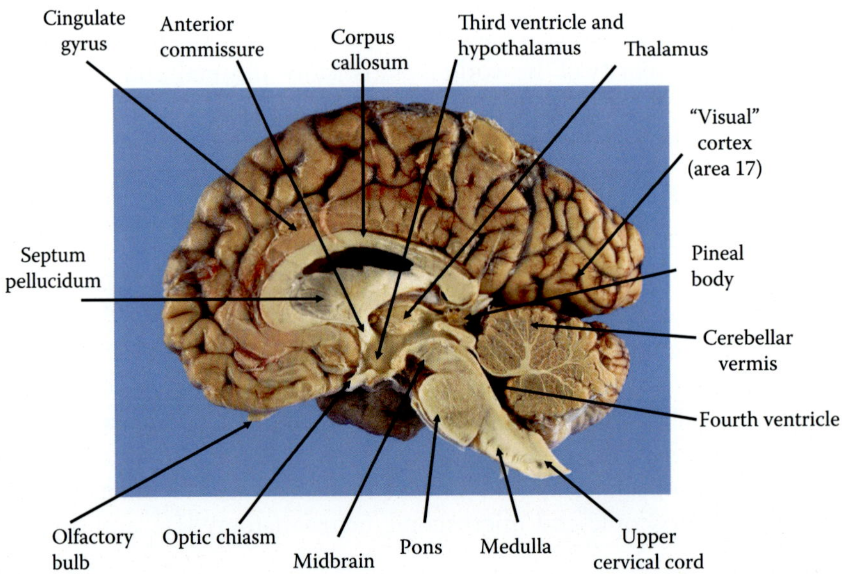

Figure 3.2 This photograph of the midsagittal plane of the brain illustrates midline structures of importance. The extensive corpus callosum extends from the frontal part of the brain (genu) to the posterior parts of the brain (splenium), ending just above the pineal body. The lateral ventricles are separated by the septum pellucidum. The posterior portion of the thalamus (pulvinar) lies below a thickened portion of the septum pellucidum, the fornix, which is part of the limbic system of the brain. The hypothalamus borders the third ventricle, which lies just above the optic chiasm and pituitary (not included). The cingulate gyrus courses above the corpus callosum and is part of the limbic system. The "visual" cortex lies in the midline of the occipital lobe (calcarine gyri) and constitutes the conscious visual perception area (area 17 of Brodmann). The brain stem is composed of the midbrain, pons, and medulla. The midline of the cerebellum displays the cerebellar vermis with the fourth ventricle just below. The fourth ventricle drains into the subarachnoid space via the midline foramen of Magendie just above the caudal medullar and above the upper cervical cord.

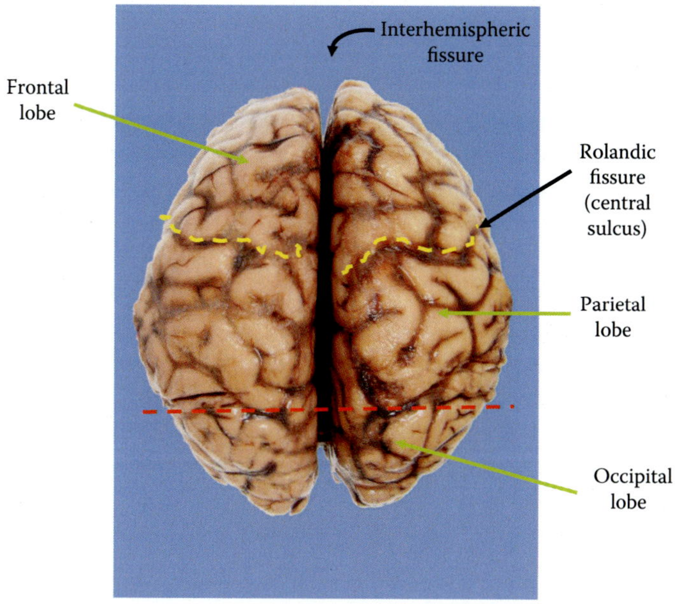

Figure 3.3 This photograph of the vertex of the brain in a fixed specimen illustrates the major landmarks visible from this view. The interhemispheric fissure where in life the falx is positioned, and in the deep shadow is the corpus callosum. The central sulcus (Rolandic fissures) are traced in yellow. Anterior to these fissures lie the main motor areas of the brain, and posterior to them lie the main sensory areas both with a somotopic localization of function. At the most rostral portion and into the midline are areas that serve the lower extremities, bladder and bowel functions. Laterally the shoulder, arm, then the face, and hands.

fan-shaped arrangement of small gyri called the Heschel's gyri (the primary auditory sensory area). The central sulcus (fissure of Rolando) can usually be identified on the most common dominant (left) hemisphere by the fissure that originates near the mid-top of the brain branches the least and terminates in a blind sulcus at the Sylvian fissure. This important sulcus delimits the motor (anterior) from the sensory (posterior) areas. On the non-dominant hemisphere (usually the right), sometimes it is difficult to delineate this sulcus. The parietal lobe is more complex in its organization and a neuroanatomy text or atlas is helpful in finding one's way to identify various lobules that have eloquent functions for language. In the midline posterior is a fissure that delimits the occipital lobe from the parietal lobe, the occipital–parietal fissure. Deep and posterior to this in the midline is a horizontal fissure that defines the primary visual perception area (Area 17 or the calcarine region).

Inside the brain, each gyrus sends myelinated nerve fibers (axons) to the neighboring gyri ("U" fibers). There are also fibers of long passage that connect anterior to posterior portions of the brain. The two hemispheres are joined in the midline by a thick band of myelinated nerve fibers, the corpus callosum running from the deep frontal region to the posterior parietal–occipital region. This structure contains fibers that originate in all areas of the cerebral cortex and communicate with the opposite hemisphere. In a fixed brain specimen when thicker sections are simply torn apart manually, the courses of these fibers can be easily visualized [12,13]. Other side-to-side fiber connections that tether the two hemispheres together, although in a much less physical manner are the anterior and posterior commissures.

The surface of the brain undulates in convolutions and sulci and is referred to as the cerebral cortex. The cortex contains a large percentage of the brain's neurons that are arranged into six horizontally apparent layers or lamellae, although the true functional organization of the cortex is in vertical columns of neurons. The structure of the cortex is not uniform and has a different architecture for nearly every cortical location. The individual characteristics of a particular area can, with some difficulty, permit identification microscopically of where the cortical sample has been taken. There are many texts and articles on cortical architectonics, a discipline pioneered by Vogt and Vogt [14] and refined by many others including Brodmann [15] and Bailey and von Bonin [16]. Depending upon the function of the given region of the cortex there may be special histological features such as in the motor area (Area 6) where large pyramidal neurons populate the middle lamellae; in the primary visual perception area (Area 17) of the occipital lobe in the calcarine gyri where a double row of rather symmetrical neurons populate the middle lamellae, and of course the hippocampal formation of the medial temporal region where the unique structure of the Ammon's horn is located (see Figure 3.4). It is important to stress that every population of neurons may have differing forms, metabolic pathways and nutritional requirements, and neurotransmitter systems operating. Each population may not respond to the same stresses in the same manner. The functional importance of most cortical areas have been mapped, owing to the work of Penfield and his colleagues, and others, who performed electrical stimulation studies on

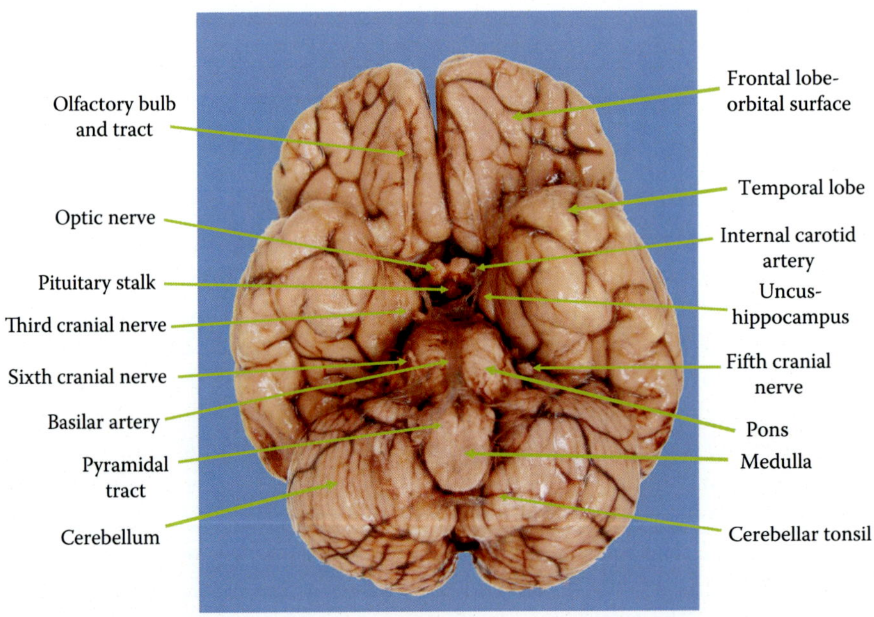

Figure 3.4 This photograph of the base of the brain in a fixed specimen illustrates some of the major easily visible landmarks. The inferior surfaces of the frontal and temporal lobes and uncus, beneath which is the hippocampus, and brain stem and cerebellum are easily noted. A few of the cranial nerves are noted (I, olfactory; II, optic; III, oculomotor; V, trigeminal; VI, abducens). Others are less visible or have been torn away. The basilar artery, which receives two short portions of the vertebral arteries, and the internal carotid arteries, with their posterior communicating arteries, are also shown. The brain stem is also shown but the midbrain is not visible but lies rostral to the third cranial nerves.

the brain in conscious subjects [17]. In the center of the cerebrum lie the paired lateral ventricles and their choroid plexuses. The lateral ventricles fuse to form the third ventricle lying between the hypothalami and join with the cerebral aqueduct (iter) in the upper midbrain for the egress of cerebrospinal fluid.

The cerebellum, lying in the posterior fossa below the tentorium is joined to the brain via the brain stem by the superior, middle, and inferior cerebellar peduncles. These fiber bundles connect the cerebellum to rostral and caudal centers. The largest of these bundles, the middle cerebellar peduncle, connects the cerebellar hemispheres to each other via the basis pontis (Figure 3.2). The cerebellar cortex has a unique morphology with much smaller convolutions (folia) that the cerebrum. The divisions of the cerebellar cortex are not as immediately obvious as in the cerebrum, but some structures are easily identified. In the midline where the two hemispheres join is the cerebellar vermis, which when visualized resembles the body of a caterpillar. At the base of the cerebellum where this structure impinges upon the foramen magnum are the two cerebellar tonsils.

The volume of the cerebellum is about 162 mm^3 and its weight is between 136 and 169 grams [18] in the adult or about 10.63% of the weight of the brain as a whole, but in the infant it constitutes 5%–6% of brain mass. Histologically, in the infant, there is an external granular layer (Obersteiner's layer) of small neurons that usually by 12–14 months of age have disappeared. The small neurons of the adult inner granular layer of the cerebellar cortex exceed the number of cortical neurons in the cerebrum. The deeper layer of the cerebellar cortex is populated by large branching neurons, Purkinje cells. Below this side-by-side uniform layer is the internal granular layer of small neurons admixed with various glial cells. There are between 15 million and 25 million Purkinje cells in the cerebellar cortex in adults, each with between 600,000 and a million synaptic dendritic connections on each neuron [19].

In the deep cerebellar white matter are paired serpentine collections of large neurons called the dentate nuclei. These cells and the Purkinje cells are particularly sensitive to hypoxia and ischemia. In the center of the cerebellum lies the fourth ventricle. This chamber empties via two lateral foramina (Luschka) and a single midline foramen (Magendie) at the cerebellopontine angle into the subarachnoid space. The fourth ventricle also contains paired choroid plexuses that generate cerebrospinal fluid.

The brain stem is composed of the midbrain, pons, and medulla. The midbrain joins with the diencephalon–hypothalamus, which is in turn intimately connected to the thalamus–pulvinar, globus pallidus, putamen, and caudate nuclei. These deep neuronal masses are collectively called the basal ganglia. Each structure has its own morphology and metabolic profile and functions. The midbrain is about 1 cm in length; the pons, about 2.5 cm in length; and the medulla, about 3 cm in length [18].

The most rostral brain stem structure, the midbrain, contains the cerebral aqueduct (iter) that conducts cerebrospinal fluid from the lateral ventricles of the cerebrum into the fourth ventricle. It also houses the cerebral peduncles, mostly composed of the descending pyramidal (motor) tracts, and in the midline, there are important populations of neurons called the brain stem reticular formation. These subserve consciousness and when damaged result in an unconscious–comatose victim. Just deep to the cerebral peduncles are paired pigmented nuclei, the substantia nigra, which are affected in Parkinson's disease, and also the red nuclei, important in motor control. In the midline of the midbrain are cranial nerve nuclei that control pupillary function, and nuclei and fiber bundles that connect and control conjugate eye movements (the media longitudinal fasciculus).

The midbrain blends with the pons via the superior cerebellar peduncle that houses descending fibers involved in coordination. The large bulge in the central pons is composed of fibers connecting the two cerebellar hemispheres intermingled with bundles of fibers of the descending pyramidal tract. The deep pons (tegmentum), like the midbrain, contains parts of the reticular activating system and other portions of the reticular formation that help to control respiration. There are also cranial nerve nuclei that subserve many functions including conjugate eye movements. The lower pons is composed of the interior cerebellar peduncle that contains fibers communicating with lower centers and the medulla and tracts that ascend to higher centers.

The medulla is the brain stem's most immediate connection to the spinal cord. It is the locus of control for respiration, balance, swallowing and mouth movements, and coordination. There is a reticular formation here as well but it is not intimately involved with consciousness, but is important in control of respiration. The pyramidal tract coalesces here in the medullary pyramids in the anterior medulla. Like other portions of the CNS each nucleus of neurons has a different morphology and cellular composition [11]. The neural connections of all these nuclei here and higher up are complex and amply illustrated in all neuroanatomy texts and atlases. Details on the neuroanatomy and physiology of respiratory control are discussed in detail in Chapter 9.

Vascular Anatomy

The brain is normally perfused by arterial supply from the two internal carotid arteries and the two vertebral arteries that communicate via the circle of Willis by means of the anterior communicating and posterior communicating arteries. Figure 3.5 illustrates the perfusion territories of the anterior cerebral artery (midline of the brain), the middle cerebral artery (lateral surface of the brain), and the posterior cerebral artery (the base of the brain). Because of these vascular territories topography perfusion is often shared at border zones of the various vessels, referred to as "watersheds." It is in these border zones that perfusion deficits may occur in hypoxic and/or ischemic states, which may result in infarctions. One of the most common "watersheds" is a crescent shaped zone on the upper lateral surface of the cerebral hemispheres depicted later in the text in Figure 3.30. Other "watersheds" exist where perfusion territories meet in the brain stem, and spinal cord (see Chapter 5) that sometimes can be misinterpreted as spinal cord injury, when it is in fact part of the respirator brain phenomenon.

Venous drainage of the brain is illustrated in Figures 3.6 and 3.7 shown in the lateral and midline sagittal views. Cortical venous drainage mostly proceeds to the superior sagittal sinus via numerous bridging veins. There is some redundancy in anatomoses so that obstruction to possibly several cortical veins may not produce serious obstructions and venous infarcts. Important in this regard to the two major anastomotic veins (the vein of Trolard and the vein of Labbé). If these vessels become nonpatent, the risk of venous infarction rises dramatically. The bulk of venous outflow finds its way via the straight and transverse sinuses into sinuses of the basal dura and thence into the jugular system. The medical surface of the brain also has a rich venous drainage into the superior and inferior sagittal sinuses, via the paired internal cerebral veins that drain the basal ganglia into the great vein of Galen and thence to the basal dural sinuses into the jugular system. It is important to examine the venous sinuses at autopsy to detect possible thromboses of these channels.

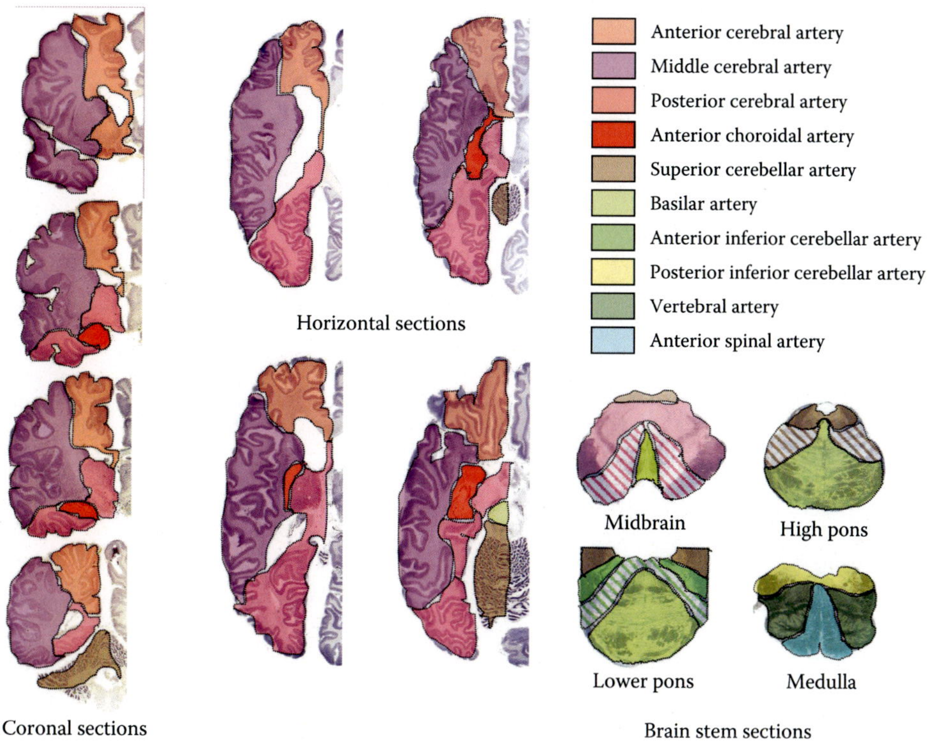

Figure 3.5 This montage depicts (left) vascular perfusion territories in the hemicoronal plane. In the center vascular perfusion territories as seen in horizontal partial sections are illustrated. In the lower right, perfusion territories for the brainstem are illustrated. In the upper right are color codes for the various major vascular territories. Cross hatched regions represent shared perfusion zones that are anatomically quite variable from individual to individual.

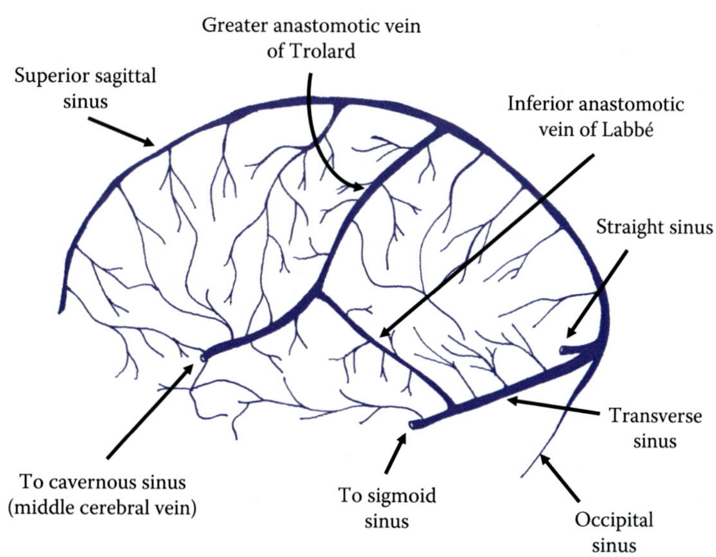

Figure 3.6 Diagramatically illustrated here are the major cortical venous drainage patterns for the surface of left cerebral hemisphere (frontal is left and occipital is right).

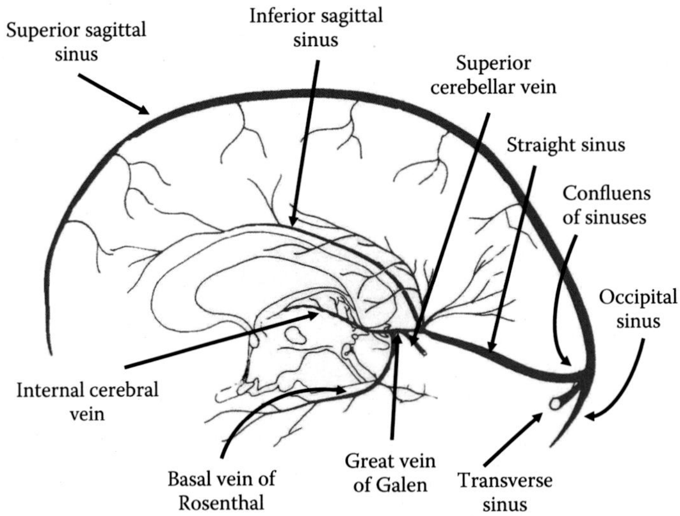

Figure 3.7 Diagramatically illustrated here are the major draining veins for the medial surface of the cerebral cortex with frontal region in the left and occipital region on the right.

Forensic Neuropathology in the Adult

The prevalence of natural disease processes in the nervous system of those adult individuals coming to autopsy in a general hospital or a forensic setting is very high, and it is almost a rare case in which the brain is truly without pathological diagnosis that may or may not play in the basic cause/manner of death determination. Most individuals past middle age will commonly show one or more of the following: manifestation of atherosclerosis in their cerebral vessels, buildup of lipofuscin pigment in many of the neurons, a few lacunar infarcts in the basal ganglia, accumulation of corpora amylacea in the subpial regions, mineralization of their choroid plexuses and pineal body, and quite probably the odd neurofibrillary tangle or senile plaque in the cerebral cortex. Incidentally, small unruptured "berry" aneurysms, cryptic vascular anomalies, small asymptomatic meningiomas, or unrecognized acoustic Schwannomas may be discovered. Generally, such findings are not unexpected and would ordinarily have little impact on the interpretation of the neuropathology in a forensic setting; however, in occasional cases recognition and proper interpretation of naturally occurring disease processes in the brain will have significant impact on the forensic investigation. These cases fall into two groups: those in which there is a sudden or unexpected death in which systemic pathology is lacking and it is hoped the cause (and manner) of death will be revealed by an intracranial examination, and those in which the presence of intracranial pathology may have influenced events prior to the victim's death or combined with external events to cause the death. So that an informed analysis of such cases can be made, a brief review of the general neuropathology of those processes and disease conditions that can be of importance to the forensic pathologist is undertaken to provide background and a context within which elements of a given case may be interpreted.

Intracranial Pathology as a Cause of Death

The most commonly encountered conditions that regularly occur on a forensic pathology service and are responsible for, or are intimately involved in, unexpected deaths, and thus are of forensic concern include stroke, infectious diseases, neoplasms, malformations, degenerative diseases, and epilepsy [20–25]. All of these issues and several others will be discussed in this chapter.

Strokes, which include the entities of cerebral infarction, spontaneous intracerebral hemorrhage, ruptured cerebral aneurysm, and vascular malformation, are chiefly diseases of adulthood, but they can also occur in childhood and cause forensic problems. These types of pediatric cases are discussed in Chapter 4, as are most of the common infectious processes, which include bacterial meningitis and brain abscess as well as viral encephalitis and a host of less common diseases most commonly found in children.

Neoplasms, such as primary tumors such as glioblastoma and other glial tumors, cystic cerebellar astrocytoma, and other posterior fossa tumors, brain stem gliomas, and colloid cysts of the third ventricle may occasionally pose forensic concerns. Metastatic tumors are also important and are frequently undiscovered until autopsy and may cause death by relatively sudden decompensation with increased intracranial pressure or seizures or may cause neurological deficits that might lead to an accidental death in the victim.

Brain malformations may be discovered in the adult autopsy and may be responsible for the death, either primarily or in some other fashion. Most of these and related conditions are found in infants and children and, as such, will be discussed in Chapter 4 or in Chapter 9 (complex neural functions).

Neurodegenerative diseases such as Alzheimer's disease (AD), Parkinson's disease, motor neuron disease, and multiple sclerosis (MS) have few forensic considerations apart from those that might bear on cognitive ability and might contribute to death by suicide or accident, or they might involve challenges to wills or testaments. Forensic issues quite often arise in connection with disabled individuals who require institutionalization and where care may be substandard, leading to injuries or deaths from falls, malpositioning, or poor restraint practice in bed with attendant injury or death, or where elder abuse may have occurred.

Functional diseases such as epilepsy, the behavioral disorders, and the neurosensory diseases such as blindness and deafness, as well as perceptual disorders such as aphasia, the apraxias, and related conditions, may have considerable forensic importance and be directly related to correct determination of the cause and manner of death. Many of these conditions will be discussed separately in Chapter 9.

Every physician associates several intracranial disease processes with a fatal outcome, but it is a common failing, even among pathologists, to not fully understand the mechanisms by which *intracranial* pathology produces death [23–25]. There are a limited number of mechanisms by which this can occur [26,27]:

1. Cerebral neural discharges that reach cardiac autonomic nerves resulting in sudden cardiac standstill or fatal neural mediated arrhythmia as in epilepsy for example [27–30]
2. Central depression of respiratory control or disruption of pulmonary function without brain stem herniation

3. Respiratory failure with brain stem herniation and increased intracranial pressure from any cause
4. Central dysfunction of vomiting and guarding reflexes with secondary problems relating to breathing, possibly related to psychiatric disease and/or phenothiazine medications [31]
5. The neurological vegetative state
6. Neural shock associated with major trauma or disruption of basic neurological functions as in missile or blast-related wounds to the brain

Each of these is discussed below and in some cases will be discussed in greater detail in Chapter 9 or elsewhere.

A phenomenon that bears some examination is that of so-called sudden death. This term evokes an immediate sense of appreciation because for any physician, upon being pressed to define the meaning, difficulties arise, but it has been noted that about 20% of all medical examiner cases occur suddenly [22]. In general, the term *sudden* would be applied to a death that occurred within a few minutes or less from some preceding event, known or unknown [25]. For deaths that take somewhat longer to play themselves out, perhaps the term *rapid death* is preferable. Integral to both of these courses of death is the element of the unexpected, and the two terms *sudden* and *unexpected* are often used together, as in sudden unexpected death in epilepsy (SUDEP) [25]. The unexpected quality usually arises in connection with the enigma of an apparently healthy individual engaged in, or appearing to die during, presumably normal activity. Cases such as this, especially when witnessed or when the victim is found without apparent signs of foul play, very often are referred to the coroner or medical examiner for investigation and may pose a significant challenge to him or her in reaching a proper determination of the cause and manner of death. Another category that surrounds these kinds of deaths is the unexplained aspect to many of them. The majority of sudden/unexpected deaths after an autopsy has been performed and circumstantial and historical information has been considered can be explained, although not always anatomically (see Table 3.3). Such cases usually involve some physiological mechanism of death, such as cardiac arrhythmia, that may have no immediately obvious anatomic representation. Cases that have no apparent anatomic cause of death are relatively common and comprise probably between 4% and 8% of all medical examiners' cases [25].

Table 3.3 Autopsy-Proven Causes of Death in Cases of Sudden Unexpected Death in a Forensic Autopsy Population

Disease Process	Percentages
Heart and aorta	56.1 (±7.4)
Respiratory	14.5 (±6.4)
Brain or meninges	15.8 (±2.4)
Digestive/urogenital	8 (±1.7)
Miscellaneous	9.5 (±8.9)

Source: Adapted from the data of Kuller L, *J Chron Dis* 19, 1192, 1966 and Kuller L et al., *Medicine* 46, 341–61, 1967.

Neurally Mediated Mechanisms of Death

Cardiac suppression via neural discharge is not usually invoked as an immediate cause of death in the presence of intracranial pathology; however, this mechanism has been postulated for many years as an explanation for the sudden deaths observed during epileptic seizures [27,29,30], and is discussed in detail in Chapter 9. Briefly, however, it is possible that neural discharges originating within higher centers in the brain, via the hypothalamus and brain stem autonomic centers, may reach the heart in the form of sympathetic or parasympathetic discharges. Parasympathetic (vagal) impulses may stop the heart for short periods of time and could possibly cause death if the interval of stoppage were long enough or occurred in combination with cardiac pathology, but generally the heart, through its own inherent pacemaker, will override vagal stimulation and beat on its own eventually. In the case of sympathetic discharges, the heart rate will increase, stroke volume will increase, and a variety of arrhythmias may supervene, the most serious of which is ventricular fibrillation, which may result in a fatal outcome [30]. The situations in which these mechanisms may be invoked are probably relatively few: death in connection with epileptic seizure, sudden death associated with fright, so-called voodoo deaths, and sudden deaths in Oriental groups (*bangungut*, *pokuri*, *Laotian* [H'mong] sudden deaths) [32,33], sudden trauma to the brain or brain stem, and probably, although only rarely, sudden or proximate death during stroke. In the latter situation, it appears that some stroke cases suffer previously unrecognized ECG abnormalities, including arrhythmias. Because the cause of death in any of the above is physiological, pathological findings may be scant or absent entirely [23].

Disorders of Respiratory Control

Acting alone or in conjunction with disorders of cardiac function, a disorder of central respiratory control may be responsible for some cases of sudden death. It is well known that lesions at various levels of the brain, brain stem, and cord will produce alterations in the patterns of respiration; thus, knowledge of any premortem respiratory difficulty may help to localize the lesion. The anatomy of physiology of respiratory control is discussed in detail in Chapter 9. At the highest cortical level, when large areas of the frontal cortex are compromised, as in massive infarction or metabolic encephalopathy, respiration may exhibit periods of apnea, especially after a period of hyperventilation [34]; however, such lesions will rarely cause death by themselves. Another related type of breathing pattern seen frequently is Cheyne–Stokes breathing (alternating hyperpnea and apnea). It is often seen in persons who have suffered destructive or disruptive lesions deep to the cortex, as in large basal ganglia or subcortical infarcts, closed head trauma (perhaps due to diffuse traumatic axonal injury) [34], diffuse hypoxia or metabolic encephalopathy, or diencephalic or upper brain stem injury [34]. The pattern of breathing may be due to exaggerated or disconnected responses to arterial PCO_2. Hyperventilation may be seen with upper brain stem injuries [35], but clear-cut neuropathological and neuroanatomical correlations in most cases are lacking. In any case, such respiratory dysfunctions usually cannot cause death by themselves. Other patterns of abnormal breathing include apneustic breathing (inspiratory stoppage associated with mid–lower pontine lesions involving the nucleus parabrachialis) [34], ataxic breathing (irregular, spastic breathing caused by dorsal–medial medullary lesions) [34], and apnea. The latter is clearly the most frightening and may be the explanation for sudden infant death syndrome (SIDS) [36,37]. Total respiratory failure, in the absence of brain stem herniation, can be seen in cases of Leigh disease (subacute necrotizing encephalopathy), narcotic and analgesic overdose, brain stem trauma, or destruction in which neural shock presumably shuts down respiratory centers. Acute spinal cord injury in which the upper cervical spinal cord is injured or destroyed may also cause respiratory failure, owing to loss of the motor impulses to the primary and secondary muscles of respiration. The same can be said for acute poliomyelitis and Landry-Guillain-Barré syndrome.

Respiratory failure and death due to pulmonary edema that is apparently neurally mediated (so-called neurogenic pulmonary edema) may occur especially following head trauma with or without subarachnoid hemorrhage (SAH) and can develop extremely rapidly. As was thought at one time, pulmonary edema and trauma occurred apparently in the absence of cardiac failure [38,39] by mechanisms that were presumed to be neurogenic and which were notoriously refractory to the usual therapy. Over the years the apparent absence of myocardial dysfunction has been shown to be incorrect, with the greater percentage of patients showing various degrees and types of myocardial failure but by mechanisms that are still unclear [40]. Such neurogenic pulmonary edema and congestion are also commonly found in otherwise anatomically negative autopsies of victims of sudden death in epilepsy [41–44].

Respiratory Depression with Herniation

In the presence of increased intracranial pressure, brain stem and tonsillar herniation often occurs and usually leads to unconsciousness and eventually to some degree of respiratory failure, especially when accompanied by so-called upward cerebellar herniation [45]. Cerebellar tonsillar herniation is probably the most common mechanism for death due to acute or subacute neurological disease. The conditions that cause increased intracranial pressure are legion and include any condition that produces a mass effect, be it a neoplasm in a critical CSF pathway (subependymoma, colloid cyst, cerebellar astrocytoma, etc.), intracerebral hematoma, SAH, or cerebral edema from whatever cause (metabolic, hypoxic, toxic, traumatic, neoplastic, or inflammatory).

Many of the above conditions can occur in circumstances that may have a great deal of forensic and legal relevance, such as death occurring during arrest or incarceration, or during a presumably minor altercation or accident. Case examples are found later in this chapter and a full discussion of possible mechanisms of death due to mass effects and intracranial equilibrium dysfunction can be found in Chapter 5.

Failure of Guarding Reflexes and Vomiting

Although aspiration of vomitus and the attendant infectious and chemical bronchitis that results commonly accompany many serious illnesses, the cause of the vomiting and sometimes the death that results is usually not primarily neurogenic. Vomiting and aspiration can, however, follow strokes, subdural hemorrhages, SAHs, and migraine. Vomiting in the absence of nausea (so-called projectile vomiting) is a common symptom of brain tumors, especially in children, but likewise is rarely a fatal event, even though the failure to recognize the vomiting as being due to intracranial causes may lead to death, as in the case of colloid cyst of the third ventricle [46]. There are some circumstances in which vomiting with massive aspiration can be the cause of sudden death, for example, in some cases of sudden death in epileptics and in psychiatric patients receiving large doses of phenothiazine tranquilizers [31,47]. In such cases, presumably the guarding reflex that closes the epiglottis while vomiting is overwhelmed or absent, and the entire gastric contents may be aspirated with no apparent warning or distress.

The Neurological Vegetative State

Under circumstances where there has been global brain damage, regardless of its cause and associated conditions (trauma, asphyxia, cardiorespiratory arrest, gunshot wounds, drowning, prolonged hypoglycemia, etc.), it often occurs that the affected individual will be maintained for long periods of time on life support yet remain unconscious and in coma. The depth and functional aspects of the coma are subjects with great diversity of opinion. The victim may be able to be weaned off a respirator but is generally completely dependent upon outside care for nutrition, respiratory, toilet, bladder, and bowel functions. Inactivity generally leads to muscular atrophy and flexion contractures, pressure sores, and ulcerations. The presence of a urinary catheter is a constant source for potential urinary tract infections. Aspiration of food or secretions poses a constant threat of pneumonia. It is generally these conditions, almost all of which lead to bacterial sepsis, that cause the immediate death of the individual. Pulmonary thromboembolism from deep vein thrombosis is another perpetual threat to continued existence.

The issues that surround the persistent vegetative state are many—medical, scientific, forensic, philosophical, sociological, moral, ethical, and legal [48,49]. All have been amply illustrated in the cases of Karen Anne Quinlan [50] and, most recently, Terri Schiavo [51]. All of these important considerations will be explored in detail in Chapter 9.

Vascular Diseases of the Nervous System

The finding of some form of cerebral vascular disease is so common on any autopsy service that pathologists have come to expect it in any individual more than 40 or 50 years of age. In the forensic setting, natural disease processes may overshadow or complicate the analysis at hand, where some violent act, accident, or unusual set of circumstances may have interacted with underlying disease processes to produce death, and it is incumbent upon the pathologist to make a judgment about their interaction. Examples of this are the differentiation between a hypertensive basal ganglion hemorrhage and a traumatic intracerebral hemorrhage where a known hypertensive individual may have fallen or has been found dead under circumstances in which abrasions may be found on the face or scalp or a traffic accident case where there may be an issue as to whether a lesion was the effect or cause of an accident. There is much guesswork involved in this task, and often no firm conclusions can be drawn. Other circumstances where vascular disease may be important in the forensic environment are when neurological deficits caused by vascular disease may have been responsible for an accident or some other event. The role of vascular disease in dementing illness may also assume importance, not so much in a typical forensic autopsy, but later in litigation that may involve a will contest or in a malpractice action for failure to diagnose and treat a condition. Another issue involving vascular disease of the nervous system is the phenomenon of delayed posttraumatic apoplexy or other delayed effects of trauma on vessels [52–55].

The following descriptions of various diseases, whenever possible, will present points of differentiation between natural and external events or highlight situations of forensic significance that may arise.

Cerebral Atherosclerosis

The basic underlying pathogenesis of cerebral atherosclerosis is probably no different from that in any other artery, and the risk factors that have been recognized, including smoking, hyperlipidemia, diabetes, obesity, and hypertension, probably apply as well to brain vessels as any other [56–61]. Precisely how these various risk factors produce cerebrovascular disease is still the subject of research that involves how genetics and environmental factors interact. There is much recent interest in the role of inflammation/infection [62–63], phospholipid metabolism and free radicals [64], lipid and apolipoprotein metabolism, and cerebrovascular disease. The assumption that the process of atherosclerosis is equal in every vessel system is brought into question by the undeniable fact that atherosclerosis is not a uniform process, and there is often great disparity between the degrees of atherosclerosis found in the aorta, peripheral vessels, coronary arteries, and the cerebral vessels. Cerebral atherosclerosis is not usually as severe as in systemic vessels but rarely may be far more severe than elsewhere. There is no universally agreed-upon classification for cerebral atherosclerosis, but most neuropathologists, after observing the various permutations and combinations of cerebral vascular disease in their autopsy material, have developed some broad categories into which a given case can be placed. The following arbitrary divisions may prove useful as a way of thinking about cerebral atherosclerosis.

Probably the most common pattern of cerebral atherosclerosis, seen with increasing severity over the age of 50 in both sexes is that in which the arteries of the circle of Willis are of normal external diameter and, except for focal plaques that may or may not appear to limit flow, the lumens are of normal caliber. Often, the neck vessels are far more severely involved than those in the circle of Willis. Probably most individuals with vessels such as these never suffer a major or significant infarctive stroke, but when they do, they may have an infarct of any form, such as progressive evolving strokes or transient ischemic attacks (TIAs), depending on associated extracranial vessel pathology and the presence of a myocardial infarction, atrial fibrillation, and other cardiac pathology that can produce thromboemboli [61,65,66].

Another far less common situation exists when the circle of Willis arteries are inherently of small delicate caliber and in which very little atherosclerosis is required to compromise the circulation. Plaques may be nodular and literally turn the affected vessels into bead-like strings. Virtually all the named vessels are affected, as are peripheral brain vessels. Persons with such vessels usually have severe atheromatous disease in other vessels and may have numerous major strokes over many years. They may be virtually incapacitated by the ever-present danger of a catastrophic stroke and may suffer progressive loss of neurological function, leading to dementia on a vascular or multi-infarct basis [67].

Of intermediate occurrence are those individuals in which the circle of Willis arteries are much larger than normal and are often calcified, having rather flat, ulcerated, or excavated intimal plaques (so-called calcified–dilated form), and may show an S-shaped deformity of the basilar artery (so-called atherosclerotic or cirsoid aneurysm). This form is more commonly associated with so-called lacunar infarcts and TIAs than large-territory infarctions. At times the vessels may become so large that they indent the pons or other structures and may cause neurological (cranial nerve) symptoms.

Why such diversity in cerebral vascular disease exists is completely unknown, but serves to complicate the nature of lesions produced and their interpretation.

Arterial Hypertension

There is no more universally accepted risk factor for cerebral vascular disease than arterial hypertension, yet considerable argument still exists on precisely how hypertensive disease produces its pathology [68,69]. The high prevalence of this disease in the United States, Europe, and other affluent societies is clearly a major public health problem. This is especially true among African Americans who perhaps suffer the ravages of this disease more than any other group. Hypertension has been blamed as the major developmental factor in cerebral atherosclerosis, aneurysms, spontaneous nontraumatic intracerebral hemorrhage, and cerebral infarction [68,69]. That some form of endothelial damage from whatever cause leads to a focal lesion and so-called fatty streak below the endothelium and eventually forms a nidus for atheroma formation, medial damage, and potential weakness of the vessel wall, is now well accepted [60,61]; however, a complete understanding of the process is far from complete despite many decades of research. In forensic autopsy, it is very common to detect lacunar state and prominence of small subcortical vessels (white matter lacunes or *etat lacunaire*) in individuals not suspected of having hypertensive disease, yet when the heart is examined, it is heavier than normal, and other organs, such as the kidneys, may show the early changes typical for hypertension. Thus, there is probably a vast "iceberg" of pathology due to hypertension that does not correlate with the clinically recognized form of the disease.

Not all workers, however, agree that hypertension by itself is the cause of strokes, especially of the acute intracerebral hemorrhage type. Nevertheless, it appears that as hypertension has become recognized as the serious disease it is and public awareness has been kindled toward screening and treatment even of mild hypertension, the incidence of hypertensive intracerebral hemorrhage has been progressively falling over the past 20 years. Perhaps as an artifact of changing patterns of hospitalization in the United States, the declining tendency to autopsy hospital deaths, and the sudden and unexpected quality of deaths due to hypertensive cerebral hemorrhage, these lesions are commonly seen by forensic pathologists in coroner's or medical examiner's facilities, where they make up a significant proportion of cases signed out as a natural manner of death. Therefore, the observations made by forensic pathologists have added significance as monitors of trends in public health statistics.

Cerebrovascular Accident/Stroke

The most common consequence of cerebral vascular disease is a clinical syndrome known historically as apoplexy and more recently as cerebrovascular accidents (CVAs), or stroke. Stroke is typically a sudden unexpected intracranial catastrophe that may render the victim unconscious, paralyzed, mute, or uncomprehending and may cause prompt, but rarely sudden or immediate, death. Stroke is commonly divided pathologically into four entities that produce this syndrome: cerebral aneurysm with rupture and SAH; intraparenchymal, hypertensive hemorrhage with subarachnoid and intraventricular hemorrhage; bleeding of a vascular malformation; and cerebral infarction.

The symptoms produced by each of these pathological processes depend on the location of the lesion, its extent, what neurological function had been subserved by the damaged brain region, the chronicity of the lesion, whether hemorrhage was contained or dissected to ventricles or subarachnoid spaces, whether cranial nerves were involved or compressed, and whether vital centers were involved early on in the evolution of the lesion. Each process has been classically described symptomatically, and it is beyond the scope of this discussion to enumerate the points of clinical differentiation between each of the entities. For those readers whose needs require specific points of differentiation, there are several useful references, the most recent among them being the monograph by Wiebers [70].

Stroke is one of the most common diseases of the nervous system worldwide. The incidence varies between 0.31 and 1.24 cases per 1000 population as of the year 2000 and affected at least 1.8 million persons in the United States in 1977 [71] of which more than 750,000 represented new cases [71]. It is estimated that stroke is the third most common cause of death in the United States, but this rate has declined over the last 10 years [72]. Strokes of all types result in death in roughly 15% of cases and produce sufficient disability in 50% of survivors that they are unable to return to their occupations when released from the hospital. Strokes are seen increasingly with age and account for at least 50% of hospital admissions for neurological diseases in the United States. Risk factors identified over the years include obesity, smoking, being male, being African American, diabetes, hypertension, hypercholesterolemia, and hyperlipidemia or a previous myocardial infarction [60,61,70].

The relative occurrences of various types of stroke are estimated from several population studies to be thromboembolic brain infarction (56%–89%, with the lowest incidence occurring in Japan and the highest in the United States); intracerebral hemorrhage, regardless of cause (8%–30%, with the lowest incidence in the United States and the highest in Japan); SAH, presumably due to ruptured aneurysm (3%–14%, with the lowest incidence in the United States and the highest in Japan); and ill-defined or unspecified stroke, which occurs in 10%–40% in some series. These etiologies are often based on clinical presentation rather than pathological information; therefore, the assignment of causality (especially between stroke due to thrombosis and that due to embolism) would be open to debate, and the true incidence of each category is also subject to error (Table 3.4). Nevertheless, cerebral infarct remains the most common form of stroke.

Table 3.4 Etiologies of Fatal and Nonfatal Strokes in a Large Cooperative Study

Type of Stroke	Incidence (% of cases)
Thrombotic stroke	57
Embolic stroke	15–20
Hypertensive hemorrhage	4
SAH (due to aneurysm or vascular malformation)	10–12
TIA (lacunar infarct)	8–10
Miscellaneous forms	1–3

Source: Adapted from Sahs AL et al., eds., *Aneurysmal Subarachnoid Hemorrhage: Report of a Cooperative Study*, Baltimore: Urban & Schwarzenberg, 1981.

The source of the statistics in any epidemiological study can have a major effect on the accuracy of figures. A study [73] that compared the diagnoses on the death certificates in a controlled population (Framingham, Massachusetts) with subsequent autopsy findings has revealed that over a 30 year period, of the cases certified as having died of a stroke, 21% of these showed no evidence of the disease at autopsy, and 40% of those with positive autopsy evidence of a major stroke had no mention on the death certificates of that disease. In general, the more acute the illness and death, the greater the accuracy of the death certificate, but when the illness lasted more than 30 days, the error rate rose to nearly 60% of false negative certifications. These and other figures relating to correspondence between clinical and pathological diagnoses illustrate the importance of autopsy studies in amassing accurate public health data.

Spontaneous Subarachnoid Hemorrhage

SAH is a common finding in the forensic autopsy, and in a study by Helpern and Rabson [55] of 2030 cases of sudden and unexpected death, SAH was present in nearly 5% and made up 26% of cases where the cause of death involved CNS pathology [21–24,74,75]. It is important to separate SAH into those due to a traumatic event and those that are spontaneous. The traumatic causes of SAH are discussed in Chapter 6.

Occurrences of the various etiologies of SAH according to sex and age are listed in Table 3.5. In nonfatal cases of SAH, bleeding aneurysms were by far the most common cause (more than 50%); various forms of hypertensive and atherosclerotic disease and vascular causes account for another 25% of cases; and no known cause could be found in about 20 to 25% of spontaneous nonfatal SAH [74–76].

Sequelae of Subarachnoid Hemorrhage

As mentioned above, the most common symptoms of free blood in the subarachnoid space are meningeal irritation manifested by a painful stiff neck, headache, nausea, vomiting, and usually unconsciousness. The precise cause of this irritation is not known but may be related to the fact that erythrocytes contain a higher concentration of potassium than extracellular fluid and may lyse when in contact with CSF, producing irritation of free nerve endings in the meninges or in the walls of vessels in much the same manner as the pain reported during intravenous therapy with potassium solutions. Other possibilities

Table 3.5 Age and Sex Distribution (%) for Various Causes of Spontaneous SAH

	Age Groups (years)				Sex	
Type	0–20	21–40	41–60	>60	Male	Female
All SAH	4	22	52	22	46	54
Aneurysm	<2	16	55	27	41	59
AVM	15	44	34	7	54	46
Other SAH	<3	13	46	38	50	50

Source: Adapted from Locksley HB, Natural history of subarachnoid hemorrhage: Intracranial aneurysms and arteriovenous malformations. Based on 6368 cases in the cooperative study, in Sahs AL, Perret GE, Locksley HB, Nishioka H, eds., *Intracranial Aneurysms and Subarachnoid Hemorrhage: A Cooperative Study*, Philadelphia: Lippincott, 1969, pp. 35–108.

include the release of prostaglandins and leukotrienes as well as other inflammatory mediators contained in platelets and other blood elements, which may cause vasoconstriction. How hemorrhage causes death may also involve local rise in potassium concentration or interaction with CNS tissues by products of inflammation, especially when subarachnoid blood enters the fourth ventricle and comes in contact with the brain stem nuclei just beneath its floor. Furthermore, SAH may develop so rapidly that it produces a diffuse mass effect that cannot be compensated by efflux of CSF, and the bleeding itself may interfere with CSF flow and reabsorption. With rising intracranial pressure and combined toxic effects of free blood in the CSF, brain stem function becomes compromised, resulting in loss of consciousness, eventual respiratory paralysis, possibly circulatory arrest, and death. The progression of these mechanisms rarely occurs in minutes and generally takes hours or even days to cause death. When medical assistance, including ventilatory support, is not available or sought, death usually occurs within 1 or 2 hours from the onset of massive bleeding. Bleeding may not reach the subarachnoid space to a major degree but may accumulate in the form of a hematoma within the brain. The effects of this phenomenon will be discussed under hypertensive [77], as previously mentioned, is irritative and will promote an inflammatory response eventually. The effects of this inflammatory reaction can lead to scarring of the arachnoidal membrane and produce thickened, opalescent meninges that can be easily peeled off the fixed brain in contradistinction to normal arachnoidal membranes, which are difficult to remove. This scarring reaction may also adversely affect the arachnoid granulations (villi) and arachnoid trabecular vessels and superficial brain vessels where at least some CSF is thought to be reabsorbed (see Chapter 5), leading to a communicative hydrocephalus that may or may not be clinically evident. Scarring and obliteration of the subarachnoid space are seldom so severe following hemorrhage that flow of CSF is totally inhibited, but the impedance to flow may be sufficient to produce a so-called low-pressure hydrocephalus. Leptomeningeal fibrosis may also be caused by a prior infectious or inflammatory process, but there is little in the histological features of the scarring, especially when remote, to indicate the exact cause.

A feared complication of SAH is cerebral vasospasm that may occur promptly or after a variable interval, days or more, after hemorrhage. The consequences of vasospasm result in often profound neurological deterioration in a previously recovering patient. Spasm may be sufficient to produce infarctions and damage far more severe than the original cause of the SAH. The causes of hemorrhage-induced vasospasm have been investigated for many years and may include products of inflammation and inflammatory mediators, failure/inhibition of nitric oxide synthetase in the region, dysfunction of ion channels in vessels and brain, and many other mechanisms, all of which have therapeutic strategies with varying degrees of effectiveness [78–80].

Other immediate complications of SAH are neurogenic pulmonary edema and cardiac failure through mechanisms that are not fully understood or appreciated [43,81]. The mortality and morbidity of seizures can also complicate SAH.

Of practical importance when evaluating acute SAH by the pathologist in the fresh autopsy specimen is the need to gently examine the brain grossly before placing it in formaldehyde. The source of the bleeding should be sought, and if found at the base of the brain, the basal arachnoidal membranes should be gently removed with a small forceps under a gentle jet of running water. This procedure will allow inspection of the circle of Willis for a possible aneurysm or tear in the major vessel. The adhesions between the frontal lobes and those bridging the inferior Sylvain fissure should also be gently split to allow examination of the anterior cerebral and anterior communicating vessels and the middle cerebral vessels to the point of trifurcation. The washing away of fresh blood at the time of autopsy during a preliminary examination prevents the rock-hard fixation of the blood over delicate structures, which can easily be destroyed when trying to dissect the fixed blood clot later on. Intracerebral hematomas should not be washed out, only superficial blood, generally at the base. Of course, prior to washing away blood, if documentation is required, photographs should be taken or diagrams drawn. The brain may then be safely placed in fixative until a more complete and thorough examination can be made. If one is confident that the brain was removed without laceration or tearing of any circle of Willis vessel, it is possible to search for tiny aneurysms or rents in vessels by perfusing the basal vessels with water, saline, or fixative under 100 mmHg pressure. Although it is technically challenging, actual dissection of vessels of the circle of Willis and others can be accomplished and may reveal injuries to the lumen of vessels that would ordinarily be missed [54].

Intracranial Aneurysms

Cerebral vascular aneurysms can be divided into saccular (berry aneurysms), atherosclerotic, mycotic, traumatic, and dissecting aneurysms, and microaneurysms. All can produce a stroke-like syndrome. The most common form of aneurysm is the so-called berry aneurysm. Cerebral berry aneurysms are typically saccular, bleb-like outpouchings occurring at the branching points of named intracranial cerebral arteries. They may vary in size from less than a millimeter to a centimeter or more in diameter, may be spherical or multilobate, single or multiple. It is estimated that at least 2% of the population have cerebral aneurysms that are asymptomatic [76,82–84], encountered usually during routine autopsies or during angiography for some other purpose [85,86], and usually less than 6 mm in diameter. Such asymptomatic aneurysms have a characteristic distribution within the population by age and sex (Table 3.5) as well as in anatomic location (Table 3.6), with about 90% occurring in the anterior circle of Willis and lying within a 2-cm radius of the junction of the internal carotid artery with the circle in people mostly between ages 41 and 60 years [76,85]. When one aneurysm is present, there is a significant likelihood that others also exist. In women this likelihood is about 20% of cases, but in men it is about 12% [87].

Asymptomatic aneurysms are those found incidentally at autopsy or angiography and were apparently without symptoms in life. Symptomatic berry aneurysms are those that

Table 3.6 Locations of Intracranial Aneurysms by Mode of Discovery (%)

Location	Asymptomatic	Symptomatic	Bleeding
Anterior communicating	35	5	35
Internal carotid	25	80	36
Middle cerebral	30	10	21
Posterior cerebral or communicating	11	~5	~5
Basilar or vertebral	5	~5	~5

Source: Adapted from Locksley HB, Natural history of subarachnoid hemorrhage: Intracranial aneurysms and arteriovenous malformations. Based on 6368 cases in the cooperative study, in Sahs AL, Perret GE, Locksley HB, Nishioka H, eds., *Intracranial Aneurysms and Subarachnoid Hemorrhage: A Cooperative Study*, Philadelphia: Lippincott, 1969, pp. 35–108.

produce symptoms such as localized, sometimes pulsatile, headache; palsy or dysfunction of an adjacent cranial nerve, including the optic nerve, caused by pressure; paralysis; dizziness; seizures; pituitary dysfunction; or some other localizing signs or symptoms by virtue of their mass effect and not by the patient's having bled. These aneurysms also have a characteristic anatomic distribution that is different from the asymptomatic berry aneurysms (Table 3.6). Bleeding aneurysms are those located about the internal carotid artery or anterior communicating artery at the circle of Willis and appear different by location than other aneurysms [76].

Asymptomatic (unruptured) aneurysms do not inevitably bleed, but the bleed rate is about 1.3% per year, influenced by a number of factors that include aneurysm size, age at discovery (inverse survival with respect to age), and whether the individual is hypertensive and smokes [87,88] or has multiple aneurysms. Many unruptured aneurysms may be obliterated by organizing clot or atheromata naturally.

The symptoms associated with rupture of an aneurysm are typically stroke-like. The patient may complain of a sudden severe headache, with nausea and vomiting, severe pain and stiffness in the neck, or loss of consciousness. Death due to the accompanying acute SAH and its complications rarely occurs within minutes but, rather, may occur over many days or even years from chronic complications or new ruptures in other aneurysms. About 10%–15% of deaths occur by about 24 hours after rupture, with a rapid increase in mortality rate between 24 hours and 10 days post-rupture, at which time about 50% of patients have died. The death rate after this is much more gradual, so that by 3 years post-rupture about 70% of patients will have died [76]. Improvements in aneurysm survival have occurred because of better neurosurgical and endovascular treatments of the aneurysm itself as well as better means of controlling vasospasm and other morbidity factors [83,89]. Because of the sudden and unexpected nature of aneurysm rupture, these types of cases often come to the coroner/medical examiner's services. Rapid or immediate death due to rupture of an aneurysm, which is not usually the case, can occur, as has been discussed in the classic paper on sudden unexpected death by Moritz and Zamcheck [24] and by others [22,23].

Relationship of Rupture to External Events

From a cooperative multicenter study on SAH, cases of bleeding aneurysms have been analyzed. The circumstances of bleeding are listed in Table 3.7, which illustrates the relationship of aneurysmal rupture to external events. These data are derived from a study of some 2288 cases of bleeding aneurysms, reported by Locksley [76] in 1969. The prominent occurrence during sleep suggests that rupture may be completely independent of any physical activity; however, the association of a significant number of cases with straining or emotion suggests that increased heart rate and blood pressure or raised venous pressure, as during a Valsalva-like circumstance, may be important. It is possible that circadian rises in blood pressure during sleep, possibly associated with dreaming or nightmares, produce a stressful hemodynamic state favoring rupture.

In the forensic setting, the issue of causality or aggravation (stress) leading to rupture of a previously undetected aneurysm is frequently raised. Common circumstances include aneurysmal rupture following a fight, robbery attempt, rape attempt, sexual activity, or on-the-job trauma [76,90,91]. When rupture occurs in direct proximity to the antecedent event (immediately or within a few hours), a connection appears attractive but fundamentally unprovable, but when rupture occurs some days or weeks later, the causal connection

Table 3.7 Circumstances Related to Aneurysm Rupture in 2288 Cases

Circumstances of Rupture	Percentage of Cases
During sleep	36
While lifting or bending	12
Emotional stress	4.4
While defecating, coughing, or urinating	8.4
During sexual activity	3.8
Associated with physical trauma	2.8
During surgery or childbirth	0.8
No known association	32

Source: Adapted from Locksley HB, Natural history of subarachnoid hemorrhage: Intracranial aneurysms and arteriovenous malformations. Based on 6368 cases in the cooperative study, in Sahs AL, Perret GE, Locksley HB, Nishioka H, eds., *Intracranial Aneurysms and Subarachnoid Hemorrhage: A Cooperative Study*, Philadelphia: Lippincott, 1969, pp. 35–108.

obviously becomes even more tenuous. These are cases that involve careful analysis and thought, and an interpretation of causality or noncausality can be successfully argued either way, depending upon individual circumstances. Aneurysm and vascular malformation rupture after or while riding amusement park roller coasters continue to be a significant civil litigation and forensic problem [92,93].

Etiology and Pathogenesis of Berry Aneurysms

For many years, it was believed that most aneurysms were congenital, but numerous autopsy studies have shown that significant numbers of aneurysms do not occur until into the second decade of life and that they hardly ever occur in children [85,94,95]. In one series of 3000 cases, only 58 occurred in the first two decades, and none were found at less than 7 years of age [96]. Perhaps the youngest case of typical berry aneurysm yet reported occurred in a 19-day-old infant [97]. Several authors state that aneurysms in children almost always have a traumatic or inflammatory etiology [95,98] and, as such, may not be typical or classic berry aneurysms.

The congenital factors in the pathogenesis of cerebral aneurysms are probably medial muscular or elastica defects in the walls of the vessels [99–102], which, in the face of stresses including systemic hypertension, cause outpouching of the vessel wall at the weakened point after many years. It is possible that such defects are inherited or acquired in the very early embryonic process of vessel remodeling so that at the branching points of vessels about the circle of Willis, "mistakes" are made and gaps in the reinforcing structures of the vessels occur [99]. Some authors suggest that so-called intimal pads, another congenital defect, disrupt the laminar flow of blood in the vessel, resulting in turbulence and increased stress at certain points [84] where aneurysms may ultimately develop. Another possibility is that aneurysms occur at infundibula, or outpouchings of vessels at the apex of which a smaller vessel, possibly a residual one, exists and provides a point of weakness [94]. In any case, because of the special architecture of intracranial arteries (thin media, only one elastic lamina, and minimal adventitia as compared with systemic arteries) and possible congenital weaknesses, small aneurysms may tend to form and will tend to enlarge with time. As they increase in diameter, the tendency for further increase grows greater as the tension in the wall of the aneurysm sac increases, owing to the physical principle embodied in the law of Laplace, which describes the relationship between tension in the wall of a vessel and its radius [100]. The tendency, then, is for a gradually increasing diameter with increasing tension in a vicious cycle until rupture occurs.

Several factors may interfere with rupture; these include scarring of the sac wall (reinforcement), development of atheromatous plaques in the wall, thrombosis with organization, abatement of the intravascular pressures acting upon the damaged vessel, and, of course, medical or surgical intervention. It is nevertheless striking to observe the histological appearance of an aneurysm wall and how few cells may be interposed between the lumen and the adventitia of the vessel, even in unruptured aneurysms.

Aneurysms may be associated with a variety of systemic pathology such as congenital polycystic renal disease [101], coarctation of [94]. It should be pointed out that the role of hypertension in the pathogenesis of aneurysms and their ultimate rupture is controversial and is not conclusive. An association of aneurysm with cerebral arteriovenous malformation (AVM) has been repeatedly suggested [74,102], and multiplicity of aneurysms is said to occur in 10 to 25% of cases [74]; familial occurrences have also been reported [103].

Pathology of Aneurysms

The gross pathological appearance of SAH caused by a small saccular aneurysm of the anterior cerebral artery at the anterior communicating artery is illustrated in an unfixed specimen in Figure 3.8. Much of the blood has been washed away to reveal the aneurysm prior to fixation, a technique that should always be followed. Not all cases of ruptured aneurysms result in typical basal SAH. When the fundus of the aneurysm is embedded in the brain or totally enclosed or compressed by the opposing cerebral hemispheres, as

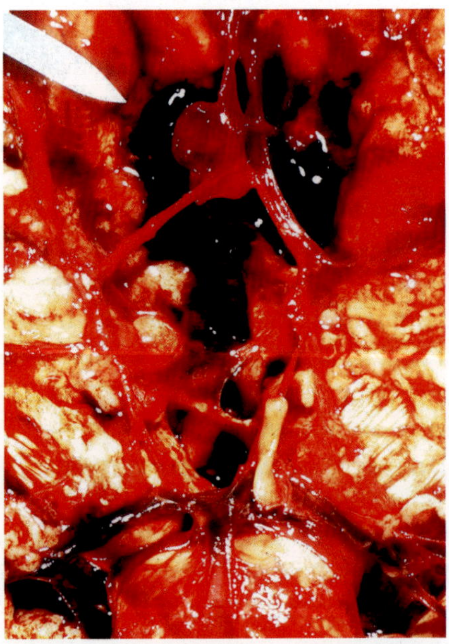

Figure 3.8 This basal view of the unfixed brain with a massive SAH reveals a relatively small aneurysm of the anterior cerebral–anterior communicating artery (white arrow).

in anterior communicating artery aneurysms, hemorrhage may be contained and not leak into the subarachnoid space. Thus, when rupture occurs in these two circumstances, the course of blood "jetting" from the fundus may dissect into the brain, producing a hematoma that may or may not communicate with the subarachnoid space and cause an obvious SAH (Figure 3.9). In unusual circumstances the stream of arterial blood may be conducted along the corpus callosum to a remote portion of the brain where either subarachnoid bleeding, intraventricular bleeding, or localized hematoma may occur [104]. The jet lesions into brain parenchyma often resemble in cut section the parabolic course of water as if from a fire hose. The jet may have such force that it dissects its way into the ventricle and produces an intraventricular hemorrhage and may mimic clinical, radiographic, and pathological appearances of an acute intracerebral hypertensive hemorrhage, producing SAH only secondarily by way of the CSF pathway to the basal cisterns. In such cases it is important to properly recognize the source of the bleeding, and the true nature of the process.

The gross pathological appearances of berry aneurysms vary considerably from a single spherical bleb to a mulberry-like or group of irregular outpouchings. In aneurysms of long standing, there is usually an atheromatous plaque within the fundus, probably caused by turbulence within the sac and intimal injury. As previously mentioned, most aneurysms are found at the branching points of vessels in a distribution described above.

When one aneurysm is found, the examination cannot be considered complete until all the major vessels, especially of the portion of the circle of Willis anterior to the internal carotid junctions, have been exposed and viewed completely on all sides. Multiple aneurysms are not uncommon and may be symmetrical, as is often seen in cases of congenital polycystic renal disease, as shown in Figure 3.10 [101]. Sometimes as many as six or eight subsidiary aneurysms may be found, most of which are unruptured.

Occasionally, very large aneurysms may be discovered, especially of the basilar artery (Figure 3.11), that indent the pons with their mass effect. Sometimes long-standing unruptured aneurysms behave like tumors, causing cranial nerve injury such as might occur with a Schwannoma (Figure 3.12). Owing to the large size of these aneurysms, rupture usually is a rapidly fatal event, but sometimes the fundus may be largely replaced by a thrombus, which may lead to multiple secondary embolic infarctions [105,106]. The

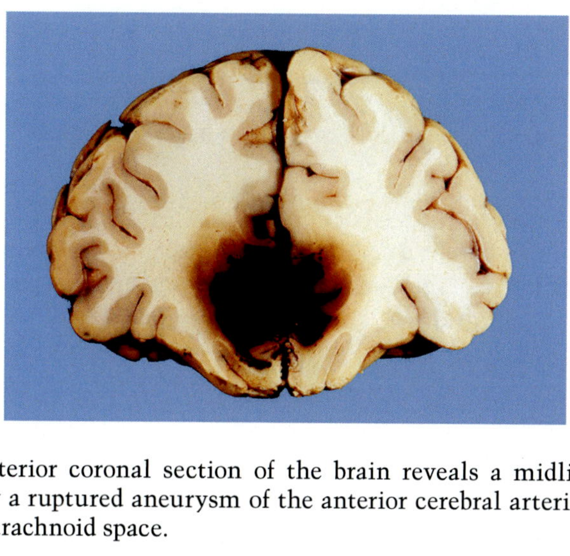

Figure 3.9 This anterior coronal section of the brain reveals a midline interhemispheric hematoma caused by a ruptured aneurysm of the anterior cerebral arterial system with some leakage into the subarachnoid space.

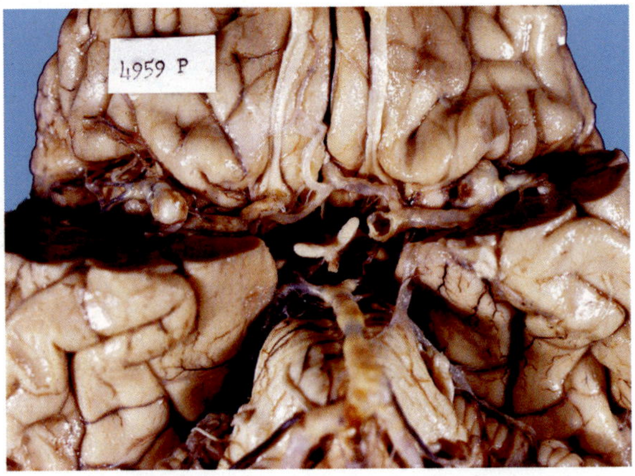

Figure 3.10 This basal view of the brain with temporal lobe tips removed reveals two aneurysms of the middle cerebral arteries in a patient with polycystic renal disease and long standing hypertension.

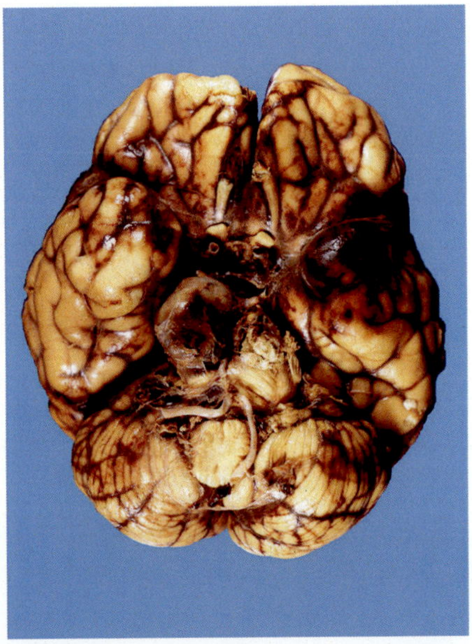

Figure 3.11 This basal view of the brain shows a huge largely thrombosed basilar artery aneurysm.

pathogenesis of such large aneurysms is not known, and it is not immediately clear if they arise by different mechanisms than smaller, more classic aneurysms elsewhere in the circle of Willis. Direct complications of aneurysm leakage, or rupture, include an associated infarction usually in one or more of the vascular territories served by the affected vessels, often due to vasospasm. The etiology of this complication may be the irritative action of subarachnoid blood on the muscle of the vessel wall or a neurogenic response to the tearing of the vessel itself, which causes vascular spasm. This complication may occasionally be seen following surgical clipping of the aneurysm's neck or some of the newer endovascular treatments for such aneurysms.

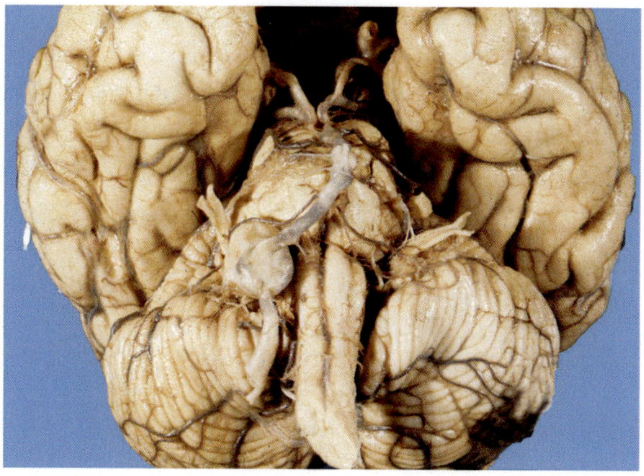

Figure 3.12 This basal view of the brain shows a 1.5-cm unruptured aneurysm of the right vertebral artery discovered incidentally in the autopsy of an 80-year-old woman who died of unrelated conditions but who apparently had a facial paralysis and some other possible cranial nerve symptoms on the right side, but had not been worked up for them. Her death occurred before widespread use of the CT scanning.

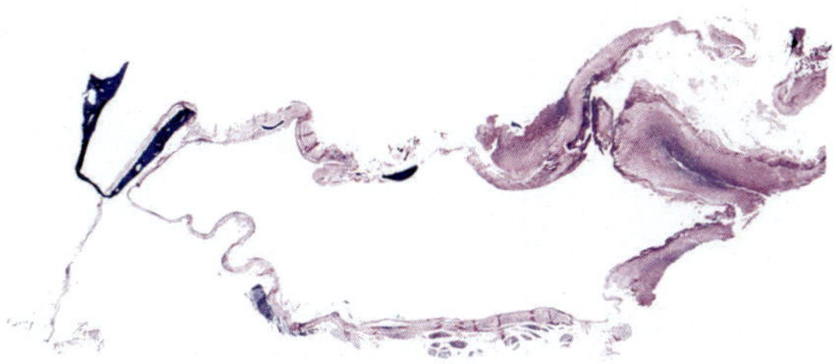

Figure 3.13 This low power photomicrograph illustrates the fundus of an intracranial aneurysm and reveals the extreme thinness of portions of its wall.

Microscopic examination of aneurysms often reveals how thin portions of the fundus are often only a few cell layers thick (Figure 3.13). If the proper connective tissue stains are used, it is very common to find breaks and absence of the elastic fibers of the media that should be present. Such elastic fiber loss is commonly encountered in people with aneurysms at the branching points of arteries at the circle of Willis where there is no aneurysm.

Atherosclerotic Aneurysms

The term *atherosclerotic aneurysm*, when applied to brain vessels, is probably a special case, and some would argue that the label is inappropriate because rupture of an atheromatous vessel occurs only rarely. Nevertheless, what is described in authoritative works as an atherosclerotic aneurysm is usually a dilatation and elongation of the basilar or other arteries, so that instead of taking a straight course from the posterior circle of Willis to the vertebral arteries, it becomes "S" shaped [107,108]. The misshapen vessel is often mineralized and may reach nearly 1 cm in diameter along its entire length, but it is rarely obstructed by atheromatous plaques. The dilatation of this vessel is not localized and, in fact, may involve virtually all the major named vessels of the circle of Willis, so that all the vessels resemble a nest of snakes. The convexities of the vessels may indent neighboring structures with their imprints, and small tributaries may be elongated. These dilated vessels usually have their own designation as a special form of cerebral arteriosclerosis, which might properly be referred to as the calcified-dilated or ectatic form of cerebral arteriosclerosis. In such conditions dissection into the arterial wall may occur.

Mycotic Aneurysms

Contrary to what the name implies, most mycotic aneurysms are not caused by fungal infections [109–111] but, rather, are sequelae of bacterial infections, including infective endocarditis and meningitis. Such aneurysms may be saccular or fusiform, are usually multiple, and affect branches of the middle cerebral artery [112], the crucial point of differentiation being that they occur in locations other than typical berry aneurysms. Histologically, evidence of infection is usually obvious, with inflammation and necrosis of the vascular wall. Histological demonstration of the infecting organism is usually possible. In the case of fungi, the Grocott's methenamine-silver stain is recommended. From an etiological and forensic perspective, mycotic aneurysms of cerebral vessels generally occur in immunosuppressed or immunoincompetent individuals, intravenous drug addicts, diabetics, persons who have congenital cyanotic heart disease, those who have had recent cardiac surgery, those who suffer from infective endocarditis, or those who have an autoimmune inflammatory disease [113,114].

Dissecting Aneurysms

Dissecting aneurysms (sometimes called pseudoaneurysms) of intracranial vessels are rare, with only eight new cases reported between 1968 and 1980 [115,116] and apparently only thirty cases reported in the world literature prior to 1968. A great many additional cases now too numerous to cite have been reported. There may be difficulty in separating aneurysmal dissections from simple vascular dissections, although the consequences are similar or identical. They affect persons in their second and third decades but have also been reported in infants. Dissections tend to present suddenly with a stroke-like syndrome and no antecedent history. Vessels affected are most commonly the larger intracranial vessels such as the internal carotids, middle cerebral, and vertebrobasilar system. The etiologies of the dissections have been reported to include syphilis, congenital defects of vessels, Marfan's syndrome, allergic arteritis, cerebral or cervical trauma, therapeutic manipulations of the neck, and a host of other conditions and circumstances [21,117–121]. Pathologically, dissecting aneurysms usually reveal a rent in the intima with dissecting hemorrhage into the subintima or media, with fusiform enlargement of the vessel wall. When the dissection persists for some time, a layered thrombotic structure may be seen in the wall.

Traumatic Aneurysms

The term *traumatic aneurysm* should not be confused with traumatically induced rupture of a preexisting berry aneurysm, as discussed above; rather, the term denotes trauma as being the primary cause for the aneurysm. Such aneurysms could be a special form of dissecting aneurysm because most show rents in the intima and subsequent dissection in the vessel wall, with either immediate rupture or more protracted evolution of a fusiform aneurysm containing clotted and often organized blood. The term *pseudoaneurysm* has also been applied to them [115]. Most such aneurysms involve extracranial portions of the internal carotid artery and are associated with basilar skull fractures, but when intracranial vessels are involved, they are usually the anterior circle of Willis vessels. Less commonly involved are the posterior cerebral, superior cerebellar, or basilar arteries. When rupture has been acute, differentiating a traumatic aneurysm or traumatic division of a vessel from a ruptured small berry aneurysm may be very difficult and requires patience and good luck. Sometimes small peripheral arteries on the surface of the brain are damaged by trauma, especially when adjacent to the falx or beneath fracture lines on the convexity of the skull, and may show aneurysmal dilatation [116].

Intracranial Hypertensive Hemorrhage

This form of cerebral hemorrhage of usually massive proportions accounts for at least 52% of fatal cases of SAH but has been decreasing over the past 20 years; in fact, the rate of decrease has now flattened out [77,122–124]. The fatality rate is high (90% of victims die within 72 hours of onset of symptoms), and only a small percentage survive even in the face of surgical treatments. Persons affected are generally older than 40 years (more than 75%), with about 25% of cases occurring in each succeeding decade. Males and females are about equally affected. Cerebral hemorrhages that occur in young people appear to have a slightly different demographic than in older victims [125]. Typical symptoms of acute intracerebral hemorrhage are usually stroke-like, sudden, and occur at all times of the day and in association with all forms of activity, in much the same pattern as rupture of berry aneurysms. There may be an associated sudden headache, an urge to vomit or use the toilet (many victims are found in the bathroom), a rapidly progressing hemiparesis, and rapid loss of consciousness. Death rarely occurs within 1 hour and can be protracted if the victim is transported to the hospital and ventilatory support provided.

Surgical treatment of hypertensive hemorrhages, with the exception of those with cerebellar hemorrhages [126,127] who have stabilized, is generally not rewarding. In some cases of basis pontis hemorrhage, protracted coma in the locked-out state may occur [34,128] with little chance that a surgical intervention is useful. The common locations for such hypertensive hemorrhages are first and foremost (about 80% of cases) within the basal ganglia (usually in the lateral ganglionic region involving the globus pallidus and external capsule region), followed in about equal amounts (about 10% each) by hemorrhages in the basis pontis [129] and in the cerebellar hemispheres involving the dentate nucleus. Multiple hemorrhages or hemorrhages in other locations will probably have an etiology other than hypertension, which should be investigated.

In so-called lateral ganglionic hemorrhage, as illustrated in Figures 3.14 and 3.15, the site of origin of the hemorrhage appears to be within either the external globus pallidus, the putamen, or the external capsule–claustrum, deep to the insula. The hemorrhage then appears to push the remaining basal ganglia toward the midline and then to dissect upward along the path of least resistance, through the white matter over the caudate nucleus, into the lateral ventricle, or to dissect forward or backward until another ventricular chamber is reached. Occasionally, the primary hemorrhage may occur within the internal capsule

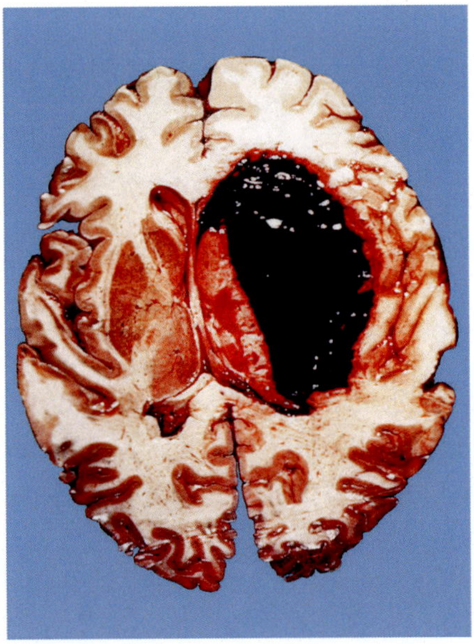

Figure 3.14 This horizontal section of an unfixed brain with a typical "hypertensive" lateral ganglionic hemorrhage illustrates the huge hematoma that has arisen in the external capsule-claustrum region and pushed the basal ganglionic structures toward the midline and ruptured into the anterior ventricular system.

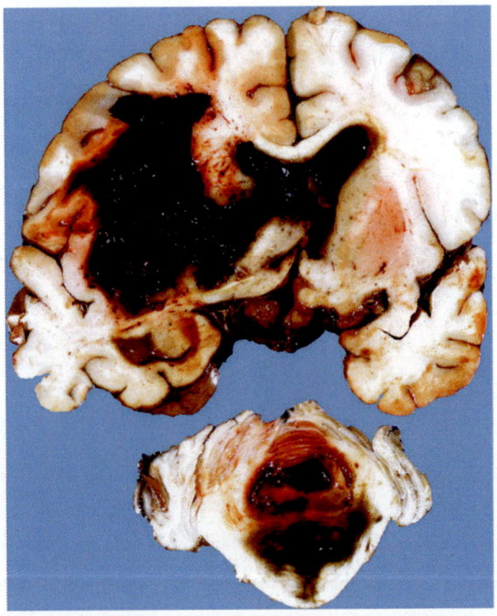

Figure 3.15 This coronal section of a case similar to that shown in Figure 3.14 again illustrates the lateral ganglionic region of the "hypertensive" hemorrhage with ventricular rupture and an associated secondary upper brain stem hemorrhage ("Duret" hemorrhage) due to herniation.

or thalamus and rupture directly into the lateral ventricle or third ventricle. On rare occasions, the hemorrhage may be circumscribed and fail to dissect into the ventricle. In this circumstance, the individual may survive and, when coming to autopsy for another or related cause even years later, will show a smooth-walled, brownish or yellow cystic space at the site of the old hemorrhage, as illustrated in Figure 3.16.

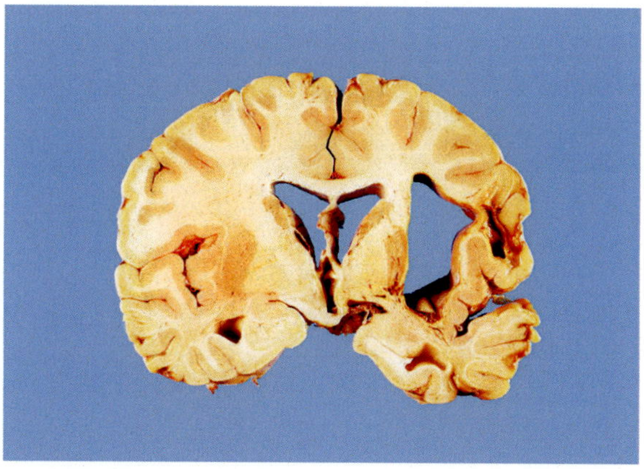

Figure 3.16 This coronal section of the brain of an individual who has suffered a lateral ganglionic "hypertensive" hemorrhage some years before death and survived without surgical removal of the hemorrhage illustrates the smooth-walled cystic space left after the hemorrhage was gradually absorbed. Such instances are very uncommon.

Histological examination of the hematoma itself generally is unrewarding; however, adjacent to the hemorrhage or in the opposite basal ganglia, one can usually find the stigmata of hypertensive microvascular disease in the form of sclerotic, tortuous small arterioles within a space that contains a few macrophages or siderophages. Sometimes mineralization or profound collagenization of the perivascular space is seen. Old or recent perivascular hemorrhage (bleeding globes) apart from the main hematoma may also be visible, and occasionally what appear to be true saccular microaneurysms (as described by Charcot and Bouchard in 1868) [130] may be found. It is usually obvious that chronic microvascular disease, not radically different from the typical hypertensive arteriolar sclerosis in the kidneys, is present in several locations. Lacunar infarcts (*etat lacunaire*) and similar perivascular microinfarcts in the subcortical white matter (*etat crible*) are also commonly associated.

Commonly associated with ganglionic hemorrhage is a separate hemorrhage in the upper brain stem that results from herniation, often referred to as a Duret hemorrhage (see Figure 3.15), although this is probably a misnomer [131]. This hemorrhage most likely occurs when unilateral rapidly developing mass lesions lead to brain stem herniation [132]. Sometimes bilateral mass lesions can produce Duret hemorrhages, but in these cases the evolution of the mass lesions is probably not uniform or in synchrony. A more complete discussion of this lesion can be found in Chapter 5. The hemorrhage may evolve within 30 minutes of the initial catastrophe. Duret hemorrhages are irreversible and mean that restoration of consciousness regardless of treatment is impossible, because the brain stem reticular formation has usually been destroyed. However, vegetative existence may be maintained for some time if ventilatory assistance is available. Survivals from Duret hemorrhages have been reported [133]. An unusual example of an individual who survived a Duret hemorrhage but remained in a vegetative state (locked out) is illustrated in Figure 3.17. The usual course of events, once Duret hemorrhage has occurred and a respirator is in use, is the development of the respirator brain (discussed in greater detail in Chapter 5).

Hypertensive hemorrhages that involve the deep cerebellar gray matter (dentate nucleus) tend to evolve suddenly and often result in relatively prompt loss of consciousness,

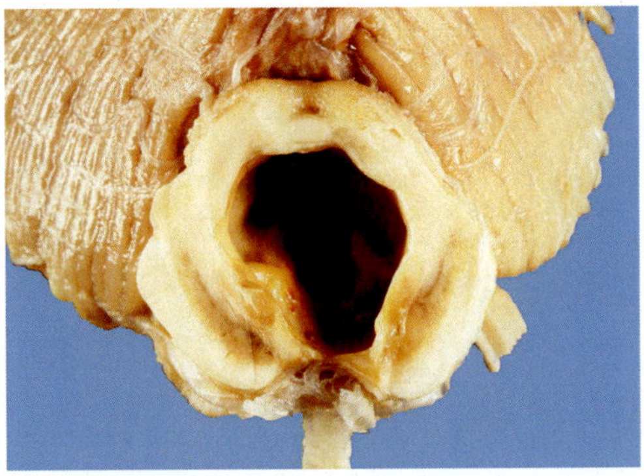

Figure 3.17 This cross section of the midbrain near the cerebral aqueduct from a rostral position illustrates a "chronic" Duret hemorrhage of the midline midbrain in which the victim survived, albeit in coma and a vegetative state for many months. The basis for the coma was the destruction of the midline reticular activating system of the brain stem. Such surviving Duret hemorrhage cases are quite rare.

owing to proximity to the brain stem reticular formation. Likewise, hemorrhages to the base of the pons cause a rapid loss of consciousness by the same mechanism. Cerebellar hemorrhages produce a mass effect that not only produce tonsillar herniations but may also produce upward herniation of the rostral cerebellar vermis through the tentorial notch, as illustrated in Figure 3.18. Cerebellar hemorrhages may rupture into the fourth ventricle and sometimes into the subarachnoid space. These hemorrhages have a high mortality

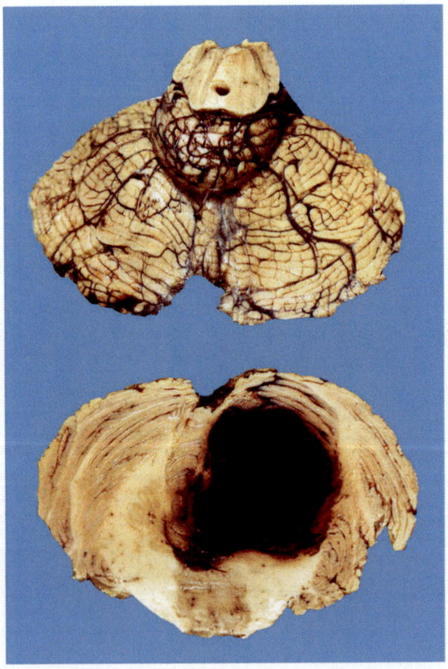

Figure 3.18 This horizontal section of the cerebellum and midbrain illustrate a dentate nucleus "hypertensive" hemorrhage. The mass effect of this hemorrhage that appears to have ruptured into the fourth ventricle has caused an "upward" herniation of the rostral vermis through the tentorial notch.

rate, but prompt neurosurgical intervention with evacuation of the clot may be life saving, although neurological deficits may persist.

Primary hemorrhages of the pons involve the basis pontis, as illustrated in Figure 3.19. Such hemorrhages are almost always fatal, but when survivals are prolonged, the individual is usually comatose but may show so-called alpha coma, wherein waking–sleeping EEG patterns may be observed although the victim is deeply comatose [128]. In unusual cases where the hemorrhage is in the distal basis pontis and mass effect or hemorrhage has not damaged the reticular formation, victims of pontine hemorrhages may be conscious but unable to move the extremities or to speak—the so-called locked-in state [34].

Occasionally, it is important in the forensic environment to differentiate between hypertensive hemorrhages and intracerebral hemorrhage due to trauma or some other condition. A practical guide in this situation is that nonhypertensive intracerebral hematomas do not usually occur in the locations where hypertensive hemorrhages are seen (lateral ganglionic region, basis pontis, dentate nucleus of cerebellum). Furthermore, such traumatic hematomas usually underlie the cortical ribbon and are generally smaller than hypertensive bleeds, but they may also be multiple. In apparently traumatic hemorrhages, there may be associated cortical contusions and other evidence of inner brain trauma, such as streak or punctate hemorrhages about the cerebral aqueduct or in the white matter, which should be distinctive. For further discussion of these points regarding physical injury etiologies, see Chapter 6. Forensic issues may arise in cases with cerebral hemorrhages that occur during pregnancy and delivery (with and without eclampsia), with anticoagulation, and in association with drugs of abuse, notably cocaine and amphetamines [125,134,135].

It should be borne in mind that individuals with amyloid vascular disease of the brain, a condition whose commonness in elderly individuals [136–139] with or without AD has been recognized in recent years, may be more vulnerable to traumatic cerebral hemorrhage than other individuals. In fact, it may well be that many of the cases of posttraumatic intracerebral hemorrhages, especially in elderly individuals, are actually cases of amyloid vessel disease that suffered sufficient trauma to cause the affected vessels to bleed (Figure 3.20).

Amyloid angiopathy has been known for many years and was thought to be uncommon or rare [136,140]. The condition appears to be caused by the apolipoprotein E (APOE) e-2

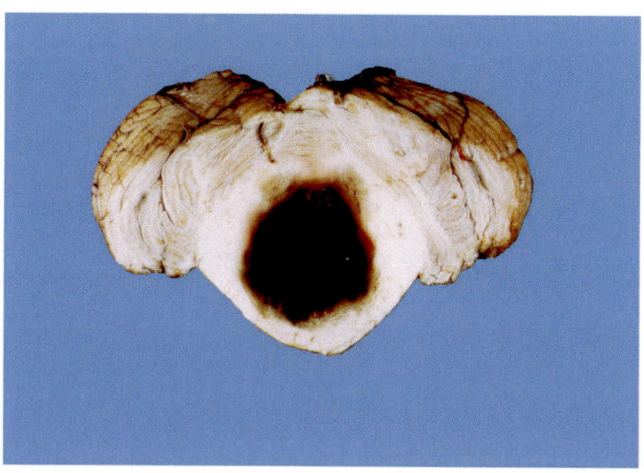

Figure 3.19 This horizontal section through the cerebellum and mid-pons illustrates a "hypertensive" basis pontis hemorrhage.

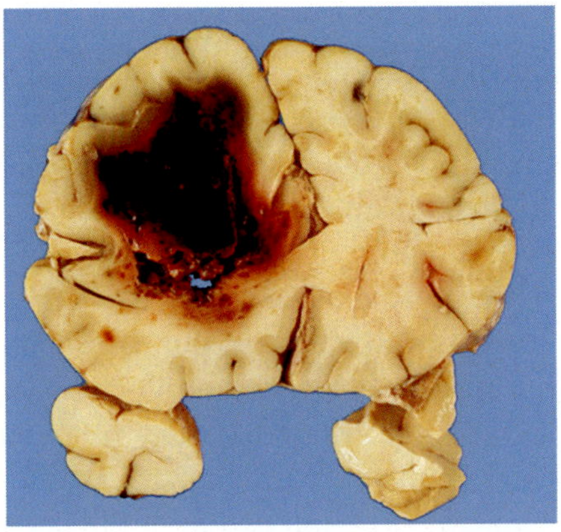

Figure 3.20 This coronal section of brain illustrates a subcortical hemorrhage due to amyloid vascular disease. Although this hemorrhage may dissect into the ventricles or rupture to the subarachnoid space, the location of this hemorrhage is topographically different from the typical hypertensive hemorrhage.

allele, which causes deposition of B-amyloid in arteriolar walls in the brain but apparently not in other organs of the body. Grossly, if one is suspecting amyloid angiopathy, affected cortical arterial branches may appear somewhat silvery, but generally gross observations are insufficient to make the diagnosis. Microscopic examination of affected vessels shows a thickening of the media and adventitia with a hyaline material (Figure 3.21) that stains positively with Congo red and thioflavine dyes (with ultraviolet microscopy). Sometimes in the center of a hemorrhage due to amyloid vessel disease, one can find a mass of amyloid material (amyloidoma) and evidence of previous hemorrhage and reactions. Usually,

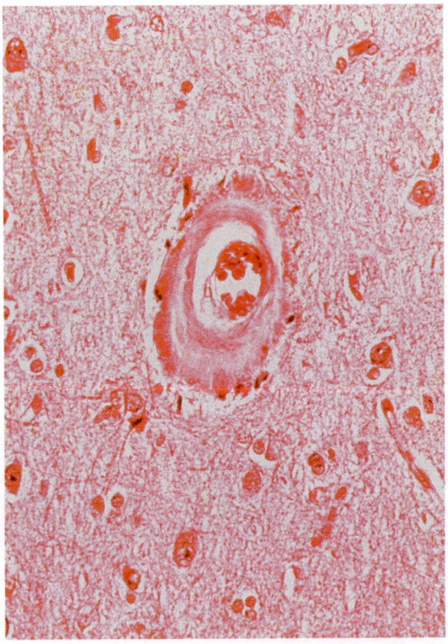

Figure 3.21 This photomicrograph of a small cerebral arteriole affected with amyloid deposition in its wall. Congo red dye staining with polarizing microscopy would show an apple green fluorescence in the hyaline material in the vessel wall.

surrounding nonhemorrhagic regions will show affected arterioles as well. Affected individuals may hemorrhage many times and sometimes require surgical evacuation of the hematomas, but there is no cure for the condition.

Hemorrhage due to Blood Dyscrasias and Other Diseases

When massive intracerebral hemorrhage not connected with head trauma has occurred and is multifocal or not located in one of the typical sites (lateral ganglionic region, basis pontis, or cerebellar hemisphere) for hypertensive hemorrhage, one of a multitude of other causes must be suspected. The most common of these are diseases of the blood, which include leukemia, polycythemia, hemophilia, thrombocytopenia, disseminated intravascular coagulation (DIC), and sickle cell disease (plus the many heterogeneous hemoglobinopathies), and overmedication with anticoagulant medications. Other conditions causing similar hemorrhages include delayed deaths in intoxication; fat, bone marrow, and amniotic fluid embolism; disseminated fungal infections (aspergillosis and the other mycelia infections); metastatic choriocarcinoma; melanoma and other neoplasms; cerebral malaria; amyloid vessel disease; and cryptic telangiectatic and other vascular malformations.

Regardless of the underlying disease, the pattern of bleeding is remarkably similar. Especially in leukemia, where a blastic crisis has occurred, hemorrhages are multiple and often lie in the subcortical location in the cerebrum but may involve deep nuclear structures of the basal ganglia, cerebellar white matter, and occasionally the brain stem. The perivascular character of the hemorrhages can often be appreciated on coronal section, where even though the hematoma may be large, it is actually a confluent hemorrhage made up of many adjacent perivascular hemorrhages represented as discrete ball-like bleeds that blend into one another. The basis for such a form of bleeding is massive multifocal destruction of several vessels. Microscopic examination of the transitional zone between normal brain and hemorrhage may reveal the cause of the vessel pathology, be it leukemic infiltration, metastatic tumor, vascular malformation, sickled red blood cells, or intravascular platelet–fibrin thrombi, as in DIC or related conditions. In the case of hemophiliac hemorrhages, microscopic appearances are not especially helpful except to rule out more obvious etiologies.

Vascular Malformations

Vascular malformations of the nervous system seem best divided into the groups suggested by McCormick [141,142]: telangiectases, varices, cavernous malformations, arteriovenous (A–V) malformations, and venous malformations. Each form is a general descriptive category, and there may be some overlap between groups. All of the lesions are considered maldevelopmental in origin, and most show growth potential throughout life, which suggests that these malformations may be neoplasms or hamartomas in a special sense. Because a familial basis may be involved, discovery of a cavernous or telangiectatic anomaly in the brain of a patient or victim should lead to informing the family of their potential risk and suggesting a genetic counselor.

In infancy, vascular malformations may be encountered that are small and which enlarge with time and, like aneurysms, seem to require many years to grow large enough to produce symptoms [143,144]. The symptoms that may appear include primary SAH with or without a fatal result; focal neurological signs and symptoms; epileptic seizures;

generalized neurological symptoms, including dementia, personality, and behavioral abnormalities; disturbances of consciousness; and systemic symptoms that may include heart failure (from massive A–V shunting) [143,145]. Many smaller vascular anomalies are asymptomatic and found only at autopsy. Because tissue destruction may be massive when rupture occurs, the malformation itself may be destroyed or overshadowed by the hemorrhage that results [146]. This phenomenon is a common problem when interpreting intracerebral hemorrhages that occur in locations not usually affected by hypertensive hemorrhages. This mechanism is also invoked to explain the phenomenon of so-called delayed traumatic intracerebral hemorrhage (Spät-Apoplexie), as briefly mentioned above [53,55] and discussed in detail in Chapter 6.

Telangiectatic Vascular Malformations

Telengiectatic vascular malformations are best defined as capillary or end-vessel (arteriolar or venular) anomalies that may be small, focal, but generally rather circumscribed lesions that may represent a persistence of the embryonic feltwork of small vessels that once represented the background of developing neural tissue (*rete mirabile*). These are probably the most common form of vascular anomaly and are frequently found incidentally at autopsy [141,142]. They can occur anywhere in the CNS but seem to occur most commonly in deeper portions of the brain in and about the basal ganglia and thalamus, in the brain stem, and even in the spinal cord. They are only rarely superficial and visible on the surface of the brain or ventricles. There are usually no large feeding or draining vessels, and they may be invisible even on angiography owing to their small size. The natural history of these lesions in the CNS is gradual slow enlargement and probably only rarely overt rupture [147–149], but systemic manifestations of similar malformations may bleed and overshadow the CNS lesions. A number of genetic mutations have been reported under these circumstances, many of which appear to be autosomally dominant [150].

Grossly, telangiectases may appear as a dark stain on the cut surface of the brain specimen or clearly have a sponge-like microvascular appearance (Figure 3.22), which shows

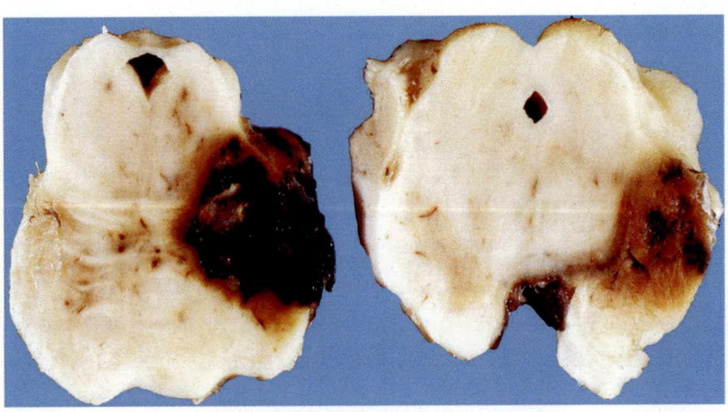

Figure 3.22 This cross section of the pons and midbrain show a telangiectatic vascular malformation that was discovered incidentally at autopsy. The neurological history in this case is vague but it was thought that this person might clinically have had a form of cerebral palsy. Histologically this lesion was composed of a complex pattern of small vessels, many of which were sclerosed and surrounded by siderophages and gliosis.

chronic leaking and deposition of blood pigments and sometimes mineralization. The usual size of the lesions is a few millimeters to a centimeter or two in diameter.

In the forensic setting, these small, usually asymptomatic, lesions have been blamed for large fatal brain hemorrhages following head trauma that may not have been especially severe, and even trivial, referred to above as Spät-Apoplexie [52,55]. Sometimes these small lesions are located in subcortical locations or hippocampal–amygdaloid regions where they can act as epileptogenic foci (Figure 3.23). They may also occur in the brain stem or spinal cord, where they produce symptoms that may have led to a misdiagnosis of MS [151] or a neurological degenerative disease.

Microscopically, they are usually composed of very small vessels that are dilated and trap normal neural elements between the vascular channels (Figure 3.24). There is usually

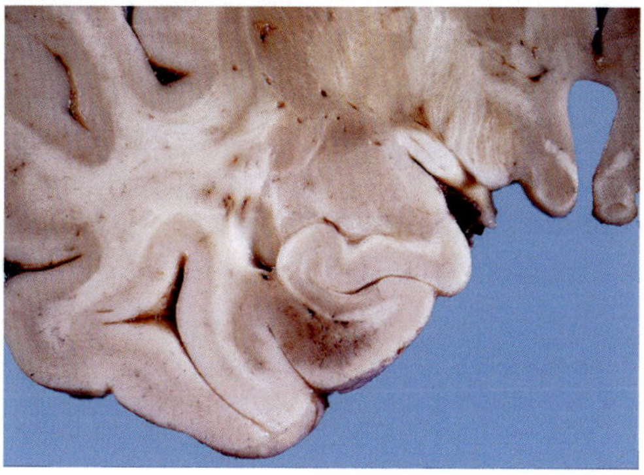

Figure 3.23 This photograph of the hippocampal–amygdala region of the temporal lobe shows a small, dark discoloration that represents a cryptic telangiectatic vascular anomaly. Such an anomaly in this location may represent an epileptogenic focus.

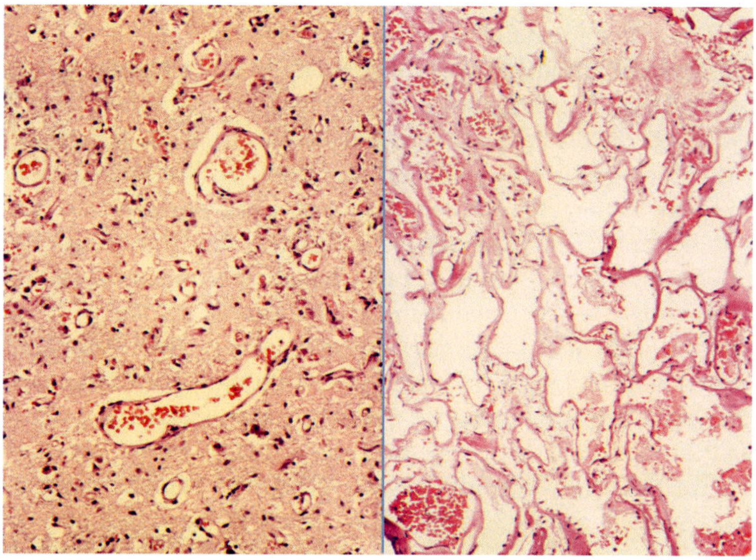

Figure 3.24 A telangiectatic vascular malformation composed of many tiny vascular channels appears in the left panel. A cavernous angioma composed of a sponge-work of thin-walled capillaries with no intervening neural tissue appears in the right panel.

evidence of numerous prior episodes of minimal hemorrhage, and the vessels of intervening tissue may be mineralized. There is often an intense glial reaction, sometimes containing Rosenthal fibers in the entrapped or adjacent neural tissue. In some lesions there may be larger vessels and dilated spaces, which cause some problems of classification with the other forms of vascular anomaly. This issue arises only occasionally, and there is no generally agreed-upon resolution of this problem among neuropathologists.

Varices

In its simplest form, the CNS varix is a single, tortuous, dilated venous vessel, usually on the surface of the brain, spinal cord [152], or meninges. The varix may be composed of more vessels in a more tangled mass, however, and again may cause problems of classification [142,143,145]. They may also lie beneath the cortical surface in the white matter and, although usually small, may reach large proportions, as in the case of vein of Galen malformations, which may also involve arterial feeders and, as such, are probably better classified as A–V malformations [153,154]. The basic differentiating features of these lesions are that they are relatively simple, composed of thin-walled venous structures, and generally not mineralized. When they rupture, hemorrhage may be massive and catastrophic. Such ruptures have sometimes also been associated with or invoked as an explanation for delayed posttraumatic apoplexy. When located on the surface of the brain or cord, surgical removal may be relatively simple with very few sequelae. Vein of Galen malformations are a different story and pose difficult challenges for their management.

Cavernous Angiomas

As with other forms of vascular malformations, the classification of cavernous angiomas is often arbitrary and difficult. Nevertheless, there appears to be a series of low-flow, primarily venous malformations that are complex masses of dilated larger vessels that are different enough from other anomalies to warrant a special designation [141]. As previously mentioned, these lesions, although likely congenital, do not generally make their appearance symptomatically by bleeding until into adult life. They are inherited by an autosomal dominant mode, and the genetics of the condition has been the subject of considerable investigation [155,156]. These lesions are usually found in the cerebral hemispheres but may occur anywhere in the CNS and can be multiple. Radiographically, they do not tend to show up in angiograms, but if they have bled, computerized tomography (CT) and magnetic resonance imaging (MRI) scanning easily pinpoint them but may not provide a specific diagnosis. Grossly, they are usually single, circumscribed, filled with blood, and thus have a dark purple, grape-like appearance. Microscopically, the vessels are thin or thick walled but are venous, not arterial. The thicker channels do not contain elastica and are thus not arteries, although they appear to be so. There may or may not be entrapped neural tissue between the loops of the vessels making up the malformation, but most lesions have little or no space between adjacent loops of vessels (Figure 3.24). The vessels have no elastic connective tissue in them compared with AVMs. Many of the vessels may be thrombosed completely or partially. Evidence of prior hemorrhage is usually present, and mineralization is often prominent. These lesions may rupture spontaneously with fatal result but more likely remain relatively indolent, producing a variety of neurological symptoms and signs, depending upon their location.

Arteriovenous Malformations

AVMs are the form of vascular anomaly with which pathologists are most familiar and, apart from the numerically more common telangiectatic malformations, are the most common vascular malformation of clinical and pathological significance, accounting for between 1% and 4% of all intracranial masses [157].

As the name implies, the malformation is composed of both arteries and veins of all sizes and calibers. The lesions are presumed to have arisen from embryonic vessels that have persisted in much the same manner as telangiectasis, although no direct connection between the two lesions has been conclusively established. AVMs can occur anywhere in the CNS but most commonly are found in the territory of the middle cerebral artery, laterally over or in the cerebral hemispheres (Figure 3.25). When they occur in the spinal cord [153] (as either telangiectatic AVMs or larger A–V malformations) or in association with a dural vascular anomaly, they may be associated with a progressive necrotizing and hemorrhagic transverse myelopathy known as the Foix–Alajouanine syndrome [57,158]. AVMs occur about twice as often in males as in females. They often do not become clinically evident until the second decade of life or later, when, because of increasing size and tendency to leak, they produce a seizure focus, a focal neurological sign or symptom. The most common presenting symptom (in about 40% of cases) is that of SAH, which, in the majority of cases, is not fatal; in fact, probably fewer than 10% ever die of this lesion [159]. Treatment may be nonsurgical, involving embolization or some other endovascular procedure, stereotactic radiosurgery, or operative removal of the lesion, all offering excellent results [145,160–162]. Nearly 70% of persons with AVMs will lead normal or relatively normal lives, but about 30% will suffer some, often disabling, neurological deficit.

As illustrated in Figure 3.25, the typical AVM lies on the surface of the brain but invades beneath the cortical surface, presenting a sponge-like mass on cross section (Figure 3.26) and a tangled jumble of vessels much like a ball of snakes before sectioning. There are usually one or more major arterial feeder vessels that, when clamped, cause the AVM to collapse. A special form of AVM may involve the great vein of Galen in the posterior portion of the brain in the region of the pineal body, as mentioned above. These lesions can occur in adults but may be seen more frequently in children. They take the form of huge dilated

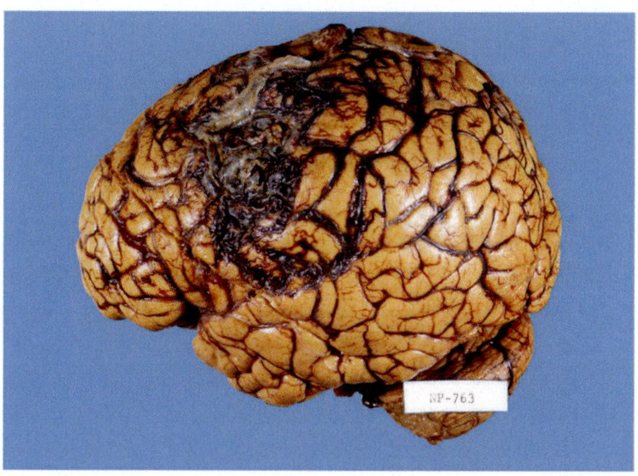

Figure 3.25 This left lateral view of the brain illustrates a large AVM involving the region of the Rolandic fissure. The malformation is typical in that large, dilated draining veins are visible along with thickened meninges.

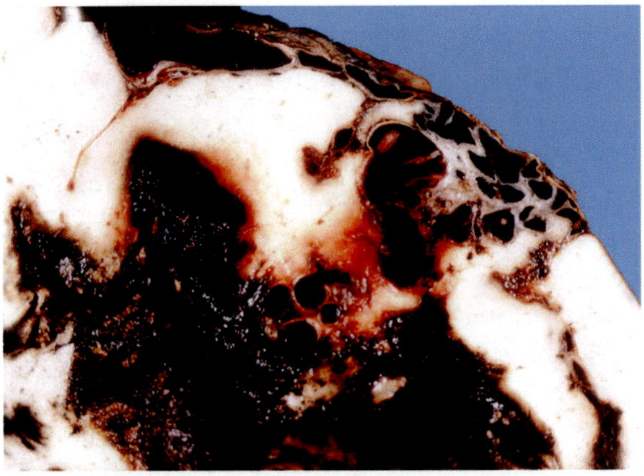

Figure 3.26 This macrophotograph of a portion of an AVM of the brain reveals dilated vascular channels (likely veins distended by exposure to shunted arterial blood) and in intracerebral hemorrhage caused by rupture of one or more vascular channels.

vessels that may push into the ventricular chambers, causing obstructive hydrocephalus, or possibly hydrocephalus on the basis of high venous pressure, and overproduction of CSF by the engorged choroid plexuses. In some cases, the A–V shunting in these and other AVMs is so great that heart failure may result [154]. Surgical treatment of vein of Galen malformations is nearly impossible unless the feeder arteries can be easily reached and ligated or endovascular technology employed [153].

Microscopically, the typical AVM shows vessels of all calibers and forms, both arteries and veins, although probably most of the vessels, even though they appear arterial, are veins; when higher than normal pressures occur in veins, they become arterialized; that is, they become thickened by deposition of collagen in their walls. The true nature of these vessels can be appreciated when elastic connective tissue stains are done and they fail to reveal elastica elements in the walls. Sometimes it may be rather difficult to identify arteries in larger malformations without careful sampling of the tissue. Thrombosis, mineralization, evidence of prior leakage of blood, and all sorts of blood pigments are found in the lesions. There is usually entrapped neural tissue, mostly showing reactive gliosis, between the dilated abnormal vessels [141,142].

The forensic significance of these lesions may lie in the production of symptoms such as epileptic seizures, headache, dizziness, and personality or behavioral changes that do not immediately suggest the diagnosis and may result in misinterpretation about the relationship between head trauma and rupture of the malformation with fatal result. There is no obvious consistent relationship between head trauma and leakage or rupture in most circumstances. Most reported cases of alleged traumatic injury to AVMs are poorly described or documented [163].

Infarction in the Central Nervous System

Cerebral infarction, the most common form of stroke, has many forms and causes, the most basic of which is deprivation of arterial circulation to a portion of the brain. Interruption—incremental, transient, or permanent—of the blood supply can occur as a result of ischemic injury in the affected brain. The most common mechanisms are the following: thrombotic occlusion, *in situ*, of an arterial branch or main vessel; embolic occlusion by thromboembolus, air embolus, fat embolus, atheromatous, or other embolic material; direct occlusion of an artery by an atherosclerotic plaque, an inflammatory or infectious process, external compression of the vessel, or vasospasm; venous obstruction; and hypoperfusion. Infarction, however, may occur in the presence of adequate blood flow, both venous and arterial, and in these circumstances, the cause is an inadequate concentration in the blood of glucose or oxygen, or both. Ultimately, the lack of either or both of these vital nutrients is the basis for all forms of infarction, whatever the original basis.

The most common preexisting lesion for an infarct is atherosclerosis, in which an atheromatous plaque presumably produces disruption in the pattern of laminar flow, leading to eddies, turbulence, and deposition of a thrombus in the vessel. Such lesions can certainly occur in the vessels of the circle of Willis but probably occur much more commonly in atheromas of the neck vessels, where they can obstruct the carotid or vertebral artery. Not all infarctive strokes occur in older individuals with atherosclerosis; they are also associated with younger people, even infants [164,165].

Thrombotic–Embolic Strokes

The cause for most infarctions is thrombotic or thromboembolic occlusion of an artery, although the precise proportion caused by one or the other is still debated. One school of thought espouses the point of view that only between 5% and 20% of all brain infarctions are caused by thromboemboli and that most of the remainder result from *in situ* thrombosis [56,57], whereas others [166–168] feel that half or more of all infarcts are due to thromboemboli. Probably part of the difficulty lies in the problem of defining each of the conditions and whether the definitions are clinical or pathological.

Clinically, distinctions have been drawn between thrombotic and embolic strokes and so-called TIAs. The thrombotic infarction may present in a rather vague manner and show evolution of neurological symptoms over several hours, days, or even weeks. The embolic infarct characteristically produces sudden, dramatic neurological deficits, whereas the TIA may produce minimal or very transient symptoms, most of which resolve over hours or days. The pathological basis for each of these forms of occlusive stroke is not always clear, but sometimes a well-developed thrombus can be found in the carotid artery, which shows layering and firm attachment to the arterial wall with histologic evidence of organization. In this circumstance it is often difficult to say that the evolution of symptoms was not due to shedding of small terminal emboli and that the final symptoms were not due to obstruction. In the case of a sudden-onset stroke, sometimes a source of emboli can be found in the neck or heart, and there is no evidence of organization in the obstructed vessel [60,66]. In the case of TIAs, lesions found at autopsy include thrombosis of a major vessel, a source of microemboli as in valvular vegetations, or ulcerated plaques in the vessels of the neck or the circle of Willis vessels associated with some degree of atheroma formation.

Perhaps it is best to acknowledge that precise classification may not be possible or even relevant, as has been voiced by Yates and Hutchinson [169], who wrote: "cerebral infarction has rarely a single cause and usually the result of a combination of systemic disease and stenosis of extracranial and intracranial arteries, or both (the extracranial arteries being more often associated with infarction than the intracranial)" and that a combination of thrombosis and embolization probably characterizes the typical major infarction. This analysis seems to reflect the experience of this neuropathologist.

Another challenging problem is the proper interpretation of brain infarcts in which no thrombus or embolus is demonstrated grossly in any of the vessels of the circle of Willis. This situation is often encountered in strokes in younger individuals where an explanation such as oral contraceptive use (see below) or some other cause is invoked. The fact is that infarctive strokes do occur in young people and even children [164]. The lack of a demonstrable embolus is analogous to the nagging problem of acute myocardial infarction and its cause, in the face of fewer than 25% of cases that have a thromboembolus in a coronary vessel demonstrable at autopsy [170,171]. In these circumstances the hypothesis is often invoked that vascular spasm is the mechanism of infarction. Such a mechanism is impossible to corroborate by morphological methods but also cannot be easily disproved. Nevertheless, some support for the rarity of this mechanism can be found in the results of very careful autopsy studies on stroke victims, which reveals that probably 90 to 95% of major brain infarctions show thrombi/emboli on careful microscopic examination [168–172]. Further corroboration can be found in several postmortem angiographic studies [173], which showed obstructions in more than half of brain infarction cases. Vasospasm of cerebral vessels can cause infarction, especially when there is SAH, and is a dreaded complication of aneurysm rupture [89].

Hypoxic/Ischemic Brain Lesions

Hypoxia refers to a less-than-optimal delivery of oxygen to an affected area. Ischemic damage refers to deprivation of circulation to a region and the damage to tissues and cells that results by two mechanisms: insufficient delivery of oxygen and glucose to the target tissue and lack of blood flow to remove metabolites from the target area. It has long been recognized that when an area of brain is perfused, even though the blood is hypoxic, damage is generally less than if there is blood flow stasis. Where tissue hypoxia and ischemia intersect, and depending upon the time and degree of deficits, the degree of neural damage will vary. As previously mentioned, there are regional differences of circulatory deprivation in the brain, and equal degrees of deprivation of circulation (and the oxygen it carries) will not result in identical pathological lesions. For example, in adults, gray matter, in general, and large neurons seem more vulnerable than small ones; white matter and glial cells are less vulnerable than neurons. It is a general principle that ischemic lesions are distinguishable from infarcts by gross and microscopic characteristics. An hypoxic/ischemic lesion does not generally result in the large-scale destruction of both gray and white matter seen in an infarct, in which there is breakdown of the structure of the tissue with liquefaction and eventual cyst formation. In an hypoxic/ischemic lesion, there will be death of neurons and a repair reaction in the glial cells of the affected region eventually, but the lesion may not be apparent from the external surface and might only be appreciated microscopically. Most acute hypoxic/ischemic lesions appear to affect the cortex only, and on cut section the cortex may appear congested or darker than normal and sometimes show pseudolaminar or laminar necrosis (Figure 3.27). When the process is more global, the basal ganglia in addition to the cerebral cortex may be affected (Figure 3.28). In the more chronic or older hypoxic/ischemic lesion, the affected region will have a characteristic shrunken or wilted appearance externally, often called ulegyria, as illustrated in Figure 3.29 [174]. When such a brain is sectioned, laminar necrosis will be very evident, represented by a tan or brown shrunken cortex and sometimes deeper damage as well. Physiologically, perhaps the distinction between the conditions that produce ischemic (partial) lesions and those that produce

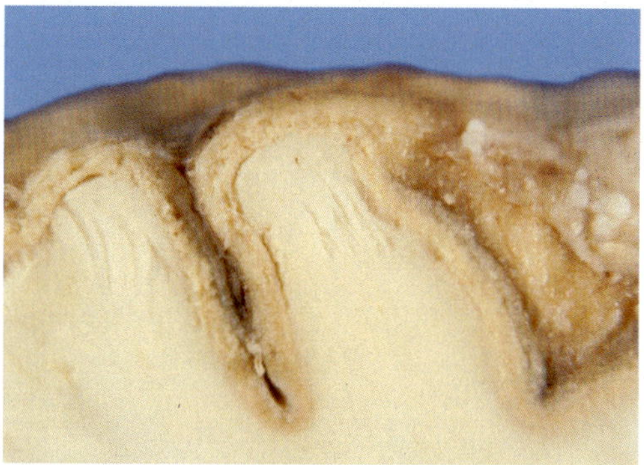

Figure 3.27 This macrophotograph of a portion of cerebral cortex shows laminar necrosis (separation of cortical ribbon from underlying white matter). This process can result from ischemia, hypoxia, and sometimes hypoglycemia or combinations of these. The "watershed" zone of the cerebrum will tend to show such lesions before other parts of the cortex do, but if the insult is global, and for a sufficient period of time, more widespread, cortical necrosis can occur. Laminar necrosis may take several days or longer after the insult to become this grossly evident.

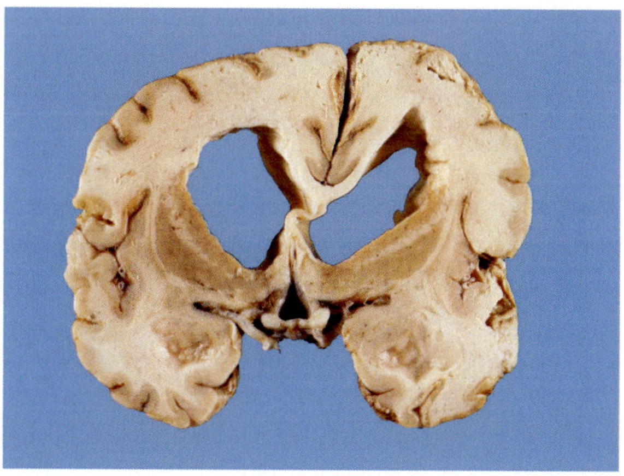

Figure 3.28 This coronal section of the brain shows many areas of cortical necrosis and ischemic necrosis of the basal ganglia that had been present for many months. Note the symmetrical enlargement of the lateral ventricles, which is a reflection of volumetic tissue loss (hydrocephalus *ex vacuo*).

infarctions involves the duration of absent or low blood flow, the status of arterial oxygen tension, the previous state of health of the region in question, the degree of local acidosis allowed to develop, the impact of other metabolites or substances released by injured cells, and probably many local hemodynamic factors. The level of blood glucose during a stroke may also influence its extent. This issue has recently been raised to explain the tendency for larger infarcts in diabetics [175]. Sometimes there may be a delay in development of an ischemic lesion for reasons that are unclear. This can have forensic significance in cases where attempted suicidal hanging or attempted homicidal strangling with resuscitation has occurred with apparent survival but later deterioration [176,177].

Microscopically, hypoxic/ischemic lesions show no gross cavitation, only loss of neurons, perhaps microcavitation, and extensive reactive fibrillary gliosis. Sometimes, the

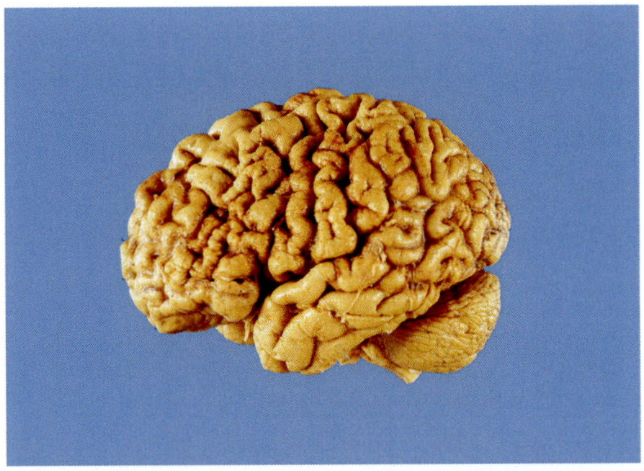

Figure 3.29 The photograph of the left hemisphere of the brain shows the wrinkled, atrophic appearance of ulegyria, the result of a global ischemic/hypoxic process. The appearance requires many months or longer of attempted tissue reactions and repair to produce this change.

laminar separation of the cortex seen in ischemic damage is obvious only microscopically and will also show loss of neurons, often the larger ones, with microcavitation and extensive gliosis and sponge-like appearance. The sequence of development of neuronal and glial changes is similar, if not identical, to that described below for an infarct.

A special form of regional ischemia, sometimes referred to as a watershed lesion, can result from severe main vessel cerebral atherosclerosis with or without atherosclerosis in the neck vessels or in other circumstances where global perfusion of the brain is insufficient. In this situation the end-vessel perfusion territories of the major vessels receive less than optimal blood flow, resulting in acute or chronic deprivation of these regions, with eventual death of neurons and sometimes the underlying white matter in affected areas. Ischemic watershed-type lesions can occur in the cerebrum, brain stem, and other CNS structures from a multitude of intrinsic and extrinsic processes, which can include the following: cardiac arrest where low cardiac output is associated with low general or regional cerebral blood flow (made worse by cerebral atherosclerosis); hypoglycemia/hypoxia with some disorder of perfusion; severe anemia or blood loss; mechanical obstruction of blood flow in the neck (strangulation, compression, injury); profound and sustained shock; and embolic states [178,179].

In the most common instance, when global perfusion of the brain is diminished because of cardiac output failure, or shock, only the territories nearest the major vessels may receive adequate perfusion, and the more remote end-vessel regions, often referred to as boundary zones (*die letzte Wiese*—"the last meadow"), may receive little or no blood flow. An analogy here might be the phenomenon of experiencing sudden loss of water pressure in an apartment building when someone uses a lot of water on a lower floor. Another cause of injury may be due to showers of tiny platelet emboli, perhaps caused by alterations in blood coagulability during ischemia or hypoxemia [179]. The watershed region for the cerebrum, illustrated in Figure 3.30, represents the junction of perfusion among the anterior cerebral artery field, the middle cerebral artery field, and the posterior cerebral artery field. When perfusion is diminished for only a short period of time, the damage may be slight and virtually undetectable grossly, may eventually show cortical shrinkage or ulegyria, or may be so severe that a frank infarction, anemia or hemorrhagic, may be seen.

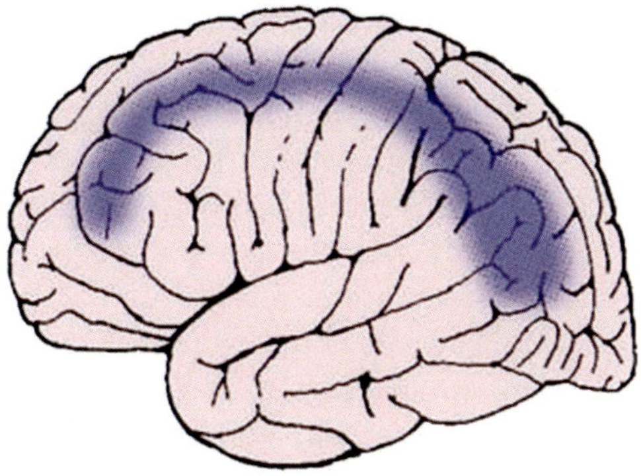

Figure 3.30 This diagram illustrates the crescent shaped cerebral "watershed" zone, which represents the end vessel perfusion territories of the anterior, middle, and posterior cerebral arteries that is vulnerable when global ischemia/hypoxia occurs with variable preservation of cortex that had better vascular perfusion.

The more severe changes of watershed ischemia occur in the depths of the sulci and the subjacent white matter rather than at the gyral surface, because these regions are perfused by arteriolar terminations rather than larger branches. Whether any given individual will suffer a watershed infarction is highly variable, dependent upon circle of Willis anatomy, the degree of collateral circulation to the brain, and probably a host of other factors.

Another important lesion, which is a part of a broader issue that involves the uneven and unequal vulnerability of neurons to hypoxic/ischemic insult, is the classic Ammon's horn lesion in the hippocampus of the medial temporal lobe that occurs with hypoxia/ischemia. The structure of the hippocampus has been studied for more than 100 years and has been recognized as a unique and important part of the brain [180]. Illustrated in Figure 3.31, the hippocampal formation is composed of V-like fascia dentata and various areas whose morphology is distinct, labeled CA1 to CA4 (CA = *Cornu ammonis*). The area most typically, but not universally, affected in global hypoxia/ischemia is the CA1

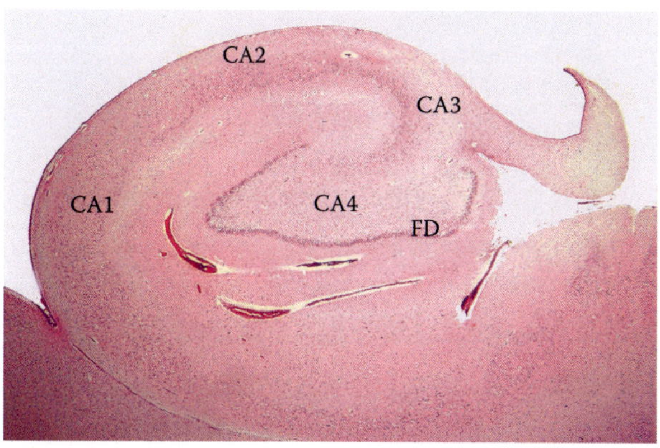

Figure 3.31 This macrophotomicrograph of the hippocampus illustrates the various anatomic areas, CA-1-4, and the fascia dentate (FD). The CA1 (Sommers' sector) section is the most vulnerable to global hypoxia/ischemia.

region, in which usually an obvious transition between viable neurons and pale, red, or absent neurons is evident. If the neurons have been absorbed, there is almost a laminar form of necrosis and microcavitation evident in CA1. Other areas of the hippocampus can be affected but appear more resistant than the CA1 portion. This local vulnerability to hypoxia/ischemia has been referred to as selective vulnerability [181], a phenomenon that has been studied exhaustively. This phenomenon, as indicated above, deals with the nonuniform vulnerability of populations of the neurons to a global and presumably equal insult. The most vulnerable populations are the CA1 section of the hippocampus, Purkinje cells, larger cortical neurons, and neurons of the basal ganglia. The thalamic neurons and motor neurons in the spinal cord are much more resistant to hypoxia/ischemia. The reasons for this variable vulnerability are not fully understood [69,181–183].

The Anemic (Pale) Infarction

When circulation to a portion of the brain is completely removed or exists at a level below a critical threshold, caused by one or more of the above processes, the process of infarction proceeds (see Figure 3.32). In the case of a so-called anemic infarct, once the obstruction to blood flow has occurred, little or no circulation ever reestablishes itself in the damaged region despite lysis or removal of the obstruction. This process, the no-reflow phenomenon [184], apparently occurs because the capillary bed has been damaged to such a degree that impedance to flow exceeds perfusion pressure such that passage of blood, regardless of the pressure, is not possible.

Most brain infarctions are of the anemic type and occur in all locations, although those territories that receive the bulk of the cerebral blood flow are the most likely to suffer infarctions. The middle cerebral artery territory in any or all of its branches is the most commonly affected. Most clinically significant cerebral infarcts affect large territories in which both the cerebral cortex and underlying white matter are often affected to some

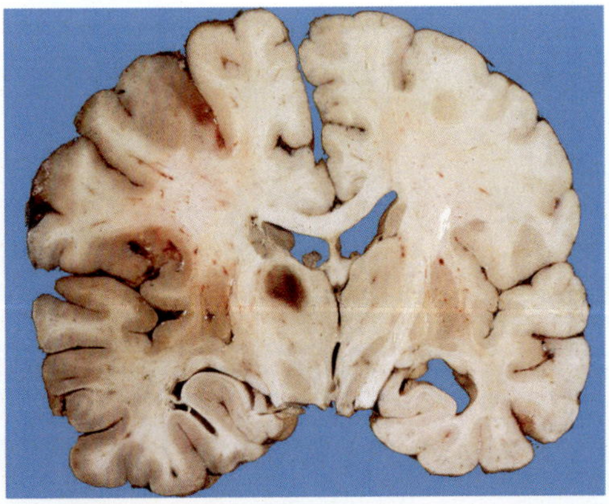

Figure 3.32 This coronal section of left middle cerebral arterial territory infarction in its early stages (about 24 hours) illustrates that the superior frontal convolution and cingulated gyrus appear spared (anterior cerebral arterial territory). The most medial temporal lobe structures appear less affected also. In the thalamus is a focal hemorrhagic area of the infarction probably due to fact of a embolic event that attended the middle cerebral arterial occlusion. There is some shift of the midline structures to the right from cerebral edema.

depth. The pattern of any infarction depends on several factors, which include the distribution of atherosclerotic plaques within the vessel and its branches; the patterns of blood flow, which are determined by collateralization with other circle of Willis vessels; and whether the main arterial supply to the circle of Willis by carotid and vertebral vessels is fully functional. In less than 50% of the normal population is a completely symmetrical circle of Willis found, and probably 40% of the population has a major asymmetry [185]. In many individuals there is functional separation of the anterior from the posterior circle of Willis circulation because of anatomical variants in which there is elimination or only minimal representation of posterior communicating arteries. Furthermore, absence of one vertebral artery is quite common, which places an added responsibility on the remaining vessel(s). Lack of adequate anterior communicating artery anastomosis is less common but may also serve to isolate a segment of the circle of Willis to one main perfusing vessel. Thus, should anything happen to a critical vessel in the face of some anatomical variation of the circle of Willis, the territory of an infarct may be far greater than what would appear obvious for an occlusion of a single internal carotid or vertebral artery.

When infarctions occur in the brain stem, owing to obstruction of a single vessel, a variety of neurological syndromes may be produced that often bear the names of those who described them, e.g., Wallenberg's syndrome and Brown-Sequard syndrome. The anatomical and clinical features of each of these syndromes, well known to clinical neurologists, can be found in most neuroanatomy and clinical texts [186–188].

Infarctions may also occur in the spinal cord, but the patterns of infarction are highly variable owing to the complexity of the spinal cord vascular supply and its anatomic variability [58]. Infarctions of the cord may occur when there is interruption of blood supply in the aorta and subclavian arteries, vertebrals, intercostals, radicular arteries, or intrinsic vessels of the cord, such as the anterior spinal and posterior spinal arteries. The massive involvement of the aorta in atherosclerosis would seem to be a logical cause of spinal cord infarction, but, in fact, such is rarely the case [189,190]. The most common aortic disease responsible for infarction of the cord is dissecting aneurysm, which may compromise intercostal or lumbar arteries that feed the cord [191,192]. Occasionally, thoracic trauma may also result in spinal cord infarction by aortic dissection, and neck trauma (perhaps including chiropractic manipulation) [193] may also compromise the vertebral artery supply to the cervical cord, resulting in infarction [189]. Likewise, surgical resection and grafting for aortic aneurysm [43] may occasionally result in secondary infarction of the cord, as can portocaval shunt procedures for relief of portal hypertension in cirrhosis.

Therapeutic misadventures most commonly in connection with spinal epidural steroid injections penetrate the dura or become injected intravascularly with catastrophic results and inevitable litigation [194,195]. Many physiatrists, anesthesiologists, and others who perform epidural steroid or analgesic injections recommend doing so under fluoroscopic visualization and often employ a small instillation of contrast material to check positioning before injecting the steroids or analgesics. Cord infarctions can occur also with spinal angiography [196,197] and have been reported with cocaine use [198] and illicit use of amphetamines [199,200]. Occasionally, attempted and poorly performed cervical and supposedly lumbar punctures will result in penetration of the cord or lower brain stem. Often the consequences are limited, but sometimes severe deficits may result. Although the basic pathology is not infarction but, rather, inhibition of axonal transport and neural toxicity [201,202], ill-advised intrathecal injection of mitotic spindle inhibitors or the vinca-periwinkle plant (vinblastine and vincristine) [203] and of cholchicine [204] has resulted in near-total necrosis and atrophy of the cord and portions of the brain stem [205]. These drugs should never be administered by this route.

The clinical manifestations of spinal cord infarction usually are a transverse myelopathy syndrome and paralysis below the level affected, but lesser and partial lesions may occur. Pathologically, the reactions in the cord are little different from those in the brain, except that descending (corticospinal) and ascending (dorsal column) myelin degeneration of tracts may be seen, giving a clue to the level of the lesion. In the unfortunate circumstance when the spinal cord has not been taken at autopsy but in retrospect should have been examined, a clue to these conditions may sometimes be discovered in the stump of the high cervical cord. Here demyelination in the more medial portions of the dorsal columns reliably denotes damage to the cord caudally.

Pathological Changes

The sequence of events that transpires after occlusion of a cerebral vessel in which little or no reflow [184] of blood occurs and in which there is little or no hemorrhagic component to the infarction, results in liquefaction of the affected segment with a macrophage response like any infarct in the brain. In much the same manner as the evolution of the infarct in the heart, the brain shows a similar temporal progression; that is, once the obstruction of blood flow causing the infarct is established, time is required for the pathological changes to evolve revealing its existence. Generally, a period of about 8 hours or longer of survival is required before the classic infarct is detectable grossly. The basis of detection is not always visual. In the fresh specimen, the affected area in an acute infarct may appear congested, darker in color than surrounding brain externally and on cut section and also softer and more fragile than unaffected tissue. The preferred method of examination is in the fixed specimen, which may show the infarcted area to have slight darkening of color (Figure 3.32) but more characteristically reveals a softer texture to the touch than does normal brain. This underscores the necessity in gross neuropathological examination to be cognizant of the tactile feeling of a specimen and the way it cuts.

Microscopically, the very acute infarct may be difficult to identify; the most important early feature of its boundaries is the tendency toward eosinophilia in the larger neurons [69,167]. This change, which is generally regarded to occur about 6 or more hours after an infarct, ischemic, or hypoxic episode, has been classically referred to as Spielmeyer's ischemic cell change or, more popularly and simply, red neurons. It is not known with accuracy how early red neurons can occur and what factors other than ischemia or hypoxia may influence the development of the eosinophilia. Basically, the change involves an early evanescent phase, perhaps akin to cloudy swelling in systemic pathology, which rapidly and progressively (by hematoxylin and eosin [H&E] staining) leads to reddening of the cytoplasm, darkening and blurring of the cell nucleus, and a gradual shrinkage of the cell with loss of its rounded contours, as illustrated in Figure 3.33. Such a cell, even though it may exist in the red state for many days and possibly even weeks, is moribund or lifeless, with no possibility for recovery.

In some circumstances, it appears that red neurons can evolve in as little as an hour or two and possibly slightly less. These circumstances seem to involve very acute ischemic episodes in previously healthy individuals, as in a suicidal or accidental (e.g., autoerotic) hanging with prompt rescue and attempted but failed resuscitation, acute cardiac arrest with attempted resuscitation and then death within a known short interval, anesthetic

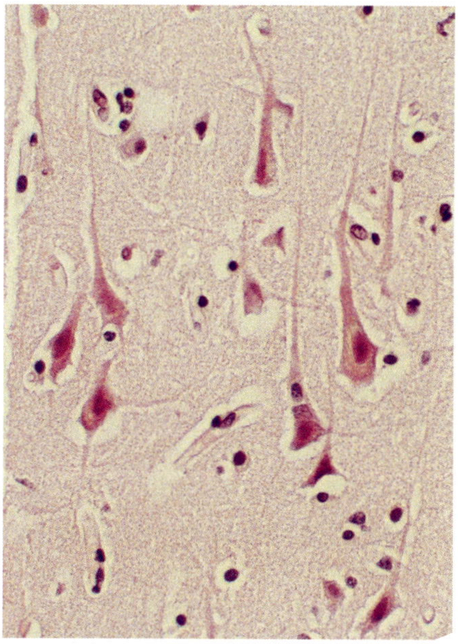

Figure 3.33 This photomicrograph illustrates the appearance of "red" neurons in H&E-stained paraffin section. Note the obvious eosinophilic cytoplasm, which should normally be basophilic. The nuclei are also eosinophilic and shrunken with obscured features. Such "red" neurons are indicative of hypoxic/ischemic and sometimes other vital cellular insults and connote a dead and functionless neuron, which will over a number of days, if vital signs persist, dissolve and disappear or sometimes become mineralized (ferruginated) and persist for years.

accidents, and other acute events. Similar early red changes can be seen in experimental animals subjected to middle cerebral artery ligations [69]. The basis for this unusually fast development may have something to do with the tendency for normal brains to autolyze more rapidly than chronically ill brains, a phenomenon described in several papers by Lindenberg [182,183,206,207]. In cerebellar Purkinje cells (Figure 3.34), it appears that the

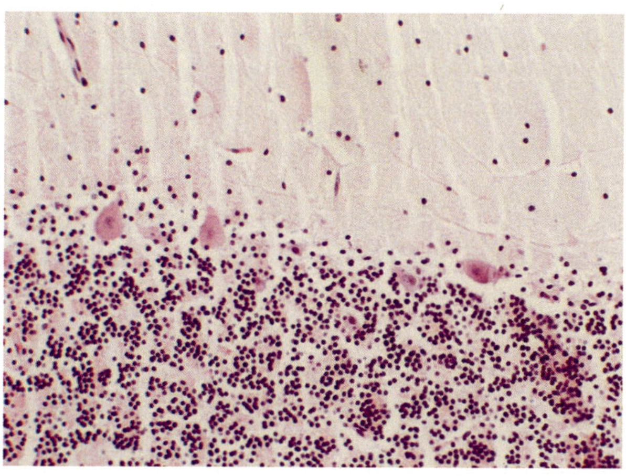

Figure 3.34 This photomicrogaph of the cerebellar cortex illustrates the same "red" neuronal change in Purkinje cells with preservation of the granule cell layer.

development of red neurons occurs more rapidly than elsewhere, especially in perinatal hypoxia, where the phase may be so evanescent as to escape detection, the neurons appearing to dissolve and disappear without passing through this phase. There is forensic importance to red neurons because their presence, concentration, and distribution may provide potentially valuable aging and dating information to the pathologist; however, a systematic study of this phenomenon in man has apparently not been undertaken, and thus conclusions should be made cautiously [208].

The period during which the red neurons may persist in the brain is unknown, but it appears that in some cases, as mentioned above, they may persist for weeks after the ictus or disappear rather rapidly, even in a few days. In some circumstances red neurons may remain *in situ* for even longer periods and attract minerals, eventually becoming encrusted with calcium and iron to form ferruginated neurons that may remain in place for years [209]. The mechanism by which this occurs is unclear but may involve the failure of outward-directed calcium pump function before cell death, with development of a nidus that eventually becomes completely mineralized. How iron enters into this process is not known.

By about 12 hours after interruption of the blood supply, in addition to congestion, swelling of the infarct may be evident grossly. This swelling continues to become more and more evident until 2 to 3 days have passed and then may gradually diminish over the next several days. Microscopically, at 12 to 24 hours, there may be some pallor by H&E staining of the infarcted area, compared to nearby normal tissue, even though all cellular elements are still present and may appear deceptively normal [69]. There may be the subtle appearance of small vacuoles in the neuropil, and there may be more vacuolation at the junction of infarct with normal tissues. The zone of pallor extends into the white matter in a rather irregular outline to the limits of the normal perfusion zone of the affected vessel. Occasionally, there may be a transient influx of polymorphonuclear leukocytes into the transitional zone by about 24 hours, but this is never as obvious as the acute inflammatory infiltration in a myocardial infarction.

By 3 to 4 days after infarction, the gross appearance of the infarcted area is more obvious and is generally easily delimited from normal brain. A dusky, gray-brown color is evident, and injection of small pial capillaries is typical. Microscopically, the previously described changes are more and more evident, with altered staining and the appearance of increased "preparation artifacts" (pericellular vacuolation, bubbling, and vacuolation of the neuropil, exaggerated perivascular spaces, cracks and rips in the tissue, as well as irregular and spotty staining). Numerous red neurons are seen, and some may be fading from view. Careful examination by H&E will reveal axonal degeneration and swelling. These changes are more easily seen with Bodian and other axon stains. It becomes obvious that cellular activity is occurring about capillaries in the form of round cell activity and macrophage activation, and capillary proliferation becomes more prominent (Figure 3.35) [69].

By about 7 days after infarction, degeneration of the area is obvious and the affected area is clearly soft and easily fragmented before or after fixation. The process of liquefaction is evolving. On the cut section (Figure 3.36), there is a crumbly or mushy appearance of the tissue, which continues to develop to a maximal state over the next week, when the infarct clearly breaks away from unaffected tissue. Microscopically, between days 7 and 14, the macrophage response is maximal. This is evident by the appearance of rounded phagocytic cells that become engorged with foamy material, which is strongly stained by Oil

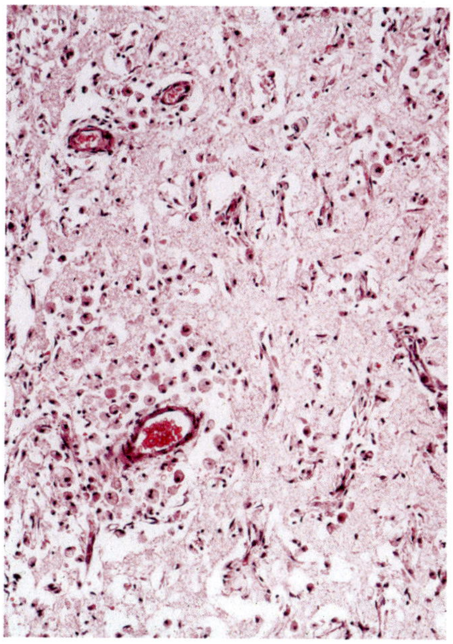

Figure 3.35 This photomicrograph illustrates a cerebral infarction of 7 days duration. Vessels have become prominent and capillary proliferation is evident as is the collection of macrophages about vessels and looseness and vacuolation of the neuropil. Virtually no neurons are visible in the field. Some astrocytes are beginning to swell, but little proliferation is noted.

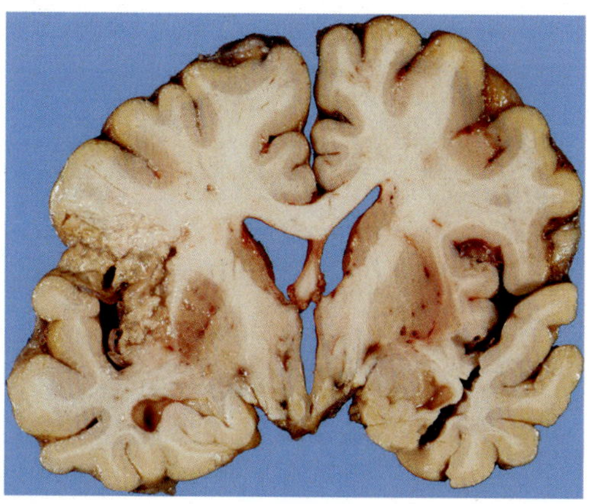

Figure 3.36 This is a gross photograph of a left middle cerebral artery infarction that is 7–10 days old. Note the crumbly/mushy appearance of the affected insular region. In time this area would have become multicystic.

Red O and other sudanophilic fat stains. These are the scavenger cells, sometimes referred to as gitter cells (from the German *Gitterzellen*) [210]. PAS and Luxol Fast Blue staining of macrophages are also obvious at this point (they contain polysaccharide moieties and phospholipid products of myelin degradation). Macrophages may cluster about capillaries, which are very prominent at this phase, as they migrate in and out of the vessels. In the body of the infarct, only the shadows of neurons and other cells are visible, and the picture is one of coagulative and liquefactive necrosis. By about 2 weeks after infarction, capillary proliferation and hypertrophy are obvious, and some early reactions in astroglia appear primarily in the boundary of the infarct. The change in the astroglia is usually one of swelling. Fibrillary hypertrophy does not become evident until about 2 weeks after infarction, and then only in the border zones of the infarct. Fibrillary gliosis then continues to develop over many months, if not years. One can usually also see axonal balloons (retraction bulbs) in the border zones of the infarct, which represent transected axons of passage that were interrupted and in which axoplasmic transport may have continued for a while. These balloons, which will eventually disappear, are eosinophilic and contain granular material. Although they can be stained immunohistochemically for B-APP, this reaction does not imply a particular pathogenesis other than some disturbance of axonal transport during the production of the lesion [211,212].

The process of liquefaction is maximal during the 2- to 3-week postinfarct period, after which, as more and more of the necrotic material is removed, the infarct becomes grossly more and more sponge-like and gradually takes on a cohesiveness and substance that resists fragmentation. At the margin of the resolving infarct, the macrophage response is still active and glial hypertrophy is more and more evident, as is the frequent influx of lymphoid cells that may cuff nearby penetrating vessels [210]. Fibroblastic responses are rare in contrast to the repair reaction seen in the heart or other visceral organs at this stage.

About 2 months seem to be required to remove the necrotic debris in a cubic centimeter of brain in most cases, but the process trails on for many months in a manner only detectable microscopically. In fact, even in infarctions many months or even years old, macrophages can usually be found, and some evidence of a continuing process of reaction and repair may be seen. In the healed infarct, the gross appearance is one of a filmy, sponge-like, sometimes sunken area (Figures 3.37 and 3.38). Well-circumscribed, cystic spaces are rarely seen and, when present, usually indicate that a major hemorrhagic component or frank hematoma had been present. The infarct is usually tan or brown owing to residual hemosiderin contained in macrophages, which once was the blood trapped in damaged vessels at the time of the original infarct or leaked into the neuropil in the first few days. The territory of the infarct can usually be defined rather easily in the fixed specimen at this phase.

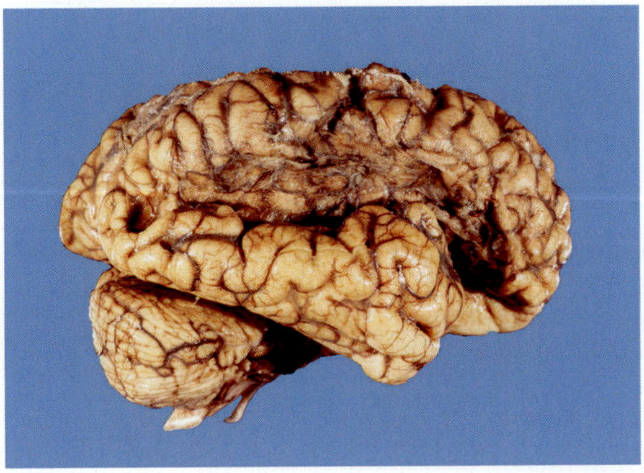

Figure 3.37 This gross photograph of the right side of the brain illustrates an old cavitary middle cerebral arterial infarction. This man lived about 20 years after his infarction and was able to work despite a left hemiplegia that was surprisingly mild considering the size of this infarct.

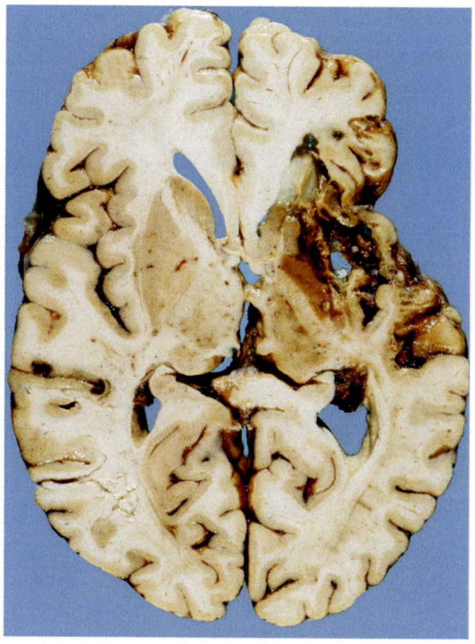

Figure 3.38 This tangential section of the brain illustrates large old right middle cerebral arterial infarction. Note that there is no single cavity, rather a sponge-work left behind, stained brown and yellow from the persistent hemosiderin-laden macrophages that remain years after this infarct occurred.

Microscopically, the old infarct mirrors the gross appearance, being composed of a sponge-like network of capillaries, thin fibrous cords, thin ropes of astroglial fibers, residual inflammatory cells and macrophages, and clear spaces (filled with low-protein-content fluid removed during preparation). At the margin, the astroglial proliferation is clearly evident, and sometimes Rosenthal fibers are present [213]. Mineralization is not very common, and fibrosis is very rare except in the walls of some sclerotic vessels in the border zone. Beyond the final stages of repair, aging and dating of infarcts from the gross microscopic specimen become very difficult and unreliable. One can attempt to estimate the volume of the infarct and then divide this volume (in cubic centimeters) by 2 (months) to yield its age, provided some macrophage response is still evident. Historical information provides a much better clue, however.

Reperfusion Injury

In the course of thrombotic and/or embolic strokes, perfusion may be disturbed but then restored naturally or after anticoagulant therapy. Another important scenario is the individual who suffers a cardiorespiratory arrest with a variably long interval between loss of circulation to the brain and then restoration by CPR and then perhaps normal sinus rhythm. The same situation arises when extracorporeal membrane oxygenation (ECMO) or similar technologies are used in open cardiac surgery [214]. The consequence of such reperfusions is a cascade of events that may produce focal perivascular infarctions, which are often hemorrhagic and may lead to multifocal lesions resembling traumatic contusions and/or SAHs [214]. The process first involves primary endothelial injury [214–216] with attendant blood–brain barrier damage, instigation of release and activation of free radicals and inflammatory mediators via cyclo-oxygenase pathways that act upon polyunsaturated fatty acids and other substrates [217]. All of these substances (leukotrienes, cytokines, nitric oxide, and others) are vasoactive and set into motion a chain of reactions that may expand the basic lesion extensively [218–220]. Leading, as mentioned above, to perivascular hemorrhage, edema, and damage to nearby neuropil, which may perpetuate the process after it is injured also. The process may lead to loss of vascular autoregulation function and the so-called no-reflow phenomenon [221].

The temporal sequence of events has mostly been studied in small animals and the critical time intervals of lack of brain perfusion with reperfusion for man are not well established nor are collateral events [222,223]. The forensic importance of reperfusion arises when an individual, perhaps a victim of an assault or other potentially criminal act, is found pulseless and not breathing with no precise notion of how long the victim was in this state or the time conditions that preceded it. Even though the victim appears clinically dead, the police or other responders often proceed with CPR that may include chest compressions. Often these efforts continue for many minutes or longer until resuscitation efforts are abandoned. During this interval of attempts at restoring circulation and ventilation the brain and other organs receive at least putative circulation with presumably oxygenated blood. This period of reperfusion may lead to pathological changes in the brain and other organs that might be misinterpreted at autopsy as representing premortem injuries when in fact they are actually intramortem or postmortem processes.

The following are examples of these scenarios:

A young woman is assaulted by a former boyfriend in her apartment. The attack apparently occurred about midnight. She is discovered by her roommates about 2:00 am lying face down in her bed apparently lifeless. CPR is administered first by the persons at the scene and later by EMT personnel who intubate the victim and continue chest compressions for at least 30 minutes before abandoning their efforts. The victim has clearly suffered trauma to her face but at autopsy apart from soft tissue injuries no skull fracture, subarachnoid or subdural hemorrhage is found. There were scattered small petechial intracortical hemorrhages in many areas of the brain that were interpreted as diffuse traumatic brain injury. Investigation revealed that the victim had been drinking heavily for some hours when last seen, and had a history of taking prescribed amphetamines. It appeared that the victim had lain face down on a pillow after the assault in bed which was stained with blood, secretions and possibly vomitus before being found. The main forensic issue in this case was not that she had suffered a beating, but precisely how she died: a direct consequence of her beating from brain injury; or suffocation contributed to by the beating, alcohol intoxication, possibly drug effects, and artifactual injuries to her brain caused by reperfusion of an essentially dead of dying brain by CPR.

Another case example which is not uncommon involves the discovery of an infant in its crib cyanotic and not breathing. It is usually not known for what duration the infant was in this moribund condition. CPR is instituted by caregivers and later EMT personnel with or without any significant return of vital functions. Resuscitative efforts may have continued for more than 30 minutes before being abandoned. The child may or may not reach hospital where efforts are continued. At autopsy the child may have bruises about the face, scalp, chest and extremities. Vascular access sites are often multiple. There may be bruises to the lips and tears in the frenula. There are usually no significant subgaleal hemorrhages unless IV access had been attempted using scalp veins. There may a thin subdural hemorrhage. There may be "contusions" reported in the cerebral cortex that are interpreted as being of traumatic origin. There may be rib fractures, and retinal hemorrhages. It is not uncommon for such a case to be called a death due to child abuse (often due to alleged shaking) when in fact the case actually represents SIDS (or "missed" SIDS) in which most if not all of the pathologies found represent effects of resuscitation of a dead child and may involve reperfusion injuries.

The Hemorrhagic "Red" Infarct

An alternative process to the anemic or bland infarction is hemorrhagic or red infarction, in which the territory of the infarct is hemorrhagic (Figure 3.39). This can be produced by obstruction of a draining vein, or it may follow intermittent ischemia or loss of blood flow that occurs with later reperfusion of the damaged vascular territory but before the processes responsible for no-reflow [184] have fully developed. Thus, hemorrhagic infarction can occur only during a window in time [224,225]. The temporal dimensions of that window in humans are not precisely known; however, from clinical–pathological correlations it appears that some time within the first 30 minutes of profound ischemia or total lack of blood flow may represent the beginning of the window, and probably about 2 hours of ischemia represents the outlines of the end of the window, after which anemic infarction will result. This probably represents the so-called no-reflow phenomenon. Support for this concept can be found in experimental infarctions in animals and in human observations [184,225].

When the proper set of circumstances are present to produce a red infarction, leakage from small vessels occurs and blood spreads into the surrounding tissue. The process is usually limited to the cerebral cortex of the brain and may occur in association with embolic events, herniations, or compressions of vessels, as in the typically red infarct in the medial occipital lobe, which follows extensive uncal herniation (compression of branches of the posterior cerebral artery by the edge of the tentorium). In this latter circumstance, which in many ways illustrates the conditions that produce these lesions, blood flow may wax and wane as compression of the vessel varies with the excursions of intracranial

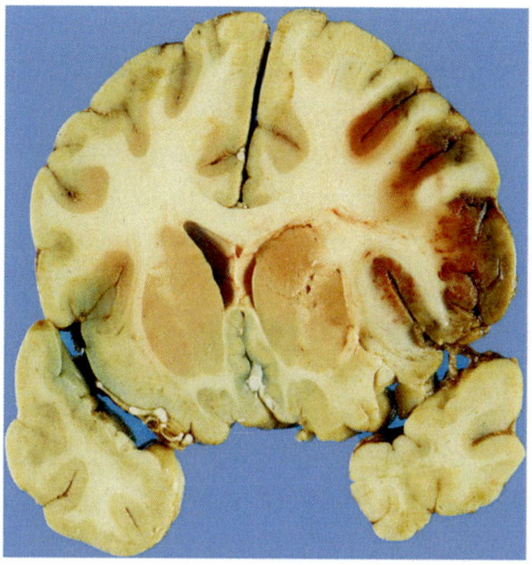

Figure 3.39 This coronal section of the brain illustrates a typical hemorrhagic infarction in the right lateral hemisphere. While they can involve deep gray matter as well as cortex, hemorrhagic infarctions typically are mostly confined to the cortical ribbon. The etiology is intermittent obstruction of blood flow, often by an embolic process. As in this case, mass effect from edema is evident and represents the most immediate threat to life.

pressure. This repeated ischemia during a short period of time, which may be an important etiologic mechanism for this lesion, also occurs in watershed infarcts, which are usually totally hemorrhagic or have hemorrhagic portions [226]. The mechanism in force here is that peripheral collateral flow from a less affected major vascular territory may enter a deprived region normally perfused by another major vessel and produce a localized intracortical hemorrhage or microembolization [179].

The repair reaction for red infarction is similar to that for any infarct, except that hemosiderin-laden macrophages are more prominent, and when the lesion has aged, its gross appearance will be browner in color than the anemic infarction because hemosiderin tends to linger in old hemorrhagic lesions. Because the red infarct tends to involve mostly the cortex, it will appear depressed and shrunken. The subcortical white matter may be damaged in varying degrees and show reactive gliosis and occasionally microcystic cavitation. Even in nearly every anemic infarction, there will be some degree of perivascular hemorrhage in border zones of the infarct or if the vascular obstruction was intermittent or partial.

Venous Infarction

Infarction of brain may occur when venous outflow from a territory is obstructed by whatever means (compression, injury, thrombosis, etc.). Such an obstruction is only rarely distant, because there is much collateralization of venous drainage in the brain, even if a major outflow sinus or vein is physically compressed. Venous infarcts may occur with total sagittal sinus obstruction, straight sinus obstruction, vein of Galen obstruction, and sometimes obstruction of other major venous sinuses [227,228]. Venous infarctions can also occur in the spinal cord in association with vascular malformations [189]. On rare occasions cerebral venous outflow can be obstructed externally and produce a venous infarct. The author has encountered a possible example of this in a suicidal hanging in which the ligature about the neck probably slipped and apparently occluded venous outflow more than arterial inflow, resulting in bilateral venous infarction (great vein of Galen) of the pulvinar. Most commonly, however, occlusion occurs in connection with intrinsic occlusion of venous drainage by thrombosis produced by dehydration, malnutrition, high fever (especially in babies), right heart failure, bacterial meningitis, sinusitis–mastoiditis, leukemia, polycythemia, amniotic fluid embolism, increased intracranial pressure, and occasionally head trauma. Seen relatively infrequently in adults, most affected individuals are children younger than 1 year [227,229]. The venous channels most often obstructed by thrombosis, due to one of the above causes, are the superior sagittal sinus or lateral sinuses, with or without extension of the thrombosis into adjacent cortical veins. Sometimes cortical vein thrombosis will also produce a venous infarction, but curiously, cavernous sinus thrombosis will only rarely produce an infarction, no doubt because of collateral drainage.

The mechanism of venous infarction is stasis of blood under high pressure. Most venous infarcts are hemorrhagic, and in view of the origin of most commonly being the superior sagittal sinus, the infarcts tend to be paramedian (Figure 3.40) but may not necessarily be extensive. When the lateral sinuses are obstructed or the great vein of Galen occluded, infarctions tend to be posterior median and may involve the posterior median thalamus and pulvinar. Venous infarcts are especially dangerous because of the potential for severe edema and mass effects.

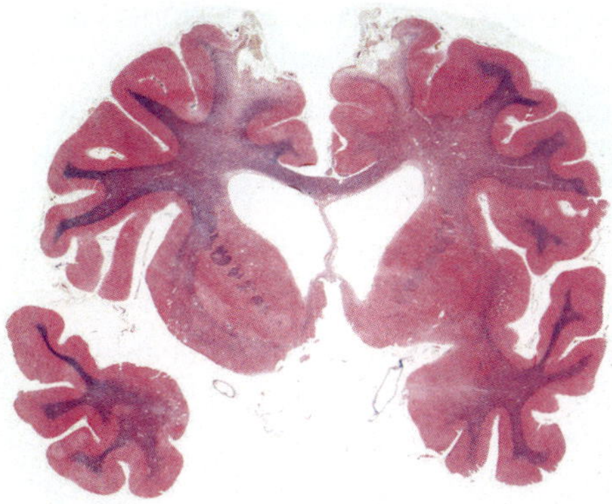

Figure 3.40 This large "window pane" paraffin section of a coronal section of the brain illustrates the superior paramedian effects of a superior sagittal sinus thrombosis and venous infarction. The degree of damage is highly variable ranging from sometimes a localized infarct to extensive hemorrhagic infarctions.

The Lacunar Infarct and Related Conditions

There are several forms of minor infarctions that may be associated with TIAs and hypertension and may evolve in a vague manner over years but produce a constellation of troublesome neurological syndromes, such as dementing illness, rigidity, and tremor reminiscent of Parkinson's disease, and choreaform and athetoid movements in an elderly individual [112,230]. These small infarctive lesions are commonly said to represent part of the spectrum of neuropathology caused by arterial hypertension [231,232] and generally occur in two locations: in deep gray masses such as the basal ganglia, thalamus, and basis pontis, and in the subcortical white matter (Figure 3.41). All of these lesions have a small arteriole at the center of a widened perivascular space, which is usually visible grossly as a small hole having a brownish discoloration. Usually small lacunar infarcts (lacunes) are multiple and involve the globus pallidus and putamen with greater regularity than the caudate nucleus, or portions of the thalamus or basis pontis, and have been referred to in the continental

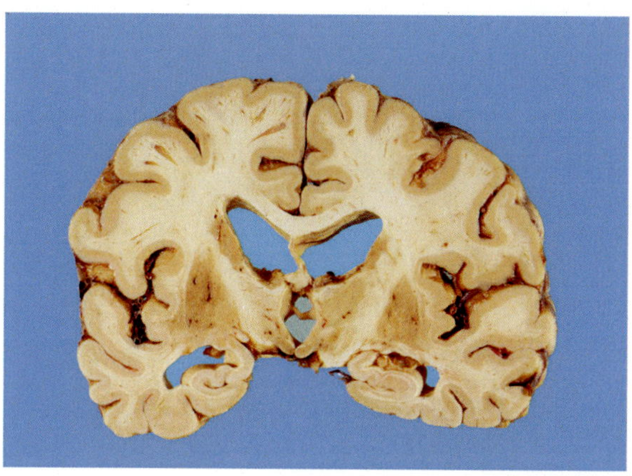

Figure 3.41 This coronal section of the brain illustrates both a number of lacunar infarcts in the basal ganglia (dark small cavities) and extensive subcortical lacunes sometimes referred to as *etat crible*. Such individuals may be demented due to extensive disconnection of axons from the cortex by the necrotic lesions.

literature as *etat lacunaire* (lacunar state). These lesions may become larger than a few millimeters or appear confluent and even cystic. Lacunes may abut on the internal capsule or exist in the basis pontis to produce transient or permanent hemiparesis and other symptoms. When widespread in the thalamus, as compared with other basal ganglionic structures, a dementing illness may result for reasons that have yet to be fully understood.

When lacunes occur in the subcortical location, a condition that is often ignored in most current works on neuropathology and clinical neurology, they produce a curious microcystic or fan-like pattern of small holes (Figure 3.41) referred to, again in the French literature, as *etat crible* (cribriform state). These lesions, also thought to be related to arterial hypertension, have the same basic structure as the classic basal ganglionic lacunes. Microscopically, both have a small arteriole as their center, about which the neuropil is pulled away to form an exaggerated perivascular space. The vessel at the center is sclerotic, or mineralized, and is surrounded by a few macrophages filled with hemosiderin and a few lymphocytes and often will be bounded by reactive astrocytes. Sometimes intact red blood cells will be found. The pathogenesis of the process is not known, but it appears that these small vessels are damaged by either the direct effect of hypertension or a failure in circulatory autoregulation, resulting in repeated stasis of blood flow, which injures the vessel so that plasma proteins exude or transude into the vessel wall, where they eventually become collagenized or mineralized [69,233]. Another etiology of microembolization takes place with fibrin/platelet thrombi (Figure 3.42) that produces the same perivacular lesion. The perivascular tissue is deprived of circulation and seems to pull away from the vessel, perhaps because of edema that at one time was present. Some element of bleeding undoubtedly occurs, as evidenced by the ubiquitous presence of siderophages in the lacunar space. If a section passes fortuitously longitudinally along one of these damaged vessels, which are often found to be tortuous or corkscrew-like and may show focal microaneurysm formation (Charcot-Bouchard microaneurysms), focal perivascular hemorrhages (bleeding globes), or various degrees of sclerosis [232]. Regardless of where they lie, subcortically or deep in the gray matter, lacunes usually show pallor of myelin about them. This may be especially prominent in subcortical locations in which rather profound demyelination may

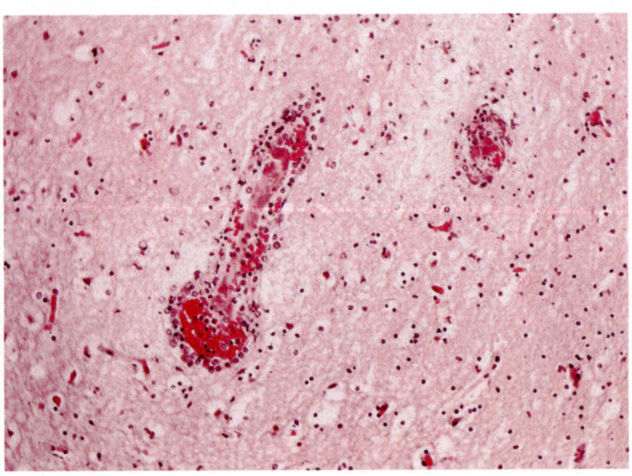

Figure 3.42 This photomicrograph illustrates a microvascular thrombus with perivascular edema, hemorrhage, and ischemic changes in the surrounding neuropil. This lesion can produce a "lacune" and may clinically be part of TIAs.

be seen. This finding forms the pathological basis for a syndrome described by Binswanger in which there is progressive subcortical myelin loss associated with dementia (Binswanger disease) [234,235]. In this case, the dementia probably results from massive disconnection by axonal damage of cortical association fibers caused in turn by ischemia, microinfarction, or damage by perivascular edema due to small-vessel disease. Why lacunes form in some but not all hypertensive patients is not known, but they seem especially prominent in the basal ganglia and basis pontis in the so-called calcified-dilated form of cerebral atherosclerosis. Experimental observations by Nag and associates [233,236] have provided some insight into the pathology of hypertensive disease on the brain.

Stroke and Oral Contraceptive Agents

With the widespread use of oral contraceptive agents (OCAs) in the mid-1960s and onward, many concerns were raised about the apparent occurrence of thromboembolic disease and stroke in patients using this form of medication. At the time, there was a great deal of controversy and litigation over the issue of whether OCAs were causal. Pathologists were drawn into this controversy by having performed autopsies on young women not normally expected to be felled by a stroke [237,238], whose attorneys claimed associations between the underlying pathology and the use of OCAs, or by having been called upon to render expert testimony in connection with litigation of the case. Because this has been an important issue, which in the minds of some is still not resolved, a review of the issue may be of value. Although venous thrombosis and embolism (usually pulmonary embolism) have been the major focus of attention with OCAs, this discussion will be limited to an alleged association between OCAs and cerebral thrombosis–embolism.

With the introduction of OCAs in Europe and other Western countries in the early 1960s and their immediate popularity, many physicians quite rightly wondered when the downside of this revolutionary approach to contraception would occur and what it would be. Some 7 years later, the first of a series of papers appeared that suggested a link between thromboembolic disease and OCAs. In the first account, Inman and Vessey [237], working in the United Kingdom, reported on the retrospective analysis of 385 married women aged 20 to 44 who died in 1966 in Great Britain. Selection of the cases was based upon death certificate data that indicated that some form of thromboembolic disease was involved (pulmonary, coronary, cerebral). Medication histories were obtained and a statistical correlation was performed that indicated that the use of OCAs in those women dying of pulmonary embolism was four times higher than in age-matched non-OCA users; in cases of cerebral thrombosis, the incidence of OCA use was about three times higher than that of controls; and no significant differences were observed in cases of coronary thrombosis. From these data, Inman and Vessey [237] concluded that there was a strong association between the use of OCAs and the death differences they observed. Several other retrospective studies [239,240] followed, with similar results and conclusions.

The conclusions of the several retrospective studies were challenged on the grounds of sampling bias, case collection methods, and the inherent problem of implying causality after examining statistical correlations [241–244]. The problem of implying causality from a superficial analysis, which at first glance may appear quite reasonable, can be illustrated humorously by an example [244] in which a reported 50% decrease in the number of storks in a portion of Germany occurred at the same time there was a reported decrease in the birth rate of the same amount. Goldzieher has pointed out the attractive, but fallacious, implication from these data—that storks brought babies, and that by analogy the interpretation of causality by OCAs of thromboembolic disease may be just as fallacious. This all-too-human propensity has been classically named the *post hoc ergo propter hoc* fallacy (that which preceded something is the cause of it).

In response to the above criticisms and to suggestions by many investigators, several prospective epidemiological studies were conducted, as were a number of population surveys regarding any changes in cause of death in women in the pre- and post-OCA era [245–247]. The population studies showed no increase in thromboembolic disease with the introduction of OCAs. Of the several prospective studies that were undertaken, many of which have been subsequently criticized on methodological or statistical grounds [243], probably the study most accepted by strong critics was published by Fuertes-de La Haba et al. [248]. This careful analysis was conducted in Puerto Rico on nearly 10,000 women and concluded that there was no correlation between use of OCAs and death due to pulmonary embolism, coronary thrombosis, or cerebral thrombosis in the absence of any predisposing medical condition. Despite the weight of carefully analyzed evidence that does not support a positive connection between OCA use and thromboembolic disease, many still did not accept this conclusion and alleged that there were specific vascular lesions produced by OCAs that could lead to thromboembolic events, including strokes [249,250]. The flaws in these papers include lack of reliable medical historical and medication data, small statistical sample size, lack of case randomization and blinding, potential investigator bias, and the overshadowing problem of statistical analysis of arbitrary factors that imply causality. It was clear that a careful pathological analysis of the possible effects of OCAs on systemic and cerebral vessels needed to be done to resolve the persistent controversy that surrounded this issue.

Eventually, from very carefully controlled studies, it emerged that stroke was likely not associated with OCAs only but that stroke was a risk outcome for those who smoked and used OCAs. It appears that a more likely linkage exists between solitary use of OCAs and venous thromboses, including sagittal sinus thrombosis, when there is smoking as well, though dissenting voices existed and still exist on these conclusions [251–254].

Cerebral Embolic States

There are many types of emboli (thromboemboli, fat and air emboli, bone marrow emboli, foreign body emboli, etc.), any of which may occlude a major artery or terminal arteriole, producing an ischemic or infarctive lesion in the brain. The variability of pathological change produced by the various emboli is considerable, and many of these conditions have important forensic implications.

Thromboembolism

The most common embolic event involving cerebral vessels is thromboembolism, the sequelae of which are discussed above. Such emboli may originate most commonly in extracranial vessels (carotids, aortic arch) or from within the heart in connection with atrial fibrillation, mural thrombus formation, and infectious or nonbacterial thrombotic endocarditis [255]. Occasionally, paradoxical thromboembolism may occur when an intraventricular or interatrial septal defect or patent foramen ovale is present [256,257]. Another condition, disseminated intravascular coagulation (DIC) [258–262] of whatever etiology, may involve cerebral vessels with myriad thromboemboli (Figure 3.43). The phenomenon of DIC is a complex one, and excellent reviews of the subject should be sought for a complete discussion [260–261]. DIC affecting the CNS [262] may be seen in any of the conditions that cause it but regularly appears in bacteremic shock, especially in infants, in connection with puerperal maternal deaths (presumably in connection with DIC caused by amniotic fluid embolism) [23], in mucin-secreting and other neoplasms [263], and in head trauma [264–266], where its presence is a contributor to a poor clinical outcome. The clinical appearance of DIC is that of diffuse encephalopathy with obtundation, sometimes with seizures, coma, and death.

Pathologically, the brain may be swollen, and petechiae may occasionally be seen on the cortical surface. The cut section may or may not show gross lesions, but when present, the cortex may appear injected or show petechiae or more confluent lesions, suggesting an embolic state or hemorrhagic infarction. The subcortical white matter often shows small hemorrhages, but streak hemorrhages, petechiae, or more extensive hemorrhages may be seen in the white matter and deep nuclear masses (Figure 3.36). Microscopically, the main lesion is perivascular hemorrhage of some degree or perivascular blanching and edema. An extensive search may be required to locate a fibrin–platelet thrombus in a small vessel (Figure 3.42), but this search is aided if the PTAH (phosphotonastic acid hematoxylin) or PAS stain is employed. In infants, histological examination of the choroid plexus is often rewarding in demonstrating the intravascular microthrombi. In cases that survive several weeks, the residual lesions resemble patchy demyelinating diseases with a moth-eaten white matter appearance, sometimes a diffuse cortical destructive process with multiple small gliotic lesions, or possibly old viral encephalitis. Clinical laboratory correlation or diagnosis of DIC may be unappreciated by noting only the common parameters of clotting ability, such as platelet counts, prothombin time (PT), and partial thromboplastin time (PTT), which may be only mildly abnormal. Probably the most reliable and sensitive measure of coagulopathy is evidence of consumption of fibrinogen and split products of fibrin degradation (D-dimer etc.) [266].

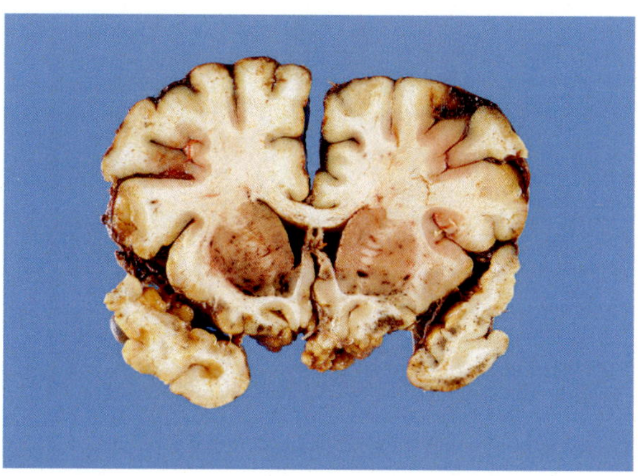

Figure 3.43 This coronal section of the brain of a victim of disseminated intravascular coagulation shows an irregular disseminated pattern of cortical and basal ganglia focal hemorrhages. Microscopically, these lesions often show fibrin/platelet thrombi in the small vessels.

Fat Embolism

Fat embolism is an enigmatic and complex problem that has been reported to follow significant traumatic injuries, especially fractures of the long bones, abdominal trauma, liposuction, blast injury, head injury, subarachniod hemorrhage, childbirth, and a host of other conditions [267–269]. Occasionally, only a minimal traumatic history is obtained. Sometimes evidence of alcoholism and severe fatty liver is found. Curiously, the fatty embolization usually does not occur immediately after the injury but, more commonly a few days to a week later, and, classically makes its appearance with respiratory distress, petechial skin hemorrhages, encephalopathy that can lead to profound clinical deterioration, and multiple organ failure [269]. The clinical syndromes associated with fat embolization are graded from a rather mild condition that involves petechial hemorrhages in the skin to a more generalized and serious situation in which skin petechiae are still present, but there is extensive embolization of the lung, kidney, and brain. Clinically, cerebral fat embolism presents as a diffuse encephalopathy showing agitation, fatigue, lethargy, occasional paralysis, cranial nerve paralysis, coma, and death [270,271]. Imaging studies, generally with MRI, will show multiple, rather diffuse white matter lesions with surrounding edema [271,272].

Grossly, the brain may be swollen and even show the changes of a respirator brain (see Chapter 5). There may be petechiae on the cortical surface, and the cut section usually shows a spectrum of cortical and white matter petechial hemorrhage and edema (Figure 3.44). Histological examination with standard methods may miss the acute fatty emboli, and usually frozen sections of fixed or fresh tissue with neutral fat staining (such as Oil Red O) will demonstrate fat globules in the vessels (Figure 3.45). After some days, it is likely that intravascular fat will have dissipated, leaving microvascular and perivascular pathology in the brain that may or may not be recognized for what it is [272–276].

The consequence of intravascular fat is obstruction of blood flow at the capillary level, with congestion and perivascular bleeding into the surrounding brain tissue. If recovery occurs, the sequelae may be global, with aphasias, dementia, depression, and a persistent obtundation. Fat embolization has even been suggested as an etiology for MS, although

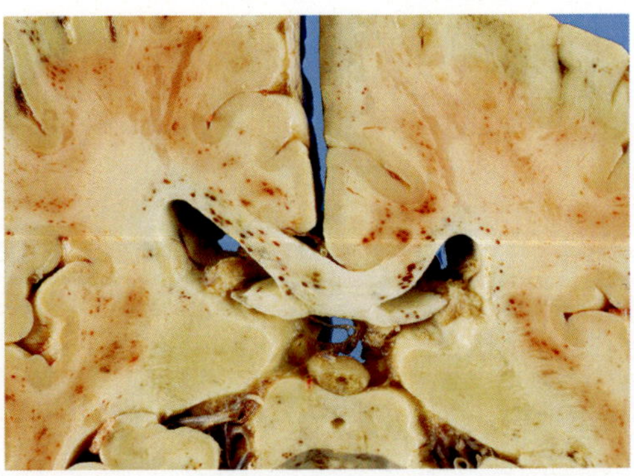

Figure 3.44 This portion of a coronal section from a brain of a victim of fat embolism due to extensive soft tissue and skeletal trauma illustrates numerous punctuate perivascular hemorrhages in the subcortical white matter, centrum semiovale, corpus callosum, and occasionally in the gray matter. Some areas of the white matter are becoming necrotic.

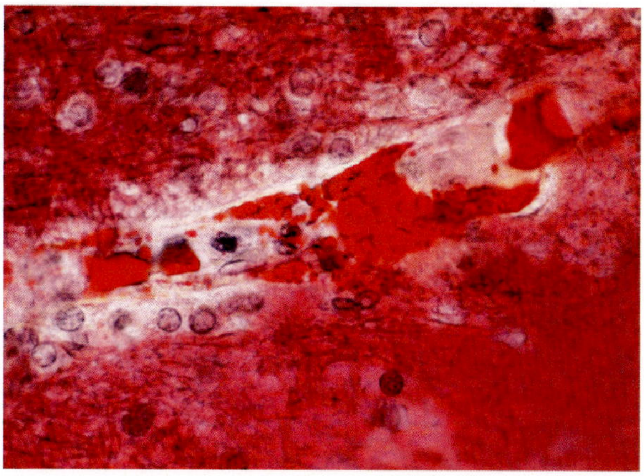

Figure 3.45 This photomicrograph of a portion of the brain from a case of fatal cerebral fat embolism stained with Oil Red O in frozen section illustrates the bright red lipid material within the lumen of a small capillary in the white matter. Paraffin-embedded material will not demonstrate intravascular fat owing to the solvents used in preparation of the blocks and the paraffin sections. Frozen (cryostat) sections are required.

this suggestion is not taken seriously by most workers. The exact pathophysiological basis for fat embolization is still being debated. The most obvious mechanism is physical transmission of fat globules into vessels at the site of injury. More intriguing possibilities include the direct intravascular precipitation of fat globules due to altered lipoproteins and chylomicrons, perhaps in response to stress (corticosteroids, catecholamines), and a host of other biochemical factors [277].

Air or Gas Embolism

Air or gas embolism involving the brain or spinal cord may occur in connection with neurosurgical procedures (burr holes, surgery in sitting position, placement of subdural or intracerebral cannulae or shunt tubes); barotrauma and diving accidents; thoracic, abdominal, pelvic, or rectal surgery; childbirth or abortions; radiographic procedures (arteriography, venography, barium enema, peritoneal or retroperitoneal gas contrast studies); stab wounds, chest trauma, and gunshot wounds; and many more unusual circumstances [278–281]. Cerebral embolism, regardless of the portal of entry of air or gas, results from transmission of the gas into the intracranial arterial blood supply via the heart, likely through a patent foramen ovale or other defect [282]. During a therapeutic procedure where the risk of air embolism is well known, the anesthesiologist usually carefully monitors by Doppler detection or direct auditory monitoring of the heart for the first sign of embolism [281]. Usually corrective action can be taken to withdraw aerated blood from the right atrium immediately, with little risk of significant damage. Only when significant amounts of air reach the left side of the heart will tissue damage result. The mechanism is basically microembolic in the brain, where collateral circulation will not have had time to occur [283]. The clinical signs of air embolism may be subtle, especially when under anesthesia. Cerebral symptoms include loss of consciousness, seizures, paralysis, paraplegia, paresthesias, and blindness. Demonstration of air embolism in the postmortem specimen may be challenging, and various methods have been suggested to detect it, including opening the chest cavity underwater and opening the heart underwater. Many forensic pathology texts suggest that the cranium should not be opened before the chest, to prevent accidental and factitious introduction of air when sawing the skull and opening the venous sinuses. When the brain is removed and care is taken to observe the cortical surface *in situ*, air bubbles may be directly visualized in the large cortical vessels. Recently, the use of postmortem advanced imaging techniques (so-called virtopsy) has addressed the radiological diagnosis of air or gas embolism [284]. Microscopically, there is usually no sign of damage, but in chronic cases there may be perivascular petechial hemorrhages and edema present. Areas of the brain that have been deprived of circulation because of the air embolism will show classic appearances of ischemic damage if time is allowed for them to develop.

Foreign Body and Other Unusual Emboli

A variety of foreign objects may become lodged in intracranial or neck vessels and may directly occlude the vessel or may form the nidus for a thrombus, which may secondarily embolize the brain and produce infarctive lesions. Examples of this include bullets or missile fragments lodged in the lung, heart, or other locations that enter venous or arterial vessels and perhaps via traumatic A–V shunts or right–left shunts in the heart find their way to the brain [285,286]. Occasionally, intra-arterial catheters or portions of them may produce intracranial embolization, as can fragments of endovascular catheters, glues, and fibers, and metallic coils as well [287–290]. It is not surprising that some of these unusual emboli will have forensic or, at the very least, medical–legal significance. Unusual forms of tissue embolization may also occur, usually in connection with trauma. Examples include brain embolization, usually to the lungs in newborns in connection with vigorous forceps delivery or head trauma [291,292], atheroma emboli (in association with endarterectomy or cardiac procedures), bone marrow embolization (rarely seen following cardiopulmonary resuscitation), bone embolization (following extensive fractures or surgical procedures), or tumor embolization from cardiac myxoma or other tumors. When emboli are radiodense, a variety of imaging technologies can be employed to locate and identify them [284].

Tumors of the Nervous System

Brain Tumors and the Forensic Pathologist

At first thought it might appear that brain tumors would have little impact on forensic medicine, but issues regarding brain tumors arise frequently enough in the forensic setting that a brief visit to the subject is justified. The forensic pathologist and neuropathologist may become involved separately or jointly in the following circumstances: brain tumor as a cause of sudden unexpected death; prior head trauma as an alleged etiology for a brain tumor, and litigation in connection with this contention; a tumor as the cause of irrational and violent behavior in which prosecution or defense attorneys have much interest in expert opinion; environmental exposure as an alleged or possible cause of brain tumor or the risk of brain tumor; brain tumors as precipitating causes of accidents, accidental death, or injury to another; and litigation involving misdiagnosis or lack of proper treatment of neoplasms of the brain. Because there are many reliable encyclopedic works on the neuropathology and biology of brain neoplasms, an in-depth discussion of the pathology of specific brain neoplasms will not be undertaken here. The reader is referred to the text of Burger, Scheithauer, and Vogel for general surgical neuropathology of brain neoplasms [293], to the excellent monograph of Schiffer [294], and, for WHO classifications, to Kleihues et al. [295], Louis et al. [296], and Nakazato [297]. For overviews of the clinical aspects of brain tumors and their treatment, the reader is directed to Berger et al. [298], Baehring and Piepmeier [299], and Greenberg et al. [300]. There are a number of more targeted books to which the reader is referred. These include monographs on glioblastoma [301], brain lymphoma [302], and germ cell tumors of the nervous system [303]. An excellent and encyclopedic work on meningioma by Kepes is still relevant [304].

With the declining rate of hospital autopsies, a greater burden is placed upon the forensic pathologist in the coroner's or medical examiner's service to generate a death certificate in cases that are probably due to natural causes but occur outside the care of a physician who can or will sign the death certificate. This unenviable position will inevitably bring the forensic pathologist into contact with unsuspected diseases, including brain tumors that escaped diagnosis or occurred under circumstances potentially affecting the public health, such as in cluster cases [305]. Brain tumors and sudden or unexpected death are not as uncommon as might be expected from reports on the rate of occurrence of various lesions in cases of sudden unexpected death [21–24], as shown by Huntington et al. [306], who analyzed 109 cases in which the fatality was due to a primary brain tumor in Kern County, California, between 1950 and 1962. Of these 109 cases, in 40 the diagnosis of brain tumor was made only after autopsy examination in a general hospital, where the clinical diagnoses ranged from stroke to subdural hemorrhage to suspected brain tumor. There were nineteen cases that were autopsied during the same period by the coroner. All these cases were undiagnosed prior to autopsy and died often after minimal head trauma, with behavioral abnormalities, in connection with possible workplace toxic exposure, or suddenly and unexpectedly with no clue as to the cause. The most common tumors (all primary brain tumors) found were gliomas (glioblastomas, astrocytomas, ependymomas, or oligodendrogliomas), but also included were medulloblastomas, hemangioblastoma, lipoma, and lymphoma. Similar figures have been reported by others [307].

Another primary tumor that has occasionally been reported to cause sudden death is colloid cyst of the third ventricle (Figure 3.46) [308–312]. Other sporadic reports involve even nerve sheath tumors as a part of von Recklinghausen disease [313]. Secondary tumors involving the brain are probably a more common problem in unexpected deaths because brain metastases are such a common accompaniment to carcinoma of the lung, which itself is so common. Because 20% or more of lung cancer cases present with brain metastases, it is inevitable that some of these will experience some neurological symptom that may cause an accident, or suffer trauma, which will cause hemorrhage into the tumor and only be discovered at the autopsy table.

The mechanisms by which a tumor, primary or secondary, may cause death, sudden or otherwise, involve death by accident or suicide or death by some sudden dramatic mass effect of the tumor [314]. Accidental fatal injury caused indirectly by a brain tumor can be illustrated by the following case that was autopsied at the Cook County Medical Examiner's Office.

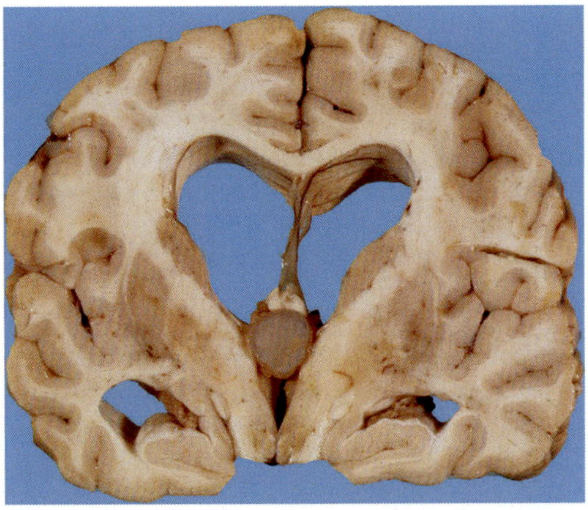

Figure 3.46 This coronal section of the brain illustrates a colloid cyst of the third ventricle. Typically the cyst is filled with mucoid material that coagulates upon fixation and is generally less than 15 mm in diameter, lying within the foramen of Munro. It is not unusual to find some degree of obstructive hydrocephalus in victims of this condition who may die suddenly and unexpectedly as was the case with this individual.

An 82-year-old white female was struck by a truck while crossing the street during the day. The driver reported that the victim stopped at a crosswalk, appeared to look both ways, then walked directly into the path of his truck, which could not stop in time to avoid hitting her. The woman died soon afterward in an emergency room, having suffered massive thoracic and skeletal trauma. Autopsy revealed a huge pituitary adenoma, which undoubtedly had produced, at the very least, bitemporal hemianopsia, so that victim was unable to perceive objects in her lateral visual fields. There is no evidence that medical attention had ever been sought in connection with visual difficulty or any other related complaint. This case is not uncommon, and similar situations can involve drivers of automobiles who may have visual difficulty because of a tumor, or who suffer epileptic attacks for the same reason and cause an accident.

Occasionally, an undiscovered brain tumor will produce chronic headaches and systemic malaise to such a degree that the victim may commit suicide in the throes of depression or to escape the unremitting discomfort for which they know no cause. More commonly, deaths due to tumors will occur in connection with medical mismanagement, neglect, or failure to communicate. The following cases illustrate some examples.

A 34-year-old white female had visited a local clinic 2 weeks before death complaining of headaches, which were diagnosed as being due to allergies. A few days before death she returned to the clinic complaining of worsening of the headaches and "ringing in the ears." The physician who examined her told her there was nothing wrong with her. On the day of death the woman had such a severe headache that she called the fire department ambulance, which took her to a nearby emergency room, where she received a shot and was sent home at 4:00 a.m. At 1:50 p.m. the same day she was found unresponsive in bed, breathing irregularly and in a labored fashion. The fire department ambulance was again called, and she was brought to an emergency room DOA. The general autopsy revealed no obvious cause of death, but the brain, shown in Figure 3.47, revealed an edematous, low-grade, rather diffuse astrocytoma of the right temporal lobe.

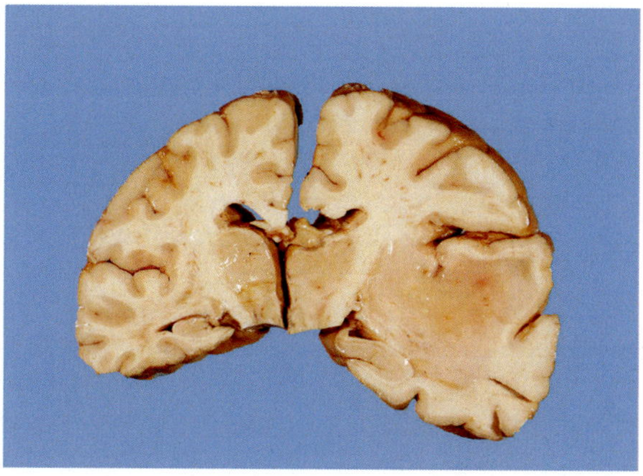

Figure 3.47 This coronal section of the brain reveals a large edematous diffuse low grade astrocytoma of the right temporal lobe that was never diagnosed in life and found at autopsy. (Courtesy of Dr. Y. Konakci, Office of the Medical Examiner, Cook County, IL.)

A 39-year-old African American man was found dead in his bed. At some time in the past a possible brain tumor had been diagnosed but apparently not treated. Autopsy revealed a large hemorrhagic–necrotic tumor of the right temporal region (Figure 3.48) that proved to be a glioblastoma multiforme.

A 41-year-old African American man, after some weeks of severe headaches, was admitted to a hospital. He was diagnosed as depressed but was found to be ataxic and have muscular weakness. Disc disease or multiple sclerosis was considered, but few diagnostic studies were performed. The patient discharged himself against medical advice 3 weeks after admission claiming nothing was being done for him. A few days later he was found dead in bed. The general autopsy was nonrevealing, but the brain showed a huge edematous brain stem glioma extending upward into the diencephalon and hypothalamus.

An elderly man with long-standing diabetes was admitted to the hospital because of failing vision. The man had cataracts, and visualization of the fundi was difficult. Visual loss was ascribed to diabetic retinopathy, but one observer had commented that the optic discs

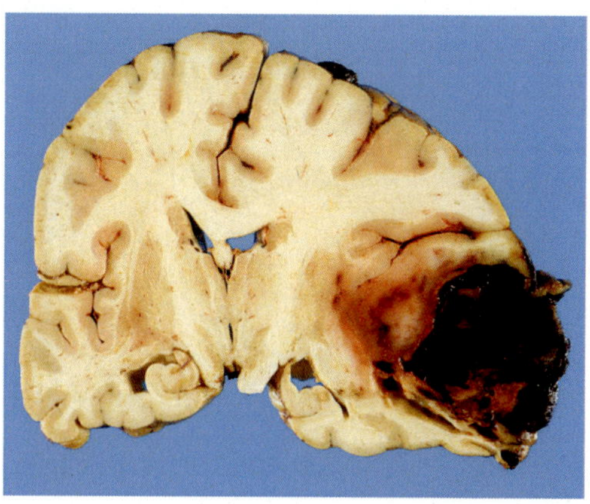

Figure 3.48 This coronal section of the brain reveals a large hemorrhagic tumor of the right temporal region that has produced a right to left shift of the midline. This tumor, which had apparently been diagnosed clinically but apparently never treated, proved to be a glioblastoma multiforme. The man was found dead at home in bed. (Courtesy of Dr. Shaku Teas, Office of the Medical Examiner, Cook County, IL.)

appeared pale, suggesting optic atrophy. The man died from cardiovascular disease at home and was autopsied at a coroner's facility. The autopsy revealed many manifestations of diabetes, including severe cardiovascular disease, which was the cause of death, but examination of the brain revealed a huge olfactory groove meningioma, shown in Figure 3.49.

Brain tumors may cause death in circumstances that would appear, at first examination of the facts, to be due to other causes. This phenomenon is illustrated by the following cases.

A 19-year-old woman had delivered a baby normally 3–4 days before complaining of severe headache and vomiting. She had had a history of these same symptoms in the past. She died at home 5 days after the delivery. The visceral autopsy revealed no anatomic cause of death. Examination of the brain revealed a right cerebellar hemisphere cystic lesion with a mural nodule with compression of the fourth ventricle and enlargement of the lateral ventricles (Figure 3.50). The histology of the tumor was a benign juvenile pilocytic astrocytoma. This woman must have had this tumor for many years. If it had been discovered and operated upon, it is very likely she would have been cured of the tumor and not died from a sudden decompensated hydrocephalus and increased intracranial pressure.

A 50-year-old white man who had not missed a day of work in many years fell backward off a step ladder while changing a light bulb at the factory where he was employed. He apparently only fell a few feet but was unconscious when found by coworkers. He died without regaining consciousness a few hours later in a hospital emergency room. The autopsy was at first nonrevealing as to the cause of death. The brain, however, showed a large hemorrhagic metastatic lesion in the right temporal lobe. There was massive midline shift with uncal and tonsillar herniation as well as an extensive Duret hemorrhage of the pons and midbrain. Histologically, the tumor was a poorly differentiated adenocarcinoma, which prompted a review of the lung tissue and the discovery of a very small primary tumor in the periphery of the lung, which had been overlooked during the initial examination.

A 46-year-old white female who was suffering from advanced ovarian carcinoma was involved in an automobile collision while driving along a narrow suburban city street. She struck an oncoming automobile nearly head-on with the left front of her car but at a low rate

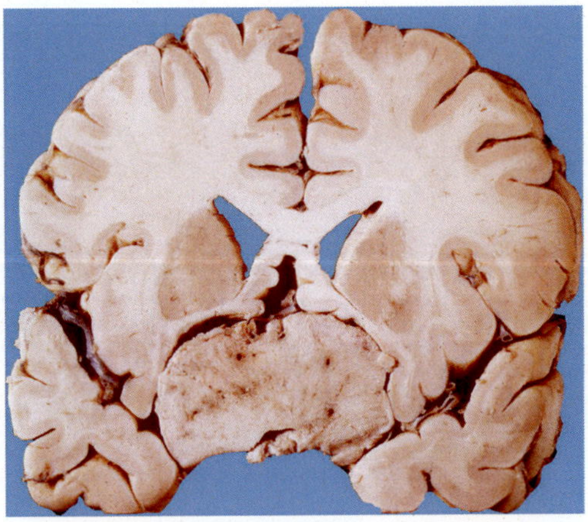

Figure 3.49 This coronal section of the brain reveals a large olfactory groove meningioma that pushed the optic nerves laterally and almost totally compressed them. This tumor was not suspected in life. (Courtesy of the Department of Pathology, DC General Hospital, and the Armed Forces Institute of Pathology, Washington, DC.)

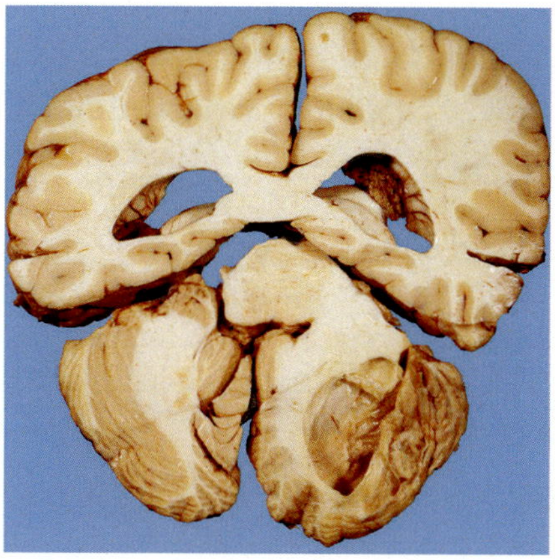

Figure 3.50 These combined coronal and horizontal sections of the brain of a 19-year-old woman who died at home 5 days after having given birth reveal a large cystic lesion with a mural tumor nodule in the right lobe of the cerebellum that compressed the fourth ventricle and caused hydrocephalus. Histologically, this lesion was a "juvenile" pilocytic astrocytoma. (Courtesy of Dr. E, Choi, Office of the Medical Examiner, Cook County, IL.)

of speed. Her forehead struck the windshield, but she did not lose consciousness, and she was able to drive her damaged car home. She reported that she had "not even seen" the other car when she struck it. A few days later she was admitted to the hospital complaining of headache, nausea, and vomiting, which had begun a few hours following the accident. Examination revealed numerous dermal, visceral, and brain metastases. A progressive downhill course resulted in her death in coma 2 weeks later. Autopsy confirmed the diagnosis and the brain showed metastases in the right frontal lobe (less than 1 cm diameter) and a 1.5-cm metastasis in the superior lip of the calcarine gyrus at its midportion on the right side, with a 1-cm zone of edema about it. This lesion corresponded functionally to the left lower lateral visual field but, because of the surrounding edema, would have been expected to produce a left homonymous hemianopsia. It is likely that this lesion was the reason why she was unable to see the vehicle that she struck.

These preceding cases illustrate instances where a cause for death may be an unsuspected condition or head trauma that under ordinary circumstances would produce minimal or no sequelae, but with a tumor present, hemorrhage may occur within the tumor or further disruption of the blood–brain barrier near the tumor may take place, so that the mass effects of the neoplasm are magnified beyond the capacity of the brain to compensate, resulting in brain stem herniation, coma, and eventual respiratory failure. It is often difficult to explain how individuals with such massive or extensive intracranial pathology can be unaware of it and apparently pursue normal activities until the fatal moment, but the brain is a clever computer that is able to reroute and reprogram around functional loss, especially if there is sufficient time for it to do so. Furthermore, the power of human beings to deny and rationalize their illnesses plays an important role. In some cases, one can be left only with the conclusion that certain individuals seem impervious to pain or functional loss in themselves and that some individuals associating with obviously ill and poorly functioning people seem oblivious to their dysfunction and never bring it to their attention.

The importance of a correct analysis in cases such as these for potential defendants or parties involved in the settlement of insurance or malpractice claims speaks for itself.

Whenever particularly violent public acts are carried out by apparently previously normal individuals, it is not surprising that the news media and the public attempt to seek an explanation for such aberrant behavior by those who set about murdering those nearby, often continuing until being shot down by the police or, when cornered, committing suicide. When these horrid events occur and the public seeks answers for such horrific behavior, the notorious case of mass murderer Charles Whitman, in Austin, Texas, is invariably brought to mind [315,316]. This case is discussed in detail in Chapter 9.

Etiology of Brain Tumors

Brain tumors occur spontaneously in nearly every species of higher animal, with some species, such as rats, having the highest incidence of all. The cause of human brain tumors is not known, but evidence gleaned from experimentation on animals and epidemiological studies has provided a number of possibilities. Some of the most intriguing arise from study of so-called cancer clusters, in which a greater-than-expected number of individuals are affected by one form of cancer in an area or in which a particular age group may be affected. Studies of such clusters almost inevitably provide interesting possibilities for etiology but almost never offer definitive demonstration of a particular cause [317,318]. Apparent brain tumor clusters have occurred among laboratory workers, but analysis of these phenomena often reveals that the tumors were of different types, possible exposures to a carcinogenic agent appear too short, or some of the individuals did not actually work with chemicals. As with most neoplasms, modern advances in molecular genetics have shown that neoplasms arise from differentiated cells and not from embryonic rests. Transformation occurs mostly by failure of tumor suppressor genes by mutational events from various exogenous circumstances or by an interplay with inheritance [293,319,320]. A number of important genes seem to be involved, among them, the genes coding for P-53 [321], and the list continues to grow.

Chemical Neurooncogenesis

Neurocarcinogens can be classified into the following groups: polycyclic aromatic hydrocarbons (methylcholanthrenes, benzopyrenes, dibenzanthracenes, and aminofluorenes); the N-nitroso compounds (methyl- and ethylnitrosoureas and nitrosamines); triazines; hydrazines; salts of heavy metals (thorium, uranium, mercury); radiation; RNA and DNA viral agents (papovaviruses, adenoviruses, retroviruses); and various mycotoxins and lectins [322]. All have been shown to produce a varying yield of brain tumors of all types in animals. Most carcinogens appear to act by damaging DNA or its repair process. The most important experimental chemical carcinogens are the N-nitroso compounds. The importance of the N-nitroso compounds is that they act primarily and most efficiently *in utero* to produce a high incidence of brain tumors in the offspring of the treated pregnant animal [322]. They act during neural development and produce tumors at a later date after maturation. The implications for all heavily industrialized nations with increasing pollution of the environment by organic compounds are obvious and have been the subject of intensive study over many years [319,323], the results of which are not decisive but raise the concern of increased risk to women of childbearing age with respect to their offspring as well as risks of hydrocarbon exposure to young children from the environment in heavily industrialized areas.

Occasionally "clusters" of cases of brain tumors arise, sometimes in and around chemical plants or other locations where organic chemical exposure could occur. In evaluating these cases it is important to realize, that with the exception of the N-nitroso compounds/intra uterine exposure, most known chemical carcinogens take a very long time in an adult animal to produce a brain tumor. Thus, as attractive as it may be, the causes of such "clusters" remain unknown.

Oncogenic Viruses

The viral etiology of brain tumors has been reinforced by recent experimentation with the DNA viruses of papovavirus and adenovirus groups and with several RNA viruses (avian sarcoma viruses, murine sarcoma viruses). Of interest to human neurooncology is the implication that the virus of progressive multifocal leukoencephalopathy (PML), the so-called J-C papovavirus, which in common experience is the cause of an opportunistic infection of the brain in immune-deficient persons, might cause human neoplasms. J-C virus DNA has been recovered from some cases of brain lymphoma [324] and has been found in, and potentially was the cause of, two cases of astrocytoma of man [325] and in various visceral neoplasms [326,327]. Whether this virus is the actual cause of the tumors is open to argument, but when taken with experimental evidence in animals, which has shown that this agent can induce brain tumors, the implications are clear.

Radiation

Ionizing radiation has been blamed for an occasional human brain tumor and, to some workers is the most compelling of oncogenic causes [320]. These cases usually involved therapeutic radiation for a brain tumor, such as a pituitary adenoma or other lesions of the face and head, with a long interval of sometimes 20 years elapsing before a tumor developed [320,322]. Furthermore, human primary brain lymphomas have developed following chemotherapy for visceral cancers and in the course of immunosuppression to prevent rejection reactions to transplanted organs [328]. It remains to be seen what the impact of increasingly successful treatment of cancer and organ failure by transplantation will yield 20 or 30 years hence for the survivors of these treatments.

Electromagnetic radiation, such as is most commonly found in cellular telephones, has been suggested as a cause of brain tumors [329]. At one time there were a number of pending lawsuits regarding this possibility. A considerable literature exists regarding the effects on DNA of electromagnetic fields (often at wavelengths employed by cellular phones), which can cause DNA breakage. Perhaps in certain individuals the combination of certain genetic defects and a superimposed event that damages critical portions of the genome may result in formation of a neoplasm. The linkage, however, is theoretical and has not been proven. The issue, especially with the prevalence of cell phone and other wireless device use, continues to draw scrutiny.

Heredity

There are many reports of the familial occurrence of various brain neoplasms. Numerous typical examples of glioma families have been reported, with a variety of apparent genetic defects [330–332]. Families that have greater than the expected incidence of pituitary adenomas, usually prolactinomas, have also been reported [333]. Other classical examples of expected familial brain tumor occurrence include the phaecomatoses, such as von Hippel–Lindau disease [334], tuberous sclerosis [335], von Recklinghausen's syndromes (NF I and II and variants) [336], and retinoblastoma [337].

Trauma as an Etiology for Brain Tumors

The traumatic etiology of glial and nonglial brain tumors has been debated for many years since the first publications appeared in the literature suggesting the possibility [338]. The contention that previous head trauma, often with implantation of foreign bodies, or trauma in other parts of the body resulted in the later appearance of a tumor is regularly raised in connection with workers' compensation litigation and veterans' benefit claims [339]. As absurd as it might seem, there are probably legitimate instances in which trauma or the consequences of trauma have caused a tumor, most commonly a meningioma, to form. Harvey Cushing [340], one of the founders of American neurosurgery, explored this possibility and reported several cases in which he thought trauma the likely etiology of the tumor he removed. Probably the most notable and convincing case is that of Reinhardt [338], who reported in 1928 the case of a 58-year-old man who suffered a head injury following an explosion that implanted metallic foreign bodies in his brain that were found surrounded by a meningioma some 20 years later. Other cases of a similar type involving meningioma have been reported or referenced [304,341–343]. Other types of neoplasms alleged to be linked to trauma include development of an astrocytoma or glioblastoma in the previous site of prefrontal leukotomy [344] or at the site of a previous penetrating brain injury as few as 5 or 6 years, but more commonly 10 or more years, after injury [345–347].

The role of trauma and an etiology of brain tumors are controversial enough [339,348] that criteria have been formulated that some authors feel should probably be fulfilled to reasonably consider the traumatic etiology valid [349]. They are the following:

1. The site of injury should correspond to the site of the tumor.
2. The trauma should be sufficiently severe and not incidental.
3. The area of trauma must have been shown free of tumor at the time of the injury.
4. The time interval between injury and tumor discovery must be significant.
5. There must be continuity in the pathological changes of the wounded areas from the time of the injury to the appearance of the tumor.
6. There has to be microscopic proof of the tumor diagnosis.

Cushing [340] felt that evidence of open head injury, with or without implantation of foreign materials or bone fragments, constituted another important criterion. The author advocated the use of these or similar criteria to test any such cases that come to analysis. In our experience, of the several cases coming for consultation that have been alleged to have been caused by trauma, not one met these requirements and could not reasonably be judged to be related in any etiologic manner to preexisting trauma.

Epidemiology of Brain Tumors

Like any other statistic, it is subject to sampling error and bias, but general trends in several large series [293,347,350–353], when combined, indicate that brain tumors are found in about 1.2% of all autopsies, affect 4 to 5 persons per 100,000 per year in the North American population, and account for about 1.5% of all new primary cancers. They kill at least 15,000 persons each year in the United States and represent about 2.4% of cancer deaths each year. All age groups can be affected, but the peak incidence is between 60 and 70 years. For about the past 30–40 years, it appears that brain tumor incidence has been increasing for reasons that are not clear [354,355]. Some have suggested increasing urbanization of the American population and environmental degradation, with increasing exposure to environmental hydrocarbons that might be carcinogenic.

Classification of Brain Tumors

The classification and nomenclature of brain tumors have a confused past and remain unsettled. One problem is that some tumors with the same cell of origin and histologic pattern have different behaviors and prognoses, depending upon their location, and now, with respect to genetic mutations, can be probed for in tissue specimens. Another problem is that some tumor classifications make use of terms that may be equivalent or that have subtle shades of meaning only to the experienced neuropathologist. To be sure, the histological and biological variability of the gliomas makes the task more difficult, but recent classification approaches facilitate learning and minimize confusion. The historical classifications have largely been supplanted by the so-called World Health Organization (WHO) classification, which is now employed worldwide and apparently constantly updated [293,295–297]. Probably little of this has much forensic significance except when incorrect diagnoses and inappropriate therapeutic decisions are made on the basis of faulty or erroneous information. Litigation regarding such issues will almost certainly involve a tumor neuropathologist, who presumably is familiar with the latest standards and diagnostic issues.

Infections of the Nervous System

Infectious disease of the nervous system is not usually an immediate common concern of the forensic pathologist and generally is a side issue to the primary concern of determining the cause and manner of death. However, as one of the guardians of the public health, the forensic pathologist acting for the coroner or medical examiner may be the first to recognize unusual infections that might herald naturally occurring epidemics, such as West Nile virus encephalitis, or that are part of a terrorist action that threatens the public and necessitates notification of the responsible health and governmental officials, such as anthrax. Examples of real or potential infection scenarios include meningococcal meningitis [356], Legionnaires' disease [357], anthrax [358], plague [359], tularemia [360], smallpox [361], the arthropod-borne viral infections such as West Nile, the equine encephalitides, Japanese encephalitis, and other viruses of similar character that cause hemorrhagic fevers [362,363]. Many of these diseases are only rarely encountered and may first be detected on a forensic service; thus, it behooves forensic pathologists to familiarize themselves at least basically about these diseases.

There are a number of infectious diseases for which reporting is mandatory but which unfortunately are commonly ignored. CNS infections may have medical-legal significance, especially in malpractice litigation involving operative infections and their complications, vaccination and inoculation reactions, and product liability. Not all forms of infectious disease will be covered here—only those that commonly occur on a forensic service or have forensic import. The viral and bacterial infections that are important to the hospital neuropathologist, with some exceptions, have little importance in the forensic arena. Therefore, only selected diseases and general infectious processes will be discussed below. Some of the entities have been discussed in Chapter 4 on pediatric forensic neuropathology and will be only superficially discussed here. For general information about CNS infections, the reader is referred to the recent text by Scheld et al. and other texts and chapters [364–367].

Subdural Empyema

Subdural empyema is a suppurative form of inflammation, usually involving pyogenic bacterial organisms, that results in collection of pus in the cranial or spinal subdural compartment, as illustrated in Figure 3.51 [368]. Probably more children suffer from this dreaded infection than adults owing to the prevalence of sinus and ear infections in this age group. In adults [369] subdural empyema is associated with open head trauma (fracture, gunshot, stab wounds, or missile wounds), a neurosurgical procedure such as craniotomy or laminectomy [370], or a complication of acupuncture, injections for pain management, catheter or pressure monitor insertion, paranasal sinus infection, otitis media, dental surgery and tooth extractions, or head injury with basilar skull fracture. Because external contamination is virtually always the source of the organisms, they are typically skin flora such as *Staphylococcus albus* or *Staphylococcus aureus*, streptococcal species, and coliforms. Occasionally, if the scalp or head wound is contaminated with earth, clostridial infection may occur. Calvarial osteomyelitis may become a complication, along with meningitis, cerebritis, and systemic sepsis. Treatment is surgical incision, and drainage, intensive antibiotic therapy, and correction of any entryway for infection to the area. Complications may include generalized sepsis, meningitis, cavernous, and nearby venous sinus thrombosis, and all of the tertiary complications that can arise from these problems [371].

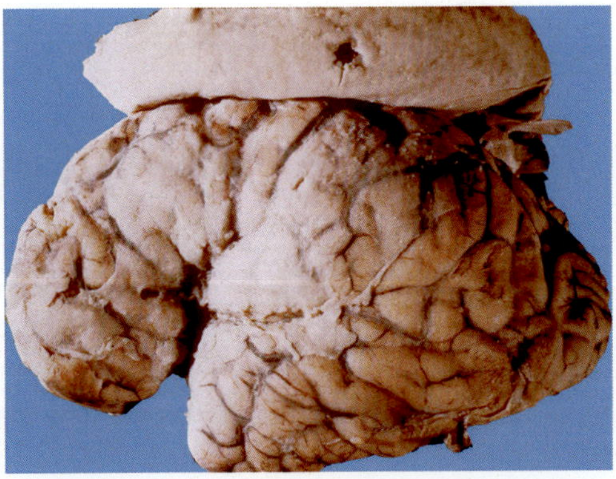

Figure 3.51 This gross photograph of the left cerebral hemisphere and its dura illustrates a Staphylococcal subdural empyema. This was a victim of head trauma who sustained a basilar skull fracture and subdural hematoma (drained via the burr hole in the dura that is visible). The basilar skull fracture traversed a paranasal sinus, which may have been the source of the infection and caused the later development of the empyema. Likewise, contamination could have occurred via the burr hole.

From a forensic point of view, subdural empyema may or may not have been recognized clinically or in life; thus, when bacterial meningitis or bacterial brain abscesses are known or discovered, attempts should be made to determine the source and pathway by which this process occurred. Such an investigation should include attempts to culture the organism, stripping the basal skull dura and opening the sinuses, and may involve some exploration of the basal venous sinuses and sagittal sinus.

Bacterial Meningitis

Often referred to simply as meningitis [372–375], bacterial infection most commonly affects the leptomeninges (the pia and the arachnoidal membranes) and the subarachnoid space of the CNS. All manner of bacteria have been reported to cause meningitis, but there are age groups in which meningitis tends to be almost predictable etiologically, as discussed in Chapter 4. In the neonatal and perinatal period, bacterial meningitis is almost always due to Gram-negative rods (*Escherichia coli*, *Pseudomonas*, *Flavobacterium*, *Serratia*, *Listeria*, and the coliforms) [372]. This disease is virulent in most neonatal cases, and there is a very high mortality rate despite antibiotic therapy [376]. The causes of neonatal meningitis include placentitis and infections of the birth canal, delivery under unsanitary conditions, contamination of the nursery, contamination of milk and formula, and contamination of the stump of the umbilical cord. The latter etiologies are more common than the former.

Bacterial meningitis in the toddler age group is quite commonly due to *Haemophilus influenzae* and *Streptococcus pneumoniae*. The usual portals of entry for the organisms are upper respiratory, sinus, and ear infections common in this age group. The impact of immunizations against these organisms has dramatically reduced the incidence of meningitis in this age group, as has effective antibiotic therapy. The mortality rate is low, and morbidity, when it occurs, includes deafness and hydrocephalus [377,378].

Meningitis in the teen and young adult age group, compared with that in younger children, is rather uncommon, and in the past the most frequent organism was *Neisseria meningitidis* (meningococcus), followed by *Streptococcus pneumoniae* (pneumococcus) and a host of other organisms. In recent years, there has been a trend to fewer cases of meningococcal meningitis and predominance of pneumococcal meningitis and other forms [356,374,378]. Meningitis in this age group presents a greater diagnostic and treatment challenge than in the toddler group, and there is a greater incidence of complications and likelihood of a fatal outcome. The causes of meningitis in this age group are more varied than in infants and include, as before, upper respiratory infection, sinusitis, mastoiditis, otitis, dental infection, and congenital heart disease but also, now, intravenous narcotic use, systemic traumatic injury with infection, basal skull fracture with paranasal sinus involvement with or without CSF rhinorrhea, penetrating injury to the brain, burns, immune suppression or incompetence, diabetes, and a host of other conditions encountered with increasing age. In the case of meningococcal disease, no definite predisposing cause other than proximity to others of the same age group who may harbor the organism is involved [356].

Clinical presentations of meningitis in this age group are similar to those in younger individuals and, as mentioned above, may be more subtle, and dependent upon the coexisting conditions. Headache, fever, lethargy, focal neurological signs, and seizures are common. As before, stiff neck and evidence of meningeal irritation are often diagnostic. Diagnosis is still confirmed by lumbar puncture with Gram staining and culture of the CSF. Gross and microscopic pathological appearances are no different from the appearances described and illustrated in Chapter 4. There may be a greater tendency for cortical involvement (cerebritis or encephalitis) and for inflammatory thrombosis or vessels with focal infarctions in this age group, owing to the greater chance of infection by virulent and aggressive organisms such as staphylococci. Sequelae tend to be more severe and frequent in survivors, and mortality rates are greatly increased [375].

In the over-40 age group, bacterial meningitis (especially in alcoholics and diabetics) presents a special and diverse category of etiologies and coexisting conditions. For relative commonness, *Streptococcus pneumoniae* is still the most common organism causing meningitis, but it is closely followed by other streptococci, staphylococcal species, many Gram-negative bacillary infections, and, last, individual uncommon pathogens [374]. Still important as underlying causes are paranasal, dental, and upper respiratory infections; trauma (cranial and systemic); diabetes; debilitating illnesses and disorders of immunity; and complications of cancer therapy. Meningitis in the middle-aged or older adult is a dangerous illness with many complications and often a high mortality rate [364]. Clinical presentations are similar to those in the other age groups, as is the pathology, both gross and microscopic. In this age group there is a tendency for the infection not to be limited to the subarachnoid space and for cortical erosion, focal abscess formation, ventriculitis, and, in general, more extensive disease to be seen. In the elderly, symptoms may be masked, even in the face of overwhelming disease. The forensic importance of these conditions is obvious.

The Meningococcal Syndrome

At one time, it may have been appropriate to consider meningococcal (*Neisseria meningitidis*) infections mostly within the context of bacterial meningitis, but over the past 30 to 40 years, for reasons that are not clear but probably include increased awareness, meningococcal infections have broadened their pathology to involve other organs and to produce a clinical and pathological pattern of disease most properly dealt with conceptually as a syndrome [379,380]. This awareness is particularly crucial to the forensic pathologist, who may be in a key position to pick up patterns of an epidemic and to properly interface with public health and other officials, not to mention the general public, whose fears may be quickly mobilized by rumor or ill-informed news accounts of an "epidemic of meningitis." True epidemics of meningococcal disease rarely occur on a public-wide scale but, rather, are limited to collections of susceptible people, usually students or military recruits [356].

The organism is ubiquitous and can be cultured from the nasopharynx in about 10% of the normal adult population. During epidemics, which in the past have occurred every 15 to 20 years, the incidence of positive nasopharyngeal culture increase in unaffected individuals rises to 60% or greater. Clinical presentation of a meningococcal syndrome is that of a systemic illness, often initially mistaken for influenza, with fever, headache, nausea and vomiting, myalgia, and malaise. Symptoms may evolve slowly at first and then progress with startling rapidity to stupor, appearance of purpuric skin rash, prostration, coma, and death in a few hours after the first realization of significant illness.

The autopsy findings in most recent cases include the effects of disseminated intravascular coagulation (DIC) with purpura of the skin; petechial hemorrhages on visceral surfaces, pericardium and epicardium, conjunctiva, and mucous membranes; and adrenal medullary hemorrhage (Waterhouse–Friderichsen syndrome). Where one would expect a typical purulent meningitis, there may be no sign of exudate on the brain. The most common findings are those of congestion of the surface, brain edema, and herniation. Microscopic examination of the brain may reveal slight acute inflammatory exudate in the leptomeninges, sometimes stigmata of DIC, but most commonly edema and vascular congestion. Significant changes may be seen in the heart, where a diffuse acute myocarditis or frank myocardial necrosis may be seen [381,382]. Meningococcus can usually be demonstrated by culture of blood, CSF, and affected tissues. It is probably the combination of DIC and myocardial damage that is responsible for the sudden and fulminant death associated with meningococcal sepsis—hence one of the more preferred terms for the syndrome, fulminant meningococcemia.

Bacterial Brain Abscess

Brain abscess caused by bacteria may occur in any age group but has a peak incidence in the fifties and sixties [369,372,383]. The causes of brain abscess are most commonly bloodborne infection from an infected site somewhere else in the body (about 50% of cases), such as in the lung, urogenital system, bone, skin, or heart. Other important causes are congenital cyanotic heart disease (in young victims), dental or paranasal sinus infection, skeletal trauma, head trauma with skull fracture or open head injury, a recent surgical procedure, intravenous drug abuse, diabetes mellitus, and immunosuppression or incompetence. Organisms reach the brain by arterial or venous routes, direct extension, or implantation [365]. An abscess evolves from a sequestrated septic focus, usually an embolus, which comes to rest in most cases at the junction of the gray and white matter or just beneath the gray matter in the cerebrum. The most common area, in proportion to its volume of perfusion, is the territory of the middle cerebral arteries. As has been demonstrated in experimental animals and correlated with empirical observations in humans, once the septic focus is established and not immediately inactivated by host defense mechanisms, bacterial growth proceeds, with destruction of the capillary in which the embolus lies and egress of organisms into the surrounding neuropil, where little defense is present. Growth proceeds in an ever-expanding pattern along the path of least host resistance—the white matter. The gray matter, which is much more vascularized, presents an effective barrier to growth. The developing infection does not immediately form a classic suppurative focus but, rather, spreads diffusely outward in a roughly spherical fashion, producing what is commonly referred to as cerebritis, as illustrated in Figure 3.52. Acute inflammatory cells and macrophages gradually become mobilized and attempt to organize a defense to the invading bacteria. The process proceeds in a clinically silent manner, often for several weeks, until sufficient cortex is undermined and enough white matter connections are compromised and irritated that symptoms of a focal neurological nature may appear (seizures, headache, paralysis) [384].

At about 3 to 5 weeks postinfection, the host defenses have sufficiently mobilized that necrosis of the infected tissue has occurred, and the process of isolation by vessels and fibroblasts in their walls, as well as astroglia, has usually developed. At this point, several critical events may take place. The walling-off process may have evolved sufficiently to limit the expansion of the process, which has now progressed from cerebritis to an abscess, and the expanding destructive process and liquefaction may have carried the lesion in proximity to the ventricular wall before the capsule of the abscess could contain it (Figure 3.53). Leakage or rupture of the abscess into the ventricle may now take place. This is attended by a severe worsening of the clinical condition of the patient, and death may follow rapidly once rupture has occurred. More often, there is leakage of infected material into the subarachnoid space or ventricle, which causes the sudden development

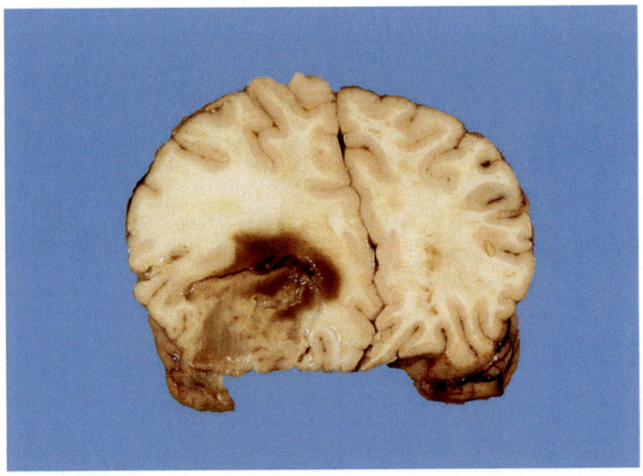

Figure 3.52 This coronal section of the brain illustrates in the inferior frontal lobe a large area of cerebritis. There is necrosis of the brain with focal hemorrhage and incipient abscess cavity formation. This stage, preceding the actual abscess formation, may be present for weeks before symptoms are evident or spread of the infection from within the brain to the subarachnoid space (meningitis) or rupture into the ventricle, which is usually a fatal event.

of meningitis and ventriculitis, alerting clinicians to the seriousness of what might have been only slightly symptomatic before. Complete rupture of infected material into the ventricle is usually a fatal event caused by a mechanism probably very similar to that of acute intraventricular hemorrhage, i.e., volume and mass effect, as well as toxic materials or pharmacologically active products of inflammation in contact with hypothalamic or brain stem centers [365].

The organisms that most commonly cause bacterial brain abscesses are the so-called peptostreptococci (mouth and upper gastrointestinal [GI] streptococci), which are either anaerobic or microaerophilic and generally of low pathogenicity. These organisms are often difficult to culture, especially when there has been previous antibiotic therapy, and when

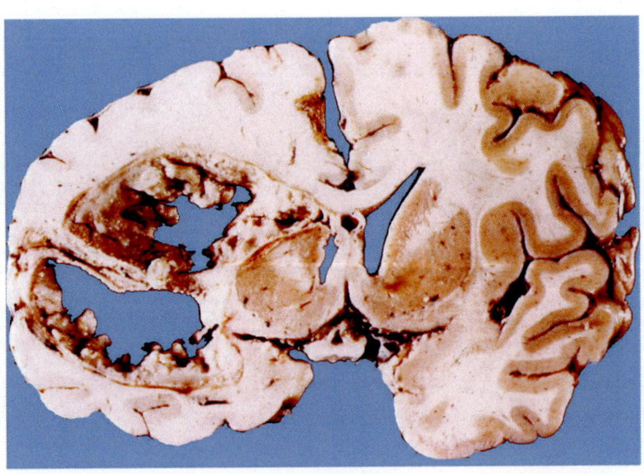

Figure 3.53 This section is from a diabetic derelict found comatose in an alleyway. He had a gangrenous leg that was infested with maggots. This biloculated abscess was caused by *Proteus* organisms. Note the rime-like capsule and the area of rupture into the lateral ventricle just below the corpus callosum. (Courtesy of the Department of Pathology, DC General Hospital, and the Armed Forces Institute of Pathology, Washington, DC.)

attempting to demonstrate the causative organism in brain abscesses, special care and devotion by the microbiologist may be necessary to recover an organism. *Staphylococcus*, *Proteus*, *Pseudomonas*, and other Gram-negative organisms are also frequently seen. Mixed floral infection is not uncommon, accounting for perhaps 15% of cases. Unfortunately, so-called sterile abscesses occur in nearly 25% of cases, presumably because of prior antibiotic therapy or inadequate recovery techniques [372,383].

Grossly, areas of cerebritis (prior to abscess formation) are edematous, often focally hemorrhagic, and discolored (yellow or green) and generally lie below the gray matter in the white matter of the cerebrum or elsewhere (Figure 3.52). Histologically, the pattern is diffuse inflammation with relatively easy demonstration of the organism by Gram stain of the tissue. Once the abscess has evolved, it shows breakdown of tissues and coalescence into a classic suppurative focus. Multiple abscesses are said to occur clinically in about 15% of cases but are found in almost half of autopsied cases. Histologically, the wall and other components of the abscess are logically composed of necrotic material and pus at the center, a zone of foamy macrophages, a collagenized and vascular wall, a zone of lymphoid cells, and an outer zone of reactive gliosis. Some abscess walls develop so fully that the abscess is completely isolated by dense collagenous tissue and even bone.

The classic treatment for abscesses at one time was incision, excision, and drainage. When this was not done or the abscess was missed, the mortality rate was nearly 100%, but with this treatment, survival approached 70%. In recent years there has been a tendency for surgeons to treat abscesses with massive antibiotic therapy with success that rivals or surpasses a surgical approach. When lesions are multiple, this approach is especially attractive.

The problem of bacterial brain abscess may confront the forensic pathologist in the form of a complication to a previous head injury or gunshot wound, where death may occur in a victim weeks or even months after the criminal assault. In such cases, etiological connection of the complication to the initial event is a vital aspect to adjudication of the case. A proper and complete understanding of the dynamics and mechanisms of formation and evolution of brain abscesses should prepare the forensic pathologist for his task as the consultant for the court. Abscess may also complicate medical and surgical therapy and, as such, may be important in malpractice litigation. No consistent guidelines for such cases can be presented here because circumstances may be highly variable. Nevertheless, a careful analysis of what facts exist and a knowledge of the processes involved will facilitate a proper medical opinion. As has been already mentioned in the context of subdural empyema, a portal of entry for the infection should be sought. This should include stripping of the basal dura and opening the paranasal sinuses.

Mycobacterial Infections of the Nervous System

The two most common mycobacteria that produce disease in the nervous system are *Mycobacterium tuberculosis* and *Mycobacterium leprae*. Both diseases are more common in undeveloped and impoverished countries but are to be found in virtually every country of the world. The most important, at least to Western countries, is tuberculosis, which, after being controlled quite successfully for many years, is emerging again as a threat to the public health owing to the emergence of multiple antibiotic-resistant strains of the organism [385].

Tuberculosis (TB)

Tuberculosis continues to be a major public health problem worldwide, accounting for more than 1.2 million deaths each year [2]. Current rates of new TB infections in the United States average 50 to 60 per 100,000, but among minorities concentrated in large cities, these rates are often doubled. In American Indian and black populations, tuberculosis is especially virulent, owing to an inherent lack of resistance to the organism as well as the high incidence of poverty, poor nutrition, often-crowded living conditions that foster its spread, and the emergence of antibiotic-resistant strains [385,386,388]. Forensic pathologists are in a better position than most to encounter tuberculosis in its many forms, including CNS tuberculosis. Occasionally, TB can account for sudden and unexpected deaths (without TB history), and in some parts of the country TB meningitis and other forms of CNS TB are commonly seen in children, as in the early days of the century [389].

Tuberculosis of the nervous system is usually caused by human tubercle bacilli but can be caused by *Mycobacterium avium*, *Mycobacterium bovis*, or a host of atypical tubercle bacilli (groups I–IV photochromogens, scotochromogens, nonchromogens, and rapidly growing forms), especially in susceptible and compromised hosts [390]. The CNS is involved usually only after pulmonary infection has first occurred. The infection may spread in a fulminant manner to the CNS initially or may be involved in miliary spread at a later time, in connection with reactivation of an old primary focus. This may occur spontaneously or following steroid therapy, immunosuppression, or acquired immunoincompetence. Tuberculous meningitis is most commonly seen in children, but all ages are susceptible [391]. Tubercle bacilli react in the CNS via the blood in virtually all cases and may gain access to the subarachnoid space by leakage of organisms from a small tubercle established in or near the cerebral or cerebellar cortex (so-called Rich focus) or, less commonly, from a tubercle established in the choroid plexus [392]. TB meningitis is a complication of miliary disease in 70 to 80% of cases, and evidence of the disease elsewhere in the body is the rule. The meningitic process is chiefly evident in the basal meninges, where a diffuse, fibrosing, gray or greenish exudate, which is sometimes nodular and tubercle-like in character, is seen, but the pattern is very similar to that of fungal meningitides. The usually intense granulomatous inflammation surrounds cranial nerves and vessels and may obstruct the foramina, leading to hydrocephalus. Infection and reaction in vessels (both arteries and veins) may lead to thrombosis and infarction or hemorrhage. Cranial nerve lesions are common and are usually permanent. The organisms can usually be demonstrated with the Ziehl-Neelsen (acid-fast) stain, but sometimes the atypical or modified infections are poorly acid-fast, and more reliable detection of the organisms can be accomplished using the fluorescent stain Auramine. The treatment of tuberculous meningitis involves systemic chemotherapy with a variety of drugs, including rifampin, isonicotinic hydrazide, streptomycin, and para-aminosalicylic acid, often in combination. The earlier the treatment, the better the chance of limiting complications. Recently, greatly resistant strains of TB have arisen, posing a major challenge in treatment of public health practices [393].

Tuberculomas [394] are space-occupying lesions that, in the older brain tumor series such as Cushing's, contributed one of the largest categories, but now in most well-developed countries are only infrequently seen. These localized forms of TB may occur anywhere in the CNS, generally at the gray–white matter junctions, but seem to occur most commonly in the cerebellum and brain stem in children (Figure 3.54) and in the cerebrum in adults (Figure 3.55). They vary in size from only a few millimeters to several centimeters and

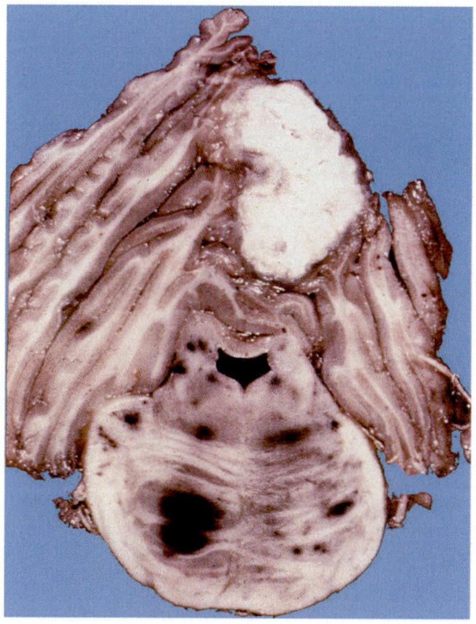

Figure 3.54 This section through the upper pons and adjacent rostral cerebellar vermis reveals a white caseous tuberculoma in a child. Such lesions in the past were often associated with tuberculous lymphadenitis (scrofula) when drinking unpasteurized milk and bovine tuberculosis was common. Such lesions may cause sudden unexpected deaths.

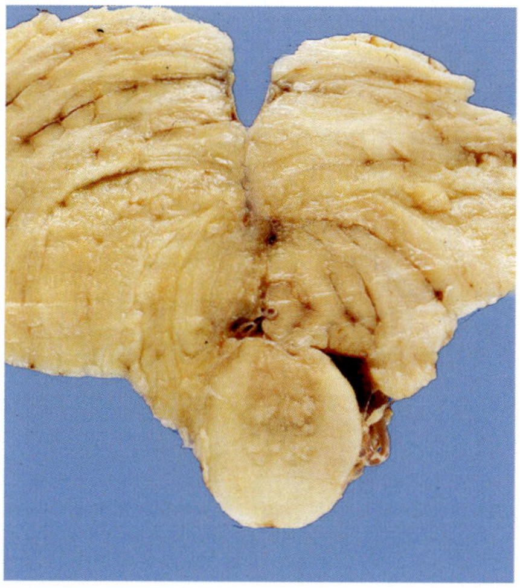

Figure 3.55 This section of the cerebellum including the medulla shows a granular mass in the midline of the medulla filling the lower fourth ventricle. This was a man in his mid-30s incarcerated for drug-related offenses who was found dead in his jail cell. Autopsy revealed a mass in the medulla, which proved to be tuberculoma caused by *Mycobacterium avis*. It is likely that the deceased was suffering from HIV infection probably related to IV illicit drug use. (Courtesy of Dr. Shaku Teas, Office of the Medical Examiner, Cook County, IL.)

usually are not purely spherical but, rather, have a lobate shape. In cut section they may show typical caseous (cheesy) contents and may be quite well circumscribed or calcified, depending on their age. In early forms, they are indistinguishable from bacterial embolic microabscesses. There may be considerable surrounding edema in early tuberculomas, which may cause intraoperative deaths during attempted resection, especially of deeply lying cerebellar or brain stem lesions, due to uncontrollable brain swelling with herniation and fungation through the operative site. Histologically, the typical appearance of any TB granuloma is well known to every pathologist, but sometimes the host response to the organisms is unusual and can give rise to a mostly collagenous response, which produces dense, rubbery masses that appear almost like solid rubber balls, in which the organisms may be very sparse. Much less commonly the tissue response will be purulent, almost like that appropriate for a bacterium, with massive numbers of tubercle bacilli everywhere, even free in the tissue. In this case, the gross appearance will resemble cerebritis or bacterial brain abscess.

Other classic forms of TB affecting the nervous system include spinal TB osteomyelitis with epidural cold abscess formation, which may compress the cord. Here, the spinal column becomes weakened and may collapse, compressing the cord and producing transverse myelopathy.

Fungal Diseases of the Nervous System

Fungal infections of the nervous system [365,395,396] tend to occur in individuals past middle age, but in any age group they tend to affect those who are immunocompromised, debilitated, or have undergone some sort of invasive procedure or injection that introduced the organism [397,398]. With the increasing longevity of organ transplant patients and survivors of various cancers who have been treated with numerous chemotherapeutic agents, and with individuals being treated for many serious diseases with corticosteroids that may produce some suppression of the immune mechanisms and other individuals who are compromised in some way, there is a huge population who are candidates for fungal diseases. Any or all of these classes of individuals may present clinically in unusual ways and may die suddenly and unexpectedly in circumstances that will bring the case to the attention of a coroner or medical examiner. The variability of each individual's reaction to this class of organisms makes for difficult analysis and diagnosis at times and adds to the challenge to the forensic pathologist, who may not always have access to detailed clinical records or history and must by necessity approach the case "cold," having to use his or her skill and observational powers to develop all the information he or she needs to come to a conclusion.

There are certain generalizations concerning fungal infections that may be helpful to remember when analyzing such cases. Even though fungi will reveal all potential forms (mycelia and hyphae, yeast and cyst forms, fruiting bodies, etc.) on the culture plate, growth in tissues limits the expression of these forms and will, to some extent, affect the tissue response to infection. Basically, fungi exist in tissues, the brain included, in either hyphal (mycelial) or yeast-like forms. The most common organisms making hyphae are *Aspergillus* sp. and *Mucor-Rhizopus* sp. Those displaying yeast forms are *Cryptococcus* sp., *Coccidioides* sp., *Blastomyces* sp., and *Histoplasma* sp. Organisms that may display features of both and that have correspondingly complex tissue reactions include *Candida*, *Actinomyces*, and *Nocardia* [395].

The hyphal-mycelian organisms (*Aspergillus* and *Mucor*) tend to proliferate in the blood vessel walls, leading to thrombosis, infarction, and hemorrhagic lesions, rather than meningitis and abscess formation (Figures 3.56 and 3.57) [399]. In the case of *Aspergillus* species, there is most often a lung focus of infection except when direct implantation of the

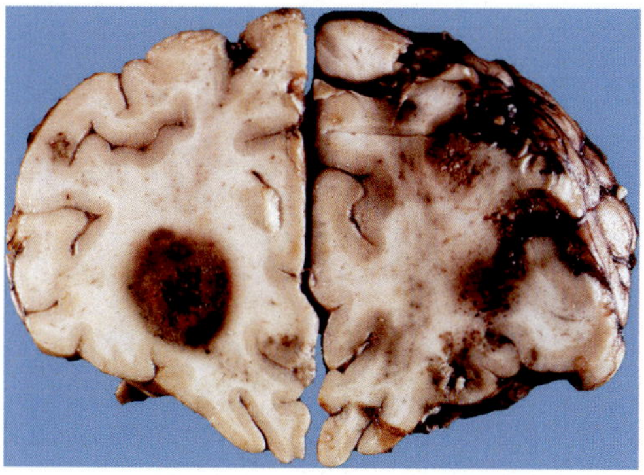

Figure 3.56 This coronal section of the frontal lobes illustrates numerous hemorrhagic abscess foci of cerebral aspergillosis. The organism most likely was blood-borne from a lung focus, but instances of similar cases can occur following contamination during brain surgery, cardiac surgery with valve replacements, contaminated instruments and graft materials, and in immune deficiency states. The hemorrhagic character of the lesions occurs because hyphae of the fungus affect the walls of vessels and may thrombose and weaken them.

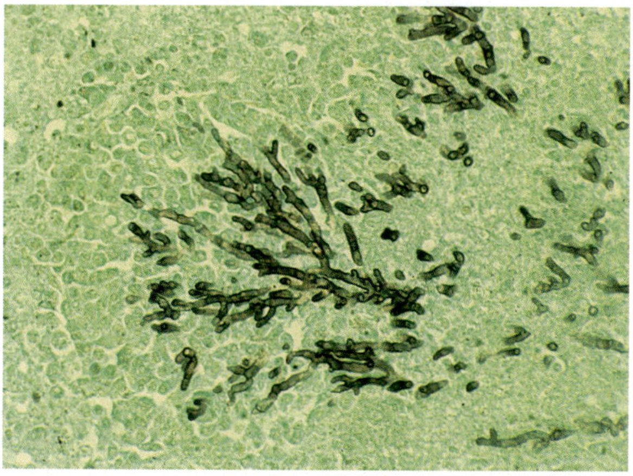

Figure 3.57 This methenamine silver (Grocott) stain illustrates the typical septate branching hyphae of *Aspergillus* species fungi in tissue.

organisms has occurred [400]. There is an extensive literature of case reports and series that detail common and unusual circumstances for *Aspergillus* infections in the nervous system. With respect to *Mucor* and related fungal infections, the portal of entry may be by way of the paranasal sinuses, or the cribriform plate especially (Figures 3.58 and 3.59) in diabetics, leading to necrotizing vasocentric infections in and near the base of the brain [401–403]. *Mucor* infections are notoriously difficult to treat and mortality is high [404]. Identification of the hyphal fungal organism involved can usually be accomplished histologically with the aid of periodic acid-Schiff (PAS) or Grocott's methenamine silver (GMS) staining of paraffin sections. In the case of *Aspergillus*, the hyphae are branching and septate (Figure 3.57). In the case of *Mucor*, hyphae [395] are very large and nonseptate, sometimes being mistaken for capillaries (Figure 3.59). There is usually an inflammatory reaction, with both types of organisms composed of neutrophils, mononuclear cells, and

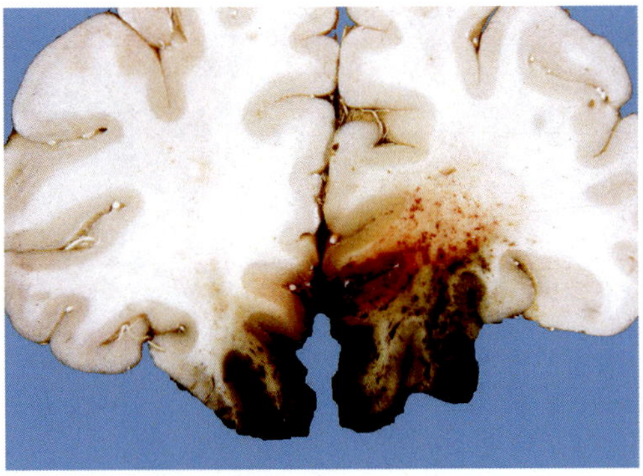

Figure 3.58 This frontal coronal section illustrates a case of mucormycosis, which apparently entered the brain via the cribriform plate in a diabetic individual. Note the hemorrhagic character of the lesion.

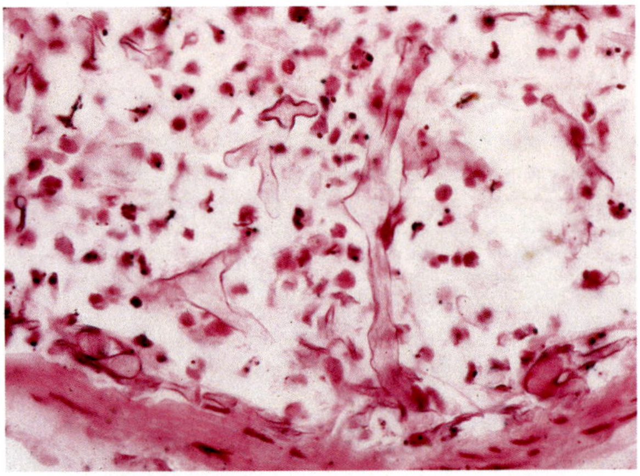

Figure 3.59 This H&E-stained section of meninges contain the large nonseptate hyphae of *Mucor* fungi. The large size of these hyphae may sometimes be mistaken for capillaries.

blood, which surround the affected vessel that may be thrombosed. The degree of inflammatory reaction is variable, dependent upon the capacity of the host to mount a defense, and there may be little or no reaction in some victims.

The yeast-forming organisms (*Cryptococcus* etc.) may elicit a diffuse basal meningitis much like tuberculous meningitis or form multiple cyst-like abscesses in tissue, often the gray matter [396]. When meningitis occurs, there is usually a cloudy, opaque thickening of the basal meninges, not a purulent exudate, which distinguishes it from typical bacterial meningitis (Figure 3.60). Again, the response of the host is variable but is generally intense in the cases of coccidioidomycosis and blastomycosis and more bland in the case of cryptococcosis [405]. When abscesses are formed, they are usually multiple and may have the appearance of foamy spongy cysts in the brain. Histologically, at least in the case of cryptococcosis, the most common yeast infection of the nervous system, there is little or no reaction, and organisms may lie free in the tissue. Cryptococcal yeasts are characterized by their wide capsule and variable spherical shape (Figure 3.61), especially well illustrated

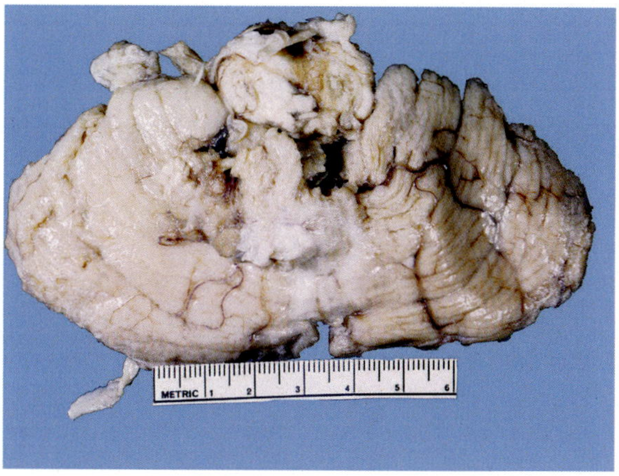

Figure 3.60 This rostral view of the cerebellum from a case of cryptococcal meningitis illustrates the typical creamy thickening of the meninges caused by this organism. From a gross perspective any of the yeast-type fungi can produce a meningitis that is very similar.

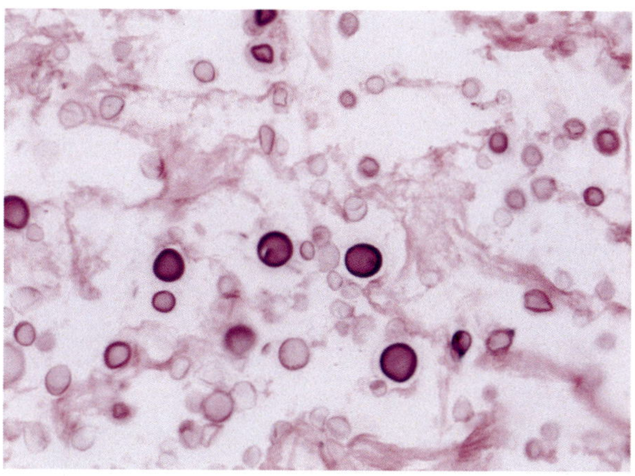

Figure 3.61 This PAS stain demonstrates the typical forms of *Cryptococcus* species fungi in tissue.

in India ink preparations made of suspensions of exudate or CSF [395]. Blastomycosis and coccidioidomycosis also have distinctive appearances, with sporangia filled with microspores being most typical [395]. Histoplasmosis, which is quite common as a benign infection of the lung, is rarely encountered in the brain, where it behaves much like tuberculosis by causing meningitis or, very rarely, brain abscesses [406,407]. It is not always possible to determine viability of the organisms, which is a common question after amphotericin B therapy, and inactivated or dead yeasts may be shed for months into the CSF in a controlled infection, giving the false impression of refractoriness. Detection of yeasts by lumbar CSF examination or culture is often unsuccessful, and cisternal puncture or surgical biopsy of the meninges may be required in life for diagnosis.

Infections with *Candida* species, even though they are not strictly considered fungi taxonomically, are contracted like most of the other fungi, via the respiratory tract, contaminated fluids, drugs, implanted materials, catheters, or instruments, and may or may not occur in the immunocompromised host [397,408]. *Candida* seems to combine features of both the yeasts and hyphal fungi where an abscess may appear grossly little different from a bacterial abscess and may become hemorrhagic. In addition, organisms can infect the walls of arteries, leading to mycotic aneurysms (Figure 3.62). *Candida* species appear to make hyphae but have modified colonial forms and at least morphologically bridge the gap between the yeasts and the purely hyphal organisms and produce abscesses (usually resembling bacterial more than fungal ones), mycotic aneurysms of cerebral and other vessels, and meningitis. Identification of these organisms in ordinary H&E preparations may be difficult, and the organisms are easily missed unless PAS or GMS staining is employed (Figure 3.63) [395].

The sequelae of fungal infection of the nervous system are usually significant (seizures, mental retardation, dementia, hydrocephalus, global or focal neurological deficits, and cranial nerve palsies or blindness), and fatalities are common [396]. The common drugs employed to treat fungal infections are amphotericin B and related compounds. Most of these drugs have potentially severe side effects that include renal, bone marrow, and lung toxicity, which must always be taken into account when anticipating therapy. Many unusual and special circumstances may surround fungal infections in the event that they infect valve prostheses, intravenous tubing, and catheters and implanted materials. Recently an epidemic of fungal meningitis involving hundreds of patients

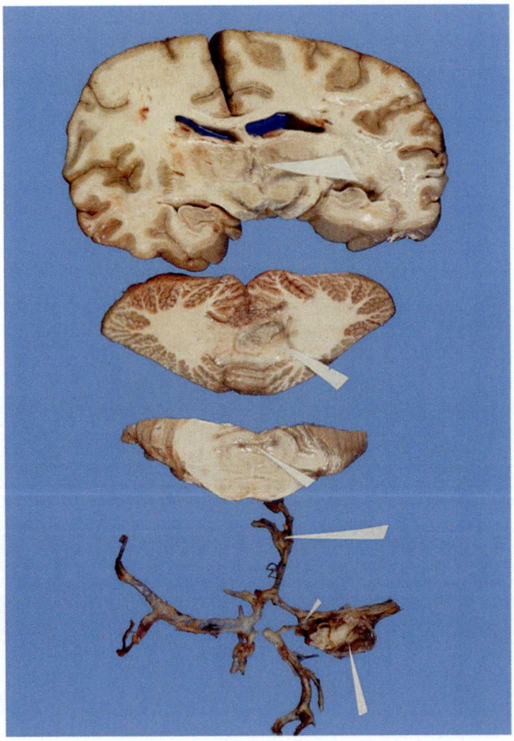

Figure 3.62 This composite gross photograph of the brain and circle of Willis of a victim of *Candida* sepsis illustrates in the brain sections (arrows) multiple abscesses, and in the vessels (arrows) true mycotic aneurysms.

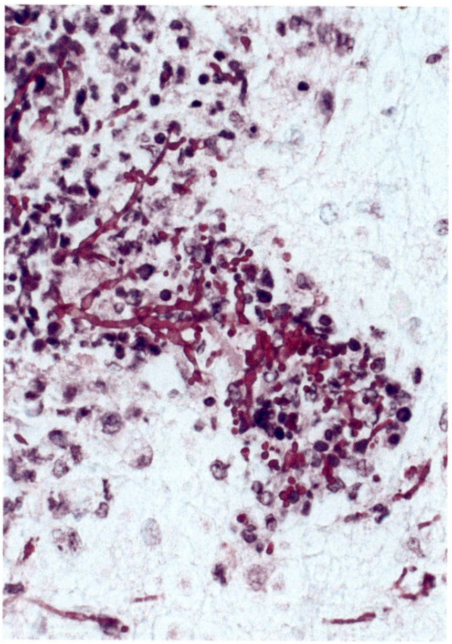

Figure 3.63 This photomicrograph of a focal *Candida* abscess in the brain stained with the PAS stain illustrates the mixed acute and chronic inflammatory response and the complex branching hyphae of the organism with numerous apical blebs, which may appear more or less numerous than the hyphae depending upon the plane of the section.

in several states has been traced to spinal epidural steroid injections with formulations contaminated with *Exserohilum rostratum* and other fungi [398,409,410]. The impact of this incident will have enormous economic consequences and will eventually involve litigation.

Protozoal and Metazoal Diseases

Some of these diseases are discussed in Chapter 4 because they primarily affect children, such as amoebic encephalitis, or have special forensic significance in that age group. Others that affect both infants/children and adults are discussed both in Chapter 4 and below.

Toxoplasmosis

Toxoplasmosis is a far more common disease than generally realized, although systemically, it follows a benign course in most individuals and is seldom diagnosed except in AIDS victims. The typical systemic case is a nonspecific illness resembling influenza or infectious mononucleosis, with fever, lymphadenopathy, and hepatomegaly. The disease is caused by *Toxoplasma gondii*, a protozoan, which is a common parasite of rodents and a frequent resident of the GI tracts of cats and other household pets, from whom humans may contract the disease. Inadequately cooked meat and game animals may also be a source of the organism. The most common form of human toxoplasmosis involves the developing

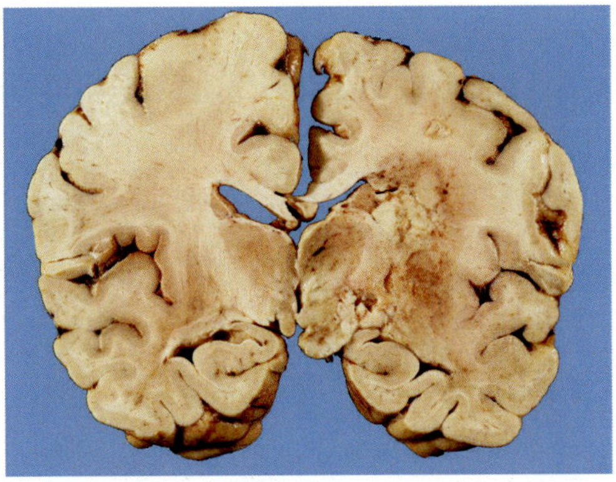

Figure 3.64 This coronal section of the brain of an AIDS victim affected by toxoplasmosis illustrates the typically necrotizing unifocal or multifocal lesions, which, on brain imaging studies, can appear "ring-enhancing" and may mimic brain lymphoma, abscesses, or other conditions.

fetus, usually during the first and second trimesters [411] and has different behavior and manifestations than in the adult.

In the adult who is not immunologically compromised, CNS sequelae are uncommon and rarely diagnosed as toxoplasmosis, but encephalitis, meningitis, and retinitis may be seen. By far, the most common adult host for toxoplasmosis is the AIDS victim. Confusion, both clinically and pathologically, can occur with related or similar organisms that appear very similar to toxoplasmosis, specifically sarcocystis and microsporidiosis [366]. When the CNS of adults is affected, toxoplasmosis will produce multifocal, necrotic, radiologically ring-enhancing cerebral lesions. This latter form is most common and can be devastating in the immunoincompetent person, especially in victims of AIDS [412,413].

In adult cases, the disease is usually a multifocal, hemorrhagic, and necrotizing encephalitis. Imaging studies show ring-enhancing necrotizing lesions that may be difficult to differentiate from primary CNS lymphoma, gliomas, bacterial abscess, and other conditions (Figure 3.64). Often stereotactic biopsy is the most efficient means of obtaining a definitive diagnosis. Histologically, the lesions are necrotizing and sometimes granulomatous, with chronic inflammatory cells in the lesion and cuffing nearby vessels. If they can be found, the so-called cysts are diagnostic [412]. Sometimes, Giemsa stains will reveal organisms free in the tissue, although they are most commonly found in macrophages. An example is illustrated in Figure 4.51 in Chapter 4.

Malaria

Malaria is the most important parasitic disease affecting man in the world. It affects between 200 million and 500 million people and causes 1 million to 3 million deaths each year, mostly in children. The regions most affected are north-central South America, sub-Saharan Africa, and southern Asia and the Indo-Pacific region [414,415]. Virtually every country in the world has malaria victims; sometimes they have contracted the disease locally, but most brought the disease with them when they immigrated or upon returning from foreign travel in epidemic zones. The most serious form of malaria is from the *Plasmodium falciparum* organism, although *Plasmodium vivax*, *Plasmodium ovale*, and *Plasmodium malariae* and occasionally other genera may cause disease, which is usually less severe. The parasites are spread by mosquitoes, usually of the *Anopheles* genera, that carry the sporozoites of the parasite in their salivary glands, the secretion of which enters the victim during biting. The mosquito originally acquires its infestation by biting a parasitized human. Rarely, malaria is contracted through transfusions of parasitized blood [416].

Once the parasitic sporozoites enter the blood, they rapidly infect the liver, where they multiply over a period of a week or two, usually without symptoms. At the end of this time, infected hepatocytes rupture, releasing merozoites, which then infect erythrocytes, where further multiplication and secondary infestation of other red blood cells in several cycles occur, causing the classical symptoms of malaria: fever, sweating, malaise, joint and muscle pain, vomiting, and possibly prostration and seizures. Complications and morbidity arise from hemoglobinuria and renal damage, anemia, and damage to viscera and cerebral vessels by rather complex mechanisms [417,418] that produce ischemia and edema that may prove fatal or leave the victim neurologically compromised [418].

The diagnosis of malaria in a clinical setting involves examination of a blood smear that may reveal parasitized red cells, or various serological and molecular genetic probes may be used [419]. Autopsy examination usually reveals enlarged, congested, and sometimes necrotic liver and spleen with focal hemorrhage. The kidneys may show congestion and tubular necrosis with hemoglobin casts. Grossly, the brain in cases of cerebral malaria will be swollen, congested, and often with petechial hemorrhages at the gray–white matter junctions and in the white matter and microscopically a vasocentric hemorrhage, edema, and necrosis can be seen, as illustrated in Figure 3.65 [420]. Vessels are usually filled with parasitized red cells (Figure 3.66). Those that survive will often have an encephalopathy, movement disorders, seizures, and mental impairment.

From a forensic point of view, in developed countries, malaria is yet another "traveler" that may strike nonimmigrants who have contracted the disease during foreign travel, only to return home after the latent interval of weeks or longer to develop the disease and perhaps die, without a diagnosis being made [421]. Others may have contracted the disease locally in endemic foci, from blood transfusions [416], from shared needles in drug addicts, and from more exotic circumstances [422].

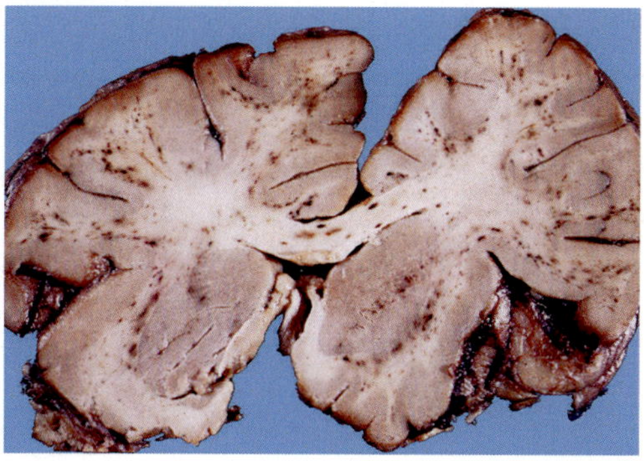

Figure 3.65 This photograph of a coronal section of the frontal region of the brain of a victim of *Plasmodium falciparum* malaria in its cerebral form. Note the innumerable perivascular hemorrhages in the white matter and in the subcortical regions. Sometimes the lesions involve gray matter masses in the cortex of basal ganglia as they do here. The appearance is similar to microembolic phenomenon such as fat and air embolism.

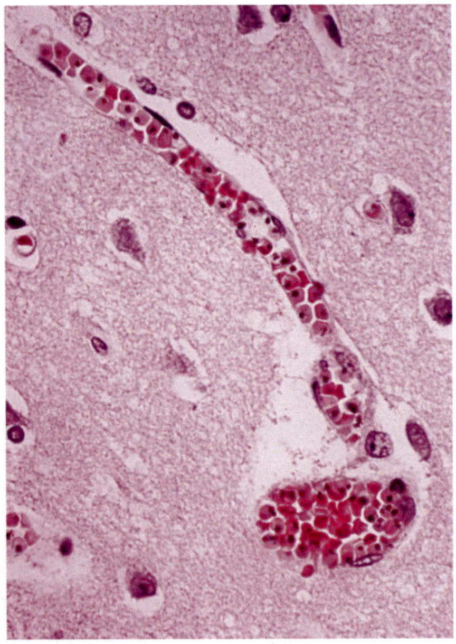

Figure 3.66 This photomicrograph of the cortex of the cerebrum of a victim of *Plasmodium falciparum* malaria. Note the capillary that is distended with parasitized erythrocytes adherent to the vessel wall and, in the lower part of the photograph, which have bled into the perivascular space.

Helminthic and Other Parasitic Diseases

CNS parasites are far more common in less developed parts of the world than in the United States, and it therefore often comes as a surprise when a case is encountered. Probably the most common form of parasitic disease that affects the nervous system in the United States is cysticercosis [423], but occasionally other less common helminthic infections, such as echinococcosis [424], schistosomiasis [425], and paragonimiasis [424], will affect the nervous system, although other organ systems are more classicially and commonly affected. The helminthic diseases ordinarily do not affect native-born residents, and most cases are found in individuals who have recently come to North America or have traveled to portions of the world in which these diseases are common. Given the vast number of immigrants from all corners of the globe who come to live in North America and Western Europe, it is probably only a matter of time before every pathologist encounters one or more of these "tropical" diseases. Because of its often cryptic character, neuroparasitism may be discovered by a forensic pathologist in cases of unexpected death and sometimes in accidental deaths.

Cysticercosis

Cysticercosis is produced by the larval form (*Cysticercus cellulosae*) of the pork tapeworm, *Taenia solium* [426]. The organism is not contracted by eating infected pork but, rather, by ingesting matter contaminated by feces of swine and other animals that have the tapeworm and that are shedding proglottids of the worm from their GI tracts or by autoinfection. The

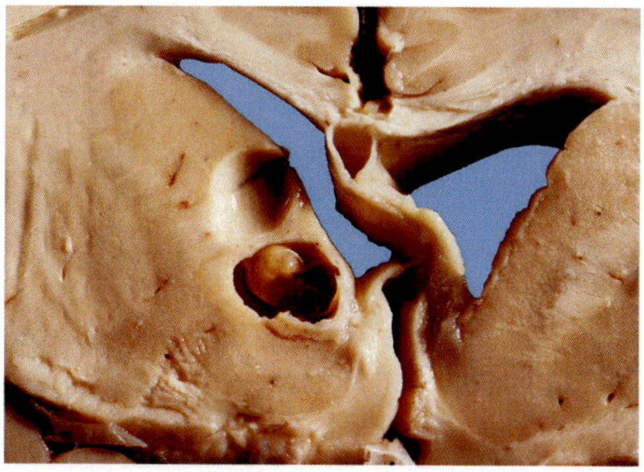

Figure 3.67 This photograph of the ventricular chambers and basal ganglia of a victim of cysticercosis infestation of the brain. There are characteristically many cysts throughout the brain, brain stem, and sometimes the cord, ventricular cavities, and even the meninges. In this instance, remains of the parasite are found in the lower cyst.

ingested parasites enter the GI tract, develop, and penetrate the wall of the gut to enter the systemic circulation, carrying the larvae to all parts of the body, including skeletal muscle and brain [423,427].

The developing larvae may be found within the brain (Figure 3.67), meninges, or ventricular cavities. When in the brain, the larvae produce multiple small cysts with inverted scolexes and a cuticular wall, which eventually become isolated by a glial and fibrous tissue reaction in the brain. Often the parasite is fragmented, but portions of the cuticle remain and are strongly PAS positive [424]. Apparently little inflammation or reaction is obvious until the parasite dies, at which time inflammatory responses and attendant edema magnify the functional size of the lesion and cause symptoms, which can be those of a brain or spinal tumor, or meningitis or encephalitis, and include headache, seizures, and focal or generalized neurological signs [428]. Cases of sudden unexpected death have been reported due to cysticercosis [429]. When the meninges or ventricles are involved, the parasites form opaque globular or grape-like (racemose) clusters of organisms 3 to 10 mm in diameter, which may obstruct CSF flow, causing hydrocephalus, or may impinge on the brain stem or spinal cord. Involvement may be diffuse and produce a spectrum of local and generalized symptoms. Treatment usually involves surgical removal of the most troublesome cysts, but a number of antihelminthic drugs may also be employed, although there are complications from these agents [430].

Viral Infections of the CNS

The viruses that affect the nervous system are numerous, and a complete discussion of all the issues involved in viral pathogenesis is left to other sources. Most of the relevant specific viral infections are discussed in Chapter 4 and will not be redescribed here.

Pathogenesis of Viral Infections in the CNS

Viruses may enter the nervous system by many routes, some of which are novel and unique to the nervous system [367,431]. The most familiar routes are via the respiratory tract and the GI or urogenital tracts, where initial replication of the agent may take place in local lymphoid tissues, as in the enterovirus infections (poliovirus etc.), which replicate in the upper GI or pharyngeal–tonsillar lymphoid tissues. They may also enter the blood in a viremic phase or inside macrophages and other inflammatory cells and enter the brain via the choroid plexus and CSF, or they may infect endothelial cells and gain entrance to the extracellular space of the brain by that route and eventually infect susceptible cells (neurons or glia). Direct inoculation of the virus into the blood by an insect or tick vector may occur, as in the so-called arboviruses (arthropod-borne viruses), which produce the equine encephalitides, tick fever, La Crosse encephalitis, West Nile encephalitis, and similar diseases [432,433]. Other mechanisms include traumatic inoculation of the infecting virus into tissue (as in rabies) by means of an animal bite, with local replication and infection of nerve terminals, followed by retrograde transport of the virus intra-axonally by axoplasmic transport to the dorsal root ganglia and spinal cord, where another phase of replication may occur, followed by further spread cell to cell or via extracellular space to other cells [434]. An even more novel means of infection is found in herpes simplex virus infections, where a previous infection has implanted latent viral genomes in the dorsal root ganglion or cranial nerve ganglia, which will periodically awaken in response to stress, other infection, ultraviolet irradiation of the skin, and immunosuppression to cause a new outbreak of viral replication and pathology [435]. The process of viral replication and the events that must occur if infection is to take place are highly complex and only partially understood. They first involve the process of adsorption of the virus to the cell membrane of the target cell, then envelopment by phagocytosis or endocytosis. Once the virus is inside the host cell, uncoating and interaction of the various protein, glycoprotein, and nucleic acid components with cell organelles occur, leading to control of the host cell metabolism. Conversion to viral component synthesis then takes place. Eventually, assembly of the viral components, transport to the cell surface, envelopment and packaging of the viral particle, and budding or release of the infectious particle into the environment occur [367].

The replicative process is usually far from efficient, and many errors can arise, leading to failure to release organisms or release of defective particles. One of the effects of inefficiency, which may approach 90% in some infections such as herpesvirus infections (herpes simplex, cytomegalovirus, varicella-zoster virus, etc.), is the formation of inclusion bodies, which are welcome aids in diagnosis to the pathologist. Other errors in viral replication may result in abortive or latent infections or to viral persistence, as in subacute sclerosing panencephalitis (SSPE—measles), or herpes simplex [431]. Sometimes the interaction of host defenses in the form of interferon production, complement reactions, or cellular or humoral immune reactions will modify or magnify the effects of the viral infection, further confusing an already complex process. Why certain cells or systems of cells are preferentially or exclusively infected and killed by the virus, as in the tropism for the motor system neurons by the poliovirus, is not well understood but frequently observed in CNS virus infections [367].

Pathological Reactions to Viral Infection in the CNS

Viruses can cause infection anywhere in the nervous system and produce meningitis, polioencephalitis–myelitis (involvement of the gray matter) or leukoencephalitis (involvement of the white matter), neuritis, radiculitis, or panencephalitis (all elements of the brain affected). The most common neural tissue reaction to viral infection is a chronic inflammatory infiltrate in the area and perivascular cuffing of lymphoid cells. Another common reaction, which is very helpful in suggesting viral etiology, is the formation of the glial nodules or inflammatory nodule (sometimes also called glial star, or Babes nodes) [367]. This is a small cluster of inflammatory cells or reactive glial cells that can be found in gray or white matter (Figure 3.68). Usually inflammatory nodules contain viral antigens and probably represent a focus of reaction to viral concentration. The inflammatory nodule is not specific for any particular virus but can be seen with infections produced by virtually all of them and in rickettsia infections as well. Inflammatory nodules may persist in the brain for years after the obvious pathology has long since faded, which implies that some viral replication is still going on but to a limited degree. Inclusion bodies, discussed briefly above, which are a helpful diagnostic aid, may be produced in the cytoplasm (typically rabies virus—Negri body, as illustrated in Figure 4.46 in Chapter 4) or in the nucleus (typically in herpesvirus infections, SSPE, and papovavirus infections, as illustrated in Figure 4.45 in Chapter 4). The changes in neural tissue in addition to, or apart from, focal inflammation may be virtually nonexistent and result in severe destruction and cavitation or more subtle changes, such as spongiosus, neuronal loss, or demyelination. Viral infections can produce malformations in developing neural tissue (see Chapter 4) and may even produce tumors [324,326,413]. The following diseases are reviewed for their relevance to the forensic pathologist and are by no means the only important viral infections of the nervous system.

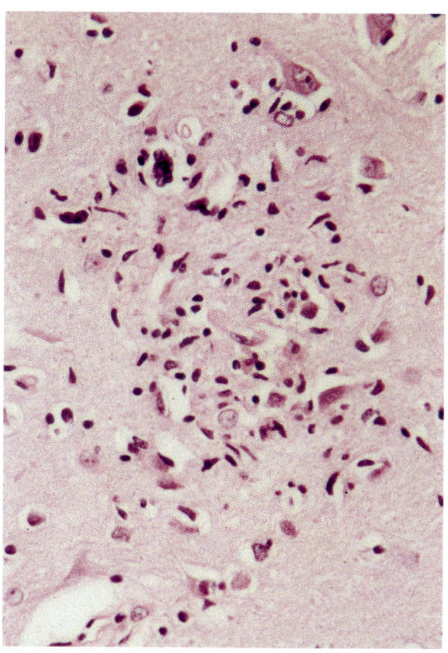

Figure 3.68 This photomicrograph is taken from the brain of a victim of AIDS and illustrates the frequent finding of "glial" or inflammatory nodules in the brain, in this case, gray matter. The nodule is composed of activating microglial cells and astrocytes with often a minor capillary component and usually a scattering of lymphoid cells and sometimes fused inflammatory cells. Such nodules are not specific for any particular viral disease, having been seen in many of them that affect the brain. In this case, it cannot be known if the HIV agent is responsible or a superinfection by another virus.

Human Immunovirus and Acquired Immune Deficiency Syndrome

This condition, shown to the satisfaction of most scientists, is caused by an RNA-containing virus, a so-called retrovirus, now referred to as HIV (HIV-1 and HIV-2, with the most common and virulent being HIV-1), that eventually in most cases effectively destroys the cellular immune system (CD4+ T cells) and allows opportunistic infections of many types to affect the victim. Many organ systems can be affected, but the nervous system is one of the most damaged by the condition and its complications.

First recognized in 1981, the number of cases recorded in 1984 was in excess of 3000 confirmed victims, and by 1986, probably more than 13,000 were known to be suffering from the disease in the United States. As of 2006, the Joint United Nations Program on HIV/AIDS had estimated that in the United States about 1.2 million persons are living with HIV infection, with 70% or more receiving antiretroviral therapy. It is estimated that about 2.8 million persons have died of the disease worldwide and that between 33 million and 46 million persons are afflicted with HIV but have not yet died. AIDS is found in every country of the world but is especially concentrated in Namibia, Botswana, and neighboring countries in Africa, where infection rate estimates may have reached 50% of the populations. The impact on these societies is devastating.

The individuals at greatest risk for HIV infection in most Western countries are homosexual or bisexual men who may or may not be intravenous drug users and who are between 20 and 30 years of age. In Africa, on the other hand, most cases appear to affect heterosexual individuals, their spouses, and their children. Although transfusions and accidental infections of health care workers occasionally occur, such cases are relatively uncommon. The widespread HIV testing and multidrug antiretroviral treatment regimens, when they are available and employed, have significantly altered the formerly nearly fatal outcome of HIV infection, especially in Western countries, with large numbers of individuals living nearly normal lives, and some appear to have completely cleared themselves of the HIV agent [413].

When HIV status is not discovered and AIDS develops, it presents insidiously, often with a rather bland illness consisting of lymphadenopathy, fever, malaise, and other minimal symptoms, which, clustered together, are now known as the AIDS-related complex. AIDS itself usually begins with a chronic pneumonia due to *Pneumocystis carinii* (more than half the cases), with the signs of Kaposi sarcoma (26% of cases) or with an encephalitis, myelitis, or retinitis caused by herpes simplex, herpes zoster, cytomegalovirus, toxoplasmosis, papovaviruses, tuberculosis, or fungal infection, and probably many others [412,436]. Because of virally induced lack of function of CD4+ T (helper) lymphocytes and an unopposed function of T-suppressor lymphocytes, an effective humoral immune response cannot be mounted. Work on determining the etiological agent(s) since 1981 has resulted in determination of the genome of the virus and a great deal of knowledge about how it produces disease. The agent appears to have originated in the Congo, with cases as far back as 1959 having been shown to contain the agent [437].

The viral agent apparently has a low virulence and can be inactivated by sterilization and common disinfecting solutions, including benzalkonium chloride (Zephiran®) and hypochlorite [412]. In performing an autopsy on an AIDS victim, one should exercise the same caution as in an infectious hepatitis case or a case of Creutzfeldt–Jakob disease and be very conscious of technique to avoid accidental injury.

The neuropathology of AIDS and related disorders appeared to rest until recently with the complication, already mentioned, of opportunistic viral, fungal, mycobacterial, and

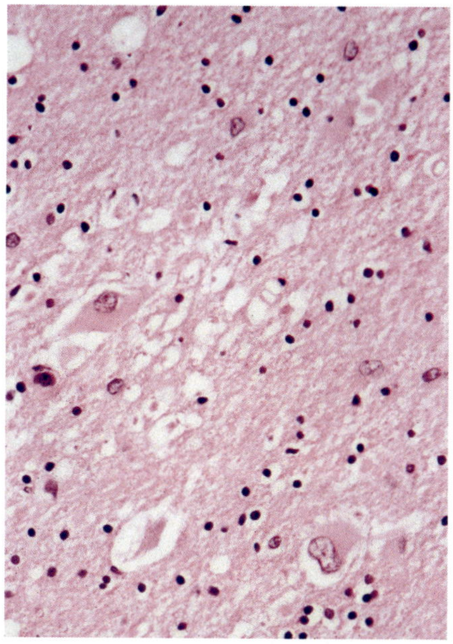

Figure 3.69 This high-power photomicrograph of the white matter in an AIDS victim shows a focal lesion in which HIV may be demonstrated and presumably caused by the agent. Typically seen are foci of vacuolating edema, hypertrophic astrocytes, scattered microglia, and sometimes small giant cells. Axons that are injured by the lesion will show ballooning as they do here.

parasitic infections, which are discussed above and below. It now appears that the brain is directly infected by the AIDS virus (illustrated in Figures 3.68 and 3.69) [413,438], possibly leading to complex neurological dysfunctions mediated by microglia and secreted inflammatory mediators [435]. This commonly leads to dementia of some degree. Direct infection has also been implicated in a demyelinating condition of the spinal cord. A hallmark of AIDS in the brain appears to be accumulation of inflammatory giant cells in perivascular sites in the brain.

The forensic implications of AIDS are many. When HIV infection apparently occurs in conjunction with medical treatments, such as transfusions, immunizations, or drug administration with contaminated needles or other devices; by accident or design of a health care worker perpetrator; by intentional or wanton infection in a correctional institution by another inmate; or by infection during a crime, the forensic pathologist may become involved in the legal process. Owing to the delay in appearance of symptoms and manifestations of AIDS, the autopsy may only confirm the obvious, yet these cases must be analyzed carefully and professionally. On rare occasion, deaths may occur because of the complications or effects of AIDS, in which case the forensic pathologist may be called upon to elucidate the circumstances of death and may require the advice and counsel of a neuropathologist.

Herpes Simplex Encephalitis

Herpes simplex virus type I is a relatively common cause of viral encephalitis in the adult population. Usually the affected individual has had numerous episodes of cold sores in

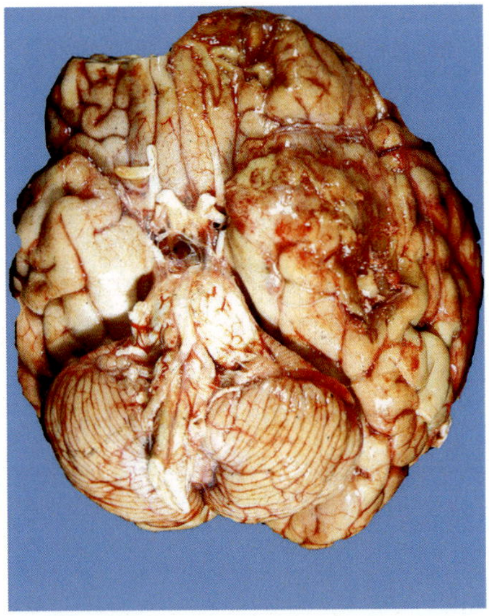

Figure 3.70 This gross photograph of the brain of a victim of herpes simplex encephalitis illustrates the necrotizing and hemorrhagic character of this "lobar" encephalitis.

the past. Occasionally, the individual may be immunocompromised by virtue of an HIV infection but may also have been treated with steroids for a variety of diseases, or, most commonly, there is no particularly significant antecedent event. The disease may begin with or without dermal herpes and may present as a nonspecific illness with headache and other relatively nonspecific neurological symptoms, which may progress rapidly to a typical encephalitis picture, with prostration and seizures. The disease tends to localize to one or more lobes of the brain, typically the temporal lobes, where a hemorrhagic and necrotizing infection is manifest (Figure 3.70). Microscopically infected neurons and glia may contain typical intranuclear Cowdry type A inclusions. In recent years, prompt diagnosis and treatment with acyclovir and its variants have resulted in a higher percentage of survivors than in the past, in which the disease was either fatal or devastated the victim with disabling neurological sequelae. Because of the often bilateral temporal lobe destruction, sufferers may become victims of the Kluever–Bucy syndrome, in which no new long-term memory can be stored [367,431]. A further discussion of herpes simplex infections can be found in Chapter 4.

Epstein–Barr Virus Infection

Epstein–Barr virus infection is most commonly encountered in infectious mononucleosis, Burkitt lymphoma, and apparently in some nasopharyngeal carcinomas. At least 50% of individuals older than 18 years of age have antibodies to the agent, and despite this immunity, there is evidence that once infected, an individual harbors the virus for life [439]. The infection may be spread by kissing and other intimate interpersonal contact but can also be transmitted via infected mononuclear cells in blood transfusions. Neurological involvement with Epstein–Barr virus (EBV) is uncommon but has been implicated in the Landry–Guillain–Barré syndrome, in Bell palsy, and in rare cases of myelitis and encephalitis [440]. It is possible that at least some of the CNS pathology in AIDS is due to EBV. Fatalities are rare, and most neuropathologists have little experience with the pathology of the EBV-induced neurological disease. The diagnosis is usually made serologically and sometimes virologically with recovery of the agent.

Progressive Multifocal Leukoencephalopathy

PML, first described by Åstrøm, Mancall, and Richardson in 1958 [440,441], is caused by a DNA-containing group B papovavirus commonly referred to as the J-C virus, which was predicted but not recovered from case material until 1971 [442]. The disease occurs usually as an opportunistic infection in immunosuppressed or debilitated hosts, usually lymphoma patients and now most recently in AIDS patients. PML does occur occasionally in apparently normal individuals and may be mistaken for a brain tumor radiologically, grossly, and microscopically. The clinical onset of the disease is usually insidious, without fever or any of the usual signs of infection. Early symptoms may be confusion, dementia, aphasia, cortical blindness (usually with denial or lack of appreciation of visual difficulty—Anton's syndrome), ataxia, and behavioral abnormalities. Sometimes there are signs of increased intracranial pressure, headache, and seizures. The CSF is usually normal, and the CT scan may or may not show multifocal lesions of the white matter. The diagnosis of PML may be suspected clinically but frequently is only made at operation or postmortem examination.

Lesions of PML may be found anywhere in the nervous system, with a lesser involvement of the brain stem and cord. The lesions are relatively confined to the white matter, which has a moth-eaten or crumbly granular appearance (Figure 3.71), and the size of the lesions varies from multiple, small, barely visible foci to devastated large areas of the cerebral white matter (centrum ovale). Particularly severe or long-standing lesions may be cavitary. In large myelin-stained paraffin or celloidin sections of the brain, the multifocal character of the lesions is very evident. Histologically, the most prominent reaction is a bizarre transformation of astroglia into pseudoneoplastic cells (Figure 3.72). Sometimes intense inflammation with mononuclear cells, a macrophage response, and usually numerous grossly enlarged oligodendroglia bearing red or purple intranuclear inclusions without a perinuclear halo, as seen in Cowdry type A inclusions, are found. The meninges may show lymphoid infiltrates, and the gray matter is usually only incidentally

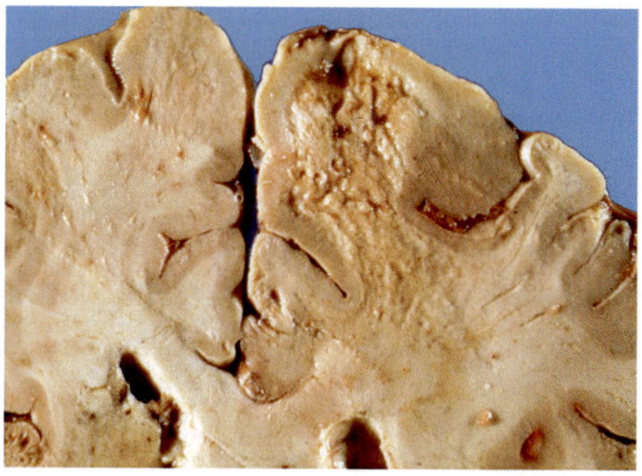

Figure 3.71 This photograph is of a portion of the vertex of the brain in an AIDS victim with PML. Note the typical crumbly or "moth-eaten" appearance of the white matter and only focally the cerebral cortex.

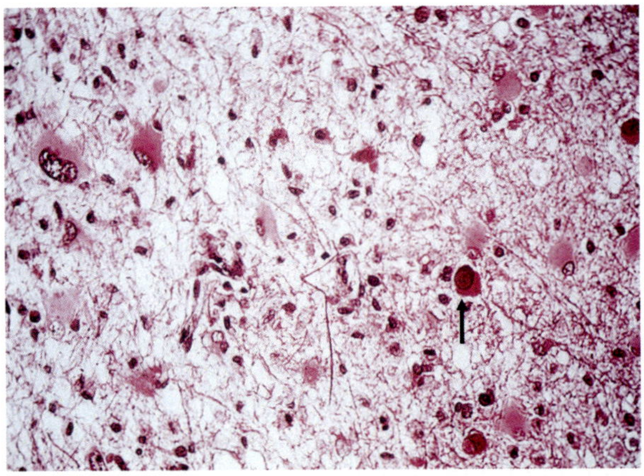

Figure 3.72 This photomicrograph of a PML lesion illustrates one of the many histological appearances that the lesions can have depending upon their age. In this case, bizarre reactive astrocytes with nuclear atypicalities as well as more typical "gemistocytic" astrocytes are common. Very commonly seen, and a helpful diagnostic feature, are the large swollen oligodendrocytes whose nuclei are distended with viral components (arrow).

affected, with most of the changes found in the white matter. Ultrastructural examination usually reveals the characteristic paracrystalline arrays of virions, first described by Zu Rhein [442]. In some older cases, inclusions may have to be searched for but can usually be located. The disease may persist for weeks or months but is usually a final fatal complication of the underlying neoplastic disease. The J-C virus is an oncogenic virus in animals and has been implicated in a few cases of human primary brain lymphoma [325] and in a few unusual cases of multifocal astrocytomas associated with PML lesions [367]. In the forensic setting, especially in cases of AIDS, PML is often an unexpected finding, but this disease is so unique that it should be known to most pathologists. Clinical–pathological correlations may often be possible to explain antemortem neurological deficits. The disease is not thought to be dangerous to personnel because the agent, J-C virus, appears to be ubiquitous in the environment, anyway, and most individuals have antibodies to it by middle age.

Infections by Unconventional Agents

The concept of unconventional or atypical infectious agents that all produce a spongiform encephalopathy has developed with the discovery that several animal and human degenerative diseases appear to be caused by agents, the molecular biology of which are unusual. The transmissible character of these diseases was first established in Kuru, a disease for the Fore people in Papua New Guinea that appears to be have been spread by ritual cannibalism [443]. These agents, which have come to be known as prions and to cause the spongiform encephalopathies, are physically very small, probably composed of a relatively simple molecule or molecules of low weight (on the order of 60,000 to 100,000, or even smaller) without any nucleic acids [444,445]. Recent data suggest that genes for the prion proteins (now referred to as PrP) exist in apparently normal cells, but little is known about how they got there and what controls the expression of protein replication, the replicative protein apparently being infectious in an unconventional and novel way [431,446,447].

The animal disease most commonly associated with an unconventional agent infection is scrapie, an infection in sheep and goats. Aleutian mink disease, thought for a time to be a separate disease, is probably simply scrapie in the mink, contracted by feeding infected sheep carcasses to minks [446]. Most recently, bovine spongiform encephalopathy (BSE; mad cow disease) [448] and chronic wasting disease in deer and elk [449,450] have been shown to be caused by the same PrP infections. Human counterparts of prion disease include Kuru, Creutzfeldt–Jakob disease (CJD), Gerstmann–Sträussler–Scheinker syndrome [451], familial fatal insomnia [452], and what appears to be crossover BSE or variant CJD [453,454]. What at one time were an arcane disease of cannibals in New Guinea (Kuru) and a rare dementing disease in Germany and elsewhere (CJD) have almost become household words with the discovery of BSE and human crossover cases. Episodic discovery of BSE in domestic American and Canadian cattle remains a mystery and is responsible for an impact on beef and meat product exports.

Creutzfeldt–Jakob Disease

Since the original descriptions of Creutzfeldt–Jakob disease in 1921, most neuropathologists in all parts of the world have come to know the disease well from their own case material [454]. Creutzfeldt–Jakob disease (CJD; not to be confused with J-C virus of PML) is characterized clinically by the insidious onset of dementia, which progresses rapidly and may be associated with weakness, visual difficulties, ataxia, and, in the late phase of the disease, myoclonic jerks, and a bedfast vegetative state. There is considerable clinical variability from case to case, leading some to question the validity of CJD as an entity. The course may be as brief as a few months or as long as several years, the average being less than 12 months. There are no symptoms of inflammation, fever, meningitis, or encephalitis, and the disease resembles a degenerative disease. Laboratory studies are usually within normal limits.

There is no obvious visceral pathology, and the gross findings in the brain are subtle, perhaps only slight convolutional atrophy and on cut section a tendency for atrophy and a brownish discoloration of the caudate nucleus and putamen. Sometimes the cerebellum is atrophic as well. The microscopic finding now most commonly associated with CJD is a spongiform encephalopathy (Figure 3.73) of the gray matter with neuronal dropout and replacement gliosis in the cerebral cortex of the frontal and temporal lobes, caudate, putamen, and other basal ganglia structures. This appearance is very similar to that of the other spongiform encephalopathies. Nuclear masses in the upper brain stem and cerebellum may be similarly affected. Amyloid deposits may be found in some forms of the disease. The major histological change has given rise to a descriptive name for CJD and related diseases—subacute spongiform encephalopathy—which many now find more attractive than the eponym. Spongiosus is not always demonstrable, however, and many of the early cases did not show this feature [454]. Ultrastructural examination in such cases, however, will usually demonstrate vacuolization in neuronal cell bodies and dendrites. There is usually no inflammation, and at times neuronal loss may be subtle. There are no inclusion bodies or other characteristic bodies in neurons, such as the Lewy body of Parkinson's disease or the neurofibrillary tangle of AD. Occasional cases of CJD may show amyloid (Kuru) plaques in the cerebellum and elsewhere [455].

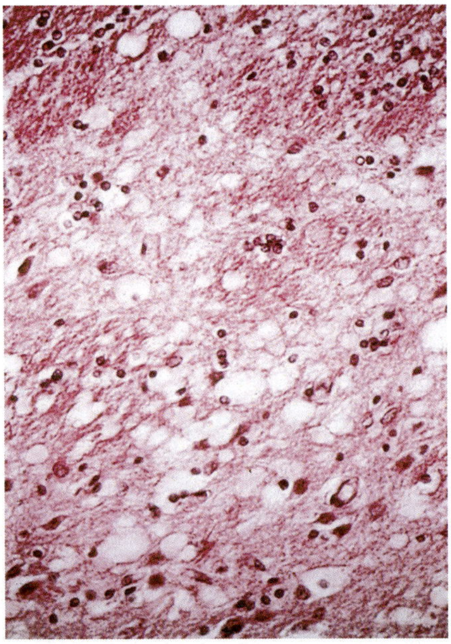

Figure 3.73 This photomicrograph of a portion of the brain of a victim of Kuru illustrates the spongiform character of the histopathology of the condition and differs little between the various other spongiform encephalopathies such as Creutzfeldt–Jakob disease and its subtypes, or BSE. Amyoid plaques may also be seen in all of these conditions but are not depicted here. (Courtesy of Dr. D.C. Gajdusek and Dr. J. Gibbs, National Institutes of Health, Washington, DC.)

The most important aspect of CJD to the forensic pathologist is its mode of transmission, or if it was spontaneous, if this can be known or discovered. Genetic sequencing of PrP has revealed a number of specific codons that seem to correlate with the form of the disease [446,447]. Features of the infectious agent raises several medical–legal issues and concerns among morticians, pathologists, dieners, and laboratory workers regarding possible work-related contraction of the disease [456,457]. In any case, the material isolated and extracts of tissues from CJD cases indicate that the prions are not readily inactivated by formalin or routine sterilization and are found in all organs of the body, but they are most concentrated in neural tissues [456–458]. Excreta, secretions, hair, and skin from victims are apparently not infectious. The mode of transmission of the disease is not known, but about 10% of cases appear to be familial. CJD has reached the public consciousness through reports of now more than 400 tragic cases involving iatrogenic, primarily human-to-human transmission of the disease, generally in connection with implantation of banked tissues that were contaminated [459]. The first incident of this type involved transmission of CJD from a victim to the recipient of a corneal transplant about 2 years after the operation [459]. Apparently, the physicians who obtained the eyes from the donor had no knowledge of CJD and unwittingly performed an experiment of nature. Additional incidents involved transmission of the disease to several patients in Switzerland via the reuse of cerebral electrodes that had been thought sterilized by formalin vapor after studies had been performed on a CJD patient [460,461]. The use of postmortem-derived pituitary glands for the extraction of human growth hormone has been halted because of apparent contamination of these pooled tissues by CJD agents. There have been some fears expressed for transmission of the disease by transfusions [461]. These cases corroborate the experimental findings in animals concerning resistance of the agent to sterilization, the infectivity of neural tissues, and implantation of inoculation as a mode of transmission of the disease [458].

There is widespread concern among pathologists, technicians, nursing personnel, and morticians about handling CJD material, which has extended to a fear about handling tissue from any dementing or unclassified neurological disease. These fears appear to be groundless because those individuals who have the greatest exposure to cases of this sort—neuropathologists, neurosurgeons, and neurologists—have not been known to be affected by the disease. Most neuropathologists have examined scores of CJD and related types of cases with no known ill effect. Furthermore, there does not appear to be any greater-than-expected incidence of CJD among health care workers, either. Thus, refusal to autopsy a suspected CJD case is not only scientifically unfounded but also an abrogation of professional responsibility. A protocol of precautions [462] for handling and disposing of CJD and suspected CJD material has been developed and consists of care in performing the autopsy, analogous to the care used in an infectious hepatitis case (wearing gowns, gloves, and masks), care not to spill or spread blood and other tissue materials, and careful cleaning of instruments and table after the autopsy. Instruments and materials coming into contact with blood and tissues of CJD patients should be soaked and washed in a dilute solution of hypochlorite (common laundry bleach or Clorox), which rapidly inactivates the agent. Care should be taken not to leave the instruments for several hours or more in hypochlorite solutions, as corrosion may result. Ordinary sterilization is not effective, but longer times, higher temperatures, and higher pressures than normally employed in steam sterilizers will sterilize instruments. Formalin may decrease infectivity but will not eliminate it; thus, brain crocks, when reused, should be cleaned with hypochlorite solution. Tissue may be retained in formalin, but when it is discarded, it should be labeled as infectious and incinerated. Paraffin blocks may be infectious, and care should be taken in cutting and trimming them to avoid cuts. A prudent measure would be to avoid doing frozen sections of suspected CJD tissues and to process CJD tissues separately from other autopsy materials and then to wash containers with hypochlorite. One should avoid the possibility of exposure to CJD material by refraining from eating, drinking, or smoking around microtomes, autopsy instruments, or other potentially contaminated items, because the greatest danger lies in the unsuspected case [462]. It might also be prudent to section paraffin blocks and stain sections at the end of the workday and then discard solutions and to clean containers, microtomes, and work areas with hypochlorite solution as a precaution. It seems unlikely, but it is possible, that prepared and stained sections might retain infectivity, although there would seem little danger in handling or storing such materials.

Parainfectious Brain Diseases

A number of conditions that accompany or appear to accompany infections may affect the nervous system. At one time, before vaccines for rabies and some other diseases were perfected, immune reactions could devastate the nervous system, but these issues have been ameliorated by elimination of foreign antigens and more modern vaccine technology. There are examples of diseases that, although relatively uncommon or rare, may from time to time come to the attention of the forensic services.

Acute Hemorrhagic Encephalitis of Hurst

Acute hemorrhagic encephalitis of Hurst is a fulminating, usually fatal disease now considered to be a CNS manifestation of a generalized Schwartzman reaction but that may be directly related to an infectious organism itself. The syndrome may follow mild upper respiratory infection, influenza, viral enteritis, Epstein-Barr virus infection, an attack of ulcerative colitis, acute glomerulonephritis, immunization, treatment with sulfa or other drugs, or exposure to other environmental allergens [463–467]. At a variable interval after a prior infection or other circumstance listed above, there is an abrupt onset of fever, lethargy, prostration, unconsciousness, coma, and death. These symptoms may evolve in a matter of hours. Grossly, the brain is swollen, with punctate or larger hemorrhages on the surface, and there may be SAH. All these changes may be seen in various imaging studies as well [466]. Cut section reveals a diffusely hemorrhagic, flea-bitten appearance in the white matter mostly that resembles acute fulminant herpes simplex encephalitis. Microscopically, the hemorrhages are perivascular and affect smaller vessels. There may be intravascular coagulation and thrombosis, but inflammation is minimal or absent. The mechanism of this process is thought to be mediated via endotoxin activation of the complement chain, producing a toxic necrosis of endothelium, and can be duplicated in experimental animals by two intravenous injections of bacterial endotoxins 24 hours apart. Another possible mechanism involves a so-called hyperacute cellular immune response [467].

Landry–Guillain–Barré Syndrome

Landry–Guillain–Barré (LGB) syndrome is characterized by rapid or slowly progressive, usually ascending paralysis of limbs, and the muscles of respiration, the face, and the eyes may also be affected. The progression usually abates after 2 to 3 weeks, and recovery begins a week or two afterward, with a descending recovery of function. The symptoms are usually motor only, but sensory loss may also occur. The disease may or may not be febrile. The cerebrospinal fluid (CSF) usually shows high and rising protein but a low cell count. Consciousness is not lost unless there is respiratory failure with no external support. Some patients have autonomic dysfunctions that include tachycardia, cardiac arrhythmias, hypotension or hypertension, and vasomotor disturbances. Reflexes are absent, and all clinical signs are thought to be due to peripheral nerve involvement, not CNS involvement [469]. Sometimes the disease is confused with acute poliomyelitis. Treatment is symptomatic and may include steroid therapy, with some improvement but also a greater likelihood of relapse than in untreated individuals. Recently, plasma exchange seemed to benefit some victims. The mortality rate is between 2% and 6%, and about 15% of cases suffer some neurological deficit after recovery [470]. Complications of LGB include respiratory paralysis and failure, decubitae, pulmonary embolism, genitourinary and respiratory tract infections, peptic ulcer, fluid electrolyte imbalances, and other consequences of being bedfast and immobilized.

The disease tends to occur more in the winter than other times of the year and is most likely to affect individuals 40 years of age and older, with no gender difference. The incidence is up to 2 cases per 100,000 population, and thousands of cases have been reported or discussed in the literature [469–471]. About 75% of cases have a history of a recent prior infection, usually viral, but antecedent events may include bacterial infection (mycoplasmal, *Campylobacter*, and others), vaccination or immunization, trauma or surgical procedures, collagen-vascular disease, and systemic malignancy [470,471]. Most recent public awareness of LGB syndrome has come as a result of alleged complications of the 1976 and later immunization programs to protect against an anticipated swine flu or avian flu epidemic that may or may not be factitious [472,473]. The disease is thought to be caused by cellular immunity to peripheral nerve gangliosides (GM1, GM1b, GD1a, and others) from similarities in bacterial components to nerve components [474].

There is no obvious gross pathology in most cases of LGB because most individuals will die of infection or complications of respiratory paralysis or respirator dependence. Microscopically, the lesions may be very hard to demonstrate or may include diffuse lymphoid infiltrates around vessels and within nerves and patchy demyelination or evidence of remyelination in spinal or cranial nerve roots, in dorsal root ganglia, or at any segment of the intraspinal or extraspinal peripheral nerves. In some cases where repeated episodes of immune-mediated demyelination and repair have occurred, "onion bulbs" or myelin whorls may be seen. To be sure that lesions are present, sometimes extensive dissection of the spinal cord, its roots, and attached plexuses and peripheral nerves is necessary, with numerous histological sections employing not only H&E but also nerve fiber stains (Bielschowsky, Bodian, etc.) and myelin stains (Luxol Fast Blue or Woelcke) in cross- and longitudinal sections [475]. Electron microscopy of nerves may also be helpful. The workup of suspected LGB cases is complex and time-consuming but must be thorough. Professional neuropathological consultation should be sought.

Degenerative Diseases of the Nervous System

Neurological degenerative diseases are the most enigmatic of CNS diseases because there is great clinical and pathological diversity, complexity, no unifying etiology, and usually no treatment other than symptomatic therapy for any of the conditions. The concern of the forensic pathologist for these conditions is indirect, because they form a group of natural conditions that may cause death. Generally, such natural deaths do not lead the forensic pathologist to an in-depth pathological analysis of the cases; rather, a goal-directed approach is used to answer the questions at hand, the cause and manner of death. At times other considerations arise that may impose upon the pathologist the burden of understanding more about the case than might initially be appreciated. Litigation may occur where functional capabilities of the decedent or relationship of the disability to some antecedent event may have legal importance. Examples are the following: the relationship of a degenerative disease to an episode of trauma, drug treatment or abuse, therapeutic misadventure, or unconventional therapy; the basis for the decision to terminate life support, whether to allow organ donation, and the determination of informed consent for surgical procedures or medical treatment; the determination of mental competence and responsibility relating to financial decisions, such as in will contests; whether neglectful treatment occurred while under nursing home or medical care; questions of euthanasia and mercy killing; questions relating to suicide and accidental death; and questions of environmental hazards. An in-depth discussion of all these issues cannot be undertaken here, but when pertinent and when personal experience in some of the issues is relevant, it will be presented for emphasis. In recent years, considerable experimental and clinical research has been devoted to understanding these diseases more fully, and major strides have been made in discovering their causes and the development of therapeutic strategies.

Some of these have been abandoned because of severe side effects during clinical trials. For in-depth expositions of the various neurodegenerative diseases, the reader is referred to standard neuropathology and other texts [475,476].

Characteristics of Neurodegenerative Diseases

The general characteristics of the neurological degenerative diseases are that they have no known etiology and tend to be progressive illnesses, sometimes following a familial pattern (although the precise genetics are not well known in most of them). They are noninflammatory and nonfebrile illnesses that result usually in the death of neurons organized into functionally related systems within the CNS, such as the motor system and the extrapyramidal system. Usually, there is little other than a glial reaction to the death of neurons, and often there is some abnormality of the cytoskeleton of the affected neurons in the form of an accumulation of proteinaceous material inside neurons (Lewy bodies, neurofibrillary tangles, Pick bodies, Hirano bodies, etc.) related to one or more of the major structural proteins (tubulin, actin, neurofilament, tau proteins, and other intermediate filament or associated proteins) [477]. Most degenerative conditions affect adults or elderly persons, but infantile and childhood degenerative syndromes occur, sometimes quite commonly, such as Rett's syndrome, which is said to be second only to Down syndrome in incidence [478,479]. Other degenerative conditions include infantile motor neuron disease (Werdnig–Hoffmann disease) [480] and Alpers' disease [481]. In general, the diagnosis of these types of diseases rests on a wedding of clinical observations of the symptomatology, the neurological examination, imaging, familial genetic investigations, and the course of the illness with the pathological features as seen at autopsy or brain biopsy. The analysis of the neuropathological material generally involves attention not only to the lesions that occur in the brain but also to their distribution and topography. At times, a multitude of special stains (myelin stains, axon stains, fluorescent tags, fat stains, amyloid stains, immunochemical stains for structural proteins like tau, and carbohydrate stains) is required to complete an analysis. A number of genetic probes exist for known or suspected genetic abnormalities, but these often require access to the resources of research laboratories. Nevertheless, there are laboratories that are capable and often willing to undertake extensive analyses of interesting or rare cases on request. Such laboratories generally exist at the larger academic medical centers in major cities or the National Institutes of Health in the United States and similar institutions in Europe and Japan.

The degenerative diseases in adults can be roughly classified into those that affect the cerebral cortex, the basal ganglia and brain stem, the cerebellum, the spinal cord and peripheral nervous system or muscle, or combinations of these. Examples of the cerebral forms include the following: AD, Pick's disease, and progressive supranuclear palsy (Steele–Richardson–Olszewski syndrome) corticobasal degeneration. Important clinical manifestations of the cerebral diseases are dementia and disorders of behavior, which are discussed separately in Chapter 9. The basal ganglionic and brain stem diseases include Parkinson's disease, Huntington's chorea, and striatonigral degenerations. The cerebellar and brain stem syndromes include olivopontocerebellar degeneration, various forms of primary cerebellar degenerations, and a number of eponymic conditions reported on a case-by-case basis. The spinal diseases, which often involve other anatomical regions, include amyotrophic lateral sclerosis (ALS) and related motor neuron diseases, Charcot–Marie–Tooth disease, the spinocerebellar degenerations, and Friedreich ataxia. The peripheral nervous diseases include pandysautonomia, hereditary sensory neuropathy, and other rare conditions. Muscular degenerative diseases include the muscular dystrophies such as Duchenne, Becker, and myotonic dystrophy, as well as a host of mostly congenital myopathies.

Alzheimer's Disease

Alois Alzheimer in 1906 presented the clinical and pathological study of a 51-year-old woman who displayed symptoms of progressive dementia (memory loss, disorientation), depression, and hallucinations that led to her death after a 5-year course. The pathological findings consisted of cerebral atrophy and the microscopic findings of "senile" amyloid plaques that others had noted in demented patients, as well as the new finding, which bears Alzheimer's name, an exaggerated network of neurofibrils in the cytoplasm of cortical neurons now referred to as Alzheimer's neurofibrillary tangles. In the years since this original description, the entity has been well studied and characterized [482–484]. It was once thought to be an isolated and rare disease but is now appreciated to be a major public health hazard and the major cause of dementia (rather than so-called arteriosclerotic dementia) in the aged. It has been estimated that more than 4.5 million persons in the United States suffer from AD and that by the year 2050, more than 14 million will be affected [483], accounting for more than 100,000 deaths each year in the United States alone. Although AD often does not appear on the death certificate as a cause of death (usually the proximate cause is pneumonia, heart failure, or cachexia), it is responsible for the conditions that lead to death and, as such, is probably the fourth or fifth leading cause of death in the United States, after heart disease, cancer, stroke, and accidents. The disease is as yet unpreventable and has a major impact on the population, which will soon include more aged individuals than ever before, because to some AD is synonymous with aging in the brain.

The clinical and pathological features of AD tend to occur in three settings: in persons younger than 65 years of age (an arbitrary cutoff regarded developmentally as the presenile period or presenium) who become progressively demented and nonfunctional, usually dying within 5 years of the onset of symptoms (classic AD); in individuals older than 65 who show a similar progressive dementia and characteristic pathological changes (senile dementia of the Alzheimer type [SDAT]), and those elderly individuals who do not show an incapacitating degree of forgetfulness and are regarded within the normal spectrum of mental function for their age group. At autopsy, some of these individuals will show, albeit to a limited degree, the clinical features of AD (benign senile forgetfulness or "normal" aging). The perplexing issues that are raised by this apparent disease spectrum are whether these three conditions are identical, whether they are variants of a unitary disease process, or whether there is a relationship to normal aging so that AD might be considered abnormal or accelerated aging. The answers to these questions are not yet clear and are the subject of much debate and research [483,484]. There is an interplay between cerebral vascular disease (usually many subcortical manifestations of small-vessel disease such as lacunar infarcts) and Alzheimer's pathology that together produce dementia and often pose challenges for a proper clinical and pathological diagnosis [485–488].

Regardless of the clinical form of the disease, many general principles apply both clinically and pathologically, the major differences in the various forms being the rate of acceleration of symptoms and the density of pathological changes. The salient clinical features of AD are the gradual deterioration in the ability to recall recent events and the evolution of difficulties with orientation as to time and place. During this phase of the disease, which may evolve over several years or more rapidly, the individual displays many of the characteristics that most have come to expect of aged persons but which in middle-aged individuals are out of place and soon become obviously abnormal. This gradual loss of high-order functioning often leads to disorientation, especially at night or when driving, which may cause the individual to become lost and confused. A deterioration in grooming and dressing habits may occur. Emotional drive and spontaneity may decline, and the individual may have signs of depression and emotional lability, with wide mood swings. During this phase, accidents may happen owing to inattention, confusion, or misuse of objects. Alzheimer's patients may wander away from residences and become lost, sometimes in bad weather, and may die. It is here that the forensic pathologist may first come in contact with the Alzheimer's patient, sometimes before a clinical diagnosis has been made. Examples of accidental deaths include those due to exposure, drowning, automobile or pedestrian–vehicular accidents (ignored stop signs, traffic lights, one-way street signs, etc.), burns (smoking while using gasoline to clean objects or forgotten smoking materials about the house), falls (from ladders, while attempting to repair the house or trim trees, or down stairs), accidental poisonings due to drinking cleaning solutions and other items, and accidental medication overdose due to forgetfulness. The Alzheimer's patient may injure others unintentionally, especially when driving an automobile. Careful investigation will often reveal evidence of recent failing behavior from the spouse, relatives, or friends and help to place a given case in perspective, especially when current behavior does not match past behavior of the individual months or years prior to death [489,490].

As the first phase of the disease evolves, more significant and obvious neurological deficits appear, mostly of high-order association in the form of loss of knowledge of the names of objects and what they are used for (apraxia, aphasia, agnosia), loss of ability to understand spoken and written words, and the loss of ability to recognize sons, daughters, spouses, and even photographs of themselves. These deficits, coupled with a declining ability of the individual to recognize that he or she is incapacitated, make for severe limitations in function within society and in anything other than a highly controlled environment. As the dementia evolves, further additional symptoms and signs may appear, including seizures, extrapyramidal signs, and a tendency toward symptoms of the Kluever-Bucy syndrome (visual agnosia, hypersexuality, hyperoralism, and lack of ability to retain new information) as well as prolonged crying, moaning or screaming, and agitation [489]. At this late stage of the illness, whether middle-aged or elderly, the victim cannot care for himself or herself and requires more or less constant care or even restraint. Even when care is available, the victim may become cachectic or wasted, develop decubitae, and give the appearance of someone not cared for. In this situation, persons who have not seen the victim for some time may be shocked by the individual's appearance and allege maltreatment. This may lead to litigation or accusations that will involve the police and ultimately the medical examiner or coroner. The appearance of maltreatment (cachexia, decubitae, sometimes evidence of injuries) does not necessarily mean that this has occurred, for victims may become agitated and, free from restraints, may fall from their beds, bang their heads repeatedly against the bed frame, or otherwise cause injury to themselves in their demented state [489].

When death occurs, it is usually due to pneumonia with or without aspiration, urinary tract infections, and sepsis [491]. Occasionally, GI bleeding and coronary artery disease are responsible. In many cases, the actual anatomic cause of death cannot be determined with certainty. As mentioned above, many, if not most, death certificates do not list AD or senile dementia as the primary cause of death. This tendency on the part of physicians is regrettable because accurate public health statistics cannot be collected and the seriousness and prevalence of diseases such as this may escape the public consciousness. Grossly, the brain of most AD patients shows cortical atrophy of the major association areas (frontal, temporal, and parietal lobes), and brain weight is significantly lower than normal due to loss of neurons and neuronal arborizations (dendrites) (Figure 3.74).

It appears that AD and SDAT have no obvious pattern of inheritance, but statistical analysis has shown that siblings of Alzheimer's patients have the highest incidence of AD (about 3% of cases), whereas the parents of the victim have a high incidence of SDAT (about 2.8%). Offspring of Alzheimer's victims have an incidence of about 1.6%. With respect to victims of SDAT, there seems to be a close relationship of incidence in siblings, offspring, and parents (2.22 to 3.4%) for SDAT, and offspring have a higher incidence of AD (2.16%) than siblings (0.43%) [492]. These figures suggest that the diseases are separate but that persons who have AD tend to have parents with SDAT, and persons with SDAT will tend to have offspring with a higher-than-expected incidence of both SDAT and AD. In recent years, a number of genetic loci have been scrutinized for having a role in the disease; prominent among them in allelic alterations is the gene for APOE [493].

A practical problem for the pathologist or neuropathologist is clinical–pathological correlation or estimation of functional status from an autopsy brain specimen. This quest has been facilitated by the many studies comparing the brains of aged, nondemented individuals with those of victims of AD from many perspectives [494]. In recent years a number of cooperative studies have been undertaken to systematize the diagnosis of AD microscopically and topographically according to the degree of dementia and to attempt

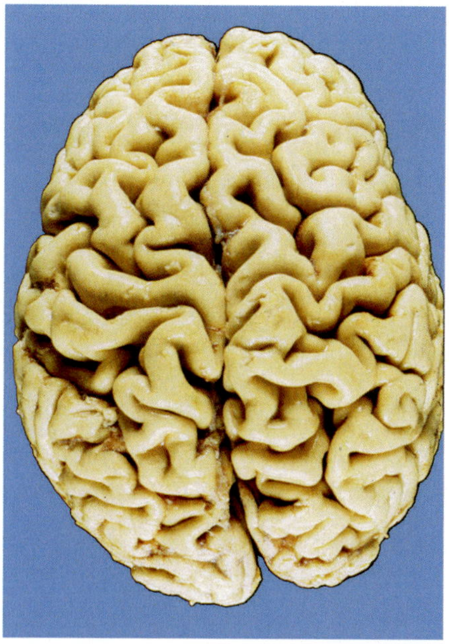

Figure 3.74 This photograph is a rostral view of the brain of a victim of AD and shows moderate convolutional atrophy with relative preservation of the occipital lobes. (Courtesy of Dr. J.D. Balentine, Medical University of South Carolina.)

to chart the course of the disease with considerable success [495–499]. The three major systems that have been employed are the Consortium to Establish a Registry for AD (CERAD) [498], the system of Braak and Braak [494,495], and the National Institute of Aging and Reagan Institute working group (NIA-Reagan) [499]. An older, now largely supplanted protocol was that of Khachaturian [500]. The methods and results of these protocols have been compared and analyzed by Alafuzoff et al. [497] with respect to the likelihood of dementia due to AD and topography of neurofibrillary pathology using various histological methods (see below).

There is a variety of technical methods to demonstrate neuritic pathology and neurofibrillary tangles that include many of the classical silver methods, like the Bielschowski, Bodian, Holmes, Gallyas, or similar methods (Figures 3.75 and 3.76). Chemical methods may also be employed that recognize hyperphosphorylated tau proteins or amyloid proteins [499,501].

It appears that although amyloid plaques abound in the AD brain and are associated with a surrounding halo of abnormal neurites, morphologically the amyloid plaques do not appear to have the linkage with dementia that neurofibrillary (tangle) or neuritic plaque pathology does. Topographically, the mesial temporal lobe cortex is the region affected earliest with neurofibrillary pathology and whose density correlates best with dementia using most of the protocols and employing reasonable technical controls for the methods used [501]. As a general rule, when neuritic plaque density is greater than three or more than six neurofibrillary tangles are seen per ×100 field, there is a strong likelihood that AD and dementia are present. When neurofibrillary pathology spreads beyond the mesial temporal lobe, often in an ever-expanding pattern to reach all parts of the cerebral cortex, the

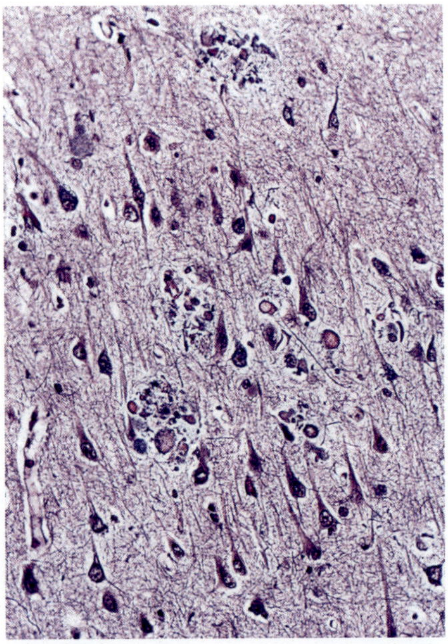

Figure 3.75 This Bodian silver stained paraffin section from the cerebral cortex in the hippocampus illustrates both neuritic ("senile") plaques and neurofibrillary tangles. The globular masses with lavender staining nodules are the neuritic plaques and the lavender material is amyloid. In affected neurons, usually the apical dendrite has a string-like quality and contains condensed neurofilaments.

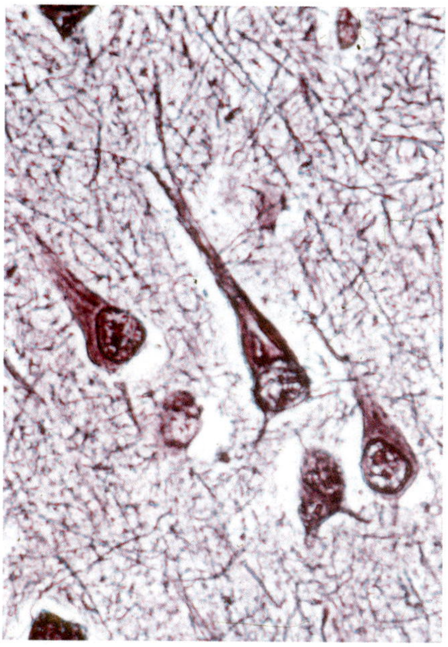

Figure 3.76 This Bodian silver–stained preparation illustrates several neurofibrillary tangles in neurons of the hippocampus. Typical are strands of argyrophilic material that extend often in a spiral pattern upward into the apical dendrite of the affected neuron.

dementia is usually profound and there is little doubt about the diagnosis. At this stage the brain usually shows frontal–parietal convolutional atrophy and weighs about 1000 grams or less. The brain mass loss is probably due to loss of neuronal dendritic arborizations, because Golgi impregnation studies have shown that, perhaps more significant than simple neuronal loss, which does occur, many cortical neurons become simplified and lose many of their dendritic branches, thus limiting the contacts between cortical neurons and causing axonal volume loss [502].

It is interesting to note that studies on aging of the brain in a number of very different animals have shown a tendency to neuronal loss and the development of amyloid plaques, but not neurofibrillary pathology, which appears to be a singularly human trait [502]. In an effort to differentiate between cases that have varying proportions of pathological lesions, the Alzheimer-type dementias have been divided into seven groups by Constantinidis as quoted by Alafuzoff et al. [496]:

I. Many SP (senile plaques), high density of NFT (neurofibrillary tangles) in hippocampus, diffuse high density of NFT in cerebral cortex
II. Moderate density of NFT in the cerebral cortex
III. Low density of NFT in cerebral cortex
IV. Moderate or high density of NFT in hippocampus, no NFT in frontal or occipital cortex
V. Low density of NFT in hippocampus
VI. Many SP in the cortex but no NFT
VII. No NFT or SP found

This subdivision is of historical interest, but from a practical and correlative point of view, the newer histological protocols are more useful (Tables 3.8–3.10) [497,498].

Evaluator consistency was somewhat variable using the CERAD protocol. Although all cases were known to be demented for whatever reason (AD or other), all pathologists (either seven or eight) agreed on four of thirteen cases as being definite AD and that one

Table 3.8 CERAD Protocol Semiquantitative Microscopic Assessment Using Bielschowsky Method (Silver-Stained Paraffin Sections of Brain) Applied to Cases of Demented Individuals

Frequency of Plaques	Age at Death (50–75 years)	Age at Death (>75 years)
None (0)	0	0
Some (1–2)	Probable AD	Probable AD
Moderate (3–10)	Definite AD	Probable AD
Severe (>11)	Definite AD	Definite AD

Source: National Institutes of Health, Consensus recommendations for the postmortem diagnosis of Alzheimer's disease. The National Institute on Aging, and Reagan Institute Working Group on Diagnostic Criteria for the Neuropathological Assessment of Alzheimer's Disease, *Neurobiol Aging* 18(Suppl), S1–2, 1997.

Note: Thirteen areas in the temporal lobe were examined for senile/neuritic plaques at ×100 magnification, using six to eight evaluators [499]. The magnification of ×100 is derived by multiplying the magnification of the ocular of the microscope, by whatever internal lens system might exist, by the magnification of the objective lens. In most microscopes, this means that a ×6–×10 objective lens will yield to the eye about a ×100 image.

Table 3.9 Braak and Braak Staging [494–496] Using the Gallyas Silver Staining Method

Braak and Braak Stage	Severity
Stage 0	None
Stage I–II	Some (1–5)
Stage III–IV	Moderate (6–10)
Stage V–VI	Severe (>11)

Note: This study was performed on the same case material as in Table 3.8 but evaluated frequency of neurofibrillary tangles in the temporal lobe cortex, not neuritic plaques.

Table 3.10 NIA-Reagan Protocol [497,499] Using Combined Evaluations from CERAD and Braak and Braak

CERAD Protocol	Braak and Braak Protocol	Likelihood of AD
None	0	None
Possible AD	II–II	Low
Probable AD	III–IV	Intermediate
Definite AD	V–VI	High

Note: The NIA-Reagan protocol [499] was employed using the same case material to determine the likelihood that the dementia in the victims was due to AD lesions using combined evaluations from CERAD and Braak and Braak.

case showed no pathology. However, in three more cases, whereas seven pathologists classified these as definite, one pathologist classified them as probable; thus, eight of thirteen cases' agreement was close among the pathologists. Troublesome was the fact that there were five cases in which the classification ranged from no pathology to definite.

Agreement among the evaluating pathologists using the Braak and Braak protocol was nearly random, with only three cases being unanimously classified by all pathologists as being stages V–VI. With respect to the one case judged unanimously negative using the CERAD protocol, seven of eight of the reviewers in this study also felt the case was negative for Alzheimer's pathology. The remainder was scattered among other categories.

The method embodied by the NIA-Reagan protocol resulted in the best concordance among the evaluating pathologists, resulting in six of eight agreeing on five cases as having a high likelihood of AD and one case having no likelihood. The remaining cases resembled the results of the CERAD protocol, with narrow or wide variations among evaluators.

The issues that may explain the variations in evaluations include variances in the methods of fixation, embedding, sectioning, and staining methods that can clearly impact the precision of any histological evaluation and appear to have done so in this study. Nevertheless, if anything can be taken away from this study, it is that, at this point in time, it appears the best correlations with dementia may result from attempting to determine the density of neuritic (senile) plaques rather than the density of neurofibrillary tangles, at least in the temporal lobe. Clearly, the extent of occurrence of either lesion away from the temporal lobe of the brain is important and does correlate with dementia scores, and the likelihood is very high that in the face of decreased brain weight and obvious atrophy, and the presence of plaques or tangles in regions well away from the temporal lobe in other regions of the cerebral cortex, the individual's dementia is due to AD, and some estimates may be made of its functional significance. There is no doubt that cooperative, broad, coordinated studies of the kind attempted by Alafuzoff and colleagues [496,497] offer a laudable beginning to a protocol that anyone can use with confidence.

The neuropharmacological basis for the dementia in AD is complex but most probably related to disruption of cholinergic terminals to the cortex from lower centers and disconnection of large areas of cerebral cortex by loss of dendritic branching and synaptic connections; the disruptive and disconnecting effect of intracortical SPs; and associated disruption of cholinergic connections of the basal nucleus of Meynert and other apparently important nuclei [502,503].

Pick's Disease and the Frontotemporal Dementias

At one time, Pick's disease was regarded as an extreme rarity but has now become included in a broader group of dementias united by mutations in the tau genes mostly centered about chromosome 17q. These include Pick's disease, frontotemporal dementia, primary progressive aphasia, corticobasilar degeneration, and progressive supranuclear palsy (Steele–Richardson–Olszewski syndrome) [504–507]. Linkages with Parkinson's disease and related conditions have also been suggested [508]. Tau proteins exist in neurons and glia, appear to be associated with microtubule function, and are a component of a number of neurofilamentous inclusions in neurons in various degenerative diseases, including AD.

Pick's disease, like the other frontotemporal degenerations, is a dementing illness not unlike AD, which may have some clinical features of its own, but the end result is a profoundly demented victim with a correspondingly exceptionally atrophic brain. The pattern

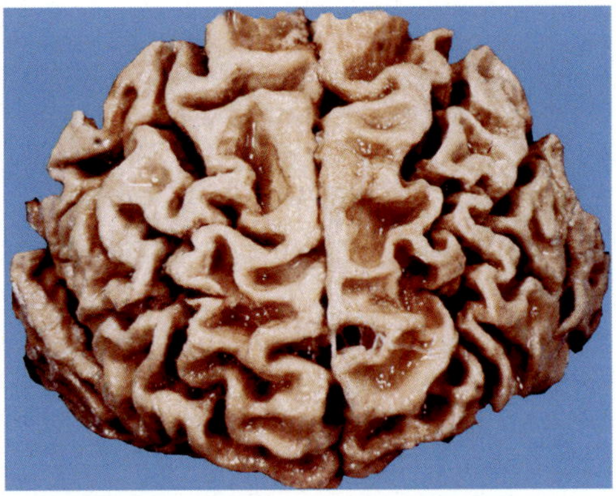

Figure 3.77 This view of the frontal lobes of a victim of Pick's disease illustrates the profound cortical atrophy typically found in this condition. Classically this atrophy is much more severe than is seen in AD.

of atrophy is primarily in the frontal lobe and the superior temporal gyrus of the temporal lobe, although in advanced cases, atrophy may be generalized (Figure 3.77). Histologically, in classical Pick's disease there are argyrophilic globular inclusions in neurons known as Pick's bodies without neurofibrillary tangles or neuritic plaques, but some cases seem to have features of both Pick's pathology and Alzheimer's pathology.

Progressive supranuclear palsy (Steele–Richardson–Olszewski syndrome) [507] has a characteristic clinical presentation of dementia in which, although the victim is demented, often with stimulation, rather high-order cognitive tasks can be performed. Other clinical features are apraxia of speech, spasticity, and weakness, and some cases have parkinsonian symptoms. The disease is unremitting but generally does not result in significant brain atrophy. The pathology is mostly subcortical, in that neurons in the basal ganglia and brain stem, rather than the cerebral cortex, house globular (globose) neurofibrillary tangles [507].

Parkinson's Disease

Several neurological syndromes show the phenomenon of parkinsonism (an involuntary, resting, three-to-five-per-second "pill-rolling" tremor, usually of the hands, which is abolished on movement; "cogwheel" muscular rigidity; and poverty of movement and facial expression, with no loss of underlying emotional affect), which results from lesions in the nigral–striatal system or pathway, due to functional–pharmacological [508] or anatomical disruption in the case of trauma [509,510]. The classic disease, described in 1817 and typified by parkinsonism, is paralysis agitans or idiopathic (sporadic) Parkinson's disease [511]. It is a disease that probably arises from an interplay of genetic and environmental factors, although apparently inherited cases are known in an autosomal dominant pattern [512]. Genetic factors in the disease may be associated with mutations in the a-synuclein and so-called parkin genes. The latter, a protein that appears to be related to ubiquitin, is important to survival of nigral neurons [512].

In recent years a broader view of Parkinson's disease has evolved from simply being a disease of the substantia nigra and its pathways to the striatum. Rather, this pathology, as Langston points out, may only be the tip of the iceberg [513]. It now appears that well before Lewy body proteins appear in the substantia nigra, they appear in various nuclei of the brain stem and olfactory bulb [514]. Often Lewy bodies or Lewy proteins can be immunochemically demonstrated in various areas of the cerebral cortex before the substantia nigra is affected [515], and Lewy bodies may be found in the cortex quite commonly in typical Parkinson's victims. A variety of symptoms, many noted in the original description of the disease, give credence to later neuropathological observations of a much more widely and sometimes subtly expressed pathology than was classically thought. Autonomic dysfunction is quite common, as are disorders of olfaction, constipation, trouble sleeping, and cognition in many patients [513,515].

Sporadic (classical) Parkinson's disease usually starts in the fifties but may begin at a younger or older age and is usually heralded by the gradual development of parkinsonism. The disease may appear bilaterally or unilaterally and progresses to full force over several years. The classic untreated Parkinson's patient presents a sad, droopy, dull countenance, and sits in a hunched-over attitude with the hands folded in the lap in constant rolling motion, as though something were being manipulated by the fingers. When walking, the patient tends to tilt forward, and to experience difficulty in initiated movement. The gait is propulsive, with small steps on the tips of the toes, and often causes the individual to move with small, jerky steps that come faster and faster until the victim falls or has to grasp an object to halt the accelerating motion. The difficulty in initiating movement or speech may also involve thought (bradyphrenia) and may appear as a symptom to others long before the victim himself or herself appreciates he or she is experiencing any difficulty [516,517]. The disease may progress slowly over many years and eventually leads to a bedfast state in which rigidity, tremor, a poverty of voluntary movement, and often a terminal dementia render the victim to fatal bacterial infection and inanition [515]. Some studies indicate a greater-than-expected incidence of neoplasms in Parkinson's patients, for which no cause has been found [518].

The pathology of the classical form of the disease is centered in the substantia nigra of the midbrain (Figure 3.78). The gross appearance of the substantia nigra and locus ceruleus in Parkinson's disease is pronounced pallor, sometimes so severe that it resembles the prepubescent appearance of virtually no visible pigmented cells. Pigment loss may be

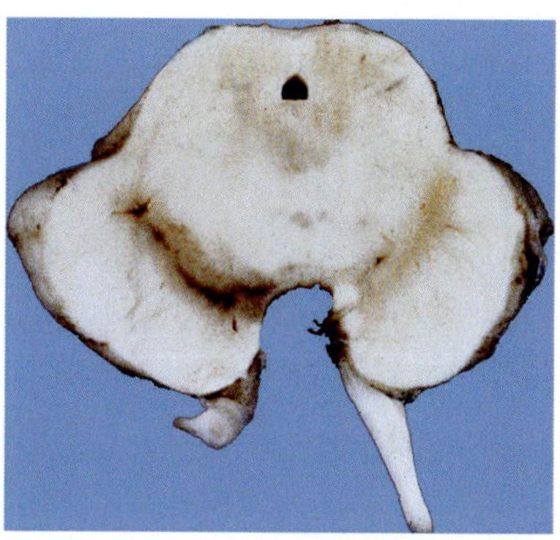

Figure 3.78 This cross section of the midbrain with a segment of the third cranial nerves visible illustrates profound depigmentation of the substantia nigra primarily on one side in a victim of Parkinson's disease. The depigmentation is due to loss of neuromelanin-pigmented neurons.

bilateral or unilateral. The brain may appear slightly atrophic and the ventricles somewhat enlarged. The basal ganglia may appear brownish in color.

Microscopically, there is profound loss of pigmented (neuromelanin) neurons and replacement gliosis, most severe in the zona compacta portion of the nucleus. Remaining neurons may contain spherical or ovoid cytoplasmic inclusion bodies (Lewy bodies, as in Figure 3.79), which are easily visible as eosinophilic or basophilic objects in H&E stain. Various other special stains, including immunochemical reactions for Lewy proteins, may highlight them somewhat better. Lewy bodies and neuronal loss are usually also seen in the other major pigmented brain stem nucleus, the locus ceruleus in the pons. Free pigment is often found in the neuropil or in macrophages around vessels, but no signs of inflammation or other obvious abnormalities are noted. Lewy bodies are often encountered incidentally (4 to 5% of cases over 65 years of age) in otherwise normal aged brains. It is unclear what significance this may have [515]. As noted above, Lewy bodies and Lewy proteins are very commonly noted in nonnigral regions of the brain and probably correlate with symptoms involving those areas [519,520].

Cases in which Lewy bodies predominate in the cerebral cortex, often with neurofibrillary pathology, may constitute a special group of dementing illnesses, often referred to as cerebral Lewy body disease [519–522].

The discovery of the pathophysiology and neurochemistry of the disease represents one of the most notable advances in neurological diseases and has led directly to a therapeutic strategy for symptomatic management of parkinsonism but not of the underlying disease, which probably progresses despite the treatment. To summarize very briefly, the substantia nigra neurons synthesize dopamine from tyrosine and transport it via their axons to the caudate nucleus and putamen (the corpus striatum), where it acts on striatal

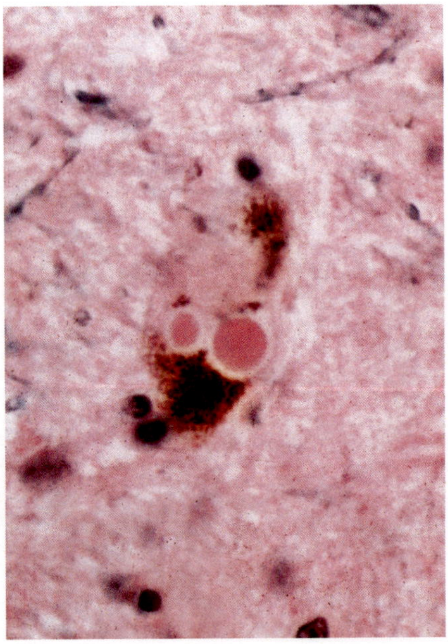

Figure 3.79 This H&E-stained paraffin section shows a substantia nigra neuron containing two spherical Lewy bodies, typical for Parkinson's disease. Such bodies may also be found in the locus ceruleus of the pons.

neurons in concert with cholinergic influences to modulate muscle tone and movement via interconnections with the thalamus via the globus pallidus. When insufficient dopamine is supplied to the striatal neurons because of death of nigral neurons, there is an unbalanced relative excess of cholinergic influence, which acts to release the thalamus from the influence of the striatum, apparently causing the oscillatory tremors that are so classic for parkinsonism [523].

The therapeutic strategy that has developed into the most effective means of treating the disease's symptoms involves supplying the striatum with l-dopa, which is able to pass across the blood–brain barrier and is not metabolized as quickly as dopamine would be in the general circulation, where it is converted to dopamine by an enzyme (L-aromatic amino acid decarboxylase) that is found in many neurons, in contradistinction to tyrosine hydroxylase, which is found almost exclusively in catecholamine-synthesizing neurons such as in the substantia nigra. Once dopamine is synthesized in target neurons, it is incorporated into secretory vesicles and can perform its neuropharmacologic function as though the dopamine had been supplied via anatomical connections that have now been diminished or lost. Other strategies involve suppression of catabolic enzyme systems that degrade dopamine and prolong the presence of dopamine vesicles at the synaptic cleft or at receptor sites or stimulate reuptake [524]. There are a number of complications and complexities in the L-dopa or analog treatment for parkinsonism that cannot be predicted or controlled with confidence; these generally result from an imbalance between dopamine and acetylcholine in the striatum. This imbalance produces athetoid and choreaform movements more characteristic of Huntington's chorea than parkinsonism. A number of other drugs can produce either choreaform–athetoid or parkinson-like movements, especially the phenothiazine tranquilizers, although the mechanisms are not always clear [524,525]. New treatments for parkinsonism involve deep brain stimulation with electrodes, various deep brain lesions done neurosurgically or radiosurgically, and implantation of dopamine-secreting or stem cells. These newer methods have achieved some notable, although often short-lived, successes, along with major complications [526].

Several years ago, in connection with a most tragic circumstance, an analog of meperidine (Demerol®) was synthesized by a drug-addicted chemist and found its way onto the street market for recreational drugs [527]. This compound, known as MPTP, is able to cross the blood–brain barrier, where it is metabolized by monoamine oxidases to a toxic substance that binds tenaciously to dopaminergic neurons in the substantia nigra and elsewhere and kills them. The net effect of this toxicity is to produce a chemically induced form of Parkinson's disease that is incurable but treatable with the usual anti-Parkinson's drugs. To date, several hundred drug addicts, including the chemist who originally synthesized this compound, have been affected by its use. Study of some human patients has demonstrated that although MPTP produces a reliable and reproducible animal model for parkinsonism, it does not reproduce the complexities of the true disease [528]. It also appears that MPTP or possibly some analogs are not important in the pathogenesis of Parkinson's disease.

From a forensic perspective, Parkinson's disease, like AD, may make its appearance on a forensic service, probably most often in connection with accidental deaths from the neurological disability and its complications and from deaths from neglect or abuse in care facilities of disabled victims. In unusual circumstances, there are attempts to correlate disability and cognition with morphological and histological features in the brain. This may be a daunting task and often is imprecise, but some protocols exist for diagnosing the disease and its consequences [521]. Although it seems bizarre, some individuals treated with drugs for parkinsonism may display so-called restless legs as well as impulse disorders and may compulsively gamble or engage in other seemingly obsessive behaviors [529].

Postencephalitic Parkinson's Disease

The symptoms of Parkinson's disease have been known to follow episodes of viral encephalitis, especially a form of encephalitis that has apparently not occurred since the 1920s—von Economo's encephalitis lethargica—but may follow other forms of encephalitis that inflict damage on the substantia nigra [530]. It appears that von Economo's encephalitis appeared before the great influenza epidemics in the early years of the twentieth century; thus, it may not have been involved in the pathogenesis of so-called postencephalitic Parkinson's disease [531], which still remains an enigma [532–534]. In recent years the similarity of various forms of influenza have given rise to concerns about the consequence of a pandemic beyond the inevitable deaths that would occur and the longer-term sequelae, namely, Parkinson's disease [534]. The clinical appearance of postencephalitic Parkinson's disease may differ slightly from idiopathic Parkinson's disease, but the pathology is quite distinctive and different in both forms of the disease. In postencephalitic Parkinson's disease and progressive supranuclear palsy, complex globose neurofibrillary tangles are found in the substantia nigra, locus ceruleus, and other subcortical nuclei, rather than the Lewy bodies in typical Parkinson's disease. Occasionally, old inflammatory nodules or glial scars are found, which suggest that a viral infection was once present. Because of the clinical and pathological overlap (include supposed disorders of tau proteins—tauopathies) between what has been called postencephalitic Parkinson's disease and other degenerative conditions, such as corticobasilar degeneration, progressive supranuclear palsy [535,536], ALS, the ALS-Parkinson's-dementia complex in Guamanians, and even AD [537], many consider these conditions related [538–540].

Huntington's Disease

From a neuropharmacological standpoint, Huntington's chorea occupies a special niche along with Parkinson's disease, because the symptoms of both diseases revolve around disturbances in the balance of cholinergic and dopaminergic influences on the striatum (caudate nucleus and putamen) [541]. In Parkinson's disease, the pathology is in the nigrostriatal system, which supplies dopamine to the striatum, resulting in too little [542] dopamine and a relative excess of acetylcholine. In Huntington's chorea, due to pathology in the striatum, there is a paucity of acetylcholine and an excess of dopamine and disturbances in glutamate metabolism [543]. The result is the appearance of choreaform and athetoid movements. The disease is autosomally dominantly inherited but does not usually manifest itself until the adult years, between 25 and 45 years of age. The disease tends to appear earlier in males, who inherited the disease from their fathers rather than their mothers, and there is a tendency for earlier and earlier occurrence with each generation in some families [544]. There are concentrations of the disease in some countries (Venezuela, for example), where inbreeding may be responsible for the exceptional prevalence [544,545]. Recent work has discovered that the probable genetic factor responsible for the disease is trinucleotide (CAG) repeats within the genome that result in an aberrant protein called "huntingtin" and polyglutamine strands that are toxic to the affected neuronal systems.

The length of the repeat sequences appears to correlate with early age of onset and severity of the disease [545,546].

The clinical features of the disease are the gradual appearance of subtle involuntary "extra" movements of the hands, arms, shoulders, and upper trunk or face, which may be interpreted as mannerisms or nervous tics. These movements may evolve over many years but invariably grow more severe until obvious choreaform and athetoid movements are seen with facial grimacing. As the movement disorder becomes evident, behavioral changes become manifest and include irritability, emotional lability, depression, paranoia, confusion, and loss of memory [547]. An awareness of the process of deterioration, coupled with depression, results in a very significant risk of suicide in the Huntington's disease patient. Not every victim of Huntington's disease displays all the signs of the disease, and some sufferers show very little choreaform activity. Nevertheless, the disease progresses relentlessly, resulting in death in 5 to 10 years after onset of symptoms. At death, the victim is bedfast and demented, usually succumbing to pneumonia or another form of infection [543].

The gross appearance of the Huntington's brain is diffuse cerebral atrophy, but not as obvious or severe as in AD. The coronal sections reveal an obvious shrinkage and brownish discoloration of the caudate nuclei and the putamen with corresponding enlargement of the lateral ventricles (see Figure 3.80). Microscopic changes consist mainly of neuronal loss, especially of the smaller neurons, with replacement gliosis in the striatum and, to a lesser extent, in the globus pallidus. By counting the large and small neurons in the striatum, one can develop a ratio, which normally is about 40 small to 1 large, for comparison with doubtful or problem cases. Neuronal loss and gliosis can also be found, but with some difficulty, in the thalamus, diencephalon, upper brain stem, and cerebellum, which indicates that this disease, like most other degenerative diseases, has diffuse pathological manifestations, but with a concentration of lesions to particular locations. Areas of neuronal loss are very difficult to identify, but gliosis may be easier to find, especially when highlighted by stains for glial fibers such as the Holzer stain or immunocytochemical stain for glial fibrillary acidic protein (GFAP), which can be performed on paraffin sections and is reliable.

The treatment for Huntington's chorea is not as effective as for Parkinson's disease because the neurons that project to the thalamus from the striatum, upon which dopamine

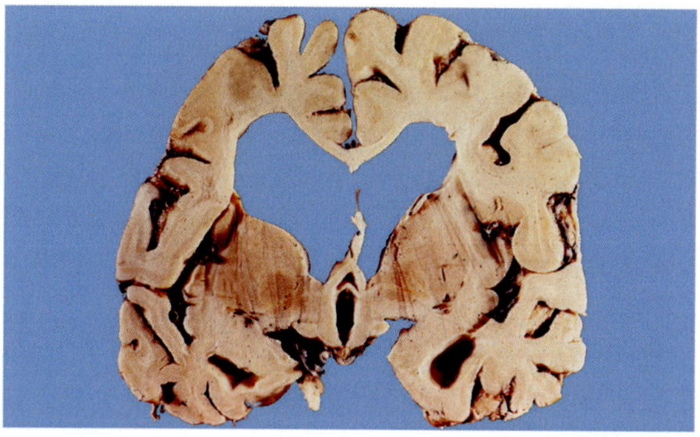

Figure 3.80 This coronal section of the brain of a victim of Huntington's chorea illustrates the typically enlarged ventricles and nearly absent caudate nuclei. Some element of cortical atrophy is also typically present.

and acetylcholine act, are lost in this disease. Furthermore, it is not possible to manipulate the intrastriatal neurotransmitter environment for acetylcholine as easily as for dopamine. Symptomatic treatment for depression and minimal treatment for the movement disorder are possible but do not affect the course of the disease. Recently, major efforts have been directed to discovering genetic markers and genetic probes for the disease so that carriers can be identified before they show the disease and can be counseled against transmitting the gene by not having children. Additional developments in amniocentesis have been applied to detecting the Huntington's gene in utero as a guide for elective abortion of affected fetuses [546].

Motor Neuron Disease

The classic example of motor neuron system disease in the adult is ALS, but other named diseases such as Werdnig-Hoffmann disease (infantile motor neuron disease) [480] and Kugelberg-Welander disease (juvenile motor neuron disease) form other members of this family but affect younger individuals [549]. There are numerous case reports of variants of these main forms, most of which have not been named. All these conditions have in common basic confinement of the pathology and clinical findings to the motor system, although minor involvement may be seen in other systems in some cases [550]. ALS can have familial variants, but most cases are considered sporadic. Not all conditions are clearly inherited, but examples of inheritance can be found in all forms. The etiology of the diseases is not known, but several hypotheses have been advanced, which include infectious, nutritional, environmental toxic, biochemical, and genetic causes [551]. There is no treatment at present for any of the diseases.

Amyotrophic Lateral Sclerosis

ALS is not an uncommon neurological disease in that it probably affects 10,000 to 15,000 persons in the United States at this time and about 4 to 6 persons per 100,000 of population on a worldwide scale, and it has been publicized most recently by the fact that several persons of national and international prominence have suffered from it. It begins with subtle symptoms of clumsiness in the hands, progressing to muscular weakness in limbs, trunk, and neck, with fibrillations and fasciculations in affected muscles. Muscular atrophy develops, and difficulty in swallowing, in talking, and with respiration develops early or evolves eventually. ALS patients do not lose mental capacity, and appropriate behavior is maintained, even with full insight into the nature and prognosis of the disease. Extraocular muscles and bladder function are usually not affected. The disease may begin at any age but generally does not do so before age 30 years, peaking during the forties and fifties. The course of the disease is variable but generally claims most victims within 10 years of onset. The cause of death is usually respiratory complications and pneumonia or sepsis arising from a bedfast state [550].

Most ALS cases are sporadic, but about 10% seem to have a familial pattern [551]. Males are affected about four times as frequently as females, and there is a greater-than-expected tendency for victims to have been competitive athletes in high school or college, to have worked in environments where heavy metals were used, to have lived in areas where high levels of manganese or selenium are found in the environment, or to have regularly drunk milk as adults [552]. Some individuals who have suffered from poliomyelitis as children develop a progressive motor neuron disease in adult life [553]. On the Pacific island of Guam, one ethnic group, the Chamorro people, have an extraordinary incidence of a complex disease that has some features of ALS (the so-called ALS–Parkinson dementia complex), discussed above.

The basis for the disease is a loss of motor nerve cells, most obviously in the anterior horns of the spinal cord, but neuronal and axonal loss may be traced all the way to the motor strip in the cerebral cortex. Motor neuron loss in the brain stem is most severe in the nuclei of cranial nerves XII and XI and to a lesser degree in the nuclei of cranial nerves VII and V. The classic gross pathology is that of a slightly atrophic cord, with obvious shrinkage of the motor roots in comparison to the intact sensory roots (Figure 3.81). There is usually no cerebral atrophy. The microscopic appearances consist of profound motor neuron loss in the anterior horns, shrinkage and sometimes swelling of remaining neurons, and degeneration of the pyramidal tracts with loss of myelin staining. Apparent involvement of the corticospinal tract decreases rostrally and cerebral changes (internal capsule) are inapparent by normal methods. In rare cases, degeneration and dropout of Betz cells may be demonstrated in the motor areas. No inflammation or evidence of viral infection is found. The muscular pathology is typical for neurogenic atrophy, showing group lesions and homogenization of muscle fiber types by ATP-ase histochemistry due to a tendency for terminal axonal sprouting and cross-innervation by surviving motor fibers in the muscle as other fibers atrophy. The clinical result of this neural plasticity is that late

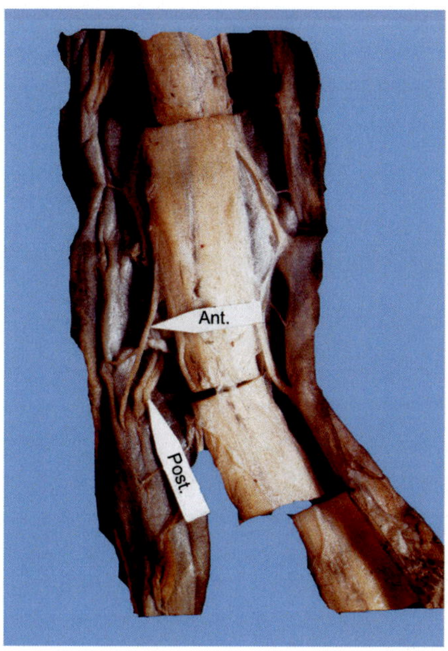

Figure 3.81 This gross photograph of a segment of spinal cord with roots and dura from a case of ALS illustrate the profound and obvious atrophy of the anterior (ventral, motor) roots as compared with the dorsal sensory roots, which are not atrophic. The cord is not externally altered, but with cross-sectioning, it may be possible to observe a whiteness of the lateral corticospinal (pyramidal) tracts, which are very obvious microscopically even in H&E preparations. Myelin stains provide dramatic evidence of the deterioration of the pyramidal tracts at any level of the cord or brain stem.

in the disease, as neurons die, they take with them an ever-increasing number of muscle fibers and produce a pronounced step-like decline more obvious than early in the disease.

It appears that the molecular/neurochemical basis for at least some cases of ALS is a mutation in the code for Cu/Zn superoxide dismutase (SOD-1) or for the gene for dynactin, a protein integral to proper functioning of retrograde axonal transport. A malfunction of the latter could account for failure of signaling to the motor neuron that its nerve ending exists, leading to eventual shutdown and death of the neuron [549].

The forensic implications or considerations with the motor neuron diseases in recent years have centered about initiatives taken by some individuals to seek euthanasia or assisted suicide and enlist a medical professional or relative at some point, not necessarily at the end stages of ALS. The most notorious case is of Dr. Jack Kevorkian (now deceased), a pathologist in Michigan who participated in the videotaped assisted suicide of a number of people, including several with ALS, and who was convicted of murder and served an 8-year prison sentence [554–556]. The issue of assisted suicide in this and often other neurological degenerative diseases, including Alzheimer's, is a very difficult one socially, ethically, morally, and legally [556], and the forensic pathologist may find himself or herself involved in such a case where issues of mental capacity, severity of the disease, and other issues may arise. On the other side of this difficult problem is an example of a man almost totally incapacitated by ALS, yet managing to survive and even painfully authoring best-selling books with the aid of various devices, computers, and devoted caregivers—the cosmologist Stephen Hawking [557].

Diseases of White Matter

For want of a better classification, such as one based upon etiology, there is a group of nervous system diseases whose effect is primarily on the white matter of the brain and specifically on the myelin sheath or the oligodendrocyte, which produces myelin in central axons. Often, these diseases are called demyelinating diseases, a term that presupposes that myelin had formed normally in the first place and that some subsequent event caused dissolution or loss by a mechanism that is presumably selective for the myelin sheath and not for the axon, as would be the case in a coexistent process like infarction or viral infection. It is also common to refer to the former groups of demyelinating diseases, such as in primary demyelination, and the latter groups, as would be seen after severance of axons as in spinal cord injury or infarction, as secondary demyelination. The most important primary demyelinative disease in terms of its impact on society and prevalence is MS, of which the etiology has still not been proven. Another group, which is composed primarily of diseases of childhood or infancy, the leukodystrophies, has been exhaustively studied biochemically and has been identified as being the result of specific inherited enzymatic defects that mostly affect infants and children, and this group is therefore discussed in Chapter 4.

Multiple Sclerosis

MS is a frequent visitor to the forensic service and perhaps may be encountered more frequently there than on most hospital autopsy services, owing to changes in hospital admissions policies, length-of-stay limitations, evolution of the hospice movement, and the declining autopsy rate in the United States and elsewhere. In addition, MS is one of the great masqueraders in neurology and can mimic a variety of symptoms of other diseases and even appear as full-blown pathological cases in individuals who apparently never realized they suffered from the disease [558]. MS may also play a role in accidental deaths, suicides, and occasionally so-called assisted suicides, or mercy killings. Furthermore, occasionally various external events have been alleged to precipitate or cause MS, such as irradiation to the head or brain, exposure to toxic substances, viral infections, allergies, head trauma, and fat embolism. Such instances are usually in the form of single case reports that must be evaluated individually against known observations and experimental science as to potential merit.

MS is a geographically delimited disease, occurring in about one of every 1000 people who live north of the 36th parallel in the northern hemisphere and affecting about twice as many females as males. In the region between 36° north and 36° south, the incidence is less to much less, such that in sub-Saharan Africa, MS could be considered rare. In the deep southern latitudes of Australia and New Zealand, the incidence is comparable to that in some parts of Europe and the southern United States. Certain geographic regions have a remarkably high incidence, such that some have referred to MS in the Faeroe Islands of the North Atlantic Ocean as epidemic [559]. It appears that if one is born and lives for the first 15 years of life in a high-incidence zone for MS and moves to a lower incidence zone, one carries with him or her the incidence of his or her place of birth. Why this phenomenon occurs is as yet unproven. For more detailed epidemiological information, the reader is referred to the excellent online (Internet) review of Kurtzke [560,561].

The presentation of the disease is so variable that it is often ignored or misdiagnosed. Common symptoms, however, include relatively sudden onset of painless diplopia, blurred vision, vertigo and incoordination, tremor or ataxia with nystagmus, vague sensory phenomena such as paresthesias or numbness, dysphagia or speech difficulty, hemiplegia or hemiparesis, alterations in mood or behavior, and rarely seizures. Sometimes dementing illness or severe behavioral illness is seen, Babinski signs and other pathological reflexes may be elicited, and the disease may appear to present as an intracerebral, brain stem, cerebellar, spinal, or mixed multifocal disease. One of the most typical aspects of the disease is that it pursues an exacerbating and remitting course over many years [562,563].

MS has been divided into several categories based upon the onset and progression, or lack thereof, of attacks. The most common form is the so-called relapsing–remitting pattern that categorizes the initial pattern of the disease in 60%–90% of patients. This typical form shows unpredictable attacks alternating, sometimes with gaps of years, with remissions that may or may not be recovered from, with life span at risk but not necessarily shortened in mild forms. The remainder of patients may be categorized as suffering from progressive forms of MS. These may begin with attacks and remissions but then progress, sometimes without apparent attacks, in an unremitting deteriorating course. Others seem, after their first attack, to steadily decline to die of the disease. This form of the disease is often referred to as Marburg variant MS [564]. There are apparent variants of MS with and without familial connections. The time span for all of these forms is highly variable and unpredictable. Why such variability in the course of MS occurs is not known.

Within the general categories of MS, there are several forms where the brunt of the illness will fall on one particular region—the brain stem or cerebellum, the cerebrum, or the spinal cord—or will affect the CNS diffusely, with symptoms that are appropriate to each area affected. The peripheral nervous system is not generally involved in the disease, but a number of cases of MS and diffuse hypertrophic neuropathy have been reported. A relationship of MS to retrobulbar or optic neuritis has been alleged for many years, with a relatively small percentage of victims going on to a more typical form of MS. Recently, this connection seems more remote, and it appears that the two conditions are related but separate. Some support for this idea lies in the fact that tissue histocompatibility typing seems to indicate that persons with MS tend to have one or two particular HLA forms, whereas bulbar neuritis patients have others [565].

The pathology of MS is highly variable, as are the clinical variations. The classic MS lesion is the demyelinated plaque grossly visible on cut section in fixed or fresh tissue, and the lesions have sharp boundaries, often appearing more pale or translucent than the surrounding normal creamy white matter. Classic cerebral plaques are found near the edge of the lateral ventricles beneath the corpus callosum and have crescent-shaped or irregular outlines (Figure 3.82). In other locations, the plaques can occur in any part of the white matter, can spill over into the gray matter where myelinated fibers also exist, do not respect tract boundaries or vascular territories, and may affect any area of the deep nuclei, brain stem, or spinal cord. Occasionally, MS may be confined to the immediate subcortical region, in which case the victim may present with seizures or dementia (Figure 3.83). Especially in the brain stem, plaques may be very irregular, but there is a tendency for them to be 1 to 2 cm in diameter, roughly spherical or crescent, and to have sharp boundaries both grossly and microscopically. Precisely what the earliest lesion in MS is was debated for years until a few fortuitous brain biopsies managed to glimpse acute plaques. Later, when stereotactic brain biopsies became common, the pathology of the acute plaque was revealed as an often very inflammatory, even necrotizing process, sometimes visible as a ring-enhancing, space-making lesion [566]. In what once were regarded (usually at autopsy) as early plaques, only myelin was lost, with good preservation of axons that pass through the lesion unhampered. In older plaques, axons were said to be gradually lost, so that the plaque is composed of rarified tissue, mostly capillaries, and astroglial processes without cyst formation, as would be expected in an infarct. It is this lack of necrosis that further characterized the MS plaques before a more complete temporal view of them was achieved. Recently, a more thorough understanding of the role of inflammation and inflammatory mediators in the MS plaque has evolved, such that the prospects for remyelination in a

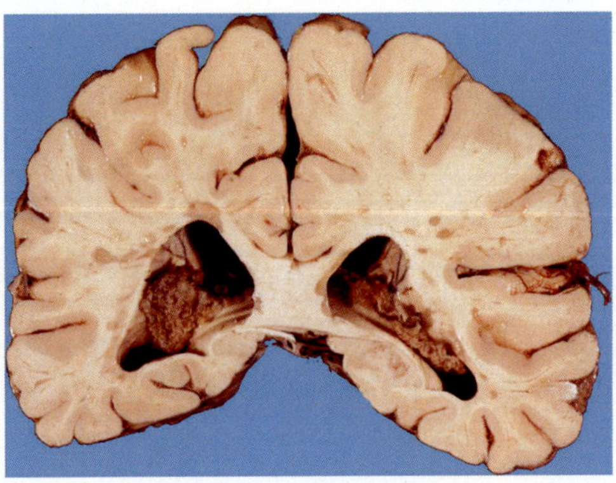

Figure 3.82 This coronal section of the posterior part of the cerebrum illustrates typical "sentinel" MS plaques about the ventricles as well as a number of relatively small plaques scattered through the white matter.

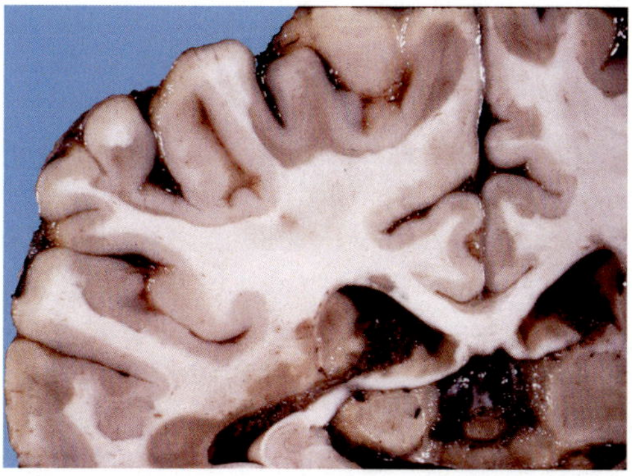

Figure 3.83 This photograph illustrates more MS plaques involving the corpus callosum and periventricular white matter but note that virtually all the immediately subcortical white matter is starkly highlighted against the deeper white matter. In this case, there is diffuse subcortical MS plaque formation, which effectively cuts off the cortex from the rest of the brain. In this case, the victim was demented as a result. Note also in the left superior convolution, the MS plaque extends to involve the cortex.

lesion may in fact be dependent upon some aspects of the inflammatory reaction in the plaque. A special, rare, and enigmatic possible form of MS in which remyelination is prominent and shows concentric rings of remyelination is Balo's concentric sclerosis [567].

What it is that triggers the demyelinating process in the first place has been the subject of much investigation over the years and remains as enigmatic now as it was more than 100 years ago, when Charcot made his classic observations on the disease [562]. The more popular mechanisms hypothesized today are (1) the viral theory of MS, (2) the immunological theory, and (3) other diverse theories that impute nutritional, genetic, embolic, toxic, and other mechanisms. The viral theories take several forms and include the following possibilities: that direct viral replication by a classic or unconventional virus causes myelin breakdown; that remote viral infection has altered myelin membranes and made them vulnerable to later insult via another viral infection, immunological response to a virus, or other organism; or that an immune response to a new viral infection produces local effects that unintentionally "hit" nearby myelin (innocent bystander effect). The immune hypotheses involve some mechanism like that in experimental allergic encephalomyelitis, where sensitization to myelin basic protein and an autoallergic reaction occur, which may be triggered by a viral infection or some other process. Another possibility is that there is a failure on the part of the individual to recognize his or her own myelin as "self." Some theories make use of combined viral infection and immunological mechanisms in various permutations and combinations. Suffice it to say that there is considerable controversy over these hypotheses, and there is a great deal of experimental evidence to support any or all of them. The relationship of MS to other diseases of the nervous system is sometimes troublesome, and many classify diseases such as Devic's disease and some forms of diffuse white matter disease, like Schilder's, as variants of MS. There are valid reasons for doing this, but the fine points of these arguments are not appropriate in this discussion.

The forensic importance of MS and related conditions, like the neurodegenerative diseases, is that victims often commit suicide, may die in accidents facilitated or caused by their disease, may die at home from unknown causes, or may die in custodial or care facilities from complications of their disease and sometimes neglect or homicide. It may fall to the pathologist to attempt to correlate the pathological lesions with some measure of functional state of the victim for various purposes, which sometimes involve litigation. It would be wise in such circumstances for the forensic pathologist to seek the advice and counsel of an experienced neuropathologist who may be able to assist in these tasks.

A number of cases of misdiagnosis of MS as a brain neoplasm or other mass-making lesion have occurred that have resulted in lawsuits against pathologists, even neuropathologists, radiologists, neurosurgeons, and radiation oncologists. These occasionally invariably arise because the radiological picture of a ring-enhancing, mass-making lesion immediately calls to mind the diagnosis of brain tumor (primary or secondary), abscess, or another lesion [568–571]. When or if a biopsy is taken, owing to the small amount of tissue and sometimes the worrisome cellularity and gliosis of the specimen, as well as the presence of sometimes-bizarre macrophages that may possess mitotic figures, macrophages are frequently mistaken for neoplastic glial cells by the pathologist, who may be inexperienced or led astray by the radiographic appearance of the lesion that strongly suggests a neoplasm, and the lesion may be wrongly diagnosed as such (Figures 3.84 and 3.85). Treatment may then proceed as if the lesion were a neoplasm (radiation and chemotherapy), which may or may not be discovered to be in error, often with disastrous consequences for the patient [572]. There appears to be little doubt that irradiation of MS is not helpful and may worsen the course of the disease with or without radiation necrosis. Litigation in such cases is common.

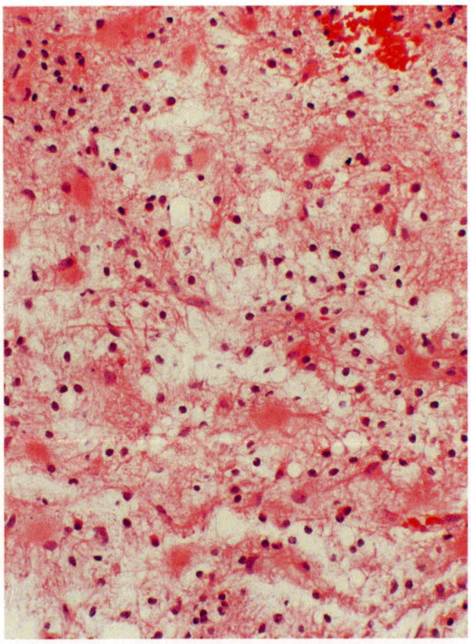

Figure 3.84 This photomicrograph from a stereotactic brain biopsy of a victim of rapidly progressive (Marburg variant) MS illustrates a typical necrotic appearance of a plaque in such a case. Note the many star-shaped gemistocytic reactive astrocytes and the background of macrophages (small round dark nuclei surrounded by halos).

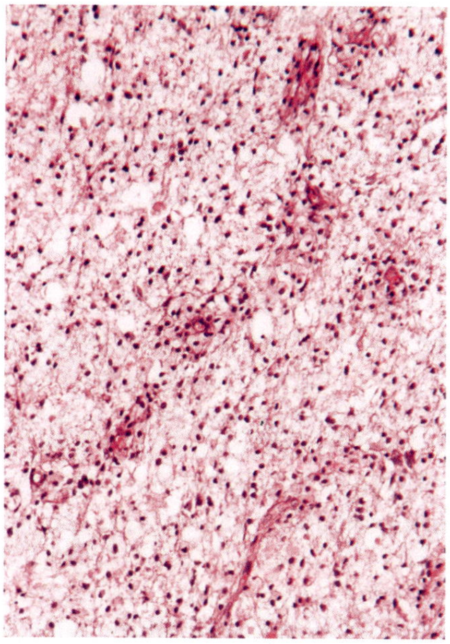

Figure 3.85 This photomicrograph from another stereotactic brain biopsy from an individual who presented with seizures and a ring-enhancing lesion of the subcortical white matter. This rather cellular lesion has few, if any, gemistocytic astrocytes and shows prominent capillaries and clustering of cells about them. There have been many instances in which biopsies such as this one have been misinterpreted as being gliomas, when, in fact, they represent acute MS plaques filled with all stages of macrophage activation.

Toxic and Miscellaneous Conditions

There are a great many toxins, chemical, radiological, and biological, that affect the nervous system. Neurotoxicology, once a restricted and esoteric subspecialty within the broader field of toxicology or neuroscience, has become a burgeoning field in recent years, attracting scientists from all disciplines of biology and medicine. Evidence of increasing interest is that several journals are now devoted entirely to neurotoxicology alone, and substantial portions of toxicology journals, as well as brain research and neuroscience journals, are devoted to some aspect of neurotoxicology and its role in experimental models or as probes for studying cellular and molecular processes in the nervous system. Because there are so many forms of neurological injury that can result from ingestion, inhalation, or other exposure to a wide range of common as well as esoteric substances and chemicals, it behooves the active forensic pathologist as well as the neuropathologist to be aware of, at the very least, the most important of these and the general principles by which exogenous substances produce neurological injury and how such injuries can he recognized or characterized. Most recent texts of forensic pathology highlight the most important and common toxic conditions [573–575], and there are a number of excellent texts on neurotoxicology by itself to which the reader is referred [576–579]. The following will be an abbreviated discussion of some of the most common and important toxic conditions affecting the nervous system of practical importance to the forensic pathologist.

From a conceptual point of view, the simplest and most logical approach to the pathology of toxic injury of the nervous system is to examine those substances that affect a specific portion of the nervous system, such as the peripheral nerve (its neuron, axon, nerve ending, or myelin sheath), the central neurons in perikaryon, axon, dendrites, or processes, the glial cells, the vessels, or other specialized structures within the brain or cord. One might extend such a division downward to the subcellular level by specifying those substances that affect the cell membrane (its ionic channels, synaptic specializations, or junctions) or that affect the cytoskeleton (neurotubules, neurofilaments, etc.), endoplasmic reticulum, Golgi apparatus, ribosomes, lysosomes, mitochondria, or cell nucleus [578,579]. One could also continue to the molecular level of toxic interaction in some cases. Another approach might be to associate the various toxic substances with their power to disrupt given neural functions, such as in the blood–brain barrier, so as to produce cerebral or neural edema, alteration of neural conduction or synaptic transmission, or more complex functions that may produce alterations of neural development and behavioral abnormalities, induce seizures, produce ataxia and sensory disturbances including blindness, or cause paralysis.

Still another approach might be to separate the various toxic agents by type (heavy metals; organometallic compounds; aliphatic, aromatic, and complex organic compounds, including many drugs, natural plant products, animal and plant venoms, toxins, etc.), but there is no uniform effect by any of these types of toxic substances, and the pathology of each class may be quite diverse. Each form of intoxication now has monographs devoted almost solely to these areas [578–582].

The nervous system relies on a variety of barrier functions to preserve its highly sensitive homeostatic environment. The most important of these barriers is the so-called blood–brain barrier (see Chapter 5), but others include the blood–CSF barriers and blood–nerve barriers. There are many processes that disrupt these barrier functions and lead to edema or transudation; these include hypoxia/ischemia, thermal injury, physical injury, neoplasia, metabolic imbalances, and toxic exposure. Edema may result when brain vessels are injured (because the endothelium is probably the most important and sensitive element in the blood–brain barrier system). Brain endothelium may be injured by toxic substances in a variety of ways that may compromise the so-called tight intercapillary junctions or compromise the energy metabolism of the endothelial cell and thus the membrane processes, including various transport and membrane functions so vital to its barrier function. Such toxins may physically disrupt the cell membrane by virtue of a solubilizing effect (hydrocarbons), damage subtle membrane functions such as ion channels or receptor sites (ouabain, marine toxins, heavy metals), or poison enzyme systems within the membranes or within the cells (cyanide, carbon monoxide, heavy metals, azides, etc.). As is typical among the toxic agents, there are many more examples known in experimental animals than in humans, and most human examples have been discovered in connection with accidental exposures, most often associated with industrial or environmental accidents.

Substances that, as a part of their pathology, appear to disrupt, in some fashion, various neural barrier systems in the brain or nerves include the following: lead, mercury salts, hexachlorophene, triethyl tin, aluminum, nickel, arsenic, tellurium, bismuth, manganese, phosphorus, gold, various alcohols, radiographic contrast media, vitamin A, cyanides, cardiac glycosides, 6-aminonicotinamide, isonicotinic acid hydrazide (INH), cycloleucine [581–588]. Only some of these have been observed clinically to poison man, and most have been discovered to have this effect only in experimental animals. The consequence of disruption of blood–brain barrier function by these or other agents is the production of increased intra- or extracellular water, which in the brain leads to increased intracranial pressure, possibly herniation, stupor, coma, and death (discussed in detail in Chapter 5).

In the peripheral nerve, edema may lead to degeneration of the myelin sheath or axon if it is protracted. The resulting neuropathy may cause motor, sensory, or combined symptoms.

Toxicity Affecting Axonal Transport

The process of intracellular transport is found in all cells but is highly specialized within the nervous system, where the cellular processes (neurites) of most nerve cells are far more voluminous and extensive than virtually any other cell in the body. This process of neuroplasmic transport (axonal transport) is necessary to provide the cytoplasmic extensions of nerve cells with nutrients and to return exhausted organelles and metabolites to the cell body for degradation, because comparatively little synthetic or degradative activity exists in peripheral neuronal processes.

The most common substances that affect neuroplasmic transport are the so-called mitotic spindle inhibitors, of which colchicine, vinblastine, and vincristine are the most common, certainly to the experimental neuroscientist [578,579,589–591]. A variety of other substances interfere with neuroplasmic transport as well, either by probable interaction with the cytoskeletal apparatus or by interfering with what appear to be membrane-associated neuroplasmic transport mechanisms. These include various ketones (methyl *n*-butyl ketone, methyl ethyl ketone), the hexacarbons (*n*-hexane, 2,5-hexanedione, cyclohexanone), aluminum salts, fluorinated organic compounds (fluoroacetate, fluorocitrate), acrylamide, triorthocresyl phosphate, doxorubicin (Adriamycin), zinc pyrinethione, *p*-bromophenyl-acetylurea, diethyldithiocarbamate, iminodipropionitrile (IDPN), and probably many others [592–596].

The biological impact of some disruption in intracellular transport, including neuroplasmic transport, is varied, depending on the precise locus of injury to this complex mechanism. Nevertheless, disruption of this process usually results in the eventual degeneration of one or more portions of the neuron or its processes but has little immediate effect on electrical conduction. The toxic effects of the axonal transport block often mimic interruption of the axon as far as the neuron is concerned and set into motion a series of reactions known as the axonal reaction. In most cases, the peripheral nervous system neuron and its processes are involved, but occasionally central neurons may be affected. The result of injury to the peripheral nervous system is motor or sensory dysfunction or both. This damage may be temporary (repairable) or permanent.

Case examples of therapeutic misuse of mitotic spindle inhibitors have found their way into the courts by way of wrongful death litigation. Examples of these are inappropriate intrathecal administration of vincristine and colchicine that resulted in widespread damage to the spinal cord and death to the victims (Figures 3.86 and 3.87) [590].

Toxicity Affecting Neural Membrane Function

The majority of these agents are animal, plant, or microorganism toxins and thus often have complex chemical compositions [597]. Some of these toxins are rather esoteric, rarely producing human morbidity or mortality, and of interest primarily to researchers, whereas others occupy a prominent position in human toxicology by virtue of either their commonness or their potency. Some other toxic agents that can be included in this group are relatively simple organic chemical compounds that have been commonly used as pesticides or for vermin control.

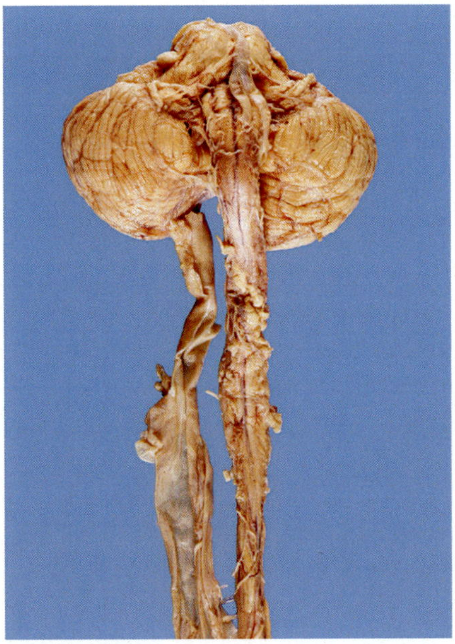

Figure 3.86 This gross photograph of the brain in continuity with the spinal cord illustrates severe atrophy of the cord that followed an unfortunate intrathecal injection of colchicines in a patient with spondylitis. The route of administration for colchicine is contraindicated. (Courtesy of the Office of the Medical Examiner, Cook County, IL.)

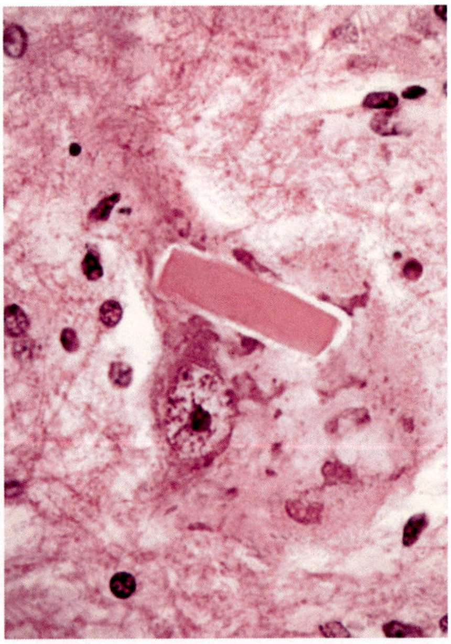

Figure 3.87 This photomicrograph illustrates a spinal anterior horn neuron from another unfortunate case of an individual with leukemia who received an intrathecal administration of vincristine that caused destruction of the cord and the death of the patient. The crystal is precipitated tubulin. (Courtesy of Dr. S. Schochet, Armed Forces Institute of Pathology, Washington, DC.)

The most well known of the so-called membrane-active neurotoxins are the marine toxins, tetrodotoxin (TTX), saxitoxin (STX), and ciguatoxin (CTX) [578,597–599]. TTX is the toxin found in the ovaries of the puffer fish (blowfish) and is responsible for occasional incidents of poisoning in Japan, where the puffer fish is consumed as a delicacy. This toxin seems to have a high degree of specificity for the membrane sodium channel that it disrupts. The biological effect of this disruption is neuronal dysfunction, which leads to paralysis, coma, and death in some cases.

The Alcohols

There is probably no class of compounds generally available that causes more neuropathology than the alcohols, specifically ethanol, although in the usual context of neurotoxicology the exposure to this compound is unique because it is uncommonly accidental. Rather, its use has been so completely incorporated into human lifestyle that one could consider it a foodstuff. However, most enlightened individuals recognize the drug-like attributes of ethanol, not to mention the potential it has for the production of human disease. Ethanol and other alcohols are common industrial solvents and are used widely, and human contact is widespread. Environmental exposure and unwitting consumption of methanol and some of the higher alcohols regularly cause death and debility, at least to some extent as a result of neurotoxicity and the neurological complications of poisoning.

Methanol, or so-called wood alcohol, is a common solvent in use in myriad applications in industry and in the home, in lacquer and paint thinners and solvents, and as an antifreeze and fuel. Accidental exposures, especially in industry, almost always involve inhalation of the vapors of methanol or, less commonly, absorption through the skin, whereas in civilian environments intoxications almost always result from accidental or willful oral consumption as a substitute for ethanol. Methanol is commonly used as a denaturant, along with isopropyl alcohol (rubbing alcohol), for ethanol and, as such, is frequently consumed unwittingly by alcoholics in search of a substitute for beverage alcohol.

The symptoms of methanol intoxication at first are no different from intoxication with ethanol, and the intoxicated individual appears typically inebriated. However, within a few hours to 24 hours after consumption, the victim becomes violently ill, with nausea, vomiting, abdominal pain, and visual disturbances including blindness, and may lapse into a coma from which he or she may not recover [601–603]. Not everyone will display these symptoms or even become ill, and some may even be able to tolerate chronic consumption of methanol. In large-scale poisonings, fatalities may reach 25%, with the remainder showing a variety of residua [603].

Methanol is metabolized to formaldehyde and then to formic acid, which leads to systemic metabolic acidosis. Methanol levels in blood and various tissues can be measured reliably, as can formate levels [580]. The combination of high levels of formate and acidosis is probably responsible for edema in the optic nerve and the brain, although the exact pathogenesis of brain and nerve lesions is not known.

Neuropathologically, the brain will usually be edematous and show petechial hemorrhages over the meninges and within the brain. There will usually be evidence of diffuse neuronal toxicity, as seen by many red neurons, or small depopulated or microcystic changes in the cortex where neurons have dropped out. Occasionally, laminar necrosis of the cerebral cortex may be seen as well as necrosis of the globes pallidus or striatum, which may lead to a parkinsonian state [603]. The microscopic changes often reflect the duration of the terminal course in that the longer the individual has survived, the greater chance there is for histological changes to develop. The changes of the respirator brain may also be superimposed on the above. Within the eye there may be degeneration of the retina and optic atrophy [604]. Experimental methanol intoxication has not been as thoroughly studied as many of the other neurotoxins, and much remains to be learned about the pathogenesis of neural injury due to this alcohol.

Ethanol or grain alcohol is a common industrial and laboratory chemical used in many solvents, lacquers, inks, dyes, and paints; in gasohol as a fuel additive; in medicinal preparations such as cough syrups, elixirs, and tinctures; and in cosmetic preparations such as aftershave lotions, mouthwashes, colognes, and perfumes; and it is probably most widely consumed as beverage alcohol in beers, wines, and liquors. Only rare examples of workplace intoxication due to inhalation occur, and, as mentioned above, ethanol is not thought of as an industrial toxin but, rather, a social one, in which vast numbers of persons worldwide are incapacitated as a result of its use. The morbidity, mortality, and total costs to society associated with alcohol use are enormous. The systemic pathology and forensic aspects of alcohol use and abuse will not be discussed here and are adequately covered in most standard forensic pathology texts. Rather, only the main neuropathological aspects of alcohol use and abuse will be presented.

Acute Ethyl Alcohol Intoxication

It is well known that the tolerance for ethyl alcohol is highly variable and depends largely on the regularity of its consumption, which induces appropriate hepatic enzymes for its degradation [580]. Apparently, there is little or no definite measurable effect on brain morphology from short-term consumption of alcohol in adults, although one often hears various vocal proponents of abstinence preach that, in effect, each drink may cause the loss of millions of nerve cells. If one were to challenge such individuals to produce a credible scientific study to support this contention, they would be unable to do so, because none exist, and it is unlikely that any study of this kind could ever be done that would be credible. It appears that whatever effects are observed in an acutely intoxicated individual eventually pass away, although they may leave an unpleasant residue in the form of a hangover. The nature of this aftermath of alcohol use has never been universally agreed upon, although there is some evidence that accumulation of acetaldehyde in brain and other tissues is responsible [605]. In the short term, there appears to be little effect of this metabolic residue, which eventually is resolved, but there is no doubt that repeated and prolonged consumption of alcohol can have a major impact on brain function and can produce a series of pathological conditions, which are discussed below.

Acute alcohol intoxication in a naive individual, such as a child or young person, or extreme excess consumption in an experienced alcohol user can occasionally be fatal. Such consumption may occur in conjunction with drinking contests, initiation ceremonies or hazing exercises, or exhibitions of braggadocio and may occasionally occur accidentally when an unwitting individual is forced or induced to drink beverages containing alcohol, not realizing how much he or she is imbibing until he or she loses control over his or her actions. Under these conditions, the individual may become rapidly intoxicated and lose consciousness. During unconsciousness the individual may vomit and aspirate with immediate or delayed fatal effect, may fall and seriously or fatally injure himself or herself, or may drown. Occasionally, highly intoxicated individuals may become entangled in clothing or other material and may strangle themselves. On other occasions, the intoxication may be so acute and intense that central respiratory depression may occur alone or in combination with acute cerebral edema to produce fatal respiratory or cardiac arrest. This combination of circumstances is often observed in situations where an individual may consume a whole bottle of spirits (vodka, whiskey, gin, etc.) within a short period of time, as in "chug-a-lug" contests. When autopsies are done on such individuals, the brain will usually appear swollen and show evidence of uncal and tonsillar herniation and will often, in the fresh state, have a frankly alcoholic or fruity (ketone) smell. Blood alcohol levels in such cases may be as little as 200 mg% but usually are much greater. The precise levels of blood alcohol that will produce a fatal outcome are highly variable from individual to individual and cannot be reliably predicted [606].

Chronic Alcohol Abuse

There is no doubt whatsoever that in some, but not all, individuals chronic alcohol use affects brain function and can produce a series of well-known alcohol-related or alcohol-caused diseases of the nervous system. Whether these are the result of the direct toxic effects of alcohol or its metabolites, or of associated nutritional or other secondary conditions, they are, and have been, a constant source of disagreement among scientific workers, and several of them are controversial as to etiology. The following neurological conditions have been associated with chronic alcohol use: Wernicke's disease (and Korsakoff's syndrome) [607,608]; alcoholic cerebellar degeneration [609]; alcoholic myopathy; alcoholic polyneuropathy or effects of Antabuse treatment [610,611] Marchiafava–Bignami disease; chronic brain syndrome, presumably due to alcohol and alcoholic cerebral atrophy; transverse myelopathy; cerebral trauma; accidental carbon monoxide intoxication; accidental or homicidal injuries, including gunshot wounds; hepatic encephalopathy; central pontine myelinolysis (CPM) [612–615]; PML; subacute combined degeneration of the cord; sudden unexpected death; alcohol withdrawal seizures and delirium tremens; and accidental poisoning with lead, ethylene glycol, methanol, and other adulterants or substitutes for ethanol. Toxic interactions with alcohol and various drugs, including Antabuse (disulfuram), may also occur [610]. Although many of these are somewhat indirect effects of alcohol abuse, they are nonetheless part of the pathology of alcoholism and form a substantial part of the workload of the forensic pathologist.

Wernicke's Disease

The first cases described by Wernicke in 1881, and by others in succeeding years, did not apparently involve alcohol abuse but were then mostly seen in connection with systemic neoplasia, nutritional disorders, pernicious anemia, and chronic GI diseases [607,611]. Since that time it has been recognized that chronic alcohol abuse is also an important cause, if not an accompaniment, to the syndrome, perhaps acting alone by direct toxic effect in some individuals or, more likely, causing primary or secondary thiamine deficiency or malutilization in the brain [611], and thus is related to Leigh encephalopathy. Clinically, the syndrome may be acute, subacute, or chronic and is characterized by disorientation, confusion, loss of memory, ataxia, nystagmus, paralysis of the oculomotor and trochlear nerves (extraocular muscle palsy, meiosis, depressed pupillary reflexes), and peripheral

Central Pontine Myelinolysis

CPM is a condition that can occur in chronic alcoholics but, like Wernicke's disease, is not limited to this group. It has been reported in a variety of poor nutritional states, severe hyponatremia, and chronic lung or liver disease; as a remote effect of neoplasia or peptic disease; and in other conditions [612–615]. CPM, oddly enough, displays no specific clinical findings but may be associated with signs of Wernicke's disease, quadriplegia, pseudobuibar palsy, and polyneuropathy and is generally only diagnosed at autopsy. Improved methods of tomographic and MRI may demonstrate the lesion in life. Neuropathologically, the lesion is seen grossly as a gray or faded triangular plaque involving the area of the mid-pons directly beneath the pontine tegmentum in the central basis pontis, but it may include virtually the entire basis pontis (Figure 3.90). The lesion is rarely necrotic in appearance or cavitary and can be easily missed or dismissed as an artifact of fixation. Microscopically, the most striking findings emerge when the pons is subjected to myelin stains, which show virtually total absence of myelin but preservation of neurons in the affected area. Sometimes identical lesions can be seen focally in other portions of the brain. Myelin breakdown products can often be found in macrophages, and minimal lymphoid reactions are occasionally seen in the lesions. Older lesions may show reactive gliosis, and sometimes so-called Alzheimer type II gliosis can be noted, which is most commonly a feature of hepatic encephalopathy. The cause of CPM is not clear but has been associated with severe hyponatremia and too-rapid rehydration [615].

Carbon Monoxide Poisoning

The effects of carbon monoxide (CO) intoxication on the nervous system are striking and variable and are regularly observed on any active forensic pathology service. Thus, it demands a thorough understanding by all who are called upon to pass judgment in potential cases. Despite widespread public awareness of the dangers of CO, large numbers of individuals die or are incapacitated by it each year, and this can be expected to continue.

Carbon monoxide, a colorless, tasteless, odorless gas, was first discovered by Priestley in 1799, but it was not until 1860 that Claude Bernard discovered that the mechanism of its toxicity occurred because of its more competitive binding (250 times) to hemoglobin than

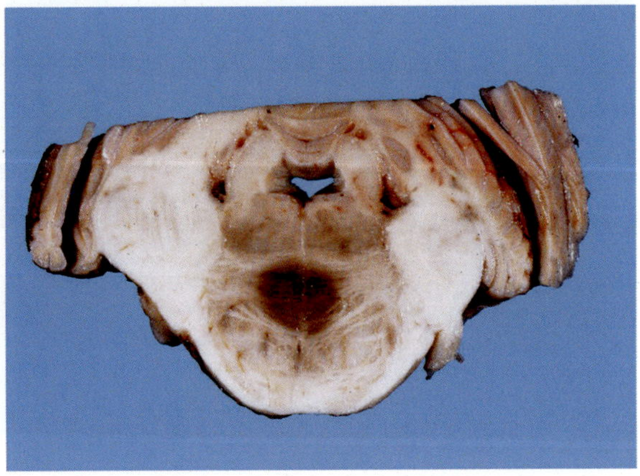

Figure 3.90 The section of the mid-pons illustrates the phenomenon of CPM. The lesion may be larger or smaller but typically occupies this central location.

oxygen. Carbon monoxide also interferes with oxidative enzymes, such as cytochrome oxidase in cells, and thus has secondary effects beyond those inherent in the lack of oxygen-carrying capacity of the blood [616,617].

Carbon monoxide normally exists in the atmosphere in concentrations of about 1 part per 100,000 and is increased in urban environments, especially during thermal inversions and whenever the air is highly polluted due to automobile or industrial emissions. Odd as it might seem, plants produce CO in addition to oxygen, and concentrations in forests and jungles are somewhat higher than in nonforested areas. Virtually any combustion process involving organic matter produces carbon monoxide because of incomplete oxidation of carbon or its compounds, and it cannot be assumed that its production in automobile emissions or furnace emission is necessarily due to faulty design or malfunction, though malfunctions or poor adjustments in these types of equipment may result in higher-than-normal outputs of the gas. Ordinary automobile exhaust emissions contain 7% to 12% CO, even under the best of circumstances [616,618].

Human intoxication by CO can occur under many diverse circumstances, and it is said that about 50% of such instances are accidental and 50% are intentional (suicidal). Accidental intoxication may occur when furnaces or space heaters are operated without proper ventilation or are malfunctioning, when automobile exhaust systems are plugged or leaky and allow seepage into the passenger compartment, or when automobiles or other engines are operated in closed spaces such as workrooms or garages without adequate ventilation. When fireplaces or charcoal braziers are operated without proper ventilation, dangerous concentrations of CO may also occur. Occasionally, CO gas may be drawn into ventilation systems in buildings or mines with serious toxic results, or CO may be produced by machinery that may contaminate air conditioning or air suppliers. Such is sometimes the case in scuba air compressors or surface air supplies for divers, in which inappropriate oil has been used to lubricate the compressor, improper filters have been used, or oil has contaminated cylinders or lines that may then become partially oxidized to yield CO in harmful concentrations. At one time in the United States, city gas (illuminating gas) contained substantial concentrations of CO (which is combustible), but since the introduction of natural gas rather than manufactured coal gas, very little, if any, CO is found in municipal or bottled gas. In some parts of the world, because of a shortage of natural gas and a dependence on artificially produced gas, CO may be present in significant concentrations to cause problems to humans. Every fire or combustion process produces CO, and the dangers to fire victims and firefighters from this source are well known. In the case of suicidal exposure to CO, everyone is familiar with the method usually employed—that of operating an automobile engine in a closed garage [616,631].

It has been presumed that a concentration of CO below 1 part per 10,000 in air is not dangerous to most healthy persons, but individuals with heart or respiratory diseases may be harmed by this level. An important phenomenon in regard to CO, because of its tenacity in binding with hemoglobin, is that relatively low concentrations in air can rapidly result in accumulation of carboxyhemoglobin (HbCO) in the blood. At 1:10,000 CO concentration in air, within relatively few minutes a human being will equilibrate to a steady-state blood concentration of about 10% HbCO, which, in most people, will not produce symptoms. In fact, an individual accustomed to smoking (and inhaling) a pack or more of cigarettes per day will probably carry a HbCO concentration of 5 to 10% at all times. Similar concentrations are also regularly observed in persons who are surrounded by automobile traffic in their work environment, such as traffic policemen.

Table 3.11 Relationship between CO Concentrations and Symptoms

CO Concentration in Environment	HbCO Concentration in Blood (%)	Symptoms/Outcomes
1:10,000	10	No symptoms, no danger
1:5000	20–30	Nausea, headache
1:3000	30–40	Headache, confusion; +– residual effects
1:1000	40–50	Delirium, coma; +– fatalities; + residual effects
1:500	60–70	Death in 4–5 hours; ++ residual effects with survival
1:20	>80	Death in 15 minutes; +++ residual effects with survival

Source: Adapted from Camps FE et al., eds., *Gradwohl's Legal Medicine*, Bristol: A. John Wright, 1976.

The relationships among environmental CO concentrations, blood concentrations of HbCO, and symptomatology are given in Table 3.11.

Although this table gives some relative indications of outcomes by environmental concentration of CO, there are many variables that enter into ultimate outcomes of CO exposures. These include individual factors and responses and the time of actual exposure versus concentrations of CO during exposure, as well as any treatment given. As previously mentioned, it is possible to develop fatal concentrations of HbCO very rapidly with very few breaths in heavily contaminated air. For example, in an atmosphere of 10% CO, it is possible to attain a 60% HbCO level in 1 minute. Furthermore, to spontaneously "blow off" accumulated CO may take a protracted period of time if normal room air is breathed, but blow-off is accelerated if pure oxygen is respired. Further acceleration can be achieved if the victim is placed in a hyperbaric oxygen environment. The consequence of the tenacious binding of CO with hemoglobin in which 50% or more of the hemoglobin is in the form of HbCO rather than HbO is that the brain and other organs are subjected to a special form of hypoxia in which blood flow is preserved. The effects on the nervous system of this form of cellular hypoxia, combined with whatever special direct toxic effects CO has on cellular oxidative enzymatic functions, are a series of clinical and pathological states that are commonly recognized as associated with CO poisoning but may not ultimately be unique for this condition.

In acutely fatal CO intoxication, consciousness is never restored and the victim dies before any major reaction can be observed in the brain beyond the expected cherry red color of the unfixed specimen due to HbCO in the tissue and some degree of cerebral congestion and edema. Microscopic examination of such a specimen may reveal little or nothing of note, but if there has been survival of some hours, red neurons and evidence of edema may be seen in the hippocampus, the pallidal, and the striatum as well as in middle laminae of the cerebral cortex. In other individuals who survive longer, perhaps due to aggressive and prompt treatment or less severe exposure, there will be a period of unconsciousness that may or may not clear. More often than not, consciousness is never restored. At autopsy the brain will probably have lost the cherry red color of acute intoxication, may appear entirely normal, and may be swollen or even show changes typical for the respirator brain, depending on many preterminal factors. In such brains, however, one is usually likely to observe some degree of necrosis of the cerebral cortex in a lamellar pattern (laminar necrosis or pseudolaminar necrosis), most typically in the hippocampal regions (about 50% of the time) but possibly also scattered in other cortical areas (Figure 3.91). In

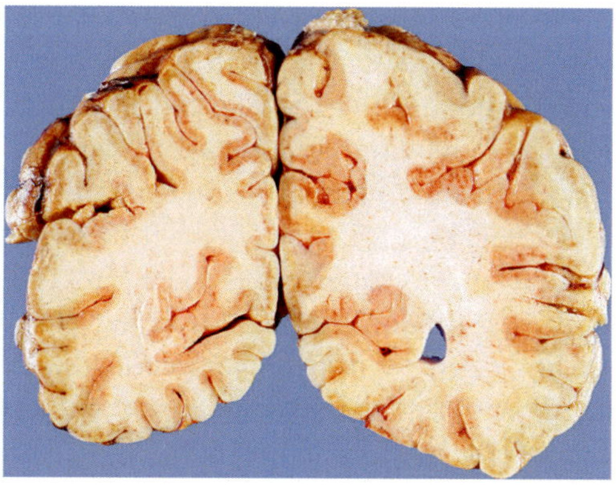

Figure 3.91 This coronal section of the brain of a victim of carbon monoxide intoxication who survived for about a week after exposure illustrates widespread cortical necrosis.

addition, it is very common to observe necrosis of the globus pallidus alone or in combination with striatal necrosis, or necrosis of other deep nuclear masses in a patchy fashion (Figure 3.92) [618].

Depending on the duration of the intoxication and the length of time the lesions have had to develop, necrosis may be minimal and early or obvious and cavitary. In individuals who have remained in coma for protracted periods of time, the affected structures may be completely destroyed and are represented as brown, cavitary outlines of the former nuclei. The pattern of destruction corresponds to roughly the same areas affected in pure hypoxia and illustrates the phenomenon of selective vulnerability. Microscopically, the necrotic areas are suffused with macrophages and differ little from the changes expected in an infarction. There is nothing in the microscopic appearance that is specific for CO poisoning.

In rare individuals who either have been treated early or were exposed to a borderline dose of CO, a biphasic clinical course may occur [618,619]. The individual is usually in coma for a period of days or weeks, during which there may be convulsions, periods of decerebrate posturing, and hypertonia or hypotonia, with respiratory or vasomotor

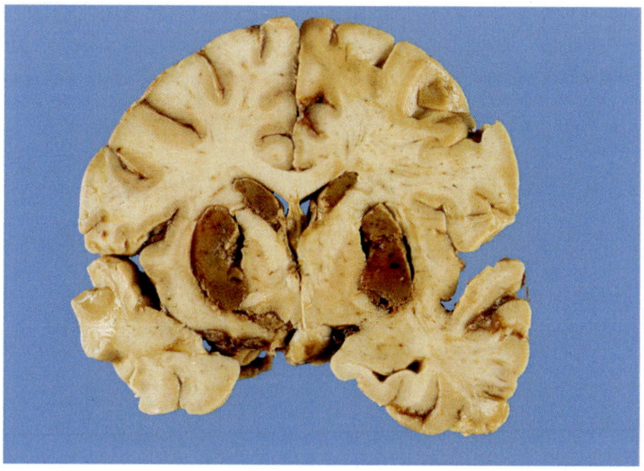

Figure 3.92 This coronal section of the brain of a carbon monoxide intoxication victim who survived several weeks reveals bilateral necrosis of the basal ganglia without apparent other lesions grossly. This same pattern may be seen in individuals who suffer heroin or barbiturate overdoses and/or sometimes insulin overdose and its attendant severe hypoglycemia.

instability. However, eventually the coma clears and the victim gradually appears to recover, but in most cases incompletely. However, occasionally recovery may be nearly complete. An interval of nearly normal functioning may take place, but within 10 to 30 days a progressive encephalopathy recurs in which individuals may become demented and akinetic, show muscular rigidity, and drift into a stuporous or comatose state from which they do not recover. The neuropathological examination of such victims reveals one or more patterns of injury. If the deterioration was rapid and the lucid interval short, the brain may be swollen externally, but on the cut section the deep draining veins of the white matter will appear enormously dilated and show perivenous hemorrhages. Such a case is illustrated in Figure 3.93. There may or may not be associated necrosis of the pallidum and other deep nuclear areas. In cases that survive longer and may have a more protracted interval of consciousness, the brain may appear entirely normal externally, but the cut section presents the appearance of diffuse white matter degeneration, resembling that seen in the leukodystrophies. Here the white matter has a gray or creamy color. There is sparing of the subcortical myelinated U fibers, and the entire centrum ovale as well as the cerebellar white matter will show demyelination. Hemorrhages in the white matter may or may not be seen.

This latter form of CO poisoning is uncommon but has been known for many years and is often referred to as Grinker myelinopathy [618,619]. The pathogenesis of this unusual lesion appears to be due to a delayed effect of CO on cerebral microcirculation, specifically on venules in the white matter rather than on some form of unusual delayed reaction in oligodendroglia. This hypothesis is supported by clinical observations in humans such as have been illustrated above and also in the experimental laboratory, where identical lesions have been produced in dogs and other animals [620]. In these experiments it has been shown that cerebral arterial pressure and perfusion are decreased, whereas venous pressure drastically increases, perhaps due to intracerebral mechanisms as well as to a more generalized rise in venous pressure, possibly due to an element of cardiac failure. Other theories suggest that hypoxia and perhaps CO itself incite a particularly damaging form of edema which then results in white matter necrosis. Support for these theories can be found in pathological lesions similar to those of CO poisoning, where hypoxia and dehydration and too-rapid rehydration have occurred without the presence of CO.

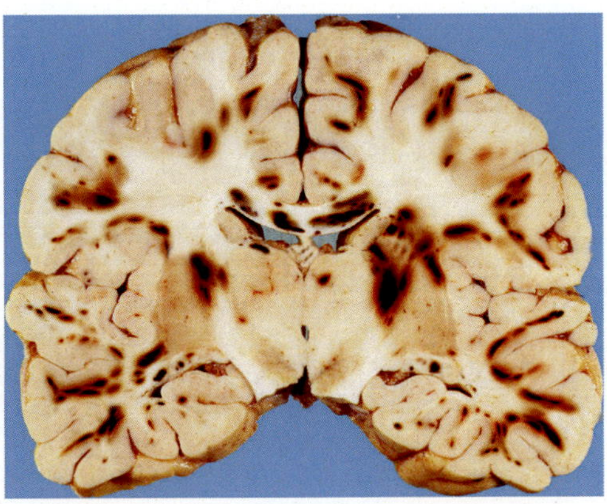

Figure 3.93 This coronal section of the brain of a victim of carbon monoxide intoxication illustrates Grinker myelinopathy. This victim survived for several weeks in coma and then died. The entire white matter of the brain and cerebellum showed extensive perivenous hemorrhage and necrosis. (Courtesy of the Office of the Medical Examiner, Cook County, IL.)

Oxygen Toxicity

It may appear paradoxical that one of the most important elements to the metabolism of the brain and the other organs, when delivered in excess, would have a deleterious effect, but this fact was appreciated, although not understood, even in the 1800s. Pulmonary toxicity was first noted, and later CNS toxicity (the Paul Bert effect) became known [621]. This toxicity to the brain was first recognized when animals were exposed to higher-than-atmospheric pressures of pure oxygen and suffered convulsive seizures. Later, Bean [621] found that in addition to convulsions, permanent neurological deficits (forelimb paralysis and rigidity) could be produced in rats that were repeatedly exposed to hyperbaric oxygen. The importance of these observations to humans has arisen only relatively recently in conjunction with the aerospace program and the rapidly advancing technology of deep-sea diving, as well as hyperbaric medicine's application for treating decompression sickness (the bends), clostridial infections, neoplasia, and other conditions. A further human consideration has arisen in connection with the burgeoning field of neonatology, where the complications of oxygen therapy have had the greatest impact (hyaline membrane disease and retrolental fibroplasia) [622].

The study of experimental oxygen toxicity in the nervous system has revealed that necrotizing lesions can be produced in the brains of animals probably by a multifaceted toxic effect on the enzymes of cellular respiration, of various cellular organelles including mitochondria, and of cell membranes by means of free radical and peroxide formation [621]. However, it is heartening to learn that such necrotizing lesions have not yet been reported in humans. The only important CNS effects that have been reported are convulsions, which can be fatal, and retrolental fibroplasia in the retinas of infants treated with high concentrations of oxygen for prolonged periods of time. The pathology and pathogenesis of retrolental fibroplasia have recently been reviewed by Terry [622].

Diseases of Peripheral Nerve

Peripheral nerve diseases [593,623,624] can be divided into those in which the primary disease process is in the myelin sheath provided by the Schwann cell, which invests the nerve fiber, and those conditions where the major problem is in the nerve fiber. Because both structures are interdependent, degeneration of one usually results in degeneration of the other; hence, peripheral nerve diseases are rarely simple and often involve both primary and reactive pathological changes at the same time. Peripheral neuropathies have many causes and can, for convenience, be divided into the following general groups:

I. Metabolic neuropathies: Diabetic neuropathy; neuropathies due to avitaminosis of the B complex group; neuropathy in uremia, porphyria, hypothyroidism, and as a remote effect of systemic cancer; neuropathies in connection with inherited metabolic disorders such as metachromatic leukodystrophy, Refsum's disease, Fabry's disease, and Krabbe's disease; amyloidosis

II. Degenerative neuropathies: Charcot–Marie–Tooth disease; Dejerine–Sottas disease; Friedreich's ataxia; hereditary sensory neuropathy, pandysautonomia; the motor neuron diseases

III. Toxic neuropathies: Alcoholic neuropathy; drug-caused neuropathy (vincristine, nitrofurantoins, isoniazid, disulfiram, dapsone, phenytoin, and others); solvent neuropathies (*N*-hexane, methyl *n*-butyl ketone, 2,5-hexanedione, carbon disulfide, trichloroethylene); various organic chemical neuropathies (acrylamide, kepone, cresyl phosphates, hexachorophene, triethyltin); heavy metal neuropathies (lead, thallium, mercury, arsenic)

IV. Vascular neuropathies: Arteriosclerosis; rheumatoid disease, the collagen vascular disease, and arteritides

V. Infectious or inflammatory neuropathies: Landry–Guillain–Barré syndrome; leprosy; allergic neuritis; diphtheritic neuropathy

VI. Traumatic neuropathies: Entrapment neuropathies; compression neuropathies; fracture injuries; laceration and repair reactions

The etiologies and pathologies of many of these conditions speak for themselves and will not be discussed here except to note that diabetes mellitus, alcoholism, and neuropathic remote effects of cancer are by far the most commonly associated conditions, especially in the forensic context. Medical–legal issues may arise with these diseases, but mostly within the context of civil litigation, workers' compensation, and related issues [625]. The interested reader is referred to several recent texts and monographs on peripheral nerve disease for a complete discussion of each of the entities. A noteworthy reference in this regard is the two-volume work by Dyck [593].

Diseases of Skeletal Muscle

Diseases of skeletal muscle take many forms, most of which do not immediately occupy the forensic pathologist. The conditions that may be of concern are those that occur as a result of poisoning, parasitic infection, trauma, stress, and dehydration, or as a reaction to anesthetics or other drugs, as in the neuroleptic malignant (malignant hyperthermia) syndrome. The following brief review of these conditions as well as the more common classic diseases provides background and a source of preliminary information for the forensic pathologist should he or she encounter one of them. For in-depth treatment of the clinical and pathological aspects of muscle disease, the reader is referred to a number of recent books and monographs [626–628].

Muscular Dystrophy and Myopathies

Muscular dystrophy and myopathies constitute a class of diseases that are the muscular degenerative disease counterparts to neurological degenerative diseases in that their etiology is unknown, they are usually familial, they involve degeneration of apparently normal preexisting elements generally without inflammation, and they have few effective treatments other than rehabilitation and genetic counseling. Most of these diseases affect children and are discussed at least in brief in Chapter 4. Those conditions affecting adults or which may have forensic aspects are discussed below.

Myotonic Dystrophy

This distinctive disease is inherited as autosomal dominant and generally makes its appearance usually not earlier than the teen years. Individuals with the disease may never be clinically diagnosed. It occurs with different frequencies in various countries but is usually 2–5 per 100,000 people, or about the same occurrence rate as Duchenne's dystrophy [628,629].

The typical victim of the disease has characteristic facies, those of an elongated dour-appearing face with a drooping mouth. Males tend to have obvious frontal pattern baldness. There is some degree of muscle wasting, with weakness that generally does not tend to progress. In addition to muscle weakness and unsteadiness, victims experience myotonia, or the tendency to not be able to release certain muscles, especially the grip. There may be a degree of kyphosis. What sets this disease apart from other degenerative muscle diseases is that there are a number of nervous system and systemic pathologies. These include testicular atrophy, cataracts, cranial hyperostosis, mental deficiency, cardiac arrhythmias and sudden cardiac failure [630–633], and hypoventilation from diaphragmatic dysfunction. There may also be a dysfunction of smooth muscle that may lead to GI symptoms. Many victims have abnormal glucose tolerance responses, and many have a mild form of immune compromise as well [538]. Persons with myotonic dystrophy are at increased risk for untoward reactions to anesthetic agents and other drugs, sometimes displaying malignant hyperthermia and fatal rhabdomyolysis during or after surgical procedures [634].

Recent work has shown that there are genetic alterations, sometimes in the form of trinucleotide repeats, in the DMPK gene located on chromosome 19 [632,633]. Other alterations that include toxic RNA transcripts appear to explain abnormal glucose utilization and other disorders in the condition.

The pathology of myotonic dystrophy varies with how long the disease has been manifested. In the early stages, usually evaluated by biopsy, there may be a very mild and subtle increase in the number of muscle cell nuclei distributed throughout the fiber in cross section and in longitudinal section long rows of nuclei may form. Eventually, there is variation in fiber caliber and histochemical stains for ATPase showing that type I fibers are more likely to be smaller or atrophic than type II fibers. Some fibers will be disorganized, and so-called ring fibers and target fibers are common. Fiber degeneration and regeneration can be seen, but generally only in advanced cases [626–629].

Myositis

Inflammatory diseases of muscle can be divided into those due to the following: infectious agents such as viruses (influenza and Coxsackie A and B viruses), bacteria, or parasites (such as *Trichinella*, *Cysticercus*, and *Toxoplasma*); allergic or chronic inflammatory conditions such as polymyositis, dermatomyositis, granulomatous myositis, inclusion body myositis, and myositis associated with the collagen vascular and granulomatous diseases; and reactive or traumatic myositis. Only a few forms of inflammatory myopathy are likely to be of interest or concern to the forensic pathologist, either because of their ability to incapacitate and kill rapidly, because they have some public health significance, or because litigation may result from some action or inaction on the part of a physician or medical care institution [626,627].

Clostridial Myositis

Clostridial myositis or gas gangrene is a relatively uncommon complication of deep penetrating wounds of the extremities but may occur when injuries are sustained in a dirty environment, such as a barnyard, refuse facility, or battlefield. The condition results from implantation of spores of *Clostridium* sp. (commonly found in excreta of horses and other large farm animals) into the wound, which are then relatively deprived of oxygen. The bacteria are anaerobes that release many toxins with properties as collagenases or hyaluronidases and also release gases that facilitate spreading of the organisms and produce necrosis of the muscle and fascia. Clostridial infection proceeds rapidly, leading to discoloration of the extremity; a foul, sickly sweet, or putrescent odor; and the rapid development of wet gangrene. Treatment includes administration of antitoxin, hyperbaric oxygen therapy, extensive surgical resection of necrotic and affected tissues, and penicillin. If recognized and treated promptly and aggressively, 80% of victims will survive [627,629].

Trichinosis

Trichinosis is one of the more well-known parasitic diseases, although it is relatively uncommon. Cluster outbreaks of the disease are reported periodically in the media and generally involve homemade sausage fests or picnics where poorly cooked pork has been served. The infestation is caused by the nematode *Trichinella spiralis*, which most commonly infects swine fed on garbage or excrement, and is rather uncommon in grain-fed animals [626,627]. The larvae of the worm infest the skeletal muscle of pig and are contracted by humans when infected pork is poorly cooked or eaten raw, as is the custom in some ethnic groups. On rare occasions, the disease can be contracted from poorly cooked predatory or scavenging game animals such as raccoons and bears [635]. Trichinosis is a disease that is reportable to public health officials when encountered, and generally about 100 cases are reported each year in the United States.

The disease presents with abdominal cramps and diarrhea within a day or two of eating infected meat. At this stage, the worms are reproducing and producing larvae in the intestine, which invade the blood and lymph vessels, eventually reaching the skeletal muscles, where the infection produces muscle aches and pains; fever; skin rash; elevation of the leukocyte count with prominent eosinophilia; muscular weakness, including diplopia; lethargy; stupor; and, in some cases, coma and death. Involvement of the brain and heart may be seen in fatal cases. In some cases where infection is minimal, symptoms may be evanescent or not recognized. At about 2 weeks after infection, larvae may be found in the stool. The third week after infection, the main phase of the disease is in the skeletal muscles, which are sore and swollen. If muscle tissue is examined histologically at this stage, numerous worms can be found coiled in the muscle surrounded by variable inflammatory infiltrates that include eosinophils. Later the worms may become mineralized and encysted. Most persons infected with *Trichinella* survive without major impairment, but despite past infection, permanent immunity is rarely achieved and reinfection can occur. The diaphragm is one of the more common muscles infected and one of the best sites to demonstrate the organism [635].

Rhabdomyolytic Syndromes

Necrosis of skeletal muscle with release of myoglobin into the bloodstream may occur in connection with several conditions, as mentioned above; these include malignant hyperthermia [634,636] in connection with general or local anesthesia, acute polymyositis, crushing injuries of the extremities, following drug reactions (neuroleptic malignant syndrome) [637–639] or excessive alcohol intake, dehydration and heat stroke, excessive exercise, or, in some individuals, for no apparent reason [636–639]. The precise pathogenetic mechanisms for all of these conditions may vary, but all lead to massive release of myoglobin into the blood. Myoglobin is rapidly filtered by the kidney and produces a red-colored urine, sometimes resembling wine. When myoglobinuria is massive, precipitation within the renal tubules may occur, with eventual renal failure.

Malignant Hyperthermia and the Neuroleptic Malignant Syndrome

First recognized in the 1960s, malignant hyperthermia has gradually become well known, in which an individual receiving general anesthesia suddenly develops an inexorably rising body temperature, sometimes as high as 44°C, experiences diffuse rhabdomyolysis and myoglobinuria, and may die suddenly with heart failure or die later with renal failure [636]. Untreated, the condition is nearly uniformly fatal. Because the first anesthetics for surgical procedures usually are given in childhood for tonsillectomy, appendectomy, dental procedures, or reduction of fractures, most victims are young. The propensity for development of this syndrome is inherited most commonly as a dominant gene and can be precipitated by exposure to most of the commonly employed inhalational anesthetics, especially halothane. Most of the common muscle relaxants, such as succinyl choline, may also precipitate an attack, as can local anesthetics on occasion. The mechanism of the syndrome is probably an idiosyncratic reaction by the anesthetic agents or muscle relaxants on the sarcotubular system of the muscle, which severely alters membrane channels, resulting in disruption and lysis of the sarcoplasm.

Family histories are often obtained that are positive for myotonic dystrophy or myotonia congenita or one of the congenital myopathies. Other conditions associated with the syndrome include arthrogryposis and scoliosis. There is no consistently obvious muscle biopsy pathology prior to an attack, and most individuals show what would ordinarily be interpreted as a normal biopsy. However, occasionally subtle changes that include slight variation of fiber size, some central nucleation, splits in fibers, and occasional target or targetoid or spotted fibers are noted. Sometimes the distribution of fiber types by ATPase histochemistry is abnormal and suggestive of neuropathic changes [640]. What is generally conceded to be the most reliable means of predicting malignant hyperthermia is to obtain a muscle biopsy prior to an anticipated surgical procedure using a special form of general anesthesia consisting of fentanyl and thiopental as well as oxygen and nitrous oxide; the anesthesiologist should be prepared to treat the syndrome according to an established protocol should any signs of hyperthermia develop. The biopsy, in addition to the usual histological workup, should be subjected to *in vitro* exposure to halothane and caffeine, which is a method often employed but not completely reliable. Exposure of the biopsy specimen to these substances in the individual who will develop malignant hyperthermia will show retraction bands, evidence of swelling, degeneration, and other changes that differ from the reactions to control muscles. This test can be performed only in laboratories with considerable experience with the procedure and in some cases may give false-positive and false-negative results [640]. Postmortem examination of muscle in individuals suspected of having died with malignant hyperthermia may require extensive sampling of muscles to demonstrate pathological changes (moth-eaten fibers, degenerating fibers, retraction bands, cores, and target-like fibers). In general, paraffin embedding and standard H&E stains are not adequate, and better results are obtained when frozen sections or plastic-embedded (methacrylate or epoxy) specimens are examined. Even so, the diagnosis may be difficult to substantiate on histological grounds alone, although the clinical history and the finding of myoglobin in the urine or in the renal tubules speak highly for the condition.

A very similar, if not identical, disease alluded to above, widely known by the ungainly label of neuroleptic malignant syndrome [638], is a fulminant and devastating rhabdomyolitic condition that may be associated with virtually any of the so-called neuroleptic drugs, such as the phenothiazines and related compounds; the butyrophenones, such as haloperidol; and other drugs not of these types, such as cocaine [641,643]. Typical presenting features of this disease are severe hyperpyrexia, tachycardia, delirium, muscular rigidity, dyspnea, tachypnea, severe sweating and salivation, uncontrolled movements, and other symptoms. Laboratory studies usually show elevated muscle and liver enzymes, coagulopathy, elevated white blood cell count and platelet count, acidosis, myoglobinuria, and proteinuria. Unless recognized and immediately treated, there is a high mortality rate [641]. Pathologically, a spectrum of lesions may be found, depending upon the course of the disease and its complications. The kidneys will likely show myoglobin casts in the renal tubules and varying elements of renal necrosis. The liver may have focal areas of necrosis. Skeletal muscle will be pale and flabby and microscopically will show severe fiber lysis and degeneration. The brain may be swollen and show perivascular hemorrhages and areas of neuronal necrosis and edema, or there may be hemorrhages typical for hypertension (basal ganglia, cerebellar, or pontine). The heart may show elements of myolysis and fiber degeneration as well.

The propensity for reacting to neuroleptic drugs in this manner is said to be dominantly inherited and involving the *RYR*-1 (ryantidine) gene that has been localized to chromosome 19q [644,645]. The gene codes for a receptor in skeletal muscle that is integral to muscle excitation–contraction and to proper calcium ion regulation in muscle cells [645]. Individuals with myopathies of myotonia and central core and multicore disease are more susceptible to this syndrome [644], although most victims have no known muscle pathology. The *RYR*-1 gene anomalies can be screened for, as can other mutations that may produce the syndrome.

Myasthenia Gravis

Myasthenia gravis is an autoimmune disease that produces antibodies that attack the postsynaptic acetyl choline receptor or muscle tyrosine kinase proteins (MuSK) at the neuromuscular junction in voluntary muscle, resulting in varying degrees of muscular weakness or paralysis [646]. Autoantibodies explain the majority of cases, but antibody-negative cases are not uncommon. The reason for this is not clear, but 25% of victims have a thymoma, the removal of which may improve or cure the myasthenic syndrome [647,648]. Recently, aberrant reactions to various drugs have been demonstrated to produce a myasthenic syndrome. Notable among these is telithromycin [649,650].

In myasthenia gravis, the first muscular weakness is often manifested in facial muscles and eyelids but can progress, sometimes suddenly, to a profound generalized weakness, including the muscles of respiration. When this occurs, the affected individual may suffer respiratory embarrassment or death unless ventilation support and other treatments are instituted [651].

In life, when myasthenia gravis is suspected, the so-called Tensilon (edrophonium) test may unmask the symptoms and essentially confirm the diagnosis; however, serological studies are also useful in determining if there are autoantibodies to the acetyl choline receptor or MuSK [646]. Treatment for the disease often involves the use of anticholinesterases, immunosuppression, plasmaphaeresis, and if a thymoma is present, its removal [648].

The epidemiology of the disease is that it generally affects women younger than 40 years of age and both genders after age 60 years. It does not appear to be inherited or caused by an infectious agent. The prevalence in the United States is reported to be about 20/100,000 population, according to the Myasthenia Gravis Foundation of America. Although most cases are diagnosed in life, the condition may lead to sudden, unexpected, or unexplained deaths [652,653]. Such deaths can occur in infants of myasthenic mothers as well as in adults with or without a relevant history. In most of these cases, myasthenia appears also to affect the myocardium, in which varying degrees of myopathic changes can be found at autopsy [651,652]. The microscopic pathology in skeletal muscle is usually subtle, but if special methods are employed that display the motor end plates, they are often dystrophic and larger and more complex than normal [626,628].

McArdle's Disease

One of the disorders of glycogen metabolism, McArdle's disease (glycogen storage disease type V) results from muscle phosphorylase deficiency, which renders the victim unable to mobilize stored muscle glycogen for metabolism, resulting in exercise intolerance, myalgia, cramping, and sometimes prostration and death [626–628]. The disease is inherited as an autosomal recessive trait. The genetic defect is in the myophosphorylase gene located on chromosome 11 [654,655]. From a forensic point of view, the disease may be unsuspected and may first come to light in young adults who are engaged in vigorous physical activity to which they are unaccustomed, such as in an informal competitive activity, military boot camp, hazing situations, or emergencies where extreme physical activity may be required. The victim may collapse while others are experiencing no difficulty, and they are often the brunt of jokes, harassment, or abuse that may prompt the victim to exert himself or herself further, to his or her detriment. In its worst form, the disease may lead to rhabdomyolysis, renal failure, and death.

Pathologically affected muscles in fatal cases or in muscle biopsies of affected persons may show muscle fiber degeneration and fiber myolysis with loss of cross-striations and repair reactions. In nonnecrotic fibers, there is increased glycogen easily visualized using the PAS stain. The concentration of PAS-positive granules is easily differentiated from those in normal muscle [626–628]. It is possible to diagnose the disease by gene probes.

Familial Periodic Paralysis

Like McArdle's disease, there are other inherited conditions that may produce sudden and sometimes catastrophic muscular weakness. In this instance, the dominantly inherited autosomal defect involves an ion-gated calcium channel in the muscle membrane [626–628,656,657]. Often a hypokalemic state in sensitive individuals can provoke this weakness, but in others even a normokalemic state may result in weakness. Attacks tend to occur in the second decade of life and decline thereafter. They usually occur, like McArdle's disease, with vigorous exercise or hours or longer afterward. They may occur at night after the period of exercise and manifest as profound all-extremity weakness that may begin in the upper extremities and extend to the lower extremities. Usually, the victim is able to speak but not move about. In severe attacks, respiratory weakness may also occur. Cardiac involvement may occur, resulting in arrhythmia or death. The attack may pass in a few hours or days, with full return of muscle strength. Sometimes injury to the muscle will occur with residual weakness and damage.

Pathologically affected muscle by biopsy or at autopsy usually will show central vacuolation that by electron microscopy is filled with regular tubular profiles [626–628,656].

References

1. U.S. Department of Health and Human Services, Centers for Disease Control. *National Vital Statistics Reports*. 2012.
2. Lozano R, Naghavi M, Foreman K, Lim S, Shibuya K, Aboyans V et al. Global and regional mortality from 235 causes of death for 20 age groups in 1990 and 2010: A systematic analysis for the Global Burden of Disease Study 2010. *Lancet* 2013;380(9859):2095–128.
3. England MA WJ. *Color Atlas of the Brain and Spinal Cord*. 2nd ed. Philadelphia: Mosby Elsevier, 2006.
4. Nolte J, Angevine JB Jr. *The Human Brain in Photographs and Diagrams*. 3rd ed. Philadelphia: Mosby Elsevier, 2007.
5. Haines DE. *Neuroanatomy: An Atlas of Structures, Sections, and Systems*. 8th ed. Philadelphia: Lippincott Williams & Wilkins, 2012.
6. Waxman SG. *Clinical Neuroanatomy*. 26th ed. New York: McGraw Hill-Lange, 2010.
7. Gould DJ, Breuckner, JK. *Sidman's Neuroanatomy: A Programmed Learning Tool*. 2nd ed. Philadelphia: Lippincott Williams & Wilkins, 2008.
8. Snell RS. *Clinical Neuroanatomy*. 7th ed. Philadelphia: Lippincott Williams & Wilkins, 2010.
9. Afifi AK, Berman RA. *Functional Neuroanatomy*. New York: McGraw Hill, 1998.
10. Kretschmann H-J, Weinrich W. *Cranial Neuroimaging and Clinical Neuroanatomy: Atlas of MRI Imaging and Computed Tomography*. 3rd ed. New York: Thieme, 2004.
11. Olszewski J, Baxter D. Cytoarchitecture of the human brain stem. Philadelphia: Lippincott, 1954.
12. Komaromy L. *Dissection of the Brain*. Budapest: Akademiai Kiado (Hungarian Academy of Sciences), 1966.
13. Rosett J. *Interecortical Systems of Thee Human Cerebrum: Mapped by Means of New Anatomic Methods*. New York: Columbia University Press, 1933.
14. Vogt C, Vogt O. Die vergleichend-architektonische und die vergleichend-reiz-physiologische Felderung der Grosshirnrinde unter besonderer Beruecksichtigung der menschlichen. *Naturwissenschaften* 1926;14:1190–94.
15. Brodmann K. Beiträge zur histologischen Lokalisation der Grosshirnrinde. 1. Miteilung: Die Regio Rolandica. *J Psychol Neurol* 1903;2:79–107.
16. Bailey P, von Bonin G. *The Isocortex of Man*. Urbana: University of Illinois Press, 1951.
17. Penfield W, Rasumussen T. *The Cerebral Cortex of Man*. New York: MacMillan, 1950.
18. Blinkov SM, Glezer IP. *The human Brain in Figures and Tables: A Quantitative Handbook*. New York: Basic Books, Plenum, 1968.
19. Kandel ER, Schwartz JH, Jessell TM. *Principles of Neural Science*, 4th edition. New York: McGraw Hill, 1991.
20. Andrion A, Colombo A, Mollo F. Sudden and unexpected death in adults: Autopsy study of 1901 autopsy cases in Turin (1949–1978). *Pathologica* 1982;74:47–56.
21. Kuller L. Sudden and unexpected non-traumatic death in adults: A review of epidemiological and clinical studies. *J Chron Dis* 1966;19:1192.
22. Kuller L, Lilienfeld A, Fisher R. An epidemiological study of sudden and unexpected deaths in adults. *Medicine* 1967;46:341–61.

23. Luke JL, Helpern M. Sudden unexpected death from natural causes in young adults. *Arch Pathol* 1968;85:10–7.
24. Moritz AR, Zamcheck N. Sudden and unexpected deaths of young soldiers: Diseases responsible for such deaths during World War II. *Arch Pathol* 1946;42:459–94.
25. Leestma JE. Sudden unexpected death associated with seizures: A pathological review. In Lathers CM, Schraeder PL, eds., *Epilepsy and Sudden Death*. New York: Marcel Dekker, 1990, pp. 61–88.
26. De Villiers J. Unexpected natural death of cerebral origin in mediocolegal practice. *Foren Sci Int* 1975;5:11–9.
27. Lathers CM SP, Bungo MW, Leestma JE, editor. *Sudden Death in Epilepsy: Forensic and Clinical Issues*. New York: CRC Press, 2011.
28. Lathers CM, Leestma JE. Psychoactive agents, epilepsy, arrhythmia, and sudden death. In Lathers CM, Schraeder PL, eds., *Epilepsy and Sudden Death*. New York: Marcel Dekker, 1990, pp. 447–84.
29. Lathers CM, Schraeder PL, eds. *Epilepsy and Sudden Death*. New York: Marcel Dekker, 1990.
30. Lathers CM, Schraeder PL. Autonomic dysfunction in epilepsy: Characterization of autonomic cardiac neural discharge associated with pentylenetetrazol-induced epileptogenic activity. *Epilepsia* 1982;23:633–47.
31. Leestma JE, Koenig KL. Sudden death and phenothiazines: A current controversy. *Arch Gen Psych* 1969;18:137–48.
32. Baron RC, Thacker SB, Corelkin L, Vernon AA, Taylor WR, Choi K. Sudden death among Southeast Asian refugees. An unexplained nocturnal phenomenon. *JAMA* 1983;250:2947–51.
33. Dimsdale JE. Emotional causes of sudden death. *Am J Psychiat* 1977;134:1361–6.
34. Plum F, Posner JB. *The Diagnosis of Stupor and Coma*. Philadelphia: F. A. Davis, 1982.
35. Plum F, Swanson AG. Central neurogenic hyperventilation in man. *Arch Neurol Psychiatr* 1959;81:535–49.
36. Kinney H, Filiano J. Brain research in sudden infant death syndrome. In Byard R, Krous H, eds., *Sudden Infant Death Syndrome: Problems, Progress & Possibilities*. London: Arnold, 2001, pp. 118–37.
37. Byard R, Krous H, eds. *Sudden Infant Death Syndrome: Problems, Progress & Possibilities*. London: Arnold, 2001.
38. Graf CJ, Rossi NP. Pulmonary edema and the central nervous system: A clinico-pathological study. *Surg Neurol* 1975;4:319–25.
39. Simmons RL, Heisterkamp CA 3rd, Collins JA, Bredenburg CE, Martin AM. Acute pulmonary edema in battle casualties. *J Trauma* 1969;9:760–75.
40. Bahloul M, Chaari AN, Kallel H, Khabir A, Ayadi A, Charfeddine H, Hergafi L, Chaari AD, Helly HE, Ben Hamida C, Rekik N, Bouaziz M. Neurogenic pulmonary edema due to traumatic brain injury: Evidence of cardiac dysfunction. *Am J Crit Care* 2006;15:462–70.
41. Terrence CF, Rao GR, Perper JA. Neurogenic pulmonary edema in unexpected, unexplained death of epileptic patients. *Ann Neurol* 1981;9:458–64.
42. Lathers CM, Schraeder PL. Stress and sudden death. *Epilepsy Behav* 2006;9:236–42.
43. Oppenheimer S. Neurothanatology-clinical significance of cerebrally induced cardiac changes. *Postgrad Med J* 1990;66:591–4.
44. Grunsfeld A, Fletcher JJ, Nathan BR. Cardiopulmonary complications of brain injury. *Curr Neurol Neurosci Rep* 2005;5:488–93.
45. Cuneo RA, Caronna JJ, Pitts L, Townsend J, Winsestock DP. Upward transternorial herniation. *Arch Neurol* 1979;36:618–23.
46. Leestma JE. Sudden unexpected death caused by neuroepithelial (colloid) cyst of the third ventricle. *J Foren Sci* 1981;26:486–91.
47. Jay GW, Leestma JE. Sudden death in epilepsy. A comprehensive review of the literature and proposed mechanisms. *Acta Neurol Scand Suppl* 1981:82:1–66.
48. Kinney HC, Samuels MA. Neuropathology of the persistent vegetative state. A review. *J Neuropathol Exp Neurol* 53:548–58.

49. Jennett B. Thirty years of the vegetative state: Clinical, ethical and legal problems. *Prog Brain Res* 2005;150:537.
50. Kinney HC, Korein J, Panigrahy A, Dikkes P, Goode R. Neuropathological findings in the brain of Karen Ann Quinlan. The role of the thalamus in the persistent vegetative state. *New Engl J Med* 1994;330:1469–75.
51. Wolfson J. The rule in Terri's case: An essay on the public death of Theresa Marie Schiavo. *Stetson Law Rev* 2005;35:39–47.
52. Baratham G, Dennyson WG. Delayed traumatic intracerebral hemorrhage. *J Neurol Neurosurg Psychiatry* 1972;35:698–706.
53. Kaufman H. Delayed traumatic intracerebral hematomas. *Neurosurgery* 1984;14:784–85.
54. Krauland W. *Verletzungen der Intrakraniellen Schlagadern*. Berlin: Springer-Verlag, 1982.
55. Morin MA, Pitts FW. Delayed apoplexy following head injury ("traumatische spät-apoplexie"). *J Neurosurg* 1970;33:542–7.
56. Jörgensen L, Torvik A. Ischeamic cerebrovascular diseases in an autopsy series. 1. Prevalence, location and predisposing factors in verified thromboembolic occlusions, and their significance in the pathogenesis of cerebral infarction. *J Neurol Sci* 1966;3:490–509.
57. Jörgensen L, Torvik A. Ischaemic cerebrovacular diseases in an autopsy series. Part 2. Prevalence, location, pathogenesis, and clinical course of cerebral infarcts. *J Neurol Sci* 1969;9:285–320.
58. Torvik A, Svindland A, Lindboe CF. Pathogenesis of carotid thrombosis. *Stroke* 1989;20:1477–83.
59. Kannel WB. High-density lipoproteins: Epidemiological profile and risks of coronary artery disease. *Am J Cardiol* 1983;52:9B–12B.
60. Mohr JP, Caplan LR, Melski JW, Goldstein RJ, Duncan GW, Kistler JP, Pessin MS, Bleich HL. The Harvard Cooperative Stroke Registry: A prospective registry. *Neurology* 1978;28:754–62.
61. Mohr JP. Anticoagulation for stroke prevention: Yes, no, maybe. *Cleveland Clin J Med* 2004;71 Suppl 1:S52–6.
62. Elkind MS. Inflammation, atherosclerosis, and stroke. *Neurologist* 2006;12:140–8.
63. Morita A, Nakayama T, Soma M. Association study between C-reactive protein genes and ischemic stroke in Japanese subjects. *Am J Hypertens* 2006;19:593–600.
64. Tsimikas S, Aikawa M, Miller FJ, Torzewski M, Lentz SR, Bergmark C, Heistad DD, Libby P, Witztum JL. Increased plasma oxidized phospholipid: Apolipoprotein B-100 ratio with concomitant depletion of oxidized phospholipids from atherosclerotic lesions after dietary lipid-lowering: A potential biomarker of early atherosclerosis regression. *Arterioscler Thromb Vasc Biol* 2006;27:175–81.
65. Baumgartner RW, Sidler C, Mosso M, Georgiadis D. Ischemic lacunar stroke in patients with and without potential mechanism other than small-artery disease. *Stroke* 2003;34:653–9.
66. Wolf PA, Dawber TR, Jr, Thomas HE Jr, Kannel WB. Epidemiologic assessment of chronic atrial fibrillation and risk of stroke: The Framingham study. *Neurology* 1978;28:973–77.
67. Micieli G. Vascular dementia. *Neurol Sci* 2006;27(Suppl 1):S37–39.
68. Caplan LR. Stroke treatment: Promising but still struggling. *JAMA* 1998;279:1304–6.
69. Garcia JH, Mena H. Vascular diseases. In Garcia JH, Budka H, McKeever PE, Sarnat HB, Sima AAF, eds., *Neuropathology: The Diagnostic Approach*. St. Louis: Mosby, 1997, pp. 266–320.
70. Wiebers DO, Feigin VL, Brown RD., eds. *Handbook of Stroke*. Philadelphia: Lippincott Williams & Wilkins, 2006.
71. Carandang R, Seshadri S, Beiser A, Kelly-Hayes M, Kase CS, Kannel WB, Wolf PA. Trends in incidence, lifetime risk, severity, and 30-day, mortality of stroke of the past 50 years. *JAMA* 2006;296:2939–46.
72. Kotila M. Declining incidence and mortality of stroke? *Stroke* 1984;15:255–59.
73. Corwin LI, Wolf PA, Kannel WB, MacNamara PM. Accuracy of death certification of stroke: The Framingham study. *Stroke* 1982;13:818–20.
74. Sahs AL, Nibbelink DW, Torner JC, eds. *Aneurysmal Subarachnoid Hemorrhage: Report of a Cooperative Study*. Baltimore: Urban & Schwarzenberg, 1981.

75. Helpern M, Rabson SM. Sudden and unexpected natural death: General considerations and statistics. *NY State J Med* 1945;45:1197–201.
76. Locksley HB. Natural history of subarachnoid hemorrhage: Intracranial aneurysms and arteriovenous malformations. Based on 6368 cases in the cooperative study. In Sahs AL, Perret GE, Locksley HB, Nishioka H, eds., *Intracranial Aneurysms and Subarachnoid Hemorrhage: A Cooperative Study*. Philadelphia: Lippincott, 1969, pp. 35–108.
77. Kennady JC. Investigations of the early fate and removal of subarachnoid blood. *Pacific Med Surg* 1967;75:163–8.
78. Gallia GL, Tamargo RJ. Leukocytes-endothelial cell interactions in chronic vasospasm after subarachnoid hemorrhage. *Neurol Res* 2006;28:750–8.
79. Pluta RM. Dysfunction of nitric oxide synthases as a cause and therapeutic target in delayed cerebral vasospasm after SAH. *Neurol Res* 2006;28:655–71.
80. Wartenberg KE, Mayer SA. Medical complications after subarachnoid hemorrhage: New strategies for prevention and management. *Curr Opin Crit Care* 2006;12:78–84.
81. Urbaniak K, Merchant AI, Amin-Hanjani S, Roitberg B. Cardiac complications after aneurysmal subarachnoid hemorrhage. *Surg Neurol* 2007;67:21–8; discussion 28–9.
82. Bremer JL. Congenital aneurysm of cerebral arteries: Embryological study. *Arch Pathol* 1943;35:819–31.
83. Brisman JL, Song JK, Newell DW. Cerebral aneurysms. *N Engl J Med* 2006;355:928–39.
84. Sheffield EA, Weller RO. Age changes at cerebral artery bifurcations and the pathogenesis of berry aneurysms. *J Neurol Sci* 1980;46:341–52.
85. McCormick WF, Nofzinger JD. Saccular intracranial aneurysms (an autopsy study). *J Neurosurg* 1965;22:155–9.
86. Keedy A. An overview of intracranial aneurysms. *McGill J Med* 2006;9:141–6.
87. Kaminogo M, Yonekura M, Shibata S. Incidence and outcome of multiple intracranial aneurysms in a defined population. *Stroke* 2003;34:16–21.
88. Juvela S, Porras M, Poussa K. Natural history of unruptured intracranial aneurysms: Probability and risk factors for aneurysm rupture. *Neurosurg Focus* 2000;8 (5).
89. Maira G, Albanese A, Pentimalli L, Tirpakova B. Treatment of intracranial aneurysms. *Clin Exp Hypertens* 2006;28:371–76.
90. Lecomte D, Fornes P, Nicolas G. Stressful events as a trigger for sudden death: A study of 43 medico-legal autopsy cases. *Forensic Sci Int* 1996;17:1–10.
91. Lovas JG, Silver MD. Coincident rupture of berry aneurysm and aortic dissection during sexual intercourse. *Arch Pathol Lab Med* 1984;108:271–2.
92. Braksiek RJ, Roberts DJ. Amusement park injuries and deaths. *Ann Emerg Med* 2002;39:65–72.
93. Pelletier AR, Gilchrist J. Roller coaster related fatalities, United States, 1994–2004. *Inj Prev* 2005;11:309–12.
94. Sahs AL. Observations on the pathology of saccular aneurysms. In Sahs AL Perret GE, Locksley HB, Nishioka H, eds. *Intracranial Aneurysms and Subarachnoid Hemorrhage: A Cooperative Study*. Philadelphia: Lippincott, 1969, pp. 22–34.
95. Stehbens WE. Intracranial berry aneurysms in infancy. *Surg Neurol* 1982;18:58–60.
96. Housepian EM, Pool JL. A systematic analysis of the intracranial aneurysms from the autopsy file of the Presbyterian hospital, 1914–1956. *J Neuropath Exp Neurol* 1982;17:409–23.
97. Lipper S, Morgan D, Kirgman MR, Staab EF. Congenital saccular aneurysm in a 19-day old neonate: Case report and review of the literature. *Surg Neurol* 1978;16:161–5.
98. Østergaard JR, Voldby B. Intracranial arterial aneurysm in children and adolescents. *J Neurosurg* 1983;58:832–7.
99. Suzuki J, Ohara H. Clinicopathological study of cerebral aneurysms. Origin, rupture, repair and growth. *J Neurosurg* 1978;48:505–14.
100. Milnor WR. Cardiovascular system. In Mountcastle VB (ed). *Medical Physiology*, St. Louis: CV Mosby, 1980, pp. 1022–3.
101. Ditlefsen EM, Tiinjum AM. Intracranial aneurysms and polycystic kidneys. *Acta Med Scand* 1960;272:954–1003.

102. Cronqvist S, Troupp H. Intracranial arteriovenous malformation and arterial aneurysms in the same patient. *Acta Neurol Scand* 1966;43:307–66.
103. Ullrich DP. Familial cerebral aneurysms including one extracranial internal carotid aneurysm. *Neurology* 1960;10:288–94.
104. Mohr G, Ferguson G, Malloy D, Watts R, Benoit B, Weir B. Intraventricular hemorrhage from ruptured aneurysm. Retrospective analysis of 91 cases. *J Neurosurg* 1983;58:482–87.
105. Gelal F, Vidinli BD, Yurt A, Cakir Y, Uygur M. Giant fusiform basilar artery aneurysm causing obstructive hydrocephalus. *Skull Base* 2002;12:197–200.
106. Levati A, Tommasino C, Moretti MP, Paino R, D'Aliberti G, Santoro F, Meregalli S, Vesconi S, Collice M. Giant intracranial aneurysms treated with deep hypothermia and circulatory arrest. *J Neurosurg Anesthesiol* 2007;19:25–30.
107. Nakayama Y, Tanaka A, Kumate S, Tomonaga M, Takebayashi S. Giant fusiform aneurysm of the basilar artery: Consideration of its pathogenesis. *Surg Neurol* 1999;51:140–45.
108. Pessin MS, Chimowitz MI, Levine SR, Kwan ES, Adelman LS, Earnest MP, Clark DM, Chason J. Stroke in patients with fusiform vertebrobasilar aneurysms. *Neurology* 1989;39:16–21.
109. Chun JY, Smith W, Halbach VV, Higashida RT, Wilson CB, Lawton MT. Current multi-modality management of infectious intracranial aneurysms. *Neurosurgery* 2001;48:1203–13.
110. Peters PJ, Harrison T, Lennox JL. A dangerous dilemma: Management of infectious intracranial aneurysms complicating endocarditis. *Lancet Infect Dis* 2006;6:742–48.
111. Yamakawa H, Hattori T, Tanigawara T, Enomoto Y, Ohkuma A. Ruptured infectious aneurysm of the distal middle cerebral artery manifesting as intracereberal hemorrhage and acute subdural hematoma. *Neurol Med Chir* (Tokyo) 2003;43:541–5.
112. Frazee JG, Cahan LD, Winter J. Bacterial intracranial aneurysms. *J Neurosurg* 1980;53:633–41.
113. Fauci AS, Haynes B, Katz P. The spectrum of vasculitis: Clinical, pathologic, immunologic and therapeutic considerations. *Ann Intern Med* 1978;89:660–76.
114. Hughes JT, Brownell B. Granulomatous giant-celled angiitis of the central nervous system. *Neurology* 1966;16:293.
115. Grosman H, Fornasier VL, Bonder D, Livingston KE, Platts ME. Dissecting aneurysm of the cerebral arteries. Case report. *J Neurosurg* 1980;53:693–97.
116. Paul GA, Shaw CM, Wray LM. True traumatic aneurysm of the vertebral artery: Case report. *J Neurosurg* 1980;53:101–5.
117. Yakushiji Y, Haraguchi Y, Soejima S, Takase Y, Uchino A, Koizumi S, Kuroda Y. A hyper-dense artery sign and middle cerebral artery dissection. *Intern Med* 2006;45:1319–22.
118. Arnold M, Bousser MG, Fahrni G, Fischer U, Georgiadis D, Gandjour J, Benninger D. Vertebral artery dissection: Presenting findings and predictors of outcome. *Stroke* 2006;37:2499–503.
119. Chung YS, Han DH. Vertebrobasilar dissection: A possible role of whiplash injury in its pathogenesis. *Neurol Res* 2002;24:129–38.
120. Smith WS, Johnston SC, Skalabrin EJ, Weaver M, Azari P, Albers GW, Gress DR. Spinal manipulative therapy is an independent risk factor for vertebral artery dissection. *Neurology* 2003;60:1424–28.
121. Yoshii F, Shinohara Y, Takeoka T. Two autopsy cases with ruptured dissecting aneurysm of the intracranial vertebral artery. *Eur Neurol* 1986;25:388–95.
122. Kotila M. Declining incidence and mortality of stroke? *Stroke* 1984;15:255–59.
123. Numminen H, Kotila M, Waltimo O, Aho K, Kaste M. Declining incidence and mortality rates of stroke in Finland from 1972 to 1991. Results of three population-based stroke registers. *Stroke* 1996;27:1487–91.
124. Avendano M, Glymour MM. Stroke disparities in older Americans: Is wealth a more powerful indicator of risk than income and education? *Stroke* 2008;39:1533–40.
125. Ruiz-Sandoval JL, Romero-Vargas S, Chiquete E, Padilla-Martinez JJ, Villarreal-Careaga J, Cantu C, Arauz A, Barinagarrementeria F. Hypertensive intracerebral hemorrhage in young people: Previously unnoticed age-related clinical differences. *Stroke* 2006;37:2946–50.

126. Segal R, Furmanov A, Umansky F. Spontaneous intracerebral hemorrhage: To operate or not to operate, that's the question. *Isr Med Assoc J* 2006;8:815–18.
127. Zuccarello M, Brott T, Derex L, Kothari R, Sauerbeck L, Tew J, H VL, Yeh HS, Tomsick T, Pancioli A, Khoury J, Broderick J. Early surgical treatment for supratentorial intracerebral hemorrhage: A randomized feasibility study. *Stroke* 1999;30:1833–39.
128. Hughes J, Cayaffa J, Leestma J, Mizuno Y. Alternating "waking" and "sleep" EEG patterns in a deeply comatose patient. *Clin Electroencephalogr* 1972;3:86–93.
129. Ferro JM. Update on intracerebral haemorrhage. *J Neurol* 2006;253:985–99.
130. Sutherland GR, Auer RN. Primary intracerebral hemorrhage. *J Clin Neurosci* 2006;13:511–7.
131. Alexander EJ, Kushner J, Six EG. Brainstem hemorrhages and increased intracranial pressure: From Duret to computed tomography. *Surg Neurol* 1982;17:107–10.
132. Parizel PM, Makkat S, Jorens PG, Ozsarlak O, Cras P, van Goethem JW, van den Hauwe L, Verlooy J, de Schepper AM. Brainstem hemorrhage in descending transtentorial herniation (Duret hemorrhage). *Intensive Care Med* 2002;28:85–8.
133. Fujimoto Y, Aguiar PH, Freitas AB, de Andrade AF, Marino Junior R. Recovery from Duret hemorrhage: A rare complication after craniotomy—Case report. *Neurol Med Chir* (Tokyo) 2000;40:508–10.
134. Bateman BT, Schumacher HC, Bushnell CD, Pile-Spellman J, Simpson LL, Sacco RL, Berman MF. Intracerebral hemorrhage in pregnancy: Frequency, risk factors, and outcome. *Neurology* 2006;67:424–29.
135. Qureshi AI, Mohammad Y, Suri MF, Braimah J, Janardhan V, Guterman LR, Hopkins LN, Frankel MR. Cocaine use and hypertension are major risk factors for intracerebral hemorrhage in young African Americans. *Ethn Dis* 2001;11:311–19.
136. Yamada M. Cerebral amyloid angiopathy. An overview. *Neuropathology* 2000;20:8–22.
137. McCarron MO, Nicoll JAR, Ironside JW, Love S, Alberts MJ, Bone I. Cerebral amyloid angiopathy-related hemorrhage. Interaction of APOEe2 with putative clinical risk factors. *Stroke* 1999;30:1643–46.
138. Dada MA, Rutherford G. Medicolegal aspects of cerebral angiopathy. A case report. *Am J Foren Med Pathol* 1993;14:319–22.
139. Zhan RY, Tong Y, Shen JF, Lang E, Preul C, Hemplemann RG, Hugo HH, Buhl R, Barth H, Klinge, Mehdorn H. Study of clinical features of amyloid angiopathy hemorrhage and hypertensive intracerebral hemorrhage. *J Zhejiang Univ Sci* 2004;5:1262–69.
140. Soffer D. Cerebral amyloid angiopathy—A disease or age-related condition. *Isr Med Assoc J* 2006;8:803–6.
141. McCormick WF. Pathology of vascular malformations of the brain. In Wilson CB, Stein BM, eds., *Intracranial Arteriovenous Malformations*. Baltimore: Williams & Wilkins, 1984, pp. 44–63.
142. McCormick WF. The pathology of vascular ("arteriovenous") malformations. *J Neurosurg* 1966;24:807–16.
143. Stein BM, Wolpert SM. Arteriovenous malformations of the brain. I. Current concepts and treatment. *Arch Neurol* 1980;37:1–5.
144. Takashima S, Becker LE. Neuropathology of cerebral arteriovenous malformations in children. *J Neurol Neurosurg Psychiatry* 1980;43:380–85.
145. Mohr JP. Neurological manifestations and factors related to therapeutic decisions. In Wilson CB, Stein BM, eds., *Intracranial Arteriovenous Malformations*. Baltimore: Williams & Wilkins, 1984, pp. 1–11.
146. Prakash B, Beohar PC, Misra RC. Low flow (cryptic) arteriovenous malformation and spontaneous haematoma. *Acta Neurochir* (Wien) 1983;69(1–2):61–7.
147. McCormick WF, Nofzinger JD. "Cryptic" vacular malformations of the central nervous system. *J Neurosurg* 1966;24:865–75.
148. Fernandez L-A, Sanz-Rodriguez F, Blanco FJ, Bernabeu C, Botella LM. Hereditary hemorrhagic telangiectasia, a vascular dysplasia affecting the TGF-beta signaling pathway. *Clin Med Res* 2006;4:66–78.

149. Lenato GM, Guanti G. Hereditary haemorrhagic telangiectasia (HHT): Genetic and molecular aspects. *Curr Pharm Des* 2006;12:1173–93.
150. Wang QK. Update on the molecular genetics of vascular anomalies. *Lymphat Res Biol* 2005;3: 226–33.
151. Stahl SM, Johnson KP, Malamud N. The clinical and pathological spectrum of brain stem vascular malformations. Long-term course stimulates multiple sclerosis. *Arch Neurol* 1980;37:25–9.
152. Antoni N. Spinal vascular malformations (angiomas) and myelomalacia. *Neurology* 1962;12: 795–804.
153. Blount JP, Oakes WJ, Tubbs RS, Humphreys RP. History of surgery for cerebrovascular disease in children. Part II. Vein of Galen malformations. *Neurosurg Focus* 2006;20(6).
154. Lasjaunias PL, Chng SM, Sachet M, Alvarez H, Rodesch G, Garcia-Monaco R. The management of vein of galen aneurysmal malformations. *Neurosurgery* 2006;59(Suppl 3):S184–94.
155. Felbor U, Sure U, Grimm T, Bertalanffy H. Genetics of cerebral cavernous angioma. *Zentralbl Neurochir* 2006;67:110–16.
156. Laurans MS, DiLuna ML, Shin D, Niazi F, Voorhees JR, Nelson-Williams C, Johnson EW, Siegel AM, Steinberg GK, Berg MJ, Scott RM, Tedeschi G, Enevoldson TP, Anson J, Rouleau GA, Ogilvy C, Awad IA. Mutational analysis of 206 families with cavernous malformations. *J Neurosurg* 2003;99:38–43.
157. Perret F, Nishioka H. Arteriovenous malformations. An analysis of 545 cases of craniocerebral arteriovenous malformations and fistulae reported to the cooperative study. In Sahs A, Perret GE, Locksley HB, Nishioka H, eds. *Intracranial Aneurysms and Subarachnoid Hemorrhage: A Cooperative Study*. Philadelphia: Lippincott, 1969, pp. 200–22.
158. Mishra R, Kaw R. Foix-Alajouanine syndrome: An uncommon cause of myelopathy from an anatomic variant circulation. *South Med J* 2005;98(5):567–9.
159. Luessenhop AJ. *Natural History of Cerebral Arteriovenous Malformations*. Baltimore: Williams & Wilkins, 1984.
160. Du R, McDermott MW, Dowd CF, Young WL, Lawton MT. Neurosurgery at the crossroads: Integrated multidisciplinary management of 449 patients with brain arteriovenous malformations. *Clin Neurosurg* 2005;52:177–91.
161. Sirin S, Kondziolka D, Niranjan A, Flickinger JC, Maitz AH, Lunsford LD. Prospective staged volume radiosurgery for large arteriovenous malformations: Indications and outcomes in otherwise untreatable patients. *Neurosurgery* 2006;58:17–27; discussion, 17–27.
162. Pollock BE, Gorman DA, Brown PD. Radiosurgery for arteriovenous malformations of the basal ganglia, thalamus, and brainstem. *J Neurosurg* 2004;100:210–14.
163. Wilson C, Stein BM, eds. *Intracranial Arteriovenous Malformations*. Baltimore: Williams & Wilkins, 1984.
164. deVeber G. Stroke and the child's brain: An overview of epidemiology, syndromes and risk factors. *Curr Opin Neurol* 2002;15:133–38.
165. Martin P, Enevoldson P. Causes of ischaemic stroke in the young. *Postgrad Med* 1997;73:8–16.
166. Harrison MJG, Dyken ML, eds., *Cerebral Vascular Disease*. London: Butterworths, 1983.
167. Adams RD, Fisher CM. Pathology of cerebral arterial occlusion. In Fields W, ed., *Pathogenesis and Treatment of Cerebrovascular Disease*. Springfield, IL: Charles C. Thomas, 1961, pp. 126–47.
168. Torvik A, Jörgensen L. Thrombotic and embolic occlusions of the carotid arteries in an autopsy series. I. Prevalence, location and associated diseases. *J Neurol Sci* 1964;41:24–39.
169. Yates PO, Hutchinson EC. *Cerebral Infarction: The Role of Stenosos of the Extracranial Cerebral Arteries*. Vol. 300. London: Privy Council, Medical Research Council, 1961.
170. Edwards BS, Edwards JE. *Pathology of Sudden Cardiac Death: An Illustrated Guide*. Malden, MA: Blackwell/Futura, 2006.
171. Fineschi V, Baroldi G, Silver MD. *Pathology of the Heart and Sudden Death in Forensic Medicine*. Boca Raton, FL: CRC Press/Taylor & Francis, 2006.
172. Adams RD, Vander Eecken HM. Vascular diseases of the brain. *Ann Rev Med* 1953;4:213–52.

173. Riishede J. Cerebral apoplexy: Statistical considerations. *Acta Psychiat Neurol Scand* 1956;108 (Suppl):347–61.
174. Kim HI, Lee MC, Lee JS, Kim HS, Kim MK, Woo YJ, Kim JH, Jung S, Palmini A, Kim SU. Bilateral perisylvian ulegyria: Clinicopathological study of patients presenting with pseudobulbar palsy and epilepsy. *Neuropathology* 2006;26:236–42.
175. Plum F, Pulsinelli WS, Petito CK. Glucose levels as a factor influencing the outcome of ischemic damage. In Reivich M, Hurtig HI, eds., *Cerebrovascular Disease*. New York: Raven Press, 1983, pp. 195–97.
176. Dooling EC, Richardson EPJ. Delayed encephalopathy after strangling. *Arch Neurol* 1976;33:196–99.
177. Ginsberg MD, Hedley-Whyte ET, Richardson EP Jr. Hypoxic-ischemic leukoencephalopathy in man. *Arch Neurol* 1976;33:5–14.
178. Bogousslavsky J, Regli F. Unilateral watershed cerebral infarcts. *Neurology* 1986;36:373–77.
179. Torvik A, Skullerud K. Watershed infarcts in the brain caused by microemboli. *Clin Neuropathol* 1982;1:99–105.
180. Braak H. *Architectonics of the Human Telencephalic Cortex*. Vol. 4. Berlin: Springer-Verlag, 1980.
181. Schade J, McMenemey WH, eds. *Selective Vulnerability of the Brain in Hypoxaemia*. Oxford: Blackwell, 1963.
182. Lindenberg R. Patterns of CNS vulnerability in acute hypoxemia, including anaesthesia accidents. In Schade J, McMenemey WH, eds., *Selective Vulnerability of the Brain in Hypoxaemia*. Oxford: Blackwell, 1963, pp. 189–209.
183. Lindenberg R. Systemic oxygen deficiencies. In Minckler J, ed., *Pathology of the Nervous System*. Vol. 2. New York: McGraw Hill, 1971, pp. 1583–617.
184. Ames IA, Wright RL, Kowada M, Thurston JM, Majno G. The no-reflow phenomenon. *Am J Pathol* 1968;52:437–53.
185. Fisher CM. The circle of Willis: Anatomical variations. *Vasc Dis* 1965;2:99–105.
186. Haymaker W. *Bing's Local Diagnosis in Neurological Disease*. St. Louis, MO: C. V. Mosby, 1969.
187. Ropper A, Brown R, eds. *Adams and Victor's Principles of Neurology*. New York: McGraw Hill, 2005.
188. Blumenfeld H. *Neuroanatomy Through Clinical Cases*. Sunderland, MA: Sinauer Associates, 2002.
189. Hughes J. *Pathology of the Spinal Cord*. London: Lloyd-Luke, 1966.
190. Jacobs MJ, de Mol BA, Elenbaas T, Mess WH, Kalkman CJ, Schurink GW, Mochtar B. Spinal cord blood supply in patients with thoracoabdominal aortic aneurysms. *J Vasc Surg* 2002;35:30–7.
191. Lipton HL, Teasdall RD. Acute transverse myelopathy in adults. A follow-up study. *Arch Neurol* 1973;28:252–57.
192. Matsuda H, Ogino H, Saito S, Sasaki H, Minatoya K, Kobayashi J, Yagihara T, Kitamura S. Monoparesis after graft replacement of non-ruptured abdominal aortic aneurysm. *Ann Thorac Cardiovasc Surg* 2006;12:376–78.
193. Easton JD, Sherman DG. Cervical manipulation and stroke. *Stroke* 1977;8:594–97.
194. Ludwig MA, Burns SP. Spinal cord infarction following cervical transforaminal epidural injection: A case report. *Spine* 2005;30:E266–68.
195. Hodges SD, Castleberg RL, Miller T, Ward R, Thornburg C. Cervical epidural steroid injection with intrinsic spinal cord damage. Two case reports. *Spine* 1998;23:2137–42; discussion, 2141.
196. Pathak M, Kim RC, Pribram H. Spinal cord infarction following vertebral angiography: Clinical and pathological findings. *J Spinal Cord Med* 2000;23:92–5.
197. Furman MB, Giovanniello MT, O'Brien EM. Incidence of intravascular penetration in transforaminal cervical epidural steroid injections. *Spine* 2003;28:21–5.
198. Schreiber AL, Formal CS. Spinal cord infarction secondary to cocaine use. *Am J Phys Med Rehabil* 2006;86:158–60.
199. Gofton TE, Barber PA. Anterior spinal artery infarction at the cervicomedullary junction. *Can J Neurol Sci* 2006;33:418–20.

200. Goldstein LH, Mordish Y, Abu-Kishak I, Toledano M, Berkovitch M. Acute paralysis following recreational MDMA (ecstasy) use. *Clin Toxicol* (Phila) 2006;44:339–41.
201. Karlsson JO, Sjøstrand J. Transport of neurotubular protein and the effect of colchicine on axonal transport. *Acta Physiol Scand Suppl* 1970;357:11–2.
202. Wisniewski H, Terry RD. Experimental colchicine encephalopathy. I. Induction of neurofibrillary degeneration. *Lab Invest* 1967;17:577–87.
203. Schochet S, Lampert P, Earle K. Neuronal changes induced by intrathecal vincristine sulfate. *J Neuropathol Exp Neurol* 1968;27:645–57.
204. Leestma J. *Forensic Aspects of Neurotoxicology: Forensic Neuropathology*. New York: Raven Press, 1988, pp. 380–81.
205. Jacobs JM, Cavanagh JB, Chen FC. Spinal subarachnoid injection of colchicine in rats. *J Neurol Sci* 1972;17:461–80.
206. Lindenberg R. Morphotropic and morphostatic necrobiosis; investigations on nerve cells of the brain. *Am J Pathol* 1956;32:1147–77.
207. Lindenberg R. Anoxia does not produce brain damage. *Japan J Legal Med* (Nihon Hoigaku Zasshi) 1982;36:38–57.
208. Itabashi H, Andrews JM, Tomiyasu U, Erlich S, Sathyavagisawaran L. *Forensic Neuropathology. A Practical Review of the Fundamentals*. San Diego, CA: Academic Press, 2007.
209. Leestma J, Martin E. An electron probe and histochemical study of the "ferruginated" neuron. *Arch Pathol* 1968;86:597–605.
210. Oehmichen M, Eisenmenger W, Raff G, Berghaus G. Brain macrophages in human cortical contusions as indicator of survival period. *Foren Sci Int* 1986;30:281–301.
211. Kaur B, Rutty GN, Timperley WR. The possible role of hypoxia in the formation of axonal bulbs. *J Clin Pathol* 1999;52:203–9.
212. Oehmichen M, Meissner C, Schmidt V, Pedal I, König HG, Saternus KS. Axonal injury—A diagnostic tool in forensic neuropathology? A review. *Foren Sci Int* 1998;95:67–83.
213. Torvik A, Svindland A. Is there a transitional zone between brain infarcts and the surrounding brain? A histological study. *Acta Neurol Scand* 1986;74:365–70.
214. Iijima T, Bauer R, Hossmann KA. Brain resuscitation by extracorporeal circulation after prolonged cardiac arrest in cats. *Intensive Care Med* 1993;19(2):82–8.
215. Lowenthal A, Maimon N, Waldman S, Almog Y. Sub-arachnoid hemorrhage following cardiopulmonary resuscitation. *Resuscitation* 2004;63(2):221–23.
216. Adams JA. Endothelium and cardiopulmonary resuscitation. *Crit Care Med* 2006;34(12 Suppl):S458–65.
217. Boyle EM, Jr., Pohlman TH, Cornejo CJ, Verrier ED. Endothelial cell injury in cardiovascular surgery: Ischemia-reperfusion. *Ann Thorac Surg* 1996;62(6):1868–75.
218. Caceres MJ, Schleien CL, Kuluz JW, Gelman B, Dietrich WD. Early endothelial damage and leukocyte accumulation in piglet brains following cardiac arrest. *Acta Neuropathol* 1995;90(6):582–91.
219. Brait VH, Jackman KA, Walduck AK, Selemidis S, Diep H, Mast AE et al. Mechanisms contributing to cerebral infarct size after stroke: Gender, reperfusion, T lymphocytes, and Nox2-derived superoxide. *J Cereb Blood Flow Metab* 2010;30(7):1306–17.
220. Jung JE, Kim GS, Chen H, Maier CM, Narasimhan P, Song YS et al. Reperfusion and neurovascular dysfunction in stroke: From basic mechanisms to potential strategies for neuroprotection. *Mol Neurobiol* 2010;41(2–3):172–79.
221. Bottiger BW, Krumnikl JJ, Gass P, Schmitz B, Motsch J, Martin E. The cerebral "no-reflow" phenomenon after cardiac arrest in rats—Influence of low-flow reperfusion. *Resuscitation* 1997;34(1):79–87.
222. Trummer G, Foerster K, Buckberg GD, Benk C, Heilmann C, Mader I et al. Successful resuscitation after prolonged periods of cardiac arrest: A new field in cardiac surgery. *J Thorac Cardiovasc Surg* 2010;139(5):1325–32, 1332.e1–2.

223. Miller CL, Lampard DG, Alexander K, Brown WA. Local cerebral blood flow following transient cerebral ischemia. I. Onset of impaired reperfusion within the first hour following global ischemia. *Stroke* 1980;11(5):534–41.
224. Miller CL, Lampard DG, Alexander K, Brown WA. Local cerebral blood flow following transient cerebral ischemia. I. Onset of impaired reperfusion within the first hour following global ischemia. *Stroke* 1980;11:534–41.
225. Miller CL, Lampard DG, Brown WA, Griffiths R. Local cerebral blood flow following transient cerebral ischemia. II. Effect of arterial PCO2 on reperfusion following global ischemia. *Stroke* 1980;11:542–8.
226. Torvik A, Svindland A. Is there a transitional zone between brain infarcts and the surrounding brain? A histological study. *Acta Neurol Scand* 1986;74:365–70.
227. deVeber G, Andrew M, Adams C, Bjornson B, Booth F, Buckley DJ, Camfield CS, David M, Humphreys P, Langevin P, MacDonald EA, Gillett J, Meaney B, Shevell M, Sinclair DB, Yager J, Ischemi C-C. Cerebral sinovenous thrombosis in children. *N Engl J Med* 2001;345:417–23.
228. Fluss J, Geary D, Deveber G. Cerebral sinovenous thrombosis and idiopathic nephrotic syndrome in childhood: Report of four new cases and review of the literature. *Eur J Pediatr* 2006;165:709–16.
229. Sebire G, Tabarki B, Saunders DE, Leroy I, Liesner R, Saint-Martin C, Husson B, Williams AN, Wade A, Kirkham FJ. Cerebral venous sinus thrombosis in children: Risk factors, presentation, diagnosis and outcome. *Brain* 2005;128:477–89.
230. Mohr JP. Lacunar stroke. *Hypertension* 1986;8:349–56.
231. Fisher CM. Lacunar strokes and infarcts: A review. *Neurology* 1982;32:871–76.
232. Fisher CM. Lacunes: Small, deep cerebral infarcts. 1965. *Neurology* 1998;50:841.
233. Nag S, Kilty DW. Cerebrovascular changes in chronic hypertension. Protective effects of enalapril in rats. *Stroke* 1997;28:1028–34.
234. Caplan LR, Schoene WC. Clinical features of subcortical arteriosclerotic encephalopathy (Binswanger's disease). *Neurology* 1978;28:1206–15.
235. Fisher CM. Binswanger's encephalopathy: A review. *J Neurol* 1989;236:65–79.
236. Nag S. Cerebral endothelial mechanisms in increased permeability in chronic hypertension. *Adv Exp Med Biol* 1993;331:263–66.
237. Inman WH, Vessey MP. Investigation of deaths from pulmonary, coronary, and cerebral thrombosis and embolism in women of child-bearing age. *Br Med J* 1968;2:193–99.
238. Janaki S, Baruah JK, Jayaram SR, Saxena VK, Sharma SH, Gulati MS. Stroke in the young: A four-year study, 1968 to 1972. *Stroke* 1975;6:318–20.
239. Sartwell PE, Masi AT, Arthes FG, Greene GR, Smith HE. Thromboembolism and oral contraceptives: An epidemiologic case-control study. *Am J Epidemiol* 1969;90:365–80.
240. Vessey MP, Doll R. Investigation of relation between use of oral contraceptives and thromboembolic disease. A further report. *Br Med J* 1969;2:651–57.
241. Drill VA. Oral contraceptives and thromboembolic disease. I. Prospective and retrospective studies. *JAMA* 1972;219:583–92.
242. Drill VA, Calhoun DW. Oral contraceptives and thromboembolic disease. II. Estrogen content of oral contraceptives. *JAMA* 1972;219:593–96.
243. Goldzieher JW, Moses LE, Averkin E, Scheel C, Taber BZ. A placebo-controlled double-blind crossover investigation of the side effects attributed to oral contraceptives. *Fertil Steril* 1971;22:609–23.
244. Goldzieher JW, Dozier TS. Oral contraceptives and thromboembolism: A reassessment. *Am J Obstet Gynecol* 1975;123:878–914.
245. Illis L, Kocen RS, McDonald WI, Mondkar VP. Oral contraceptives and cerebral arterial occlusion. *Br Med J* 1965;2:1164–66.
246. Jennett WB, Cross JN. Influence of pregnancy and oral contraception on the incidence of strokes in women of childbearing age. *Lancet* 1967;1:1019–23.

247. Schoenberg BS, Whisnant JP, Taylor WF, Kempers RD. Strokes in women of childbearing age. A population study. *Neurology* 1970;20:181–89.
248. Fuertes-de la Haba A, Cuevas JO, Pelegrina I, Bangdiwala I. Deaths among users of oral and nonoral contraceptives. *Obstet Gynecol* 1970;36:597–602.
249. Irey NS, Norris HJ. Intimal vascular lesions associated with female reproductive steroids. *Arch Pathol* 1973;96:227–34.
250. Irey NS, McAllister HA, Henry JM. Oral contraceptives and stroke in young women: A clinicopathologic correlation. *Neurology* 1978;28:1216–19.
251. Ciccone A, Gatti A, Melis M, Cossu G, Boncoraglio G, Carriero MR, Iurlaro S, Agostoni E. Cigarette smoking and risk of cerebral sinus thrombosis in oral contraceptive users: A case-control study. *Neurol Sci* 2005;26:319–23.
252. Lidegaard O. Smoking and use of oral contraceptives: Impact on thrombotic diseases. *Am J Obstet Gynecol* 1999;180:S357–63.
253. Burkman RT. Venous thromboembolism and oral contraceptives: Current status and clinical implications. *Treat Endocrinol* 2002;1:143–47.
254. Zimlichman E, Mandel D, Mimouni FB, Wartenfeld R, Huerta M, Grotto I, Kreiss Y. Oral contraceptive use and smoking habits in young Israeli women: A cross-sectional study. *Isr Med Assoc J* 2004;6:546–49.
255. Biller J, Challa VR, Toole JF, Howard VJ. Nonbacterial thrombotic endocarditis. A neurologic perspective of clinicopathologic correlations of 99 patients. *Arch Neurol* 1982;39:95–8.
256. Aslam F, Shirani J, Haque AA. Patent foramen ovale: Assessment, clinical significance and therapeutic options. *South Med J* 2006;99:1367–72.
257. Holmes D Jr, Cohen H, Katz WE, Reeder GS. Patent foramen ovale, systemic embolization and closure. *Curr Probl Cardiol* 2004;29:56–94.
258. Fan KJ, Scott-Cora JW. Disseminated intravascular coagulation involving the brain: A topographical study. *J Natl Med Assoc* 1982;74:457–60.
259. Voves C, Wuillemin WA, Zeerleder S. International Society on Thrombosis and Haemostasis score for overt disseminated intravascular coagulation predicts organ dysfunction and fatality in sepsis patients. *Blood Coagul Fibrinolysis* 2006;17:445–51.
260. Mammen EF. Disseminated intravascular coagulation (DIC). *Clin Lab Sci* 2000;13:239.
261. Saba HI, Morelli GA. The pathogenesis and management of disseminated intravascular coagulation. *Clin Adv Hematol Oncol* 2006;4:919–26.
262. Schwartzman RJ, Hill JB. Neurologic complications of disseminated intravascular coagulation. *Neurology* 1982;32:791–97.
263. Rogers LR. Cerebrovascular complications in cancer patients. *Neurol Clin* 2003;21:167–92.
264. Stein SC, Smith DH. Coagulopathy in traumatic brain injury. *Neurocrit Care* 2004;1:479–88.
265. Chiaretti A, Pezzotti P, Mestrovic J, Piastra M, Polidori G, Storti S, Velardi F, DiRocco C. The influence of hemocoagulative disorders on the outcome of children with head injury. *Pediatr Neurosurg* 2001;34:131–37.
266. Selladurai BM, Vickneswaran M, Duraisamy S, Atan M. Coagulopathy in acute head injury—A study of its role as a prognostic indicator. *Br J Neurosurg* 1997;11:398–404.
267. Aydin MD, Kotan D, Aydin N, Gundogdu C, Onder A, Akcay F. Mechanism of cerebral fat embolism in subarachnoid hemorrhage: An experimental study. *Neuropathology* 2006;26:544–49.
268. Taviloglu K, Yanar H. Fat embolism syndrome. *Surg Today* 2007;37:5–8.
269. Habashi NM, Andrews PL, Scalea TM. Therapeutic aspects of fat embolism syndrome. *Injury* 2006;37(Suppl 4):S68–73.
270. Bontross AR, Henry CE. Electrocerebral silence associated with adequate spontaneous ventilation in a case of fat embolism. A clinical and medicolegal dilemma. *Arch Neurol* 1982;39:314–16.
271. Butteriss DJ, Mahad D, Soh C, Walls T, Weir D, Birchall D. Reversible cytotoxic cerebral edema in cerebral fat embolism. AJNR *Am J Neuroradiol* 2006;27:620–23.
272. Ryu CW, Lee DH, Kim TK, Kim SJ, Kim HS, Lee JH, Choi CG, Suh DC. Cerebral fat embolism: Diffusion-weighted magnetic resonance imaging findings. *Acta Radiol* 2005;46:528–33.

273. Cammermeyer J. Cerebral fat embolism with focal siderosis and pericapillary hemorrhages after intraperitoneal injection of oil in cats terminally fixed by perfusion. *Exp Neurol* 1977;55:690–708.
274. von Hochstetter AR, Friede RL. Residual lesions of cerebral fat embolism. *J Neurol* 1977;216:227–33.
275. McTaggart DM, Neubürger KT. Cerebral fat embolism: Pathologic changes in the brain after survival of 7 years. *Acta Neuropathol* (Berl) 1970;15:183–87.
276. Kamenar E, Burger PC. Cerebral fat embolism: A neuropathological study of a microembolic state. *Stroke* 1980;11:477–84.
277. McNamara JJ, Molot M, Dunn R, Burran EL, Stremple JF. Lipid metabolism after trauma. Role in the pathogenesis of fat embolism. *J Thorac Cardiovasc Surg* 1972;63:968–72.
278. Easton JD, Sherman DG. Management of cerebral embolism of cardiac origin. *Stroke* 1980;11:433–42.
279. Gempp E, Blatteau JE. Neurological disorders after repetitive breath-hold diving. *Aviat Space Environ Med* 2006;77:971–73.
280. Cole AJ, Griffiths D, Lavender S, Summers P, Rich K. Relevance of postmortem radiology to the diagnosis of fatal cerebral gas embolism from compressed air diving. *J Clin Pathol* 2006;59:489–91.
281. Engelhardt M, Folkers W, Brenke C, Scholz M, Harders A, Fidorra H, Schmieder K. Neurosurgical operations with the patient in sitting position: Analysis of risk factors using transcranial Doppler sonography. *Br J Anaesth* 2006;96:467–72.
282. Schlimp CJ, Loimer T, Rieger M, Lederer W, Schmidts MB. The potential of venous air embolism ascending retrograde to the brain. *J Foren Sci* 2005;50:906–9.
283. van Hulst RA, Klein J, Lachmann B. Gas embolism: Pathophysiology and treatment. *Clin Physiol Funct Imaging* 2003;23:237–46.
284. Plattner T, Thali MJ, Yen K, Sonnenschein M, Stoupis C, Vock P, Zwygart-Brugger K, Kilchor T, Dirnhofer R. Virtopsy-postmortem multislice computed tomography (MSCT) and magnetic resonance imaging (MRI) in a fatal scuba diving incident. *J Foren Sci* 2003;48:1347–55.
285. Ronsivalle J, Statler J, Venbrux AC, Arepally A. Intravascular bullet migration: A report of two cases. *Mil Med* 2005;170:1044–47.
286. da Costa LB, Wallace MC, Montanera W. Shotgun pellet embolization to the posterior cerebral circulation. *AJNR Am J Neuroradiol* 2006;27:261–63.
287. Shannon P, Billbao JM, Marotta T, Terbrugge K. Inadvertent foreign body embolization in diagnostic and therapeutic cerebral angiography. *AJNR Am J Neuroradiol* 2006;27:278–82.
288. Henkes H, Lowens S, Preiss H, Reinartz J, Miloslavski E, Kuhne D. A new device for endovascular coil retrieval from intracranial vessels: Alligator retrieval device. *AJNR Am J Neuroradiol* 2006;27:327–29.
289. Shilling K, Uretsky BF, Hunter GC. Entrapment of a cerebral embolic protection device—A case report. *Vasc Endovascular Surg* 2006;40:229–33.
290. Chapot R, Wassef M, Bisdorff A, Rogopoulos A, Merland JJ, Houdart E. Occlusion of the middle cerebral artery due to synthetic fibers. *AJNR Am J Neuroradiol* 2006;27:148–50.
291. Clement R, Bresson C, Marcorelles P, Rodat O, Lagarde N. Cerebellar-pulmonary embolism, cause of death in the newborn. *J Clin Foren Med* 2006;13:361–65.
292. Ogilvy CS, McKee AC, Newman NJ, Donnelly SM, Kiwak KJ. Embolism of cerebral tissue to lungs: Report of two cases and review of the literature. *Neurosurgery* 1988;23:511–16.
293. Burger PC, Scheithauer BW, Vogel FS. *Surgical Pathology of the Nervous System and Its Coverings.* New York: Churchill Livingstone, 2002.
294. Schiffer D. *Brain Tumor Pathology: Current Diagnostic Hotspots and Pitfalls.* Dordrecht: Springer, 2006.
295. Kleihues P, Burger PC, Scheithauer BW, Zülch KJ. *Histological Typing of Tumours of the Central Nervous System.* Berlin: Springer-Verlag, 1993.
296. Louis DN, Ohgaki H, Wiestler OD, Cavenee WK, Burger PC, Jouvet A et al. The 2007 WHO classification of tumours of the central nervous system. *Acta Neuropathol* 2007;114(2):97–109.

297. Nakazato Y. [Revised WHO classification of brain tumours]. *Brain Nerve* 2008;60(1):59–77.
298. Berger MS, Prados MD, Al-Mefty O, eds. *Textbook of Neuro-Oncology*. Philadelphia: Elsevier-Saunders, 2005.
299. Baehring JM, Piepmeier JM, eds. *Brain Tumors: Practical Guide to Diagnosis and Treatment*. New York: Informa Healthcare, 2007.
300. Greenberg H, Chandler WF, Sandler HM. *Brain Tumors*. New York: Oxford University Press, 1999.
301. Markert J. *Glioblastomas Multiforme*. Sudbury, MA: Jones & Bartlett, 2005.
302. Batchelor T, ed. *Lymphoma of the Nervous System*. Amsterdam, Butterworth-Heinemann, 2004.
303. Sawamura Y, Sirato H, de Tribolet N, eds. *Intracranial Germ Cell Tumors*. New York: Springer, 1998.
304. Kepes JJ. *Meningiomas. Biology, Pathology, and Differential Diagnosis*. New York: Masson, 1982.
305. Rachet B, Partanen T, Kauppinen T, Sasco AJ. Cancer risk in laboratory workers: An emphasis on biological research. *Am J Ind Med* 2000;38:651–65.
306. Huntington RW Jr, Cummings K, Moe TI, Wybel HV. Discovery of fatal primary intracranial neoplasms at medicolegal autopsies. *Cancer* 1965;18:117–27.
307. Vougiouklakis T, Mitselou A, Agnantis NJ. Sudden death due to primary intracranial neoplasms. A forensic autopsy study. *Anticancer Res* 2006;26:2463–66.
308. Buettner A, Winkler PA, Eisenmenger W, Weis S. Colloid cysts of the third ventricle with fatal outcome: A report of two cases and review of the literature. *Int J Legal Med* 1997;110:260–66.
309. Leestma JE, Konakci Y. Sudden unexpected death caused by neuroepithelial (colloid) cyst of the third ventricle. *J Foren Sci* 1981;26:486–91.
310. Shaktawat SS, Salman WD, Twaij Z, Al-Dawoud A. Unexpected death after headache due to a colloid cyst of the third ventricle. *World J Surg Oncol* 2006;4:47.
311. McDonald JA. Colloid cyst of the third ventricle and sudden death. *Ann Emerg Med* 1982;11:365–67.
312. Hamlat A, Pasqualini E, Askar B. Hypothesis about the physiopathlogy of acute deterioration and sudden death caused by colloid cysts of the third ventricle. *Medical Hypoth* 2004;63:1014–17.
313. Chow LT, Shum BS, Chow WH. Intrathoracic vagus nerve neurofibroma and sudden death in a patient with neurofibromatosis. *Thorax* 1993;48:298–99.
314. Bailey O. Notes from the medical examiner. Unexpected death due to intracranial tumors. *New Engl J Med* 1949;24:988–89.
315. The Texas Sniper. *Life*, Aug. 12, Time Life, Inc., 1966.
316. The madman in the tower. *Time*, Aug. 12, Time Life Inc., 1966, vol. 88.
317. Jacquez GM, Kaufmann A, Meliker J, Goovaerts P, AvRuskin G, Nriagu J. Global, local and focused geographic clustering for case-control data with residential histories. *Environ Health* 2005;4:4.
318. Houben MP, Coebergh JW, Birch JM, Tijssen CC van Duijn CM, McNally RJ. Space-time clustering patterns of gliomas in the Netherlands suggest an infectious aetiology. *Eur J Cancer* 2005;41:2917–23.
319. Fang Z, Kulldorff M, Gregorio DI. Brain cancer mortality in the United States, 1986 to 1995: A geographic analysis. *Neuro-Oncology* 2004;6:179–87.
320. Ohgaki H, Kleihues P. Epidemiology and etiology of gliomas. *Acta Neuropathol* (Berl) 2005;109:93–108.
321. Kleihues P, Aguzzi A, Ohgaki H. Genetic and environmental factors in the etiology of human brain tumors. *Toxicol Lett* 1995;82–83:601–5.
322. Jänisch W, Schreiber D, eds. *Experimental Tumors of the Central Nervous System*. Kalamazoo, MI: The Upjohn Co., 1977.
323. Wogan GN, Hecht SS, Felton JS, Conney AH, Loeb LA. Environmental and chemical carcinogenesis. *Semin Cancer Biol* 2004;14:473–86.
324. Del Valle L, Enam S, Lara C, Miklossy J, Khalili K, Gordon J. Primary central nervous system lymphoma expressing the human neurotropic polyomavirus, JC virus, genome. *J Virol* 2004;78:3462–69.

325. Castaigne P, Rondot P, Escourolle R, R'badeau dumas JL, Cathala F, Hauw JJ. [Progressive multifocal leukoencephalopathy and multiple gliomas]. *Rev Neurol* (Paris) 1974;130(9–10):379–92.
326. Hori R, Murai Y, Tsuneyama K, Abdel-Aziz HO, Nomoto K, Takahashi H, Cheng CM, Kuchina T, Harman BV, Takano Y. Detection of JC virus DNA sequences in colorectal cancers in Japan. *Virchows Arch* 2005;447:723–30.
327. Murai Y, Zheng HC, Aziz HO, Mei H, Kutsuna T, Nakanishi Y, Tsuneyama K, Takano Y. High JC virus load in gastric cancer and adjacent non-cancerous mucosa. *Cancer Sci* 2006.
328. Henry JM, Heffner RR, Jr., Dillard SH, Earle KM, Davis RL. Primary malignant lymphomas of the central nervous system. *Cancer* 1974;34:1293–302.
329. Moulder JE, Foster KR, Erdreich LS, McNamee JP. Mobile phones, mobile phone base stations and cancer: A review. *Int J Radiat Biol* 2005;81:189–203.
330. Fountaine T, Lind CR, Law AJ. Primary glioblastomas and anaplastic astrocytoma in a glioma family. *J Clin Neurosci* 2006;13:497–501.
331. Lossignol D, Grossman SA, Sheidler VR, Griffin CA, Piantadosi S. Familial clustering of malignant astrocytomas. *J Neurooncol* 1990;9:139–45.
332. Dimopoulos VG, Fountas KN, Robinson JS. Familial intracranial ependymomas. Report of three cases in a family and review of the literature. *Neurosurg Focus* 2006;20(1).
333. Daly AF, Jaffrain-Rea ML, Ciccarelli A, Valdes-Socin H, Rohmer V, Tamburrano G, Borson-Chazot C, Estour B, Ciccarelli E, Brue T, Ferolla P, Emy P, Colao A, DeMaris E, Lecomte P, Penfornis F, Delemer B. Bertherat: Clinical characterization of familial isolated pituitary adenomas. *J Clin Endocrinol Metab* 2006;91:3316–23.
334. Fisher C, Rajpurkar M, Alcasabas P, Curtis M. Central nervous system hemangioblastoma and von Hippel-Lindau syndrome: A familial presentation. *Clin Pediatr* (Phila) 2006;45:456–62.
335. Sharma MC, Ralte AM, Gaekwad S, Santosh V, Shankar SK, Sarkar C. Subependymal giant cell astrocytoma—A clinicopathological study of 23 cases with special emphasis on histogenesis. *Pathol Oncol Res* 2004;10:219–24.
336. Friedman JM, Gutmann DH, McCollin M, Riccardi VM, eds. *Neurofibromatosis: Phenotype, Natural History and Pathogenesis*. Baltimore: Johns Hopkins University Press, 1999.
337. Wilson WG, Serwint JR. Retinoblastoma. *Pediatr Rev* 2007:28:1–37.
338. Reinhardt G. Trauma-Fremdköper-Hindgeschwülst. *Münch Med Wochenschr* 1928;75:399–401.
339. Dunsmore RH, Roberts M. Trauma as a cause of brain tumor: A medicolegal dilemma. *Conn Med* 1974;38:521–23.
340. Cushing, H, Eisenhardt L. *Meningiomas: Their Classification, Regional Behavior, Life History and Surgical End Results*. New York: Hafner, 1962.
341. Walsh J, Gye R, Connelley TJ. Meningioma: A late complication of head injury. *Med J Aust* 1969;1:906–8.
342. Whatmore WJ, Hitchcock ER. Meningioma following trauma. *Br J Surg* 1973;60:496–98.
343. McGonigal LJ, Riggs JE Jr, Schochet SS, Ortiz O. Posttraumatic meningioma: Explanation of an epidemiologic dichotomy. *Mil Med* 1995;160:92–4.
344. Heyck H. Glioblastom nach Leukotomie. *Wschr Psychiat Neurol* 1954;128:180–88.
345. Cusick JF, Bailey OT. Association of ossified subdural hematomas and meningioma. Case report. *J Neurosurg* 1972;37:731–34.
346. Manuelidis EE. Glioma in trauma. In Minckler J, ed., *Pathology of the Nervous System*. Vol. 2. New York: McGraw Hill, 1971.
347. Russell DS, Rubinstein LJ. *Pathology of Tumors of the Nervous System*. Baltimore: Williams & Wilkins, 1977.
348. Ewing J. Modern attitude toward traumatic cancer. *Arch Pathol* 1935;19:690–728.
349. Auster LS. The role of trauma in oncogenesis: A juridical consideration. *JAMA* 1961;175:946–50.
350. Annegers JF, Schoenberg BS, Okazaki H, Kurland LT. Epidemiologic study of primary intracranial neoplasms. *Arch Neurol* 1981;38:217–19.
351. Schoenberg BS, Christine BW, Whisnant JP. The resolution of discrepancies in the reported incidence of primary brain tumors. *Neurology* 1978;28:817–23.

352. Davis FG, Malinski N, Haenszel W, Chang J, Flannery J, Gershman S, Dibble R, Bigner DD. Primary brain tumor incidence rates in four United States regions, 1985–1989: A pilot study. *Neuroepidemiology* 1996;15:103–12.
353. Davis FG, Kupelian V, Freels S, McCarthy B, Surawicz T. Prevalence estimates for primary brain tumors in the United States by behavior and major histology groups. *Neuro-Oncology* 2001;3:152–58.
354. Chakrabarti I, Cockburn M, Cozen W, Wang YP, Preston-Martin S. A population-based description of glioblastoma multiforme in Los Angeles County, 1974–1999. *Cancer* 2005;104:2798–806.
355. Deorah S, Lynch CF, Sibenaller ZA, Ryken TC. Trends in brain cancer incidence and survival in the United States: Surveillance, Epidemiology, and End Results Program, 1973 to 2001. *Neurosurg Focus* 2006;20(4):E1.
356. Butler KM. Meningococcal meningitis prevention programs for college students: A review of the literature. *Worldviews Evid Based Nurs* 2006;3:185–93.
357. Pendlebury WW, Perl DP, Winn WW Jr, McQuillen JB. Neuropathologic evaluation of 40 confirmed cases of *Legionella* pneumonia. *Neurology* 1983;33:1340–44.
358. Inglesby TV, Henderson DA, Bartlett JG, Ascher MS, Eitzen E, Friedlander AM, Hauer J, McDade J, Osterholm MT, O'Toole T, Parker G, Perl TM, Russell PK, Tonat K. Anthrax as a biological weapon: Medical and public health management. Working Group on Civilian Biodefense. *JAMA* 1999;281:1735–45.
359. Inglesby TV, Dennis DT, Henderson DA, Bartlett JG, Ascher MS, Eitzen E, Fine AD, Friedlander AM, Hauer J, Koerner JF, Layton M, McDade J, Osterholm MT, O'Toole T, Parker G, Perl TM, Russell PK. Plague as a biological weapon: Medical and public health management. Working Group on Civilian Biodefense. *JAMA* 2000;283:2281–90.
360. Dennis DT, Inglesby TV, Henderson DA, Bartlett JG, Ascher MS, Eitzen E, Fine AD, Friedlander AM, Hauer J, Layton M, Lillibridge SR, McDade JE, Osterholm MT, O'Toole T, Parker G, Perl TM, Russell PK. Tularemia as a biological weapon: Medical and public health management. *JAMA* 2001;285:2763–73.
361. Henderson DA, Inglesby TV, Bartlett JG, Ascher MS, Eitzen E, Jahrling PB, Hauer J, Layton M, McDade J, Osterholm MT, O'Toole T, Parker G, Perl T, Russell PK, Tonat K. Smallpox as a biological weapon: Medical and public health management. Working Group on Civilian Biodefense. *JAMA* 1999;281:2127–37.
362. Sidwell RW, Smee DF. Viruses of the Bunya- and Togaviridae families: Potential as bioterrorism agents and means of control. *Antiviral Res* 2003;57:101–11.
363. Borio L, Inglesby T, Peters CJ, Schmaljohn AL, Hughes JM, Jahrling PB, Ksiazek T, Johnson KM, Meyerhoff A, O'Toole T, Ascher MS, Bartlett J, Breman JG, Eitzen EM Jr, Hamburg M, Hauer J, Henderson DA et al. Hemorrhagic fever viruses as biological weapons: Medical and public health management. *JAMA* 2002;287:2391–405.
364. Scheld WM, Whitley RJ, Marra CM, eds. *Infections of the Central Nervous System*. Philadelphia: Lippinicott Williams & Wilkins, 2004.
365. Kirkpatrick JB. Neurologic infections due to bacteria, fungi and parasites. In Davis RL, Robertson, DM, eds., *Textbook of Neuropathology*. Baltimore: Williams & Wilkins, 1991, pp. 719–803.
366. Lindsay DS, Weiss LM, eds. *Opportunistic Infections: Toxoplasma, Sarcocystis, and Microsporidia*. Boston: Kluwer Academic Press, 2004.
367. Leestma JE. Viral infections of the nervous system. In Davis R, Robertson DM, eds., *Textbook of Neuropathology*. Baltimore: Williams & Wilkins, 1991.
368. Osborn MK, Steinberg JP. Subdural empyema and other suppurative complications of paranasal sinusitis. *Lancet Infect Dis* 2007;7:62–7.
369. Bernardini GL. Diagnosis and management of brain abscess and subdural empyema. *Curr Neurol Neurosci Rep* 2004;4:448–56.
370. van Aals J, Beuls EA, Cornips EM, Vanormelingen L, Vandersteen M, Weber JW, Vles JS. Anatomy and surgery of the infected dermal sinus of the lower spine. *Childs Nerv Syst* 2006;22:1307–15.

371. Kamouchi M, Wakugawa Y, Okada Y, Kishikawa K, Matsuo R, Toyoda K, Yasumori K, Inoue T, Ibayashi S, Iida M. Venous infarction secondary to septic cavernous sinus thrombosis. *Intern Med* 2006;45:25–7.
372. Bell WE, McCormick WF. *Neurologic Infections in Children*. Philadelphia: W.B. Saunders, 1975.
373. Frosch M. *Akute Bakterielle Meningitis*. Bremen: Uni-Med, 2003.
374. Tunkel AR. *Bacterial Meningitis*. Philadelphia: Lippincott Williams & Wilkins, 2001.
375. Schoenfeld H, Helwig H, eds. *Bacterial Meningitis*. Vol. 45. Basel: Karger, 1992.
376. Sáez-Llorens X Jr, McCracken GH Jr. Bacterial meningitis in neonates and children. *Infect Dis Clin North Am* 1990;4:623–44.
377. Kutz JW, Simon LM, Chennupati SK, Giannoni CM, Manolidis S. Clinical predictors for hearing loss in children with bacterial meningitis. *Arch Otolaryngol Head Neck Surg* 2006;132:941–45.
378. Husain E, Chawla R, Dobson S, Dele Davies H. The Paediatric Investigators Collaborative Network on Infections in Canada. Epidemiology and outcome of bacterial meningitis in Canadian children: 1998–1999. *Clin Invest Med* 2006;29:131–35.
379. Souza de Morais J, Munford RS, Risi JB, Antezana E, Feldman RA. Epidemic disease due to serogroup C *Neisseria meningitidis* in Sao Paulo, Brazil. *J Infect Dis* 1974;129:568–71.
380. Hardman JM. Fatal meningococcal infections: The changing pathologic picture in the '60s. *Mil Med* 1968;133:951–64.
381. Hardman JM, Earle KM. Myocarditis in 200 fatal meningococcal infections. *Arch Pathol* 1969;87:318–25.
382. Sandler MA, Pincus PS, Weltman MD, Naude GE, Kallenbach JM, King PC, Zwi S. Meningococcaemia complicated by myocarditis. A report of 2 cases. *S Afr Med J* 1989;75:391–93.
383. De Louvois J, Gortvai P, Hurley R. Bacteriology of abscesses of the central nervous system: A multicenter prospective study. *BMJ* 1977;2:981–84.
384. Ingham H. *Pyogenic Neurosurgical Infections*. London: Edward Arnold, 1991.
385. Hopwood DA. How do antibiotic-producing bacteria ensure their self-resistance before antibiotic biosynthesis incapacitates them? *Mol Microbiol* 2007;63:937–40.
386. Varkey P, Jerath AU, Bagniewski SM, Lesnick TG. The epidemiology of tuberculosis among primary refugee arrivals in Minnesota between 1997 and 2001. *J Travel Med* 2007;14:1–8.
387. American Lung Association. *Trends in Tuberculosis Morbidity and Mortality*. New York: American Lung Association, 2006.
388. Minion J, Gallant V, Wolfe J, Jamieson F, Long R. Multidrug and extensively drug-resistant tuberculosis in Canada 1997–2008: Demographic and disease characteristics. *PLoS One* 2013;8(1).
389. Wilkinson HA, Ferris EJ, Muggia AL, Cantu RC. Central nervous system tuberculosis: A persistent disease. *J Neurosurg* 1971;34:15–22.
390. Davidson P. A treatment of infections due to atypical mycobacteria. In Remington S, Schwartz MN, eds., *Current Clinical Topics in Infectious Disease*. New York: McGraw-Hill, 1982, pp. 160–76.
391. Thurtell MJ, Keed AB, Yan M, Gottlieb T, Spies JM, Halmagyi GM. Tuberculous cranial pachymeningitis. *Neurology* 2007;68:298–300.
392. Dannenberg AM. *Pathogenesis of Human Pulmonary Tuberculosis: Insights from the Rabbit Model.* Washington, DC: ASM Press, 2006.
393. Marais BJ, Mlambo CK, Rastogi N, Zozio T, Duse AG, Victor TC, Marais E, Warren RM. Epidemic spread of multidrug-resistant (MDR) tuberculosis in Johannesburg, South Africa. *J Clin Microbiol* 2013; e-publication ahead of print (April 3).
394. Damergis JA, Leftwich EI, Curtin JA, Witorsch P. Tuberculoma of the brain. *JAMA* 1978;239:413–15.
395. Kauffmann CA, ed. *Atlas of Fungal Infections*. Philadelphia: Springer/Current Medicine, 2007.
396. Richardson M, Warnock DW. *Fungal Infection: Diagnosis and Management.* Malden, MA: Blackwell, 2003.
397. Wingard JR, Anaissie EJ, eds. *Fungal Infections in the Immunocompromised Patient.* Boca Raton, FL: Taylor & Francis, 2005.

398. Wilson LE, Blythe D, Sharfstein JM. Fungal meningitis from injection of contaminated steroids: A compounding problem. *JAMA* 2012;308(23):2461.
399. Manuel RJ, Kibbler CC. The epidemiology and prevention of invasive aspergillosis. *J Hosp Infect* 1998;39:95–109.
400. Munoz P, Guinea J, Bouza E. Update on invasive aspergillosis: Clinical and diagnostic aspects. *Clin Microbiol Infect* 2006;12:24–39.
401. Szalai G, Fellegi V, Szabo Z, Vitez LC. Mucormycosis mimicks sinusitis in a diabetic adult. *Ann NY Acad Sci* 2006;1084:520–30.
402. Bouza E, Munoz P, Guinea J. Mucormycosis: An emerging disease? *Clin Microbiol Infect* 2006;12:7–23.
403. Eucker J, Sezer O, Graf B, Possinger K. Mucormycoses. *Mycoses* 2001;44:253–60.
404. Weprin BE, Hall WA, Goodman J, Adams GL. Long-term survival in rhinocerebral mucormycosis. Case report. *J Neurosurg* 1998;88:570–75.
405. Bradsher RW, Chapman SW, Pappas PG. Blastomycosis. *Infect Dis Clin North Am* 2003;17:21–40, vii.
406. Bradsher RW. Histoplasmosis and blastomycosis. *Clin Infect Dis* 1996;22(Suppl 2):S102–11.
407. Kauffmann CA. Histoplasmosis: A clinical and laboratory update. *Clin Microbiol Rev* 2007; 20:115–32.
408. Pfaller MA, Diekema DJ. Epidemiology of invasive candidiasis: A persistent public health problem. *Clin Microbiol Rev* 2007;20:133–63.
409. Multistate fungal meningitis outbreak—Interim guidance for treatment. *MMWR Morb Mortal Wkly Rep* 2012;61(41):842.
410. Kerkering TM, Grifasi ML, Baffoe-Bonnie AW, Bansal E, Garner DC, Smith J et al. Early clinical observations in prospectively followed patients with fungal meningitis related to contaminated epidural steroid injections. *Ann Intern Med* 2013;158(3):154–61.
411. Stegmann BJ, Carey JC. TORCH infections. Toxoplasmosis, other (syphilis, varicella-zoster, parvovirus B19), rubella, cytomegalovirus (CMV), and herpes infections. *Curr Womens Health Rep* 2002;2:253–58.
412. Lechtenberg R, Hollenberg Sher J. *AIDS in the Nervous System*. New York: Churchill Livingstone, 1988.
413. Rosenblum ML, Levy RM, Bredesen D, eds. *AIDS and the Nervous System*. New York: Raven Press, 1988.
414. National Center for Infectious Diseases. *Malaria. Geographic Distribution*. Atlanta, GA: CDC, 2004.
415. Greenwood BM. The epidemiology of malaria. *Ann Trop Med Parasitol* 1997;91:763–69.
416. Marcucci C, Madjdpour C, Spahn DR. Allogeneic blood transfusions: Benefit, risks and clinical indications in countries with a low or high human development index. *Br Med Bull* 2004;70:15–28.
417. Hunt NH, Golenser J, Chan-Ling T, Parekh S, Rae C, Potter S, Medana IM, Miu J, Ball HJ. Immunopathogenesis of cerebral malaria. *Int J Parasitol* 2006;36:569–82.
418. Medana IM, Turner GD. Human cerebral malaria and the blood-brain barrier. *Int J Parasitol* 2006;36:555–68.
419. Mens PF, Schoone GJ, Kager PA, Schallig HD. Detection and identification of human *Plasmodium* species with real-time quantitative nucleic acid sequence-based amplification. *Malar J* 2006;5:80.
420. Peoc'h MY, Gyure KA, Morrison AL. Postmortem diagnosis of cerebral malaria. *Am J Foren Med Pathol* 2000;21:366–69.
421. Stoppacher R, Adams SP. Malaria deaths in the United States: Case report and review of deaths, 1979–1998. *J Foren Sci* 2003;48:404–8.
422. Gonzalez Garcia JJ, Arnalich F, Pena JM, Garcia-Alegria JJ, Garcia-Fernandez F, Jimenez-Herraez C, Vazquez JJ. An outbreak of *Plasmodium vivax* malaria among heroin users in Spain. *Trans R Soc Trop Med Hyg* 1986;80:549–52.

423. Shandera WX, Kass JS. Neurocysticercosis: Current knowledge and advances. *Curr Neurol Neurosci Rep* 2006;6:453–59.
424. Garcia LS. *Diagnostic Medical Parasitology*. Washington, DC: ASM Press, 2007.
425. Roberts M, Cross J, Pohl U, Lucas S, Dean A. Cerebral schistosomiasis. *Lancet Infect Dis* 2006;6:820.
426. Crompton DWT. *Handbook of Helminthiasis for Public Health*. Boca Raton, FL: CRC Press, 2007.
427. John DT, Petri WA, Markell EK, Voge M. *Markell and Voge's Medical Parasitology*. St. Louis, MO: Saunders Elsevier, 2006.
428. Ahmad FU, Sharma BS. Treatment of intramedullary spinal cysticercosis: Report of 2 cases and review of literature. *Surg Neurol* 2007;67:74–7.
429. Verma SK, Agarwal BB, Agarwal G. Sudden death in neurocysticercosis by trauma. *Foren Sci Int* 1998;95:23–6.
430. Bogitsh BJ, Carter CE, Oeltmann TN. *Human Parasitology*. Amsterdam: Elsevier Academic Press, 2005.
431. Johnson R. *Viral Infections of the Nervous System*. New York: Raven Press, 1982.
432. Centers for Disease Control and Prevention: Arboviral encephalitides. *MMWR* 1994;43:385–7.
433. Goudsmit J. *Viral Fitness: The Next SARS and West Nile in the Making*. New York: Oxford University Press, 2004.
434. Fu SF, ed. *The World of Rhabdoviruses*. New York: Springer, 2005.
435. Kleinschmidt-DeMasters BK, Gilden DH. The expanding spectrum of herpesvirus infections of the nervous system. *Brain Pathol* 2001;11:440–51.
436. Zhu T, Korber BT, Nahmias AJ, Hooper E, Sharp PM, Ho DD. An African HIV-1 sequence from 1959 and implications for the origin of the epidemic. *Nature* 1998;391:594–97.
437. Martin LS, McDougal JS, Loskoski SL. Disinfection and inactivation of the human T lymphotropic virus type III/lymphadenopathy-associated virus. *J Infect Dis* 1985;152:400–3.
438. Gray F, Adle-Biassette H, Chretien F, Lorin de la Grandmaison G, Force G, Keohane C. Neuropathology and neurodegeneration in human immunodeficiency virus infection. Pathogenesis of HIV-induced lesions of the brain, correlations with HIV-associated disorders and modifications according to treatments. *Clin Neuropathol* 2001;20:146–55.
439. Hojberg L, Sondergard E, Pedersen C. A case of Epstein-Barr virus infection complicated with Guillain-Barre syndrome involving several cranial nerves. *Scand J Infect Dis* 2005;37:522–24.
440. Åstrøm KE, Stoner GL. Early pathological changes in progressive multifocal leukoencephalopathy: A report of two asymptomatic cases occurring prior to the AIDS epidemic. *Acta Neuropathol* (Berl) 1994;88:93–105.
441. Padgett BL, Walker DL, ZuRhein GM, Eckroade RJ, Dessel BH. Cultivation of papova-like virus from human brain with progressive multifocal leucoencephalopathy. *Lancet* 1971;1:1257–60.
442. Zu Rhein GM, Chou S. Papova virus in progressive multifocal leukoencephalopathy. *Res Publ Assoc Res Nerv Ment Dis* 1968;44:307–62.
443. Bolton DC, McKinley MP, Prusiner SB. Molecular characteristics of the major scrapie prion protein. *Biochemistry* 1984;23:5898–906.
444. Prusiner SB. Prions: Novel infectious pathogens. *Adv Virus Res* 1984;29:1–56.
445. Priola SA, Caughey B, Wehrly K, Chesebro B. A 60-kDa prion protein (PrP) with properties of both the normal and scrapie-associated forms of PrP. *J Biol Chem* 1995;270:3299–305.
446. Prusiner SB, McCarty M. Discovering DNA encodes heredity and prions are infectious proteins. *Annu Rev Genet* 2006;40:25–45.
447. Legname G, Nguyen HO, Peretz D, Cohen FE, DeArmond SJ, Prusiner SB. Continuum of prion protein structures enciphers a multitude of prion isolate-specified phenotypes. *Proc Natl Acad Sci USA* 2006;103:19105–10.
448. Harris DA, ed. *Mad Cow Disease and Related Spongiform Encephalopathies*. New York: Springer, 2004.

449. Miller MW, Williams ES. Chronic wasting disease of cervids. *Curr Top Microbiol Immunol* 2004;284:193–214.
450. Xie Z, O'Rourke KI, Dong Z, Jenny AL, Langenberg JA, Belay ED, Schonberger LB, Petersen RB, Zou W, Kong Q, Gambetti P, Chen SG. Chronic wasting disease of elk and deer and Creutzfeldt-Jakob disease: Comparative analysis of the scrapie prion protein. *J Biol Chem* 2006;281:4199–206.
451. Liberski PP, Budka H. Gerstmann-Sträussler-Scheinker disease. I. Human diseases. *Folia Neuropathol* 2004;42(Suppl B):120–40.
452. Gambetti P, Parchi P, Petersen RB, Chen SG, Lugaresi E. Fatal familial insomnia and familial Creutzfeldt-Jakob disease: Clinical, pathological and molecular features. *Brain Pathol* 1995;5:43–51.
453. Laprevotte I, Henaut A. The new variant of the Creutzfeldt-Jakob disease accounts for no relative increase of the Creutzfeldt-Jakob disease mortality rate in the United Kingdom; this fits ill with the new variant being the consequence of consumption of food infected with the agent of bovine spongiform encephalopathy. *BMC Public Health* 2003;3:25.
454. Kirschbaum WR. *Jakob-Creutzfeldt Disease*. New York: Elsevier North Holland, 1968.
455. Liberski PP. Amyloid plaques in transmissible spongiform encephalopathies (prion diseases). *Folia Neuropathol* 2004;42(Suppl B):109–19.
456. Davidson SS, Benjamin WH Jr. Risk of infection and tracking of work-related infectious diseases in the funeral industry. *Am J Infect Control* 2006;34:655–60.
457. Brown P, Gibbs JCJ, Amyx HL, Kingsbury DT, Rohwer RG, Sulima MP, Gajdusek DC. Chemical disinfection of Creutzfeldt-Jakob disease virus. *N Engl J Med* 1982;306:1279–82.
458. Brown P, Brandel JP, Preece M, Sato T. Iatrogenic Creutzfeldt-Jakob disease: The waning of an era. *Neurology* 2006;67:389–93.
459. Tullo AB, Buckley RJ, Kelly T, Head MW, Bennett P, Armitage WJ, Ironside JW. Transplantation of ocular tissue from a donor with sporadic Creutzfeldt-Jakob disease. *Clin Exp Ophthalmol* 2006;34:645–49.
460. Sutton JM, Dickinson J, Walker JT, Raven ND. Methods to minimize the risks of Creutzfeldt-Jakob disease transmission by surgical procedures: Where to set the standard? *Clin Infect Dis* 2006;43:757–64.
461. Hewitt PE, Llewelyn CA, Mackenzie J, Will RG. Creutzfeldt-Jakob disease and blood transfusion: Results of the UK Transfusion Medicine Epidemiological Review study. *Vox Sang* 2006;91:221–30.
462. Jeffries Dl. Decontamination and CJD: The latest guidance. *J Perioper Pract* 2006;16:555–60.
463. Hofer M, Weber A, Haffner K, Berlis A, Klingel K, Kruger M, Kandolf R, Volk B. Acute hemorrhagic leukoencephalitis (Hurst's disease) linked to Epstein-Barr virus infection. *Acta Neuropathol* (Berl) 2005;109:226–30.
464. Olgar S, Ertugrul T, Nisli K, Aydin K, Caliskan M. Influenza A-associated acute necrotizing encephalopathy. *Neuropediatrics* 2006;37:166–68.
465. Akiyoshi K, Hamada Y, Yamada H, Kojo M, Izumi T. Acute necrotizing encephalopathy associated with hemophagocytic syndrome. *Pediatr Neurol* 2006;34:315–18.
466. Gibbs WN, Kreidie MA, Kim RC, Hasso AN. Acute hemorrhagic leukoencephalitis: Neuroimaging features and neuropathologic diagnosis. *J Comput Assist Tomogr* 2005;29:689–93.
467. Graham DI, Behan PO, More IA. Brain damage complicating septic shock: Acute haemorrhagic leucoencephalitis as a complication of the generalised Shwartzman reaction. *J Neurol Neurosurg Psychiatry* 1979;42:19–28.
468. Haymaker W, Kernohan JW. The Landry-Guillain-Barré syndrome. A clinicopathologic report of fifty fatal cases and a critique of the literature. *Medicine* 1949;28:59–141.
469. Server AC, Johnson RT. Guillain-Barre syndrome. In Remington JS, Swartz MN, eds., *Current Clinical Topics in Infectious Disease*. New York: McGraw-Hill, 1982, pp. 74–96.
470. Leneman F. The Guillain-Barre syndrome. Definition, etiology, and review of 1100 cases. *Arch Intern Med* 1966;118:139–44.

471. Hughes RA, Cornblath DR. Guillain-Barre syndrome. *Lancet* 2005;366:1653–66.
472. Sencer DJ, Millar JD. Reflections on the 1976 swine flu vaccination program. *Emerg Infect Dis* 2006;12:29–33.
473. Hughes RA, Charlton J, Latinovic R, Gulliford MC. No association between immunization and Guillain-Barre syndrome in the United Kingdom, 1992 to 2000. *Arch Intern Med* 2006;166:1301–4.
474. Kuwabara S, Kuwabara S. Guillain-Barre syndrome. *Curr Neurol Neurosci Rep* 2007;7:57–62.
475. Graham DI, Lantos PL, eds. *Greenfield's Neuropathology*. New York: Arnold, 2002.
476. Beal MF, Lang AE, Lodolph AC, eds. *Neurodegenerative Diseases: Neurobiology, Pathogenesis, and Therapeutics*. New York: Cambridge University Press, 2005.
477. Iqbal K, Grundke-Iqbal I. Discoveries of tau, abnormally hyperphosphorylated tau and others of neurofibrillary degeneration: A personal historical perspective. *J Alzheimers Dis* 2006;9(Suppl):219–42.
478. Armstrong DD. Neuropathology of Rett syndrome. *Ment Retard Dev Disabil Res Rev* 2002;8:72–6.
479. Renieri A, Meloni I, Longo I, Ariani F, Mari F, Pescucci C, Cambi F. Rett syndrome: The complex nature of a monogenic disease. *J Mol Med* 2003;81:346–54.
480. Towfighi J, Young RS, Ward RM. Is Werdnig-Hoffmann disease a pure lower motor neuron disorder? *Acta Neuropathol (Berl)* 1985;65:270–80.
481. Gordon N. Alpers syndrome: Progressive neuronal degeneration of children with liver disease. *Dev Med Child Neurol* 2006;48:1001–03.
482. Hansen LA, Terry RD. Position paper on diagnostic criteria for Alzheimer disease. *Neurobiol Aging* 1997;18(Suppl):S71–73.
483. Yaari R, Corey-Bloom J. Alzheimer's disease. *Semin Neurol* 2007;27:32–41.
484. Hyman BT. The neuropathological diagnosis of Alzheimer's disease: Clinical-pathological studies. *Neurobiol Aging* 1997;18(Suppl):S27–32.
485. Chui HC, Zarow C, Mack WJ, Ellis WG, Zheng L, Jagust WJ, Mungas D, Reed BR, Kramer JH, Decarli CC, Weiner MW, Vinters HV. Cognitive impact of subcortical vascular and Alzheimer's disease pathology. *Ann Neurol* 2006;60:677–87.
486. Etiene D, Kraft J, Ganju N, Gomez-Isla T, Gemelli B, Hyman BT, Hedley-Whyte ET, Wands JR, De La Monte SM. Cerebrovascular pathology contributes to the heterogeneity of Alzheimer's disease. *J Alzheimers Dis* 1998;1:119–34.
487. Jellinger KA. Clinicopathological analysis of dementia disorders in the elderly—An update. *J Alzheimers Dis* 2006;9(Suppl):61–70.
488. Duckett S, de La Torre J, eds. *Pathology of the Aging Human Nervous System*. New York: Oxford University Press, 2001.
489. Morris J, Galvin JE, Holtzman D, eds. *Handbook of Dementing Illnesses*. New York: Taylor & Francis, 2006.
490. Herholz K, Perani D, Morris C, eds. *The Dementias: Early Diagnosis and Evaluation*. New York: Taylor & Francis, 2006.
491. Katzman R, Terry RD, Bick KL, eds. *Alzheimer's Disease: Senile Dementia and Related Disorders*. New York: Raven Press, 1978.
492. Bertram L, McQueen MB, Mullin K, Blacker D, Tanzi RE. Systematic meta-analyses of Alzheimer disease genetic association studies: The AlzGene database. *Nat Genet* 2007;39:17–23.
493. Berg L Jr, Miller JP, Storandt M, Rubin EH, Morris JC, Baty J, Coats M, Norton J, Goate AM, Price JL, Gearing M, Mirra SS, Saunders AM. Clinicopathologic studies in cognitively healthy aging and Alzheimer's disease: Relation of histologic markers to dementia severity, age, sex, and apolipoprotein E genotype. *Arch Neurol* 1998;55:326–35.
494. Braak H, Braak E. Neuropathological stageing of Alzheimer-related changes. *Acta Neuropathol* (Berl) 1991;82:239–59.
495. Braak H, Alafuzoff I, Arzberger T, Kretzschmar H, Del Tredici K. Staging of Alzheimer disease-associated neurofibrillary pathology using paraffin sections and immunocytochemistry. *Acta Neuropathol* (Berl) 2006;112:389–404.

496. Alafuzoff I, Iqbal K, Friden H, Adolfsson R, Winblad B. Histopathological criteria for progressive dementia disorders: Clinical-pathological correlation and classification by multivariate data analysis. *Acta Neuropathol* (Berl) 1987;74:209–25.
497. Alafuzoff I, Pikkarainen M, Al-Sarraj S, Arzberger T, Bell J, Bodi I, Bogdanovic N, Budka H, Bugiani O, Ferrer I, Gelpi E, Giaccone G, Graeber MB, Hauw JJ, Kamphorst W, King A, Kopp N, Korkolopoulou P, Kovacs. Interlaboratory comparison of assessments of Alzheimer disease-related lesions: A study of the BrainNet Europe Consortium. *J Neuropathol Exp Neurol* 2006;65:740–57.
498. Mirra SS, Heyman A, McKeel D, Sumi SM, Crain BJ, Brownlee LM, Vogel FS, Hughes JP, van Belle G, Berg L. The Consortium to Establish a Registry for Alzheimer's Disease (CERAD). Part II. Standardization of the neuropathologic assessment of Alzheimer's disease. *Neurology* 1991;41:479–86.
499. National Institutes of Health. Consensus recommendations for the postmortem diagnosis of Alzheimer's disease. The National Institute on Aging, and Reagan Institute Working Group on Diagnostic Criteria for the Neuropathological Assessment of Alzheimer's Disease. *Neurobiol Aging* 1997;18(Suppl):S1–2.
500. Khachaturian ZS. Diagnosis of Alzheimer's disease. *Arch Neurol* 1985;42:1097–105.
501. Newell KL, Hyman BT, Growdon JH, Hedley-Whyte ET. Application of the National Institute on Aging (NIA)-Reagan Institute criteria for the neuropathological diagnosis of Alzheimer disease. *J Neuropathol Exp Neurol* 1999;58:1147–55.
502. Terry RD. Alzheimer's disease. In Davis RL, Robertson DM, eds., *Textbook of Neuropathology*. Baltimore: Williams & Wilkins, 1985, pp. 824–41.
503. Ashford JW, Sherman KA, Kumar V. Advances in Alzheimer therapy: Cholinesterase inhibitors. *Neurobiol Aging* 1989;10:99–105.
504. Singh SK, van Broeckhoven C. Frontotemporal lobar degeneration: Current concepts in the light of recent advance. *Brain Pathol* 2007;17:104–13.
505. van Swieten J, Spillantini MG. Hereditary frontotemporal dementia caused by Tau gene mutations. *Brain Pathol* 2007;17:63–73.
506. Mandelkow E, von Bergen M, Biernat J, Mandelkow EM. Structural principles of Tau and the paried helical filaments of Alzheimer's disease. *Brain Pathol* 2007;17:83–90.
507. Dickson DW, Rademakers R, Hutton ML. Progressive supranuclear palsy: Pathology and genetics. *Brain Pathol* 2007;17:17–74.
508. Cools AR. Basal ganglia and Parkinson's disease: Neurobiological and pharmacological aspects in animals and man. *Clin Neurol Neurosurg* 1984;86:178–95.
509. Nayernouri T. Posttraumatic parkinsonism. *Surg Neurol* 1985;24:263–64.
510. Factor SA, Sanchez-Ramos J, Weiner WJ. Trauma as an etiology of parkinsonism: A historical review of the concept. *Mov Disord* 1988;3:30–6.
511. Langston JW. Parkinson's disease: Current and future challenges. *Neurotoxicology* 2002;23:443–50.
512. Lev N, Melamed E. Heredity in Parkinson's disease: New findings. *Isr Med Assoc J* 2001;3:435–38.
513. Langston JW. The Parkinson's complex: Parkinsonism is just the tip of the iceberg. *Ann Neurol* 2006;59:591–96.
514. del Tredici R, Rüb U, de Vos RA, Bohl JR, Braak H. Where does Parkinson disease pathology begin in the brain? *J Neuropathol Exp Neurol* 2002;61:413–26.
515. Hughes AJ, Daniel SE, Blankson S, Lees AJ. A clinicopathologic study of 100 cases of Parkinson's disease. *Arch Neurol* 1993;50:140–48.
516. Borek LL, Amick MM, Friedman JH. Non-motor aspects of Parkinson's disease. *CNS Spectr* 2006;11:541–54.
517. Braak HK, Del Tredici K, Rüb U, RA deVos RA, Jensen-Steur EN, Braak E. Staging of brain pathology related to sporadic Parkinson's disease. *Neurobiol Aging* 2003;24:197–211.
518. Pritchard PB III, Netsky MG. Prevalence of neoplasms and causes of death in paralysis agitans. A necropsy study. *Neurology* 1973;23:215–22.

519. Weisman D, McKeith I. Dementia with Lewy bodies. *Semin Neurol* 2007;27:42–7.
520. Dickson DW. Dementia with Lewy bodies: Neuropathology. *J Geriatr Psychiatry Neurol* 2002;15:210–16.
521. McKeith IG, Galasko D, Kosaka K, Perry EK, Dickson DW, Hansen LA, Salmon DP, Lowe J, Mirra SS, Byrne EJ, Lennox G, Quinn NP, Edwardson JA, Ince PG, Bergeron C, Burns A, Miller BL, Lovestone S. Consensus guidelines for the clinical and pathologic diagnosis of dementia with Lewy bodies (DLB): Report of the consortium on DLB international workshop. *Neurology* 1996;47:1113–24.
522. Kosaka K, Yoshimura M, Ikeda K, Budka H. Diffuse type of Lewy body disease: Progressive dementia with abundant cortical Lewy bodies and senile changes of varying degree—A new disease? *Clin Neuropathol* 1984;3:185–92.
523. Sibley DR, Hanin I, Kuhar M, Skolnick P, eds. *Handbook of Contemporary Neuropharmacology*. Hoboken, NJ: John Wiley & Sons, 2007.
524. Hodaie M, Neimat JS, Lozano AM. The dopaminergic nigrostriatal system and Parkinson's disease: Molecular events in development, disease, and cell death, and new therapeutic strategies. *Neurosurgery* 2007;60:17–28; discussion, 28–30.
525. Weiner WJ. Meeting review: Advances in the diagnosis, treatment, and understanding of Parkinson's disease and parkinsonism. *Rev Neurol Dis* 2006;3:191–94.
526. Nakamura K, Christine CW, Starr PA, Marks MJ Jr. Effects of unilateral subthalamic and pallidal deep brain stimulation on fine motor functions in Parkinson's disease. *Mov Disord* 2007;22:619–26.
527. Langston JW. MPTP neurotoxicity: An overview and characterization of phases of toxicity. *Life Sci* 1985;36:201–6.
528. Snow BJ, Vingerhoets FJ, Langston JW, Tetrud JW, Sossi V, Calne DB. Pattern of dopaminergic loss in the striatum of humans with MPTP induced parkinsonism. *J Neurol Neurosurg Psychiatry* 2000;68:313–16.
529. Tippmann-Peikert M, Park JG, Boeve BF, Shepard JW, Silber MH. Pathologic gambling in patients with restless legs syndrome treated with dopaminergic agonists. *Neurology* 2007;68:301–3.
530. Torvik A, Meen D. Distribution of the brain stem lesions in postencephalitic Parkinsonism. *Acta Neurol Scand* 1966;42:415–25.
531. Casals J, Elizan TS, Yahr MD. Postencephalitic parkinsonism—A review. *J Neural Transm* 1998;105:645–76.
532. Maurizi CP. Why was the 1918 influenza pandemic so lethal? The possible role of a neurovirulent neuraminidase. *Med Hypotheses* 1985;16:1–5.
533. Litvan II, Jankovic J, Goetz CG, Wenning GK, Sastry N, Jellinger K, McKee A, Lai EC, Brandel JP, Verny M, Ray-Chaudhuri K, Pearce RK, Bartko JJ, Agid Y. Accuracy of the clinical diagnosis of postencephalitic parkinsonism: A clinicopathologic study. *Eur J Neurol* 1998;5:451–57.
534. Takahashi M, Yamada T. A possible role of influenza A virus infection for Parkinson's disease. *Adv Neurol* 2001;86:91–104.
535. Jin C, Katayama S, Hiji M, Watanabe C, Noda K, Nakamura S, Matsumoto M. Relationship between neuronal loss and tangle formation in neurons and oligodendroglia in progressive supranuclear palsy. *Neuropathology* 2006;26:50–6.
536. Dickson DW. Neuropathologic differentiation of progressive supranuclear palsy and corticobasal degeneration. *J Neurol* 1999;246(Suppl 2):116–15.
537. Maurizi CP. Postencephalitic Parkinson's disease, amyotrophic lateral sclerosis on Guam and influenza revisited: Focusing on neurofibrillary tangles and the trail of tau. *Med Hypotheses* 2002;58:198–202.
538. Lees AJ. Parkinson's syndrome associated with neurofibrillary degeneration and tau pathologic findings. *Mov Disord* 2003;(Suppl 6):S28–33.
539. Morris HR, Lees AJ, Wood NW. Neurofibrillary tangle parkinsonian disorders—Tau pathology and tau genetics. *Mov Disord* 1999;14:731–36.

540. Hof PR, Perl DP, Loerzel AJ, Steele JC, Morrison JH. Amyotrophic lateral sclerosis and parkinsonism-dementia from Guam: Differences in neurofibrillary tangle distribution and density in the hippocampal formation and neocortex. *Brain Res* 1994;650:107–16.
541. Bates G, Harper PS, Jones L, eds. *Huntington's Disease*. New York: Oxford University Press, 2002.
542. Cepeda C, Wu N, Andre VM, Cummings DM, Levine MS. The corticostriatal pathway in Huntington's disease. *Prog Neurobiol* 2006;81:253–71.
543. Walker FO. Huntington's disease. *Lancet* 2007;369:218–28.
564. Harper PS, Sarfarazi M. Genetic prediction and family structure in Huntington's chorea. *Br Med J (Clin Res Ed)* 1985;290:1929–31.
545. Andresen JM, Gayán J, Djoussé L, Roberts S, Brocklebank D, Cherny SS, The US-Venezuela Collaborative Research Group, The HD MAPS Collaborative Research Group, Cardon LR, Gusella JF, Macdonald ME, Myers RH, Houseman DE, Wexler NS. The relationship between CAG repeat length and age of onset differs for Huntington's disease patients with juvenile onset or adult onset. *Ann Hum Genet* 2006;71:295–302.
546. Kohwi Y, ed. *Trinucleotide Repeat Protocols*. Totowa, NJ: Humana Press, 2004.
547. Rosenblatt A, Leroi I. Neuropsychiatry of Huntington's disease and other basal ganglia disorders. *Psychosomatics* 2000;41:24–30.
548. Pearn J. Classification of spinal muscular atrophies. *Lancet* 1980;1:919–22.
549. Gonzalez de Aguilar JL, Echaniz-Laguna A, Fergani A, Rene F, Meininger V, Loeffler JP, Dupuis L. Amyotrophic lateral sclerosis: All roads lead to Rome. *J Neurochem* 2007;101:1153–60.
550. Mitsumoto H, Przedborski S, Gordon PH, eds. *Amyotrophic Lateral Sclerosis*. New York: Taylor & Francis, 2006.
551. Kurland LT, Mulder, DW. Epidemiologic investigations of amyotrophic lateral sclerosis. I. Preliminary report on geographic distribution, with special reference to the Mariana Islands, including clinical and pathologic observations. *Neurology* 1954;4:355–78.
552. Kurtzke JF, Beebe GW. Epidemiology of amyotrophic lateral sclerosis. 1. A case-control comparison based on ALS deaths. *Neurology* 1980;30:453–62.
553. Palmucci L, Bertolotto A, Doriguzzi C, Mongini T, Schiffer D. Motor neuron disease following poliomyelitis. Bioptic study of five cases. *Eur Neurol* 1980;19:414–18.
554. Kaplan KJ, McKeon C. Michigan versus Kevorkian. *Omega* (Westport) 1999;40:271–74.
555. Back A. Euthanasia on television: Dying Kevorkian style. *J Palliat Med* 1999;2:111–12.
556. Biggs H. Euthanasia and death with dignity: Still poised on the fulcrum of homicide. *Crim Law Rev* 1996:878–88.
557. Winter RO, Birnberg BA. Tuesdays with Morrie versus Stephen Hawking: Living or dying with ALS. *Fam Med* 2003;35:629–31.
558. Phadke JG, Best PV. Atypical and clinically silent multiple sclerosis: A report of 12 cases discovered unexpectedly at necropsy. *J Neurol Neurosurg Psychiatry* 1983;46:414–20.
559. Poskanzer DC, Terasaki PI, Prenney LB, Sheridan JL, Park MS. Multiple sclerosis in the Orkney and Shetland Islands. III. Histocompatibility determinants. *J Epidemiol Commun Health* 1980;34:253–57.
560. Kurtzke JF. Epidemiology and etiology of multiple sclerosis. *Phys Med Rehabil Clin N Am* 2005;16:327–49.
561. Alter M, Kurtzke JF. *Epidemiology of Multiple Sclerosis, Compiled and Edited by Milton Alter and John F. Kurtzke*. Springfield IL: Charles C. Thomas, 1968.
562. Confavreux C, Vukusic S. Natural history of multiple sclerosis: A unifying concept. *Brain* 2006;129:606–16.
563. Kremenchutzky M, Rice GP, Baskerville J, Wingerchuk DM, Ebers GC. The natural history of multiple sclerosis: A geographically based study 9: Observations on the progressive phase of the disease. *Brain* 2006;129:584–94.
564. Simon JH, Kleinschmidt-DeMasters BK. Variants of multiple sclerosis. *Neuroimaging Clin N Am* 2008;18:703–16.

565. Franklin R, Goldman JE. Remyelination. In Lassarini R, ed., *Myelin Biology and Its Disorders*. Amsterdam: Elsevier Academic Press, 2004, pp. 173–96.
566. Frohman EM, Racke MK, Raine CS. Multiple sclerosis—The plaque and its pathogenesis. *N Engl J Med* 2006;354:942–55.
567. Grooters GS, Visser LH, Barkhof F, van der Knaap MS, van Asseldonk JT, Nita DA. Mystery cse: Balo concentric sclerosis. *Neurology* 2013;80:71–2.
568. Nesbit GM, Forbes GS, Scheithauer BW, Okazaki H, Rodriguez M. Multiple sclerosis: Histopathologic and MR and/or CT correlation in 37 cases at biopsy and three cases at autopsy. *Radiology* 1991;180:467–74.
569. Zagzag D, Miller DC, Kleinman GM, Abati A, Donnenfeld H, Budzilovich GN. Demyelinating disease versus tumor in surgical neuropathology. Clues to a correct pathological diagnosis. *Am J Surg Pathol* 1993;17:537–45.
570. Hunter SB, Ballinger WE Jr, Rubin JJ. Multiple sclerosis mimicking primary brain tumor. *Arch Pathol Lab Med* 1987;111:464–68.
571. Paley RJ, Persing JA, Doctor A, Westwater JJ, Roberson JP, Edlich RF. Multiple sclerosis and brain tumor: A diagnostic challenge. *J Emerg Med* 1989;7:241–44.
572. Peterson K, Rosenblum MK, Powers JM, Alvord E, Walker RW, Posner JB. Effect of brain irradiation on demyelinating lesions. *Neurology* 1993;43:2105–12.
573. DiMaio VJ, DiMaio D. *Forensic Pathology*. Boca Raton, FL: CRC Press, 2001.
574. Knight B. *Forensic Pathology*. London: Arnold, 1996.
575. Spitz WU, Spitz DJ, eds. *Spitz and Fisher's Medicolegal Investigation of Death: Guidelines for the Application of Pathology to Crime Investigation*. Springfield, IL: Charles C. Thomas, 2006.
576. Massaro EJ. *Handbook of Neurotoxicology*. Totowa, NJ: Humana Press, 2002.
577. O'Donoughue JL, ed. *Neurotoxicity of Industrial and Commercial Chemicals*. Boca Raton, FL: CRC Press, 1985.
578. Spencer PS, Schaumburg HH, Ludolph AC. *Experimental and Clinical Neurotoxicology*. New York: Oxford University Press, 2000.
579. Tilson HA, Harry GJ. *Neurotoxicology*. Philadelphia: Taylor & Francis, 1999.
580. Andrews LS, Snyder R. Toxic effects of solvents and vapors. In Klaassen CD, Amdur MO, Doull J, eds., *Casarett and Doull's Toxicology: The Basic Science of Poisons*. New York: Macmillan, 1986, pp. 636–68.
581. Goyer R. Toxic effects of metals. In Klaassen CD, Amdur MO, Doull J, eds. *Casarett and Doull's Toxicology: The Basic Science of Poisons*. New York: Macmillan, 1986, pp. 582–635.
582. Krigman MR, Silverman AP. General toxicology of tin and its organic compounds. *Neurotoxicology* 1984;5:129–39.
583. Muller R, Zschiesche W, Steffen HM, Schaller KH. Tellurium-intoxication. *Klin Wochenschr* 1989;67:1152–55.
584. Ibrahim D, Froberg B, Wolf A, Rusyniak DE. Heavy metal poisoning: Clinical presentations and pathophysiology. *Clin Lab Med* 2006;26:67–97.
585. Lampert P, Garro F, Pentschew A. Tellurium neuropathy. *Acta Neuropathol* (Berl) 1970;15:308–17.
586. Ochoa J. Isoniazid neuropathy in man: Quantiative electron microscopic study. *Brain* 1970;93:831–53.
587. Pentschew A, Garro F. Lead encephalo-myelopathy of the suckling rat and its implications on the porphyrinopathic nervous diseases. With special reference to the permeability disorders of the nervous system's capillaries. *Acta Neuropathol* (Berl) 1966;6:266–78.
588. Peter AL, Viraraghavan T. Thallium: A review of public health and environmental concerns. *Environ Int* 2005;31:493–501.
589. Verstappen CC, Heimans JJ, Hoekman K, Postma TJ. Neurotoxic complications of chemotherapy in patients with cancer: Clinical signs and optimal management. *Drugs* 2003;63:1549–63.
590. Stanley MW, Taurog JD, Snover DC. Fatal colchicine toxicity: Report of a case. *Clin Exp Rheumatol* 1984;2:167–71.

591. Shelanski ML. Chemistry of the filaments and tubules of brain. *J Histochem Cytochem* 1973;21:529–39.
592. Cavanaugh JB. Mechanism of axon degeneration in three toxic "neuropathies": Organophosphorous, acrylamide and hexacarbon compared. In Smith WT, Cavanagh JB, eds., *Recent Advances in Neuropathology*. London: Churchill-Livingstone, 1982, pp. 213–42.
593. Dyck PJ, ed. *Peripheral Neuropathy*. Philadelphia: Elsevier Saunders, 2005.
594. Fornazzari L, Pollanen MS, Myers V, Wolf A. Solvent abuse-related toluene leukoencephalopathy. *J Clin Foren Med* 2003;10:93–5.
595. Towfighi J, Gonatas NK. Hexachlorophene and the nervous system. In Zimmerman H, ed., *Progress in Neuropathology*. Vol. 3. New York: Grune & Stratton, 1976, pp. 297–312.
596. Prineas J. The pathogenesis of dying-back polyneuropathies. II. An ultrastructural study of experimental acrylamide intoxication in the cat. *J Neuropathol Exp Neurol* 1969;28:598–621.
597. Russell FE. *Marine Toxins and Venomous and Poisonous Marine Animals*. New York: Academic Press, 1965.
598. Landsberg JH, Hall S, Johannessen JN, White KD, Conrad SM, Abbott JP, Flewelling LJ, Richardson RW, Dickey RW, Jester EL, Etheridge SM, Deeds JR, Leighfield TA, Zou Y, Beaudry CG. Saxitoxin puffer fish poisoning in the United States, with the first report of *Pyrodinium bahamense* as the putative toxin source. *Environ Health Perspect* 2006;114:1502–7.
599. Llewellyn LE. Saxitoxin, a toxic marine natural product that targets a multitude of receptors. *Nat Prod Rep* 2006;23:200–22.
600. Lehane L, Lewis RJ. Ciguatera: Recent advances but the risk remains. *Int J Food Microbiol* 2000;61:91–125.
601. McLean DR, Jacobs H, Mielke BW. Methanol poisoning: A clinical and pathological study. *Ann Neurol J* 1980;8:161–67.
602. Wu Chen NB, Donoghue ER, Schaffer MI. Methanol intoxication: Distribution in postmortem tissues and fluids including vitreous humor. *J Foren Sci* 1985;30:213–16.
603. Ley CO, Gali FG. Parkinsonian syndrome after methanol intoxication. *Eur Neurol J* 1983;22:405–9.
604. Lins RL, Zachee P, Christiaens M, Sandra P. Prognosis and treatment of methanol intoxication. *Dev Toxicol Environ Sci J* 1980;8:415–21.
605. Swift R, Davidson D. Alcohol hangover: Mechanisms and mediators. *Alcohol Health Res World* 1998;22:54–60.
606. Karch SB, ed. *Forensic Issues in Alcohol Testing*. Boca Raton, FL: Taylor & Francis, 2007.
607. Torvik A. Brain lesions in alcoholics: Neuropathological observations. *Acta Med Scand Suppl* 1987;717:47–54.
608. Torvik A. Wernicke's encephalopathy—Prevalence and clinical spectrum. *Alcohol Alcohol Suppl* 1991;1:381–84.
609. Victor M, Adams RD, Mancall EL. A restricted form of cerebellar cortical degeneration occurring in alcoholic patients. *Arch Neurol* 1959;1:579–688.
610. Rothrock JF, Johnson PC, Rothrock SM, Merkley R. Fulminant polyneuritis after overdose of disulfiram and ethanol. *Neurology* 1984;34:357–59.
611. Victor M, Adams RD. On the etiology of the alcoholic neurologic diseases with special reference to the role of nutrition. *Am J Clin Nutr* 1961;9:379–97.
612. Adams RD, Victor M, Mancall EL. Central pontine myelinolysis. *Arch Neurol Psychiatr* 1959;119:1195–97.
613. Bhat S, Koulaouzidis A, Haris M, Tan C. Central pontine myelinolysis. *Ann Hepatol* 2006;5:291–92.
614. Kumar S, Fowler M, Gonzalez-Toledo E, Jaffe SL. Central pontine myelinolysis, an update. *Neurol Res* 2006;28:360–66.
615. Mast H, Gordon PH, Mohr JP, Tatemichi TK. Central pontine myelinolysis: Clinical syndrome with normal serum sodium. *Eur J Med Res* 1995;1:168–70.

616. Camps FE, Robinson AE, Lucas BGB, eds. *Gradwohl's Legal Medicine*. Bristol: A. John Wright, 1976.
617. Gonzales TA, Vance MMH, Umberger CJ. *Legal Medicine Pathology and Toxicology*. New York: Appleton-Century-Crofts, 1954.
618. LaPresle J, Fardeau M. The central nervous system and carbon monoxide poisoning. II. Anatomical study of brain lesions following intoxication with carbon monoxide (22 cases). *Prog Brain Res* 1967;24:31–74.
619. Grinker RR. Parkinsonism following carbon monoxide poisoning. *J Nerv Ment Dis* 1926;64: 18–28.
620. Okeda R, Song SY, Funta N, Higashino F. An experimental study of the pathogenesis of Grinker's myelinopathy in carbon monoxide intoxication. *Acta Neuropathol* (Berl) 1983;59:200–6.
621. Balentine JD. *Pathology of Oxygen Toxicity*. New York: Academic Press, 1982.
622. Terry TL. The eye. In Balentine JD, ed., *Pathology of Oxygen Toxicity*. New York: Academic Press, 1982, pp. 149–71.
623. Bromberg M, Smith AG, eds. *Handbook of Peripheral Neuropathy*. Boca Raton, FL: Taylor & Francis, 2005.
624. Kimura J, ed. *Peripheral Nerve Diseases*. Vol. 7. New York: Elsevier, 2006.
625. Wishik J. *Medical and Legal Aspects of Neurology*. Tucson, AZ: Lawyers & Judges, 2005.
626. Carpenter S, Karpati G. *Pathology of Skeletal Muscle*. New York: Oxford University Press, 2001.
627. Karpati G, Hilton-Jones D, Griggs R, eds. *Disorders of Voluntary Muscle*. New York: Cambridge University Press, 2001.
628. Wortmann R, ed. *Diseases of Skeletal Muscle*. Philadelphia: Lippincott Williams & Wilkins, 2000.
629. Mastaglia FL, Walton J, eds. *Skeletal Muscle Pathology*. Edinburgh: Churchill Livingstone, 1982.
630. Hawley RJ, Milner MR, Gottdiener JS, Cohen A. Myotonic heart disease: A clinical follow-up. *Neurology* 1991;41:259–62.
631. Moorman JR, Coleman RE, Packer DL, Kisslo JA, Bell J, Hettleman BD, Stajich J, Roses AD. Cardiac involvement in myotonic muscular dystrophy. *Medicine* (Baltimore) 1985;64:371–87.
632. Kuyumcu-Martinez NM, Cooper TA. Misregulation of alternative splicing causes pathogenesis in myotonic dystrophy. *Prog Mol Subcell Biol* 2006;44:133–59.
633. Cho DH, Tapscott SJ. Myotonic dystrophy: Emerging mechanisms for DM1 and DM2. *Biochim Biophys Acta* 2007;1772:195–204.
634. Addonizio G, Susman VL. *Neuroleptic Malignant Syndrome: A Clinical Approach*. St. Louis, MO: Mosby Year Book, 1991.
635. Binford CH, Conner DH. *Pathology of Tropical and Extraordinary Diseases*. Washington, DC: Armed Forces Institute of Pathology, 1976.
636. Aldrete JA, Britt BA, eds. *Malignant Hyperthermia*. New York: Grune & Stratton, 1978.
637. Sheil AT, Collins KA, Schandl CA, Harley RA. Fatal neurotoxic response to neuroleptic medications. Case report and review of the literature. *Am J Foren Med Pathol* 2007;28:116–20.
638. Kasantikul D, Kanchanatawan B. Neuroleptic malignant syndrome: A review and report of six cases. *J Med Assoc Thai* 2006;89:2155–60.
639. Mann SC, Lazarus A. *Neuroleptic Malignant Syndrome and Related Conditions*. Washington, DC: American Psychiatric Publishing, 2003.
640. Guerrero RM, Shifrar KA. Diagnosis and treatment of neuroleptic malignant syndrome. *Clin Pharm* 1988;7:697–701.
641. Akpaffiong MJ, Ruiz P. Neuroleptic malignant syndrome: A complication of neuroleptics and cocaine abuse. *Psychiatr Q* 1991;62:299–309.
642. Wetli CV, Mash D, Karch SB. Cocaine-associated agitated delirium and the neuroleptic malignant syndrome. *Am J Emerg Med JT* 1996;14:425–28.
643. Brandom BW. Genetics of malignant hyperthermia. *Scientific World Journal* 2006;6:1722–30.
644. Robinson R, Carpenter D, Shaw MA, Halsall J, Hopkins P. Mutations in RYR1 in malignant hyperthermia and central core disease. *Hum Mutat* 2006;27:977–89.

645. Sambuughin N, Sei Y, Gallagher KL, Wyre HW, Madsen D, Nelson TE, Fletcher JE, Rosenberg H, Muldoon SM. North American malignant hyperthermia population: Screening of the ryanodine receptor gene and identification of novel mutations. *Anesthesiology* 2001;95:594–99.
646. Deymeer F, Gungor-Tuncer O, Yilmaz V, Parman Y, Serdaroglu P, Ozdemir C, Vincent A, Saruhan-Direskeneli G. Clinical comparison of anti-MuSK- vs anti-AChR-positive and seronegative myasthenia gravis. *Neurology* 2007;68:609–11.
647. Vincent A, Leite MI. Neuromuscular junction autoimmune disease: Muscle specific kinase antibodies and treatments for myasthenia gravis. *Curr Opin Neurol* 2005;18:519–25.
648. Yuan HK, Huang BS, Kung SY, Kao KP. The effectiveness of thymectomy on seronegative generalized myasthenia gravis: Comparing with seropositive cases. *Acta Neurol Scand* 2007;115:181–84.
649. Perrot X, Bernard N, Vial C, Antoine JC, Laurent H, Vial T, Confavreux C, Vukusic S. Myasthenia gravis exacerbation or unmasking associated with telithromycin treatment. *Neurology* 2006;67:2256–58.
650. Jennett AM, Bali D, Jastri P, Shaha B, Browning LA. Telithromycin and myasthenic crisis. *Clin Infect Dis* 2006;43:1621–2.
651. Torrey J. Acute myasthenia gravis—Post-mortem diagnosis in the case of sudden death. *Med Sci Law* 1983;23:111–13.
652. de la Grandmaison GL, Durigon M. Sudden adult death: A medico-legal series of 77 cases between 1995 and 2000. *Med Sci Law* 2002;42:225–32.
653. Hofstad H, Ohm OJ, Mork SJ, Aarli JA. Heart disease in myasthenia gravis. *Acta Neurol Scand* 1984;70:176–84.
654. Tsujino S, Shanske S, DiMauro S. Molecular genetic heterogeneity of myophosphorylase deficiency (McArdle's disease). *N Engl J Med* 1993;329:241–45.
655. Beynon RJ, Bartram C, Hopkins P, Toescu V, Gibson H, Phoenix J, Edwards RH. McArdle's disease: Molecular genetics and metabolic consequences of the phenotype. *Muscle Nerve* 1995;3:S18–22.
656. Jurkat-Rott K, Lehmann-Horn F. Paroxysmal muscle weakness—The familial periodic paralyses. *J Neurol* 2006;253:1391–98.
657. Kageyama K, Terui K, Tsutaya S, Matsuda E, Shoji M, Sakihara S, Nigawara T, Takayasu S, Moriyama T, Yasujima M, Suda T. Gene analysis of the calcium channel 1 subunit and clinical studies for two patients with hypokalemic periodic paralysis. *J Endocrinol Invest* 2006;29:928–33.

General Forensic Neuropathology of Infants and Children

4

JAN E. LEESTMA

Contents

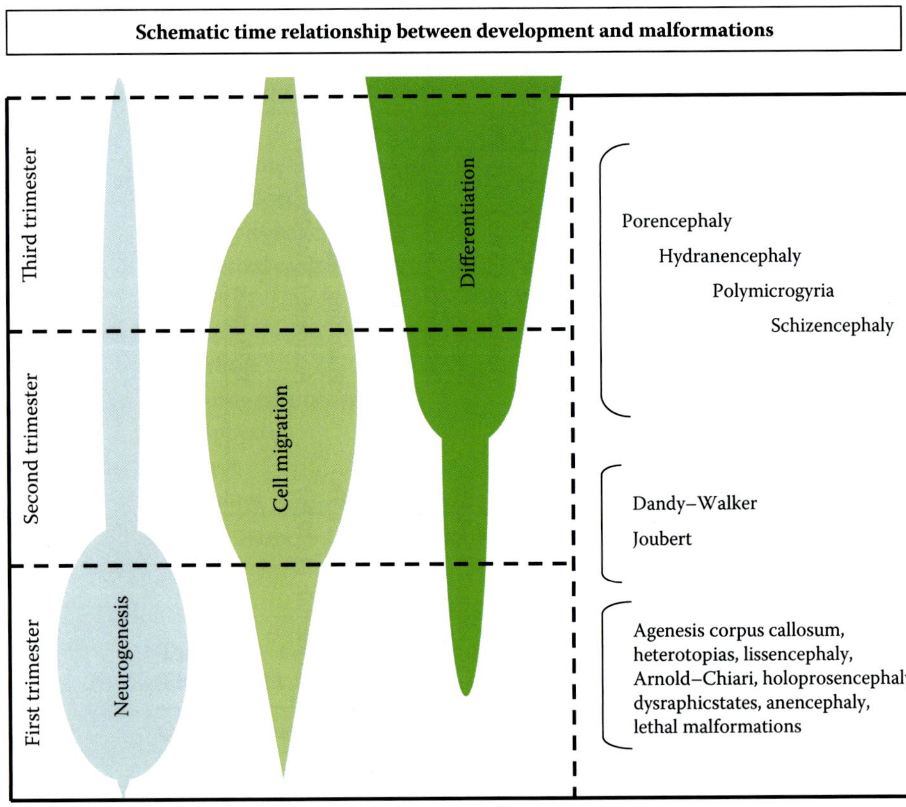

Figure 4.1 Major neurodevelopmental phases in which a teratogenic event may lead to a malformation. (Derived from a number of sources.)

occasionally possible, from examining the malformation, to determine its precise cause. Rather, a more useful exercise is to consider when in gestation a given malformation is likely to have happened. This can often be accomplished by bearing in mind the time course of brain embryology and development.

A practical approach to central nervous system (CNS) embryology and teratogenesis is to consider five time periods that are critical: the first 27 days, days 28 to 50, 51 days to 5 months, 6 to 9 months, and the postnatal period. In the first 27 days the neural tube forms and fuses. During the next 23 days the cerebral and cerebellar hemispheres begin developing. The ventricular system with cerebrospinal fluid (CSF) production is completed, the olfactory and optic systems develop, and vascular anatomy is organized. After 5 months the cells of the brain continue to differentiate and migrate to their final destinations, and the commissures develop. In the final trimester of gestation, differentiation and maturation of cells continue and myelination commences. After birth, neuronal migration continues essentially only in the cerebellum, where the external granular layer (Obersteiner's layer) of the cortex eventually differentiates and disappears by about 12 months of age. The main, grossly obvious neural developmental process of childhood is myelination and increase in brain weight (Figure 4.2) [19], along with more obvious differentiation between the appearance of the white matter and the

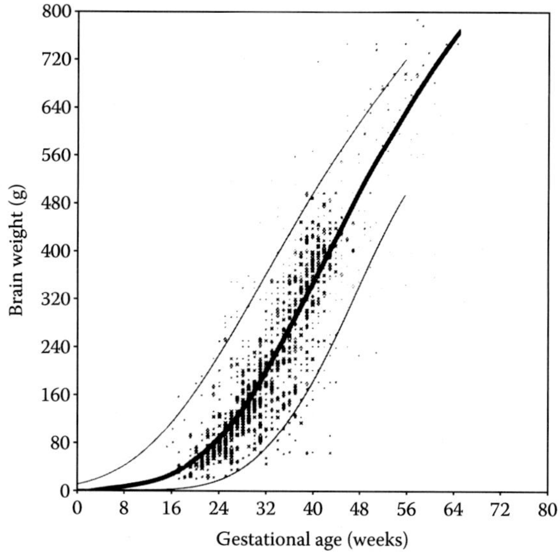

Figure 4.2 Brain weights for fetuses between gestational ages 15 and 60 weeks, based upon a study by Gilles et al. of 1233 specimens. Upper and lower 95% confidence bands are shown. (Based on Gilles FH et al., *The Developing Human Brain: Growth and Epidemiologic Neuropathology*, Littleton, MA: John Wright, 1983. Used with permission.)

gray matter. There are classic references, now many years old, which detail the patterns and rates of myelination in the human brain, which continues well into the second decade of life [18,24].

Autopsy Examination of the Developing Nervous System

When the nervous system of an infant is examined, the diseases and lesions of the rest of the body must be considered. If malformations are present in the CNS, it may also be likely that malformations will occur in other organ systems. If dehydration and sepsis are present, disorders of coagulation may also occur that can affect the brain by causing cerebral venous and venous sinus thrombosis, which in turn may lead to hemorrhagic infarctions of the brain as well as edema, subarachnoid hemorrhages, and even subdural hemorrhages [25], which might be mistakenly interpreted as being due to trauma. Inherited or conditional disorders of coagulation such as factor V, factor VIII, protein S and C deficiencies, and vitamin K deficiency must be considered, as these, too, may be misinterpreted as being due to trauma [26–32]. It is a prudent practice to save, in some manner a sample of blood for possible later analysis not thought of at the time of the autopsy.

The external examination of the body should proceed in an orderly and systematic manner so that nothing is overlooked. Photography of external lesions preserves vital evidence and documents descriptions. The examination of the head should be an inspection of the mouth for palatal malformations or injuries, the eyes for position, the state of the pupils, and any indication of direct trauma. There are now several methods than can be employed to determine if intraocular pathology is present in the deceased individual.

Postmortem indirect ophthalmoscopy (PMIO) [33,34] and endoscopy [35] provide excellent demonstrations of lesions under a variety of conditions, not just child abuse. If lesions are found and permission has been obtained to remove them, the eyes may be taken and fixed for later careful examination by qualified individuals.

Examination of the ears should include notation as to their position, shape, and the presence of hemorrhages or bruises of the pinna and surrounding tissues. The external auditory meatus should be examined for blood or pus. The nose should be examined for its position and shape, and the nares should be examined for the presence of blood or exudate. Lesions noted should be evaluated as to possible cause, especially for having been caused by medical treatment. To this end, it is a very good idea to insist that the body come to the morgue with all catheters, tubes, and instruments *in situ*. It is also a good idea to photographically document these devices before removing them and conducting the internal examination. The circumference of the head should be measured and the state of closure of the fontanels and sutures noted. Gentle percussion of the cranium may reveal a "cracked pot" sound, indicative of a closely approximated skull fracture. Palpation may also reveal masses or abnormal mobility of cranial bones. Examination of the neck should include observation of the skin of the neck and throat for any scrapes or pattern injuries and any undue mobility or crepitus on motion. The skin of the rest of the body should be carefully examined for any bruises, scrapes, lacerations, burns or scalds, or healing lesions of any sort. Their character and position must be recorded and photographed. Examination of the extremities should include palpation and an evaluation of mobility of the joints. Any lesions of the extremities should be recorded. The digits should be examined for number and position and form. If the body is that of a neonate, creases should be checked for meconium staining. When trauma is suspected, whole body radiographs including the extremities should be made and retained for later use. Traumatic skin lesions should be sampled histologically and their place of origin documented. Although it appears rather gruesome, it is sometimes necessary to make long incisions in the skin if there are numerous bruises to determine their extent and to sample them. Photographs of such dissections may be suppressed at a legal proceeding because they may be viewed as very disturbing to layperson in the jury and to parents who may be present.

A careful autopsy should be performed according to established procedures [36,37], paying particular attention to location and extent of any traumatic lesions in the viscera. When the organs have been removed, a careful inspection of the rib cage and spine should be made. Palpation of the inner circumference of the chest cavity may reveal healing or fresh fractures of the ribs, an important observation that may or may not indicate child abuse. Rib fractures should be removed and sampled histologically, recording the location of where they came from. The pelvic organs should be carefully examined, including the external genitalia, for signs of trauma. When removing the brain, special care should be taken to avoid laceration or crushing the delicate, gelatinous perinatal brain. Suggested methods have been described by Norman et al. [38]. If there is any suspicion that trauma might have been involved, the neck should be examined and opened posteriorly and the soft and hard tissues of the spine photographed. The scalp should be reflected and carefully examined for possible deep scalp injuries. Any that are found should be photographed and sampled histologically. If skull fractures are found, a histological section should be made showing the margin of the fracture from which an estimate of acuteness of the fracture might be made.

Upon removal of the brain and cord, little attempt should be made to examine it in the fresh state, as excessive handling may disrupt surface structures and produce artifacts that may be difficult to differentiate from fresh traumatic lesions [39]. The dura should be stripped from the skull cap and base of the skull and saved in fixative with the brain for later examination. If lesions are observed in the opened cranium, such as fractures or malformations, photographs are the best way to preserve this information. It is often important, especially if there has been a history of upper respiratory infection, meningitis, or brain abscess, to open the petrous bones and paranasal sinuses. Such sites are not uncommonly the nidus from which systemic or local infections emanated.

The brain should be fixed by suspension in formalin for at least a week. Some have suggested fixation in very strong formaldehyde solution to harden the brain, but the value of this is unclear. Fixation can be accomplished by suspending the brain by a string passed under the basilar artery or by adding sufficient salt to the formalin to allow the brain to float in the fixation vessel. When fixation is complete, after washing, the brain may be examined grossly. The perinatal brain is usually quite soft and easily fragmentable; thus, handling should be gentle. The use of a pancake spatula for lifting sections will avoid handling artifacts. The infant brain, although often softer than an adult's, is more easily handled and cut. In addition to searching for any surface lesions, it is important to estimate the developmental age of the brain. This can be done by noting head circumference, the weight of the brain, and the state of development of several surface features [3,19]. These include the numbers of gyri and the state of closure of the insula by the parietal and frontal opercula. One method that can aid the examiner in estimating the age of a brain between 28 and 37 weeks is to count the number of gyri above a line joining the frontal and occipital poles and passing through the middle of the temporal lobe and then add 21. The sum is an approximation of the gestational age of the infant in weeks [40]. A chart of brain weight by gestational age to aid the examiner is shown in Figure 4.2.

The gross examination should include a brief survey of surface architecture to determine if a cortical malformation is present. This may be accomplished by determining if there are superior, middle, and inferior frontal and temporal gyri; if there are a Sylvian, an interhemispheric, and a parietal–occipital fissure; and if the gyri are normal or abnormal. Are there clefts or holes in the brain? Are all the cranial nerves present at the base of the brain? Does the brain stem have a normal appearance, and is the cerebellum in its usual form? If the spinal cord is included in the specimen, its appearance should be noted along with the condition of the spinal roots and their symmetry.

When the immature brain is sectioned, it may not be possible to differentiate between cortex and white matter because of the lack of myelination and the high water content of the brain. Myelination begins *in utero* at 4 months gestation in the motor and sensory roots of the cord and then in the brain stem and cerebellar connections. At birth, myelination of the pyramidal tracts, optic radiations, commissures, acoustic radiations, and fornix has begun but is difficult to observe grossly. The process progresses into association areas and continues into the second decade [12,18,24]. In infants 3 months of age, myelination is grossly visible from the motor cortex into the cerebral peduncles and parallels clinical motor and sensory development [18]. When hydrocephalus is present, the brain often collapses with release of the ventricular fluid, making fixation and subsequent examination difficult. A number of approaches to rectifying this problem have been employed with varying degrees of success. One approach is to prepare a gelatin solution, inject it gently into the ventricular cavity, and then cool the brain or place it in cooled formalin. Another employs a somewhat watery mix of dental impression material (geltrate/alginate or similar material), which is also injected into the ventricle, and then the brain is fixed. The latter material rather rapidly forms a flexible gel that does not harden very much with fixation and can be simply included in histological blocks without difficulty. It has a rather homogeneous lavender appearance with hematoxylin and eosin (H&E) staining.

Histological samples of the brain should include several sections of cortex, with at least one section of deep nuclear structures that includes ependyma. The hippocampus, cerebellum, levels of the brain stem, and several sections of the spinal cord should be taken. Lesions should be liberally sampled. A number of texts have suggestions for such sampling [40–42]. If very detailed analysis of the brain is required, including morphometry, there are many techniques that are available. An excellent source reference for data concerning human and comparative quantitative analysis of brain anatomy is the handbook by Blinkov and Glezer [43].

Neuropathology of Perinatal Period

Pathological Reactions in the Developing Brain

The immature brain shares with other organs the basic tissue responses displayed in necrosis, repair, infarction, edema, and neoplasia. In each category of pathological processes, the immature brain may show unique reactions to injury or produce special sequelae inherent to damage in a developing system. Neurons may die in basically two ways, necrosis or apoptosis (so-called programmed cell death) [44]. The former occurs because of dysfunction of the cell membrane with failure of ion channels and mitochondria, activation of calcium-activated proteases, free radical interactions with vital cellular proteins, excitotoxicity, and cell lysis [45–47]. This form of neuronal death occurs from hypoxia or ischemia from any cause as well as from physical injury and the cascade of processes that are involved. The process is complex but results in swelling of the affected neuron, dissolution of the cytoplasm, eosinophilia of the cytoplasm, shrinkage of the nucleus, and eventual disappearance. Apoptosis may be a more deliberate or chronic process that involves a number of intracellular events such as activation of families of genes that ultimately kills the cell. A number of compounds are integral to this complex process: the caspases, BAX, bcl proteins, a number of oncogene and so-called signaling proteins, and inflammatory mediators [15,44–47]. The interplay of these and other mediators and inhibitors results in cleavage of nuclear DNA that ultimately results in shrinkage of the affected neuron and nuclear karyorrhexis. This process can be triggered by hypoxia and ischemia but can be set into motion by toxic compounds, seizures, degenerative diseases, and inflammatory/infectious conditions. The processes and mechanisms behind these two pathways have been the subject of extensive research with a large literature.

The cells most capable of a vital reaction beyond deteriorating and dying, within the central nervous system, are the astrocytes. They evolve after the second developmental period (27 to 50 days), so that insults occurring prior to 50 days of age may show no astrocytic response even in the face of profound structural alterations. Lesions occurring later may have astroglial scars in which astrocytes and their processes increase.

Myelin and Myelination

Myelin, a membrane unique to nervous tissue, is involved in specific reactions, as are its cells of origin, the oligodendrocytes (central myelin) and the Schwann cells (peripheral myelin). These reactions are referred to as demyelination, when the axon is stripped of its covering membranous lamellae because of endogenous or exogenous events, and dysmyelination, in which myelin metabolism (anabolism) is defective, usually due to an inherited enzymatic defect in lipid synthesis or degradation. Such processes can be identified histochemically by the reactions of the breakdown products of myelin to the various stains or histochemical reactions employed. For example, normally when myelin is broken down, its degradation products are stainable with various so-called neutral fat stains (Sudan dyes, Oil Red 0) and do not change the colors of certain aniline dyes (metachromasia), such as cresyl violet. However, when important degradative enzymes such as aryl sulfatases (as in metachromatic leukodystrophy) are absent, acidic sulfatides build up in tissues that stain metachromatically (change the color of blue-violet dyes to orange or red). This class of diseases is generally referred to as the leukodystrophies (see below). Chemical analysis of brain specimens can precisely identify abnormal lipids or degradation products. Genetic probes are now available that can permit identification of the precise genetic abnormality using CNS or non-CNS tissues [48,49]. Cases of these diseases and other, more obscure ones not infrequently appear on a medical examiner's service because victims may die at home. The cases generally do not pose a large forensic problem because the diagnosis is generally known; however, because death outside the immediate care of a physician may raise certain issues of how the individual died, manner of death controversies may arise.

Normal myelin formation is not complete until many years after birth [18,19,24], so that the diseases of myelin in the young brain tend to be manifested as an absence or paucity of myelin rather than destruction of it. Blunt physical trauma to the incompletely ossified skull will deform the underlying unmyelinated brain, injuring the white matter in preference to the cortex in the adult (contusional subcortical white matter tears rather than surface contusions) [50]. Occasionally, myelination within the developing brain is aberrant, as in *status marmoratus* of the thalamus and basal ganglia and in plaques fibromyelinique [5,51–53], in which astrocytic processes rather than axons become myelinated.

Disorders of Lipid Metabolism

This diverse group of often very rare inherited diseases involves an inborn error of metabolism with some aspect of lipid metabolism (synthesis or degradation) and may be classified various ways according to the product that is improperly synthesized or degraded. These diseases may be thought of as diseases of lysosomes [54,55], peroxisomes, lipid synthesis, or transport. Most of the genetic defects, of which there are often many, responsible for the diseases are now known, but it appears that almost endless variants or polymorphisms keep being reported. Most of these diseases, although there are adult variants of them, present in infancy or childhood usually as progressive psychomotor degeneration and other neurological symptoms, including blindness. Many of the diseases result in neuronal accumulation (storage) of a lipid product by which each of these diseases is categorized or named, as in the sphingolipidoses, which include Farber lipogranulomatosis, Niemann–Pick disease, Gaucher's disease, Schindler disease, and Fabry's disease. The gangliosidoses include GM-1 gangliosidoses, of which there are several variants or subtypes, and GM-2 gangliosidoses, which include Tay–Sachs disease and Sandhoff disease. The glycoprotein/glycolipidoses include fucosidosis, the mucolipidoses, and mucopolysaccharidoses (such as Hunter–Hurler's disease and variants). The ceroid lipofuscinoses include Santavuori disease, Bielschowsky–Jansky disease, Batten's disease, Batten–Spielmeyer–Vogt disease, and Kuf's disease. The so-called peroxisomal diseases include Zellweger syndrome, adrenal leukodystrophy, and Refsum's disease. The diseases that may or may not include some degree of neuronal storage but generally are thought of as leukodystrophies include metachromatic leukodystrophy, Krabbe's disease, and adrenal leukodystrophy. Other conditions primarily affecting white matter that do not easily fit into the above categorization include Pelizaeus–Merzbacher disease, Cockayne–Neel disease, and Canavan disease.

Farber lipogranulomatosis [55,56] is a group of lysosomal disorders caused by deficiency of acid ceramidases resulting in accumulation of ceramide largely in the spinal cord and brain stem, but in some forms visceral storage is seen. Neurological symptoms and painful arthritis and joint deformities are typical. The disease is caused by an autosomal recessive gene located at the p location of chromosome 8 [56].

Niemann–Pick disease has several variants affecting different age groups. Type A affects infants, causing progressive neurological deterioration and blindness, with extensive lipid (sphingomyelin) storage in affected neurons throughout the nervous system. Most affected infants die by the age of 2 years. This form of the disease was the first to be recognized. Type B affects adults and, though involving the nervous system, mostly affects the reticuloendothelial system with stored lipid [57,58]. Type C, an uncommon variant of the disease, affects adults, causing psychiatric symptoms, and has a course like many neurodegenerative diseases [59,60]. The diseases are due to autosomal recessive inheritance, with variants due to a host of mutations in the sphingomyelinase genes [58]. There is a high degree of prevalence in those of Ashkenazi Jewish heritage.

Gaucher's disease, like Niemann–Pick disease, has variants and subtypes [61,62]. This disease occurs worldwide in one of every 30,000–50,000 people [60]. Type I affects individuals of all age groups and is primarily a nonneuropathic disease, affecting the reticuloendothelial system. Type II affects infants much like Niemann–Pick disease type A does and affects both the nervous system and viscera. Type III Gaucher's disease affects juveniles and is a combined neuropathic and visceral disease with a protracted time course. All forms of the disease are autosomally inherited, with a predilection in type I for Ashkenazi Jewish families that is not seen in the other forms of the disease. All the disease forms involve accumulation of glycocerebrosides in the affected cells, which results from faulty B-glucosidase genes and mutations that appear to be located on chromosome 1 [63]. Recently, some patients with parkinsonism have been found to have a form of Gaucher's disease with a specific genetic mutation [64]. Also recently, a number of gene-based therapies have been employed in the treatment of this previously untreatable disease. Like the other common lipidoses, the lipids accumulated in the brain or other cells are periodic acid-Schiff (PAS) positive, and the material has a refractile, complex microscopic appearance different from the punctate material in Niemann–Pick cells.

Fabry's disease is the only lipidosis with an X-linked mode of inheritance [64]. The enzymatic defect is of α-galacatosidase, and the accumulated products are various ceramides and some other glycospingolipids [65]. The disease affects the nervous system, heart, kidney, and other organs that accumulate the stored product. Some patients develop subcortical white matter disease that appears somewhat like that seen in some hypertensives—the so-called *etat crible* [66].

Schindler disease is a rare autosomally inherited condition affecting infants and presenting clinically, like most of the lipidoses, with developmental retardation, seizures, blindness, and motor loss. The disease is caused by a deficiency of alpha-N-acetylgalactosaminidase, caused by defective genes for this enzyme on chromosome 22, and results in a neuroaxonal dystrophy-like pathology in neurons and their processes [67,68].

The gangliosidoses are a group of glycolipid storage diseases [69], the most important of which is Tay–Sachs disease (now called GM-2 type B gangliosidosis). These diseases resemble Niemann-Pick disease clinically and pathologically and have representations in different age groups. All are autosomal recessively inherited, and there is a preponderance for Ashkenazi Jews. GM-1 gangliosidoses are subclassified into type 1, which affects infants; type 2, which affects young children and juveniles; and type 3, which represents an adult form of GM-1 ganglioside storage and beta-galactosidase deficiency. All have neurological symptoms with few or no visceral counterparts. The GM-2 gangliosidoses, as mentioned above, include Tay–Sachs and Sandhoff disease, in which the accumulated GM-2 ganglioside resides in Figure 4.3). An interesting feature in Tay–Sachs disease and apparently in some of the other lipid storage diseases is the propensity for so-called meganeurites, usually in the initial axonal segment of cortical neurons where aberrant synapses form, that may physiologically block neural transmission from the affected cell [70]. The genetic defect affects hexosaminidases A (chromosome 15) and B (chromosome 5) and includes a number of different mutations of these genes coding for the enzyme subunits [71,72], which results in differing courses and presentations in affected individuals. Genetic testing has drastically reduced the incidence of these conditions [73].

Fucosidosis is a lysosomal storage disease in which alpha-l-fucosidase is deficient due to one or more mutations in the gene located on chromosome 1 [74] that result in storage of various glycolipids and glycoproteins. The disease is very rare and results in psychomotor retardation in young children. This disease resembles Fabry disease in many ways.

The so-called mucolipidoses constitute a list of autosomally inherited diseases that have been subclassified into at least four types, all of which are rare and involve storage of

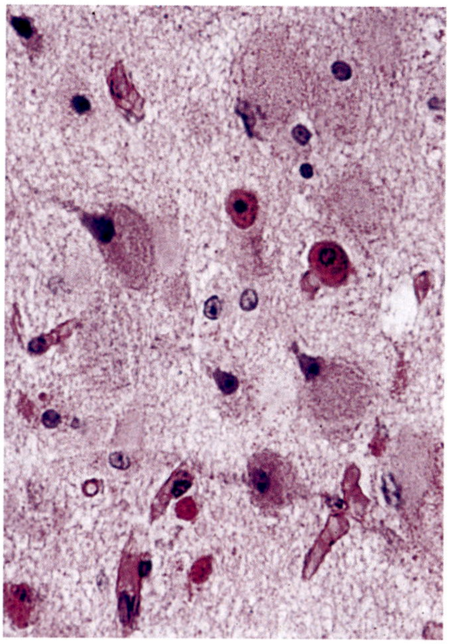

Figure 4.3 A portion of the cerebral cortex from a victim of Tay–Sachs disease showing numerous neurons distended by PAS-positive ganglioside that has pushed the nucleus up into the apical dendrite.

sialic acid–related compounds and some degree of psychomotor growth retardation and disability that may involve the musculoskeletal system and viscera [75]. Genetic testing has been established for these diseases, which have an increased prevalence among Ashkenazi Jews [76].

The ceroid lipofuscinoses constitute a group of storage diseases in which lipoid pigments (many of which have not yet been precisely characterized) accumulate largely in neurons but may spill over into some of viscera and connective tissues. In an infantile form referred to as Santavuori or Batten's disease, infants and toddlers display ataxia, progressive psychomotor retardation, and microcephaly with cerebellar atrophy and generally die before age 10 years. The disease is inherited as an autosomal recessive with localization on chromosome 1. A similar disease, Bielschowsky–Jansky disease may show cerebral atrophy and accumulation of the same type of intracellular pigment. The genetics of this disease are poorly understood beyond the fact that it is an autosomally recessive defect. Another very similar disease tending to involve slightly older children is Batten–Spielmeyer–Vogt's disease, with an apparent defect localized to chromosome 16. An adult form of the lipofuscinosis is referred to as Kuf's disease, which has been subdivided into two types. The first displays behavioral disorders, myoclonic attacks, and ataxia with dementia, and the second seems more centered on the cerebellum and extrapyramidal system. Affected neurons are filled with the same yellowish lipofuscin pigment as the other forms of this disease. The mode of inheritance may be autosomal recessive or autosomal dominant and involves mutations in several genes [77,78]. A number of animal models for this group of diseases exist.

Zellweger disease apparently results from failure of the cell to properly assemble or maintain peroxisomes [79]. In some ways, it resembles Refsum's disease and has some features similar to adrenal leukodystrophy [81] that involve disturbed metabolism of long-chain polyunsaturated fatty acids [81]. The disease displays disturbed features of neuronal migration with cortical malformations, dysplastic brain stem anatomy, periventricular white matter degeneration, and retinal degeneration. Lamellated lipidic inclusions can be seen in neuron, and some connective tissues. Its inheritance appears to be autosomal recessive.

Refsum's disease, like Zellweger disease, appears to represent a disease caused by ineffective peroxisomes. In this case, phytanic acid alpha-hydroxylase is deficient, resulting in an excess of phytanic acid in neural tissues. These causes may be seen in variants during infancy, childhood, or adulthood. Manifestations include retinitis pigmentosa, peripheral neuropathy, cerebellar ataxia, and dementia [82].

Adrenal leukodystrophy, once included in a series of leukodystrophy cases reported by Schilder, has been etiologically and pathologically separated from the other cases of Schilder that were later defined to be Krabbe's disease and metachromatic leukodystrophy [83,84]; thus, the term *Schilder* disease is no longer in use. The disease is due to an X-linked mode of inheritance that affects peroxisome function and involves accumulation of polyunsaturated fatty acids in neural and other tissues. Ultrastructurally, the lipids that are stored have a masonry-like appearance unlike any other. The cardinal feature is widespread myelin destruction, often beginning in the occipital regions and progressing forward in the brain, resulting in dementia and blindness (Figure 4.4). There is a prominent inflammatory component to the white matter degeneration, the basis of which is not yet clear but probably involves an immune component [85]. In addition to adrenal insufficiency, testicular atrophy and variable other features of the disease have been described.

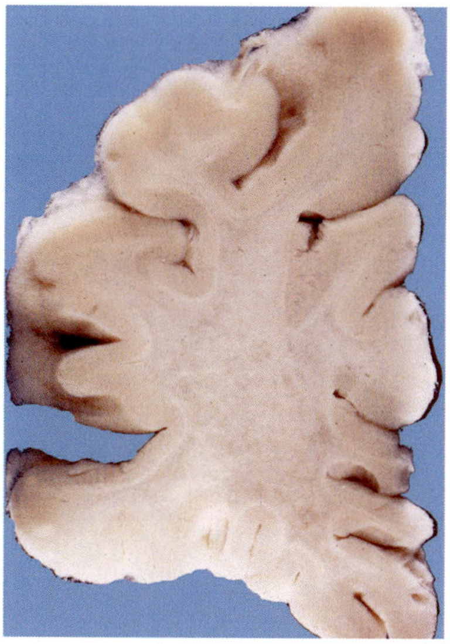

Figure 4.4 A case of adrenal leukodystrophy illustrating the moth-eaten appearance of the white matter with preservation of the subcortical "U" fibers, which remain myelinated for reasons that are unclear. This appearance is virtually the same for all of the leukodystrophies, including Krabbe's disease and metachromatic leukodystrophy.

A neonatal variant of the condition has also been described that displays dysmorphic facial features [86].

Krabbe's disease (globoid cell leukodystrophy) is an autosomally inherited deficiency of beta-galactosidase that is located on chromosome 14 and may display a number of gene deletions and polymorphisms [87] that result in accumulation of galactocerebrosides primarily in macrophages that process the deteriorating myelin and cluster about capillaries in the brain, producing the typical "globoid" cells, as shown in Figure 4.5. The classical form of the disease begins in early infancy and progresses to generally kill the affected infant before age 2 years. The brain becomes atrophic and the white matter appears "moth-eaten" but grossly is basically indistinguishable from the white matter in most of the other leukodystrophies. The symptoms of the disease are like those of most other leukodystrophies, manifested by neurological deterioration. A number of forms of the disease are known, and rare adult cases have been reported [87], as has peripheral nerve involvement [88]. A number of animal models for the condition exist, and therapeutic trials involving bone marrow transplantation show promise [89].

Metachromatic leukodystrophy is another of the leukodystrophies, resulting from deficiency in a number of types of aryl sulfatase that may involve many gene mutations that sometimes correlate with the clinical form of the disease and its age of onset [90,91]. The accumulated metabolic products are sufated glycolipids (sulfatides) that involve Schwann cells, oligodendrocytes in the white matter, renal tubules, some neurons, and connective tissues. Sulfatides, because of their acidic character, change the color of dyes such as methylene blue and toluidine blue to a red or brick color (metachromasia), a reaction that virtually ensures the diagnosis. The disease may manifest like the other leukodystrophies in infancy or may appear throughout later life, primarily as a peripheral neuropathy, a neurodegenerative disease, and dementing illness [91]. Due to the variance in genetic defects

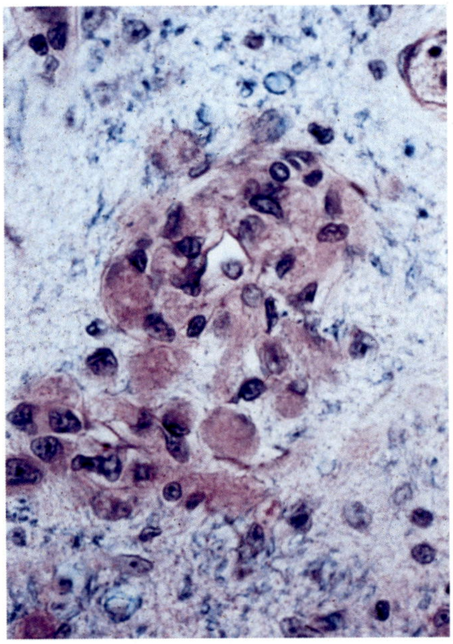

Figure 4.5 Typical globoid cells in Krabbe's disease. The swollen macrophages are filled with granular PAS-positive lipids, reflecting the abnormal lipids that have been phagocytosed from the degenerating myelin.

and unusual clinical presentations, the diagnosis may be difficult or missed [92]. Recently, a variety of animal models of the disease have been found or created and gene-based therapies are in development [93].

Pelizaeus–Merzbacher disease is a very rare, apparently X-linked inheritable condition with a number of variants and several mutations or rearrangements in genes associated with proteolipid metabolism [94,95]. An infantile form results in decreased myelin formation with cerebral atrophy that leads to psychomotor development failure and extrapyramidal signs. A juvenile form shows, in addition to the above, choreoathetoid movements.

Cockayne's disease occurs in late infancy and is caused by autosomal recessively inherited genetic defects that result in faulty DNA repair that seems to affect ubiquitin synthesis [96,97]. Affected infants show dwarfism, microcephaly, ataxia, spasticity, and photosensitivity. Pathologically, there is atrophy of the brain and decreased white matter, mineralizations in the basal ganglia, and meningeal thickening.

Canavan disease [98] generally occurs in infancy, but there are later onset cases reported. The disease is an autosomal recessively inherited defect in the gene coding for aspartoacylase, a gene restricted to the central nervous system. The disease is progressive and present as developmental decay, apathy, blindness, and motor retardation. Pathologically, the disease is characterized by a diffuse subcortical microvascuolation with prominent Alzheimer type II astrogliosis and atrophy. Hypomyelination is present.

Alexander's disease is different from the other diseases described above in that, although it results in massive destruction of the white matter (Figure 4.6) in infants and in some cases affects older individuals, it is not a disease of myelin but, rather, of astrocytes,

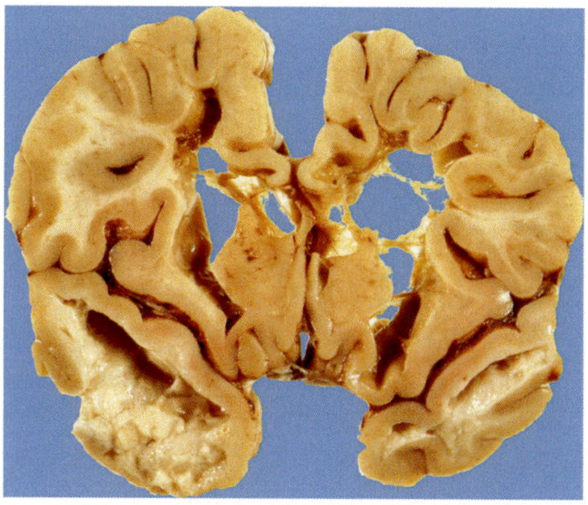

Figure 4.6 Coronal section of a case of Alexander's disease illustrating the profound destruction of the white matter with preservation of overlying cortex and basal ganglia that is seen in that condition. Although the condition is rare, it will occasionally show up on a forensic service because the affected infant died at home, with or without a diagnosis. (Courtesy of the Department of Pathology, Children's Memorial Hospital, Chicago.)

in which they accumulate massive amounts of glial fibrillary acidic protein (GFAP) and deposit it subpially, perivascularly, and subependymally (Figure 4.7). The disease presents like many of the leukodystrophies and results in profound neurological deficits and megalencephaly [99,100]. The disease, only in some adult forms, is inherited but is mostly a sporadic event resulting in mutations in the gene for GFAP [101].

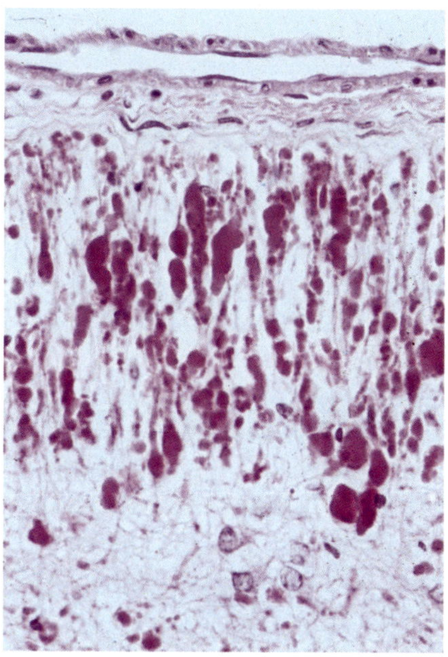

Figure 4.7 White matter and a penetrating vessel from a case of Alexander's disease illustrating the deposition of Rosenthal fibers, which is the outstanding feature of this disease. (Courtesy of Department of Pathology, Children's Memorial Hospital, Chicago.)

Prematurity and Its Consequences

The march of reproductive technology has given way to a host of unintended consequences and complications, especially in connection with low and very low birth weight babies that may have forensic consequences. These may include developmental problems and later disability, and injuries that may not have been appreciated at the time but which may suggest abusive injury later on, or conditions that might be subject to possible medical malpractice scrutiny. A recent study from Sweden [102] explored neurodevelopmental outcomes in extremely preterm infants 2½ years after birth. This study reported upon 456 infants born before 27 weeks of gestation compared with 701 controls, 366 of whom had detailed developmental information. The preterm group had statistically lower scores compared with controls for cognition (moderate disability, 5%; severe disability, 9.4%), language capability (moderate disability, 9.4%; severe disability, 6.6%), and motor abilities (cerebral palsy, 7%). The preterm group as a whole showed that 42% of the infants had no apparent disability, 31% had mild disability, 16% had moderate disabilities, and 11% had severe disabilities. From 22 weeks onward, disabilities were fewer with each succeeding week (22 weeks, 60%; 23 weeks, 51%; 24 weeks, 34%; 25 weeks, 27%; 26 weeks, 17%). The intensity of the perinatal care translated into generally better outcomes than those with less intense care. Other studies have shown comparable results with expected variations [103,104].

Neuropathologically, the disabilities vary considerably with those who have little or no apparent structural abnormality to those with obvious and typical cerebral palsy pathologies, hydrocephaly, subdural hemorrhages, and "hygromas," and other lesions that may be interpreted as derived from abuse when in fact they are the legacy of their birth circumstances. Interpretations in these infants are often challenging and require appreciation of the special circumstances each infant may have experienced.

Hypoxia/Ischemia

The reactions of the immature brain to hypoxia and ischemia also differ from those of the mature brain [2,5,105–107]. During the first half of gestation, an ischemic episode in the fetus may disturb a major portion of the developing brain with remarkably little cellular response to suggest infarction, such as in the development of a porencephalic cavity or some forms of schizencephaly. Later, cellular responses to injury by macrophages and astrocytes are more typical, but the sites of vulnerability differ from those in the adult. In the immature infant, the sites of damage in hypoxic/ischemic insults tend to be in the brain stem [108], basal ganglia, or periventricular white matter [2,109–112]. The mature infant shows lesions in adult sites of vulnerability, for example, the cerebral cortex, particularly the hippocampus and the cerebellar Purkinje cells.

Neuronal necrosis in the premature infant may be expressed as karyorrhexis or simply rapid disappearance rather than the eosinophilic cytoplasmic reaction seen in the mature neuron's response to ischemic cell damage (red neurons) [45,113]. The maturity of the brain, as well as the completeness of the ischemic insult, seems to determine the site of the infarct. For example, complete ischemia affects the brain stem (as in prolapse of the cord or cardiac arrest in the neonate), whereas a partial ischemic insult, such as shock, will produce periventricular and cortical lesions. The time course of brain ischemia may also affect the distribution of lesions observed [105,114]. Other factors, such as the levels of blood pressure and blood glucose and the presence of acidosis, will alter the pathogenesis of the lesion. It has been suggested, too, that cortical lesions in the brains of term infants tend to follow the patterns of myelination [109], for example, the functional cortical territories of the motor, sensory, auditory, and visual cortices of the hippocampi, suggesting that these actively myelinating areas may have a greater susceptibility to ischemia. Combinations of brain stem and cortical injury, such as pontosubicular necrosis [106], have been observed in term and preterm infants who have had pulmonary disease and in whom aggressive attempts have been made to correct it (oxygen therapy, respiratory assistance) [115]. In such cases, the neurons of the basis pontis and the subiculum (cortex bordering on the hippocampus) show karyorrhexis with later reactive gliosis. There may be associated lesions in the thalamus and white matter. Specific pathological states due to ischemic and hypoxic injury are discussed below.

The size and form of the head and skull depend on the normally growing brain, and during the first year of the child's life, the cranial sutures expand in response to changes in brain size. When these close, the brain is locked within a rigid encasement of bone. The importance of this developmental progression is that in the infant, if the brain should swell, it will force open the sutures of the cranium, sometimes widely, with a rapid amelioration of symptoms of increased intracranial pressure. With continued brain swelling or increase in mass effect, this compensatory mechanism is overwhelmed and herniation through the foramen magnum may result, as would be the case in the adult. Just as in the adult, there are limits to the degree of herniation before circulatory embarrassment may occur, leading to global ischemia and the "respirator" brain phenomenon (see Chapter 5).

It is clear that many congenital or perinatally acquired brain lesions may have as their etiologies some abnormality of vascular perfusion or insufficient oxygen in the blood. There are several specific pathological entities that are, in most cases, due to hypoxic or ischemic causes that may conveniently be separated from those congenital conditions in which the etiologies are multifactorial. These include conditions acquired *in utero*, such as porencephaly and hydranencephaly, as well as those that are commonly associated with prematurity or complications of delivery, including subdural hemorrhages and fluid collections, ulegyria, subependymal plate and periventricular hemorrhages, periventricular leukomalacia, and cystic encephalomalacia.

The brain of an infant responds differently to hypoxia and ischemia than does that of a child or an adult, in that the white matter may be more vulnerable than the gray, especially in premature infants. This may reflect special metabolic processes or vascular anatomy or physiology at the time that do not apply at an older age. Furthermore, hypoxia and other injuries may affect developmental processes, which are not operating in the adult, to produce special forms of brain pathology not possible at other ages, such as lesions in the basal ganglia–status marmoratus (*etát marbre*), anomalies of cortical differentiation, and neuronal migration.

With the advent of extracorporeal membrane oxygenators (ECMOs) and bypass vascular pumps, attempts to salvage previously unsalvageable babies with severe cardiac anomalies, meconium aspiration, diaphragmatic hernias, pulmonary hypertension, and other conditions became possible but ushered in a spectrum of complications because of the technology. Generally, two methods are employed for using this technology: venoarterial and venovenous. With venoarterial ECMO the right common carotid is ligated, but with venovenous ECMO it is not. It became immediately obvious that problems could and did arise with cerebral perfusion with resultant hypoxia/ischemia and embolic issues. In the study by Amigoni et al. [116], it was noted that in those infants who survived after ECMO was instituted, 8.3% of neonates and 30% of older children evaluated a year after ECMO had an unfavorable neurological outcome. Other studies have shown that from 28% to 52% of neonates treated with ECMO had abnormal brain imaging studies [117,118]. When the brains of ECMO-treated babies are examined, many display respirator brain phenomena or multifocal areas of necrosis and hemorrhage with edema. With respect to the eye, a study by Young et al. [117] reported that hemorrhagic retinopathy, usually unilateral, was discovered in 6 of 9 diaphragmatic hernia patients, 1 of 10 patients with respiratory distress syndrome (RDS), and 1 of 35 patients with meconium aspiration. The mechanism for these retinal hemorrhages is not known. The important issue here is not so much that ECMO appears to cause retinal hemorrhages and brain ischemic/hypoxic or hemorrhagic phenomena but that disorders of vascular perfusion can have widespread effects on the brain and eye that in another setting might be misinterpreted.

Infarction and Stroke

Forms of ischemic brain infarction other than hydranencephaly in the neonate may not be as devastating or as massive as in hydranencephaly. Some form of neonatal stroke is said to occur in 1 of 4000 live births [119–121], but it appears that the mortality is low, with more than 95% of victims surviving to adulthood, although they may have neurological deficits [122,123]. Stroke can occur at all ages throughout infancy and childhood. The mechanisms behind stroke are multifactorial and include primary vascular events (arterial or venous), preeclampsia, placental dysfunction, coagulopathy (inherited and acquired), hypoxia, and ischemia [122,124,125].

To most forensic pathologists, stroke in infants and young children is viewed as a rare or extremely rare event, but it is said to occur with about the same frequency as brain tumors in the age group (2.5–10 of every 100,000 individuals) [126–128]. The mortality rate depends upon the type of stroke that occurs, but overall in the infant group, the rate is about 10%, and two thirds of the survivors will have significant neurological deficits [125].

The etiologies for infant stroke can be roughly grouped into those due to embolism; thrombosis, which may be associated with congenital heart lesions; acquired cardiac or cardiac valve disease; inflammatory/infectious conditions; toxic states; coagulopathies and bleeding disorders; and trauma (accidental or inflicted) [128]. From the symptoms that are presenting, it is often difficult to determine the etiology of the stroke. With further clinical workup, including imaging studies, and laboratory examinations, which may have to be extensive, the etiology of the stroke can be determined in the majority of cases, but there remain perhaps up to 20% of cases where the causes are unclear. The forensic issues that surround infant stroke are many but generally center about whether inflicted trauma is the cause. It cannot be too strongly stressed that early impressions of abuse as an explanation may well be wrong. The differential diagnosis for causes of stroke, which may or may not have associated subarachnoid and even subdural hemorrhage as well as retinal hemorrhages, is long and the entities included may be poorly understood or obscure. However, regardless of rarity or complexity, many of these conditions, when simplistically or incompletely evaluated, masquerade as abuse. An example of infantile stroke is shown in Figure 4.8.

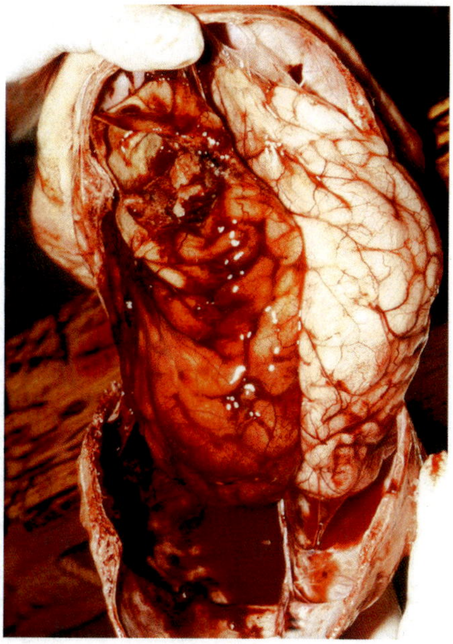

Figure 4.8 Brain of an infant who apparently suffered primarily a unilateral ischemic stroke of the left hemisphere. The presence of a subdural hematoma that was aging suggested the possibility of inflicted injury, but no injury to the neck or vessels could be found. The etiology of this stroke could not be determined. (Courtesy of Dr. Shaku Teas and the Office of the Medical Examiner, Cook County, IL.)

Periventricular (Germinal Matrix) and Intraventricular Hemorrhage

The most common cerebral lesion of the premature infant is periventricular or intraventricular hemorrhage, found in 40%–45% of babies born younger than 35 weeks' gestation and weighing less than 1500 g [129], and it occurs in from 1 to 6 per 1000 live births in the United States [122]. Periventricular lesions and hemorrhage have been demonstrated *in utero* [130]. When recognized, germinal matrix hemorrhage and associated periventricular leukomalacia are usually discovered within 24 hours of birth. A troublesome feature of this condition is that it may not be recognized at the time and treated. Up to 20% of affected infants die in the perinatal period, and 25% or more of survivors suffer permanent neurological sequelae that are often lumped into the designation of cerebral palsy but also include learning disabilities, behavioral disorders, seizures, and hydrocephalus, with or without obvious movement disorders [131]. Periventricular lesions do not occur in isolation but are often associated with pneumothorax, respiratory difficulties, and breech and other delivery issues that may involve the use of obstetrical forceps and vacuum extraction, having had prolonged labor [132,133], maternal infection, or chorioamnionitis [16,134,135]. The occurrence in connection with birth has led many to regard the cause as perinatal asphyxia, but it is more complicated than simply oxygenation deficits, however they occur [136]. In recent years, neonatal brain injury has been recognized to be basically a metabolic dysfunction that can involve transient ischemia with reperfusion issues in the damaged area, with or without a variety of inherited genetic defects that manifest near the time of birth [122,137,138]. Some of the genetic influences include defective genes coding for endothelial nitric oxide synthetase, factor VII, and others [122]. These processes lead to local tissue oxidative stress, excitotoxicity, and neuronal as well as oligodendroglial precursor death. A cascade of events is set into motion that involves activation of inflammatory mediators, free radicals, and later cell death by an apoptotic mechanism as well as local bleeding from delicate vessels within the periventricular area and germinal matrix [15]. It has recently been appreciated that damage in one part of the developing nervous system may have profound effects on more distant, apparently even unrelated parts of the nervous system, leading to cell death by apoptosis by mechanisms that are poorly understood [139]. Thus, what appears to be a focal brain injury may be more extensive than appreciated.

The diagnosis of neonatal periventricular damage can be established in life with ultrasound scanning, computerized tomography (CT), or magnetic resonance (MR) scanning, and other MR techniques, such as diffusion-weighted imaging [140,141]. The degree of hemorrhage is often graded: grade I is a hemorrhage confined to the subependymal germinal matrix zone, grade II is a hemorrhage that has ruptured into the ventricles and subarachnoid space, grade III is an intraventricular hemorrhage with dilatation of the ventricles, and grade IV is a hemorrhage with periventricular extension [141]. An example is seen in Figure 4.9.

In the more mature infant, intraventricular hemorrhage associated with prolonged labor, hypoxia, or traumatic delivery may be related to hemorrhage within the choroid plexus due to bleeding diathesis, trauma, venous thrombosis, or a vascular anomaly of the great vein of Galen. Regardless of the etiology of the intraventricular hemorrhage, it may lead to the development of hydrocephalus either acutely or after a latent period that may extend years after the birth.

The forensic implications of perinatal periventricular pathology may involve sudden, unexpected decompensation in an infant, with or without known trauma (incidental, accidental, or inflicted), and with or without a fatal outcome. Such infants often present with characteristics that include choking, respiratory arrest, seizures, vomiting, and aspiration. Examination and workup may reveal recent or old fluid collections over the brain (external hydrocephalus or subdural hygroma/hematoma) and increased intracranial pressure,

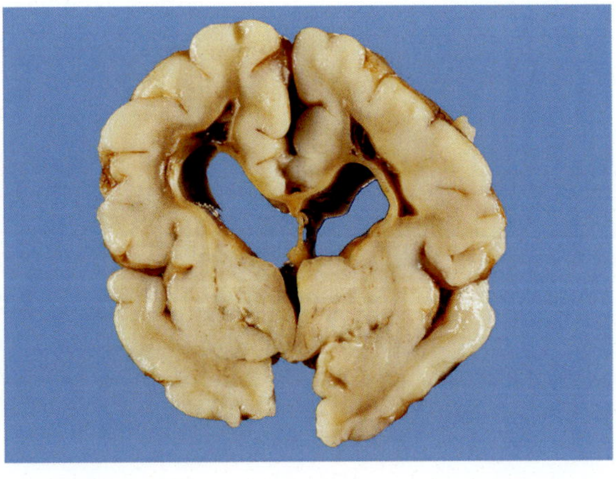

Figure 4.9 Coronal section of the brain of an infant illustrating bilateral germinal matrix subependymal hemorrhages. The infant survived for some weeks after birth, allowing the hemorrhages to become cystic and the ventricles to enlarge from tissue loss as well as some element of hydrocephalus, probably of the communicating type, as a complication of ventricular hemorrhage.

with or without a spectrum of retinal hemorrhage or other intraocular pathologies such as vitreous hemorrhage, retinal folds, papilledema, cerebral edema, and perfusion deficits in the cerebral hemispheres. Sometimes, the clinical record will have information that the head circumference of the affected infant has been increasing beyond the expected developmental curve but for an unknown reason was not acted upon or appreciated. The skull shape may be spherical and the skull may be thinned. It is not surprising that these infants may be suspected of or declared to have been the victims of abuse. Case studies relevant to these issues that may have involved mistaken diagnosis of child abuse have been reported [142–144]. A more extensive discussion of these issues in the context of trauma can be found in Chapter 6.

Multicystic Encephalomalacia

In this condition, portions of the brain are replaced by numerous loculated lacy cysts within the white matter and cortex. The distribution of lesions is in the white matter, usually in the territories of the anterior and middle cerebral arteries, with possible gross but not microscopic sparing of the temporal lobes, thalami, and other deep structures. A typical example is illustrated in Figure 4.10. An extreme example is seen in Figure 4.11 in which the infant survived in a vegetative state for many months after birth. The distribution of the lesions suggests a vascular etiology or hypoxia, possibly as a variant of perinatal hypoxia/ischemia (periventricular leukomalacia), porencephaly, or hydranencephaly, but intrauterine infection has also been suggested in some cases. In some brains with multicystic encephalomalacia, there may be lesions of ulegyria and periventricular leukomalacia that occur with differing degrees of severity [145]. The lesions often occur in twin infants and in infants born after prolonged labor with cyanosis, and seizures at birth. Death usually occurs within a few weeks of birth if the condition is widespread, but prolonged survival with lesser forms of encephalomalacia is possible, with such individuals usually requiring continuing care, attendant with a high mortality rate from aspiration and pneumonia [146].

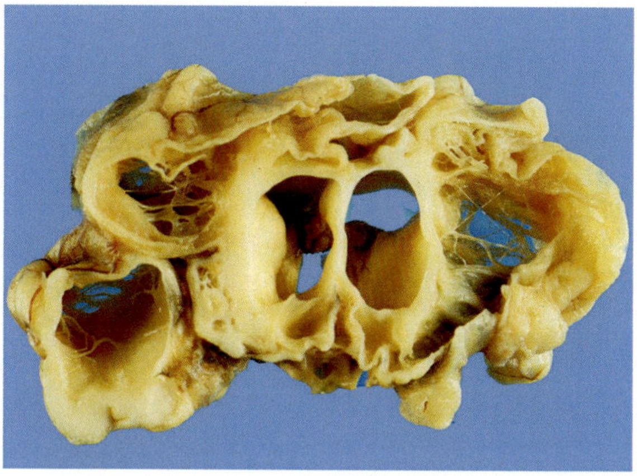

Figure 4.10 Brain of a baby who survived for several weeks after suffering periventricular leukomalacia and intraventricular hemorrhage, showing bilateral cystic cavities where the hemorrhages were. The cortex is shrunken and walnut-like. The ventricles are also significantly enlarged (hydrocephalus *ex vacuo*).

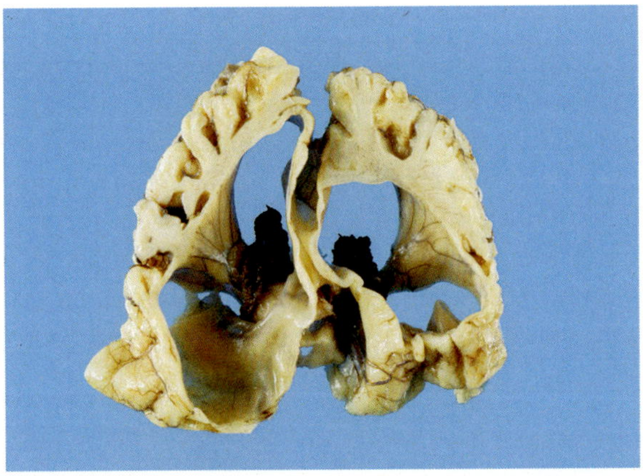

Figure 4.11 Severe multicystic encephalomalacia and hydrocephalus *ex vacuo* affects the brain of a baby who survived for many months after a profound hypoxic insult in the perinatal period.

Ischemic Lesions of the Basal Nuclei

The deep cerebral nuclei—the thalamus, globus pallidus, caudate, putamen, and hypothalamus—are frequently sites of ischemic/hypoxic injury in the "asphyxiated" or immature newborn who experiences respiratory difficulty [105]. The brain stem is also exceptionally vulnerable to asphyxia (a complex insult with alterations in blood flow, oxygen concentration, and, frequently, blood pressure). Acidosis, which also occurs, is usually vigorously treated so that the precise etiology of the deep nuclear damage is confused. It is also difficult to determine the role of toxicity of excess oxygen administration in the production of the lesions [115]. No matter how they are produced, they may be associated with periventricular cystic disease and variable cortical damage and may be indistinguishable from the basic sequence of events that unites all of these conditions: prematurity, respiratory distress, hypoxia, and probably acidosis.

The acute lesions in the deep nuclei are manifested by dissolution of cell nuclei. The chronic lesions show loss of cells, gliosis, and aberrant myelination of glial processes (*etat fibromyelinique*, *etat marbre*) to produce a marbled-appearing basal ganglia [51,53], illustrated in Figure 4.12. Survivors of this condition commonly fall into the C-P category.

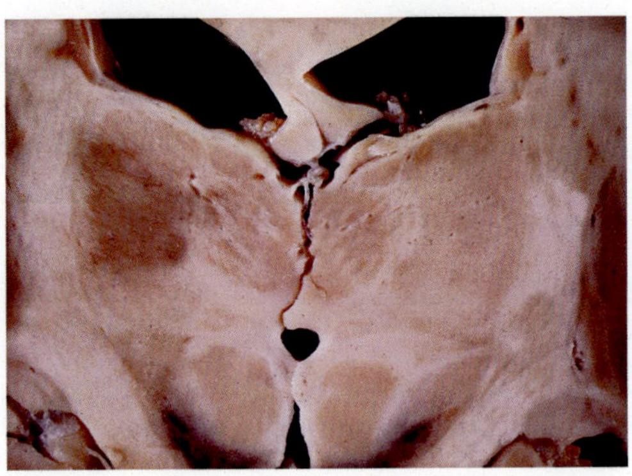

Figure 4.12 A marbled thalamus in an adult who suffered perinatal hypoxic brain damage and manifested spastic cerebral palsy throughout life. A similar picture may be seen in infants suffering from hyperbilirubinemia and kernicterus.

Cerebral Palsy

Some of the conditions listed above and others discussed below produce a clinical picture of functional disturbances that are grouped for convenience into a category of congenital, early acquired, nonprogressive brain damage known as cerebral palsy (C-P). It should be recognized that this term is not easily or specifically pathologically definable and can encompass nonfatal cortical, subcortical, deep nuclear, and brain stem lesions that leave the victim with movement disorders, such as spasticity, athetosis, paralysis, distortions of the limbs and spine, disorders of communication, sometimes mental subnormality (30% of cases), and seizure disorders (35% of cases) [147]. Some cases of C-P have their root causes developing *in utero* [6], independent of the birthing process [148–150]. Examples include placenta previa and abruptions, abnormal placental vasculature, multiple pregnancies with twin-to-twin perfusion, short cord, a cord with knots, entanglements or prolapse, bleeding disorders in the mother or fetus, anemia, uterine hyperactivity, and other conditions leading to insufficient utero-placental blood flow [6,16,151]. Postnatally acquired or expressed lesions of the brain leading to C-P also occur [152] and include inborn errors of metabolism such as glutaric aciduria (type I) [153]. The unifying issue with most of these conditions is fetal brain ischemia and local reactions and not strictly asphyxia. Other conditions are not so clearly linked with tissue hypoxia, such as low-birth-weight babies and chorioamnionitis in term or near-term infants [124].

It is often alleged that C-P's major cause is birth-related asphyxia or circulatory deficit that may involve poor or incompetent obstetrical care. Criteria for such an interpretation are often a matter of opinion that ends up being subject to litigation. The birthing process is, by all definitions, traumatic to the fetus. With uterine contractions and the movement of the fetus into the birth canal, the fetus is subjected to repeated stress, which inevitably results in episodic alterations of utero-placental blood flow and fetal circulation as well as intracranial stresses due to compression that may have circulatory counterparts as well. The interplay between maternal hypoxia and fetal hypoxia has been studied extensively [148]. The response of the fetus to these stresses results in episodic bradycardia followed by tachycardia. Alterations in fetal visceral and brain blood flow also occur, with favored perfusion of brain and heart over the viscera in an effort to insulate the brain from the circulatory events impinging on the fetus. The physiology involved in these events is complex. If circulatory stress becomes profound (severity and duration), protective mechanisms may no longer insulate the brain from injury. Paralleling brain ischemia/hypoxia and its effects are also the effects upon the fetal heart, which compound the evolving brain stress. These events are reflected symptomatically by fetal bradycardia and hypotension, often described on fetal monitoring records as "late" decelerations. Correlation between occurrence and duration of these events and brain damage is not precise or accurately predictable, even though there is a statistical correlation between extent and duration of hypoxia, ischemia, hypotension, and acidosis with brain damage [154]. The effects on neuronal survival are more severe when fetal cerebral blood flow is lowered, more than the degree of hypoxia, which probably explains the "watershed" lesions in some children.

Global ischemia/hypoxia/acidosis does not affect the fetal brain uniformly. Cortical pathology will first be displayed in the watershed zones in the brain (junctions in arterial perfusion territories of the cortex). A typical example is illustrated in Figure 4.13. The basal ganglia (striatum) will also show neuronal injury and loss with replacement gliosis but not

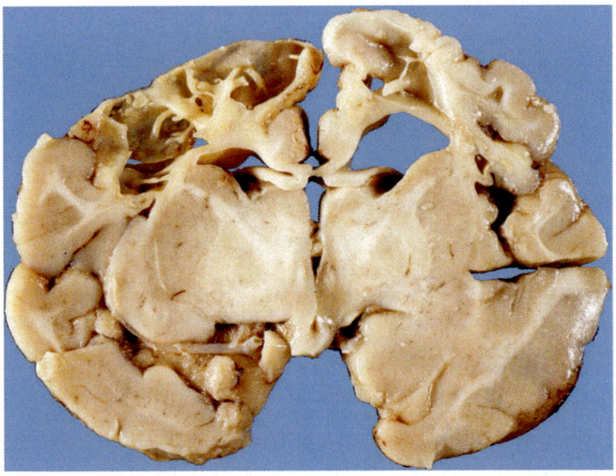

Figure 4.13 This child suffered from cerebral palsy and showed spastic plegia, worse in the lower extremities than in the upper. The child suffered from seizures and died from seizure complications in late childhood. The cystic degeneration of essentially the upper cerebral hemispheres, possibly representing a watershed lesion, is commonly observed. The basal ganglia are pale and were rubbery from replacement gliosis.

always in pace with the cortical damage. In term infants, there is a lesser likelihood for deep white matter/periventricular necrosis and hemorrhage than in the premature infant. This pathology, periventricular leukomalacia, is discussed above.

Endogenous conditions that may be discovered as likely causes in C-P infants include deficiencies of clotting factor V (Leiden) and protein C, a variety of amino acid and metabolic disorders (including glutaric acidemia) [148], mitochondrial abnormalities, and other enzymatic disorders [155–158]. A variety of neurodegenerative diseases that have a hereditary basis may be mistaken for C-P. Neuropathological correlation with clinical symptoms is possible but often difficult because of the presence of multiple neural defects [131].

In the forensic setting, C-P victims may fatally injure themselves in falls or accidents brought about by their movement disorders, difficulties in protecting their airways, communications difficulties, or seizure disorders and not infrequently are victims of violent street crimes or in childhood may suffer abuse by parents or siblings [159]. Unraveling primary external events and their interplay with inherent neural/functional difficulties may be challenging and requires care, thought, and often scholarship. Autopsy examination of some C-P individuals can be strikingly normal, despite rather severe symptoms, and at other times, from an examination of the brain (perhaps with large porencephalic cysts), it is difficult to understand how some individuals have managed to function despite their lesions. Some C-P–affected individuals have severe mental limitations but at the same time possess amazing abilities in memorization or music and might properly be called idiot savants [160–162].

Forensic Issue Surrounding Birth Injury

In recent years an important medical–legal phenomenon has developed in which parents have increasingly initiated litigation against hospitals, obstetricians, and other physicians involved in prenatal care when an infant is born with congenital malformations or suffers from some sort of perinatally discovered condition that renders the child mentally subnormal or otherwise severely incapacitated [163,164]. Another evolving phenomenon is the frequent accusation of child abuse by a caregiver when an infant or child with congenital brain malformations or conditions decompensate, and may die. Often there is a history of a difficult birth, or perinatal hypoxia associated with a low Apgar score, which is blamed for the subsequent state of the infant. It is a common practice, often unchallenged by appropriate medical expert advice and analysis, to affix blame for the sorry state of the infant and the costs connected with these consequences to the obstetrician or to a caregiver when the full extent of the infant's problems were not appreciated or even diagnosed in life according to the principle of *res ipsa loquitur* (the facts speak for themselves) argument in court. Although it cannot be denied that errors of medical and nursing care can contribute to unfortunate and tragic clinical outcomes and may be justifiably compensable, it is arguable precisely how many instances occur in which the obstetrician is responsible for an unfortunate outcome regardless of whether a caesarian section has been employed [165,166]. The hapless parent who has a brain-damaged but perhaps undiagnosed or misdiagnosed infant who suffers consequences that are interpreted precipitously as being inflicted is often presumed guilty of a crime without due process. The forensic pathologist and neuropathologist can often make the difference between precipitous and unfounded judgments when judicial processes have the benefit of informed opinion, but mistakes are commonly made.

When an infant is alive, clinical and radiological opinions, error-prone, and often dogma-driven as they are, may rule the day and result in actions against a caregiver that can include removal of the children in the family to a foster home or indictment for criminal acts by the caregiver. In instances in which an infant has died, a complete autopsy must be performed by a qualified pathologist. This may allow the demonstration of underlying diseases or conditions that affected the outcome of the case independent of any action on the part of a physician. In other circumstances, especially when no death has occurred, considerable information may be gained by an examination of the birth records, ultrasound studies, the placenta and cord, and medical and laboratory records. Review of the histological slides of the placenta/cord material may reveal abnormalities of the placenta that could have had an impact on the development of postnatally discovered problems in the infant, again independent of any medical care rendered. In any case, a review of such cases by a competent pathologist or neuropathologist may develop evidence having considerable importance to the adjudication of the case.

Birth Trauma

In the course of delivery, a variety of traumatic injuries may affect infants regardless of how they were delivered. These include skull fractures [167–169], subdural (supratentorial as well as infratentorial) [170,171] and epidural hemorrhages [172,173], scalp hemorrhages, spinal and cord injuries [37,174,175], brachial plexus injuries [176,177], and occasionally cerebral tissue embolism to the lungs [178]. These can occur during precipitous difficult deliveries in which instruments, and vacuum extraction are used inexpertly or the infant is forcefully manipulated or even during caesarian section. The most common, but least significant, is the external cranial trauma known as *caput succedaneum*, in which cranial compression by the constricting lower uterine segment or incompletely dilated cervix produces hemorrhage into the skin, usually of the vertex scalp or sometimes the face. This often obvious and alarming bruise generally decreases and disappears within a few days of birth with no sequelae. A thickened disk of scar tissue may, however, persist for months or years at the site of a caput and be misinterpreted as more recent trauma. A more serious hemorrhage is *subgaleal hemorrhage*, in which trauma has produced tears in the scalp vessels so that blood accumulates under the temporalis muscle or other connective tissue planes in the head. The condition is usually self-limited but can continue and produce hemorrhagic shock or death [179].

Hemorrhage occurring beneath the (outer) periosteum of the skull is called a *cephalohematoma*, which forms a mass limited by the sutures of the skull. It may be associated with overriding of the skull bone plates, skull fracture, with or without an epidural hematoma, in which case there is direct pressure on the brain that may cause death. Cephalohematomas are generally not life threatening but may result in deformity of the convexity of the skull, which may eventually become ossified and cause asymmetry [180]. If a subdural hematoma occurs, which is well known in the literature (see above), this may or may not give rise to immediate symptoms but can produce symptoms at a later time that might be misinterpreted as an inflicted injury.

Neonatal skull fractures are of three types: linear, depressed, or diastatic. Linear fractures are by far the most common and are simple single-line fractures that may or may not be significantly separated and may cause few or no symptoms. Depressed and diastatic fractures, on the other hand, are more serious and indicative of greater traumatic injury. Depressed fractures impinge on the brain and cause pressure effects that may be fatal unless the fracture is surgically elevated and any associated subdural or epidural hemorrhage is evacuated [168]. Diastatic fractures are those that occur through suture lines, with or without overriding edges. A common diastatic fracture occurs in the occipital region, often in association with breech deliveries, where the head is forcibly hyperextended and trapped under the symphysis pubis of the mother. This type of fracture may be difficult to observe at autopsy and requires suboccipital dissection to demonstrate hemorrhages into the soft tissues of the neck that can compress the foramen magnum externally. The radiological diagnosis of skull fractures is prone to many errors of various kinds. The fracture lines may be very narrow and are not visualized in the study performed. Anatomic variants and features such as diploic veins and interosseous Wormian bones (see Figure 6.20) lying in developing sutures are commonly to blame [181,182]. Variants in the lambdoidal mendosal suture show considerable unpredictability and may be misinterpreted as skull fractures [183,184].

In any case, fractures sustained during delivery are usually accompanied by external signs of trauma such as forceps lacerations, scalp hemorrhages, or cephalohematomas. Hospital records may or may not exist to document these lesions. This is important in cases in which very young infants are traumatized by abusing parents who claim that the lesions were birth injuries [38]. Sometimes, obstetrical forceps may injure the brain of the newborn, producing a lesion indistinguishable from so-called contusional tears [50] in the subcortical white matter. These lesions may result from "creep" of the mechanically different cortex over a more flexible white matter with a resultant hemorrhage. Deformation of the head and brain from external compression is probably the cause of this lesion. Other etiologies have been proposed to be due to cerebral edema, and ischemia [185] or a manifestation of cortical venous thrombosis [186,187].

Differentiation of forceps injuries from perinatal child abuse requires careful examination of all the evidence that is available, including hospital records that would note if forceps were used during the delivery. It is distressing that obstetrical records are often incomplete (by mistake or design) in indicating the use of forceps or vacuum extraction methods, facts that may come to light by statements of parents or other relatives who were present in the delivery or videotaped the blessed event.

Spinal Cord and Brachial Plexus Injury

In the newborn, the skull and spine are remarkably elastic and capable of absorbing considerable distortion without breakage; however, the underlying brain and cord may be less capable of surviving injury when stretching or torsional forces affect the spinal cord, as in hyperextension, twisting in connection with a difficult delivery, mishandling of the infant following delivery, or misguided attempts at repositioning the head before delivery. Nerve roots or nerve plexuses can be damaged, resulting in peripheral nerve lesions such as brachial plexus injury (Erb's palsy) [176,177,188]. Such injury can occur when the arm or shoulder is the presenting part. One center reported 0.87 lesions per 1000 live births, 80% of which showed recovery from symptoms at 1 year [37,189]. Isolated radial nerve injuries have been reported when the umbilical cord entraps an arm. Such peripheral nerve injuries may be unsuspected externally at first, but when the infant is older they may manifest as contractures, atrophy, or a flail extremity with atrophy. Damage may also result to vertebral arteries by twisting, which may cause infarction of the cord, bleeding, or pseudoaneurysm formation to occur [190].

Spinal cord injury in the infant should be suspected in all difficult or precipitous deliveries [37,174] in which the infant appears paralyzed afterward. Neuropathological examination must involve a full examination of the entire spine and cord as well as a thorough intracranial examination. Whenever there is evidence of intracranial injury, the spine should not be neglected, as it, too, may show significant trauma and may have been responsible for death due to respiratory failure because of damage to the upper cord. Case reports and small series still appear in the literature of delivery-associated spinal injuries [191,192].

Artifactual damage to the cord may occur in connection with the respirator brain phenomenon [193], discussed in detail in Chapter 5. This may occur because circulation to the upper cervical cord coming from the anterior spinal arterial vessels is insufficiently collateralized by circulation coming from "radicular" and other vessels supplying the cord from noncerebral vessels, including the aorta. This collateralization or border zone may produce necrosis in the center of the cord in patients maintained usually for many hours or days on a respirator [42]. These changes exist in the absence of evidence of spinal or paraspinal injury and have been misinterpreted as being due to shaking trauma, even in the absence of any demonstrable structural lesion in the cervical spine.

Subarachnoid Hemorrhage

Subarachnoid hemorrhage is a common condition in living neonates and is commonly seen in newborn brains at autopsy [3]. However, it becomes significant in trauma or bleeding diathesis, infection, intraventricular hemorrhage, or asphyxia when it contributes to death by producing impedance to CSF flow and absorption and raised intracranial pressure [194,195]. If an examination of the meninges is made, even some time after the event, there may be fibrous thickening, residual macrophages, and blood pigments that stain the meninges that may persist for weeks, months, or even years.

Retinal Hemorrhage in the Neonate

Just as subarachnoid hemorrhage with or without subdural hemorrhages is not uncommon in neonates, retinal hemorrhages of various kinds are also quite common and said to occur in 35% to more than 50% of cases [196–198]. There is an increased incidence of retinal hemorrhages in infants who have suffered asphyxia, difficult or prolonged births, and the use of forceps or vacuum extractions [198,199]. Increased intracranial pressure is also said to play a role in their occurrence [196]. An example of subarachnoid and subdural hemorrhages in such a case is illustrated in Figure 4.14, along with a photograph of the left eye (Figure 4.15). Retinal hemorrhages of various forms and extent usually resolve within about 2 weeks but may persist longer [197]. Most cases do not result in permanent visual

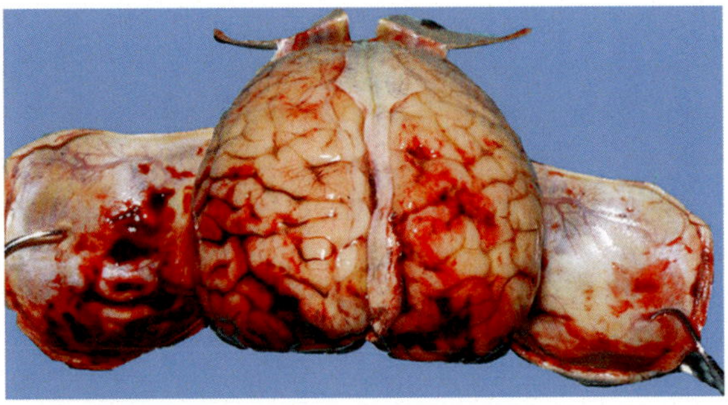

Figure 4.14 Brain of an infant who was born 3 weeks prematurely by emergency caesarian section because of fetal distress apparently due to a tight nuchal cord or a knot in the cord. Apgar scores were 0 despite major efforts at resuscitation. The infant was shown to have a patent ductus arteriosus and multiorgan failure. The infant died 2 days after birth. Autopsy revealed a fresh left frontal subdural hematoma and retinal hemorrhages. (Courtesy of Dr. Patrick Lantz, Winston-Salem, NC.)

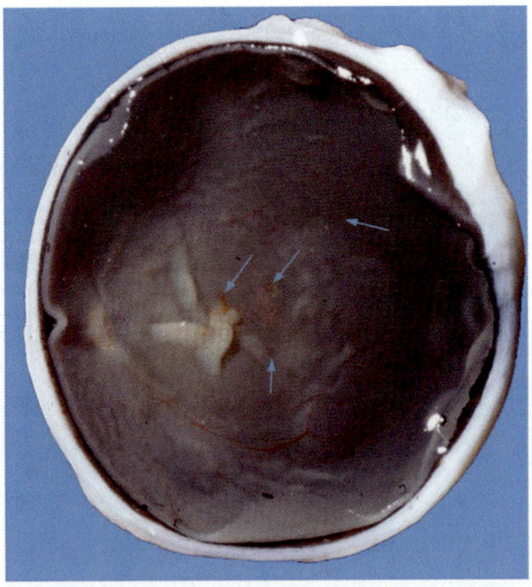

Figure 4.15 The left eye from the case illustrated in Figure 4.14 is shown here with retinal folds after formalin fixation, which is artifactual. A number of retinal hemorrhages, somewhat faded in this fixed specimen (blue arrows), are seen. (Courtesy of Dr. Patrick Lantz, Winston-Salem, NC.)

impairment. Retinal hemorrhages have been described in neonates subjected to vigorous resuscitation [200,201].

Subdural Hematoma and Subdural Effusions

Neonatal subdural hematoma is said to be uncommon to rare, with only nine cases supposedly reported as of 1978 [170], but others have indicated that subdural hematomas, often in the posterior fossa, although uncommon, are not rare [202–204]. This complication of delivery has been known for more than 100 years [171]. Most such cases occur in connection with difficult deliveries involving the use of forceps, vacuum extraction, and caesarian sections performed once the birthing process has begun [205–207]. Perhaps elongation of the cranium imposes strains upon intracranial structures, causing rents and tears with attendant hemorrhage. A typical history is a difficult delivery with the infant appearing intact at birth but then, in the course of hours or days, deteriorating. Surgical intervention may be life saving. Interestingly, there are examples of acute and chronic subdural hematomas (hygromas) in neonates with no history of obstetrical difficulties or prenatal maternal trauma [208–210].

Subdural bleeding may be acute and produce immediate symptoms, including seizures, coma, respiratory distress, and death. Sometimes, a tear into the interface between dura and arachnoid admits CSF, which can produce a pocket of fluid that may persist. Episodes of bleeding evolve slowly and only eventually (usually within a few weeks) produce symptoms, which can include all of the above as well as paralysis, abnormal movements and reflexes, nausea, and projectile vomiting. The pathogenesis of subacute and chronic subdural hematomas is discussed in detail in Chapter 6 and differs little between the infant and the adult. In addition to birth trauma and molding of the head, which can cause subdural hematomas, bleeding disorders, and sepsis, vascular anomalies may cause subdural bleeding. Cerebral cortical vein thrombosis, with or without sagittal sinus or other venous sinus thrombosis, may also lead to subdural hemorrhage or fluid collections [25,211].

Subdural effusions are collections of fluid, not necessarily blood, in the potential subdural space (border zone), which can occur as a complication of meningitis, minor trauma, or surgical procedures, or without known cause. Once a potential space has been created and fluid collects there, the same processes that cause recurrence and progression of chronic subdural hematomas are set into motion and can cause symptoms or death. Some infants may have a benign, self-limiting, subdural effusion, which can be bilateral, that eventually resolves, but other infants require surgical intervention, which can include shunting of the subdural space or irrigation to remove any blood elements to hopefully approximate the neomembranes and eliminate the fluid collection [209,212].

Traumatic Intracerebral Hemorrhage in the Neonate

Occasionally, trauma sustained during delivery will produce hemorrhages within the cerebral matter itself, alone or in combination with any of the above lesions. Such lesions are rare but take two forms: subcortical hematomas and contusional tears (discussed in Chapter 6) and deep hematomas. The contusional tear or subcortical hematoma [50] mentioned above results from deformation or indentation of the skull so that the cortical surface may buckle to a different extent than subcortical tissues, which have a different elasticity, resulting in the tearing of small vessels without any damage of the overlying cortex. These lesions may be seen only rarely in forceps deliveries [189] but most commonly in cases of intentional trauma in child abuse (see Chapter 8 for more details). Deeper hemorrhages generally occur in and around the basal ganglia and nearby white matter [16]. They are the result of shearing forces in the brain in the massively accelerated or deformed head and, as such, may be the result of child abuse (with cranial impact) rather than birth trauma. It is possible to differentiate traumatic hemorrhages from subependymal germinal plate hemorrhages on the basis that these latter hemorrhages are confined to the periventricular region and do not occur elsewhere. In addition, subependymal hemorrhages occur mainly in immature infants, whereas traumatic lesions occur in larger, mature infants.

Ulegyria and the Walnut Brain

Ulegyria results from ischemic in cortical gyri in which there is neuronal loss, cavitation, and gliosis to the depth of a sulcus, with relative preservation of the crest of the gyri giving them a shrunken, granular appearance that must be differentiated from micropolygyria [213–215]. An example in an individual who survived into adulthood is shown in Figure 4.16.

Sometimes, the whole brain will be affected, as in prolonged global hypoxia or ischemia (perinatally acquired or otherwise), with the result that the brain has a shrunken, walnut-like appearance, illustrated in Figure 4.17. The lesion is attributed to greater vulnerability of the neurons at the depth of a sulcus than at the crest to lowered blood flow (ischemia or hypotension) and some potential of repair. The implication of the morphology of the lesion in some cases is that it may have occurred at a time when the developing cortex still had some potential for growth or reaction [2,214–216]. Individuals who have such brains are usually severely compromised and may be living a vegetative existence, requiring constant care, or suffering from intractable epilepsy. Such brains are sometimes encountered on a forensic service, as affected individuals may die at home or in an institution and an autopsy is demanded by public authorities. On other occasions, malpractice litigation will bring a case to the attention of the coroner/medical examiner. Some victims of child abuse in which severe brain hypoxia/ischemia has been the result will display a walnut brain, quite often associated with a chronic subdural hematoma. In analyzing such cases, it is

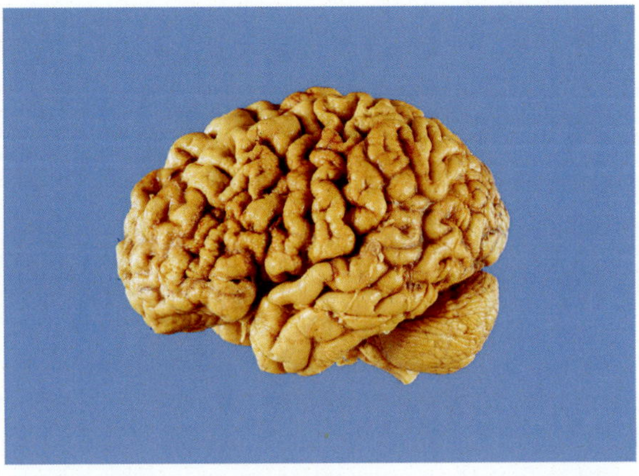

Figure 4.16 Lateral view of the brain illustrating the wrinkled atrophic cortex in ulegyria.

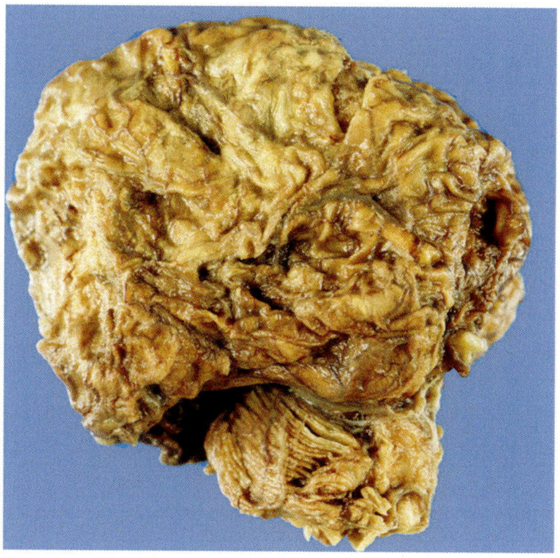

Figure 4.17 "Walnut brain" showing the profound cortical volume loss associated with a global hypoxic/ischemic insult after the neonatal period. The condition can be seen in infants and children but rarely in this form in adults. In this case, the child was brain injured at 4 months of age and remained vegetative until the age of 21 months, when she died. In coronal section, there would be little cortex left and the ventricles would be enlarged (hydrocephalus *ex vacuo*). (Courtesy of Dr. L. Beamer, Office of the Medical Examiner, Cook County, IL.)

important to consider birth and subsequent infant and family history, which may indicate likely abuse in the victim or a sibling. In those infants who are victims of abusive head injury, however it occurs, ischemic brain injury is very common in those who survive, which may result in a so-called walnut brain. Instances have occurred in which a mother apparently repeatedly injured her young babies by traumatic means and possibly by smothering, producing severely compromised infants with walnut brains who clinicians at the time considered to have an undefined inborn metabolic disease. In one particular instance known to the author, the mother was eventually tried and convicted of causing the serial deaths of three of her infant children. The analysis of such cases is often difficult.

Central Nervous System Malformations

Malformations of the nervous system may have forensic significance, especially if there is a possibility that an identifiable environmental factor or drug might be involved of if the presence of a malformation might affect a proper interpretation of a case, such as in an alleged child abuse matter. Brain malformations, at least statistically, have obvious public health impact and may be important in civil litigation related to environmental issues, management of difficult pregnancies, or the prescription of drugs during pregnancy. Occasionally, issues involving malformations might be involved in criminal prosecutions. Brain malformations are a significant cause of morbidity and mortality in the newborn in every country of the world, but statistics relating to the incidence of CNS malformations are difficult to compare [19,217–221]. They vary according to geographic region and at which period they have been compiled. For example, Japan's infant mortality due to congenital CNS malformation, among the lowest, shows about 1 death per 100,000 population, compared with that of Ireland at one time, with about 7800 deaths per 100,000. There are other countries where statistics are rarely collected or reported that might have higher incidences [22,222–224]. In response to public health initiatives, some decreases in infant mortality have been achieved, but even in advanced societies infant mortality remains a serious problem. The causes for geographic variances go beyond statistical error and must involve demographic, genetic, and probably environmental factors, most of which remain undefined [225]. A factor considered by some to be etiologically significant is environmental exposure to radiation. Sternglass [226] has reviewed this issue with respect to the impact of atmospheric nuclear testing during the 1950s and presents some thought-provoking data in this regard.

All malformations indicate that an embryotoxic event has occurred [2,3,15,22,227,228]. The initial effect may have been through cell death, reduced biosynthesis, impaired morphogenic movement, failed tissue instructions, or mechanical disruption. The numerous possible mechanisms for these events (e.g., mutations, chromosomal aberrations, altered metabolism, and interference with mitosis) will not be discussed in this survey of gross lesions, but they should be considered in defining the pathogenesis of CNS lesions, as mentioned above. The principles that apply to the development of the nervous system and its malformations also apply in general to the other organs of the body [229].

In embryology, there is a significant interdependence between tissues as they develop. The developing face is intimately related to the formation of the forebrain [17,230,231], and, consequently, facial anomalies are consistently associated with forebrain malformations such as holoprosencephaly and arrhinencephaly. In the same manner, the form of the base of the skull and posterior fossa, if abnormal, may correlate with associated malformations of basal brain structures, as in the Arnold-Chiari malformation or encephaloceles. Similarly, defects of the spine are coupled with malformed spinal cords, as in spina bifida associated with myelomeningocele [22,220]. Only some of the most common malformations are discussed below.

Anencephaly

Anencephaly is the absence of the forebrain and portions of the cranium (both membranous neurocranium and chondrocranium) and scalp with an exposed knot of disorganized vessels, meninges, and cerebral tissue (the area cerebrovasculosa situated on the residual skull). The frontal, occipital, and parietal bones show varying degrees of absence; the temporal and sphenoid bones are malformed (Figure 4.18). The face, pituitary, and hindbrain are present in term infants with anencephaly, but preterm anencephalics may lack or have hypoplastic pituitaries. The malformation is considered to be a failure of closure of the anterior neural pore during neurulation at about 25 days [220]. The malformation is common, occurring once in about 1000 live births in the United States [229]. There is an increased risk of anencephaly in pregnancies of women past the normal childbearing age and in women who have previously delivered an anencephalic infant [232]. Ultrasound studies will usually demonstrate the malformation, and amniocentesis will usually reveal increased levels of alpha-fetoprotein, acetyl cholinesterase, and other substances in the fluid [233,234]. The etiology is multifactorial—genetic and environmental [1,3]. Anencephaly is usually incompatible with life beyond several days, and death is related to absence of autonomic function or other malformations that are commonly present.

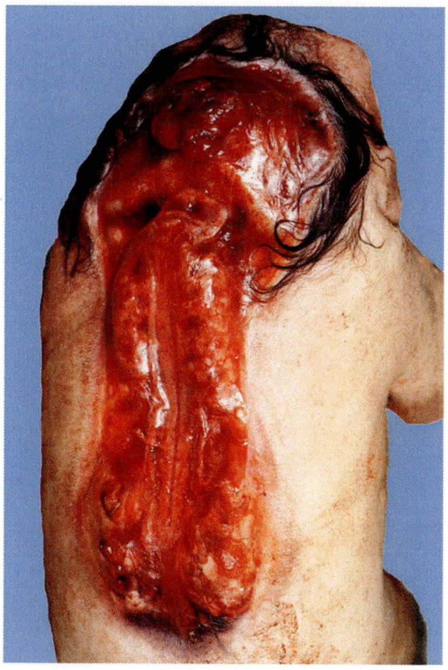

Figure 4.18 A dorsal view of a typical baby with anencephaly shows the open neural environment and near absence of a rostral brain. (Courtesy of Dr. E. N. Willey, Department of Pathology, University of Michigan, Ann Arbor, MI.)

Spina Bifida

Spina bifida is a common dysraphic malformation consisting of failure of development of the neural arches of the vertebrae [2,17,220,235] and may occur at any level of the spine, the lumbosacral being the most common [217]. Membranous closure of the spinal arches occurs normally around 40 days' gestation; chondrification and ossification take place later. If there is an interference with growth at this time, the vertebrae in the affected segments do not fuse. This fusion may be obvious and associated with defects of closure of the cord or overlying soft tissues. If only the bone is involved, the lesion is referred to as spina bifida occulta. This is the most common malformation of the spine, with an incidence of 10%–20% in the population. Occult spina bifida is common in the sacral region, where it produces no symptoms but can cause complications when a pilonidal sinus or other condition is operated on and the spinal sac is entered inadvertently or when infection from the perianal or sacral region spreads to involve the meninges. An example of a closed case of spina bifida without an obvious myelomeningocele is illustrated in Figure 4.19.

Myelomeningocele

Myelomeningocele, another common dysraphic (defect of closure) condition, occurs commonly (about 1 per 1000 live births) [217,222] and consists of a swelling along the spine that is covered or partially covered by abnormal (dysplastic) skin containing varying amounts of malformed spinal cord, spinal roots, meninges, connective tissue, vessels, or neural elements (Figure 4.20). There are numerous variations of the malformation. Sometimes, the cord is essentially normal but will have a cystic cavity at the level of the skeletal malformation (myelocystocele). The malformation may be completely open (myelocele), or the cord exists as two apparently separate hemicords (diastematomyelia), each of which may

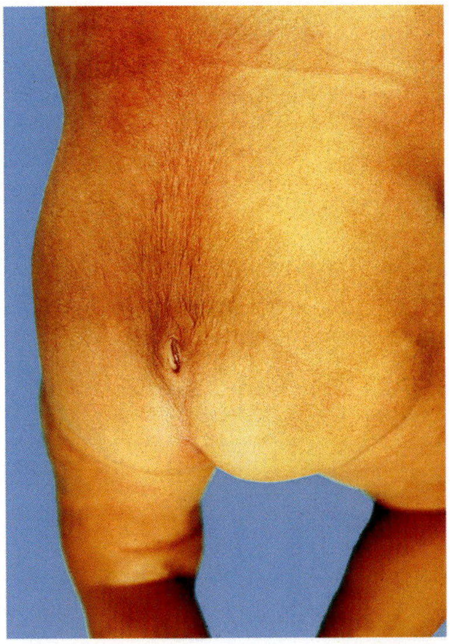

Figure 4.19 Dorsal view of a baby with spina bifida but a minimal external defect of closure that has largely healed.

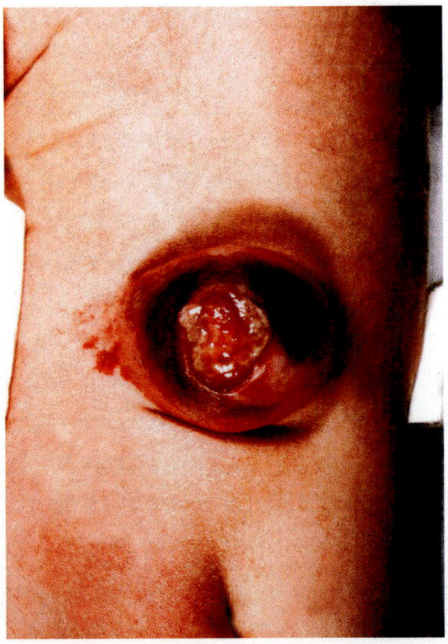

Figure 4.20 A typical myelomeningocele of the lower lumbar–sacral region in a neonate shows a thin membrane overlying the spinal defect. Uncorrected, there is a high mortality rate from meningitis.

be invested by its own dura. The more common condition is that the cord lies splayed open and dysplastic at the level of the malformation and is covered by a thin membrane that is easily broken [226] The condition develops at about 27 days of gestation when that portion of the neural canal should fuse but does not [220]. The etiology of the malformation includes genetic as well as supposed environmental factors, including folate deficiency [218,236–240]. Aggressive neurosurgical and plastic repairs of these lesions have resulted in increased survival despite lower extremity paralysis and bladder and bowel dysfunctions [241]. Associated conditions of myelomeningocele include sacrococcygeal teratomas, intraspinal lipomas, Arnold–Chiari malformations, hydrocephalus, and cortical and other malformations that decrease the salvageability of the infant. Breakdown and infection of the fragile meningocele sac pose the greatest threat to survival in the unoperated infant. Later development of severe scoliosis, epidermoid inclusion cysts in the spinal canal, and a so-called tethered cord may also complicate the course [242]. A variety of lesions can occur in the dysraphic spinal canal, such as lipomas, teratomas, Wilms' tumor, and other lesions [243,244]. Owing to remarkable advances in surgical treatment for most infants born with dysraphism, it is becoming uncommon to encounter untreated cases, and the larger percentage of victims survive to be adults.

Arnold–Chiari Malformations

Arnold–Chiari (A-C) malformation [2,3,245] is usually considered to be one of the dysraphic states (defects of closure) because of its frequent association with myelomeningocele and is one of the more common malformations of the CNS. Four types have been described. Common to all forms is some degree of bony malformation of the posterior fossa associated with platybasia, in which the volume of the posterior fossa is drastically reduced and the form of the space is flattened and funnel shaped [246]. The cerebellar tonsils and lower brain stem are situated below the foramen magnum and are severely distorted. In the simplest form, often referred to simply as the Chiari malformation or the A-C malformation (type I), herniation of the cerebellar tonsils through the foramen magnum, usually with no myelomeningocele, is seen [247]. There are no evident signs or symptoms of hydrocephalus, although this may develop in childhood or even adult life. The skull may have an unusual shape, but little functional disability results. Individuals with this form of the malformation may be asymptomatic until tonsillar herniation sufficiently compresses the fourth ventricle to cause hydrocephalus to develop, and then symptoms are often minimal until brain stem compression occurs. It is under these later circumstances that the forensic pathologist may become involved in the case, when a minor head injury, drug or alcohol overdose, or surgical procedure may cause enough cerebral edema to produce decompensation of the silently evolving hydrocephalus or cause sudden unexpected death [248–250].

The type II A-C malformation is the most common and consists of myelomeningocele (usually lumbosacral), platybasia, small posterior fossa, herniation of the cerebellar tonsils and lower brain stem through the foramen magnum, compression, and obliteration of the fourth ventricle with obstruction of CSF flow and hydrocephalus, a beak-shaped deformity of the superior colliculus (best appreciated in a midline section of the brain stem, which is illustrated in Figure 4.21), aqueductal stenosis by distortion, a kinking or buckling of the cervical cord, an elongated pons, and an upward (rather than downward) angulation of cervical nerve roots [246,251]. The cortical surface of the brain may show polygyria (many smaller than normal gyri), and it may be flattened due to hydrocephalus. There may be lacunae (or exaggerated bosselations resembling impressions of a ball peen hammer) on the inner table of the skull as well as scoliosis of the spine. This form of A-C malformation causes considerable disability due to paraplegia, complications of ventricular shunting for hydrocephalus, scoliosis and associated respiratory complications, and mental retardation. Occasionally, the diagnosis of A-C malformation is not made in life. Sudden unexpected death may occur from increased intracranial pressure in connection with a hypoxic episode, head trauma, or other condition, bringing the case to the forensic pathologist [250].

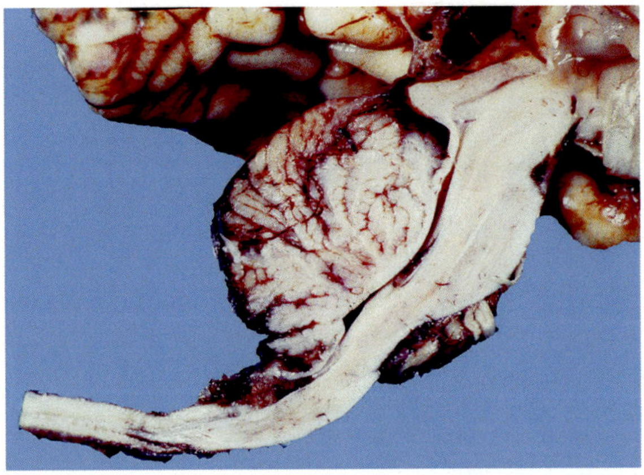

Figure 4.21 Sagittal section of the brain of a child with Arnold–Chiari type II malformation shows the typical beak-shaped quadrigeminal plate, the narrow cerebral aqueduct, and the small extruded cerebellum with a kink-like lesion at the upper cervical cord region. The pons is elongated and thin. Not shown is a hydrocephalic cerebrum.

The third type of A-C malformation shows all of the above defects of A-C type II, but in addition there is a high cervical myelomeningocele or occipital encephalocele. Such cases are rare, and the linkage with A-C in some cases has been disputed. A fourth form of A-C malformation has been suggested by Friede [2], in which there is severe hypoplasia of the cerebellum. Occasional examples can be encountered in adults [252,253].

The embryology of A-C malformation is complex and clearly involves interplay between the developing brain and spinal cord and its skeletal investment. A rather simplistic hypothesis has been proposed that the malformation is due to tethering of the developing cord in the spinal canal with subsequent traction of hindbrain and stem structures into the spinal canal, but this hypothesis is largely discredited [2]. At least one current experimental model for the A-C malformation exists [227,254], but the cause in humans remains unknown.

Dandy–Walker Malformation

The Dandy–Walker malformation [255–257] consists of a malformation of the cerebellum and posterior fossa in which the cerebellar vermis is either absent or has been pushed laterally by a cyst that arises out of the fourth ventricle compressing the cerebellum and distorting the occipital lobes of the brain (illustrated in midline section in Figure 4.22). There is usually severe hydrocephalus and an unusually shaped posterior fossa (Figure 4.23). Associated abnormalities include agenesis or destruction of all or part of the corpus callosum, micropolygyria in the cerebral cortex, heterotopic gray matter, and disorganization of medullary nuclei, including the inferior olivary nuclei [258,259]. The Dandy–Walker malformation is usually easily distinguished from the A-C malformation by the lack of myelomeningocele, basal skull abnormalities, the typical kinking and beak deformity of the brain stem, and the existence of the cerebellar vermis in the A-C malformation.

The Dandy–Walker malformation may cause death because of increased intracranial pressure and decompensated hydrocephalus; shunting will usually prevent such deaths,

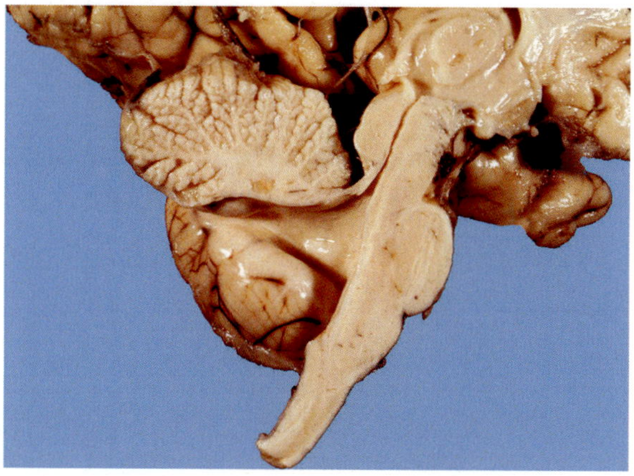

Figure 4.22 Typical Dandy–Walker malformation shown in sagittal section. Note virtual absence of the lower vermis and an exposed (thin cyst membrane has ruptured) fourth ventricle. (Courtesy of the Department of Pathology, Children's Memorial Hospital, Chicago.)

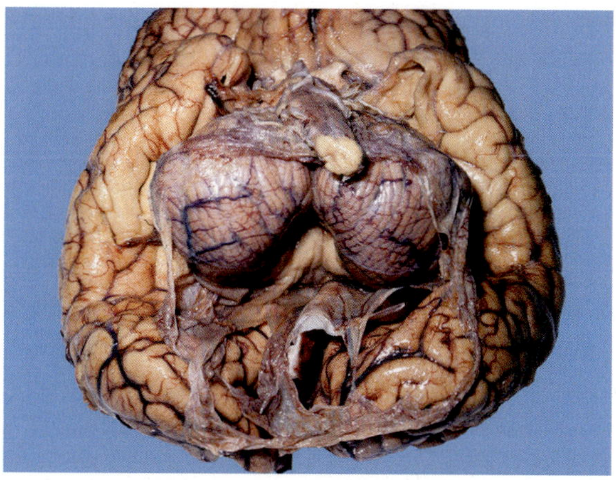

Figure 4.23 Another example of the Dandy–Walker malformation but in an adult homeless person found dead shows the remnants of the large posterior fossa cyst and absent inferior or posterior vermis with an open and smooth fourth ventricle. The brain is enlarged due to hydrocephalus. (Courtesy of the Office of the Medical Examiner, Cook County, IL.)

provided the condition is diagnosed. Occasionally, the condition is missed and discovered in a medical examiner/coroner's facility to be the cause of an unexpected death due to decompensated hydrocephalus [260,261]. The etiology for Dandy–Walker malformation is unknown, although attempts have been made to produce it in laboratory animals [258,262].

Agenesis of the Cerebellum

There are a number of conditions that affect the cerebellum and lead to some degree of atrophy. Most of these are not appreciated until later in life than childhood. These conditions, covered elsewhere, include alcoholic cerebellar degeneration, cerebellar atrophy in

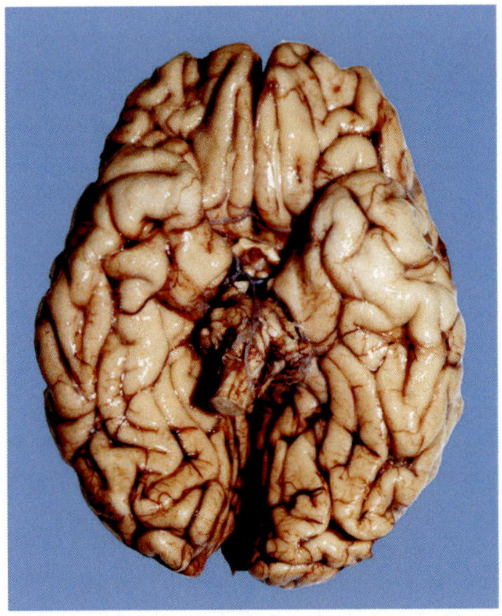

Figure 4.24 An example of near-total agenesis of the cerebellum, except for portions of the flocculonodular lobe. This adult died from an accidental electrocution. (Courtesy of the Institute of Forensic Sciences, San Juan, Puerto Rico.)

epilepsy, and the spinocerebellar degenerations. There are very uncommon syndromes, such as Marinesco–Sjøgren syndrome, Meckel syndrome [263], and Joubert's syndrome [264], that also produce some degree of cerebellar atrophy, but near-total cerebellar agenesis is very rare but can have forensic significance (Figure 4.24). In such cases the brain stem appears normal, but there is little or no cerebellum, and that which is represented appears to consist only of the flocculonodular lobes and perhaps a small amount of the vermis. Individuals who have this condition often are mentally deficient, although they seem to display little or no apparent ataxia and may come to attention of the forensic pathologist because of an accidental death [265].

Lhermitte–Duclos Disease

This unique condition, alternatively referred to as diffuse hyperplasia of the cerebellar cortex, gangliocytoma diffusum, or sometimes Purkinjeoma, manifests as a diffuse coarse rugation of the normally delicate cerebellar folia in one or portions of both hemispheres. In some ways the condition, although apparently malformative, behaves sometimes like a low-grade neoplasm gradually involving more and more of the cerebellar cortex [266–268]. Microscopically, in place of the normal folial architecture, the cortex appears inverted, with many large neurons resembling Purkinje cells and virtually no recognizable granular cell layer [2]. This distorted cerebellar cortex apparently has functional anatomic connections with cerebellar and brain stem nuclei. The forensic importance of the condition is that it may lead to a precipitous increase in intracranial pressure and decompensation much like that seen with colloid cysts of the third ventricle and may cause unexpected death. There may be associated cranial and other malformations, such as the so-called Cowen multiple hamartoma syndrome [268].

Holoprosencephaly and Arhinencephaly

Holoprosencephaly (Figure 4.25) is the most severe form of a malformation, resulting from failure of cleavage of parts of the face, forebrain, and olfactory system. The facial bones may be absent or defective; components of the nose, including the ethmoids, turbinates, vomer, sphenoids, and malar bones, may be absent or malformed; and the external appearance of the face may be grotesque [2,230,231]. The holoprosencephalic brain contains a single ventricle, one anterior cerebral artery, no olfactory nerves or tracts, and no fornix. The basal ganglia are fused, and the occipital areas are replaced by a membranous sac that communicates with the single ventricle, as illustrated in Figure 4.26 [245]. The brain caudal from the diencephalon is normal [23]. Lesser degrees of the malformation may be manifest by hypoteloric eyes; a large, flat nose with a single nostril; cleft lip or palate; absence of olfactory nerves and tracts; and perhaps a single cerebral ventricle. Occasionally, there may a single or fused eye, sometimes with a proboscis on the forehead. Defective separation of the hemispheres may be complete as in alobar holoprosencephaly or partial as in lobar holoprosencephaly. In some individuals, apart from hypotelorism and absence of the olfactory bulbs and tracts, there is no other abnormality.

The lesion forms during the fifth gestational week and usually has been associated with trisomy of the 13–15 group of chromosomes, but it can be associated also with trisomy or abnormal forms of chromosome 18 and may occur with a normal karyotype [269,270]. Malformations of the limbs and cardiac, gastrointestinal, and urogenital systems are common and are usually incompatible with survival past the perinatal period. An incomplete form of this syndrome, arrhinencephaly, is possible, in which only the olfactory bulbs and tracts are absent, with no other obvious malformation of the brain, face, or other organs. Such cases are usually found incidentally at autopsy.

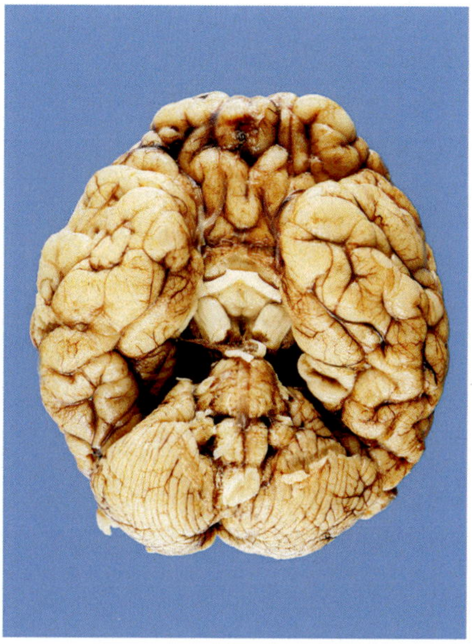

Figure 4.25 Basal view of the brain of a baby with holoprosencephaly illustrating the lack of olfactory bulbs and tracts, and a generally round shape to the brain. (Courtesy of the Department of Pathology, Children's Memorial Hospital, Chicago.)

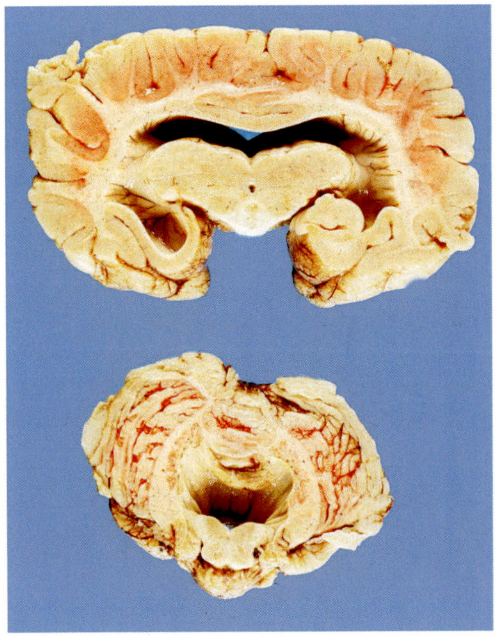

Figure 4.26 Coronal sections of a brain with holoprosencephaly showing the lack of a septum pellucidum, and a large single enlarged ventricular chamber with a large fourth ventricle in the cerebellum.

Agenesis of the Corpus Callosum

This malformation of the brain involves partial or complete absence of the corpus callosum associated with atrophy or dysgenesis of the cingulate gyri and a peculiar but distinctive appearance of the lateral ventricles, which resemble a bat's wing [271] (see Figure 4.27). The fornices and other commissures are often malformed [272,273]. As with any other CNS

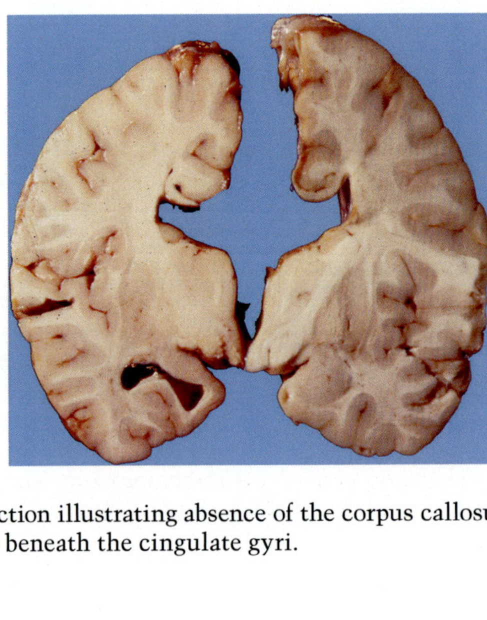

Figure 4.27 Coronal section illustrating absence of the corpus callosum, although there appear to be atrophic remnants beneath the cingulate gyri.

malformation, there may be cortical abnormalities or heterotopias as well. The clinical significance of this malformation may be subtle but usually involves mental subnormality. Individuals in families where the malformation may be inherited may show a hemispheric disconnection syndrome. Occasionally, artifacts of brain removal and dissection can produce what appears to be agenesis of the corpus callosum because of the extreme softness of the infant brain and poor handling that may disrupt the corpus callosum. In some cases of severe cortical malformations, such as schizencephaly, or with large porencephalic cysts, the axons that should have contributed to the corpus callosum do not exist or have atrophied, giving the appearance of agenesis. Imaging studies such as ultrasound examinations and later MRI or CT scans may show disappearance of the corpus callosum as encephaloclastic processes evolved.

Cavum of the Septum Pellucidum

This "malformation" is probably better considered as an anatomic variant than a lesion in most instances and involves the persistence of a space between the leaves of the septum pellucidum. In the infant, a cavum is normally present but usually disappears with maturation. Some degree of a cavum of the septum pellucidum (so-called fifth ventricle) is seen in easily 30% of adults and usually involves the anterior portion of the septum [272]. Occasionally, the space may involve the whole of the septum and extend posteriorally; then it is referred to as a *cavum vergae* [245]. The cavities formed within the septum are not true ventricular spaces and are not lined by ependymal cells but, rather, by pavemented glia. They are rarely of significance, although examples causing clinical symptoms have been described. Occasionally, a cavum may enlarge through mechanisms that are unclear, distorting or obstructing the foramina of Monro and producing obstructive hydrocephalus that leads to sudden unexpected death in much the same manner as colloid cysts. Such an example is illustrated in Figure 4.28.

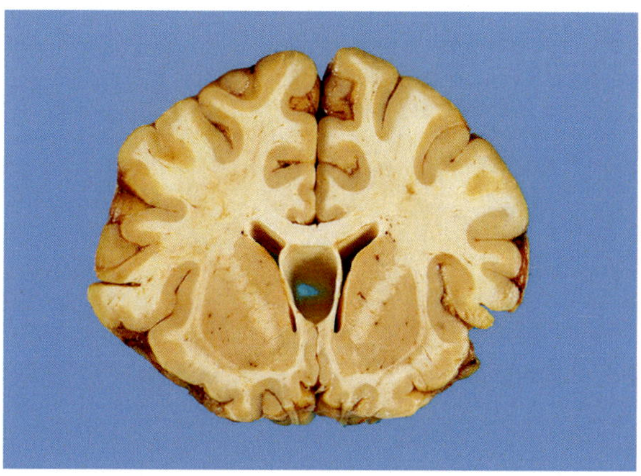

Figure 4.28 Coronal brain section illustrating a large cavum of the septum pellucidum found incidentally at autopsy. Such lesions are commonly found incidentally and generally have no clinical significance.

Agyria–Pachygyria–Lissencephaly

All of these terms refer to either complete absence of cortical gyri (agyria, lissencephaly) or a nearly smooth brain surface with only very large, coarse gyri (pachygyric convolutions) [274], as illustrated in Figure 4.29. The malformed cortex is believed to be caused by an aberration in neuronal migration and of the process that normally produces infolding of the gyri [275–277]. Until 4 months' gestation, the brain is smooth. Then infolding and gyration commence so that by 36 weeks' gestation the brain surface has all the anatomical landmarks found in the adult brain [19]. The variations in pachygyric–lissencephalic brains are considerable, but most cases show a smaller-than-normal brain, usually with a normal-appearing brain stem and cerebellum. In a cut section, the cortical mantle is usually a centimeter or more in thickness. Microscopic examination of a lissencephalic or macrogyric cortex may reveal some semblance of lamellation [278,279], which changes with depth to a columnar or finger-like pattern of neurons. Ectopic islands of cortical matter may exist below the cortex in whatever white matter exists. The corpus callosum may be absent. Not all areas of the cortex may be affected, and there is a tendency for the basal cerebral cortex, including the hippocampal formations, to be relatively normal.

Associated visceral malformations such as cardiac defects, renal agenesis, or other genitourinary malformations may be seen [280]. The causes for these malformations, like other CNS malformations, are probably multifactorial, with some cases having a familial pattern, but others are due to a chromosomal abnormality [280,281], and still others are associated with intrauterine infections. However, most cases remain unexplained. These malformations are not necessarily lethal, and many affected individuals, although mentally subnormal, may survive into adulthood. Such cases may be encountered on a forensic service because affected persons may be found dead, possibly related to sudden unexpected death in epilepsy (SUDEP; discussed in Chapter 9) [282].

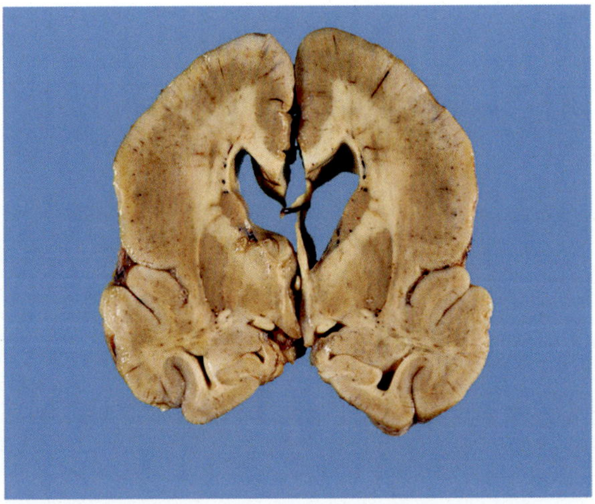

Figure 4.29 Coronal brain section illustrating a virtually smooth rostral brain (lissencephaly) with relatively normal-appearing temporal lobe architecture and basal ganglia. The affected cortex is many times the normal thickness and often contains a columnar rather than a lamellated structure. (Courtesy of the Department of Pathology, Northwestern Memorial Hospital, Chicago.)

Micropolygyria

This cortical malformation is, as the name implies, a condition where there are many small gyri. The typical appearance of micropolygyria is illustrated in Figures 4.30 and 4.31. The malformation occurs frequently in combination with other cortical malformations, including lissencephaly, schizencephaly, the Arnold–Chiari and Dandy–Walker malformations, porencephaly, and other conditions [2]. Micropolygyria (or polymicrogyria, according to individual preference) implies that the cortical neurons have at least migrated to the cortical surface but something has interfered with appropriate lamellation, and differentiation [278]. This interference may be genetically mediated, due to chromosomal abnormalities [280], or may be caused by an intrauterine infection or exposure to radiation or toxins that disrupt the orderly process of differentiation [2,283]. The lesion can be diffuse or focal. Microscopic examination reveals small, sometimes cauliflower-like, cortical gyri with abnormal lamellation or cortical organization [215]. Owing to the diversity of

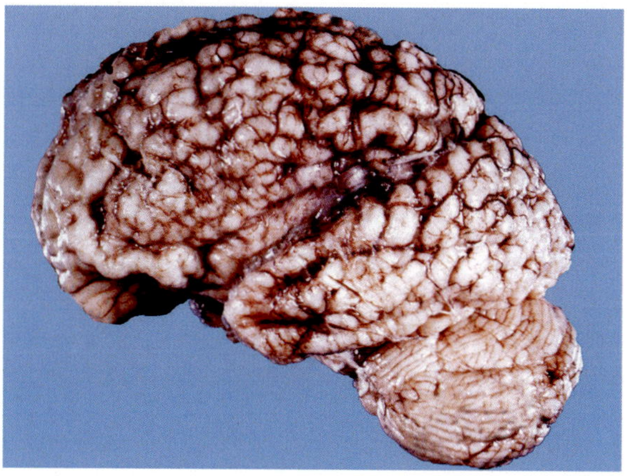

Figure 4.30 Lateral view of the brain showing an extensive pattern of micropolygyria with a smaller-than-normal brain mass compared with that of the cerebellum, which shows no abnormality.

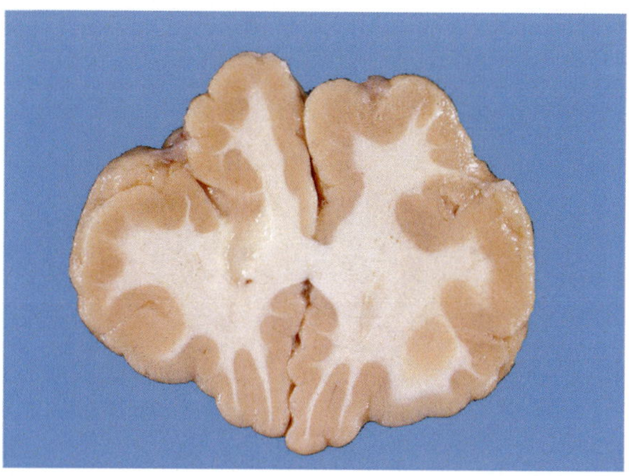

Figure 4.31 Coronal section of a brain with micropolygria illustrating the cauliflower foliations of the cortex in the affected areas more rostrally in the brain. The more inferior portions have a normal or more normal appearance.

etiology and severity of the malformation, there is no consistent clinical presentation of symptoms, although many individuals with micropolygyria suffer from mental subnormality, cerebral palsy, seizure disorders, and other neurological or functional disorders. Foci of micropolygyria may be found in apparently normal individuals, may be the cause for epileptic seizures, and may be found in individuals who experience sudden and unexpected death (see Chapter 9).

Heterotopia–Ectopia

Occasionally, masses of gray matter are found in locations where they should not normally appear and, as such, clearly indicate some disorder of neuronal migration and maturation [284]. These masses may be single small foci or may consist of multiple or even diffuse collections in many areas of the brain [2]. The most common sites are around the margins of the ventricles in the white matter of the cerebral hemispheres and below or connected with the cortex (Figure 4.32). Bilateral symmetry of ectopias is common. This may be especially evident in ectopias of the temporal lobe, where bilateral distortion of the amygdala and hippocampal formation may occur. Functional connections of these heterotopic masses with adjacent structures are probably the rule because many affected individuals suffer epileptic seizures. Such lesions may be found at autopsy in individuals who die suddenly and unexpectedly with seizures [282,285] and in victims of traffic accidents (see Chapter 9), where a seizure while driving may have caused the accident.

Megalencephaly and Hemimegalencephaly

In the strict sense of the word, megalencephaly defines a larger-than-normal brain by weight. Simple volume expansion is usually due to hydrocephalus of one form or another or may be due to cavitation of the white matter from periventricular leukomalacia and accompanying hydrocephalus, or it may be the result of massive cystic degeneration of the white matter, as in Alexander's disease [101] or Canavan disease [286]. The more traditional forms of megalencephaly involve the mass expansion beyond normal brain weights due to

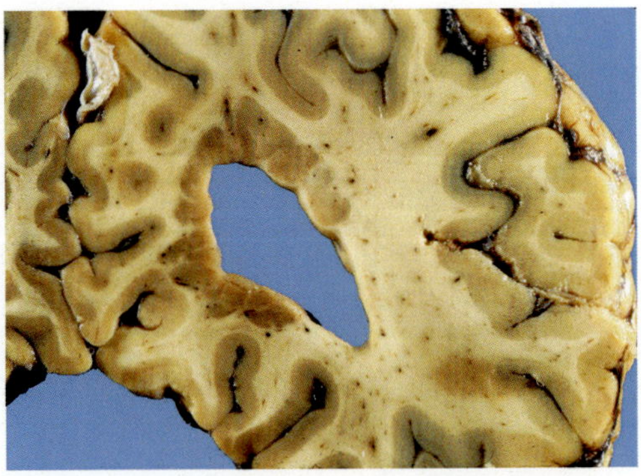

Figure 4.32 Coronal section revealing a nodular formation of ectopic gray matter near the ventricular margin. Not infrequently, the ectopias are bilateral and often are close to or involve the hippocampal/amygdaloid region. Such individuals usually have epilepsy and may die unexpectedly without obvious anatomic cause (SUDEP).

proliferation of neural elements in an organized or poorly organized manner. Some forms of megalencephaly show cortical malformations like micropolygyria, macrogyria, or even lissencephaly and often show some elements of cellular migration anomalies with ectopia of gray matter [287]. It is not unexpected that in such cases seizure disorders and mental retardation are common.

There is a body of cases in which one half of the brain appears to be normal while the other hemisphere is enlarged—hemimegalencephaly. Most such cases are discovered in infancy or childhood and are characterized by loss of developmental milestones and progressively intractable seizures [288,289]. Histologically, there may be disordered cortical architecture and other signs of migrational dysfunction [290] that seem to progress over time. Therapeutic interventions are often poorly satisfactory, and hemispherectomy has shown promise, provided all elements of the dysplastic cortex are removed [289].

The forensic importance of such conditions is that because of the prevalence of seizures in the victims of whatever form of megalencephaly is present, sudden unexpected deaths (SUDEPs) are common, as are accidental deaths in connection with seizures, such as drowning, aspiration, and trauma. Often, the conditions are not discovered until autopsy. An extensive discussion of the SUDEP phenomenon can be found in Chapter 9.

Arachnoid Cysts

Cysts of the arachnoid membrane occur at cerebral, spinal, and cerebellar sites [291,292] and are considered to be of developmental origin arising at about 3 months' gestation, when the subarachnoid space is opening and CSF pathways are developing. These are relatively frequent lesions occurring in or about the Sylvian fissure (49% of cases), cerebellopontine angle (11%), supracollicular region (10%), cerebellar vermis (9%), sellar region (9%), interhemispheric region (5%), cerebral convexity region (4%), or clival region (3%) [292,293]. Some report that arachnoid cysts always occur at or near the locations of expected cisterns and may be derived from them [291]. The cysts are thin-walled membranous sacs composed of apparently split arachnoid membranes and may increase progressively in size and indent and compress the brain wherever they occur (illustrated in Figures 4.33 and 4.34). The pressure of the cyst may produce focal neurological signs and seizures or obstruction

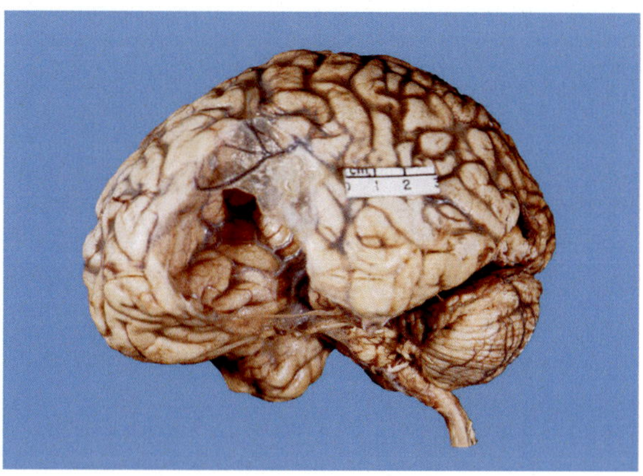

Figure 4.33 Lateral view of the brain illustrating a large arachnoid cyst involving the anterior temporal lobe/Sylvian fissure region. This lesion was found incidentally at autopsy.

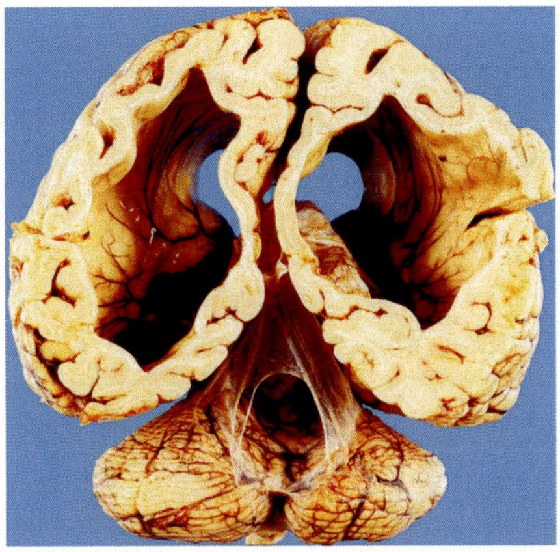

Figure 4.34 Coronal section of the brain illustrating a large arachnoid cyst that involves the pineal region and rostral cerebellum. This lesion obstructed the cerebral aqueduct and produced profound hydrocephalus. Such cases can present with sudden unexpected death or death following minor head trauma. (Courtesy of the Office of the Medical Examiner, Cook County, IL.)

to the flow of CSF, and hydrocephalus may lead to sudden unexpected death [294]. Because arachnoid cysts may represent a sequestered volume of CSF, the cyst may act like a mass lesion and cause decompensation, which may be misinterpreted as child abuse. Arachniod cysts may be associated with subdural hematomas that may have arisen with minimal trauma in children and infants [180,212,295]. When an arachnoid cyst is encountered, it usually contains watery clear fluid, but occasionally it may contain hemorrhagic fluid. Usually relatively normal-appearing, although flattened, cerebral cortex lies beneath the cyst wall. The cyst does not contain septations or divisions [295]. Sometimes, arachnoid cysts can occur with or be confused with porencephalic cysts. Although most of them are considered developmental, some may arise following inflammatory or infectious processes in the meninges where fibrosis produces loculation or where one-way valves between the lumen and the subarachnoid space have developed due to fibrosis. Familial occurrences of these cysts have also been reported [296]. Other cystic lesions of the brain that are unrelated to arachnoid cysts may include teratomatous cysts with respiratory or gastrointestinal epithelium resembling arachnoid cysts of the spinal canal [38]. Instances have been reported in which arachnoid cysts have apparently ruptured into the subdural space (border zone) and produced a subdural hematoma [212,295,297].

Hydranencephaly

This class of lesions is often referred to as encephaloclastic and may result from presumed infarctions or the devastating effects of infectious agents such as a toxoplasmosis, cytomegalovirus (CMV), and sometimes other agents. Very frequently, a precise etiology cannot be arrived at. On the one hand, if damage to the brain is restricted, the process may blend imperceptibly with malformations owing to the plasticity of the brain at the time of the injury. Some of these types of conditions are discussed below in the context of malformations, which is how they appear, such as porencephaly. Others that are more clearly massively destructive include hydranencephaly, which could be considered an extreme form of porencephaly, in which virtually the entire telencephalon (cerebral hemispheres) has

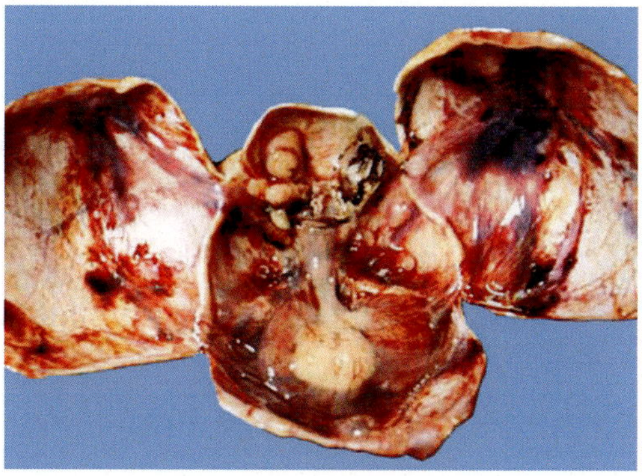

Figure 4.35 The open cranial cavity of an infant with hydranencephaly illustrates the near absence of the cerebrum due to destruction. There is some preservation of the cerebellum and brain stem structures. (Courtesy of Department of Pathology, Children's Memorial Hospital, Chicago.)

been destroyed by an intrauterine insult [2,245,298]. The brain is largely represented as a fluid-filled membranous sac that fills the skull (Figure 4.35). Sometimes, small islands of cortical tissue remain, usually in the basal portions or along the superior sagittal region of what once was the brain, giving the appearance of an empty basket, with a preserved loop of cortex appearing like a basket handle (sometimes referred to as basket brain). The basal ganglia and diencephalon, as well as the brain stem, eyes, optic nerves, and cerebellum, are usually preserved and appear relatively normal. The condition is usually lethal, discovered at or shortly after birth, but occasional examples of prolonged survival have been reported, especially if there is some preservation of the hypothalamus. The external appearance of the head may be normal or abnormal. The cause of hydranencephaly is presumed to be secondary to a massive infarction, possibly in connection with abnormal revision of the major cerebral vessels [299]. In some cases intrauterine infection due to CMV or toxoplasmosis has been demonstrated. Mineralization in surviving neural tissue may be extensive.

It is clear that hydranencephaly generally represents a near-total destructive process occurring well before birth but after the brain has formed and allowed a more-or-less normal-appearing cranium, with the process essentially completed by the time it is discovered [298]. Other circumstances result in infarction of the brain closer to birth with the resultant processes still in evolution. The expected complications of pregnancy are often the most logical explanations, such as placental abruption, placenta previa, twin fetuses with uneven shared circulation, and knotted or other problems with the umbilical cord [129,300,301].

Porencephaly

Porencephaly may be congenital or acquired, reflecting a destructive process, usually intrauterine, which has destroyed a portion of the brain, leaving a hole covered with a membrane extending to the ventricle, as illustrated in Figure 4.36. Such defects may be single or multiple and symmetrical, such that one may virtually look from side to side through the brain in the specimen or, via transillumination of the skull in the living infant, perceive increased luminescence over the defects. In most cases there is no external manifestation in the skull or head to suggest their existence in the underlying brain. These defects are probably caused by highly destructive processes (vascular accidents or infectious processes)

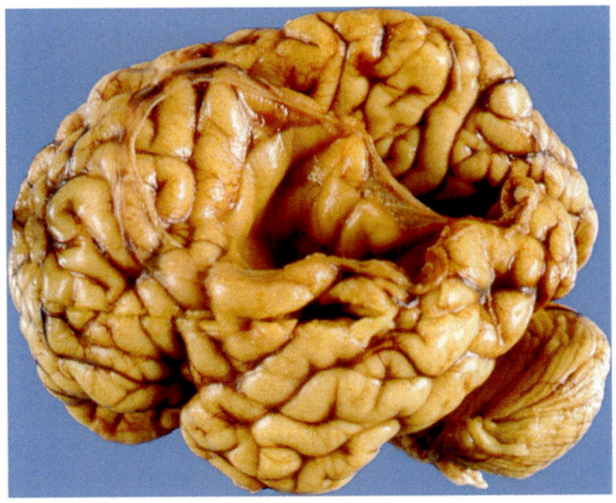

Figure 4.36 Lateral view of the brain illustrating a large porencephalic cavity that replaces a large portion of the left parietal lobe and possesses a smooth-walled margin and a partial cystic remnant of once-existent cerebral cortex.

that occur rather late in brain development (probably third trimester) and leave much of the remaining brain intact [2,112,298]. Infants with porencephaly may appear normal at birth but eventually show some abnormality of their cry, movement, or response to their environment, and in later life, should they survive, they will likely show mental and developmental retardation.

Grossly, porencephaly is represented by a rather large, laterally placed hole in the brain that is covered by a thin membrane enclosing a cavity filled with clear fluid. The cavity may or may not communicate with the ventricles and may be bilateral. Some have subclassified porencephalies according to the morphology of the clefts [245]. The margins of the cavity, usually lined by astrocytes rather than ependyma, show some remodeling of the adjacent brain and occasionally foci of micropolygyria or other cortical abnormality, but the adjacent cortex may be entirely normal, reflecting the late development of the lesion [298]. There is usually little evidence of the cause of the lesion, but occasionally residua of inflammatory or infectious process remain, such as cysts of toxoplasmosis or inclusion-bearing cells or glial nodules that suggest intrauterine CMV infection. The most commonly accepted cause of porencephaly is a prenatal cerebral infarction, perhaps due to aberrant vascular revision [112,302,303]. Cases have been reported in which porencephaly has been apparently caused by misadventures during diagnostic amniocentesis [304].

The clinical manifestations of porencephaly are highly variable, from severe mental retardation and cerebral palsy to no clinical symptoms at all. The lesions are frequently discovered incidentally at autopsy, sometimes in the forensic setting. An example of this is the following case:

> A 30-year-old derelict was found dead on the street, having apparently died of a head injury after a fall. He was known to have had a severe limp that hampered his movements. Autopsy examination revealed flexion contracture and disuse atrophy of the right arm and leg and a skull fracture with acute subdural hematoma. He also had a large porencephalic cyst of the left cerebral hemisphere. Toxicological studies were negative. From witness accounts, it emerged that the individual had apparently lost his balance while walking along a loading dock and had fallen about 6 feet to the pavement. It appeared that the disability caused by his porencephaly contributed to his fatal fall.

Schizencephaly

It is appropriate to consider brains with developmental clefts, unilateral or bilateral, as part of the spectrum that includes hydranencephaly and porencephaly because all of these conditions have some element of tissue death and repair in varying degrees. The cleft into the cerebral cortex generally occurs near the Sylvian fissure, usually in the frontal lobes, and may display a deep visible channel into or up to the ventricle (so-called open-lip schizencephaly) (Figure 4.37), or the cleft may be more narrow and the deeper recesses of the cleft not visible until the brain is sectioned (so-called closed-lip schizencephaly) [305–308]. Bordering on the cleft, there is usually dysplastic abnormal cortex showing macrogyria or micropolygyria [23,245], which are likely due to an injury to the brain in which some degree of cortical plasticity remained. Clefts are often symmetrical and bilateral (Figure 4.38). There may be varying degrees of white matter loss, cystic or not, and it is not uncommon to observe thinning of the corpus callosum due to axonal loss. Hydrocephalus is common.

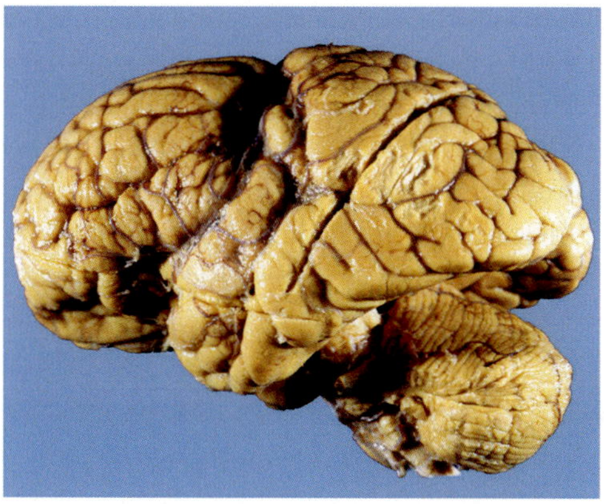

Figure 4.37 Lateral view of the brain showing a prominent schizencephalic cleft that effectively delimits the frontal from the parietal lobes. Abnormally small gyri bound the lower margins of this cleft.

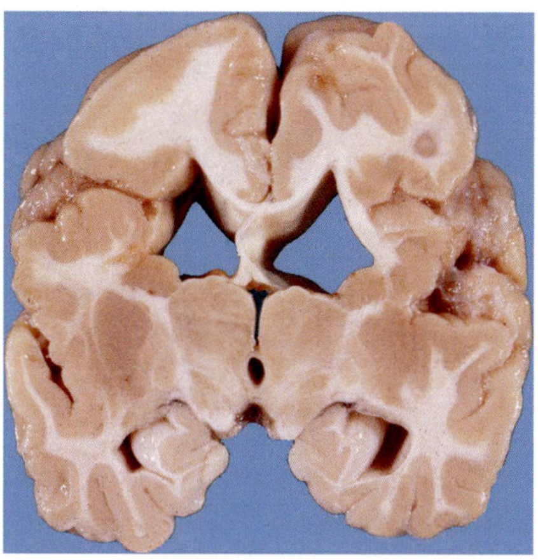

Figure 4.38 Coronal section of a brain with bilateral, roughly symmetrical schizencephalic clefts showing abnormal complex cortex at the depths of the clefts and some ventricular enlargement.

Often, until imaging studies are done, affected infants are labeled with the designation of cerebral palsy. Mental retardation and developmental delay, as well as seizures, are common. Infants, because of the lesions, may show arthrogryposis and asymmetry of extremities and deformations of the feet because there is insufficient motor innervation during development.

Various forms of schizencephaly may be found in stillborn infants, suspected SIDS cases, cases in which some form of parental abuse is suspected, and epilepsy-related deaths. Although this series of malformations is comparatively rare, they often appear on a forensic service and are not discovered until an autopsy has been done.

Hydrocephaly

Hydrocephaly is a common condition that can be congenital or acquired. When congenital, it occurs in between 0.8 and 1 case per 1000 live births in Sweden and in recent years appears to be decreasingly prevalent [309]. In the simplest sense, hydrocephalus is defined by increased ventricular volume, with or without increased intraventricular pressure [310]. In compensated hydrocephalus, the ventricles have dilated to accommodate any increases in pressure to establish equilibrium where there is little change in the CSF volume. In examining a brain with hydrocephalus at autopsy, there are two observations to be made: the first is to define the etiology of the hydrocephalus, if possible, and the second is to determine if the hydrocephalus was responsible for or contributed to death. The consequences, appearances, and physiology of the intracranial pressure/volume equilibrium and increased intracranial pressure, including hydrocephalus, are considered in detail in Chapter 5.

The etiologies of hydrocephalus [2,245,310–312] include obstruction to the flow of CSF (obstructive hydrocephalus), possible increased CSF production (as has been suggested to occur with choroid plexus papilloma or venous obstruction), conditions retarding absorption of CSF or transport of CSF (communicating hydrocephalus), or loss of tissue anywhere in the brain that has resulted in a compensatory ventricular enlargement (hydrocephalus *ex vacuo*) [245]. Time of occurrence of hydrocephaly in children appears to be prenatal in more than half of cases, with the remainder occurring in the peri-postnatal period [309].

A common form of neonatal obstructive hydrocephalus is aqueductal stenosis, which may be familial in boys [313] or may be due to intrauterine viral infection (possibly mumps), which results in damage to the ependyma and scarring of the aqueduct [314,315]. Other common causes of neonatal hydrocephalus include brain tumors, vascular malformations, the Arnold–Chiari and Dandy–Walker malformations, as well as arachnoid cysts [245,312].

In so-called communicating hydrocephalus [312], the basis of the lesion is usually impedance to the flow of CSF or to absorption by whatever mechanisms. The most common conditions giving rise to this situation are prior infection or inflammation of the meninges, such as an infectious meningitis, or subarachnoid bleeding of any cause that has led to scarring of the subarachnoid space [195] (see Chapter 5). Premature infants who have had a germinal matrix/intraventricular hemorrhage are at significant risk for later development of hydrocephalus due to scarring and reactions in the ependyma, subarachnoid space, and arachnoid granulations. This can have forensic significance when such a child has not been followed for this possibility, and then decompensates, often with findings that may suggest the possibility of abuse, sometimes in the context of a reported minor traumatic episode [142,143,316].

When hydrocephalus is associated with increased intracranial pressure, there may be changes in the skull as a result of brain expansion, such as separation of sutures; bulging fontanels; or erosion, thinning, and bosselation of the skull. If there are associated cysts or fluid-filled membranous sacs (chronic subdural hematomas—hygromas, dural effusions, or leptomeningeal cysts), these structures may compress the brain stem, cerebellum, or parts of the cerebrum. If intracranial pressures have risen rapidly and unilaterally, herniation of the brain, and Duret hemorrhage may occur (see Chapter 3) [175]. In such cases, with or without Duret hemorrhage, in rapidly evolving hydrocephalus or hydrocephalus that has reached the limits of compensation, the risks of respiratory embarrassment and sudden death are significant [143,316]. There are many consequences of rapid rises in intracranial pressure of whatever the cause that gives rise to a number of secondary and tertiary phenomena in the brain and elsewhere. These may include consequences of respirator failure: brain hypoxia and associated cerebral edema with worsening of intracranial pressure, production of seizures with its deleterious consequences, cardiac hypoxemia with cardiac failure, and multiorgan failure. By mechanisms that are poorly understood, a rapid increase in intracranial pressure may produce retinal hemorrhages, which to some strongly suggest inflicted trauma, but which is not specific for this event [317]. When an individual is hydrocephalic for whatever reason, very small incremental volume increases anywhere intracranially from any cause, perhaps as little as 1–2 ml in an infant, can cause herniation and decompensation [318–320]. Sometimes, minimal head trauma to an individual with hydrocephalus can result in collapse and even death [142,143,316].

A common, often life-saving procedure in hydrocephalus is to insert a shunt to divert CSF from the ventricles of the brain usually into the peritoneum, which has even been performed in a fetus *in utero* [321]. An unfortunate property of shunts is that they frequently become obstructed at the ventricular end by the choroid plexus or glial scar tissue, which may grow into the shunt tube openings, or if the shunt withdraws or advances into the brain. Such an event necessitates surgical revision of the shunt until it functions properly again [322]. Shunt malfunction may also occur at the distal end in the peritoneum or in the atrium of the heart if those are the sites of drainage. Infections may be transmitted via the shunt device, causing a host of complications. Because multiple surgical procedures are often required for shunt maintenance and foreign material is involved in the shunt, infection is a constant risk, which may lead to abscess formation, meningitis, peritonitis, or systemic sepsis [323].

It is not uncommon for ventricular shunts to be patent but malfunction from either too much or too little CSF flow. Complications from poor flow regulation can produce debilitating headaches, dizziness and vertigo, nausea and vomiting, and, in rare instances, when too much CSF is drained, subdural hemorrhages [323,324]. Shunt malfunctions may have serious consequences and may result in sudden and unexpected death [325].

From a forensic point of view, if a child, or for that matter an adult, who has had a venticular shunt dies under circumstances that include possible head trauma (minor or otherwise), is found dead, or dies under other circumstances apparently unrelated to an obvious other disease process, it is vital that a proper neuropathological examination be made to assess the status of a shunt (both proximal and distal) and to preserve the device, especially if there is ventricular enlargement. Persons with shunts may or may not outgrow their need for them, and when they malfunction, even after many years of apparently no problems, serious consequences may result. Decompensation may be rapid and may not be correctly diagnosed clinically [143].

Embolism, Thrombosis, and Hemorrhage

Embolism

Embolic states are mostly due to some pathology in the heart, usually of a congenital basis (cyanotic heart disease accounts for about 26% of infarction cases) [127]. Valve disease and endocarditis, as well as postcardiac surgical complications, are also common precursors. Infectious or inflammatory conditions of the vessels themselves cause a number of stroke cases, such as polyarteritis, lupus erythematosus, fungal infections, and bacterial arteritis. Other conditions, such as moya-moya, Takayasu disease, tuberous sclerosis, neurofibromatosis, vascular anomalies, and disorders of collagen/elastin, constitute a rare group of stroke etiologies. Another way of thinking about embolic/thrombotic phenomena is to consider not so much the heart or the vessels but the blood within and conditions that can cause it to clot or extravasate. Important in this regard are the hemoglobinopathies, such as sickle-cell disease (homozygous or heterzygous) [127,326], congenital clotting factor deficiencies (factors V (Leiden), VIII, IX, XIII), vitamin K deficiency, protein C and S deficiencies, platelet abnormalities, and antithrombin III deficiency [127,128]. A number of inherited metabolic defects (homocystinemia; MTHFR C677T mutation [327]), and other amino acidemias, some disorders of lipid metabolism) can be at fault [127]. An outline of the processes involved in coagulation may assist the reader in conceptualizing the complexity of the processes (Figure 4.39).

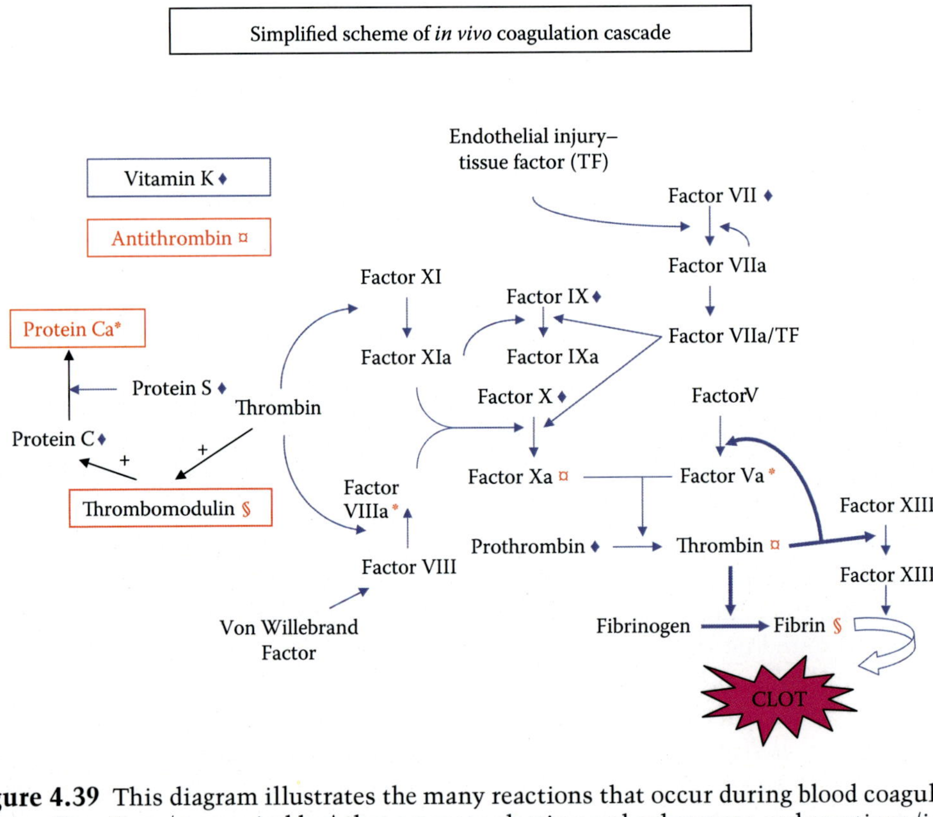

Figure 4.39 This diagram illustrates the many reactions that occur during blood coagulation *in vivo*. Reactions (arrows in blue) that promote clotting and substances and reactions (in red) that inhibit coagulation are illustrated.

Cerebral Venous and Sinus Thrombosis

Cerebral venous and venous sinus thrombosis represents a troublesome problem in infancy from both a clinical diagnostic and forensic point of view because it is often not recognized as the basis for symptoms and deaths. Common symptoms and signs are seizures (55%–58%), fever (32%), decreased level of consciousness (26%–44%), respiratory distress (29%), vomiting (19%), a variety of neurological deficits (42%), and papilledema (12%–13%) [28]. The condition is said to occur in 0.67 cases per 100,000 infants per year in Canada [25,328]. Fifty-four percent of cases affect children younger than 1 year and usually younger than 3 months. When cerebral venous thrombosis occurs in the perinatal period, it usually occurs within a week of birth [328,329]. Clinical diagnosis often rests on awareness of the phenomenon and can be confirmed using a variety of imaging techniques, such as MRI, MR venography, Doppler ultrasonography, and related methods [25,328].

Thrombosis can occur in single or multiple cortical veins alone or in combination with contiguous or separate thrombosis of portions of or the entire superior sagittal sinus. Venous sinuses at the cranial base may be affected alone or with other venous thromboses. If the occlusion of major venous channels is complete, the results can be devastating, with patterns of venous infarction in the brain that can affect paramedian cortex and white matter extensively or focally. If thrombosis of the great vein of Galen occurs, bilateral pulvinar and posterior thalamic venous hemorrhagic infarcts can occur (Figure 4.40). If the cavernous sinus is totally or partially thrombosed, pronounced orbital swelling and congestion may result, and if other basal sinuses are affected, venous infarctions of basal brain structures can result. Lesser thromboses, primarily of cortical veins, may or may not produce venous infarctions but can produce profound congestion and edema, which may be misinterpreted radiologically and grossly at autopsy for contusions and thus due to trauma (Figure 4.40). The degree of edema that may result from even a focal cortical venous thrombosis may produce decompensation, herniation, and death and may be misinterpreted for a contusion with associated edema due to trauma. It is apparently not uncommon that various patterns of retinal hemorrhage can occur with cerebral venous thrombosis, further complicating the interpretation of the case because many pathologists and clinicians regard, probably mistakenly, that retinal hemorrhages are persuasive markers for abusive head injury [330–332].

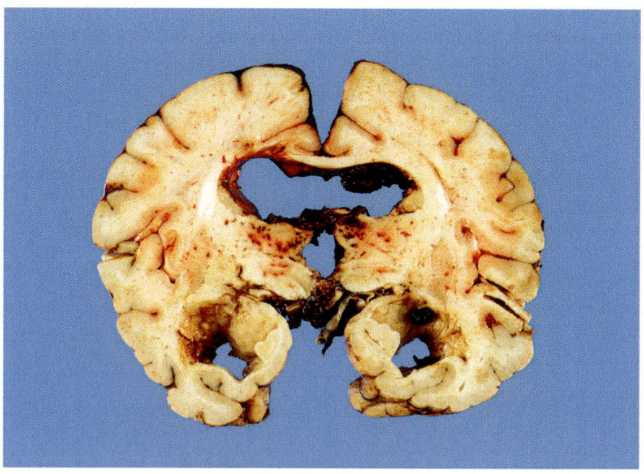

Figure 4.40 Coronal section illustrating hemorrhagic venous infarction and intraventricular hemorrhage caused by a great vein of Galen thrombosis in a child.

There are numerous conditions that can give rise to cerebral venous thrombosis in infancy. Commonly, several of the following occur together to cause thrombosis: fever, dehydration, sepsis or infection proximate to a venous sinus, and coagulopathy. Inherited disorders of clotting factors may also contribute (factor V (Leiden), factors VIII and XIII, protein S or C deficiency, and others) [25,26,28,329,333]. Any condition that produces coagulopathy can, by itself, induce cerebral venous thrombosis [333]. This surely includes ischemic/hypoxia global brain damage from any cause and diffuse brain trauma. In the infant who has brain injury of whatever cause and is sustained by mechanical ventilation because of increased intracranial pressure and brain stem dysfunction, coagulopathy is very commonly present, and it is not uncommon to discover cortical vein or sagittal sinus thrombosis at autopsy. In such cases, these findings must be carefully documented and sampled histologically so that it may be possible to age and date the thrombi. At the thrombus–vessel wall interface, inflammation, fibrinoid change, fibroblast formation, or macrophage reactions strongly support an antemortem thrombus rather than a postmortem one.

Disorders of Hemostasis

Introduction

The process of hemostasis is exceedingly complex and exists within equilibrium between the forces that cause blood to clot and those that keep it liquid and flowing. On the one hand, schemes have been proposed for blood clotting *in vitro* that certainly have applications for laboratory coagulation studies and evolution of certain concepts; on the other hand, there is a scheme that appears to represent the *in vivo* cascade. The latter is presented in Figure 4.41 as a conceptual base for the following discussion to provide a context for understanding.

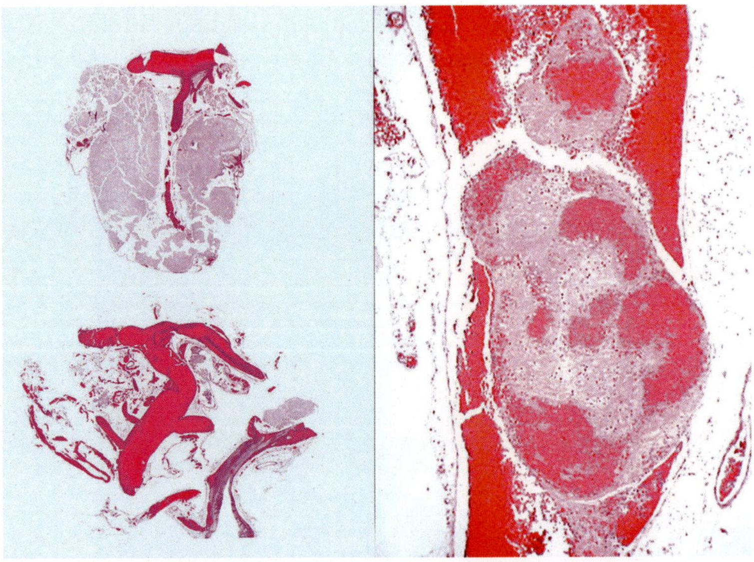

Figure 4.41 (Left) Low-power photomicrograph of obviously dilated and congested cortical veins and a vein in the right lower portion that contains an antemortem thrombus. (Right) Same but illustrated at high power.

Vitamin K Deficiency

Vitamin K is an essential fat-soluble vitamin found in green vegetables and produced in the gut by intestinal flora. It is a critical element in blood clotting and antithrombosis, interacting with factors VII, IX, X, and prothrombin as well as proteins S and C. Vitamin K deficiency in the first week of extrauterine life is quite common and has been prevented from reaching clinical significance by prophylactic administration of the vitamin in the nursery [334]. This practice widely employed in the United States is not followed in many other countries. When the deficiency leads to clinical detection (hemorrhagic disease of the newborn), it presents as bleeding from mucous membranes, skin, and sites of incision or vascular access. Retroperitoneal and intracranial hemorrhages may occur but are uncommon manifestations of the syndrome, but in one Asian country the incidence of intracranial complications with neurological deficits was reported to affect 42% of surviving babies [335]. In a study performed in Germany, 108 cases that occurred over a 10-year period revealed that males were affected about twice as often as females, with the peak being between 3 and 7 weeks of age. In this group, more than half of the cases had intracranial bleeding, with a neurological morbidity rate of 21% and a mortality rate of 19% [336]. The prothrombin time (PT) and the partial thromboplastin time (PTT) are prolonged.

Vitamin K deficiency can occur with birth or be acquired at other ages, by means of depression of gut flora by antibiotics, inadequate intake, malabsorption, hereditary defects in vitamin K utilization, or antagonists. Although anticoagulation using warfarin is rarely an issue in the neonate, it directly inhibits the action of vitamin K, as do some antibiotics directly. Inherited defects in vitamin K utilization have been reported to occur in combination with deficiencies of prothrombin and factors VII, IX, and X [32]. There are many protocols for the treatment of vitamin K deficiency [337]. The forensic importance of vitamin K deficiency is that bleeding from it may occur for a variety of reasons in infants 1–2 months of age or older, may not be suspected or immediately diagnosed, and may be misinterpreted as child abuse [338].

Factor V Deficiency

Factor V is a plasma protein that acts as a cofactor with factor Xa to activate thrombin, which in turn activates fibrin from fibrinogen. Its gene is located on chromosome 1. Like most of the other clotting factor deficiencies, many variants of factor V deficiency occur with corresponding clinical variability. Factor V (Leyden) is a defective protein caused by a number of mutations [339–341]. Factor V (Leyden) is a dominantly inherited autosomal trait said to occur in 5% of Caucasians. Severe hemorrhages, as seen in hemophilias A and B, are not commonly seen with factor V deficiencies, but hemarthrosis and intracerebral hemorrhages have been observed, usually in adults. Of interest is that factor V deficiency, alone or in combination with antiphospholipid antibodies, can lead to cerebral venous thrombosis, including sagittal sinus thrombosis in women during the puerperium and in babies in the perinatal period and later [26,342,343].

Factor VIII Deficiency (Hemophilia A), Factor IX Deficiency (Hemophilia B), and von Willebrand's Disease

Factor VIII is a plasma protein that is integral to the generation of thrombin through interactions with factors X and IX. Factor VIII is probably synthesized in the liver and reticuloendothelial systems. A distinct but related factor, von Willebrand's factor (vWF), acts to stabilize factor VIII. Its deficiency causes von Willebrand disease, a milder form of hemophilia than occurs with primary factor VIII or IX deficiency. The genes coding for factor VIII reside on the X chromosome; thus, males who lack a functional copy of these genes will suffer from a bleeding disorder referred to as hemophilia A. This genetic defect is reported to occur in one of every 5000–10,000 male births and has many genetic bases [344–347]. Deficiency of factor VIII can occur because of inhibitory antibodies [348,349].

Factor IX is a plasma protein that interacts with factor VIII to activate factor X, leading to the generation of thrombin. Like factor VIII, its gene resides on the X chromosome, and like factor VIII deficiency, it may have a variety of genetic defects that affect the severity of the disease [350]. Hemophilia B constitutes about 12% of hemophilia cases, with hemophilia A making up much of the remainder. There is a variant of hemophilia B due to genetic defects in factor IX Leiden that constitutes about 1% of hemophilia cases [351,352].

For all practical purposes, hemophilias A and B with variants can be taken as a group pathologically. Hemophilia A varies in severity, owing to the multifactorial basis for the disease, but 40%–60% of cases are severe. It is about four times more common than hemophilia B, which is due to a defect or deficiency in factor IX. Hemophilia A is six to ten times more prevalent among Caucasians than other racial groups [347]. The effects of hemophilia can be manifested at any age, depending upon the phenotype of the disease and external circumstances. The classic locus of bleeding in hemophilia is hemorrhage into a joint, which may lead to severe disability through repeated episodes of bleeding and scarring. Easy dermal bruising and unusual bleeding after a minor injury are typical and may be one of the first signs that lead to diagnostic workup. The disease may appear at birth in connection with difficult labor, use of forceps, and vacuum extraction [353,354] or occur later with known or unknown trauma. Cranial hemorrhage may manifest as epidural, subdural, subarachnoid, or intraparenchymal brain hemorrhages, which constitute the second most common cause of death in hemophiliacs after HIV/AIDS [170,202,355]. Direct analysis for factors VIII and IX is easily accomplished using blood. Treatment often involves infusion of fresh frozen or pooled plasma or administration of the individual factor. Recently, gene-based therapies have shown promise. The complications of these treatments include HIV, hepatitis B and C infections, and other viral infections, as well as the development of antibodies against the various factors.

von Willebrand disease results from insufficient levels of vWF, which is complexed with factor VIII, presumably protecting it from degradation. The gene for vWF is located on chromosome 12. A number of variants of the disease are known, as are their genetic basis; the variant known as type 1 is the most prevalent (partial deficiency), accounting for about 80% of cases [345,355,356]. Type 2 von Willebrand disease also shows partial deficiency, but type 3 has almost complete lack of the factor. Occasionally, von Willebrand disease can be acquired, usually in connection with lymphoproliferative disorders, various neoplasms, and disorders of the immune system, but these cases generally involve adults [357,358]. As with any of the hemophilias, persons with von Willebrand disease can experience intracranial and spinal hemorrhages spontaneously or in association with some form of trauma [359–361]. The ages of those affected are usually from late childhood through adulthood, but infants and even neonates can be affected [362]. Retinal and other forms of ocular hemorrhage have also been reported [363,364].

Protein C and S Deficiency

Proteins C and S are inhibitors of protease components in the coagulation cascade, chiefly acting on factors Va and VIIIa. These proteins are free in the plasma but also bound to the surfaces of platelets and endothelial cells. Their activation requires vitamin K and compounds it facilitates. These proteins function as antithrombotics and help to maintain the balance between thrombus formation and thrombolysis. Insufficiencies in either or both proteins may lead to intravascular coagulation and thrombosis. Instances of cerebral venous and other venous thromboses have been attributed in these deficiencies [25,30,365]. Protein C deficiency has been implicated in cases of retinal vein thrombosis [366]. Cases of multiple clotting factor deficiencies, including proteins C and S, are known [32].

Factor XIII Deficiency

Factor XIII, also known as fibrin-stabilizing factor, is a plasma protein that, like the alternate name suggests, acts on the fibrin clot to make it firmer and more elastic [367]. The genes coding for the protein reside on chromosomes 1 and 6. Deficiency, although rare, is usually seen when both copies of the gene are missing or defective. Heterozygotes usually do not manifest any disease, but cases of hemorrhage, including cerebral hemorrhage, have been reported [368–370]. Factor XIII deficiency can be acquired [371–373]. Deficiency, which may be difficult to prove in the laboratory, may manifest as excessive bleeding at the umbilical stump at birth or during circumcision and as soft tissue hemorrhages (pseudotumors) with or without known trauma, and intracerebral, epidural, and subdural cranial as well as spinal hemorrhages have been reported at various ages [374–376]. Deficiency may pose problems during pregnancies with abortion and uterine bleeding [29,130]. Infants who have experienced intracranial and subdural hemorrhages of unknown basis may be suspected of having been abused and may be shown to have factor XIII deficiency.

Disseminated Intravascular Coagulation

This complex condition basically involves the unregulated, excessive generation of thrombin (see Figure 4.41), which acts at many critical points in the coagulation cascade. This functional or actual excess of thrombin acts to consume fibrinogen, factor V, and factor VIII as well as to promote the aggregation and activation of platelets and the secretion of tissue plasminogen activator from endothelium-produced plasmin, an important fibrinolytic compound. This dysfunctional state promotes clotting, consumes components of the coagulation cascade, and promotes fibrinolysis, leading to both aberrant clotting and bleeding [377]. The relative amounts of thrombin and plasmin determine the manifestations of the syndrome (dominated by larger-vessel or smaller-vessel thrombosis or hemorrhage). The list of conditions that may lead to disseminated intravascular coagulation (DIC) include bacterial, fungal, mycobacterial, or viral sepsis; obstetrical complications such as abruption, amniotic fluid embolism, and a dead fetus; leukemias and lymphomas; mucus-secreting malignancies; extensive tissue injury from any cause (trauma, burns, blast, and missile injuries); dehydration; liver disease; and many others. DIC may appear in many forms; some have been referred to as compensated and uncompensated varieties [378,379]. DIC may manifest as multiorgan failure, renal failure, and respiratory distress due to multiple thromboemboli or hemorrhage. Bleeding in some form occurs in up to 90% of patients, often in sites of prior injury, surgery, or vascular access but also possibly in tissues with no apparent prior damage, such as the gastrointestinal tract, skin, lung, brain, or eye [380–382].

The diagnosis of DIC may be difficult, suspected by abnormalities in the PT, PTT, and platelet count or other standard measures of clotting, but many report that the diagnosis of DIC should not be made without increased activity of thrombin generation, elevated D-dimers, fibrin monomer, fibrin split products, or other, newer tests [377–379,383].

The forensic aspects of DIC and other disorders of coagulation always add complexity to the analysis and interpretation of what role complications of natural diseases, or enhancement of pathological changes, might have had as confounding variables in a case that may involve accidental or inflicted trauma. It is not proper to ignore such complexities simply because they are not fully appreciated or understood.

Hemoglobinopathies

Hemoglobin, the main oxygen-carrying molecular complex in the blood, is composed of four polypeptide chains (two α and two β), which are attached to and enfold the iron-containing heme molecule [384]. It appears that the genes that code for the α chain reside on the short arm of chromosome 16 and those for the β chain on short arm of chromosome 1 [385]. There are many forms of hemoglobin and the composition of the erythrocyte changes during gestation, infancy, and into adulthood. The normal adult erythrocyte contains mostly adult hemoglobin (HbA), whereas the fetus and infant also contain fetal hemoglogin (HbF) as well as variable amounts of HbA and other hemoglobins [385]. There are many mutations of hemoglobin, most of which appear to involve single amino acid substitutions usually in the β chain. These mutations and those of the α chain all carry names of the places where cases were discovered that possessed these altered hemoglobin molecules [384].

One of the most common and important of the hemoglobinopathies, sickle cell anemia (HbS), involves a single genetic miscode that results in substitution of valine for glutamic acid in the β globin chain. The miscode can affect one of the alleles producing what is known as sickle cell trait (heterozygous), but when both alleles are affected, sickle cell disease results. The prevalence of sickle cell mutations is greatest where malaria is epidemic, especially in native Africans where 5%–14% of the population harbor the genetic defect (either heterozygous or homozygous). Significant prevalence for HbS also exists in people of African descent wherever they may be (Caribbean, North Africa, South America, North America, Asia Minor, and in native non-African peoples about the Mediterranean region and elsewhere [386]. Perhaps a reason why Africans have such a high incidence of the sickle cell gene is that through natural selection, those who have the heterozygous trait are more resistant to malaria than those who do not, thus deriving a survival benefit. There are numerous polymorphisms in the affected genes in this hemoglobinopathy as well as in others, that may affect the manifestations of disease states because of the differences of the degree of oxygen binding of the specific hemoglobins and the effect of oxygen saturation of the blood on red cell morphology, which leads to sickling. This effect is the deformation of normally spherical red cells into crescent or other shapes (holly leaf, granular) that increase the possibility of aggregate formation in the blood in hypoxic and other states. Such aggregation leads to thrombosis, infarction, and hemorrhage in the affected organ (spleen, liver, extremities, brain, musculoskeleton, lung, etc.) [386]. With respect to the nervous system, sickle cell disease may produce infarctions, parenchymal hemorrhages, aneurysmal hemorrhages and rupture, and subdural hemorrhages [387–390].

Individuals with sickle cell trait (heterozygous with or without polymorphisms) generally display no symptoms or manifestations typical for homozygosity; however, under often unpredictable conditions, the spectrum of pathology of sickle cell disease can occur, even though this is uncommon to rare. These can manifest as intraocular hemorrhage [391], but some question its existence [392]. Various forms of hemorrhage and infarction can also occur, although, again, uncommonly or rarely [393–396]. Cerebral venous and sagittal sinus thrombosis may also occur [397]. The conditions under which vascular aggregations of red cells can occur even in sickle cell trait include dehydration, febrile states, any condition that may result in oxygen desaturation—hypoxia, sepsis, and pulmonary infection [386].

The forensic import of sickle cell disease, and trait, is that individuals who are not African or appear light skinned and are either not aware of an African heritage, or regard themselves as Caucasian, or apparently have no known African heritage may carry the HbS gene or other abnormal hemoglobins and may become victims of potential pathologies as a result. They may die and come to a forensic service as a result. Some cases, especially infants or children may be thought to be victims of abuse because of intracranial manifestations of the disorder. Other circumstances may present in ways that are suspicious or center about the actions or inactions of others.

Histological examination of blood either by smear or in tissue sections may or may not reveal sickled, crenated or granular red blood cells, but often a careful search will reveal these and perhaps other red cell forms (spherocytosis, acanthocytosis, ovalocytosis, etc.) that can indicate a possible hemoglobinopathy or coexistant condition that plays into the pathology. Hemoglobin electrophoresis can demonstrate various hemoglobin forms, but some polymorphisms will not be detected due to comigration with either normal or abnormal hemoglobin forms. More sophisticated technologies may be required to detect these forms.

Another relatively common hemoglobinopathy are the thalassemias. These are diseases that are inherited with defects in genes that code for either the α globin chain (α-thalassemia) or the β-globin chain (β-thalassemia). These genetic disorders are most common amongst people of Southern Italy, Sicily, Sardinia, Corsica, Greece, but are also not uncommon in Africans, and Thais [385]. The disorder is not infrequently also involving HbS polymorphisms. Both forms of thalassemia result in lower than normal amounts of HbA and increased amounts of HbF. The presence of abnormal hemoglobins result in a microcytic, hemochromic anemia due to increased fragility and destruction of red cells. Systemic manifestations of thalassemia can include hemolysis, jaundice, hypersplenism, anemia, heart failure, iron overload with cirrhosis, diabetes, and other conditions. Like sickle cell disease, there are many polymorphisms in the relevant genes that have been discovered [385].

Kernicterus

Kernicterus or nuclear jaundice [398] is a yellow staining by bilirubin of deep nuclear masses of the brain—the subthalamic nuclei, Ammon's horn, the putamen and globus pallidus, the dentate nuclei of the cerebellum, the olivary nuclei of the medulla, and many cranial nerve nuclei. Kernicterus is a feared complication of neonatal hyperbilirubinemia when serum unconjugated bilirubin levels rise above 20 mg% in the term infant and at lower levels (10–12 mg%) in premature low-birth-weight infants. The mere occurrence of high bilirubin levels is not the only cause for kernicterus [399]; rather, it must be seen in association with immaturity, ischemia, hypoxia, and acidosis. Occasionally, sepsis will also be a factor. In any case, bilirubin, which is normally excluded by the blood–brain barrier, is able to cross into the infant brain and is taken up by neuronal groups mentioned above. Neurons that absorb significant amounts of bilirubin will probably die. Kernicterus is becoming more uncommon as a result of prevention and new treatment strategies developed by neonatologists. Those infants who suffer from kernicterus display neurological sequelae that include spasticity, extrapyramidal symptoms, or hypotonia. Sometimes, hearing and vision defects are the only symptoms. Neuropathological examination will show loss of neurons and gliosis in the affected areas or an abnormal pattern of myelination reminiscent of *status marmoratus* (marbled brain) [400,401].

Fetal Alcohol Syndrome

The fetal alcohol syndrome has been well documented and widely recognized [402,403]. The cardinal features of the syndrome in infants born of alcohol-consuming mothers consist of microcephaly, short palpebral fissures, maxillary hypoplasia, prognathism, epicanthic folds, joint anomalies, palmar creases, cardiac abnormalities, and mental deficiency [404]. Although these conditions represent the pronounced cases, there is increasing evidence that even moderate alcohol use during pregnancy may cause learning disabilities in later life. For this reason, many obstetricians encourage complete abstinence from alcohol during pregnancy. The causes of fetal alcohol syndrome may be poor nutrition, pyridoxine deficiency, contaminants in the alcohol, a genetic predisposition, or the direct toxic effect of alcohol on developing neural systems. There is a 17% perinatal mortality in infants of alcoholic mothers.

Glutaric Acidemia

This autosomal recessively inherited error of metabolism affecting glutaryl-CoA dehydrogenase involves the metabolism of lysine, hydroxylysine, and tryptophan and can present as an infantile encephalopathy, the pattern of cerebral palsy with dystonia, or without symptoms [405]. Lesions of the deep gray and white matter are described, along with subdural effusions and hemorrhages with and without retinal hemorrhages [406–410]. It has been described in several Amish families [153] but may be seen in other populations where inbreeding has occurred as well as in other groups in which no apparent risk factor is evident [406]. Elevated levels of glutaric acid are found in urine and plasma, for which several assay methods are available [153]. From a forensic point of view, the presence in an infant or child of subdural hemorrhages, which may or may not be chronic, and retinal hemorrhages is a signal to some that the child was a victim of abuse. From a number of case reports and analyses, it would appear that such a precipitous intepretation in the face of this inherited toxic condition may not be warranted.

Infectious Diseases

Intrauterine Infections

Intrauterine and perinatal infections of the CNS do not form a major disease category of interest to the forensic pathologist in the same way that malformations, sudden infant death syndrome (SIDS), hypoxia, birth trauma, and child abuse do, but some conditions occasionally are important. These are neonatal meningitis, congenital syphilis, tuberculosis, and the so-called TORCH infections (toxoplasmosis, other (syphilis, varicella-zoster, parvovirus B19), rubella, CMV, and herpes simplex) [411]. Other typical infections, including those associated with acquired immune deficiency syndrome (AIDS), consist of toxoplasmosis, CMV, tuberculosis, fungal infections, and sometimes unusual infectious agents that may affect the neonate.

The TORCH Organisms

The TORCH infections include a variety of infections and agents that affect the fetus or neonate. Toxoplasmosis is a very serious infection when it occurs *in utero* and even in the neonatal period [411,412]. The organism is a protozoan that commonly inhabits the gastrointestinal tracts of house pets (cats, dogs) and other animals. The organism is ubiquitous, and most adults will have antibodies to it and never be aware of having been infected. This disease in infants is a necrotizing and destructive process and may produce near-total destruction of the brain *in utero* or later (Figure 4.42), leaving little more than a calcified shrunken brain. Microscopically the cysts and tachyzoites of the infection are generally easily found (Figure 4.43). In the adult (Chapter 3), toxoplasmosis generally affects immunocompromised individuals like those with AIDS.

Congenital rubella, another TORCH agent, and the complex of conditions it can cause usually occur in connection with maternal infection that crosses the placenta and infects the developing infant [413,414]. The consequences of intrauterine rubella are malformations of the heart, brain, and other systems that are undergoing critical steps in development at the time of the infection. In some infants destruction of periventricular gray and white matter with residual deposition of mineral is all that remains of the *in utero* infection, but in other infants damage may be extensive, causing mental retardation and symptoms of cerebral palsy and congenital cataracts [415].

CMV, still another TORCH infection, as well as toxoplasma infections tend to be much more destructive and cause more cavitation and mineralization than does rubella [411,415]. Like any of the TORCH group of infections CMV can produce congenital malformations. CMV is said to be the most common of the TORCH infections [416]. CMV infection late in the third trimester or early in the neonatal period may present with fulminant encephalitis

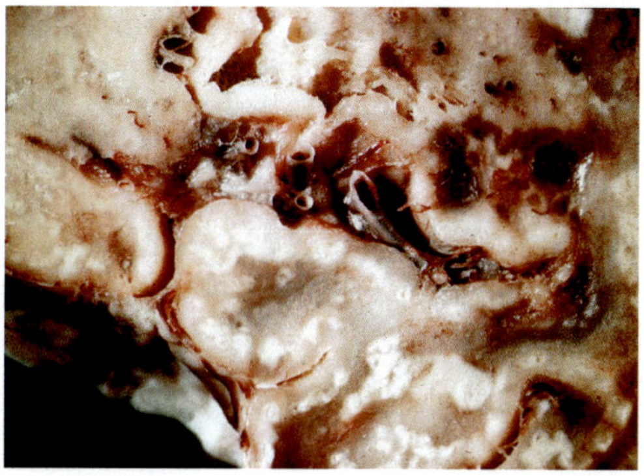

Figure 4.42 A portion of the cerebral cortex in a neonate with toxoplasmosis acquired *in utero* reveals a necrotic and shrunken cortical ribbon with extensive mineralization.

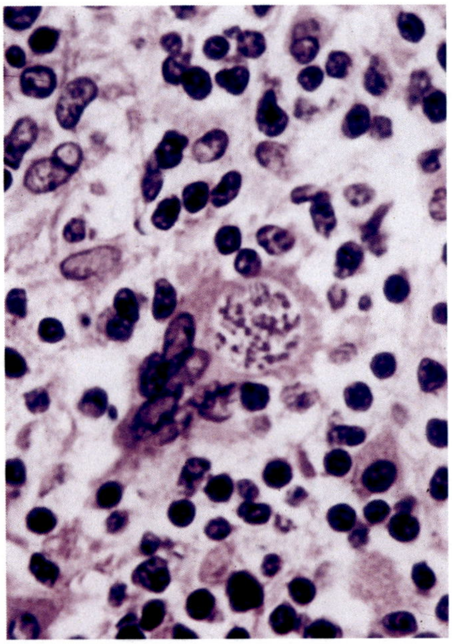

Figure 4.43 High-power H&E-stained section of a necrotizing lesion in the brain illustrating the spectrum of inflammatory infiltrate with a cyst containing tachyzoites of toxoplasmosis in an AIDS victim.

with many punctate hemorrhages in the brain and other organs, similar to those seen in systemic herpes simplex infection (Figure 4.44), or it may be more subtle, causing deafness or mental retardation [417]. Microscopically, CMV is a necrotizing encephalitis, with abundant perivascular and parenchymal chronic inflammation with large Cowdry type A inclusion bodies often found in neurons and other cells. The viscera may also show extensive inclusion body formation, especially early in the infection (Figure 4.45). When there is extensive necrosis and more time has passed before the infant has died, finding inclusions may be taxing. Immunocytochemical staining for the antigens in CMV is often helpful. The appearances of toxoplasmosis and CMV infections may be similar grossly, usually with abundant necrosis, and in the case of toxoplasmosis, abscess formation in the brain may be seen. Microscopically, a multifocal cerebritis with many areas of nodule formation is typical. Depending upon the duration of the infection, microcysts of the organisms may be seen, but often a cloud of individual organisms can be noted amidst an intense chronic inflammatory infiltrate. At times histological diagnosis is difficult, and histochemical stains are not uniformly helpful.

Herpes simplex virus, usually type I in the older patient but predominantly type II in the neonate may cause fulminant encephalitis in the newborn with extensive destruction of the brain and usually many of the viscera. Herpes simplex type II infection in the neonate is most commonly acquired during passage through the birth canal of an infected mother [418,419]. When the infection occurs in childhood or later, it is not unlike herpes encephalitis in the adult, with a local or localized pattern and predilection for the temporal lobes. Destruction of the hippocampus is common. Intranuclear Cowdry type A inclusions are helpful in the diagnosis when they can be found, but histochemical stains are usually reliable and very helpful in differentiation and diagnosis.

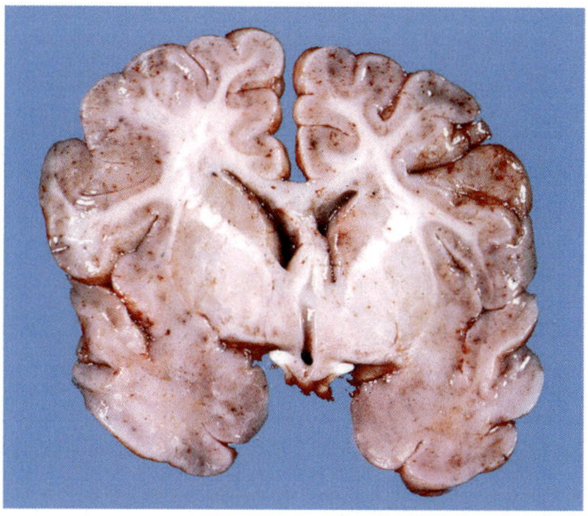

Figure 4.44 Coronal section of a neonatal brain showing many cortical punctate hemorrhages due to CMV infection.

Herpes zoster (varicella-zoster) is usually not a neonatal infection but is acquired later in connection with a chicken pox infection or after inoculation for smallpox, which was once common but is less so currently [420,422]. Immunocompromised infants and children are vulnerable to systemic infection, which may produce neurological sequelae, but some individuals develop a systemic infection that can be very destructive, resulting in death or disfigurement from loss of extremities [422]. In later life, because of the tendency for the virus to become latent in sensory ganglia, it can become reactivated and cause shingles [423].

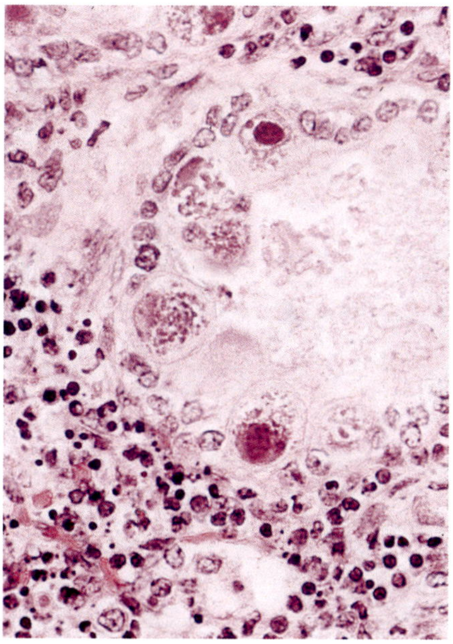

Figure 4.45 Huge Cowdry type A intranuclear inclusion bodies in renal tubular epithelium in a case of systemic CMV infection H&E stain.

Other Virus Infections

Poliomyelitis is an acute infection of primarily the anterior gray matter of the spinal cord by poliovirus, a small RNA virus and a member of the Picornaviridae family and the *Enterovirus* genus with several strains. The infection is transmitted through fecal–oral contamination and produces an acute syndrome usually within a week of infection that is flu-like, during which virions are already being shed into the feces. Up to 80% of infected individuals will not show any further progression of the disease, but the remainder will show varying patterns of the disease that result in acute infection and neuronal death, primarily in the motor neurons of the anterior spinal gray horn but possibly involving bulbar motor nuclei and even cortical motor neurons. About 2%–5% of children and 15%–30% of adults so affected will die of the paralytic effects of the infection, with those affected by bulbar poliomyelitis suffering the highest mortality rate [424].

Pathologically, the acutely infected cord shows often acute inflammatory infiltrate with neuronophagia of dying eosinophilic neurons (Figure 4.46). Other areas may show lymphocytic infiltration of the meninges, perivascular spaces, and affected neuronal populations. Necrosis with hemorrhage in affected areas may be seen. Treatment is symptomatic, and survivors often have varying degrees of paralytic symptoms.

Large-scale efforts worldwide have resulted in a profound decrease in the number of cases each year, from about 50,000 cases in 1975 to what appears to be a stable rate of infection of somewhat under 2000 cases worldwide in 2006. Epidemics periodically erupt in less developed countries but can be found anywhere when immunizations have lagged [425].

The arthropod-borne viruses (arboviruses) form a mixed group of agents belonging to the Togaviridae, Flaviviridae, and Bunyaviridae genera. They are all spread by an arthropod vector, usually a mosquito. An intermediate host, quite often a bird or perhaps a large animal

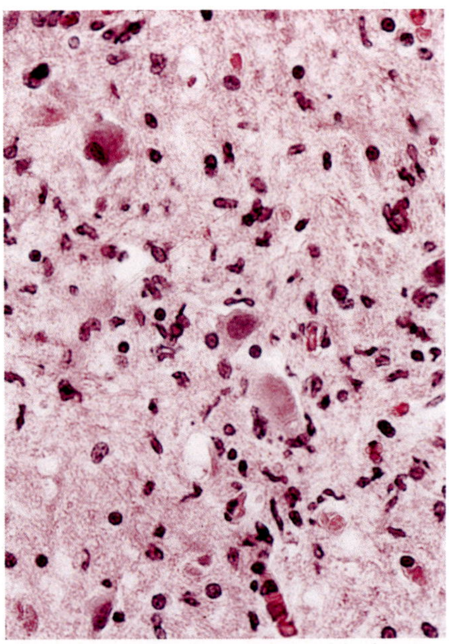

Figure 4.46 H&E-stained section of the anterior horn of the spinal cord in a child suffering from acute poliomyelitis illustrating fading and dying motor neurons surrounded by a mixed inflammatory infiltrate that may contain polymorphonuclear leukocytes.

such as a horse, may or may not harbor the agent with symptoms or ill effects. The most common arboviral infections in the United States are eastern equine encephalitis (EEE), western equine encephalitis (WEE), St. Louis encephalitis (SLE), La Crosse encephalitis, and, most recently, West Nile viral encephalitis and Dengue. All of these diseases present, when they are symptomatic, with a nonspecific flu-like illness, often with headache, myalgias, and occasionally fulminantly with prostration. The infections usually subside within a week or so after symptoms appear and leave no residua in most cases; however, probably fewer than 10% of cases involve frank encephalitis. Those most likely to succumb to encephalitis are the young and the old. Most of these illnesses have a seasonal occurrence, coinciding with breeding cycles in mosquitoes and standing water in which they can breed [414,424].

Clinical diagnosis of the infections may employ a range of immunological/serological tests, but recently specific enzyme-linked immunosorbent assay (ELISA) and monoclonal antibody-related tests are becoming more widely employed. Pathologically, when there is a fatality, the changes are usually not specific to the individual infection and cannot be grossly or microscopically diagnosed with certainty beyond the expected gross pathology of congestion, sometimes, punctate brain hemorrhages, edema, and the typical microscopic appearances that include in the brain perivascular lymphoid inflammation and scattered glial nodules in gray and white matter. None of these conditions produce an inclusion body.

Recently, an unwelcome visitor to the United States has been West Nile virus. This agent is related to Japanese encephalitis and St. Louis encephalitis (Flaviviridae) and apparently originally made its appearance in West Africa but as of 1999 became transported, probably in infected birds, to the United States. There are comparatively few states that are not now affected by the disease, which has spread countrywide in less than 8 years and is transmitted by *Culex*, *Aedes*, and *Anopheles* mosquito genera. Like most of the other arboviral infections, most cases are mild or asymptomatic, with the young and old the most vulnerable to a serious form of the disease. The pathology of the disease is little different from any of the other arboviral infections [426].

Subacute sclerosing panencephalitis (SSPE), once known as Dawson's encephalitis, is a now rare, progressive form of encephalitis due to the measles virus (Mobiliviridae). It has its onset usually 5 years or more after the victim has contracted measles, affecting usually 10- to 12-year-old children. The disease begins insidiously and causes confusion, intellectual deterioration, behavioral disturbances, and perceptual problems and leads to weakness, paralysis, seizures, and death in a vegetative state. Death usually occurs 1–2 years after onset of symptoms. There are few signs of encephalitis, with little evidence of protein or cells in the spinal fluid. Immunological studies will generally show elevated antibody levels to measles virus. Death is usually due to inanition and bacterial infection. Pathologically, the brain may be grossly normal or slightly atrophic in appearance. Upon sectioning, the white matter may appear moth-eaten, somewhat like the appearance of a leukodystrophy. Microscopically, there is neuronal loss with replacement gliosis in both gray and white matter. Large Cowdry type A intranuclear inclusion bodies are common in affected cells (Figure 4.47). Ultrastructurally, the inclusions are spaghetti-like balls of viral capsids. The disease apparently occurs because a key matrix protein is aberrant, and does not permit effective assembly of the virus, causing it to remain unreleased from the cells and pursue a protracted course [424].

At one time, the disease was thought to be due to measles live viral vaccines, but this has been largely disproven, and, in fact, widespread measles immunizations have virtually eliminated SSPE [427].

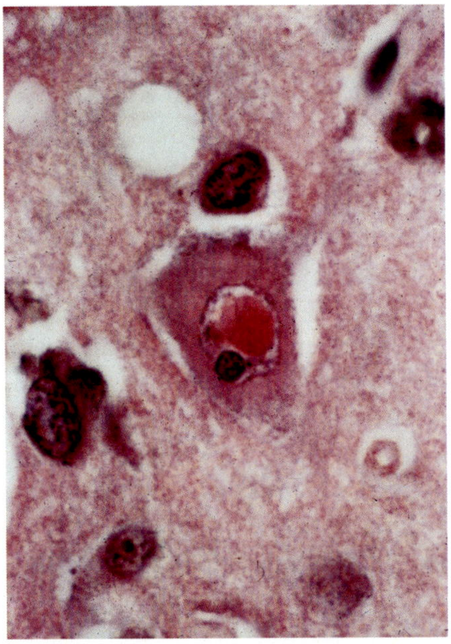

Figure 4.47 High-power H&E-stained section showing a large Cowdry type A intranuclear inclusion body in an infected cell from a case of subacute sclerosing panencephalitis (SSPE). The inclusion, if viewed with electron microscopy, would have a tangled spaghetti-like appearance of viral capsids.

Rabies is caused by a *Lyssavirus*, a member of the Rhabdoviridae family of large RNA-containing viruses. Rabies has been feared and appreciated for centuries and occurs in virtually every country in the world [424]. There are a few areas such as Hawaii that have apparently never reported an indigenous case. In the United States, although often thought of as typically being transmitted by the bite of a rabid dog, such cases are rare. More likely would be transmission by the bite of a raccoon, coyote, skunk, fox, or bat. In 2001, more than 7300 cases of rabies were reported, with major concentrations all along the states east of Ohio and Alabama, from Maine to Florida. Another concentration of cases was in Texas and in populated areas of California. The eastern U.S. cases were mostly caused by raccoon bites or from other animals who probably have been bitten by raccoons, whereas most cases in California, the Plains states, and Texas were caused by rabid skunks. In the Southwest, and Alaska, rabid foxes were most commonly responsible. Domesticated animals, usually dogs and cats, but also cattle, horses, and swine, may be infected and may transmit the disease to humans [428].

The mode of infection is almost always a bite, though inhalation of infected bat guano has been reported. The virus is shed into the saliva of the infected animal, deposited by the bite into deep tissues of the extremities, in most cases where the virus binds to nerve fibers, and transmitted by retrograde axoplasmic transport to the spinal ganglia and cord and then to the central nervous system at large. This process may take several days to reach the spinal cord, during which it may be possible to interdict the infection with timely treatment with antisera. The incubation period of the infection ranges from several days to months. Like most other viral infections, the symptoms may be flu-like, accompanied by myalgia or paresthesias in the affected limb. This period of the disease lasts from 2 to 10 days and culminates in clinical rabies with delirium, insomnia, behavioral changes, hallucinations, and prostration.

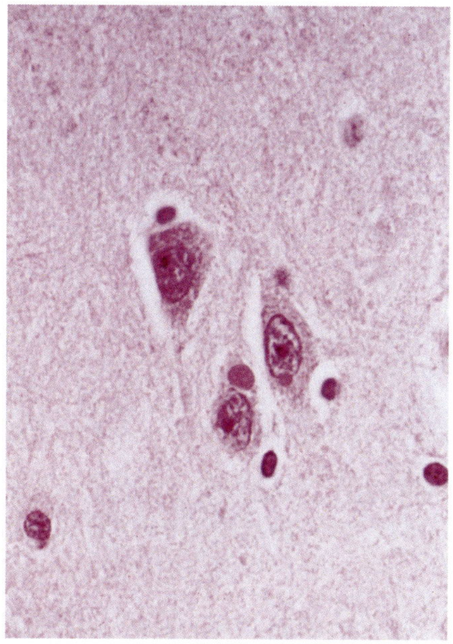

Figure 4.48 H&E-stained high-power section of the hippocampus showing intracytoplasmic inclusions and Negri bodies in a case of rabies encephalitis. Note the lack of inflammation.

Once these symptoms occur, the outcome is said to always be fatal. To date, apparently only six cases of recovery have been reported once the full syndrome has appeared [429].

The diagnosis rests on recovery and examination of the brain of a suspected animal using standard immunofluorescent or other technologies to demonstrate the virus. Serological tests in the affected individual are usually of no value until the victim is unsalvagable. Pathologically, in the animal and the victim the picture is typical, usually of intense viral encephalitis with widespread perivascular lymphoid infiltrations, glial nodules, and necrotic and hemorrhagic foci, and in neurons the presence of cytoplasmic eosinophilic inclusions called Negri bodies (Figure 4.48). There are some cases in which the encephalitis is minimal, but there may still be Negri bodies in larger neurons (motor neurons, Purkinje cells, brain stem nuclei) [424,428].

Bacterial Meningitis

Bacterial meningitis [430] in the newborn is relatively rare but is an extremely serious condition with a very high mortality rate that may approach 100%. The most common organisms producing meningitis in this age group are *Escherichia coli* and group B streptococci, and less commonly *Pseudomonas* and staphylococci [431,432]. The sources for the organism can usually be determined by the autopsy and include infection of the umbilical stump, infected vascular catheters, middle ear or pulmonary infection, and structural defects in the heart or spine (spinal myelomeningocele). Such infectious processes are especially dangerous and overwhelming in the newborn because of an immature immune system and weakened physical state. Additionally, there is great potential of complications of infection in young infants. These include venous infarction of the brain due to cortical vein and sagittal sinus thrombosis [25], DIC, brain abscess and cerebritis, ventriculitis with CSF obstruction and hydrocephalus,

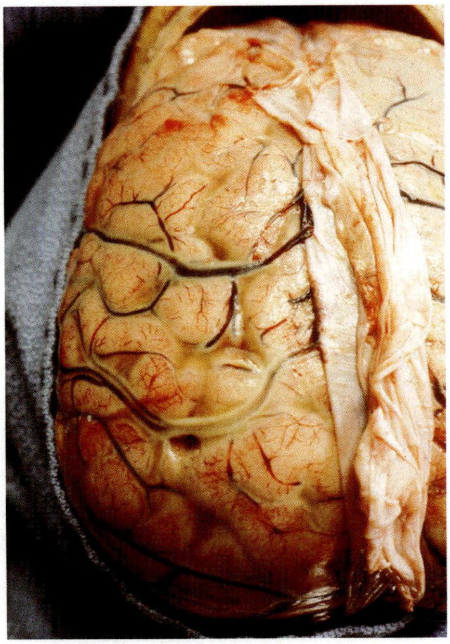

Figure 4.49 Brain surface in a case of *H. influenzae* meningitis illustrating a modest amount of purulent exudate present, along with typically congested and dilated vessels. Fatalities of meningitis from this organism are now unusual, thanks to prompt diagnosis and inclusion in many immunization schedules of antigens for this organism.

subdural effusions, meningeal fibrosis, and later hydrocephalus, interference with development, and later mental retardation or seizure disorders. Litigation is not uncommon and may involve the neuropathologist as an expert. Bacterial meningitis and its complications may masquerade as child abuse and must be borne in mind in any case analyses [433,434].

In the young child and toddler, the coliform organisms are less likely to produce meningitis than is *Haemophilus influenzae*, which accounted for about 60% of cases prior to the introduction of immunization for this organism [434]. At present, it appears that the impact of immunization has greatly diminished *H. influenzae* meninigitis so that *Streptococcus pneumoniae* now accounts for 54% of cases, group B streptococci for 13%, and *Neisseria meningitidis* for 11% of cases [408]. The mortality rate for *H. influenzae* meningitis remains very low (well below 1%), owing to the immunization and the effectiveness of antibiotics, even in the face of emerging resistance (Figure 4.49). The mortality rate for *S. pneumoniae* meningitis is about 9, and for *N. meningitidis* is about 7.5% [434,435]. Morbid conditions that affect outcome include sepsis with shock and coagulopathy, brain abscess, cerebral venous thrombosis, and cerebral hemorrhage. In children surviving meningitis, regardless of type, hearing loss is a common problem, affecting about 30% [436]. Other late complications include subdural fluid collections (hygromas), hydrocephalus, seizures, and mental retardation. *Neisseria* infections very often have only a little meningitis and produce their morbidity and mortality through the meningococcal syndrome that is characterized by DIC and purpura as well as myocarditis. The syndrome can evolve very rapidly with fatal result. In the post-toddler age group and in later years, *S. pneumoniae* is the most common causative agent for meningitis. Classically, this organism produces abundant pus formation, as illustrated in Figure 4.50.

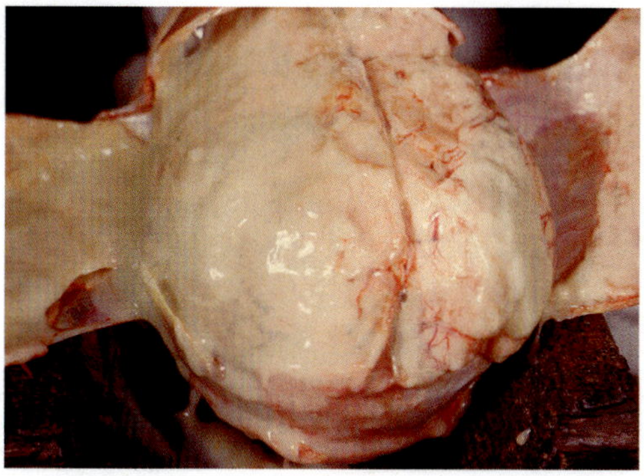

Figure 4.50 Infant with *S. pneumoniae* meningitis showing the profuse pus formation (pyocephalus) that may be seen with this organism. This child, with croup and high fever, had been untreated for several days and suddenly decompensated and died upon being transferred to a larger medical center. (Courtesy of Dr. E. N. Willey, Department of Pathology, University of Michigan, Ann Arbor, MI.)

Amoebic Encephalitis

Although uncommon, clusters of amoebic encephalitis, commonly affecting children, occur during the summer months in the United States and elsewhere throughout the world [437,438]. The organisms responsible are usually of the *Naeglaria* or *Acanthamoeba* species, but other genera may also cause the disease. These are free-living soil organisms that can become concentrated in freshwater runoff collected in ponds, stagnant streams, or excavation sites. Infection occurs when individuals, typically children, swim in these polluted

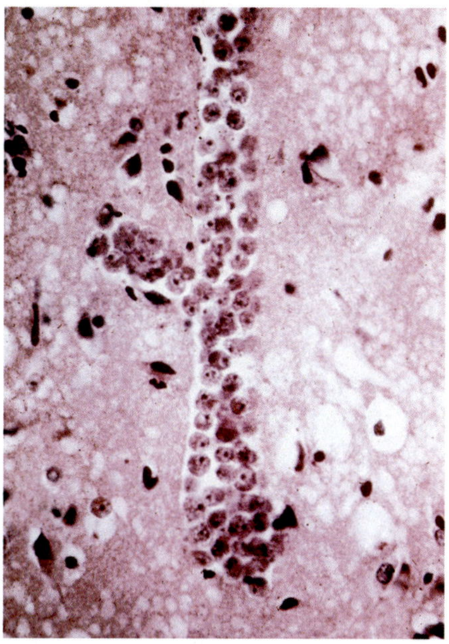

Figure 4.51 H&E-stained section of the cerebral cortex showing a Virchow-Robin space filled with uniform macrophage-like *Naeglaria* amoebic organisms. (Courtesy of the Armed Forces Institute of Pathology, Washington, DC.)

waters. The mode of infection is thought to involve entrance of contaminated water into the nasal passages, from whence the organisms may penetrate through the cribriform plate into the central nervous system. The infection proceeds rapidly, often killing the individual within days with a fulminant hemorrhagic cerebritis and meningitis that may be concentrated to the frontal lobes. Pathologically, the affected tissue is hemorrhagic and congested, and microscopically, vessels are cuffed with the organisms that closely resemble large lymphocytes or macrophages (Figure 4.51). When the organism is recognized, treatment with metronidazole (Flagyl®) or other antibiotics may be effective.

Intrauterine Trauma

Intrauterine trauma before delivery is rare because the infant is well cushioned and protected by the amniotic fluid, thick-walled uterus, abdominal wall, viscera, and skeleton of the mother. Even in massive trauma that results in the death of the mother, if the infant can be delivered by caesarian section quickly enough, there may be no damage at all. Instances of maternal pelvic trauma with fetal skull fractures have been reported and are said to result from impaction of the fetal head with the sacral promontory of the mother [167] under various circumstances—traffic accidents, assaults, falls, and a spectrum of traumatic circumstances [439]. Automobile crashes with airbag deployment appear to have a low incidence of uterine/fetal trauma [440]. Nontraumatic instances have also been reported to have occurred with large uterine leiomyomas or other tumors and severe pelvic deformations [167]. In some of these instances, the infant already at birth may have evidence of a depression in the skull that has healed. Occasionally, head or neck injuries can occur in the fetus [3,169,441]. This is especially true in penetrating or concussive injuries of the abdomen, such as gunshot wounds, bomb explosions, barotrauma, severe automobile accident trauma [442], or knife wounds. The importance of carefully documenting any such injuries is reflected in several recent successful prosecutions for murder against an offender who may or may not have killed the mother but killed the otherwise viable infant. Uterine trauma may indirectly affect the fetus by producing abruptions of the placenta [443]. Amniocentesis may occasionally result in penetration of the fetus by the aspirating needle. Brain injuries from this procedure have been reported [304].

An often unappreciated form of intrauterine "trauma" can occur from restricted intrauterine environments, and/or a short umbilical cord with or without maternal vitamin D deficiency that interferes with proper physical loading of the fetal skeleton and its proper development. These phenomena can lead to fetal and neonatal insufficient mineralization and fracatures [444,445] that may be interpreted as evidence of abusive injury.

Brain Neoplasms

Congenital or connatal brain tumors are not common, but several series have been published relating to these enigmatic lesions [446,447]. Contrary to the impression that most of these tumors should be bizarre and difficult to classify, this is not the case [448]. All the usual childhood brain tumors are represented in the expected numbers, along with a small body of primitive tumors often referred to as PNETs [449,450]. A review of a series of more than 180 brain tumors within the first 3 years of life, derived from a case study between 1951 and 1971 from the case files of the Armed Forces Institute of Pathology [449], revealed that astroglial tumors (usually in the cerebellum) were the most common, and ependymoma and medulloblastomas involving the cerebellum were about equally represented. Other tumors of the brain in this age group were pineal tumors, choroid plexus papillomas, teratomas [451], craniopharyngiomas, and a variety of hamartomatous lesions and other tumors that are rarely encountered in the adult. One of the most confusing and troublesome to neuropathologists is the so-called primitive neuroectodermal tumor (PNET) [450]. Many of these latter tumors are large, malignant growths that may involve virtually a whole hemisphere and are composed of undifferentiated cells, such as are found in medulloblastomas, but also of more differentiated elements, which suggest neuroblastic as well as glial lines [448]. Tumors that are rare in infancy and childhood compared to adulthood are the metastatic tumors and meningiomas. Neonatal brain tumors often present with hydrocephalus, which sometimes prevents normal delivery or calls for intrauterine or intrapartum shunting so that delivery can be affected. Seizures, respiratory distress, opisthotonic posturing, and vomiting can cause misinterpretation and misdiagnosis of meningitis, simple congenital hydrocephalus, idiopathic seizure disorder, or subdural hematomas [452]. Treatment involves shunting as needed, surgical removal of the tumor, and appropriate supportive measures. Irradiation, which would be helpful in older infants and children, if employed to retard or stop tumor regrowth, will almost uniformly result in severe morbidity and mental retardation when used in children under 1 year of age. Furthermore, the rate of operative and other complications is high, giving perinatal brain tumor a very poor prognosis.

The importance of these lesions to the forensic pathologist is that some such cases present with unexpected death in connection with minor illnesses, seizure deaths, alleged child abuse cases, and other circumstances that warrant the concern of the medical examiner/coroner.

The Phaecomatoses

Originally when the concept was developed, there were only a few conditions that were included in this group of inherited neurocutaneous syndromes. Now a much larger group of inherited conditions in which tissue proliferations of some kind affect multiple systems, including the nervous system, exists. For the purposes of this discussion, only the most common conditions will be presented, because they have the most common forensic implications. Uniting all of these conditions in a forensic sense is the tendency for sudden catastrophic decompensation due to sudden unexpected, possibly unexplained processes that can lead to death [453,454]. Probably the most common of these would be one of the complications of seizure disorders (SUDEP). This process will be discussed in Chapter 9 in much more physiological detail.

Tuberous Sclerosis

Tuberous sclerosis (Bourneville's disease) is usually inherited as an autosomal dominant condition that occurs in one of every 50,000–60,000 births [455,456]. It affects more males than females. The disease apparently is caused by mutations in two genes, TSC-1 and TSC-2, whose protein products, called hamartin and tuberin, produce the multifaceted features of the condition [457]. The features and symptoms of the disease generally do not manifest themselves until into childhood, when the typical acneform adenoma sebaceum skin eruption appears over the face or when the child experiences seizures and the CNS lesions become visible on scans. These lesions consist of cortical tubers and intraventricular masses. The cortical tubers show large, bizarre neuron/glial forms that obliterate the cytoarchitecture and often raise the surface of an affected convolution. These lesions are often visible grossly and are represented as rubbery nodules (Figure 4.52). The intraventricular masses are often multiple (candle gutterings) but can reach considerable size (Figure 4.53). They have been referred to as subependymal giant cell astrocytomas. Immunochemically, these tumors typically display both neuronal and glial markers. They are histologically benign. Other lesions that befall the victim include rhabdomyomas in the heart, angiomyolipomas in the kidney, subungual fibromas, and occasionally other tumorous or hamartomatous

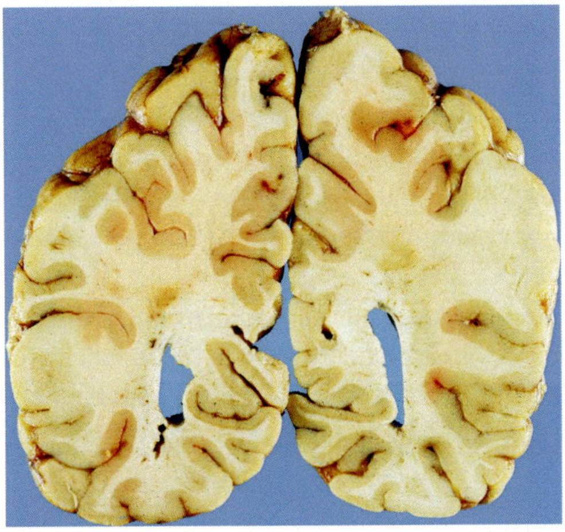

Figure 4.52 Coronal section of the brain of an individual with tuberous sclerosis showing several cortical tubers, particularly evident in the right lateral portion of the parietal lobe where the cortical gray margin is blurred and raised.

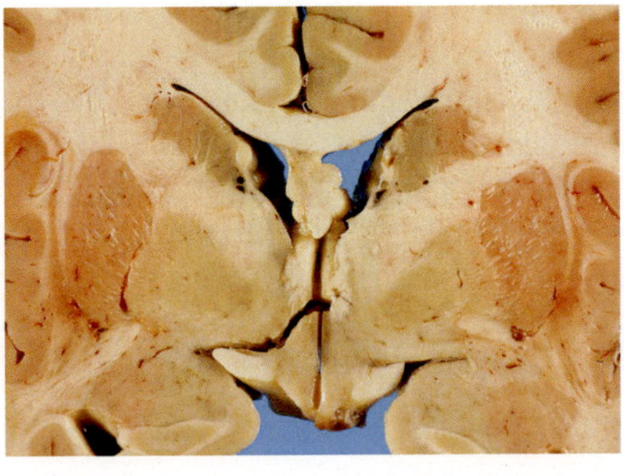

Figure 4.53 Gross photograph of a victim with tuberous sclerosis illustrating a cluster of intraventricular/subependymal tubers. These can be multiple and occasionally huge and able to obstruct the flow of cerebrospinal fluid, causing hydrocephalus and sometimes sudden death from acute obstruction.

lesions [458]. Individuals with tuberous sclerosis often die suddenly and unexpectedly from seizures, from decompensated CSF obstruction due to tumor, or from sudden cardiac decompensation due to the rhabdomyomas. It is not uncommon that a diagnosis prior to death had never been made; thus, it may fall to the forensic pathologist to make the proper primary diagnosis.

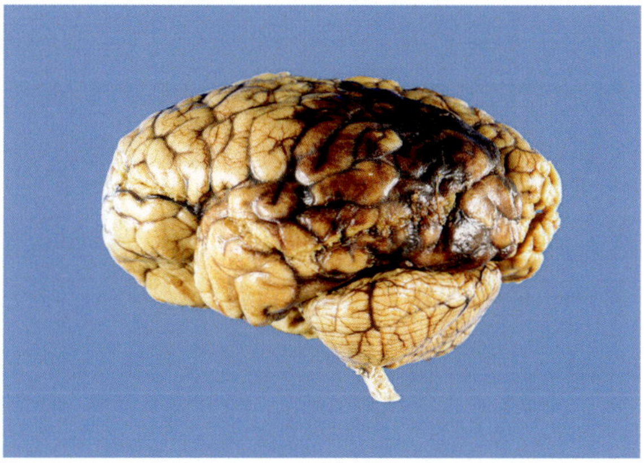

Figure 4.54 Lateral view of the cerebral hemisphere showing a dark region over much of the parietal lobe. There is local hemorrhage present, but the main lesion of Sturge–Weber disease is a feltwork of fine capillaries that fill the meninges and penetrate into the cerebral cortex.

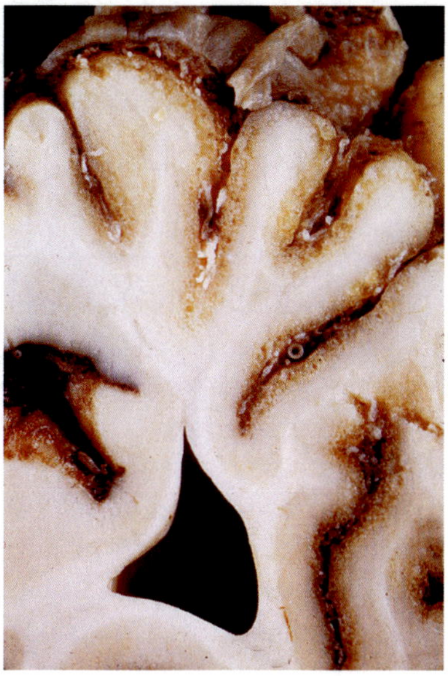

Figure 4.55 Higher power view of coronal section of victim of Sturge–Weber disease showing the cortex largely replaced by mineralized vessels and concretions. (Courtesy of Dr. W. C. Schoene, Brigham and Women's Hospital, Neuropathology Section, Boston.)

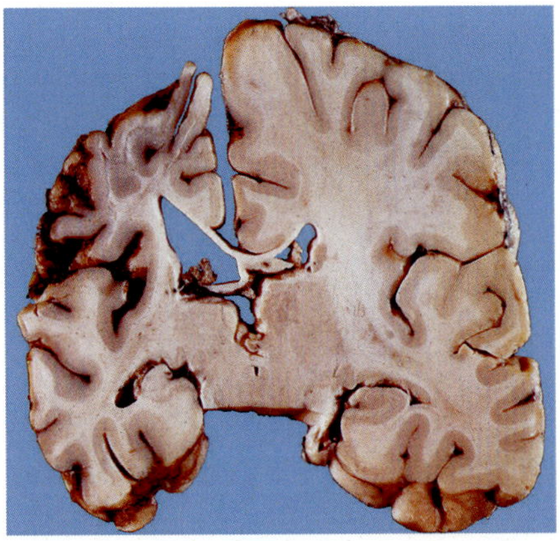

Figure 4.56 Coronal section of coronal section of the brain of a victim of Sturge–Weber disease that affected one side of the face and brain illustrating hemiatrophy of the brain that can occur in this and other conditions without Sturge-Weber disease. Quite often, such individuals have intractable seizures. (Dr. W. C. Schoene, Brigham and Women's Hospital, Neuropathology Section, Boston.)

Sturge–Weber Disease

Sturge–Weber disease [459] is an apparently nonfamilial condition, the genetics of which remain obscure. The disease manifests itself with a progressive angiomatous malformation of one side of the upper face with a corresponding vascular anomaly of the underlying cerebral cortex that shows calcifications in a tram-line pattern on plain skull films or CT scans, and it is commonly associated with hemiatrophy of the cerebral hemisphere and often contralateral atrophy of the cerebellum without angioma (Figures 4.54–4.56). Seizures are the main manifestation of the disease, which also includes mental retardation and glaucoma [460]. Deaths commonly occur in connection with the seizure disorder, which is usually intractable.

Neurofibromatosis

Neurofibromatosis (von Recklinghausen disease) is now generally divided into two major forms, so-called NF-1 and NF-2 [461]. Genes of the same name encode for neurofibromin and merlin, respectively, in which myriad mutations have been reported [462].

NF-1 is the most common, occurring in one of every 3000–4000 individuals. From 30% to 50% of affected persons acquire their disease not from inheritance but from spontaneous gene mutations, which would be transmissible as autosomal dominant if reproduction were to occur. The genetic defect is a loss of key tumor suppressor genes on chromosome 17. Affected individuals typically have multiple dermal Schwannian nodular tumors (neurofibromas), cafe-au-lait spots larger than 5 mm in children and larger than 15 mm in older individuals, and Lisch nodules of the uvea. Axillary freckles are common, and optic nerve gliomas may occur. Some individuals develop plexiform neurofibromas that appear as snake-like expansions of subcutaneous or deep neck nerves that can obstruct the mediastinum by their mass. Malignant transformation of the neurofibromas

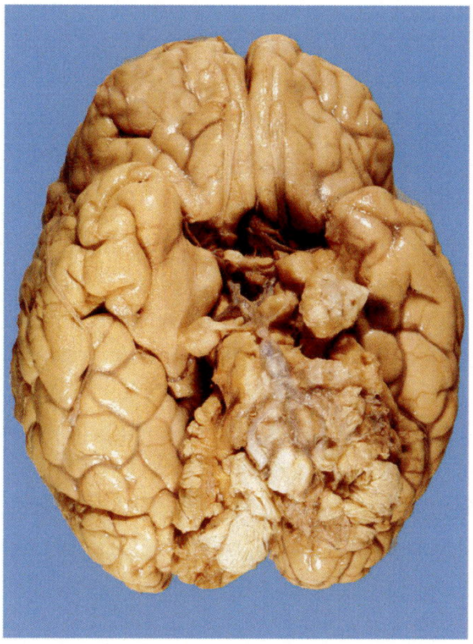

Figure 4.57 Base of the brain of a victim of neurofibromatosis type II illustrating numerous schwannomas of cranial nerves. This individual had bilateral vestibular (acoustic neuromas) schwannomas and numerous schwannomas of spinal nerve roots.

may occur. Hydrocephalus is not uncommon. Developmental deficits and learning disabilities are common. Signs of the condition generally do not appear before adolescence, and the severity of the disease is highly variable [461].

NF-2 is less common than NF-1, occurring in one of every 40,000 people. The disease is caused by loss of tumor suppressor genes on chromosome 22. This form of the disease typically involves bilateral vestibular nerve schwannomas, and many develop multiple schwannomas of the spinal roots and multiple intracranial meningiomas. There is an increased incidence of cerebral gliomas in NF-2 patients. schwannomas of cranial nerves other than the VIIIth also occur (Figure 4.57). The disease usually manifests itself in the teen years, with the appearance of cerebellopontine angle schwannomas. Morbidity and mortality are due to brain stem compression and complications of these tumors and their surgical complications. Meningiomas may also lead to profound morbidity. Microscopically, the typical schwannoma has two histological phases, Antoni A (whorled, Veocay bodies) and Antoni B (spongy tissue), which neurofibromas lack.

von Hippel–Lindau Disease

von Hippel–Lindau disease [463] is autosomal dominantly inherited, with some cases apparently occurring as spontaneous mutations. The disease generally appears in the young adult period. Most individuals have multiple cerebellar hemangioblastomas or similar tumors about the brain stem and cord that continually arise. There is a high incidence of bilateral renal cell carcinoma as well and an occasional occurrence of pheochromotocytomas. Mortality and morbidity are due to the brain tumors and renal cell cancer.

Sudden Infant Death Syndrome

In this syndrome, also known as crib or cot death, an apparently normal infant is found dead in bed [464]. The designation of SIDS is a "diagnosis" or designation of exclusion in which no obvious or defensible anatomic cause of death can be found. Some forensic pathologists decline to employ the term *SIDS*, feeling that if enough effort were made, the cause of death would be demonstrable or, because of the imprecision of the term, other designations should be employed [465]. In any case, this phenomenon at one time caused some 8000 deaths annually in the United States and represented nearly 40% of infant deaths [466], before an extensive program was launched to encourage parents to position their babies in the supine (on their backs) rather than the prone position during sleep [467]. This simple maneuver appears to have decreased the incidence of SIDS by nearly 50% [468–470]. Despite a number of initiatives against SIDS, rates vary considerably and in the United States seem to affect some Native Americans disproportionately over European-ancestry babies [471]. In other parts of the world, indigenous or native populations seem to fare no better [472] then Native Americans.

Before the program to curtail prone sleeping in infants, the mean age for SIDS was about 3 months and the range was from a few days to about 1 year. Since the sleeping position initiative, the 2- to 4-month SIDS population has decreased, whereas deaths of older victims have increased relatively [473]. Victims tend to be slightly below the norm in their growth milestones and may or may not have had any previous history of illness or episodes of apnea. Besides sleeping position, a number of other environmental and exogenous factors seem to be associated with higher SIDS rates than were they not present. These include lower socioeconomic status of the home, colder months of the year, low birth weight, smoking in the home, illicit drug use, poor prenatal care, bed sharing, soft sleeping surfaces, and overheating [465,471,472].

Autopsy findings in possible SIDS cases may occasionally disclose a serious pulmonary or cardiac malformation (hypoplastic left heart, hypoplastic lungs) or an overwhelming infection (group B streptococci of *Haemophilus influenzae) or* toxic complication (infantile botulism) that was not recognized in life, the presence of which disqualifies the case as falling into the SIDS category, which, by definition, are those cases in which autopsy findings contribute little to an understanding of the mechanism of death. Typical findings are minimal respiratory infection, minimal aspiration, congestion of organs, and sometimes cerebral edema. The spectrum of histopathological change is wide but generally not specific for a cause of death, and included changes are hyperplasia of the walls of small arterioles in the lungs, extramedullary hematopoiesis, persistence of fetal fat, and alterations in the carotid bodies [474]. Examination of the intrathoracic cavity may show petechial hemorrhages of the pleurae, in the mediastinum, and over the pericardium and thymus, which suggest an asphyxial death [464,475,476]. There are infants who have been found apneic and who have been resuscitated, perhaps many times, who may eventually die with the SIDS designation. Studies on these infants ("missed" or "near-miss" SIDS) often reveal them to have prolonged periods of sleep apnea, which suggests to some that the basic cause of SIDS is defective neural control of respiration or obstructive apnea, which may also be of neural origin [465,477–480]. In such at-risk infants, respiratory monitors and apnea alarms, as well as instructions to parents on proper methods of cardiopulmonary resuscitation, have been helpful in preventing many deaths. Generally, if an infant with a history of sleep apnea is able to survive to the age of 2 years, the risk for SIDS is minimal after that time.

Studies of the brains of SIDS victims have revealed gliosis in the medullary regions involved in the control of respiration, namely, the dorsal motor nucleus of the vagus, the nucleus tractus solitarius, and the nucleus parambiguus [108,481]. An in depth discussion of the anatomy and physiology of respiratory control can be found in Chapter 9. Naeye [478] has reported an apparent decrease in the number of neurons in the adjacent twelfth nerve nuclei in the medulla. Neurons of the medullary reticular formation have been studied using Golgi impregnation methods, and an immaturity of neuronal development has been demonstrated [466]. Furthermore, the peripheral vagus nerve in the cervical region has been shown to have an altered pattern of myelin development. A number of other neuropathological findings have been reported in SIDS cases [480]. In about 25% of SIDS cases, some degree of subcortical leukomalacia (softening) representing probable ischemia has been demonstrated [476].

These observations have prompted a unifying hypothesis by Naeye [478,479] and Steinschneider [482] for SIDS that recurrent apnea induces changes in tissue metabolism that could result in the many minor structural changes seen, for example, fat cells retaining mitochondria in their response to altered oxygen levels; circulatory responses to hypoxia involving elevation of blood pressure, which induces medial arterial wall thickening; blood-forming elements in hematopoietic organs producing blood in response to decreased oxygen levels (extramedullary hematopoiesis); and perfusion pressure alterations induced by apnea, resulting in ischemic injury to the cerebral white matter and perhaps the brain stem. This hypothesis is appealing; however, the initiating factor in the production of the apnea is not known. brain stem immaturity has been suggested and could be supported by the changes in the Golgi studies and the altered myelination of the vagus nerves; however, these changes could also be secondary to another process or hypoxia caused by apnea. For all the intriguing possible pathogenic mechanisms, SIDS remains an enigma and probably is a multifactorial process [483].

For the practicing forensic pathologist, the label of SIDS should be considered when there is a history of an apparently healthy infant who is found to have died in its crib apparently during sleep, and there are no major anatomical causes of death found at autopsy, grossly or microscopically. An investigation of the death scene is vital, as Hanzlick [484] has pointed out. Here known associated factors may be identified or alternative explanations for the death found. It is very important to try to rule out child abuse (possibly smothering) in SIDS cases, which cannot be done unless a complete autopsy is performed and postmortem radiographs made (see Chapter 8), and even then, occasional later admissions of smothering by a parent emerge to the chagrin of the pathologist. There are often very interesting and perplexing facts that come to light in the course of SIDS investigations that raise difficult scientific and philosophical issues [485]. These include the occasional finding of a familial tendency for SIDS, a history of child abuse in another child, evidence for "failure to thrive" in the affected infant or a sibling, or a history of domestic discord. To be sure, not all cases of SIDS will be associated with these problems, but the functional and developmental connection in some cases seems possible but often difficult to substantiate.

Quite often, the occurrence of SIDS will bring the forensic pathologist or even the neuropathologist into intimate contact with the family of the victim because of the shock of unexpected loss of an infant. A good deal of patience and support is often required in dealing with such families and helping them to understand what happened and to handle their loss. Valuable in this regard are various parent support groups throughout the United States and Europe dedicated specifically to this problem. Also available for at-risk infants are infant respiratory monitoring machines, about which information can usually be obtained from most children's hospitals and pediatricians.

Significant forensic and interpretive problems surround the infant who suddenly becomes apneic while being observed or discovered by a parent or caregiver. Quite often, the caregiver attempts resuscitative efforts that may be ill informed or incompetent, resulting in injuries to the infant. Medical personnel may also make mistakes in intubation, resulting in hypoxemia or injuries to the lips, tongue, and throat. Delays in proper airway restoration may also result in brain hypoxemia. Resuscitative efforts may be conducted by several different persons with variable degrees of experience and competence, sometimes over hours, and are often poorly documented in the medical charts. Attempts at securing vascular access may produce subcutaneous bleeding and hematomas that may dissect into fascial planes, simulating inflicted trauma. Misplaced venous cannulas in the groin may damage the femoral artery or penetrate the inferior vena cava, causing retroperitoneal hemorrhage that may appear to be the result of willful injury. Again, medical records are often incomplete regarding what forms of treatment were given or attempted but failed.

When infants succumb despite resuscitative efforts, one may be left with a baby that has oral injuries and scalp, facial, truncal, abdominal, and extremity bruising as the result of resuscitation and associated attempted treatments. There may be rib fractures [486], although many deny that they can occur with resuscitation [487–490]. The brain may show swelling, and there may be retinal hemorrhages [200] with or without subdural hemorrhage [491]. There may be coagulopathy and other chemical abnormalities, including a high serum glucose level. If the baby was maintained on mechanical ventilation for more than an hour or two, the respirator brain phenomenon may be present. All of these findings, observed at autopsy, may present a picture that strongly suggests inflicted injury. To differentiate SIDS-related injuries from possible inflicted injuries may be very challenging, if not impossible, and the forensic pathologist and neuropathologist involved in the case are encouraged to exercise care and prudence in their interpretations and to go no further than the evidence and science can support.

References

1. U.S. Department of Health and Human Services, CDC. *National Vital Statistics Reports*, 2012.
2. Friede RL. *Developmental Neuropathology*. Berlin: Springer-Verlag, 1989.
3. Gilles FH. Perinatal neuropathology. In Davis RL, Robertson DM, eds., *Textbook of Neuropathology*. Baltimore: Williams & Wilkins, 1985, pp. 243–83.
4. Wigglesworth J, Singer D, eds. *Textbook of Fetal and Perinatal Pathology*. Oxford: Blackwell, 1998.
5. Rorke LB. *Pathology of Perinatal Brain Injury*. New York: Raven Press, 1982.
6. Kubli F, Patel N, Schmidt WOL, eds. *Perinatal Events and Brain Damage in Surviving Children*. Berlin: Springer-Verlag, 1988.
7. Gluckman P, Heyman M, eds. *Pediatrics and Perinatology: The Scientific Basis*. London: Hodder Arnold, 1996.
8. MacDonald M, Mullett M, Seshia M, eds. *Avery's Neonatology: Pathophysiology and Management of the Newborn*. Philadelphia: Lippincott Williams & Wilkins, 2005.
9. Rennie J, Roberton N, eds. *Roberton's Textbook of Neonatology*. London: Churchill Livingstone, 2005.
10. Stocker J, Dehner L, eds. *Pediatric Pathology*. Philadelphia: Lippincott Williams & Wilkins, 2001.

11. Duckett S, ed. *Pediatric Neuropathology*. Baltimore: Williams & Wilkins, 1995.
12. Lemire RJ, Loeser JD, Leech RW, Alvord EC. *Normal and Abnormal Development of the Human Nervous System*. Hagerstown, MD: Harper & Row, 1975.
13. Naeye R. *Disorders of the Placenta, Fetus, and Neonate: Diagnosis and Clinical Significance*. St. Louis, MO: Mosby Year Book, 1992.
14. Paneth N, Rudelli R, Kazam E, Monte W, eds. *Brain Damage in the Preterm Infant*. London: Mac Keith, 1994.
15. Squier W, ed. *Acquired Damage to the Developing Brain: Timing and Causation*. London: Arnold, 2002.
16. Stevenson D, Sunshine P. *Fetal and Neonatal Brain Injury: Mechanisms, Management, and the Risks of Practice*. Toronto: Decker, 1989.
17. Arey LB. *Developmental Anatomy: A Text Book and Laboratory Manual of Embryology*. Philadelphia: W.B. Saunders, 1974.
18. Conel JL. *The Postnatal Development of the Human Cerebral Cortex*. Cambridge, MA: Harvard University Press, 1939.
19. Gilles FH, Lenton A, Dooling EC. *The Developing Human Brain: Growth and Epidemiologic Neuropathology*. Littleton, MA: John Wright, 1983.
20. Patton BM. *Human Embryology*. Philadelphia: Blakiston, 1946.
21. Tuchmann-Duplesis H. Drugs and other xenobiotics as teratogens. *Pharmacol Ther* 1984; 26:273–344.
22. Warkany J. *Congenital Malformations*. Chicago: Year Book Medical Publishers, 1971.
23. Yakovlev PI. Pathoarchitectonic studies of cerebral malformations. III. Arrhinencephalies (holotelencaphalies). *J Neuropathol Exp Neurol* 1959;18:22–55.
24. Rorke LB, Riggs H. *Myelination of the Brain in the Newborn*. Philadelphia: Lippincott, 1969.
25. deVeber G, Andrew M, Adams C, Bjornson B, Booth F, Buckley DJ, Camfield CS, David M, Humphreys P, Langevin P, MacDonald EA, Gillett J, Meaney B, Shevell M, Sinclair DB, Yager J, Ischemi C-C. Cerebral sinovenous thrombosis in children. *N Engl J Med* 2001;345:417–23.
26. Dindagur N, Kruthika-Vinod TP, Christopher R. Factor V gene A4070G mutation and the risk of cerebral veno-sinus thrombosis occurring during puerperium. *Thromb Res* 2006;119:497–500.
27. Ekelund H, Lindeberg L, Wranne L. Combined deficiency of coagulation factors II, VII, IX, and X: A case of probable congenital origin. *Pediatr Hematol Oncol* 1986;3:187–93.
28. Gunes AM, Baytan B, Gunay U. The influence of risk factors in promoting thrombosis during childhood: The role of acquired factors. *Pediatr Hematol Oncol* 2006;23:399–410.
29. Ichinose A, Asahina T, Kobayashi T. Congenital blood coagulation factor XIII deficiency and perinatal management. *Curr Drug Targets* 2005;6:541–49.
30. Koster T, Rosendaal FR, Briët E, van der Meer FJ, Colly LP, Trienekens PH, Poort SR, Reitsma PH, Vandenbroucke JP. Protein C deficiency in a controlled series of unselected outpatients: An infrequent but clear risk factor for venous thrombosis (Leiden Thrombophilia Study). *Blood* 1995;85:2756–61.
31. Thomas A, Stirling D. Four factor deficiency. *Blood Coagul Fibrinolysis* 2003;14(Suppl 1): S55–57.
32. Vicente V, Maia R, Alberca I, Tamagnini GP, Lopez Borraska A. Congenital deficiency of vitamin K-dependent coagulation factors and protein C. *Thromb Haemost* 1984;51:343–46.
33. Lantz PE, Adams GG. Postmortem monocular indirect ophthalmoscopy. *J Foren Sci* 2005;50:1450–52.
34. Lantz PE, Sinal SH, Stanton CA Jr, Weaver RG Jr. Perimacular retinal folds from childhood head trauma. *BMJ* 2004;328:754–56.
35. Davis NL, Wetli CV, Shakin JL. The retina in forensic medicine: Applications of ophthalmic endoscopy: The first 100 cases. *Am J Foren Med Pathol* 2006;27:1–10.
36. Ludwig J. *Handbook of Autopsy Practice*. Totowa, NJ: Humana Press, 2002.
37. Norman MG, Wedderburn LC. Fetal spinal cord injury with cephalic delivery. *Obstet Gynecol* 1973;42:355–58.

38. Norman MG, Smialek JE, Newman DE, Horembala EJ. The postmortem examination of the abused child. Pathological, radiographic, and legal aspects. *Perspect Pediatr Pathol* 1984;8:313–43.
39. Isaacson G. Postmortem examination of infant brains. Techniques for removal, fixation, and sectioning. *Arch Pathol Lab Med* 1984;108:80–81.
40. Pryse-Davies J, Beard RM. A necropsy study of brain swelling in the newborn with special reference to cerebellar herniation. *J Pathol* 1973;109:51–73.
41. Whitwell HL. *Forensic Neuropathology*. London: Hodder Arnold, 2005.
42. Oehmichen M, Auer R, König H. *Forensic Neuropathology and Neurology*. Berlin: Springer-Verlag, 2006.
43. Blinkov S, Glezer IP. *The Human Brain in Figures and Tables: A Quantitative Handbook*. New York: Basic Books, Plenum Press, 1968.
44. Yin X-M, Dong Z, eds. *Essentials of Apoptosis: A Guide for Basic and Clinical Research*. Totowa, NJ: Humana Press, 2003.
45. Harukuni I, Bhardwaj A. Mechanisms of brain injury after global cerebral ischemia. *Neurol Clin* 2006;24:1–21.
46. Hetz C, Vitte PA, Bombrun A, Rostovtseva TK, Montessuit S, Hiver A, Schwarz MK, Church DJ, Korsmeyer SJ, Martinou JC, Antonsson B. Bax channel inhibitors prevent mitochondrion-mediated apoptosis and protect neurons in a model of global brain ischemia. *J Biol Chem* 2005;280:42960–70.
47. Springer JE. Apoptotic cell death following traumatic injury to the central nervous system. *J Biochem Mol Biol* 2002;35:94–105.
48. Schiffmann R, van der Knaap MS. The latest on leukodystrophies. *Curr Opin Neurol* 2004;17:187–92.
49. Vanderver A. Tools for diagnosis of leukodystrophies and other disorders presenting with white matter disease. *Curr Neurol Neurosci Rep* 2005;5:110–18.
50. Lindenberg R, Freytag E. Morphology of brain lesions from blunt trauma in early infancy. *Arch Pathol* 1969;87:298–305.
51. Bignami A, Ralston HJ III. Myelination of fibrillary astrocytic processes in long term Wallerian degeneration. The possible relationship to "status marmoratus." *Brain Res* 1968;11:710–13.
52. Borit A, Herdon RM. The fine structure of plaques fibromyeliniques in ulegyria and in status marmoratus. *Acta Neuropathol* 1969;14:304–11.
53. Kinney HC. Human myelination and perinatal white matter disorders. *J Neurol Sci* 2005;228:190–92.
54. Vellodi A. Lysosomal storage disorders. *Br J Haematol* 2005;128:413–31.
55. Park JH, Schuchman EH. Acid ceramidase and human disease. *Biochim Biophys Acta* 2006;1758:2133–8.
56. Zhang Z, Mandal AK, Mital A, Popescu N, Zimonjic D, Moser A, Moser H, Mukherjee AB. Human acid ceramidase gene: Novel mutations in Farber disease. *Mol Genet Metab* 2000;70:301–9.
57. Levran O, Desnick RJ, Schuchman EH. Niemann-Pick disease: A frequent missense mutation in the acid sphingomyelinase gene of Ashkenazi Jewish type A and B patients. *Proc Natl Acad Sci USA* 1991;88:3748–52.
58. Takahashi T, Suchi M, Desnick RJ, Takada G, Schuchman EH. Identification and expression of five mutations in the human acid sphingomyelinase gene causing types A and B Niemann-Pick disease. Molecular evidence for genetic heterogeneity in the neuronopathic and non-neuronopathic forms. *J Biol Chem* 1992;267:12552–58.
59. Walterfang M, Fietz M, Fahey M, Sullivan D, Leane P, Lubman DI, Velakoulis D. The neuropsychiatry of Niemann-Pick type C disease in adulthood. *J Neuropsychiatry Clin Neurosci* 2006;18:158–70.
60. Sevin M, Lesca G, Baumann N, Millat G, Lyon-Caen O, Vanier MT, Sedel F. The adult form of Niemann-Pick disease type C. *Brain* 2006;130:120–133.
61. Niederau C, Haussinger D. Gaucher's disease: A review for the internist and hepatologist. *Hepatogastroenterology* 2000;47:984–97.
62. Morales LE. Gaucher's disease: A review. *Ann Pharmacother* 1996;30:381–88.

63. Rozenberg R, Fox DC, Sobreira E, Pereira LV. Detection of 12 new mutations in Gaucher disease Brazilian patients. *Blood Cells Mol Dis* 2006;37:204–9.
64. Brady RO, Schiffmann R. Clinical features of and recent advances in therapy for Fabry disease. *JAMA* 2000;284:2771–75.
65. Bongiorno MR, Pistone G, Arico M. Fabry disease: Enzyme replacement therapy. *J Eur Acad Dermatol Venereol* 2003;17:676–79.
66. Gavazzi C, Borsini W, Guerrini L, Della Nare R, Rocca MA, Tessa C, Buchner S, Belli G, Filippi M, Villari N, Mascalchi M. Subcortical damage and cortical functional changes in men and women with Fabry disease: A multifaceted MR study. *Radiology* 2006;241:492–500.
67. Schindler D, Bishop DF, Wolfe DE, Wang AM, Egge H, Lemieux RU, Desnick RJ. Neuroaxonal dystrophy due to lysosomal alpha-N-acetylgalactosaminidase deficiency. *N Engl J Med* 1989; 320:1735–40.
68. Desnick RJ, Wang AM. Schindler disease: An inherited neuroaxonal dystrophy due to alpha-N-acetylgalactosaminidase deficiency. *J Inherit Metab Dis* 1990;13:549–59.
69. Brady RO. Tay-Sachs disease: The search for the enzymatic defect. *Adv Genet* 2001;44:51–60.
70. Purpura D, Baker HJ. Meganeurites and other aberrant processes of neurons in feline GM1-gangliosidosis: A Golgi study. *Brain Res* 1978;143:13–26.
71. Myerowitz R, Lawson D, Mizukami H, Mi Y, Tifft CJ, Proia RL. Molecular pathophysiology in Tay-Sachs and Sandhoff diseases as revealed by gene expression profiling. *Hum Mol Genet* 2002;11:1343–50.
72. Mark BL, Mahuran DJ, Cherney MM, Zhao D, Knapp S, James MN. Crystal structure of human beta-hexosaminidase B: Understanding the molecular basis of Sandhoff and Tay-Sachs disease. *J Mol Biol* 2003;327:1093–109.
73. Leib J, Gollust SE, Hull SC, Wilfond BS. Carrier screening panels for Ashkenazi Jews: Is more better? *Genet Med* 2005;7:185–90.
74. Willems PJ, Seo HC, Coucke P, Tonlorenzi R, O'Brien JS. Spectrum of mutations in fucosidosis. *Eur J Hum Genet* 1999;7:60–67.
75. Gopaul KP, Crook MA. The inborn errors of sialic acid metabolism and their laboratory investigation. *Clin Lab* 2006;52:155–69.
76. Wreden CC, Wlizla M, Reimer RJ. Varied mechanisms underlie the free sialic acid storage disorders. *J Biol Chem* 2005;280:1408–16.
77. Kida E, Golabek AA, Wisniewski KE. Cellular pathology and pathogenic aspects of neuronal ceroid lipofuscinoses. *Adv Genet* 2001;45:35–68.
78. Cooper JD, Russell C, Mitchison HM. Progress towards understanding disease mechanisms in small vertebrate models of neuronal ceroid lipofuscinosis. *Biochim Biophys Acta* 2006;1762:873–89.
79. Santos M, Hoefler S, Moser A, Moser H, Lazarow PB. Peroxisome assembly mutations in humans: Structural heterogeneity in Zellweger syndrome. *J Cell Physiol* 1992;151:103–12.
80. Zellweger H, Maertens P, Superneau D, Wertelecki W. History of the cerebrohepatorenal syndrome of Zellweger and other peroxisomal disorders. *South Med J* 1988;81:357–64.
81. Martinez M. Abnormal profiles of polyunsaturated fatty acids in the brain, liver, kidney and retina of patients with peroxisomal disorders. *Brain Res* 1992;583:171–82.
82. Wanders R, Jansen G, Skjeldal OH. Refsum disease, peroxisomes and phytanic acid oxidation: A review. *J Neuropathol Exp Neurol* 2001;60:1021–31.
83. Sanchez JE, Lopez VF. Sex-linked sudanophilic leukodystrophy with adrenal cortical atrophy (so-called Schilder's disease). *Neurology* 1976;26:261–69.
84. Powers JM. Adreno-leukodystrophy: A personal historical note. *Acta Neuropathol* (Berl) 2005;109:124–27.
85. Powers JM, Pei Z, Heinzer AK, Deering R, Moser AB, Moser HW, Watkins PA, Smith KD. Adreno-leukodystrophy: Oxidative stress of mice and men. *J Neuropathol Exp Neurol* 2005;64:1067–79.
86. Benke PJ, Reyes PF, Parker JC Jr. New form of adrenolekodystrophy. *Hum Genet* 1981;58:204–8.

87. Xu C, Sakai N, Taniike M, Inui K, Ozono K. Six novel mutations detected in the GALC gene in 17 Japanese patients with Krabbe disease, and new genotype-phenotype correlation. *J Hum Genet* 2006;51:548–54.
88. Siddiqi Z, Sanders D, Massey JM. Peripheral neuropathy in Krabbe disease: Effect of hematopoietic stem cell transplantation. *Neurology* 2006;67:268–72.
89. Suzuki K. Globoid cell leukodystrophy (Krabbe's disease): Update. *J Child Neurol* 2003;18:595–603.
90. Berger J, Loschl B, Bernheimer H, Lugowska A, Tylki-Szymanska A, Gieselmann V, Molzer B. Occurrence, distribution, and phenotype of arylsulfatase A mutations in patients with metachromatic leukodystrophy. *Am J Med Genet* 1997;69:335–40.
91. Rauschka H, Colsch B, Baumann N, Wevers R, Schmidbauer M, Krammer M, Turpin J, Lefevre M, Olivier C, Tardieu S, Krivit W, Moser H, Moser A, Gieselmann V, Zalc B, Cox T, Reuner U, Tylki-Szymanska A, Aboul-Enein R. Late-onset metachromatic leukodystrophy: Genotype strongly influences phenotype. *Neurology* 2006;67:859–63.
92. Mancini G, van Diggelen O, Huijmans J, Stroink H, de Coo RF. Pitfalls in the diagnosis of multiple sulfatase deficiency. *Neuropediatrics* 2001;32:38–40.
93. Biffi A, Capotondo A, Fasano S, del Carrou U, Marchesini S, Azuma H, Malaguti MC, Amadio S, Brambilla R, Grompe M, Bordignon C, Quattrini A, Naldini L. Gene therapy of metachromatic leukodystrophy reverses neurological damage and deficits in mice. *J Clin Invest* 2006;116:3070–82.
94. Lee J, Inoue K, Cheung S, Shaw C, Stankiewicz P, Lupski JR. Role of genomic architecture in PLP1 duplication causing Pelizaeus-Merzbacher disease. *Hum Mol Genet* 2006;15:2250–65.
95. Woodward KJ, Cundall M, Sperle K, Sistermans EA, Ross M, Howell G, Gribble SM, Burford DC, Carter NP, Hobson DL, Garbern JY, Kamholz J, Heng H, Hodes ME, Malcolm S, Hobson GM. Heterogeneous duplications in patients with Pelizaeus-Merzbacher disease suggest a mechanism of coupled homologous and nonhomologous recombination. *Am J Hum Genet* 2005;77:966–87.
96. Sonmez F, Celep F, Ugur SA, Tolun A. Severe form of Cockayne syndrome with varying clinical presentation and no photosensitivity in a family. *J Child Neurol* 2006;21:333–37.
97. Ozdirim E, Topcu M, Ozon A, Cila A. Cockayne syndrome: Review of 25 cases. *Pediatr Neurol* 1996;15:312–16.
98. Kumar S, Mattan NS, de Vellis J. Canavan disease: A white matter disorder. *Ment Retard Dev Disabil Res Rev* 2006;12:157–65.
99. Der Perng M, Su M, Wen SF, Gibbon T, Prescott AR, Brenner M, Quinlan RA. The Alexander disease-causing glial fibrillary acidic protein mutant, R416W, accumulates into Rosenthal fibers by a pathway that involves filament aggregation and the association of alpha B-crystallin and HSP27. *Am J Hum Genet* 2006;79:197–213.
100. Gorospe JR, Meletkovic J. Alexander disease and megalencephalic leukoencephalopathy with subcortical cysts: Leukodystrophies arising from astrocyte dysfunction. *Ment Retard Dev Disabil Res Rev* 2006;12:113–22.
101. Johnson AB, Brenner M. Alexander's disease: Clinical, pathologic, and genetic features. *J Child Neurol* 2003;18:625–32.
102. Serenius F, Kallen K, Blennow M, Ewald U, Fellman V, Holmstrom G et al. Neurodevelopmental outcome in extremely preterm infants at 2.5 years after active perinatal care in Sweden. *JAMA* 2013;309(17):1810–20.
103. Ancel PY, Livinec F, Larroque B, Marret S, Arnaud C, Pierrat V et al. Cerebral palsy among very preterm children in relation to gestational age and neonatal ultrasound abnormalities: The EPIPAGE cohort study. *Pediatrics* 2006;117(3):828–35.
104. Larroque B, Ancel PY, Marret S, Marchand L, Andre M, Arnaud C et al. Neurodevelopmental disabilities and special care of 5-year-old children born before 33 weeks of gestation (the EPIPAGE study): A longitudinal cohort study. *Lancet* 2008;371(9615):813–20.
105. Brand M, Bignami A. The effects of chronic hypoxia on the neonatal and infantile brain. *Brain* 1969;92:233–54.

106. Friede RL. Ponto-subicular lesions in perinatal anoxia. *Arch Pathol* 1972;94:343–54.
107. Towbin A. Cerebral hypoxic damage in the fetus and newborn. *Arch Neurol* 1969;20:35–43.
108. Summers CG, Parker JC Jr. The brain stem in sudden infant death syndrome. *Am J Foren Med Pathol* 1981;2:121–27.
109. Azzarelli B, Meade P, Muller J. Hypoxic lesions in areas of primary myelination. *Child's Brain* 1980;7:132–45.
110. Banker BQ, Larroche JC. Periventricular leukomalacia in infancy. *Arch Neurol Psychiatr* 1962;7:386–410.
111. De Reuch J, Chattha AS, Richardson EP. Pathogenesis and evolution of periventricular leukomalacia in infancy. *Arch Neurol* 1972;27:229–36.
112. Norman RM, Urich H, Woods GE. The relationship between prenatal porencephaly and the encephalomalacias of early life. *J Ment Sci* 1958;104:758–71.
113. DeRidder MN, Simon MJ, Siman R, Auberson YP, Raghupathi R, Meaney DF. Traumatic mechanical injury to the hippocampus in vitro causes regional caspase-3 and calpain activation that is influenced by NMDA receptor subunit composition. *Neurobiol Dis* 2006;22:165–76.
114. Tanaka H, Yokota H, Jover T, Cappuccio I, Calderone A, Simionescu M, Bennett MV, Zukin RS. Ischemic preconditioning: Neuronal survival in the face of caspase-3 activation. *J Neurosci* 2004;24:2750–59.
115. Balentine JD. *Pathology of Oxygen Toxicity*. New York: Academic Press, 1982.
116. Amigoni A, Pettenzano A, Biban P, Suppiej A, Freato F, Zaramella P, Zacchello F. Neurologic outcome in children after extracorporal membrane oxygenation: Prognostic value of diagnostic tests. *Pediatr Neurol* 2005;32:173–79.
117. Young TL, Quinn GE, Baumgart S, Petersen RA, Schaffer DB. Extracorporeal membrane oxygenation causing asymmetric vasculopathy in neonatal infants. *J AAPOS* 1997;1:235–40.
118. Bulas D, Glass P. Neonatal ECMO: Neuroimaging and neurodevelopmental outcome. *Semin Perinatol* 2005;29:58–65.
119. Fullerton HJ, Chetkovich D, Wu Y, Smith W, Johnston S. Deaths from stroke in US children, 1979 to 1998. *Neurology* 2002;59:34–39.
120. deVeber G. Stroke and the child's brain: An overview of epidemiology, syndromes and risk factors. *Curr Opin Neurol* 2002;15:133–38.
121. Chalmers EA. Perinatal stroke—Risk factors and management. *Br J Haematol* 2005;130:333–43.
122. Ferriero D. Medical progress. Neonatal brain injury. *N Engl J Med* 2004;351:1985–95.
123. deVeber GA, MacGregor D, Curtis R, Mayank S. Neurologic outcome in survivors of childhood arterial ischemic stroke and sinovenous thrombosis. *J Child Neurol* 2000;15:316–24.
124. Wu YW, Lynch JK, Nelson KB. Perinatal arterial stroke: Understanding mechanisms and outcomes. *Semin Neurol* 2005;25:424–34.
125. deVeber G, Roach ES, Riela AR, Wiznitzer M. Stroke in children: Recognition, treatment, and future directions. *Semin Pediatr Neurol* 2000;7:309–17.
126. Martin P, Enevoldson P. Causes of ischaemic stroke in the young. *Postgrad Med* 1997;73:8–16.
127. Nicolaides P, Appleton R. Annotation: Stroke in children. *Dev Med Child Neurol* 1996;38:172–80.
128. Riela AR, Roach ES. Etiology of stroke in children. *J Child Neurol* 1993;8:201–20.
129. Volpe J. Current concepts in neonatal medicine. Neonatal intraventricular hemorrhage. *N Engl J Med* 1981;304:886–90.
130. Sherer DM, Anyaegbunam A, Onyeije C. Antepartum fetal intracranial hemorrhage, predisposing factors and prenatal sonography: A review. *Am J Perinatol* 1998;15:431–41.
131. Folkerth RD. Neuropathologic substrate of cerebral palsy. *J Child Neurol* 2005;20:940–49.
132. Locatelli A, Vergani P, Ghidini A, Assi F, Bonardi C, Pezzullo JC, Paterlini G. Duration of labor and risk of cerebral white-matter damage in very preterm infants who are delivered with intrauterine infection. *Am J Obstet Gynecol* 2005;193:928–32.
133. Shankaran S, Langer JC, Kazzi SN, Laptook AR, Walsh M, National Institute of Child Health and Human Development Neonatal Research Network. Cumulative index of exposure to hypocarbia and hyperoxia as risk factors for periventricular leukomalacia in low birth weight infants. *Pediatrics* 2006;118:1654–59.

134. Polam S, Koons A, Anwar M, Shen-Schwarz S, Hegvi T. Effect of chorioamnionitis on neurodevelopmental outcome in preterm infants. *Arch Pediatr Adol Med* 2005;159:1032–35.
135. Linder N, Haskin O, Levit O, Klinger G, Prince T, Naor N, Turner P, Karmazyn B, Sirota L. Risk factors for intraventricular hemorrhage in very low birth weight premature infants: A retrospective case-control study. *Pediatrics* 2003;111:e590–95.
136. Kadhim H, Khalifa M, Deltenre P, Casimir G, Sebire G. Molecular mechanisms of cell death in periventricular leukomalacia. *Neurology* 2006;67:293–99.
137. Folkerth RD. Periventricular leukomalacia: Overview and recent findings. *Pediatr Dev Pathol* 2006;9:3–13.
138. Hartel C, Konig I, Koster S, Kattner E, Kuhls E, Kuster H, Moller J, Muller D, Kribs A, Segerer H, Wieg C, Herting E, Gopel W. Genetic polymorphisms of hemostasis genes and primary outcome of very low birth weight infants. *Pediatrics* 2006;118:683–89.
139. Taylor DL, Joashi C, Sarraf C, Edwards AD, Mehmet H. Consequential apoptosis in the cerebellum following injury to the developing rat forebrain. *Brain Pathol* 2006;16:195–201.
140. Ancel PY, Livinec F, Larroque B, Marret S, Arnaud C, Pierrat V, Dehan M, N'Guyen S, Escande B, Burguet A, Thiriez G, Picaud JC, Andre M, Breart G, Kaminski M, EPIPAGE Study Group. Cerebral palsy among very preterm children in relation to gestational age and neonatal ultrasound abnormalities: The EPIPAGE cohort study. *Pediatrics* 2006;117:828–35.
141. Barkovich AJ, Westmark K, Partridge C, Sola A, Ferriero DM. Perinatal asphyxia: MR findings in the first 10 days. *Am J Neuroradiol* 1995;16:427–38.
142. Piatt JH Jr. A pitfall in the diagnosis of child abuse: External hydrocephalus, subdural hematoma, and retinal hemorrhages. *Neurosurg Focus* [Electronic resource]. 1999;7(4).
143. Papasian NC, Frim DM. A theoretical model of benign external hydrocephalus that predicts a predisposition towards extra-axial hemorrhage after minor head trauma. *Pediatr Neurosurg* 2000;33:188–93.
144. Kirschner RH, Stein RJ. The mistaken diagnosis of child abuse. A form of medical abuse? *Am J Dis Child* 1985;139:873–75.
145. Aicardi J, Goutieres F, de Verbors AH. Multicystic encephalomalacia of infants and its relationship to abnormal gestation and hydroanencephaly. *J Neurol Sci* 1972;15:357–73.
146. Ohgi S, Akiyama T, Fukuda M. Neurobehavioural profile of low-birthweight infants with cystic periventricular leukomalacia. *Dev Med Child Neurol* 2005;47:221–28.
147. Msall ME. Complexity of the cerebral palsy syndromes: Toward a developmental neuroscience approach. *JAMA* 2006;296:1650–52.
148. Hermansen M, ed. *Perinatal Causes of Cerebral Palsy*. Philadelphia: Saunders, 2006.
149. Keogh JM, Badawi N. The origins of cerebral palsy. *Curr Opin Neurol* 2006;19:129–34.
150. Gibson CS, MacLennan AH, Goldwater PN, Dekker GA. Antenatal causes of cerebral palsy: Associations between inherited thrombophilias, viral and bacterial infection, and inherited susceptibility to infection. *Obstet Gynecol Surv* 2003;58:209–20.
151. Ananth CV, Berkowitz GS, Savitz DA, Lapinski RH. Placental abruption and adverse perinatal outcomes. *JAMA* 1999;282:1646–51.
152. Lademann A. Postnatally acquired cerebral palsy. A study of the aetiology, clinical findings and prognosis in 170 cases. *Acta Neurol Scand* 1978;57:3–148.
153. Morton DH, Bennett MJ, Seargeant LE, Nichter CA, Kelley RI. Glutaric aciduria type I: A common cause of episodic encephalopathy and spastic paralysis in the Amish of Lancaster County, Pennsylvania. *Am J Med Genet* 1991;41:89–95.
154. Bax M, Tydeman C, Flodmark O. Clinical and MRI correlates of cerebral palsy: The European Cerebral Palsy Study. *JAMA* 2006;296:1602–8.
155. Yehezkely-Schildkraut V, Kutai M, Hugeirat Y, Levin C, Shalev SA, Mazor G, Koren A. Thrombophilia: A risk factor for cerebral palsy? *Isr Med Assoc J* 2005;7:808–11.
156. Costeff H. Estimated frequency of genetic and nongenetic causes of congenital idiopathic cerebral palsy in west Sweden. *Ann Hum Genet* 2004;68:515–20.

157. Menkes JH, Flores-Sarnat L. Cerebral palsy due to chromosomal anomalies and continuous gene syndromes. *Clin Perinatol* 2006;33:481–501.
158. Ueki I, Koga Y, Povalko N, Akita Y, Nishioka J, Yatsuga S, Fukiyama R, Matsuishi T. Mitochondrial tRNA gene mutations in patients having mitochondrial disease with lactic acidosis. *Mitochondrion* 2006;6:29–36.
159. Diamond LJ, Jandes PK. Child abuse in a cerebral-palsied population. *Dev Med Child Neurol* 1983;25:169–74.
160. Hermelin B, O'Connor N, Lee S. Musical inventiveness of five idiot-savants. *Psychol Med* 1987;17:685–94.
161. Treffert DA. The idiot savant: A review of the syndrome. *Am J Psychiatry* 1988;145:563–72.
162. Viscott DS. A musical idiot savant: A psychodynamic study, and some speculations on the creative process. *Psychiatry* 1970;33:494–515.
163. Mavroforou A, Koumantakis E, Michalodimitrakis E. Physicians' liability in obstetric and gynecology practice. *Med Law* 2005;24:1–9.
164. Bishop G. Cerebral palsy litigation. *JAMA* 2006;295:625–26; author reply, 626.
165. Scheller JM, Nelson KB. Does cesarean delivery prevent cerebral palsy or other neurologic problems of childhood? *Obstet Gynecol* 1994;83:624–30.
166. Stanley FJ, Blair E. Why have we failed to reduce the frequency of cerebral palsy? *Med J Aust* 1991;154:623–26.
167. Alexander E, Davis C Jr. Intra-uterine fracture of the infant's skull. *J Neurosurg* 1969; 30:446–54.
168. Dupuis O, Silveira R, Dupont C, Mottolese C, Kahn P, Dittmar A, Rudigoz RC. Comparison of "instrument-associated" and "spontaneous" obstetric depressed skull fractures in a cohort of 68 neonates. *Am J Obstet Gynecol* 2005;192:165–70.
169. Alexander JM, Leveno KJ, Hauth J, Landon MB, Thom E, Spong CY, Varner MW, Moawad AH, Caritis SN, Harper M, Wapner RJ, Sorokin Y, Miodovnik M, O'Sullivan MJ, Sibai BM, Langer O, Gabbe SG, Nat Inst Child Health Human Dev Maternal—Fetal Med Units Netw. Fetal injury associated with cesarean delivery. *Obstet Gynecol* 2006;108:885–90.
170. Blank N, Strand R, Gilles FH, Palakshappa A. Posterior fossa subdural hematomas in neonates. *Arch Neurol* 1978;35:108–11.
171. Chase W. An anatomic study of subdural haemorrhage associated with tentorial splitting in the newborn. *Surg Gynec Obstetr* 1930;51:31–41.
172. Welch K, Strand R. Traumatic parturitional intracranial hemorrhage. *Dev Med Child Neurol* 1986;28:156–64.
173. Hamlat A, Heckly A, Adn M, Poulain P. Pathophysiology of intracranial epidural haematoma following birth. *Med Hypotheses* 2006;66:371–74.
174. Byerss RK. Spinal cord injuries during birth. *Dev Med Child Neurol* 1975;17:103–10.
175. Hughes C, Harley E, Milmoe G, Bala R, Martorella A. Birth trauma in the head and neck. *Arch Otolaryngol Head Neck Surg* 1999;125:193–99.
176. Dodds SD, Wolfe SW. Perinatal brachial plexus palsy. *Curr Opin Pediatr* 2000;12:40–47.
177. Piat J. Birth injuries of the brachial plexus. *Clin Perinatol* 2005;32:39–59, v–vi.
178. Bohm N, Keller KM, Kloke WD. Pulmonary and systemic cerebellar tissue embolism due to birth injury. *Virchow's Arch* 1982;398:229–35.
179. Kilani RA, Wetmore J. Neonatal subgaleal hematoma: Presentation and outcome—Radiological findings and factors associated with mortality. *Am J Perinatol* 2006;23:41–48.
180. Gruber FH. Post traumatic leptomeningeal cysts. *Am J Roentgenol Rad Ther Nucl Med* 1969;105:305–7.
181. Weir P, Suttner NJ, Flynn P, McAuley D. Normal skull suture variant mimicking intentional injury. *BMJ* 2006;332:1020–21.
182. Wardrope J, Chennells PM. Should all casualty radiographs be reviewed? *Br Med J (Clin Res Ed)* 1985;290:1638–40.
183. Tubbs RS, Salter EG, Oakes WJ. Does the mendosal suture exist in the adult? *Clin Anat* 2005.

184. Nakahara K, Miyasaka Y, Takagi H, Kan S, Fujii K. Unusual accessory cranial sutures in pediatric head trauma—Case report. *Neurol Med Chir* (Tokyo) 2003;43:80–81.
185. Feigin I, Budzilovich GN. Laminar scars in cerebral white matter: A perinatal injury due to edema. *J Neuropathol Exp Neurol* 1978;37(3):314–25.
186. Squier W. The "shaken baby" syndrome: pathology and mechanisms. *Acta Neuropathol* 2011;122(5):519–42.
187. Keiper MD, Ng SE, Atlas SW, Grossman RI. Subcortical hemorrhage: Marker for radiographically occult cerebral vein thrombosis on CT. *J Comput Assist Tomogr* 1995;19(4):527–31.
188. McAbee GN, Ciervo C. Medical and legal issues related to brachial plexus injuries in neonates. *J Am Osteopathol Assoc* 2006;106:209–12.
189. Painter MJ, Bergman S. Obstetric trauma to the neonatal central and peripheral nervous system. *Semin Perinatol* 1982;6:89–104.
190. Yates PO. Birth trauma to the vertebral arteries. *Arch Dis Child* 1959;34:436–41.
191. Morgan C, Newell S. Cervical spinal cord injury following cephalic presentation and delivery caesarian section. *Dev Med Child Neurol* 2001;43:274–76.
192. Caird M, Reddy S, Ganley T, Drummond D. Cervical spine fracture-dislocation birth injury: Prevention, recognition, and implications for the oarthopaedic surgeon. *J Pediatr Orthop* 2005;25:484–86.
193. Leestma JE. Neuropathology of brain death. In Weijdiks, EFM, ed., *Brain Death*. Philadelphia: Lippincott Williams & Wilkins, 2001, pp. 45–60.
194. Glasser J. The cerebrospinal fluid of premature infants. *Am J Dis Child* 36:195–247.
195. Kazan S, Gura A, Ucar T, Korkmaz E, Ongun H, Akyuz M. Hydrocephalus after intraventricular hemorrhage in preterm and low-birth weight infants: Analysis of associated risk factors for ventriculoperitoneal shunting. *Surg Neurol* 2005;64(Suppl 2):S77–81; discussion, S81.
196. Bergen R, Margolis S. Retinal hemorrhages in the newborn. *Ann Opththalmol* 1976;8:53–56.
197. Lindsey A, Hughes B, May K, Talbot J, Parsons M. Incidence, distribution, and duration of birth-related retinal hemorrhages: A prospective study. *J Am Assn Ped Ophthalmol Strab* 2006;10:102–6.
198. Besio R, Caballero C, Meerhoff E, Schwarcz R. Neonatal retinal hemorrhages and influence of perinatal factors. *Am J Ophthalmol* 1979;87:74–76.
199. Anteby II, Anteby EY, Chen B, Hamvas A, McAlister W, Tychsen L. Retinal and intraventricular cerebral hemorrhages in the preterm infant born at or before 30 weeks' gestation. *J AAPOS* 2001;5:90–94.
200. Weedn VW, Mansour AM, Nichols MM. Retinal hemorrhage in an infant after cardiopulmonary resuscitation. *Am J Foren Med Pathol* 1990;11:79–82.
201. Polito A, Kah-Guan A, Repka M, Pieramici D. Bilateral retinal hemorrhages in a preterm infant with retinopathy of prematurity immediately following cardiopulmonary resuscitation. *Arch Opthalmol* 2001;119:913–14.
202. Sharma A, Diyora B, Shah S, Pandey A, Mamidanna R. An extradural and subdural hematoma in a neonate. *Indian J Pediatr* 2005;72:269–69.
203. Whitby E, Griffiths P, Rutter S, Sprigg A, Ohadike P, Davies N, Rigby A, Paley M. Frequency and natural history of subdural haemorrhages in babies and relation to obstetric factors. *Lancet* 2004;363:846–51.
204. Chamnanvanakij S, Rollins N, Perlman JM. Subdural hematoma in term infants. *Pediatr Neurol* 2002;26:301–4.
205. Towner D, Castro M, Eby-Wilkens E, Gilbert W. Effect of mode of delivery in nulliparous women on neonatal intracranial injury. *N Engl J Med* 1999;341:1709–14.
206. Hanigan WC, Morgan AM, Stahlberg LK, Hiller JL. Tentorial hemorrhage associated with vacuum extraction. *Pediatrics* 1990;85:534–39.
207. Vinchon M, Pierrat V, Tchofo P, Soto-Ares G, Dhellemmes P. Traumatic intracranial hemorrhage in newborns. *Child's Nerv Syst* 2005;21:1042–48.
208. Gunn T, Mok P, Becroft D. Subdural hemorrhage in utero. *Pediatrics* 1985;76:605–10.

209. Ney J, Joseph K, Mitchell M. Late subdural hygromas from birth trauma. *Neurology* 2005;65:517–17.
210. Hadzikanic N, Al-Habib H, Al-Ahmad I. Idiopathic chronic subdural hematoma in the newborn. *Child's Nerv Syst* 2006;22:740–42.
211. Stracke CP, Spuentrup E, Katoh M, Gunther RW, Spangenberg P. New experimental model of sinus and cortical vein thrombosis in pigs for MR imaging studies. *Neuroradiology* 2006;48:721–29.
212. Parsch CS, Krauss J, Hofmann E, Meixensberger J, Roosen K. Arachnoid cysts associated with subdural hematomas and hygromas: Analysis of 16 cases, long-term follow-up, and review of the literature. *Neurosurgery* 1997;40:483–90.
213. Norman RM. Atrophic sclerosis of the cerebral cortex associated with birth injury. *Arch Dis Child* 1944;19:111–21.
214. Norman MG. On the morphogenesis of ulegyria. *Acta Neuropathol* (Berl) 1981;53:331–32.
215. Squier W, editor. *Acquired Damage to the Developing Brain: Timing and Causation*. London: Arnold, 2002.
216. Villani F, D'Incerti L, Granata T, Battaglia G, Vitali P, Chiapparini L, Avanzini G. Epileptic and imaging findings in perinatal hypoxic-ischemic encephalopathy with ulegyria. *Epilepsy Res* 2003;55:235–43.
217. Castilla EE, Orioli IM. Epidemiology of neural tube defects in South America. *Am J Med Genet* 1985;22:695–702.
218. Frey L, Hauser WA. Epidemiology of neural tube defects. *Epilepsia* 2003;44(Suppl 3):4–13.
219. Correa-Villasenor A, Cragan J, Kucik J, O'Leary L, Siffel C, Williams L. The Metropolitan Atlanta Congenital Defects Program: 35 years of birth defects surveillance at the Centers for Disease Control and Prevention. *Birth Defects Res A Clin Mol Teratol* 2003;67:617–24.
220. Dias MS, Partington M. Embryology of myelomeningocele and anencephaly [Electronic resource]. *Neurosurg Focus* 2004;16(2).
221. Elwood JM. Anencephalus and drinking water composition. *Am J Epidemiol* 1977;105:460–68.
222. Kurtzke JF, Goldberg ID, Kurland LT. The distribution of deaths from congenital malformations of the nervous system. *Neurology* 1973;23:483–96.
223. Ananth CV, Smulian JC, Srinivas N, Getahun D, Salihu HM. Risk of infant mortality among twins in relation to placental abruption: Contributions of preterm birth and restricted fetal growth. *Twin Res Hum Genet* 2005;8:524–31.
224. Hogue CJ, Buehler JW, Strauss LT, Smith JC. Overview of the National Infant Mortality Surveillance (NIMS) project—Design, methods, results. *Public Health Rep* 1987;102:126–38.
225. Waldhoer T, Haidinger G, Wald M, Heinzl H. Non-random geographical distribution of infant mortality in Austria 1984–2002. *Wien Klin Wochenschr* 2006;118:341–47.
226. Sternglass EJ. *Secret Fallout: Low Level Radiation from Hiroshima to Three-Mile Island*. New York: McGraw-Hill, 1981.
227. Hicks S. Developmental malformations produced by radiation. *Am J Roentgenol* 1953;69:272–93.
228. Hicks S. Developmental brain metabolism—Effects of cortisone, anoxia, fluoroacetate, radiation, insulin and other inhibitors on the embryo, newborn, and adult. *Arch Pathol* 1953;55:302–27.
229. Lamire RJ, Beckwith JB, Warkany J. *Anencephaly*. New York: Raven Press, 1978.
230. Demyer W, Zeman W, Palmer CG. The face predicts the brain-diagnostic significance of median facial anomalies for holoprosencephaly (arrhinencephaly). *Pediatrics* 1964;34:256–63.
231. El-Hawrani A, Sohn M, Noga M, El-Hakim H. The face does predict the brain—Midline facial and forebrain defects uncovered during the investigation of nasal obstruction and rhinorrhea. Case report and a review of holoprosencephaly and its classifications. *Int J Pediatr Otorhinolaryngol* 2006;70:935–40.
232. Cassady G. Anencephaly. A 6 year study of 367 cases. *Am J Obstet Gynecol* 1969;103:1154–59.
233. Shoro AA. Estimation of the levels of amniotic fluid alpha fetoprotein (AFP) for the prenatal diagnosis of spina bifida and anencephaly. *Methods Find Exp Clin Pharmacol J* 1981;3:391–95.

234. Wald N, Cuckle H, Nanchahal K. Amniotic fluid acetylcholinesterase measurement in the prenatal diagnosis of open neural tube defects. Second report of the Collaborative Acetylcholinesterase Study. *Prenat Diagn* 1989;9:813–29.
235. James CCM, Lassman LP. *Spinal Dysraphism. Spina Bifida Occulta*. London: Butterworths, 1972.
236. Shaw GM, Nelson V, Olshan AF. Paternal occupational group and risk of offspring with neural tube defects. *Paediatr Perinat Epidemiol* 2002;16:328–33.
237. Vieira AR. Birth order and neural tube defects: A reappraisal. *J Neurol Sci* 2004;217:65–72.
238. Finnell RH, Greer KA, Barber RC, Piedrahita JA. Neural tube and craniofacial defects with special emphasis on folate pathway genes. *Crit Rev Oral Biol Med* 1998;9:38–53.
239. McLone DG. The etiology of neural tube defects: The role of folic acid. *Childs Nerv Syst* 2003;19:537–39.
240. Northrup H, Volcik KA. Spina bifida and other neural tube defects. *Curr Probl Pediatr* 2000;30:313–32.
241. McLone DG. Spinal dysraphism: Impact of technique and technology on expectations. *Clin Neurosurg* 2005;52:261–64.
242. Rinaldi F, Cioffi FA, Columbano L, Krasagakis G, Bernini FP. Tethered cord syndrome. *J Neurosurg Sci* 2005;49:131–35; discussion, 135.
243. La Marca F, Grant JA, Tomita T, McLone DG. Spinal lipomas in children: Outcome of 270 procedures. *Pediatr Neurosurg* 1997;26:8–16.
244. Nielsen LA, Maroun LL, Broholm H, Laursen H, Graem N. Neural tube defects and associated anomalies in a fetal and perinatal autopsy series. *APMIS* 2006;114:239–46.
245. Shaw C, Alvord EC Jr. Hydrocephalus. In Duckett S, ed., *Pediatric Neuropathologhy*. Baltimore: Williams & Wilkins, 1995, pp. 149–211.
246. Bejjani GK. Definition of the adult Chiari malformation: A brief historical overview [Electronic resource]. *Neurosurg Focus* 2001;11(1).
247. Alzate JC, Kothbauer KF, Jallo GI, Epstein FJ. Treatment of Chiari I malformation in patients with and without syringomyelia: A consecutive series of 66 cases [Electronic resource]. *Neurosurg Focus* 2001;11(1).
248. Wolf DA, Vessey SP the 3rd, Wilson SK, Adame J, Korndorffer WE. Death following minor head trauma in two adult individuals with the Chiari I deformity. *J Foren Sci* 1998;43:1241–43.
249. Makela JP. Arnold-Chiari malformation type I in military conscripts: Symptoms and effects on service fitness. *Mil Med* 2006;171:174–76.
250. Byard RW. Mechanisms of sudden death and autopsy findings in patients with Arnold-Chiari malformation and ventriculoatrial catheters. *Am J Foren Med Pathol* 1996;17:260–63.
251. Stevenson KL. Chiari type II malformation: Past, present, and future. *Neurosurg Focus* 2004;16(2).
252. Leech RW, Johnson SH, Brumback RA. Agenesis of cerebellum associated with arrhinencephaly. *Clin Neuropathol* 1997;16:90–97.
253. Ricardi VM, Marcus ES. Congenital hydrocephalus and cerebellar agenesis. *Clin Genet* 1978;13:443–447.
254. Cohlan SQ. Congenital anomalies in the rat produced by the excessive intake of vitamin A during pregnancy. *Pediatrics* 1954;13:556–67.
255. Benda CE. The Dandy-Walker syndrome of the so-called atresia of the foramen Magendie. *J Neuropathol Exp Neurol* 1954;13:14–29.
256. D'Agostino AN, Kernohan JW, Brown JR. The Dandy-Walker syndrome. *J Neuropathol Exp Neurol* 1963;22:450–70.
257. Taggart JK, Walker AE. Congenital atresia of the foramina of Luschka and Magendie. *Arch Neurol Psychiatr* 1942;48:583–612.
258. Hannaway J, Netsky M. Heterotopias of the inferior olive: Relation to Dandy-Walker malformation and correlation with experimental data. *J Neuropathol Exp Neurol* 1971;30:380–89.
259. Hart MN, Malamud N, Ellis WG. The Dandy-Walker syndrome. A clinicopathological study based on 28 cases. *Neurology* 1972;22:771–80.

260. Naidich TP, Radkowski MA, McLone DG, Leestma J. Chronic cerebral herniation in shunted Dandy-Walker malformation. *Radiology* 1986;158:431–34.
261. Osenbach RK, Menezes AH. Diagnosis and management of the Dandy-Walker malformation: 30 years of experience. *Pediatr Neurosurg* 1992;18:179–89.
262. Yamada H, Oi S, Tamaki N, Matsumoto S, Taomoto K. Congenital hydrocephalus mimicking Dandy-Walker syndrome induced by 6-aminonicotinamide injection in pregnant rat. *Neurol Med Chir* (Tokyo) 1991;31:326–29.
263. Ueda N, Sasaki N, Sugita A, Gotoh N, Yamamoto S, Yano T, Ochi H, Nishimura T, Matsuura S, Fukunishi R. Encephalocele, polycystic kidneys, and polydactyly with other defects. A necropsy case of Meckel syndrome and a review of literature. *Acta Pathol Jpn* 1987;37:323–30.
264. de Sauza N, Chaudhuri R, Bigham J, Cox T. MRI in cerebellar hypoplasia. *Neuroradiology* 1994;36:148–51.
265. Leestma JE, Vincente Torres J. Unappreciated agenesis of the cerebellum in an adult: Case report of a 38 year old man. *Am J Foren Med Pathol* 2000;21:155–61.
266. Nowak D, Trost HA. Lhermitte-Duclos disease (dysplastic cerebellar gangliocytoma): A malformation, hamartoma or neoplasm? *Acta Neurol Scand* 2002;105:137–45.
267. Rainov NG, Holzhausen HJ, Burkert W. Dysplastic gangliocytoma of the cerebellum (Lhermitte-Duclos disease). *Clin Neurol Neurosurg* 1995;97:175–80.
268. Rimbau J, Isamat F. Dysplastic gangliocytoma of the cerebellum (Lhermitte-Duclos disease) and its relation to the multiple hamartoma syndrome (Cowden disease). *J Neurooncol* 1994;18:191–97.
269. Stashinko EE, Clegg NJ, Kammann HA, Sweet VT, Delgado MR, Hahn JS, Levey EB. A retrospective survey of perinatal risk factors of 104 living children with holoprosencephaly. *Am J Med Genet A* 2004;128:114–19.
270. Warkany J, Passarge E, Smith LB. Congenital malformations in autosomal trisomy syndromes. *Am J Dis Child* 1966;112:502–17.
271. Loesser JD, Alvord EC Jr. Agenesis of the corpus callosum. *Brain* 1968;91:553–70.
272. Rakic P, Yakovlev PI. Development of the corpus callosum and the cavum septi in man. *J Comp Neurol* 1968;132:45–72.
273. Kamnasaran D. Agenesis of the corpus callosum: Lessons from humans and mice. *Clin Invest Med* 2005;28:267–82.
274. Crome L. Pachygyria. *J Pathol Bacteriol* 1956;71:335–52.
275. Dobyns WB, Reiner O, Carrozzo R, Ledbetter DH. Lissencephaly. A human brain malformation associated with deletion of the LIS1 gene located at chromosome 17p13. *JAMA* 1993;270:2838–42.
276. Jellinger K, Rett A. Agyria-pachygyria (lissencephaly syndrome). *Neuropaediatrics* 1976;7:66–91.
277. Kato M, Dobyns WB. Lissencephaly and the molecular basis of neuronal migration. *Hum Mol Genet* 2003;12:R89–96.
278. Sidman RL, Rakic P. Neuronal migration with special reference to developing human brain: A review. *Brain Research* 1973;62:1–35.
279. Takashima S, Becker LE, Chan FW. Retardation of neuronal maturation in premature infants compared with term infants of the same postconceptional age. *Pediatrics* 1982;69:33–38.
280. Dobyns WB, Stratton RF, Parke JT, Greenberg F, Nussbaum RL, Ledbetter DH. Miller-Dieker syndrome: Lissencephaly and monosomy 17p. *J Pediatr* 1983;102:552–58.
281. Elias RC, Galera MF, Schnabel B, Briones MR, Borri ML, Lipay M, Carvalheira G, Brunoni D, Melaragno MI. Deletion of 17p13 and LIS1 gene mutation in isolated lissencephaly sequence. *Pediatr Neurol* 2006;35:42–46.
282. Leestma JE, Kalelkar MB, Teas SS, Jay GW, Hughes JR. Sudden unexpected death associated with seizures: Analysis of 66 cases. *Epilepsia* 1984;25:84–88.
283. Crome L, France N. Microgyria and cytomegalic inclusion disease in infancy. *J Clin Pathol* 1959;12:427–34.
284. Gressens P. Pathogenesis of migration disorders. *Curr Opin Neurol* 2006;19:135–40.

285. Lathers CM, Schraeder PL, eds. *Epilepsy and Sudden Death*. New York: Marcel Dekker, 1990.
286. Gordon N. Canavan disease: A review of recent developments. *Eur J Paediatr Neurol* 2001;5:65–69.
287. Mirzaa G, Dodge NN, Glass I, Day C, Gripp K, Nicholson L, Straub V, Voit T, Dobyns WB. Megalencephaly and perisylvian polymicrogyria with postaxial polydactyly and hydrocephalus: A rare brain malformation syndrome associated with mental retardation and seizures. *Neuropediatrics* 2004;35:353–59.
288. Tinkle BT, Schorry EK, Franz DN, Crone KR, Saal HM. Epidemiology of hemimegalencephaly: A case series and review. *Am J Med Genet A* 2005;139:204–11.
289. Di Rocco C, Battaglia D, Pietrini D, Piastra M, Massimi L. Hemimegalencephaly: Clinical implications and surgical treatment. *Childs Nerv Syst* 2006;22:852–66.
290. Bosman C, Boldrini R, Dimitri L, Di Rocco C, Corsi A. Hemimegalencephaly. Histological, immunohistochemical, ultrastructural and cytofluorimetric study of six patients. *Childs Nerv Syst* 1996;12:765–75.
291. Little JR, Gomez MR, MacCarty CF. Infratentorial arachnoid cysts. *J Neurosurg* 1973;39:380–86.
292. Rengachary SS. Parasagittal arachnoid cyst: Case report. *Neurosurgery* 1981;9:70–75.
293. Wakisaka S, Yoneda K, Kitano I, Kinoshita K, Matsuoka S. Arachnoid cyst in the quadrigeminal cistern. *Surg Neurol* 1986;26:52–58.
294. Harsh GR 4th, Edwards MS, Wilson CB. Intracranial arachnoid cysts in children. *J Neurosurg* 1986;64:835–42.
295. Rogers MA, Klug G, Siu K. Middle fossa subarachnoid cysts in association with subdural haematomas. A review and recommendations for management. *Br J Neurosurg* 1990;4:497–501.
296. Arriola G, de Castro P, Verdu A. Familial arachnoid cysts. *Pediatr Neurol* 2005;33:146–48.
297. Albuquerque FC, Giannotta SL. Arachnoid cyst rupture producing subdural hygroma and intracranial hypertension: Case reports. *Neurosurgery* 1997;41:951–55; discussion, 955–56.
298. Friede RL. Postencephalitic porencephaly hydranencephaly or polymicrogyria. A review. *Acta Neuropathol* 1978;43:161–68.
299. Van den Bergh R, Vander Eecken H. Anatomy and embryology of the cerebral circulation. *Prog Brain Res* 1968;30:1–26.
300. Manterola A, Towbin AM, Yakovlev PI. Cerebral infarction in the human fetus near term. *J Neuropath Exp Neurol* 1966:477–88.
301. Volpe J. *Neurology of the Newborn*. Philadelphia: Saunders, 1987.
302. Lynch JK, Han CJ, Nee LE, Nelson KB. Prothrombotic factors in children with stroke or porencephaly. *Pediatrics* 2005;116:447–53.
303. Eller KM, Kuller JA. Fetal porencephaly: A review of etiology, diagnosis, and prognosis. *Obstet Gynecol Surv* 1995;50:684–87.
304. Eller KM, Kuller JA. Porencephaly secondary to fetal trauma during amniocentesis. *Obstet Gynecol* 1995;85:865–67.
305. Caraballo RH, Cersosimo RO, Fejerman N. Unilateral closed-lip schizencephaly and epilepsy: A comparison with cases of unilateral polymicrogyria. *Brain Dev* 2004;26:151–57.
306. Curry CJ, Lammer EJ, Nelson V, Shaw GM. Schizencephaly: Heterogeneous etiologies in a population of 4 million California births. *Am J Med Genet A* 2005;137:181–89.
307. Denis D, Chateil JF, Brun M, Brissaud O, Lacombe D, Fontan D, Flurin V, Pedespan J. Schizencephaly: Clinical and imaging features in 30 infantile cases. *Brain Dev* 2000;22: 475–83.
308. Hayashi N, Tsutsumi Y, Barkovich AJ. Morphological features and associated anomalies of schizencephaly in the clinical population: Detailed analysis of MR images. *Neuroradiology* 2002;44:418–27.
309. Persson EK, Hagberg G, Uvebrant P. Hydrocephalus prevalence and outcome in a population-based cohort of children born in 1989–1998. *Acta Paediatr* 2005;94:726–32.
310. Hakim S, Venegas JG, Burton JDC. The physics of the cranial cavity, hydrocephalus and normal pressure hydrocephalus: Mechanical interpretation and mathematical model. *Surg Neurol* 1976;5:187–210.

311. Shapiro K, Marmarou A, Portnoy H, eds. *Hydrocephalus*. New York: Raven Press, 1984.
312. Lourie H, Berne A. A contribution on the etiology and pathogenesis of congenital communicating hydrocephalus. *Biol Neonate* 1961;15:815–22.
313. Bickers DS, Adams RD. Hereditary stenosis of the aqueduct of Sylvius as a cause of congenital hydrocephalus. *Brain* 72;72:246–62.
314. Johnson RT, Johnson KP. Hydrocephalus following viral infection: The pathology of aqueductal stenosis developing after experimental mumps virus infection. *J Neuropathol Exp Neurol* 1968;27:591–606.
315. Johnson ML, Johnson MP. Hydrocephalus as a sequela of experimental myxovirus infections. *Exp Mol Pathol* 1969;10:68–80.
316. Rickert CH, Grabellus F, Varchmin-Schultheiss K, Stoss H, Paulus W. Sudden unexpected death in young adults with chronic hydrocephalus. *Int J Legal Med* 2001;114:331–37.
317. Ommaya AK, Goldsmith W, Thibault L. Biomechanics and neuropathology of adult and paediatric head injury. *Br J Neurosurg* 2002;16:220–42.
318. Shapiro K, Marmarou A, Shulman K. Characterization of clinical CSF dynamics and neural axis compliance using the pressure-volume index. I. The normal pressure-volume index. *Ann Neurol* 1980;7:508–14.
319. Shapiro K, Marmarou A. Clinical applications of the pressure-volume index in treatment of pediatric head injuries. *J Neurosurg* 1982;56:819–25.
320. Shapiro K, Fried A, Marmarou A. Biomechanical and hydrodynamic characterization of the hydrocephalic infant. *J Neurosurg* 1985;63:69–75.
321. Clewell WH, Johnson ML, Meier PR, Newkirk JB, Zide SL, Hendle RW, Bowes WA Jr, Hecht F, O'Keefe G, Henry GP, Shikes RH. A surgical approach to the treatment of fetal hydrocephalus. *N Engl J Med* 1982;306:1320–25.
322. Fried A, Shapiro K. Subtle deterioration in shunted childhood hydrocephalus. A biomechanical and clinical profile. *J Neurosurg* 1986;65:211–16.
323. Morissette I, Gourdeau M, Francoeur J. CSF shunt infections: A fifteen-year experience with emphasis on management and outcome. *Can J Neurol Sci* 1993;20:118–22.
324. McGirt MJ, Leveque JC, Wellons JC the 3rd, Villavicencio AT, Hopkins JS, Fuchs HE, George TM. Cerebrospinal fluid shunt survival and etiology of failures: A seven-year institutional experience. *Pediatr Neurosurg* 2002;36:248–55.
325. Emanuelson I, von Wendt L, Kyllerman M, Larsson J. Clinical outcome after near-fatal late shunt complication in hydrocephalus. *Childs Nerv Syst* 1994;10:270–74.
326. Kirkham FJ, Lerner NB, Noetzel M, DeBaun MR, Datta AK, Rees DC, Adams RJ. Trials in sickle cell disease. *Pediatr Neurol* 2006;34:450–58.
327. McGimpsey SJ, Woodside JV, Cardwell C, Cahill M, Chakravarthy U. Homocysteine, methylenetetrahydrofolate reductase C677T polymorphism, and risk of retinal vein occlusion: A meta-analysis. *Ophthalmology* 2009;116(9):1778–87.
328. Carvalho K, Bodensteiner J, Connolly P, Garg B. Cerebral venous thrombosis in children. *J Child Neurol* 2001;16:574–84.
329. Kenet G, Waldman D, Lubetsky A, Kornbrut N, Khalil A, Koren A, Wolach B, Fattal A, Kapelushnik J, Tamary H, Yacobovitch J, Raveh E, Revel-Vilk S, Toren A, Brenner B. Paediatric cerebral sinus vein thrombosis. A multi-center, case-controlled study. *Thromb Haemost* 2004;92:713–18.
330. Kivlin JD, Simons KB, Lazoritz S, Ruttum MS. Shaken baby syndrome. *Ophthalmology* 2000;107:1246–54.
331. Leestma JE. Case analysis of brain-injured admittedly shaken infants: 54 cases, 1969–2001. *Am J Foren Med Pathol* 2005;26:199–212.
332. Kaur B, Taylor D. Fundus hemorrhages in infancy. *Surv Ophthalmol* 1992;37:1–17.
333. Sebire G, Tabarki B, Saunders DE, Leroy I, Liesner R, Saint-Martin C, Husson B, Williams AN, Wade A, Kirkham FJ. Cerebral venous sinus thrombosis in children: Risk factors, presentation, diagnosis and outcome. *Brain* 2005;128:477–89.

334. Academy of American Pediatrics. Controversies concerning vitamin K and the newborn. American Academy of Pediatrics Committee on Fetus and Newborn. *Pediatrics* 2003;112:191–92.
335. Danielsson N, Hoa DP, Thang NV, Vos T, Loughnan PM. Intracranial haemorrhage due to late onset vitamin K deficiency bleeding in Hanoi province, Vietnam. *Arch Dis Child Fetal Neonatal Ed* 2004;89:F546–50.
336. Sutor AH, Dagres N, Niederhoff H. Late form of vitamin K deficiency bleeding in Germany. *Klin Padiatr* 1995;207:89–97.
337. Zipursky A. Prevention of vitamin K deficiency bleeding in newborns. *Br J Haematol* 1999;104:430–37.
338. Brousseau TJ, Kissoon N, McIntosh B. Vitamin K deficiency mimicking child abuse. *J Emerg Med* 2005;29:283–88.
339. Bertina RM, Koeleman BP, Koster T, Rosendaal FR, Dirven RJ, de Ronde H et al. Mutation in blood coagulation factor V associated with resistance to activated protein C. *Nature* 1994;369(6475):64–67.
340. Kurachi S, Furukawa M, Salier JP, Wu CT, Wilson EJ, French FS et al. Regulatory mechanism of human factor IX gene: Protein binding at the Leyden-specific region. *Biochemistry* 1994;33(6):1580–91.
341. Reijnen MJ, Maasdam D, Bertina RM, Reitsma PH. Haemophilia B Leyden: The effect of mutations at position +13 on the liver-specific transcription of the factor IX gene. *Blood Coagul Fibrinolysis* 1994;5(3):341–48.
342. Kenet G, Sadetzki S, Murad H, Martinowitz U, Rosenberg N, Gitel S, Rechavi G, Inbal A. Factor V Leiden and antiphospholipid antibodies are significant risk factors for ischemic stroke in children. *Stroke* 2000;31:1283–88.
343. Hiltunen L, Rautanen A, Rasi V, Kaaja R, Kere J, Krusius T, Vahtera E, Paunio M. An unfavorable combination of factor V Leiden with age, weight, and blood group causes high risk of pregnancy-associated venous thrombosis—A population-based nested case-control study. *Thromb Res* 2006;119:423–32.
344. Guillet B, Lambert T, d'Oiron R, Proulle V, Plantier JL, Rafowicz A, Peynet J, Costa JM, Bendelac L, Laurian Y, Lavergne JM. Detection of 95 novel mutations in coagulation factor VIII gene F8 responsible for hemophilia A: Results from a single institution. *Hum Mutat* 2006;27:676–85.
345. Weiss HJ, Pietu G, Rabinowitz R, Girma JP, Rogers J, Meyer D. Heterogeneous abnormalities in the multimeric structure, antigenic properties, and plasma-platelet content of factor VIII/von Willebrand factor in subtypes of classic (type I) and variant (type IIA) von Willebrand's disease. *J Lab Clin Med* 1983;101:411–25.
346. Cutler JA, Mitchell MJ, Smith MP, Savidge GF. The identification and classification of 41 novel mutations in the factor VIII gene (F8C). *Hum Mutat* 2002;19:274–78.
347. Soucie JM, Evatt B, Jackson D. Occurrence of hemophilia in the United States. The Hemophilia Surveillance System Project Investigators. *Am J Hematol* 1998;59:288–94.
348. Lacroix-Desmazes S, Bayry J, Misra N, Horn MP, Villard S, Pashov A, Stieltjes N, d'Oiron R, Saint-Remy JM, Hoebeke J, Kazatchkine MD, Reinbolt J, Mohanty D, Kaveri SV. The prevalence of proteolytic antibodies against factor VIII in hemophilia A. *N Engl J Med* 2002;346:662–67.
349. Lacroix-Desmazes S, Wootla B, Dasgupta S, Delignat S, Bayry J, Reinbolt J, Hoebeke J, Saenko E, Kazatchkine MD, Friboulet A, Christophe O, Nagaraja V, Kaveri SV. Catalytic IgG from patients with hemophilia A inactivate therapeutic factor VIII. *J Immunol* 2006;177:1355–63.
350. Attali O, Vinciguerra C, Trzeciak MC, Durin A, Pernod G, Gay V, Menart C, Sobas F, Dechavanne M, Negrier C. Factor IX gene analysis in 70 unrelated patients with haemophilia B: Description of 13 new mutations. *Thromb Haemost* 1999;82:1437–42.
351. Kurachi S, Furukawa M, Salier JP, Wu CT, Wilson EJ, French FS, Kurachi K. Regulatory mechanism of human factor IX gene: Protein binding at the Leyden-specific region. *Biochemistry* 1994;33:1580–91.

352. Reijnen MJ, Maasdam D, Bertina RM, Reitsma PH. Haemophilia B Leyden: The effect of mutations at position +13 on the liver-specific transcription of the factor IX gene. *Blood Coagul Fibrinolysis* 1994;5:341–48.
353. Wilson DA, Nelson MD Jr, Fenstermacher MJ, Bohan TP, Hopper KD, Tilton A, Mitchell WG Jr, Contant CF Jr, Maeder MA, Donfield SM et al. Brain abnormalities in male children and adolescents with hemophilia: Detection with MR imaging. The Hemophilia Growth and Development Study Group. *Radiology* 1992;185:553–58.
354. Rodriguez V, Schmidt KA, Slaby JA, Pruthi RK. Intracranial haemorrhage as initial presentation of severe haemophilia B: Case report and review of Mayo Clinic Comprehensive Hemophilia Center experience. *Haemophilia* 2005;11:73–77.
355. Ngo KY, Glotz VT, Koziol JA, Lynch DC, Gitschier J, Ranieri P, Ciavarella N, Ruggeri ZM, Zimmerman TS. Homozygous and heterozygous deletions of the von Willebrand factor gene in patients and carriers of severe von Willebrand disease. *Proc Natl Acad Sci USA* 1988;85:2753–57.
356. Shelton-Inloes BB, Chehab FF, Mannucci PM, Federici AB, Sadler JE. Gene deletions correlate with the development of alloantibodies in von Willebrand disease. *J Clin Invest* 1987;79:1459–65.
357. Nitu-Whalley IC, Lee CA. Acquired von Willebrand syndrome—Report of 10 cases and review of the literature. *Haemophilia* 1999;5:318–26.
358. Kumar S, Pruthi RK, Nichols WL. Acquired von Willebrand's syndrome: A single institution experience. *Am J Hematol* 2003;72:243–47.
359. Kakazu K, Ohira N, Ojima T, Oshida M, Akiyama M, Horaguchi M, Takahashi S. Extensive spinal epidural hemorrhage associated with von Willebrand's disease—A case report. *Nippon Seikeigeka Gakkai Zasshi* 1980;54:501–5.
360. Mizoi K, Onuma T, Mori K. Intracranial hemorrhage secondary to von Willebrand's disease and trauma. *Surg Neurol* 1984;22:495–98.
361. Dietrich AM, James CD, King DR, Ginn-Pease ME, Cecalupo AJ. Head trauma in children with congenital coagulation disorders. *J Pediatr Surg* 1994;29:28–32.
362. Mullaart RA, P VD, Gabreels FJ, van Oostrom C. Fetal periventricular hemorrhage in von Willebrand's disease: Short review and first case presentation. *Am J Perinatol* 1991;8:190–92.
363. Herrmann WA, Lohmann CP, Demmler-Hackenberg M, Gabel VP. Von Willebrand's disease type I as a cause for subvitreal, retinal and subretinal haemorrhages. *Graefes Arch Clin Exp Ophthalmol* 2005;243:383–85.
364. Shiono T, Abe S, Watabe T, Noro M, Tamai M, Akutsu Y, Ishikawa M, Suzuki S, Mori K. Vitreous, retinal and subretinal hemorrhages associated with von Willebrand's syndrome. *Graefes Arch Clin Exp Ophthalmol* 1992;230:496–97.
365. Ugras M, Yakinci C. Protein C, protein S and other pro- and anticoagulant activities among epileptic children using sodium valproate. *Brain Dev* 2006.
366. Gumus K, Kadayifcilar S, Eldem B, Saracbasi O, Ozcebe O, Dundar S, Kirazli S. Is elevated level of soluble endothelial protein C receptor a new risk factor for retinal vein occlusion? *Clin Exp Ophthalmol* 2006;34:305–11.
367. Duckert F, Nyman D. Factor XIII, fibrin and collagen. *Suppl Thromb Haemost* 1978;63:391–96.
368. Duckert F. Documentation of the plasma factor XIII deficiency in man. *Ann NY Acad Sci* 1972;202:190–99.
369. Larsen PD, Wallace JW, Frankel LS, Crisp D. Factor XIII deficiency and intracranial hemorrhages in infancy. *Pediatr Neurol* 1990;6:277–78.
370. Egbring R, Kroniger A, Seitz R. Factor XIII deficiency: Pathogenic mechanisms and clinical significance. *Semin Thromb Hemost* 1996;22:419–25.
371. Board PG, Losowsky MS, Miloszewski KJ. Factor XIII: Inherited and acquired deficiency. *Blood Rev* 1993;7:229–42.
372. Seitz R, Duckert F, Lopaciuk S, Muszbek L, Rodeghiero F, Seligsohn U. ETRO Working Party on factor XIII questionnaire on congenital factor XIII deficiency in Europe: Status and perspectives. Study Group. *Semin Thromb Hemost* 1996;22:415–18.

373. Tosetto A, Castaman G, Rodeghiero F. Acquired plasma factor XIII deficiencies. *Haematologica* 1993;78(Suppl 2):5–10.
374. Bhattacharya M, Biswas A, Ahmed RP, Kannan M, Gupta M, Mahapatra M, Choudhry VP, Saxena R. Clinico-hematologic profile of factor XIII-deficient patients. *Clin Appl Thromb Hemost* 2005;11:475–80.
375. Ugur S, Uzel N, Dundar K, Kaya U, Ayan I, Gedikoglu G. Intraspinal hemorrhage in a child with factor XIII deficiency. *Pediatr Emerg Care* 1991;7:231–33.
376. Nakajima M, Nakazawa T, Matsuda M, Handa J, Hayami M, Miyamoto Y, Ohta S. [Intracerebral hemorrhage associated with long-lasting deficiency of factor XIII]. *No Shinkei Geka* 1999;27:465–68.
377. Calverley DC, Liebman HA. Disseminated intravascular coagulation. In Hoffman R, Benz EJ Jr, Shattil SJ, Furie B, Cohen HJ, Silberstein LE, McGlave P, eds., *Hematology: Basic Principles and Practice*. New York: Churchill Livingstone, 2000, pp. 1983–95.
378. Taylor FJ Jr, Wada H, Kinasewitz G. Description of compensated and uncompensated disseminated intravascular coagulation (DIC) responses (non-overt and overt DIC) in baboon models of intravenous and intraperitoneal *Escherichia coli* sepsis and in the human model of endotoxemia: toward a better definition of DIC. *Hemophilia* 2005;11:193–202.
379. Mammen EF. Disseminated intravascular coagulation (DIC). *Clin Lab Sci* 2000;13:239–45.
380. Girolami A, Luzzatto G, Varvarikis C, Pellati D, Sartori R, Girolami B. Main clinical manifestations of a bleeding diathesis: An often disregarded aspect of medical and surgical history taking. *Haemophilia* 2005;11:193–202.
381. Lewis K, Herbert EN, Williamson TH. Severe ocular involvement in disseminated intravascular coagulation complicating meningococcaemia. *Graefes Arch Clin Exp Ophthalmol* 2005;243:1069–70.
382. Bick RL. Disseminated intravascular coagulation current concepts of etiology, pathophysiology, diagnosis, and treatment. *Hematol Oncol Clin North Am J* 2003;17:149–76.
383. Voves C, Wuillemin WA, Zeerleder S. International Society on Thrombosis and Haemostasis score for overt disseminated intravascular coagulation predicts organ dysfunction and fatality in sepsis patients. *Blood Coagul Fibrinolysis* 2006;17:445–51.
384. Nagel R. Disorders of hemoglobin function and stability (Chapter 52). In: Handin RI, Lux S, Stossel T, editors. *Blood: Principles & Practice of Hematology*. Philadelphia: Lippincott, 1995:1591–644.
385. Forget B, Pearson H. Hemoglobin synthesis and the thalassemias (Chapter 51). In: Handin RI, Lux AL, Stossel T, editors. *Blood: Principles & Practice of Hematology*. Philadelphia: Lippincott, 1995:1525–90.
386. Platt O. The Sickle syndromes (Chapter 53). In: Handin RI, Lux S, Stossel T, editors. *Blood: Principles & Practice of Hematology*. Philadelphia: Lippincott, 1995:1645–700.
387. Bridgers WH. Cerebral vascular disease accompanying sickle cell anemia. *Am J Pathol* 1939;15(3):353–62.5.
388. Adeloye A, Ogbeide MI, Odeku EL. Massive intracranial hemorrhage in sickle cell anemia. *Neurology* 1970;20(12):1165–70.
389. Falter ML, Sutton AL, Robinson MG. Massive intracranial hemorrhage in sickle-cell anemia. *Am J Dis Child* 1973;125(3):415–16.
390. Rothman SM, Fulling KH, Nelson JS. Sickle cell anemia and central nervous system infarction: A neuropathological study. *Ann Neurol* 1986;20(6):684–90.
391. Reynolds SA, Besada E, Winter-Corella C. Retinopathy in patients with sickle cell trait. *Optometry* 2007;78(11):582–87.
392. Nia J, Lam WC, Kleinman DM, Kirby M, Liu ES, Eng KT. Retinopathy in sickle cell trait: Does it exist? *Can J Ophthalmol* 2003;38(1):46–51.
393. Steen RG, Xiong X, Mulhern RK, Langston JW, Wang WC. Subtle brain abnormalities in children with sickle cell disease: Relationship to blood hematocrit. *Ann Neurol* 1999;45(3):279–86.
394. Riggs JE, Ketonen LM, Wang DD, Valanne LK. Cerebral infarction in a child with sickle cell trait. *J Child Neurol* 1995;10(3):253–54.

395. Partington MD, Aronyk KE, Byrd SE. Sickle cell trait and stroke in children. *Pediatr Neurosurg* 1994;20(2):148–51.
396. Reyes MG. Subcortical cerebral infarctions in sickle cell trait. *J Neurol Neurosurg Psychiatry* 1989;52(4):516–18.
397. Feldenzer JA, Bueche MJ, Venes JL, Gebarski SS. Superior sagittal sinus thrombosis with infarction in sickle cell trait. *Stroke* 1987;18(3):656–60.
398. Zimmerman HM, Yannet H. Kernicterus jaundice of the nuclear masses of the brain. *Am J Dis Child* 1933;45:740–59.
399. Gartner LM, Snyder RN, Chabohn RS, Bernstein S. Kernicterus: High incidence in premature infants with low serum bilirubin concentrations. *Pediatrics* 1970;45:906–17.
400. Ernster L, Herlin L, Zettersham P. Experimental studies on the pathogenesis of kernicterus. *Pediatrics* 1957;20:647–52.
401. Rozdilsky B. Kitten as experimental model for study of kernicterus. *Am J Dis Child* 1966;11:161–65.
402. Abel E. *Fetal Alcohol Abuse Syndrome*. New York: Springer, 1998.
403. Jones KL, Smith DW. Recognition of the fetal alcohol syndrome in early infancy. *Lancet* 1973;2:999–1001.
404. Stimmel B, ed. *The Effects of Maternal Alcohol and Drug Abuse on the Newborn*. Vol. 1. New York: Haworth Press, 1982.
405. Hedlund GL, Longo N, Pasquali M. Glutaric acidemia type 1. *Am J Med Genet C Semin Med Genet* 2006;142:86–94.
406. Funk CB, Prasad AN, Frosk P, Sauer S, Kolker S, Greenberg CR, del Bigio MR. Neuropathological, biochemical and molecular findings in a glutaric acidemia type 1 cohort. *Brain* 2005;128:711–22.
407. Gago LC, Wegner RK Jr, Capone A Jr, Williams GA. Intraretinal hemorrhages and chronic subdural effusions: Glutaric aciduria type 1 can be mistaken for shaken baby syndrome. *Retina* 2003;23:724–26.
408. Osaka H, Kimura S, Nezu A, Yamazaki S, Saitoh K, Yamaguchi S. Chronic subdural hematoma, as an initial manifestation of glutaric aciduria type-1. *Brain Dev* 1993;15:125–27.
409. Woelfle J, Kreft B, Emons D, Haverkamp F. Subdural hemorrhage as an initial sign of glutaric aciduria type 1: A diagnostic pitfall. *Pediatr Radiol* 1996;26:779–81.
410. Neumaier-Probst E, Harting I, Seitz A, Ding C, Kolker S. Neuroradiological findings in glutaric aciduria type I (glutaryl-CoA dehydrogenase deficiency). *J Inherit Metab Dis* 2004;27:869–76.
411. Stegmann BJ, Carey JC. TORCH infections. Toxoplasmosis, other (syphilis, varicella-zoster, parvovirus B19), rubella, cytomegalovirus (CMV), and herpes infections. *Curr Womens Health Rep* 2002;2:253–58.
412. Lindsay DS, Weiss LM, eds. *Opportunistic Infections: Toxoplasma, Sarcocystis, and Microsporidia*. Boston: Kluwer Academic Press, 2004.
413. Gregg NM. Congenital cataract following German measles in the mother. *Trans Ophthalmol Soc Aust* 1942;3:35–46.
414. Johnson R. *Viral Infections of the Nervous System*. New York: Raven Press, 1982.
415. Reef SE, Redd SB, Abernathy E, Zimmerman L, Icenogle JP. The epidemiological profile of rubella and congenital rubella syndrome in the United States, 1998–2004: The evidence for absence of endemic transmission. *Clin Infect Dis* 2006;43(Suppl 3):S126–32.
416. Staras SA, Dollard SC, Radford KW, Flanders WD, Pass RF, Cannon MJ. Seroprevalence of cytomegalovirus infection in the United States, 1988–1994. *Clin Infect Dis* 2006;43:1143–51.
417. Iwasaki S, Yamashita M, Maeda M, Misawa K, Mineta H. Audiological outcome of infants with congenital cytomegalovirus infection in a prospective study. *Audiol Neurootol* 2006;12:31–36.
418. Enright AM, Prober CG. Neonatal herpes infection: Diagnosis, treatment and prevention. *Semin Neonatol* 2002;7:283–91.
419. Kimberlin DW. Herpes simplex virus infections in neonates and early childhood. *Semin Pediatr Infect Dis* 2005;16:271–81.
420. Gilden DH, Cohrs RJ, Mahalingam R. Clinical and molecular pathogenesis of varicella virus infection. *Viral Immunol* 2003;16:243–58.

421. Kleinschmidt-DeMasters BK, Gilden DH. The expanding spectrum of herpesvirus infections of the nervous system. *Brain Pathol* 2001;11:440–51.
422. Chiappini E, Calabri G, Galli L, Salvi G, de Martino M. Varicella-zoster virus acquired at 4 months of age reactivates at 24 months and causes encephalitis. *J Pediatr* 2002;140:250–51.
423. Cohrs RJ, Gilden DH, Mahalingam R. Varicella zoster virus latency, neurological disease and experimental models: An update. *Front Biosci* 2004;9:751–62.
424. Leestma JE. Viral infections of the nervous system. In Davis R, Robertson DM, eds., *Textbook of Neuropathology*. Baltimore: Williams & Wilkins, 1991, pp. 804–903.
425. Oshinsky DM. *Polio: An American Story*. New York: Oxford University Press, 2006.
426. Centers for Disease Control (CDC): Arboviral encephalitides: Information on arboviral encephalitides, US Department of Health Education and Welfare, Washington, D.C., 2006.[http://www.cdc.gov/ncidod/dvbid/arbor/arbdet.htm].
427. Bellini WJ, Rota JS, Lowe LE, Katz RS, Dyken PR, Zaki SR, Shieh WJ, Rota PA. Subacute sclerosing panencephalitis: More cases of this fatal disease are prevented by measles immunization than was previously recognized. *J Infect Dis* 2005;192:1686–93.
428. Centers for Disease Control (CDC), Rabies. Washington, D.C., US Department of Health Education and Welfare, 2006 [http://www.cdc.gov/ncidod/dvrd/rabies/natural_history/nathist.htm].
429. Baer GM, ed. *The Natural History of Rabies*. Boca Raton, FL: CRC Press, 1991.
430. Bell WE, McCormick WF. *Neurologic Infections in Children*. Philadelphia: W. B. Saunders, 1975.
431. Saez-Llorens X, McCracken GH Jr. Bacterial meningitis in neonates and children. *Infect Dis Clin North Am* 1990;4:623–44.
432. Kaplan SL. Serious pediatric infections. *Am J Med* 1990;88:18S–24S.
433. James HE. Emergency management of acute coma in children. *Am Fam Physician* 1993;48: 473–78.
434. Neuman HB, Wald ER. Bacterial meningitis in childhood at the Children's Hospital of Pittsburgh: 1988–1998. *Clin Pediatr* (Phila) 2001;40:595–600.
435. Husain E, Chawla R, Dobson S, Dele Davies H. The Paediatric Investigators Collaborative Network on Infections in Canada: Epidemiology and outcome of bacterial meningitis in Canadian children: 1998–1999. *Clin Invest Med* 2006;29:131–35.
436. Kutz JW, Simon LM, Chennupati SK, Giannoni CM, Manolidis S. Clinical predictors for hearing loss in children with bacterial meningitis. *Arch Otolaryngol Head Neck Surg* 2006;132:941–45.
437. Apley J, Clarke SK, Roome AP, Sandry SA, Saygi G, Silk B, Warhurs DC. Primary amoebic meningoencephalitis in Britain. *Brit Med J* 1970;1:596–599.
438. Anderson K, Jamieson A, Jadin JB, Willaert E. Primary amoebic meningoencephalitis. *Lancet* 1973;1:672.
439. Connolly AM, Katz VL, Bash KL, McMahon MJ, Hansen WF. Trauma and pregnancy. *Am J Perinatol* 1997;14:331–36.
440. Metz TD, Abbott JT. Uterine trauma in pregnancy after motor vehicle crashes with airbag deployment: A 30-case series. *J Trauma* 2006;61:658–61.
441. Sims ME, Turkel SB, Halterman G, Paul RH. Brain injury and intrauterine death. *Am J Obstet Gynecol* 1985;151:721–23.
442. Oni OOA, Okpere EE, Tabowei O, Omu EA. Severe road traffic injuries in the third trimester of pregnancy. *Injury* 1984;15:376–78.
443. Oyelese Y, Ananth CV. Placental abruption. *Obstet Gynecol* 2006;108:1005–16.
444. Miller ME, Hangartner TN. Temporary brittle bone disease: Association with decreased fetal movement and osteopenia. *Calcif Tissue Int* 1999;64(2):137–43.
445. Miller ME. Hypothesis: Fetal movement influences fetal and infant bone strength. *Med Hypotheses* 2005;65(5):880–86.
446. Koos W, Miller M. *Intracranial Tumors of Infants and Children*. St. Louis: Mosby, 1971.
447. Cohen ME, Duffiner PK. *Brain Tumors in Children*. New York: Raven Press, 1984.
448. Leestma JE. Teaching monograph: Brain tumors. *Am J Pathol* 1980;100:243–316.

449. Leestma JE, Earle KM. Neoplasms of the central nervous system in infants 2 years of age and under. Analysis of 163 cases [Abstract]. *J Neuropathol Exp Neurol* 1973;32:154.
450. Hart MN, Earle KM. Primitive neuroectodermal tumors of the brain in children. *Cancer* 1973;32:890–97.
451. Gonzales-Crussi F. *Extragonadal Teratomas*. Vol. 18, 2nd series. Washington, DC: Armed Forces Institute of Pathology, 1982.
452. Taptas JN. Intracranial meningioma in a four-month-old infant simulating subdural hematoma. *J Neurosurg* 1961;18:120–21.
453. Kanter RJ, Graham M, Fairbrother D, Smith SV. Sudden cardiac death in young children with neurofibromatosis type 1. *J Pediatr* 2006;149:718–20.
454. Losiniecki A, Prahlow JA. Sudden infant death due to neurofibromatosis type I. *Am J Foren Med Pathol* 2006;27:317–19.
455. Devlin LA, Shepherd CH, Crawford H, Morrison PJ. Tuberous sclerosis complex: Clinical features, diagnosis, and prevalence within Northern Ireland. *Dev Med Child Neurol* 2006;48:495–99.
456. Piedimonte LR, Wailes IK, Weiner HL. Tuberous sclerosis complex: Molecular pathogenesis and animal models [Electronic resource]. *Neurosurg Focus* 2006;20(1).
457. Au KS, Williams AT, Gambello MJ, Northrup H. Molecular genetic basis of tuberous sclerosis complex: From bench to bedside. *J Child Neurol* 2004;19:699–709.
458. Raymond AA, Fish DR, Sisodiya SM, Alsanjari N, Stevens JM, Shorvon SD. Abnormalities of gyration, heterotopias, tuberous sclerosis, focal cortical dysplasia, microdysgenesis, dysembryoplastic neuroepithelial tumour and dysgenesis of the archicortex in epilepsy. Clinical, EEG and neuroimaging features in 100 adult patients. *Brain* 1995;118:629–60.
459. Alexander GL, Norman RM. *The Sturge–Weber Syndrome*. Bristol, UK: Wright, 1960.
460. Di Rocco C, Tamburrini G. Sturge-Weber syndrome. *Childs Nerv Syst* 2006;22:909–21.
461. Friedman JM, Gutmann DH, McCollin M, Riccardi VM, eds. *Neurofibromatosis: Phenotype, Natural History and Pathogenesis*. Baltimore: Johns Hopkins University Press, 1999.
462. Yohay KH. The genetic and molecular pathogenesis of NF1 and NF2. *Semin Pediatr Neurol* 2006;13:21–26.
463. Parker JN, Parker PM, eds. *The Official Patient's Sourcebook on von Hipple Lindau Disease. A Revised and Updated Directory for the Internet Age*. San Diego: Icon Health Publications, 2002.
464. Ambler MW, Naeve C, Sturner WQ. Sudden and unexpected death in infancy and childhood. *Am J Foren Med Pathol* 1981;2:23–30.
465. Byard R, Krous H, eds. *Sudden Infant Death Syndrome: Problems, Progress and Possibilities*. London: Arnold, 2001.
466. Baba N, Quattrochi JJ, Reiner CB, Andrion W, McBride PT, Yates AJ. Possible role of the brain stem in sudden infant death syndrome. *JAMA* 1983;249:2789–91.
467. Mitchell E, Aley P, Eastwood J. The national cot death prevention program in New Zealand. *Austr J Pub Health* 1992;16:158–61.
468. Hauck FR, Herman SM, Donovan M, Iyasu S, Merrick Moore C, Donoghue E, Kirschner RH, Willinger M. Sleep environment and the risk of sudden infant death syndrome in an urban population: The Chicago Infant Mortality Study. *Pediatrics* 2003;111:1207–14.
469. Hauck FR, Moore CM, Herman SM, Donovan M, Kalelkar M, Christoffel KK, Hoffman HJ, Rowley D. The contribution of prone sleeping position to the racial disparity in sudden infant death syndrome: The Chicago Infant Mortality Study. *Pediatrics* 2002;110:772–80.
470. Willinger M, Hoffman H, Hartford R. Infant sleep position and risk for sudden infant death syndrome: Report of meeting held January 13 and 14, 1994. National Institutes of Health. *Pediatr* 1994;93:814–19.
471. Burd L. Prevalence of prone sleeping position and selected infant care practices of North Dakota infants: The comparison of whites and Native Americans. *Pub Health Rep* 1994;109:446–49.
472. Hauck F. Changing epidemiology. In Byard R, Krous HF, eds., *Sudden Infant Death Syndrome: Problems, Progress and Possibilities*. London: Arnold, 2001, pp. 31–57.

Introduction

A number of equilibrated systems coexist and interact in the intracranial compartment: the various barrier systems, such as the blood–brain barrier, blood–cerebrospinal fluid (CSF) barrier, and the CSF–brain barrier; the pressure/volume equilibrium; and the process of cerebrovascular autoregulation. All function to provide a homeostatic intracranial environment. When the blood–CSF system fails, for whatever reason, hydrocephalus, cerebral edema, and/or intracranial pressure increases may result. When vascular autoregulation fails, tissue hypoperfusion and ischemia or hyperperfusion and edema result. When the brain swells, for whatever reason, or some other mass effect is present, the pressure/volume equilibrium mechanisms may or may not compensate. If these systems fail, increased intracranial pressure results, leading to a cascade of events that have untoward effects on all the intracranial systems, and may result in brain herniation, respiratory failure, and ultimately circulatory failure that terminates in so-called brain death.

An appreciation of intracranial equilibrium processes can be vital to the comprehension of many injurious phenomena affecting the brain and how they may cause decompensation and death. There are many forensic implications here. To cite one example, an individual may have a chronic subdural hematoma or be suffering from hydrocephalus, apparently without symptoms, until the individual becomes rapidly unconscious and may die following what would ordinarily be considered an episode of minor head trauma. Such a scenario is not uncommon, and may lead to an erroneous interpretation that inflicted trauma occurred. A proper forensic determination may be made with a thoughtful application of some of the principles discussed below.

Cerebral Edema and the Blood–Brain Barrier

The so-called blood–brain barrier (BBB) has been appreciated for many years, and its function is graphically illustrated in Figure 5.1. It was discovered that the brain has the ability to exclude certain molecules present in the blood from the neuropil of the brain, as in various large molecules, those with certain charge characteristics, high molecular weights, and certain polar characteristics. Molecules that can, in varying degrees, pass the BBB are lipid solvents (alcohols, ether, chloroform, and other rather short-chain hydrocarbons, as well as a host of other compounds), relatively small molecules such as most of the amino acids, inorganic salts, sugars, etc. Some drugs easily traverse the BBB, whereas others, no matter how much physicians wished otherwise, do so poorly or not at all [1–3].

It appears that the most important component of the BBB is the capillary network of the brain, followed by cells that invest the outer surface of the capillaries (astroglia and pericytes) and extracellular matrix materials. The capillaries of the brain are unlike most others in the body in that at their points of fusion as tubes, the endothelial cells meet with a very tight junction (zonula occludens) that apparently physically limits molecules from

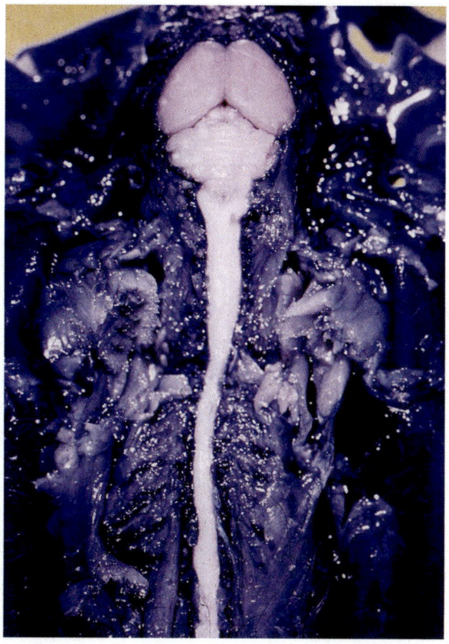

Figure 5.1 This photograph shows the appearance of a rat central nervous system in an animal that has been intravenously injected with trypan blue, a dye that is excluded by the blood–brain barrier (BBB) but penetrates every other organ. This type of experiment in the 1800s led to the evolution of the BBB concept. (Courtesy of Dr. M. Brightman, National Institutes of Health, Washington, DC.)

passing through them into the extracellular compartment of the brain [4,5]. At one time, the fact that astrocytic foot processes invest virtually the entire capillary surfaces of the brain was interpreted as having BBB significance; however, this role is probably somewhat different than originally thought. It now appears that the transport functions of astrocytes are limited and that their role in BBB function lies more likely with their participation in creating the extracellular matrix that surrounds capillaries [6]. In any case, a variety of insults can damage the BBB and cause its failure, the consequence of which is edema.

Broadly stated, cerebral edema is a state in which there is some local or diffuse increase in brain water. This increase can be determined in a variety of ways but in common practice is evaluated rather crudely by gross inspection of the fresh or fixed brain specimen, inferentially by the functional effects of brain swelling, microscopically in the tissue section, or by radiographic means, particularly magnetic resonance imaging (MRI) techniques, which reveal excess protons (hydrogen nuclei of the water molecule) in the brain [7]. In the latter method, barrier dysfunction may be enhanced by the use of enhancing agents such as gadolinium in the MRI and iodine compounds and other contrast agents in computerized tomography scanning that bind to plasma proteins that leak into the brain at points where the barrier is disrupted.

Classically, two forms of brain edema have been differentiated by gross pathological examination: so-called dry edema (brain swelling or, as it is known in the German language, *Hirnschwellung*) and so-called wet edema (brain edema, or the German term *Hirnödem*). In both cases, brain water can be demonstrated to be increased. In dry edema, the surface of the cut brain, even in the fixed state, does not exude water and appears dry.

In this instance, the excess water is presumed to be within cells, rather than in the extracellular space, and in a sense represents a compensated or controlled form of edema. In the case of wet edema, the cut surface "sweats" or shows a puddling of water upon cutting. Here, most of the excess water is probably free in the extracellular space, and only some of it lies within cells [8,9].

In some circumstances, the edematous process appears to be localized in the region of a lesion but, in fact, may be spread rather widely, even to the other side of the brain, presumably by the ability of water to extend freely into the extracellular space, limited as it is in the brain. In other instances, where the lesion is global or diffuse, the entire brain may be edematous, with little localized concentration of water. All gradations, of course, are possible and may give rise to specific clinical and pathological findings [10]. Furthermore, localization of the edematous process to the gray or white matter may take place rather selectively, depending on the injury that has occurred. It is within this context that the popular classifications, first conceived by Klatzo [8], of so-called cytotoxic and vasogenic edema, have meaning [11,12].

Vasogenic edema is primarily extracellular and tends to occur mostly in the white matter in response to injury of the vascular component of the BBB, as in tumors, traumatic injury, thermal injury, and other physically disruptive processes [8,10,13]. Vasogenic edema is classically treated with steroids [14]. Cytotoxic edema is more limited to the gray matter and is, at least initially, intracellular. This form of edema is most commonly associated with metabolic insults such as hypoxia, hyperpyrexia, hypoglycemia, seizure, and toxic states [11] and more likely will respond to osmotic therapy. It is probably too restrictive in an operational sense to attempt to think of cerebral edema only within the context of these two conceptual entities, and it may be more useful to think of edema, of whatever cause, simply as compensated or uncompensated, which after all is what matters.

Within the context of the compensated state, the excess water is mostly intracellular, probably residing mostly within astroglia and oligodendroglia as a consequence of their normal function of preserving the inner brain environment. This process is successful only to the extent that transport mechanisms are working and that the influx of water does not exceed the capacity of the cells to absorb it and transport it [15]. Once this capacity is exceeded, which is usually the case, the degree of decompensation increases and, with it, the net amount of extracellular water. It is important to think of the edema process as a dynamic one, ever shifting and changing in response to the forces that act to restore or maintain homeostasis and the forces acting to disrupt it. It is therefore reasonable to explain the rises and falls of intracranial pressure, as well as the degree of edema and its herniation and symptomatic effects, as the end result of the interplay of the two opposing aspects of one component of a very dynamic equilibrium [8,9].

The degree of cerebral edema can be influenced by a number of means, which have been exploited clinically with great success. As alluded to above, the osmotic "drawing" action of various substances such as urea and mannitol over the short term (for a few hours at a time) can rapidly and dramatically diminish the accumulation of brain water, both diffusely and locally, by dehydrating the brain. Eventually, toxicity and side effects limit the long-term usefulness of these agents. Probably the most useful and important method of treating cerebral edema, even over the long term (weeks and months), is with the use of corticosteroids, specifically dexamethasone. This compound is routinely prescribed for long-term control of edema in connection with brain tumors and other chronic sources of edema. Unfortunately, the effectiveness of corticosteroids may diminish after several months' use, allowing return of the edema and its consequences, not to mention systemic complications (weight gain, habitus change, diabetes, cataract, muscle weakness, etc.), which are well known [12].

Brain Lesions and Edema

As mentioned above, virtually every injury to the brain can produce edema. The pathological basis for edema is centered about the function of the brain capillary or the metabolism of the gray matter [15]. When any process affects the function of the capillary, edema can result (vasogenic edema). This is commonly the case with structural lesions such as tumors, both primary and secondary, any form of cerebral vascular disease, infections, or physical trauma. Quite often edema is multifactorial, and it is a forensic mistake to think of cerebral edema as being due to one factor alone. An often-neglected cause is the complication of cardiopulmonary resuscitation and poor airway access or gas transfer in a head-injured patient, which may be additive.

Edema in Connection with Neoplasms

In the case of brain tumors, especially metastatic ones, cerebral edema is a very common component. This is due to the inherent nature of the metastatic tumor and how it originates. At the inception of the metastatic lesion, an embolus of neoplastic cells must reach the capillary and must achieve an intimate relationship with the capillary cytoplasmic membrane, which is permitted by a matching of cell surface characteristics (probably glycoproteins) between cancer cell and endothelium and an evasion of defense mechanisms that are very complex and may involve a number of genetic determinants [16]. This relationship is highly variable and by no means guaranteed by the mere proximity of tumor cells and endothelium. If the tumor embolus sticks to the endothelium, it must be enclosed by the endothelium before it can grow [17,18]. Once growth occurs, the process of disruption of the BBB begins. This is brought about, in part, by the physical proliferation of the tumor cells at a greater rate than the vessel, which probably acts to elevate astroglial foot processes from their normal investing relationships, and may cause some failure of fluid or other transport. Furthermore, as the tumor grows, it may release tumor angiogenesis factors that are mitogenic to the endothelium. The stimulated endothelial cells may not form typical tight junctions with each other, thus permitting leakage of substances not ordinarily allowed to pass through the intact barrier [15]. As proliferation increases and if the blood supply is outgrown and necrosis develops, inflammatory mediators released or stimulated by the necrotizing process may be vasoactive and incite a reaction that leads to increased vascular permeability and alterations of blood flow, increasing still further the possibility of edema.

In the case of primary tumors such as astrocytomas, the process by which edema occurs is more subtle and probably relates to an altered relationship between the foot processes of the neoplastic cells and the brain capillary, although this concept is controversial [15,19]. As the tumor cells grow more and more in an unorganized fashion, there is still an attempt to maintain a relationship with capillaries, and just as in the case of metastatic tumors, there is release of tumor angiogenic factors that cause vascular proliferation. In general, the more aggressive and malignant the astrocytoma, the more angiogenic factors are released. The new vessels are very likely to have faulty tight junctions and fenestrations in the capillaries, as demonstrated by electron microscopy, which allow passage of water or serum into the extracellular space of the brain.

As a general rule, metastatic tumors produce a great deal more edema per unit volume than do primary tumors, and to a large degree the mass effect of most tumors is a combination of the true tumor mass plus the edema that it creates. Sometimes, the edema mass effect dwarfs the tumor mass effect. This is starkly illustrated in cases where one or two small metastases from a bronchogenic carcinoma produce coma and death by massive cerebral edema (Figure 5.2). The magnifying effect of tumor edema probably also explains the sudden appearance of major neurological symptoms such as epilepsy, hemiparesis, aphasia, behavioral symptoms, and coma when, on clinical examination and radiographs, it is obvious that the lesions have been present for some time. It is probably the breakdown of critical homeostatic mechanisms that have been compensating during tumor growth, but eventually collapsed at a critical point, that lead to such precipitous appearance of symptoms. This particular feature has forensic importance especially for metastatic tumors, as has been illustrated in case examples in Chapter 3. An appreciation of the mechanisms that are probably operating in such situations makes interpretation of such cases possible. A demonstration of the disrupted BBB in metastatic tumors where the liver is also affected can be seen in Figure 5.3, where elevated blood bilirubin has leaked out into the periphery of the tumor, staining, after formalin fixation, the neuropil a green color due to biliverdin.

In some extrinsic neoplasms, such as meningiomas, nerve sheath tumors, and others that do not as a rule invade the brain, cerebral edema in the margin of the tumors is common but is rarely as massive as in intrinsic tumors. The edema in such cases is probably brought about by pressure and local ischemia in the brain, which is being compressed by the advancing edge of the lesion, with perhaps some focal loss of cerebrovascular autoregulation as well as alteration of peripheral vessels by inflammatory mediators and growth factors secreted by the tumor.

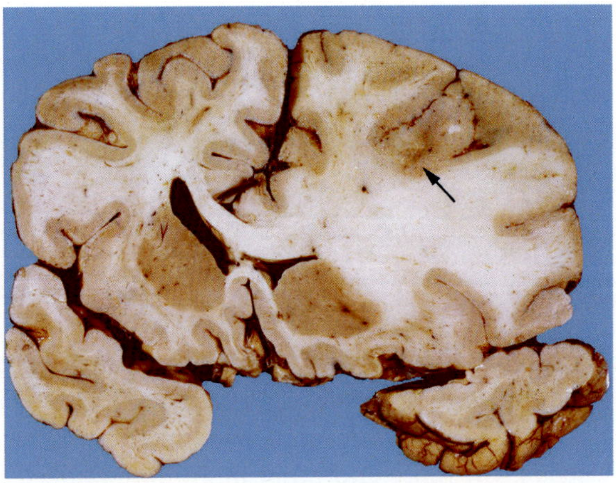

Figure 5.2 This coronal section of the brain illustrates disproportionate edema in relation to metastatic tumor size that is often seen. Here, a relatively small intracortical metastasis from a bronchogenic carcinoma (arrow) has led to extensive white matter edema with a large transfalcial herniation and effacement of lateral ventricle.

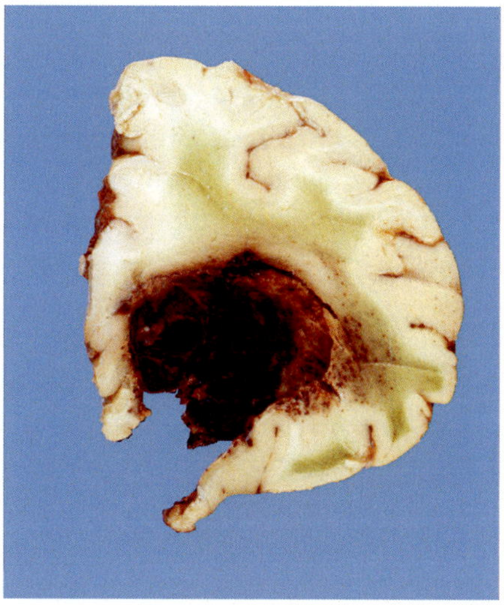

Figure 5.3 This photograph depicts a cross section of one cerebral hemisphere from an individual who died with extensive metastatic renal cell carcinoma that affected the brain, liver, and other organs. Hemorrhagic brain metastasis has disrupted the blood–brain barrier allowing bilirubin to pass into the zone of edema around the tumor. Formalin fixation converted bilirubin into biliverdin, providing green color to the zone of edema. (Courtesy of Dr. Carol Haller and the Office of the Medical Examiner, Cook County, IL.)

Edema in Connection with Physical Injury

Head trauma [20] is nearly always complicated by some degree of cerebral edema (discussed in detail in Chapter 6). Edema can occur in connection with contusions, lacerations, foreign bodies, or hemorrhages in the brain or in the subdural compartment. Cerebral edema in trauma, and its inevitable effect on intracranial pressure, is the single most important variable in patient morbidity and mortality [21,22]. Physical forces may all result in physical disruption of vessels and their immediate environment, leading to leakage of serum and often blood into the brain. In cases where there is sudden subarachnoid hemorrhage (discussed in Chapter 3), the irritating effect of blood, probably mediated by release of inflammatory mediators from platelets and endothelium or because of tissue damage, on the external walls of brain vessels may prompt an edematous reaction, which again acts to compound the mass effect of the blood and hasten a fatal outcome. It is not known why this occurs, but clearly physical disruption of the capillary–brain barrier is likely as well as chemical effects on the barriers by electrolytes such as calcium and potassium and inflammatory mediators such as those released in the course of injury, the blood coagulation cascade, and other factors [23–25].

A particularly catastrophic form of traumatic cerebral edema is occasionally observed in young children who sustain head trauma. Adults may also suffer from this condition. The trauma may be minor but is usually more significant [26–29]. A common example of such an instance is a fall from an open window to the pavement below. The fall may exceed several stories, yet the child may appear relatively uninjured and either is conscious throughout or rapidly regains consciousness. Quite often such children are taken to an emergency department, where it is ascertained that no skull fracture has occurred, minor injuries are treated, and the child is released. After a variable interval of often several hours, the child may lapse into stupor leading to coma and may be found dead in bed. These events may also occur in the hospital when there have been other injuries or when the child has been kept for observation. Autopsy reveals massive cerebral edema, with herniations, quite often with no obvious contusions, or hemorrhages in the brain or dura (see Chapters 3, 4, and 6). Frequently, therapeutic measures that are instituted to combat the cerebral edema are ineffective and the brain death phenomenon results with production of a respirator brain, discussed below.

Cerebral Edema and Inflammatory Diseases

When the nervous system is subject to injury from infectious agents that cause an inflammatory response, cerebral edema is a very common complicating factor. This is especially true in bacterial meningitis and viral encephalitis. The pathological basis for the edema is the general response by vessels to inflammation, vasoactive substances, complement reactions, inflammatory mediators including prostaglandins and leukotrienes, as well as direct cellular reactions that may disrupt blood vessels or act to alter flow in them [30–32]. There are certainly phases of the infection when whatever edema is produced is compensated for by the glial cells and probably the vessels themselves; however, eventual decompensation may result when these homeostatic mechanisms are overwhelmed.

Many of the infectious agents involve vessels directly and thus have the capacity for massive disruption of the BBB. This is clearly illustrated in the case of the more virulent bacterial meningitides, such as those caused by staphylococci, which may cause necrosis of vessel walls, or elaborate potent endotoxins that have profound vasogenic effects [33,34]. Meningococcal and other infections may also produce massive damage to vessels by means of disseminated intravascular coagulation defects leading to diffuse brain edema [35,36]. Tuberculosis and the fungal meningitides often cause thrombosis and necrosis of vessel walls, which may produce chemic or infarctive lesions, which then lead to uncompensated edema [37]. When tuberculomas in the brain occur, these lesions, because of their intense inflammation, may lead to precipitous and massive cerebral edema that causes death. This is especially true in children who have brain stem or cerebellar tubercular abscess, often of quite small dimensions. Viral infections, because they often involve vessels, may also cause massive edema and brain swelling. This effect is probably one of the major causes of acute death in encephalitis [38].

Cerebral vasculitis of whatever form or etiology may produce clinically and pathologically significant edema, especially where hemorrhagic or necrotic lesions have occurred. The mechanism for this edema is self-evident in view of the above discussion.

Pseudotumor Cerebri

Sometimes referred to as benign intracranial hypertension, pseudotumor cerebri may be anything but benign [39]. The classic case presents with signs of increased intracranial pressure, headache, papilledema, decrease in vision, and sometimes obtundation, usually in adults but sometimes in children [40]. In some cases, the syndrome waxes and wanes, with many episodes occurring over several years. The presenting symptoms do not reveal any information about the cause of the illness, and after other causes for intracranial pressure increase, such as hydrocephalus, brain tumor and other focal mass lesion, pregnancy [41], and venous sinus thrombosis [42], have been ruled out, some cases remain in which the basis for the elevated pressure remains unclear. Later careful study sometimes reveals Addison's disease, hypoparathyroidism or other hormonal dysfunction, hypervitaminosis

A, idiosyncratic reaction to a prescribed drug (including oral contraceptive agents; see Chapter 3), exposure to some toxic material, or some autoimmune process. In the latter case, from time to time immune complexes have been demonstrated in the walls of cerebral capillaries, which probably rendered them permeable and caused the edema. In other cases, the precise basis by which a diffuse but mild form of cerebral edema has occurred may remain obscure.

Edema in Connection with Vascular Diseases

When occlusion or compromise of a major vessel supplying blood to the brain occurs, two factors operate to produce cerebral edema: the effects of ischemia on the vascular bed, which will lead to vasogenic edema, and the effects of ischemia on gray matter, which leads to cytotoxic edema. The two processes become intertwined rather rapidly and are, from a practical standpoint, inseparable, although there may be special therapeutic strategies directed at both. The degree of edema that is produced by thrombosis or embolic obstruction of a vessel territory is dependent on the extent of tissue damage and the duration of the obstruction. The more complete and longer lasting the obstruction, the more likely the possibility that when the obstruction lyses or is removed, no blood flow will be reestablished (the no-reflow phenomenon) [43]. This limits, to some degree, the amount of vascular bed capable of forming the edema, which would have been much greater had blood flow been reestablished into a damaged perfusion territory before no-reflow occurred. Although there is edema to some degree attending virtually every cerebral infarction, even transient ischemic lesions, there may be delayed edema in connection with the classic anemic or pale infarction. Within a few days of the inception of the infarct, the peripheral regions of the lesion may expand to involve brain that is adequately perfused. The liberation of the products of cellular necrosis, which may include vasoactive or inflammatory substances, may produce significant amounts of edema at the periphery of the infarct. It is this secondary edema that may account for the rapidly rising mortality rates in infarct victims 4–10 days postinfarction [44].

Edema in Connection with Drugs and Chemicals

There are many compounds that produce cerebral edema, many of which have been discovered in the course of investigating industrial accidents or public health disasters. Alkyl tin (triethyltin) intoxication is such an example. In a freak occurrence in France some years ago, 100 individuals became intoxicated with this compound after ingesting it and died from severe cerebral edema [45]. Subsequently, it was found that this agent produces a rather specific form of edema of the subcortical white matter in which, in addition to the swelling of astrocytes, there is a curious accumulation of water and electrolytes, but little protein, within the myelin sheaths [46]. Additional aspects of this form of intoxication can be found in Chapter 3.

A wide spectrum of organic compounds can easily pass into the brain and interfere with neuronal metabolism and BBB functions, resulting in cerebral edema. Highly important among these are the alcohols, especially ethanol. When excessive and very rapid ingestion of ethanol-containing beverages occurs, especially in individuals who are unaccustomed to alcohol use, severe central nervous system (CNS) depression and massive cerebral edema may be fatal. In the case of other common alcohols such as methanol and isopropanol, which may be consumed willfully or by mistake, along with severe metabolic acidosis, which characterizes these intoxications, cerebral edema may also complicate the clinical picture. Furthermore, when prolonged alcohol abuse has occurred and consumption is stopped, a dangerous withdrawal syndrome may result (delirium tremens) in which seizures and other neurological dysfunctions may lead to cerebral edema on a metabolic basis (see Chapter 3).

Edema and Metabolic Processes

As already mentioned, hypoxia is a powerful and very common cause of cerebral edema, the severity of which is dependent on the severity of the hypoxia and its duration. Some degree of hypoxic edema is observed in virtually every autopsy brain because the agonal process almost invariably results in some degree of ischemia or functional hypoxia of the brain. Other metabolic events such as hypoglycemia may also induce edema, probably on the initial basis of effect on neuronal metabolism (so-called cytotoxic edema). Electrolyte abnormalities may also cause cerebral edema and include water intoxication, hyponatremia, hypernatremia, and severe and prolonged acidosis [47,48]. These edema-causing circumstances are especially important and serious in infants and children and may cause death. The issue of interpretation of suspected fluid or electrolyte abnormalities as a cause for cerebral edema often arises in cases of suspected child abuse and neglect and sometimes in connection with medical malpractice cases. Unfortunately, there are few specific features of the pathology in such cases to accurately pinpoint the basis for cerebral edema, and a final diagnosis often rests on supporting clinical or laboratory data.

Cerebral edema may complicate cases of high fever in malignant hyperthermia, heat exhaustion, or heat stroke, probably via a metabolic mechanism. By the same token, when body temperature is excessively low, as in immersion hypothermia or near drowning in very cold water, the degree of cerebral edema that occurs may be an important determiner of survival [49,50]. In such cases, there is almost always an element of hypoxia overlying the condition from which differentiation is all but impossible. Again, there is little in pathological appearances that will specify the cause of the observed edema.

Pathological Appearances of Edema

When edema is confined within cells as in so-called dry or cytotoxic edema, the process is most often diffuse rather than localized. In such a case, which is comparatively rare, the gross appearance of the brain may reflect its increased mass by showing a rounded and smooth surface, where the gyri are flattened against the inner contour of the skull and the sulci are compressed together. The brain will be increased in weight in the fresh state in proportion to the degree of edema, bearing in mind the normal weight ranges of brains with respect to race, age, and sex. When fixation takes place, the weight of the brain may fluctuate up or down during immersion in 10% formalin, depending on the osmolality of the fixative. In general, after 3 weeks of fixation, the brain will return very close to the weight in the fresh state. The process of fixation, except where osmolality of the fluid is very high, will not affect the appearance of any edema that may be present and will not obscure its pathology [51].

At the base of the brain, herniation effects may be evident as wide or deepened uncal grooves, obliteration of the CSF cisterns at the base, and a general lack of any space that is ordinarily seen. In addition, there may be expansion of the frontal lobes into the middle cranial fossa and herniation of the cerebellar tonsils through the foramen magnum with distortion of the lower brain stem. If the edema is particularly severe and uniform, additional herniation effects, described below, may be seen.

On the cut section in dry edema, roundness and swelling of the brain are evident, as is a decrease in ventricular dimensions. If the process is diffuse, there will be no obvious asymmetrical midline shift of any structures. There may be hemorrhage or necrosis where uncal grooves or tonsillar grooves are especially severe or where a vessel has been obstructed by the herniation. Although extensive dry edema may be observed from time to time, it is usually associated with wet edema of the white matter in autopsy specimens. In these cases, after cutting the brain, fluid is either immediately apparent on the cut surface or gradually sweats from the surface to puddle in the hollows of the surface. In severe edema, the white matter will have a creamy or rich yellow-green appearance and may even swell upon cutting. When there are localized lesions, which cause focal edema, the above changes may be confined to the immediate area of the lesion or may be diffuse and even involve the opposite hemisphere, although no lesion exists there. On occasion, when the patient has been jaundiced and also has a focal lesion in the brain, as would be the case in metastatic carcinoma of the lung with liver metastasis and failure, the tumor and its surrounding edematous white matter may appear yellow (in the fresh state) or green (after formalin fixation) because the BBB has allowed protein-bound bilirubin to leave the vessel and enter the extracellular space of the brain (Figure 5.3).

Histologically, depending on the duration and severity of the edema, the microscopic appearance of an edematous area is usually spongy, with numerous vacuoles in the tissue that appear different from the usual vacuolating artifact of preparation commonly seen in blood vessels and nerve cells. The neuropil may appear bubbly, and glial cells may be swollen (Figure 5.4). Sometimes the process may appear more perivascular than diffuse.

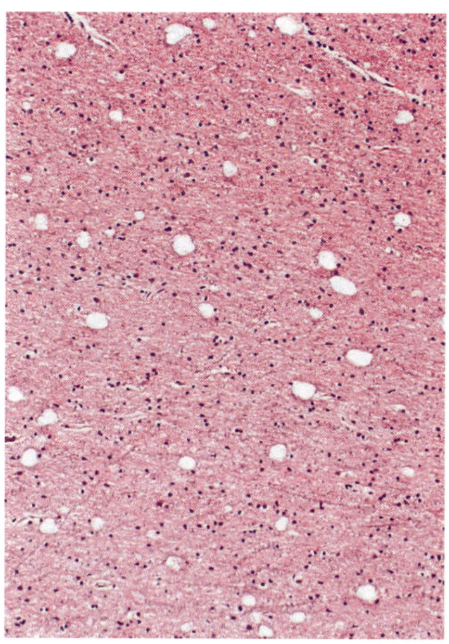

Figure 5.4 This photomicrograph shows a moderate degree of acute white matter edema with many clear vesicles. If edema is present long enough, astroglia will hypertrophy in response to edema.

If edema has been long standing, the vacuoles may be larger, and, in fact, small cysts may appear in the white matter. By employing immunohistochemical methods, which detect extravasated albumin or other serum proteins, the extent and severity of edema may be visualized in paraffin or frozen sections [52]. Occasionally, long-standing edema may lead to degeneration or necrosis of the white matter and axons. These changes are apparent in myelin and axon stains. An exaggerated variation of this process, which is rather uncommon, has been described by Feigin et al. [53,54].

Long-standing edema, of more than several weeks, may lead to reactive gliosis and the formation of larger, swollen, gemistocytic astrocytes in the affected region. Because most edema fluid is rather low in protein content, the edematous tissue usually looks paler than normal white matter in hematoxylin and eosin preparations. In those cases in which the edema-producing process has allowed high-protein-content fluid to escape into the perivascular region, it may precipitate as a pink amorphous deposit that in time will attract minerals, specifically iron and calcium, and form a concretion. This process is well illustrated in Fahr's disease, Sturge–Weber syndrome, cytomegalovirus, toxoplasmosis, and herpes simplex infections and in hypertensive small-vessel disease in the basal ganglia (see Chapters 3 and 4).

If focal cerebral edema is not present for long periods and the underlying cause has been corrected, residual fluid and electrolytes are eventually removed, restoring the neuropil to a normal state, leaving no sign of its presence. However, in longer-standing lesions, myelin pallor and some reactive gliosis may remain indefinitely [54].

Cerebrovascular Autoregulation

Cerebrovascular perfusion rests on a number of physiological processes within and outside the CNS. The cerebral perfusion pressure (CPP) is the difference between the mean arterial pressure of the blood as it enters the cranial compartment and the intracranial pressure (ICP) against which it must operate. The mean arterial pressure is a function of heart actions (cardiac output and its pressure), the characteristics and functions of the arterial tree from the heart to the brain, the viscosity of the blood, and several other incremental factors. The extent to which cerebral blood flow (CBF) changes with respect to CPP is affected by the phenomenon of cerebrovascular autoregulation, in which the vascular tree attempts to keep CBF relatively constant by means of vasodilatation or vasoconstriction in order to meet the metabolic needs of the brain, which must be satisfied constantly. This buffering capacity has limits, and when autoregulation fails, ischemia or hyperemia will result. Cerebral perfusion pressure will be reduced by arterial hypotension, hypovolemia, cardiac failure, arteriosclerosis/atherosclerosis, vascular dissection or compression or spasm, and shock [55]. Intracranial pressure may be raised and CPP lowered by a host of mechanisms that include cerebral edema, hydrocephalus, mass effects from tumors or hematomas, interference with venous outflow (cortical/sinus venous thrombosis), arteriovenous shunting, subarachnoid hemorrhage, trauma, and other mechanisms. The state of cerebrovascular autoregulation may have profound effects on clinical status and survivability after brain trauma. The mechanisms by which the cerebral vascular tree senses and then accomplishes autoregulation are incompletely understood [56,57].

Because mean arterial blood pressure in normal subjects is generally between 80 and 100 mm Hg and ICP is usually about 10 mm Hg, the normal range of CPP is 70–95 mm Hg.

Autoregulatory functions are generally capable of operating at CPP of between 50 and about 150 mm Hg. At too-low pressures, the vascular tree cannot compensate and CBF fails, leading to ischemia. At too-high pressures, compensatory vasoconstriction may fail, leading to exposure of the vascular tree to excessive pressures, which may damage the BBB and produce edema or hemorrhage (Figure 5.5) [58]. The proper management to preserve and utilize autoregulation is integral to effective management of head trauma [56,57]. One view of the relationship between CPP and vascular tone, CBF, and intracranial pressure is depicted in Figure 5.6, based on the work of Rosner and Daughton [59].

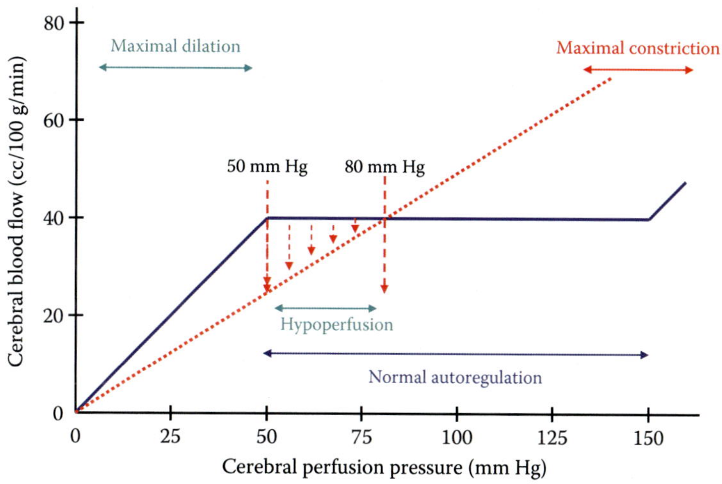

Figure 5.5 This diagram illustrates the phenomenon of autoregulation of cerebral circulation. If there were no autoregulatory processes in the brain, a change in perfusion pressure would linearly translate into a similar change in cerebral blood flow (as represented by the dotted red line). However, autoregulation yields the curve represented by the solid blue line, in which between 50 mm Hg and about 150 mm Hg perfusion pressure cerebral blood flow is constant (horizontal portion of the blue line). Below about 50 mm Hg, regulation operates but not as efficiently because vessels are essentially as dilated as is possible. Above 150 mm Hg, regulation also is inefficient because cerebral vessels are maximally constricted. In certain injury scenarios, autoregulation may "reset" to approximate the linear line as if autoregulation were not present. In this circumstance, the brain is hypoperfused. Once perfusion pressure rises to above 80 mm Hg, autoregulation can then function and restore the appropriate blood flow. (Adapted from Chesnut RM. Treating raised intracranial pressure in head injury. In Narayan RK, Wilberger JE, Povlishock JT, eds., *Neurotrauma*. New York: McGraw-Hill, 1995, pp. 445–69.)

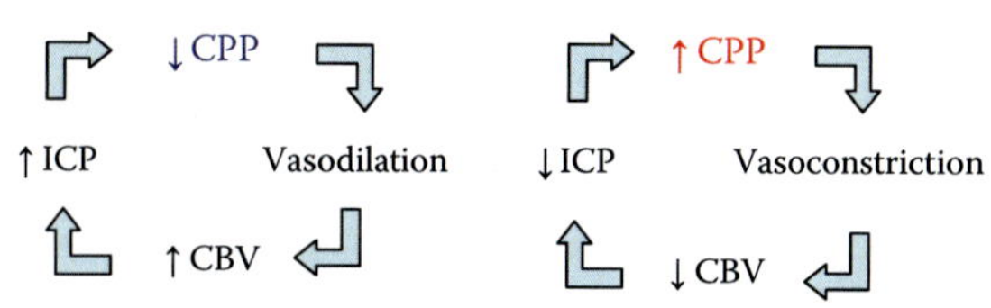

Figure 5.6 This figure illustrates in diagrammatic fashion the course of events, when cerebral vascular autoregulation is functioning, when cerebral perfusion pressure (CPP) falls (left) and when CPP rises (right). (Adapted from Rosner MJ, Daughton S, *J Trauma*, 30, 933, 1990.)

The relationship between increased intracranial pressure and CBF is not immediately predictable, although it tends to be linked [56]. In pediatric head injury patients, this lack of correlation is especially likely due to a number of complex mechanisms [60]. In general, however, patient outcome appears to be linked to keeping CPP high, even in the face of what would normally be considered fatal or near-fatal levels of intracranial pressure [61].

The importance of cerebrovascular autoregulation dynamics to forensics is not immediately clear in and of itself, because it is a physiological process that cannot be manifested or even detected after death. Nevertheless, an appreciation of the phenomenon is essential for an understanding of the intracranial environment and how it responds with the other equilibrium systems to injury, physical or otherwise. Because pathology involves the science related to how disease happens and its mechanisms, even though the mechanisms are physiological, the consequences of external and internal forces have pathological and morphological effects that can be interpreted in light of the physiological processes that exist. An example is the problem of head injury (covered in detail in Chapter 6 and briefly mentioned above) in young children, in which a child suffers what appears to be a minor head injury without loss of consciousness but then hours later develops increased intracranial pressure and may die without having an obvious mass lesion such as a subdural hemorrhage [26,28]. The mechanism that has been invoked in such cases is that for reasons not clear, the immature brain's autoregulatory function fails and permits hyperperfusion of the brain. It is likely that a number of other scenarios, possibly not involving head trauma, affect autoregulation and, although not appreciated mechanistically, may cause fatal cerebral edema and increased intracranial pressure.

Cerebrospinal Fluid: Pressure/Volume Equilibrium

The brain exists within a closed space (the cranial cavity with its extension, the spinal canal). At least in the adult, this space is constant and cannot be changed except through outside intervention. The volumetric components within the craniospinal cavities are the brain and its extracellular compartment (ECS), the blood inside the vessels of the brain and cord, and the CSF. The volume fraction of the brain that represents the extracellular compartment (sometimes referred to as α [62]) has been the subject of study for many years, and the value is a function of how the measurements are made. By electron microscopy, the ECS has been estimated to be about 5% or somewhat more [63]. Using various chemical markers that are distributed into the ECS, higher numbers in the vicinity of about 20%–25% have been estimated in the adult brain [63,64]. The immature brain appears to have a somewhat higher figure [64]. In recent years, the properties of the brain's ECS have revealed a more complex functional system, with compartmentation and functional/anatomical specializations that have been realized [62,65,66].

Cerebrospinal fluid is produced continuously, mostly by the choroid plexuses that lie in the lateral ventricles and within the fourth ventricle, but an unknown amount may arise from the brain itself via the ECS. In normal individuals, CSF is produced at a rate between 0.26 and 0.58 ml/min (or between 400 and 800 ml each day) [67], with absorption occurring at the same rate to maintain a dynamic equilibrium. Infants tend to secrete CSF at a faster rate than do adults, and CSF production tends to fall off with advancing age [68].

Cerebrospinal fluid is a water-clear fluid with usually <10 cells/mm^3 in the adult and usually fewer than 20 cells/mm^3 in infants. All of these cells should be of the lymphoid variety. The glucose concentration is usually about 20 mg% lower than the blood glucose level, with ventricular CSF having 5–10 mg% higher value than lumbar sac CSF. The protein level of CSF is 5–10 mg% in the ventricular CSF and 15–45 mg% outside the ventricles. Electrolyte levels parallel those of serum [69].

Cerebrospinal fluid is distributed within the brain ventricles, over the brain in the subarachnoid space, and in the spinal sac. Based on a study of eight normal adult subjects, Zhu et al. [70] report that lateral ventricles average 9.81 ml; the third ventricle, 2.5 ml; the fourth ventricle, 3.32 ml; and the volume of the subarachnoid space is 103 ml, for a total average of 118.63 ml. This figure corresponds closely to the figure for CSF volume, often quoted as being about 10% of brain volume, and to figures for the lateral ventricles reported by Knudsen [51], although the point is made that such formulae are arbitrary. The spinal sac holds about one-third of the total CNS cerebrospinal fluid, but is proportional to spine length and age. The CSF volume remains relatively constant throughout adult life but by the sixth decade increases gradually (Figure 5.7) and then dramatically rises to nearly twice the normal value after about age 80 years [51]. At birth, the total CSF volume is said to be about 50 ml [21].

Cerebrospinal fluid has classically been said to flow in response to intraventricular ciliary action and the small pulsations of cerebral vessels through the ventricular chambers via the foramina of Monro into the third ventricle, via the cerebral aqueduct into the fourth ventricle, and then through the two lateral foramina of Luschka at the base of the fourth ventricle at the cerebellopontine–medullary angle, and through the midline foramen of Magendie at the base of the cerebellum over the dorsal surface of the medulla into the subarachnoid space. The subarachnoid space at the base of the brain is divided into several pockets (cisternae), which normally have free access to the rest of the subarachnoid space. The subarachnoid space can be thought of structurally as the space formed between the surface of the brain, the pia, and the overlying arachnoidal membrane. The intervening space is traversed by blood vessels, strands of fine fibrous tissue, and cranial nerves that form impediments to free flow, much as might be visualized in a dense forest, where the trunks of the trees form a zone between the forest floor and the denser mat of foliage in the roof of the forest (Figure 5.8). The impedance to CSF flow in the subarachnoid space, if it

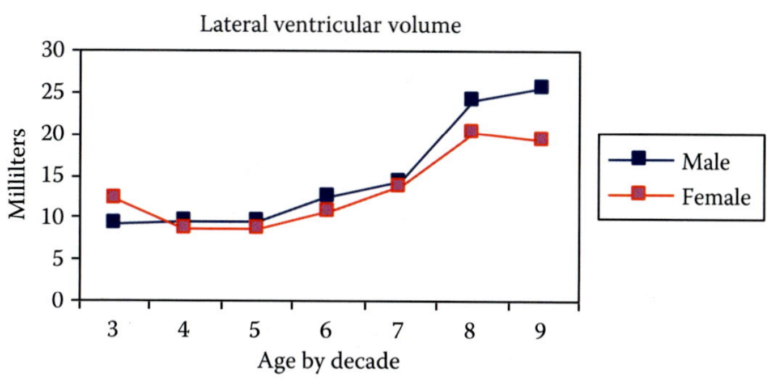

Figure 5.7 This figure shows the comparative ventricular volume of cerebrospinal fluid (CSF) of males and females by decade, which also reflects trends in total CSF volumes affected by age. (Adapted from the work of Knudsen as cited in Blinkov S, Glezer IP. *The Human Brain in Figures and Tables: A Quantitative Handbook*. New York: Basic Books, Plenum Press, 1968.)

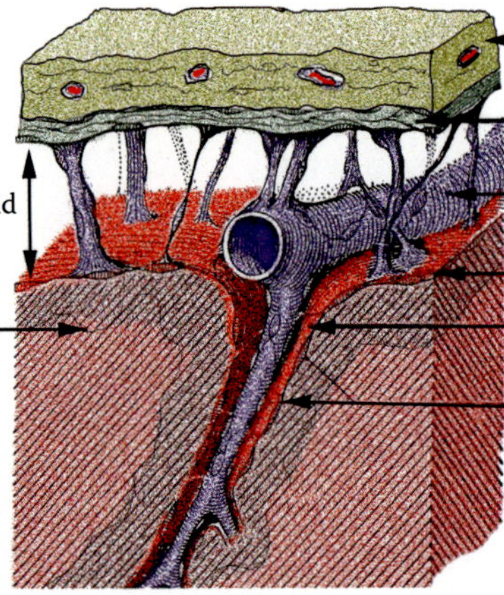

Figure 5.8 This figure illustrates the anatomy of the meninges and subarchnoid space.

plays a significant role, depends on the density of structures that traverse the subarachnoid space.

The process of CSF absorption classically was thought to occur because of bulk flow of fluid from within the ventricles of the brain, out of the basal foramina of Luschka and Magendie in the cerebellum, and over the surface in the subarachnoid space to arachnoid villi along the superior sagittal sinus and falx [71]. In recent years, the role of subarachnoid space CSF flow and the classic role of the arachnoid villi as the primary absorber of CSF have been questioned [72,73]. An alternative theory developed by Greitz and collaborators, and supported by others using magnetic resonance technologies that can monitor flow of CSF, is that CSF flow in the subarachnoid space is minimal—pulsatile—much like electrons are thought to do in an electrical circuit [74,75]. The driving force is thought to be arterial pulsations against the compliance of the arterial system in the brain as it conveys blood into the nonpulsatile venous system. In this construct, intracranial pressure (brain tissue hydrostatic pressure) is a function of arterial pulsations, capillary hydrostatic pressure, an osmotic pressure gradient in the brain created by the BBB, and dynamic movement of CSF across the foramen magnum into the spinal sac, the movement of which permits arterial-driven CSF pulsations [70,75]. CSF absorption, under these theories, is mostly accomplished by brain capillaries, the choroid plexus, and the brain itself, and not the arachnoid villi. Some have postulated that the brain has a lymphatic system that drains into the cervical lymphatic system and that it is important in CSF absorption [76]. Regardless of which theory of CSF absorption is valid, reabsorption is governed by the degree of intracranial pressure in relation to venous pressure. CSF absorption can proceed very rapidly and may exceed production by four to six times with little elevation of pressure [77,78].

Cerebrospinal fluid is the means by which most pressure/volume compensation and regulation occur over minutes, but not seconds, because it can be removed volumetrically from the intracranial compartment over time (Figure 5.9) when other volumetric components of the intracranial compartment cannot. It appears that cerebral venous blood volume plays an immediate role of pressure regulation in the very short term [22]. If there is a volumetric change in any of the intracranial components, or if a new volume such as a subdural hematoma or water due to edema is added, the pressure inside the cranium will rise above the normal homeostatic range of between 5 and about 10 mm Hg (roughly the range

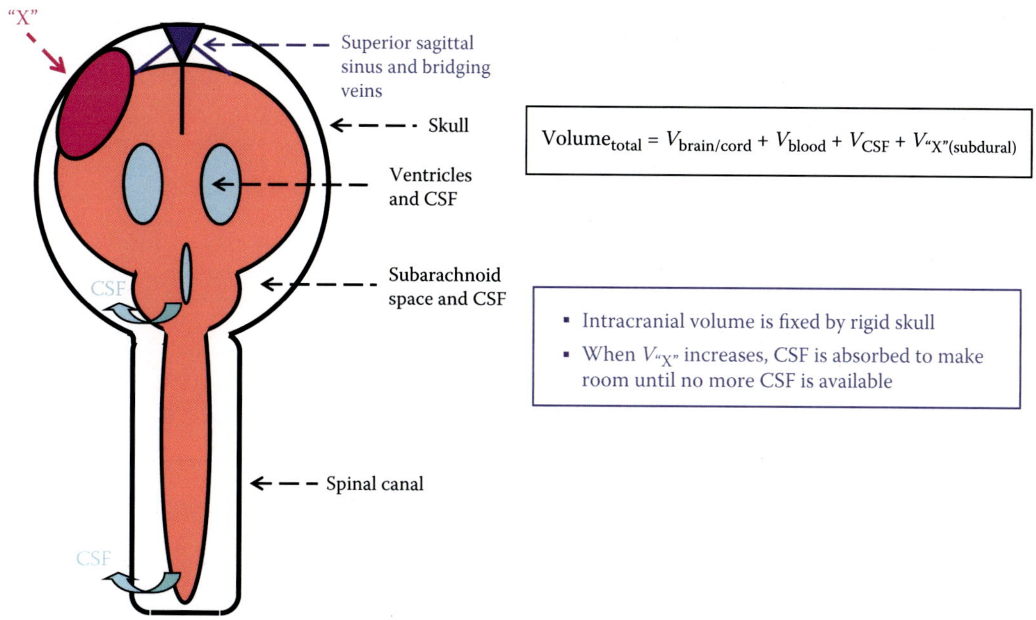

Figure 5.9 This diagram illustrates the volumetric components of the intracranial compartment as basis for understanding compensatory mechanisms to evolving mass lesions, in this case a subdural hematoma (depicted as "X"). Since in most circumstances, the cranial compartment has a fixed volume, if there is any increase in any one volumetric component, another will have to diminish to maintain equilibrium. In most cases, this changeable component is cerebrospinal fluid (CSF).

of venous pressure) [79]. With regard to the vascular contribution to intracranial pressure, it has been found that as little as a 1 ml increase in blood volume can increase intracranial pressure by 1.56 mm Hg [80]. By the same token, hypovolemia can also have effects on intracranial pressure, although less obvious. As hypovolemia may cause hypotension, it affects cerebral perfusion pressure, which, when it drops below 60 mm Hg (80 mm Hg arterial pressure), can induce increased intracranial pressure. There is a profound effect on morbidity and mortality directly related to the amount of time cerebral perfusion pressure is below 60 mm Hg and intracranial pressure is at or above 20 mm Hg [80]. Very often these factors are not considered by pathologists in coming to an understanding of causes and mechanisms of death, primarily in head-injured victims and the contributions made to the death by disorders of dynamic processes that may only be documented or inferred in the medical record.

The relationship between intracranial pressure and volume is not linear but, rather, exponential. At low pressures, the curve is relatively flat, meaning that volume changes have a relatively small effect on pressure. At higher pressures, incremental changes in volume have a much more pronounced effect. The relationship between volume and pressure is referred to as compliance ($C = \Delta V/\Delta P$). The reciprocal of this function is referred to as elastance ($E = \Delta P/\Delta V$) [80]. Measures of compliance can be assessed *in vivo* in humans by injecting or removing small volumes of CSF and creating the curve of pressure change that results over time; one can then assess and calculate a number of dynamic measures of CSF pressure regulation. The curves that result are much like that shown in Figure 5.10.

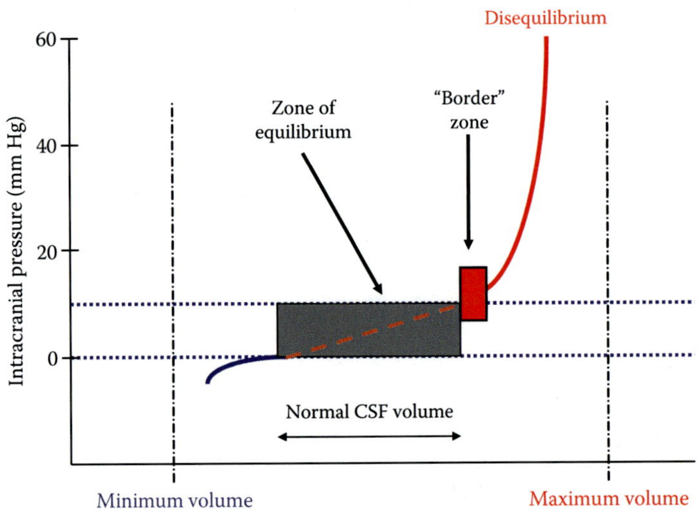

Figure 5.10 This figure illustrates the effects of volumetric brain compliance and the effect on intracranial pressure when it is overwhelmed by an evolving mass lesion. Normal intracranial pressure is usually below 10 mm Hg and is maintained in this range by absorption of CSF (zone of equilibrium). When either there is no more CSF to be absorbed or a compensatory volume cannot be transported fast enough, intracranial pressure rises precipitously and exponentially with the appearance of symptoms due mostly to brain stem herniation. Appearance of symptoms such as lethargy, vomiting, irritability, poor feeding, and other relatively nonspecific symptoms occur in the "border zone" where compensatory mechanisms are close to being overwhelmed. If compensation does not occur, even an incremental increase if volume will result in a dramatic increase in pressure (disequilibrium) and the rapid evolution of symptoms leading to respiratory failure and death. (Adapted from Friden HG, Ekstedt J, *Neurosurgery*, 13, 351, 1983. With kind permission from Springer Science+Business Media: *Intracranial Pressure IX*, Nagai H, Kamiya K, Ishii S, eds., CSF dynamics modeling in man, 1994, pp. 502–3, Friden H, Ekstedt J.)

Measures of compliance and elastance [so-called pressure/volume index (PVI) and volume/pressure response (VPR)] can be calculated and have relevance for expressing intracranial physiological compliance status primarily in head-injured patients. The PV, which seems to be the more useful measure, is defined as the volume in milliliters of fluid that, when added to the CSF compartment, results in a 10-fold increase in pressure. It can be calculated by

$$\mathrm{PVI} = \Delta V/\log(P_p/P_o)$$

where ΔV is the change in volume, P_p is final pressure, and P_o is the original pressure. The normal value for adults is about 25 ml and for children about 8–30 ml, depending on age and CSF volume [67,22]. It has been found that in head-injured patients, PVI values < 15 ml are highly correlated with increased intracranial pressure and clinical status [55].

It is obvious that age plays a role in the form of the curve, as do various disease states, including the intracerebral circulatory environment, which may determine how an individual reacts to changes in intracranial volume [80]. A number of these factors were considered by Friden [80–82] and are depicted in Figure 5.10, which views the extremes of the equilibrium and illustrates the significance of volume/pressure dynamics [67,22]. The effect of age on brain compliance is illustrated in Figure 5.11 [67]. If clinical estimates are going to be measured to assess compliance and other parameters, great care should be exercised to avoid decompensation by either removing too much or adding too much fluid to the CSF via lumbar puncture. So-called paradoxical herniation can occur if too much CSF is removed, even in the face of normal ICP [83]. This situation often occurs after craniotomy, when the basic environment intracranially is drastically altered.

During a compensatory process when a mass lesion, with or without edema, develops, the brain shifts to accommodate the new mass. Some mobility of the brain is possible simply by redistributing CSF within the intracranial space; however, when significant intracranial volume is added, in order to accommodate it and still maintain a normal ambient hydrostatic pressure, something within the brain will have to change. In children, the skull is capable of expanding by simple elasticity and by widening or "splitting" the sutures or fontanels to increase intracranial volume in response to pressure, but in the adult this is not possible. To be sure, there is a small volume to be gained by pressure on the various cerebral foramina, which have access to movable soft tissues extracerebrally, but such a space gain is incremental. In both children and adults, the intravascular blood and the CSF represent the most movable resources. Blood can be displaced into extracranial vessels and CSF can be driven out by pressure-induced absorption at the choroid plexus, ependyma, capillary surfaces in the subarachnoid space, nerve sheaths along the spinal canal, and maybe arachnoid villi [84]. Such accommodations are not instantaneous but rather rapid nevertheless. These and the following processes are illustrated schematically in Figure 5.12.

The forensic importance of the above mechanisms is that they help explain why individuals may have evolving mass lesions in their heads that may be essentially asymptomatic until their mass (volume) effect approaches or exceeds the ability of the brain to compensate either because there is insufficient CSF to be absorbed or the temporal evolution of the

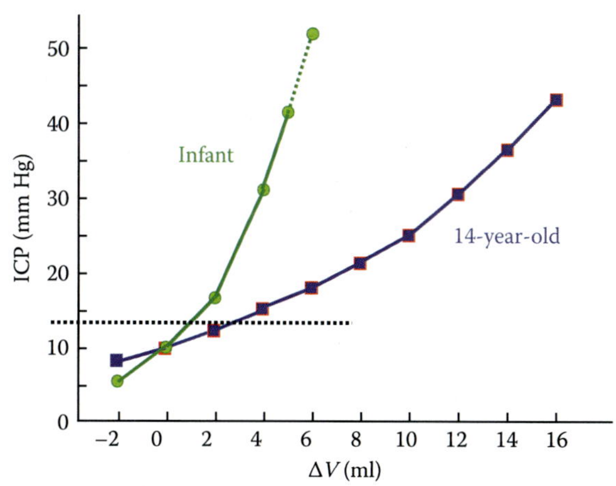

Figure 5.11 This graph depicts how small volumetric additions in CSF (ΔV) in milliliters by subarachnoid injection alter intracranial pressure in an infant and a teenage male. It is obvious that the infant brain cannot accommodate even small additions in volume before intracranial pressure (ICP) increases to levels that cannot be tolerated. (Adapted from Shapiro K et al., *Ann Neurol*, 7, 508, 1980; Shapiro K, Marmarou A, Portnoy H, eds. *Hydrocephalus*. New York: Raven Press, 1984; Shapiro K, Fried A, *J Neurosurg*, 64, 390, 1986.)

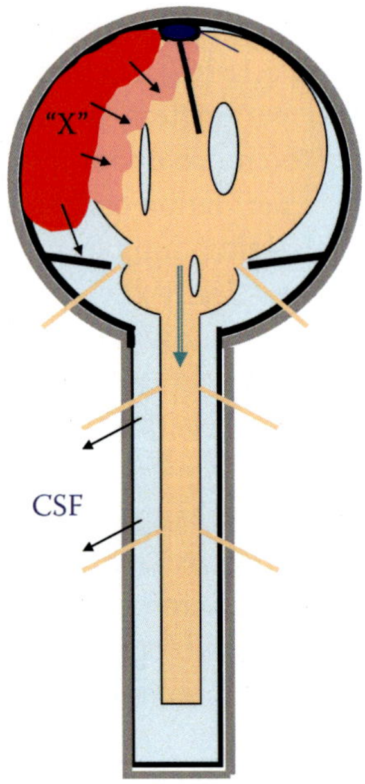

Figure 5.12 This figure illustrates a decompensated scenario caused by an expanding subdural hematoma (previously, "X" in Figure 5.10) with attendant shift of midline structures, effacement of the underlying ventricle, causing a zone of ischemia and edema beneath the expanding hematoma, and eventually brain stem herniation (green arrow). With brain stem herniation, a midline "Duret" hemorrhage may result, which is usually followed by "brain death."

mass effect is more rapid than whatever compensatory mechanism is available, at which point even an incremental increase in volume of the mass prompts an exaggerated rise in intracranial pressure and all that this portends, namely, the appearance of symptoms. These symptoms may wax and wane, but they begin as irritability, lethargy, headache, nausea, and vomiting. They may progress rapidly to decreasing levels of consciousness, leading to coma, respiratory depression and failure, seizures, decerebrate posturing, and death. This downward spiral usually reveals pupillary dilatation, eventually leading to fixed and dilated pupils that cannot react to light. If resuscitative measures are employed and treatment to address the intracranial pressure is instituted, the intracranial equilibria may be so affected that very little can be done to reverse the processes, and most such individuals will, if they survive, have significant neurological deficits or, if they die, will show the phenomena of brain herniation and brain death, discussed below [85].

Increased Intracranial Pressure and the Eye

When disturbances of the intracranial pressure/volume equilibrium occur, the brain's window to the world, the eye, often reflects changes in this equilibrium and provides to the clinician and sometimes to the pathologist insights into the nature, severity, and duration of these disturbances. To place the following discussion in the proper context, it will be necessary to review some aspects of the anatomy of the eye and its vascular supply. The vascular anatomy of the eye and orbit is complex and with considerable individual variations in man. It cannot be assumed that the vascular anatomy of the eye and orbit in animals is the same as in man, and that pathophysiology observed in experimental animals applies to man in all instances. Examples of this disparity will be discussed below [86].

Retinal and Optic Nerve Sheath Hemorrhage

The tissues of the orbit (fat, nerves, and extraocular muscles) are supplied mainly by the ophthalmic artery, which is a branch of the internal carotid artery, and branches of the external carotid artery. The ophthalmic artery most commonly arises from the internal carotid artery just after it penetrates the dura after emerging from the cavernous sinus. Rarely, the ophthalmic artery can arise from the middle meningeal artery and enter the orbit in an unusual course or even have anastomoses with both the internal carotid and middle meningeal arterial trees. Strange as it may seem, the ophthalmic artery may arise from the intracavernous internal carotid artery, middle cerebral artery, anterior cerebral artery, posterior communicating artery, and even the basilar artery [86]. The intracranial course of the artery is via the subarachnoid space on the inferior aspect of the optic nerve as it passes into the optic canal. Once inside the optic canal, the vessel may be wholly or partially within the dura but is said not to be in a subdural location. Again, considerable variation is possible. The vessel and optic nerve penetrate into the orbit through the optic foramen but occasionally can enter through the superior orbital fissure. However it enters, it generally curls around the optic nerve to occupy a superior and medial position, where it leaves the optic nerve to course forward and arborize and form the anterior ethmoidal branch, branches that supply the extraocular muscles, and continued branches of the ophthalmic artery that eventually penetrate the optic nerve and eye, forming the central retinal artery and ciliary arterial branches. There is considerable anatomic variation in the terminal courses of branches of the ophthalmic artery. Some of the orbital contents are supplied by the infraorbital and orbital branches of the middle meningeal artery (external carotid system) [86].

The venous drainage of the orbit and eye, like the arterial tree, is quite variable (even from side to side), with many anastomoses and collateral channels. The main venous channels are the superior and inferior ophthalmic veins that course near or alongside the ophthalmic artery to eventually join or enter the cavernous sinus separately [86]. The central retinal vein, which drains the retina and optic nerve and lies within the optic nerve until about halfway through its intraorbital path, exits the optic nerve, passing for a variable distance through the subarachnoid space of the optic nerve before joining the superior ophthalmic vein [87]. Along its course, the central retinal vein accepts numerous small branches from the surface of the optic nerve and may also anastomose with choroidal venous channels that provide an alternate channel for drainage. The veins of the orbit anastomose with many venous channels that drain the face and nasopharynx (facial veins; supratrochlear, nasal, and pterygoid veins) via emissary channels that may lack valves, thus allowing highly variable venous flow patterns from deep to superficial and vice versa.

Intraocular (retinal) and optic nerve sheath hemorrhages have been known to be complications of sudden increases in intracranial pressure for many years, perhaps dating back to nearly the turn of the twentieth century [88,89]. The explanation for these hemorrhages proved to be a challenge to many workers who employed human cadavers and animal material (both live and dead) in a variety of species to study the anatomy, occurrence, and presumed physiology of these hemorrhages [87,89,90]. During the course of these experiments, the differences between animal models and human material proved problematic [87]. Synthesizing the material from previous workers and performing their own studies, Muller and Deck [87] have evaluated the various theories of how retinal hemorrhages occur as well as how optic nerve sheath hemorrhages occur. A time-honored concept, that of diffusion of subarachnoid blood from the brain into the optic nerve sheath, has been shown to be unlikely or at least of lesser importance than the primary source of bleeding *in situ* in response to increased intracranial pressure [87,91]. The optic nerve sheath and associated subarachnoid space are highly trabeculated and likely present considerable impedance to significant CSF flow to or from its space [92].

The mechanism that best seems to be supported by the anatomic and physiological studies is that when intracranial pressure rises, venous drainage of the central retinal vein as it exits the globe, and at the point of a retinochoroidal anastomoses but before the central retinal vein reaches the superior ophthalmic vein, is diminished over the short distance it travels in the subarachnoid space of the optic nerve sheath. The resulting venous hypertension and stasis cause rupture of the central retinal vein or its tiny collaterals on the pia of the optic nerve. By extension, because there is no other venous drainage pathway from retinal veins at this point, they too will distend and rupture locally or into the vitreous. This process is illustrated in diagrammatic fashion in Figure 5.13. A photomicrograph of a typical optic nerve sheath hemorrhage is illustrated in Figure 5.14.

Probably, the sequence of events and their severity as well as collateral events determine the degree of hemorrhage seen, first in the optic nerve sheaths (said to be two to three times more common than retinal hemorrhage) [87] and then in the peripheral venous tree in the retina. It has been suggested that hypoxia may act along with venous distention to produce retinal hemorrhages [93]. Experiments were conducted using rat pups in which retinal hemorrhages were observed only in the animals that had been made hypoxic, inverted, and then subjected to a mechanical shaker, but no retinal hemorrhages were observed by

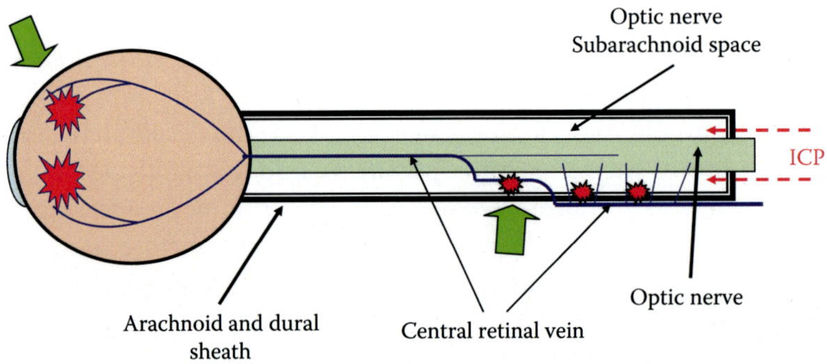

Figure 5.13 This diagram schematically illustrates the anatomy of the optic nerve sheath and describes the probable mechanism for retinal and optic sheath hemorrhages by intracranial pressure. The central retinal vein exits the eye within the optic nerve and about half-way along its course in the orbit the vein leaves the optic nerve and for a short distance passes through the subarachnoid space before penetrating the dura and accepting numerous small bridging veins from the optic nerve before it exits to the intracranial compartment. The probable site of action of increased subarachnoid space pressure (dashed red arrows) where retinal vein flow is impeded is at or near the large green arrow. While within the subarachnoid space or as the vein penetrates the dura is where optic nerve sheath hemorrhages are said to occur (small red starbursts) both in the subarachnoid and subdural spaces of the optic sheath. As venous hypertension progresses, hemorrhages can occur in the retina (large red starbursts). (Adapted from Muller PJ, Deck JH, *J Neurosurg*, 41, 160, 1974.)

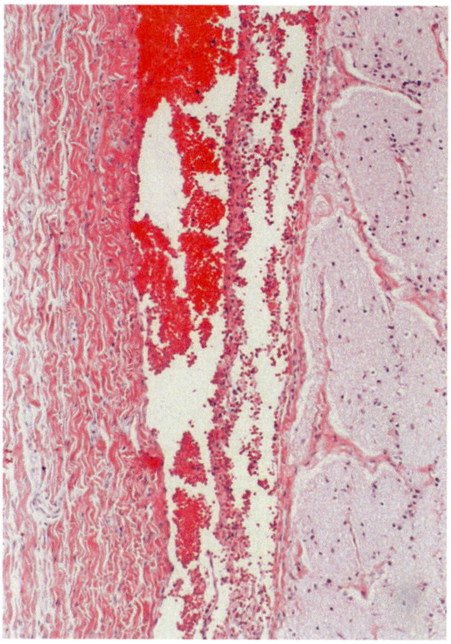

Figure 5.14 This photomicrograph of the optic nerve sheath shows on left the dural sheath with blood in the subdural space and intradurally. The thin arachnoid membrane in the middle of photograph clearly shows blood on both sides, with the optic nerve on right. This pattern of hemorrhage is the most commonly observed in fatal pediatric head injury but may also be seen under other conditions.

mechanical shaking alone. This experiment appears to reinforce the hemodynamic and hypoxic basis for retinal hemorrhages [94,95].

Retinal hemorrhages and optic nerve sheath hemorrhages are not confined to infant head trauma victims in association with the so-called shaken baby syndrome, where mechanical forces are said to be the cause of these and other intraocular lesions, such as retinal folds and detachments (these issues will be discussed in Chapters 6 and 7). In a general autopsy service population that includes individuals of all ages and causes of death (from natural diseases to homicide and accidents), various techniques have been employed to study the eye *in situ* or after fixation. Lantz has employed postmortem indirect ophthalmoscopy along with standard ophthalmic pathological methods in the study of now more than 1000 eyes (as of 2007) [96,97]. He has reported preliminary results that indicate that all manner of retinal hemorrhages, small and extensive, occur in virtually all types of death, traumatic and nontraumatic, at all ages, as do various forms of retinal folds; thus, although mechanical forces could conceivably cause some retinal pathologies, as many maintain [98], this mechanism is certainly not necessary and more likely occurs because of intracranial hypertension and probably other additive factors. Similar conclusions have been reported by Matshes in 2010 [99].

Papilledema

Swelling of the optic nerve head (papilledema) is most commonly seen via ophthalmoscopy in life but can also be observed in the fixed postmortem eye. Clinically, papilledema can be observed as a blurred optic disk margin and elevated optic nerve head above the retina. This swelling may be unilateral or bilateral and may be accompanied by streak-like or other retinal hemorrhages that may or may not radiate away from the optic nerve head. Under the microscope, the optic nerve head may be elevated quite obviously above the retina and may appear edematous. Papilledema has been classically thought to indicate chronic increased intracranial pressure significant of a brain tumor or other mass lesion or mass effect from many causes. By clinical observations of primarily head-injured patients, it has been found that although occasional cases will show papilledema in less than a week after head injury, most tend not to appear until a week or more after head injury, causing increased intracranial pressure [100,101]. At one time, papilledema was thought to represent simple edema of the optic nerve; however, Hayreh demonstrated that increased intracranial pressure that constricts the optic nerve sheath interferes with axoplasmic transport of materials from the ganglionic cell layer in the retina to their axons in the optic nerve, acting as sort of a tourniquet preventing flow [100,102,103]. The transported proteins and materials from the neurons to their axons accumulate proximal to the constriction and cause the nerve to swell. A component of axonal transport that is often referred to as "slow" is probably the component interfered with rather than the much faster "fast" component. When there is unequal pressure on an optic nerve, papilledema may be unilateral on the same basis. Very acute cases of apparent papilledema may have their basis in edema of the nerve head due to arterial or venous circulatory dysfunction [101].

The forensic significance of papilledema is one of aging and dating intracranial processes. Because it generally takes a week or more of increased intracranial pressure to produce papilledema, its presence, often with collateral observations of mass lesions or intracranial pressure increase, indicates chronicity of the process. This issue often arises in cases of alleged child abuse where injuries are thought to be acute and may not be when papilledema is encountered.

Hydrocephalus

Introduction

An important cause and effect from increased intracranial pressure is one of the many forms of acquired hydrocephalus, as differentiated from the myriad problems and manifestations of congenital hydrocephalus, discussed in Chapter 4. If one subscribes to the classic notions about hydrocephalus, it can be thought of as obstructive or communicative in etiology, can be slowly or rapidly evolving, or may have no obvious etiology. The latter circumstance can be illustrated by the problem of so-called low-pressure or normal-pressure hydrocephalus [104]. Despite having been studied for more than 100 years, there is much about hydrocephalus that remains enigmatic [71].

Communicating Hydrocephalus

Hydrocephalus may develop when there is a lack of reabsorption relative to production, with no physical obstruction to the normal flow of CSF from ventricles to subarachnoid space. In this instance, the cause of increased CSF volume usually rests with some failure of CSF absorption. Under the paradigm of Greitz and others [74,75,105], communicating hydrocephalus should be thought of in other ways. In one circumstance, the primary pathophysiology is reduced brain arterial compliance caused by inflammation, injury, or scarring in the subarachnoid space. This leads to damping of arterial-driven CSF pulsations, which leads to collapse of the capillary–venous bed and altered CBF with functional hypoxia/ischemia developing. Ventricular enlargement is said to occur because of increased intraventricular pulse pressure and decreased subarachnoid pulse pressure [74]. This process has been referred to as reduced arterial pulsation hydrocephalus [21].

In attempting to accommodate newer views on CSF dynamics with the pathological findings that have been known for many years, probably the most common cause of reabsorptive failure is said to be inflammation or scarring in the subarachnoid space due to prior hemorrhage or inflammation that affects vascular compliance, which apparently has a much more significant role than that of the arachnoid villi [106,107]. The role of scarring of the arachnoid villi is thus an epiphenomenon of the wider process. A common form of communicative hydrocephalus results days, weeks, or months after blood may reach the subarachnoid space for any reason. Even small amounts of blood may eventually cause some degree of absorptive dysfunction with a corresponding hydrocephalus. Some have reported that ferritin release from lysed red cells may contribute to villus scarring and probably injury to vessels [108,109].

The diagnosis of communicating hydrocephalus may be one of exclusion, and the pathological basis may not always be evident. Often historical information such as a history of a prior head injury, meningitis, or subarachnoid hemorrhage will be helpful circumstantially. Additionally, on gross inspection of the brain, the finding of thickening and fibrosis of the leptomeninges may give a clue to a prior hemorrhage or infection that may also have narrowed or obliterated one of the basal foramina (Luschka or Magendie). In this instance, it is generally not difficult to examine these foramina and even to take histological sections of them at autopsy. Chronic subarachnoid inflammation may have increased the impedance to CSF flow by diminishing the subarachnoid space or by causing sequestrations by fibrous tissue rather than directly scarring the arachnoid villi, which may be superfluous, anyway. The diagnosis in such cases is based on qualitative rather than quantitative information, the latter being very difficult to obtain ordinarily. It is possible to measure the various ventricles in much the same manner as neuroradiologists do; however, quite often, for the pathologist, experience as to what appears normal may well be as reliable in determining when there is ventriculomegaly as any scheme of measurement [51].

The gross appearance of communicating hydrocephalus is that of obvious enlargement, usually symmetrically, of the lateral ventricles and varying degrees of enlargement of the temporal horns of the lateral ventricle and third and fourth ventricles (Figure 5.15). It is typical that when the lateral ventricles are massively enlarged, the septum pellucidum will become fenestrated or completely destroyed. The most profound anatomic change is the loss of white matter and effacement of the convolutions of the brain. In the infant, the cortex may take on a micropolygyric appearance (see Chapter 4). In imaging studies, the periventricular white matter will have an increased water content, which is also evident by the appearance of edema microscopically. When the ventricles enlarge, the ependymal surface cannot expand or proliferate to keep the ventricular surface covered, and gaps appear that eventually become filled by a proliferated mat of subependymal glial cells that may essentially form the new ventricular covering and may overgrow and trap ependymal elements. This overgrowth may be spotty or even nodular, which is often referred to as granular ependymitis, even though there is virtually no inflammatory reaction present. The degree of collapse of the brain that may occur when shunting is done is highly variable

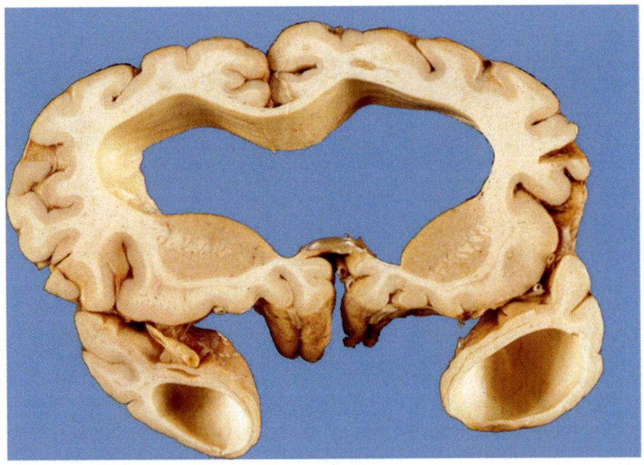

Figure 5.15 This coronal section of an adult with a communicating form of hydrocephalus shows profound enlargement of lateral ventricles with total loss of septum pellucidum and effacement of cortical convolutions.

and sometimes remarkable if the hydrocephalus has not been long standing. There is a risk, when the brain shrinks away from the dura, that a subdural hematoma may form from injured and stretched cortical bridging veins.

Obstructive, Noncommunicating Hydrocephalus

When a mass lesion, malformation, or some process or object directly impedes the flow of CSF out of the brain, the hydrocephalus that is produced is said to be of the obstructive type. This may occur at any critical point of passage of CSF, such as an obstruction at the foramina of Monro by a tumor or herniation; in the third ventricle, in the cerebral aqueduct by a tumor, herniation, arachnoid cyst, or infectious process; or, more commonly, within the fourth ventricle or the basal foramina [110]. In the latter case, any mass lesion of the posterior fossa may compress the basal foramina, leading to hydrocephalus, especially in children. Basal meningitis may block the foramina with exudate just as easily as can myriad other conditions, including the racemose form of cysticercosis. These forms of hydrocephalus are usually more easily diagnosed or confirmed than communicating types and tend to be more acutely evolving and therefore life threatening.

In any form of hydrocephalus that appears to be progressive, there is an end point at which the limits of compensation are reached and any volumetric expansion or rise in intracranial pressure at this point may be catastrophic. The final destabilizing event may be an additional element of obstruction, an increase in secretion of CSF (perhaps in response to rises in central venous pressure), a focus of cerebral edema, a small hemorrhage, an episode of cerebral hypoxia with associated edema, a minor traumatic episode, or another event. At this point, mechanisms tend to become degenerate and form vicious cycles. The mechanism of death in such circumstances involves herniation of the brain with pressure on the brain stem, interference with global or local brain perfusion, and depression of consciousness and respiration, with ultimate respiratory failure, cardiovascular failure, and death. The time during which these changes may evolve may be as short as 20–30 minutes or several hours. Occasionally, even when it is recognized that decompensation is occurring, it may be impossible to halt the progression of the process. At autopsy the brain is swollen and smooth, with ample evidence of herniation, as described above. Unremitting and progressive hydrocephalus with decompensation may be a cause of brain death and the respirator brain.

Hydrocephalus *Ex Vacuo*

This is a form of hydrocephalus that is passively formed in response to loss of cerebral tissue. In such a case, one or more ventricles will enlarge to fill the space lost due to tissue destruction or loss. This form of hydrocephalus is symptomless and under normal pressure. It is seen symmetrically in cases of cerebral atrophy and localized on the side of a large infarction or surgical defect. The process is usually not associated with evidence of herniation at autopsy. The actual mechanism for this compensatory process is unclear.

Normal-Pressure Hydrocephalus

This phenomenon has been known for many years and commonly presents in elderly patients who show ataxia of gait, evolving dementia, and urinary incontinence [104]. All of these symptoms are not specific for the condition and can be caused by many other problems; however, a significant number of individuals, when studied, may show ventricular enlargement and, when subjected to shunting, will markedly improve [111,112]. An example of normal-pressure hydrocephalus is seen in Figure 5.16. The pathophysiology of the condition is not fully understood [68], although it is thought that transependymal absorption of the CSF affects long periventricular axons of passage that mediate the gait and possibly bladder function. The forensic importance of this condition may arise when elderly individuals fall, possibly in a custodial situation where a proper diagnosis has not been made.

In this circumstance, the cerebral ventricles may be obviously enlarged radiographically, and the patient may suffer symptoms from the enlargement (apathy, dementia, ataxia,

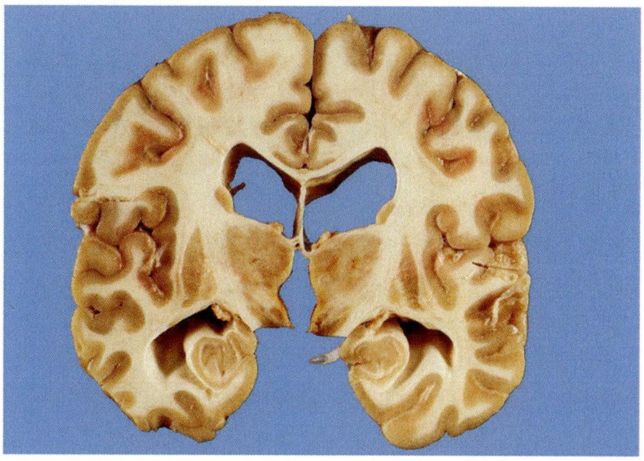

Figure 5.16 This is a coronal section of the brain of an individual who suffered from normal pressure hydrocephalus (NPH) and died of an unrelated health issue. Note the moderate symmetrical enlargement of the lateral ventricles and temporal horns with modest degree of cortical smoothing. In only rare cases is NPH a direct cause of death, although victims may suffer an accident from their diminished cognitive abilities, and gait disturbances that commonly attend the condition.

urinary incontinence) [77], yet lumbar puncture will fail to demonstrate elevation in pressure. It is possible that CSF pressure elevation is only abnormal at certain times, perhaps at night during sleep, and is related to the normal circadian rhythm of CSF production and absorption. In such persons, ventricular shunting may have a dramatic effect on improvement of clinical symptoms; however, in many cases, the condition develops so subtly that it is often not recognized clinically. This is often the case in individuals who have suffered a head injury and apparently recovered from it, only to show a slow deterioration months or years afterward. The above phenomenon is occasionally important in a forensic setting, where failure to recognize and treat the condition may form the basis of malpractice actions.

External Hydrocephalus

This condition basically involves enlargement, usually symmetrically, of the subarachnoid space over the cerebral hemispheres in infants and children. It is also discussed in Chapter 4. By way of summary, this is generally thought of as a benign condition that is often discovered when an infant's head is larger than normal by imaging studies. The external subarachnoid space can be profoundly enlarged and confused with subdural hygromas, chronic subdural hematomas, or arachnoid cysts [113,114]. The cause of this form of hydrocephalus is not known but has been associated with birth injury and intracranial hemorrhage, vitamin A deficiency, infection, and an unknown genetic condition that can lead to several members of the same family suffering from the condition. A significant complication is the risk for subdural hematoma with or without head trauma, presumably because cortical bridging veins are stretched across the widened subarachnoid space at the vertex of the brain [86,115–117]. Such cases may be misinterpreted as child abuse, especially because retinal hemorrhages may be present, which to some indicates abusive head trauma [117]. The condition may require shunting but generally resolves by age 3 years.

Shunts and Hydrocephalus

The surgical treatments for hydrocephalus, many of which with minor modifications are still in use today, parallel the evolution of neurosurgery. Walter Dandy of Johns Hopkins University is often credited with developing many of these treatments [71], which largely involved some means of diversion of CSF out of the brain. These diversions include the extracranial shunts to the peritoneal or pleural cavity, urinary tract, thoracic duct, gall bladder, and sometimes other sites, and the vascular shunts that involve diversion of CSF into the jugular, subclavian, or azygous veins; the right atrium; or the transverse dural sinus [118]. The most popular termination of the shunt is the peritoneal cavity (VP shunt). Generally, the shunt tube is fabricated out of silicone elastomer (Silastic®) tubing. The cranial end has a number of small openings, as does the termination of the shunt. There are a great many devices that are incorporated into the shunt to regulate or program the flow of CSF, with varying degrees of success.

VP shunts have many complications, the most common and serious of which is shunt infection, which often is caused by skin organisms at the time of installation, but other organisms can colonize the shunt and cause brain infections. The incidence of shunt infection can reach 30%, but the figure of about 7% is widely quoted [118]. VP shunts can also cause intra-abdominal complications, such as bowel obstructions, adhesions, abscesses, cysts, viscus perforation, and peritonitis. Shunt malfunctions from a variety of problems are common and often require replacement and revision of the shunt. Problems with drainage can occur at either end. In the cranial end, the shunt may migrate or be misplaced into the brain substance or, as commonly occurs, may approximate the choroid plexus, which can then grow into the shunt openings and obstruct them [68]. Such growth may tether the shunt tube to the choroid plexus, making removal hazardous. At the peritoneal end, omental tissues and granulation tissue may invade the shunt, plugging it.

Shunt malfunction from obstruction can be serious and lead to headaches, all the signs of increased intracranial pressure (vomiting, somnolence, irritability, seizures, etc.), and all of its consequences, including a fatal outcome. In adults, shunts may function for many years only to suddenly fail, or to fail without apparent symptoms. In such cases, it is presumed that the individual somehow stabilized his or her increased intracranial pressure and established a new equilibrium (arrested hydrocephalus) even though his or her ventricles remain enlarged. Sometimes, a shunted individual may suffer a head injury, even though minor, and decompensate or die. In such instances, the matter takes on forensic significance. It then is incumbent on the pathologist to properly examine and preserve the shunt (and whatever pressure/flow device might be attached and implanted with it) for later examination.

Another form of shunt malfunction involves overdrainage of CSF by the shunt. If overdrainage occurs, the disproportion between brain and cranium may lead to brain shifts and trapping of a ventricle, or a subdural hematoma or hygroma. Many of these issues have been ameliorated with the development of advanced programmable shunts.

Brain Herniation

Introduction

As any intracranial mass evolves, such as a subdural hemorrhage or a tumor with its peripheral zone of edema, space is made by pressure-driven egress of blood and CSF as a means of compensation. The mass may then occupy additional space by pushing adjacent brain away into cavities or corners previously occupied by CSF. This accommodation process eventually produces herniation effects. In the process of herniation, tissue may be damaged by compression against an edged anatomical structure, or its blood supply may be compromised by either diffuse or localized pressure. These phenomena give rise to the lesions described below, such as uncal grooves, notched cerebellar tonsils, third nerve compression, Duret hemorrhages, papilledema, and herniation infarcts (Figure 5.17).

At the point when as much intracerebral CSF as can be absorbed or moved in time has been driven out, the brain is still supported by CSF that lies within the spinal sac [84]. As intracranial pressure increases, this CSF may also be forced out. Presumably, this absorption takes place at the dural sheaths of the spinal nerves. As this supporting column of fluid leaves, the brain stem and cerebellar tonsils attempt to descend into the foramen magnum. As they do this, the basal foramina may become blocked and may obstruct egress of CSF, which is attempting to exit the fourth ventricle. This may exacerbate the forces of herniation, driving the brain stem further into the foramen magnum. Usually at this point, pressure has increased to such a degree on the brain stem that its neural function subserved

Forms of brain herniation

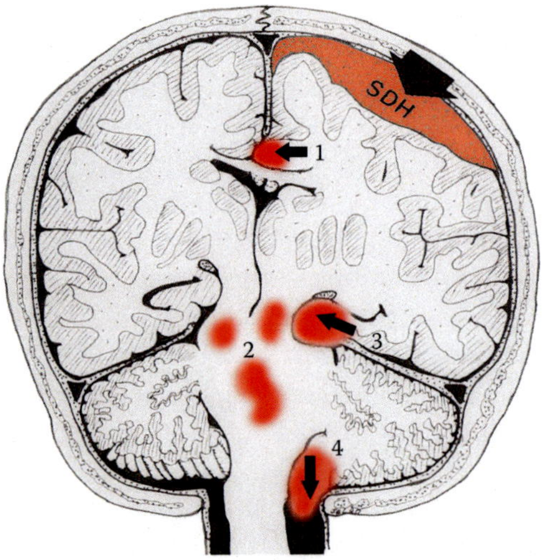

Figure 5.17 This diagrammatic picture illustrates the most common forms of brain herniation, in this example occasioned by a subdural hematoma, but any asymmetrical mass lesion (edema, tumor, hemorrhage) would act similarly: (1) shift of the cingulate gyrus across and beneath the falx with corresponding distortion of the corpus callosum; (2) pattern of midline midbrain and pontine hemorrhages often referred to as Duret hemorrhages; (3) uncal herniation of the mesial temporal lobe against the tentorium (petro-clinoid ligament); and (4) a cerebellar tonsillar herniation.

by the brain stem begins to fail because of simple pressure and also because blood flow may be compromised [119–124]. As the brain stem is distorted, the victim gradually loses consciousness, leading to stupor and eventual coma. Respiratory function also becomes altered and eventually ceases, necessitating a respirator if vital signs are to be preserved [125]. If pressure is great enough for long enough, the brain stem may be infarcted and death will result. If the herniation process is symmetrical, as in a diffuse brain swelling from hypoxia or an encephalopathy, hemorrhage in the brain stem is not likely. However, if the herniation is both rapid and asymmetrical, as in the case of an acute subdural hemorrhage, a secondary midbrain–pontine herniation hemorrhage, so-called Duret hemorrhage, may occur (Figure 5.18). When a Duret hemorrhage occurs, a large amount of the brain stem reticular activating system is destroyed, along with the medial longitudinal fasciculus (fibers connecting the vestibular nuclei with the nuclei for extraocular movement control). Loss of the reticular formation means that the individual will never regain consciousness. There are rare instances in which there has been prolonged survival after a Duret hemorrhage, as in Figure 5.19. The individual in this instance was in a vegetative state but had cortical electrical activity.

Cerebellar Tonsillar Herniation

When tonsillar herniation occurs, there is an impression made in the cerebellar tonsils with smoothing of the folia (Figure 5.20). Often this herniation is severe, and the impression of the rim of the foramen magnum on the cerebellar tonsils may be so great that local vascular perfusion may be prevented or branches of posterior inferior cerebellar artery

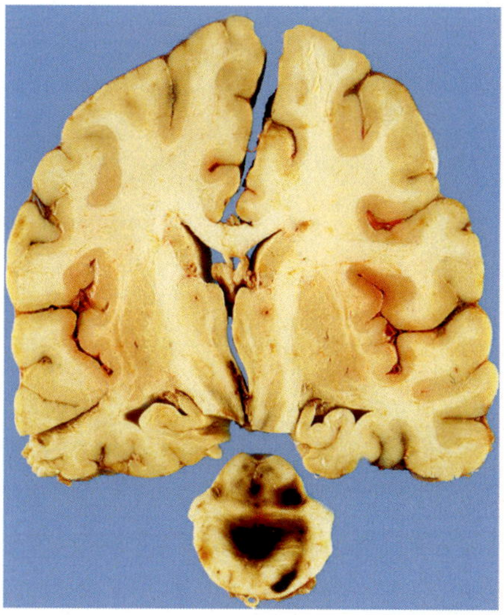

Figure 5.18 This coronal section of the brain and cross section of the pons illustrates a classic herniation hemorrhage (Duret hemorrhage). In this case, the individual suffered a left-sided "hypertensive" lateral ganglionic hemorrhage that ruptured into the lateral ventricle. The pontine hemorrhage is secondary to the asymmetrical mass effect of the higher hemorrhage.

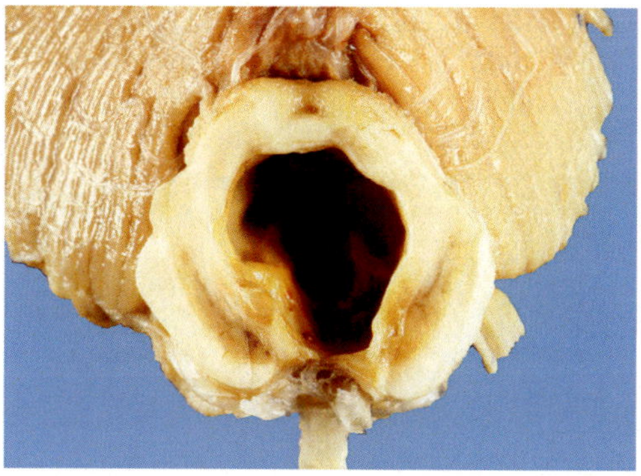

Figure 5.19 This cross section of the midbrain illustrates a rare occurrence of an individual who suffered a "Duret" hemorrhage but survived in a vegetative state for many months. Vegetative state occurred because there was near-total destruction of the reticular activating system of the brain stem.

may be obstructed. This may lead to infarction of the tonsils or parts of the medulla. The obstruction may be intermittent as intracranial pressure waxes and wanes, which may lead to hemorrhagic infarction and another source of edema that will increase the pressure to herniation. When the herniation is prolonged and occurs in the context of the respirator brain, necrotic tissue from infarcted cerebellar tonsils may shed into the CSF and fall into the lumbar sac, which, if a lumbar puncture is done, may give the false impression of inflammatory or small tumor cells in the CSF. Also in the autopsy specimen, at times the upper spinal cord may be sheathed by masses of necrotic cells resembling tumor but actually representing sloughed cerebellar material. Usually, this tissue is found in the subarachnoid space but can appear in the subdural compartment of the cord (Figure 5.21). It

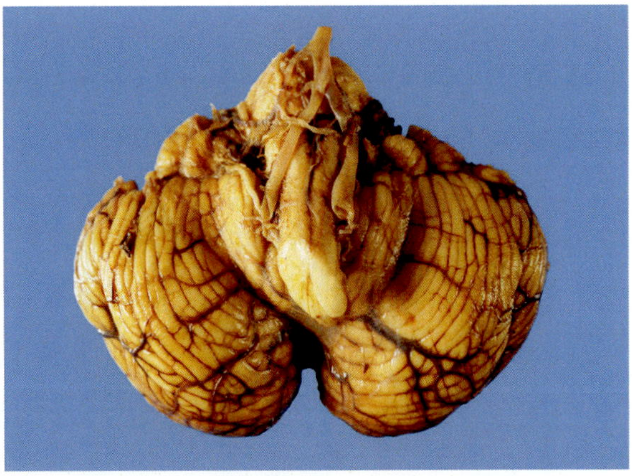

Figure 5.20 This view of the cerebellar tonsils shows an obvious circular impression of the foramen magnum with obstruction of branches of the posterior inferior cerebellar artery with focal infarction of the tonsillar folia.

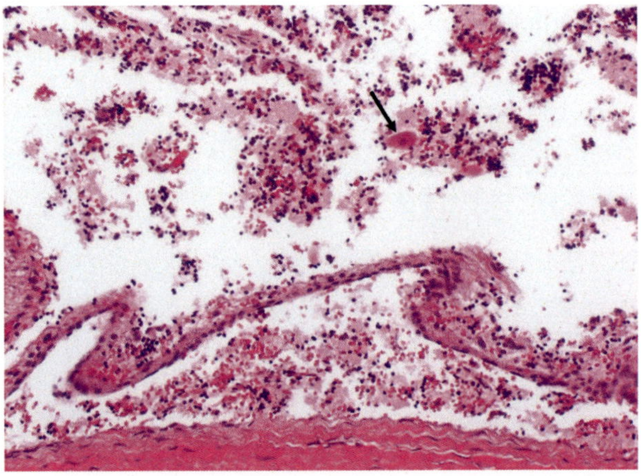

Figure 5.21 This photomicrograph of the spinal canal shows the dura on the left, which is overlain (subdural space) by a small deposit of sloughed necrotic cerebellar cortex. Sloughed material containing an eosinophilic degenerate Purkinje cell (arrow) lies also in the subarachnoid space above the spinal cord (not shown).

is not clear how this necrotic cerebellar tissue reaches the subdural compartment. The possibility of artifact should be considered.

Interpretation of the presence or degree of tonsillar herniation is sometimes difficult because the anatomy of the base of the skull varies from individual to individual and may impart varying degrees of impression in the tonsils after death and fixation. As a rule of thumb, when the tonsils are prominently molded and pushed anteriorly to warp around the medulla, herniation is real and significant even in the absence of necrosis, which is incontrovertible evidence of significant tonsillar herniation. To support this diagnosis, there is usually other evidence of brain swelling and herniation in other parts of the brain. At times, the herniation may be more unilateral and will then correlate positively with evidence of unilateral herniation above the tentorium, such as in cingulate gyral herniation and asymmetrical uncal grooves.

Upward Transtentorial Herniation

On comparatively rare occasions, a mass lesion may arise in the cerebellum that produces expected tonsillar herniation but may also, in the process of attempting to expand upward, extrude upward through the tentorial opening and be molded by it [126]. This phenomenon is illustrated in Figure 5.22. Such an event is usually very dangerous because any increase in mass effect in the posterior fossa, owing to its proximity to the brain stem, may transmit pressure there, resulting in depression of consciousness and respiration and the risk of irreversible damage to the ascending reticular formation in the upper brain stem. The conditions under which this form of herniation is observed include cerebellar tumors of childhood (astrocytoma, ependymoma, and medulloblastoma), posterior fossa subdural or epidural hematoma, Arnold–Chiari and Dandy–Walker or other malformations, cerebellar abscess or tuberculoma, and primary acute cerebellar hemorrhage.

Uncal Herniation

As supratentorial mass lesions evolve, one of the most common points where pressure due to herniation may be evident is at the mesial temporal lobes where the free edge of the tentorium lies (Figure 5.23). Herniations occur here because the basal CSF cisterns afford a potential space into which the brain can move once absorption of CSF in response to pressure has taken place. The groove that is produced by herniation may be unilateral or bilateral, depending on where the mass lesion exists above it. As is the case with tonsillar herniations, the groove may be minimal or massive and necrotic. Normally, there is a small groove that is usually symmetrical in the normal brain. As a rather arbitrary limitation, if the groove is <6 mm deep from the most mesial portion to the depths of the groove, it is said to be within normal limits and not to represent significant herniation. If it is greater, then the possibility exists that it is not artifactual and significant.

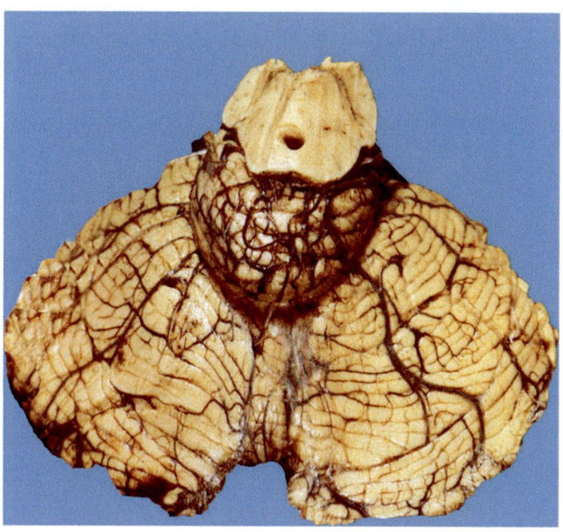

Figure 5.22 This photograph illustrates a primary cerebellar "hypertensive" hemorrhage with upward herniation of the rostral vermis through the tentorial opening.

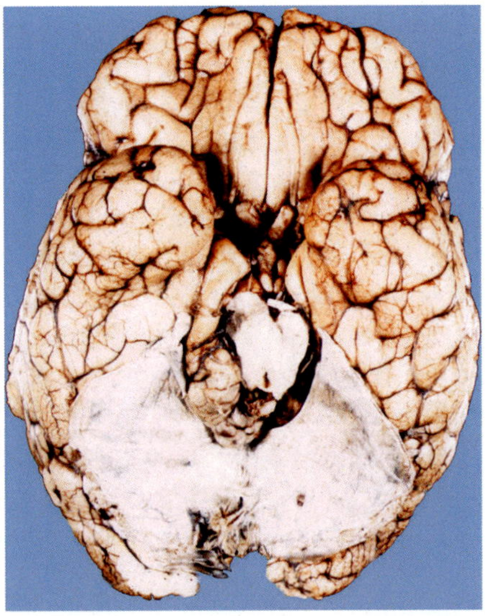

Figure 5.23 This photograph of the base of the brain with the tentorium remaining illustrates a major uncal herniation and its relationship to the tentorial notch. Note also the distortion of the midbrain by the herniation.

In most cases of significant uncal herniation, a separate but related lesion beyond the uncal groove may be produced in the third cranial nerve. The third nerve normally exits the brain stem between the posterior cerebral and superior cerebellar arteries and then crosses the tentorial edge on its way to enter the cavernous sinus. In so doing, it is very vulnerable to compression by the arteries if the brain stem is herniated and to compression against the tentorium by the herniating uncus and brain stem (Figure 5.24).

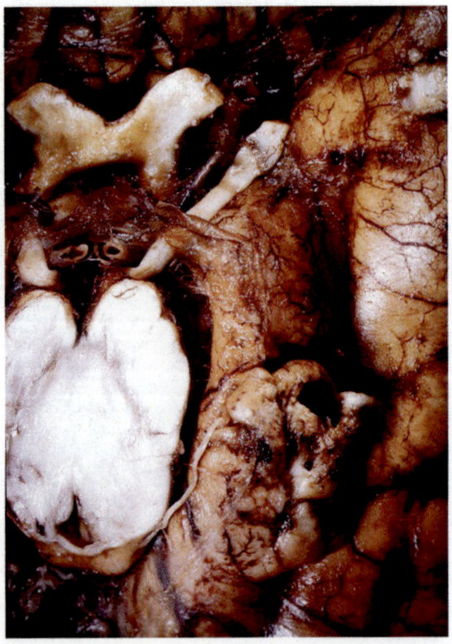

Figure 5.24 This photograph of a deep uncal herniation shows necrosis of the uncus and an obvious line of impression along the third cranial nerve that was made by the edge of the tentorium, which is not included in the specimen.

The effect of this compression is observed clinically by the fixed and dilated pupil on the side of herniation. The pupillary changes occur because the pupillary constrictor fibers occupy a peripheral location in the nerve and are the first to be injured, thus releasing the pupillary dilator influences that override constrictor function [127]. This loss of pupil function occurs before loss of oculomotor function when the nerve is further compressed. The groove formed in the third nerve is easily observed in the fixed or fresh autopsy brain. The lesion is usually reversible, and the changes in pupillary reactivity are often a valuable early indicator of elevated intracranial pressure. Although unilateral compression is most common, bilateral third nerve compression can also occur and has the same appearance.

An exaggerated example of uncal herniation may result when a very massive lesion occurs in one hemisphere, usually in the temporal lobe, which drives the uncus well past the midline and may place the opposite cerebral peduncle directly against the tentorial edge and lacerate it. The result of such massive herniation is to produce a paradoxical ipsilateral hemiparesis. This has been referred to clinically as the crus syndrome of Kernohan, or pathologically as Kernohan's notch (Figure 5.9) [128,129].

When transtentorial herniations are massive, the impression made by the tentorial edge may extend along the entire extent of the mesial temporal lobe and may indent or otherwise compress one or more branches of the posterior cerebral artery as it arborizes to supply the inferior surface of the brain and occipital lobe. This compression may result in either hemorrhagic or anemic infarction. The most common pattern of infarction is hemorrhagic, because the obstruction is often intermittent or variable. The most common area affected is the posterior inferior temporal lobe and the medial occipital lobe, often involving the primary optic cortex, area 17 (Figure 5.25). The significance of such a lesion is that vision may be affected by the herniation infarction (homonymous hemianopsia) or, if the herniation is bilateral, total cortical blindness may occur [130].

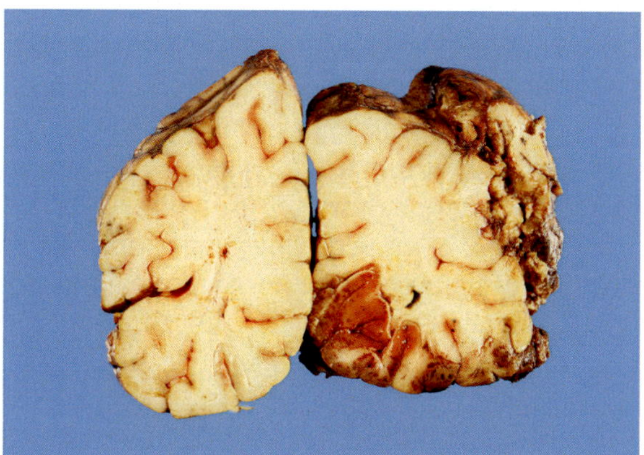

Figure 5.25 This photograph of the base of the brain with the posterior hemispheres removed illustrates a posterior uncal herniation that has resulted in compression of parts of each posterior cerebral arterial circulation with a hemorrhagic infarction that involves its perfusion territory. Such lesions may be survivable but may leave the victim cortically blind due to infarction of area 17, the calcarine gyri.

Duret Hemorrhage

One of the most feared complications of herniation is the secondary herniation hemorrhage of the midbrain and pons, also known as the Duret hemorrhage, illustrated in Figure 5.18. In most cases, the lesion is a secondary midline hemorrhage resulting from rapid, asymmetrical herniation of the brain stem downward. The lesion is most commonly found in the midline of the pons and may involve both midbrain and pons but never the medulla [131]. The morphology of the hemorrhage is highly variable—from a small streak-like discoloration in the midline pontine tegmentum to a Rorschach-like complex pattern. At times, the hemorrhage is massive, and at other times it more closely resembles a small hemorrhagic infarction.

Whatever the appearance, the lesion indicates an irreversible destruction of the brain stem reticular formation, including the oculovestibular (medial longitudinal fasciculus) fiber system and important centers for control of respiration. Most individuals who sustain a Duret hemorrhage survive only limited periods of time. If no respiratory assistance is available, death may occur in 30–60 minutes or less. If the patient is placed on a respirator, vital signs may be preserved for long periods that will allow the brain stem lesion to cavitate; however, this is rarely observed. The clinical diagnosis of Duret hemorrhage is not specific and rests only on the permanent loss of oculocephalic reflexes (doll's eye phenomenon and ocular response to caloric stimulation of the ear canals). Usually when these signs are present in two or more examinations, there is little doubt that a Duret hemorrhage is present when the mass lesion in the brain is unilateral.

The mechanism of production of the Duret hemorrhage is somewhat controversial, probably involving uneven herniation and stress on midline structures occasioned by the unequal downward pressure from the hemispheres [132]. This midline shear force may obstruct midline venous outflow, leading to stasis and venous infarction, or cause midline arterial obstruction and hemorrhage from tearing of veins or small arteries with extravasation of blood into the surrounding brain stem. There is no widespread agreement on the order and interplay of events that produce this lesion.

It appears that Duret hemorrhages can evolve fairly rapidly in cases of acute intracerebral hemorrhage or acute epidural hemorrhage, having been observed as little as 30–60 minutes after the occurrence of the mass lesion in autopsy specimens. In general, a period of about 2 hours is commonly observed, and much longer times are also common, although it can never be known precisely when hemorrhage first occurred because there is no reliable clinical means to determine its appearance as separate from the signs of severe herniation. Perhaps computerized axial tomographic or nuclear magnetic resonance scans could provide this precise information; however, it is unlikely that scans can or will be obtained under the circumstances of acute cerebral injury or vascular catastrophe.

Microscopic appearances of acute Duret hemorrhages are nonspecific and simply show fresh blood dissecting into the nervous tissue. Usually, all vascular structures within the hemorrhage are difficult to visualize, but sometimes they can be seen ringed with blood, although not obviously ruptured. At times it may be difficult to distinguish a dissecting hemorrhage from the basal ganglia that has reached the brain stem from a Duret hemorrhage or a primary pontine hemorrhage. However, when hemorrhages are primary, they are confined to the basis pontis, not the tegmental region, and the dissection hemorrhages can be traced directly to the hematoma higher up. In some instances, it is possible to discover early infarctive changes in the vicinity of the Duret hemorrhage, which indicates that some period of ischemia is probably inherent to the development of the process.

Transfalcial Herniation

When a mass lesion occurs in one of the hemispheres, the process of accommodation and herniation may drive the swollen hemisphere to cross the midline beneath the edge of the falx cerebri (Figure 5.26). To some extent, there is also shift of the falx, which, although fairly rigid, is not completely immune to lateral movement, at least inferiorly. This shift of midline may become massive and result in compression of the pericallosal branches of the anterior cerebral artery and infarction, as sometimes occurs when the tentorial edge compresses branches of the posterior cerebral artery with massive uncal herniations. The pressure on the midline cortex may produce rather minimal symptoms, which can include stupor and lethargy, paralysis of bladder or bowel function, and delirium, or blend with other signs of increased intracranial pressure. Massive midline shift may distort inner brain structures such as the fornices and may lead to an obstruction of the foramina of Monro. In congenital anomalies such as Arnold–Chiari or Dandy–Walker malformations, and where the posterior fossa architecture is abnormal, the ventricle, usually in the temporal or occipital lobe, may herniate outward and downward through an abnormal tentorial notch, producing what appears to be a ventricular diverticulum. This is a comparatively rare event and rather unlikely to be of forensic importance. In this unhappy event, intracranial pressure rises and herniation may be accelerated because CSF continues to be produced in the obstructed ventricular chamber with no means of drainage. Any mass lesion may cause transfalcial herniation, which may be an isolated finding only when the herniation is minimal; however, the process is usually reflected in another region of the brain, such as the uncus or cerebellar tonsils on the same side.

Other Forms of Herniation

On occasion, when there are mass lesions in one or both frontal lobes, there may be herniation of the frontal lobe brain matter into the middle cranial fossa, or if there are middle fossa mass effects, the opposite may occur. These events are usually linked with grooving elsewhere and are rare as isolated phenomena, for instance, where massive ventricular

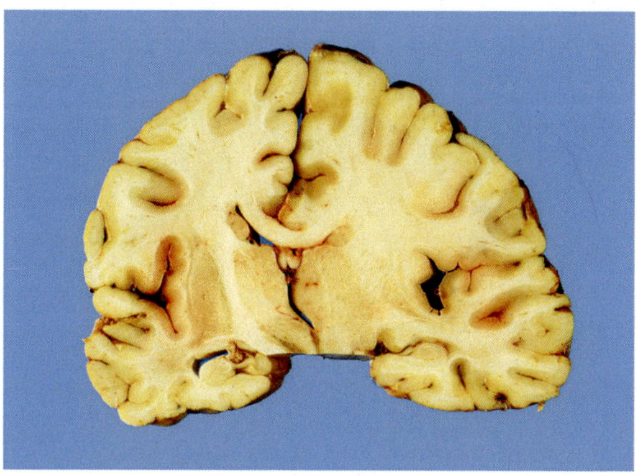

Figure 5.26 This coronal brain section shows a right-to-left transfalcial herniation of the cingulate gyrus in an individual who had an acute subdural hematoma. Note the distortion of the corpus callosum and effaced ventricles.

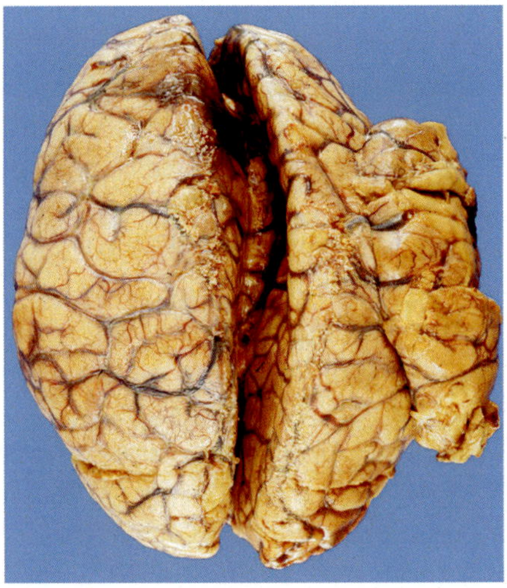

Figure 5.27 This rostral view of the brain illustrates a massive *fungus cerebri* through a craniotomy opening and a prominent transfalcial herniation from left to right due to a mass lesion within the left cerebral hemisphere.

enlargement has occurred, especially in children. Another instance of herniation, often called *fungus cerebri*, occurs when a craniotomy has been performed and the brain is severely swollen and intracranial pressure is high, as in subdural hematoma, brain tumor, or cerebral hemorrhage. In this case, in spite of all attempts to reduce intracranial pressure and edema, the brain fungates outward through a craniotomy opening, often making it impossible to replace a skull flap or at times to even close the scalp incision. This circumstance is illustrated in Figure 5.27. Usually when this happens, recovery is nearly impossible owing to the massive degree of circulatory dysfunction and ischemia in the brain.

Frequently, as a coexisting condition to increasing brain stem herniation or mass effect in the cerebellum, the fourth ventricle or cerebral aqueduct may become compressed or obstructed. This situation is often a terminal phenomenon analogous to transfalcial herniation obstruction of the foramina of Monro [133]. Because in the normal individual all CSF produced in the lateral ventricles must exit into the fourth ventricle via the cerebral aqueduct at the upper end of the midbrain and then flow out of the basal foramina of the fourth ventricle (foramina of Luschka and foramen of Magendie), any obstruction of this flow will raise intracranial pressure [134]. This rise will contribute to brain stem herniation pressures and increase the likelihood of irreversible damage to the brain stem and death.

Brain Death and the Respirator Brain

Concept of Brain Death

The phenomenon of the respirator brain and brain death is now well known, owing to the technical advances in management of critically ill individuals and the emergence of the utility of cadaver organs for transplantation; however, much misunderstanding still surrounds the phenomenon and its mechanisms, not to mention the ethical and legal controversies that surround an allied issue, that of the criteria employed for declaring death on the basis of death of the brain [124,135]. This issue, although described in 1902 by Harvey Cushing [136], became more familiar in the 1950s when mechanical ventilative support for nonbreathing patients became reliable and widely available. The use of these machines allowed the maintenance of vital signs in critically ill patients who, in earlier times, would have died when respiration failed. One of the first observations associated with continued artificial respiration was the tendency for clinical deterioration with respect to the neurological examination and the tendency for the electroencephalogram (EEG) to become flat and remain so with only occasional recovery of brain function once this condition occurred [124,135,137]. In an attempt to explore this phenomenon, many investigators began to collect relevant cases and define parameters so that there would be some criteria with which one could judge if the tiny currents observed over the head represented true physiological brain function or were artifacts [137]. The implication of these findings was that the brain can cease to function physiologically and that the lack of electrical activity, within certain limits and under defined circumstances, can be a reliable criterion for declaring death.

At first, there was the impression that in those persons maintained on a respirator for several days or longer who showed a largely softened or liquefied brain, a diffuse necrotizing process, perhaps viral, had attacked the brain, or some action of the respirator catalyzed the profound liquefaction and autolysis observed—hence, the genesis of the term *respirator brain*. Eventually, the concept evolved that in the terminal state, in the face of very high intracranial pressure, the brain becomes irreversibly damaged and the respirator merely allows but does not cause the process. The true nature of the pathogenesis of brain death began to emerge from cerebral angiography studies [138] and later from a number of studies that measured CBF or cerebral metabolism [119,120], which demonstrated that the individual who had an isoelectric or flat EEG also tended not to have any circulation to the brain and that this condition was irreversible. The basis for the irreversibility of blood flow became clearer with studies describing the no-reflow phenomenon [43].

Emerging from the observations of the mid-1950s to the 1970s came a new concept, that of brain death, as distinguished from more time-honored notions of when and what constituted death, largely based on the cardiocentric view of life [139]. No longer could a patient's having stopped breathing be regarded as sufficient to declare death, or, for that matter could the absence of a heartbeat, when artificial heart–lung machines could sustain vital signs for at least some period of time. The evolution of the need for cadaver organs to be used in transplantations forced an examination of the difficult issue of the criteria and guidelines needed for declaring death. In answer to these questions, several centers in many parts of the world attempted to formulate reasonable criteria for the declaration of death on the basis of irreversible brain damage, the most widely known at the time being the so-called Harvard criteria formulated in 1968 [140].

Briefly stated, the Harvard criteria [140] are the following:

1. The patient should show no response to even intensely painful stimuli.
2. There should be no movement or spontaneous respiration for 3 minutes when taken off the ventilator.
3. There should be no reflexes; the pupils should be fixed, dilated, and unresponsive to light; no eye movement should be elicited by turning the head (doll's eye phenomenon) or by cold water irrigation of the ears; there should be no corneal reflexes; no blinking; no postural activity, pharyngeal reflexes, and swallowing, yawning, or vocalization; no deep tendon reflexes should be present.

4. The EEG should be flat for at least 10 minutes of technically adequate recording; there should be no response to noise or pinching.
5. There should be no change in any of the above tests when repeated after 24 hours.
6. There should be no evidence of hypothermia or of CNS depressant drugs present in the blood.

When and if these criteria were met seemed to satisfy some medical authorities for declaring brain death. This was accepted in some states as a legally acceptable definition, whereas other authorities refused to accept these criteria and cited many criticisms, including anecdotal case reports where, in spite of apparently fulfilling some criteria for brain death, recovery had occurred. Some legal authorities similarly balked at the notion of brain but not somatic death, leading to a number of notorious legal trials centering about various aspects of the problem, including criminal indictments against surgeons for homicide when they removed kidneys for transplant from a person declared dead according to one or another published set of criteria. In an effort to resolve the many questions relating to the concept of brain death, a cooperative panel of experts, under the guiding force of neurosurgeon Dr. A. Earl Walker and the financial and administrative support of the National Institutes of Health (NIH), was formed in 1970 and agreed to carefully study the problem prospectively.

The study involved nine major medical centers in the United States. These centers were to study as many cases that met the following criteria as possible until about 600 cases could be collected. The admission criteria were as follows: a patient had to be deeply comatose, nonbreathing (requiring a respirator and incapable of breathing on his or her own), and with no evidence of hypothermia or drug intoxication. The patients satisfying these conditions were to be carefully evaluated by neurological examination according to a uniform protocol at regular intervals, and accompanying EEG tracings of at least 30 minutes were also to be performed. These studies were to be continued until the patient regained the ability to breathe on his or her own and then to be followed for 3 months, or until death was declared (not by a member of the study team) and ventilation discontinued, or until the cardiovascular system failed and death was determined by that basis. Autopsies were to be obtained as frequently as possible, and specimens were to be examined by a participating neuropathologist according to a lengthy standardized protocol that included gross photographs and many microscopic sections [122,123,135,141].

During the years 1971 and 1972, 503 cases were studied, of which 226 were autopsied. The analysis of these cases formed the basis for the official report of the cooperative study group and a host of other papers and monographs that reflected the special experiences of the participating institutions [141]. The data collected in the study enabled analysis of various elements of the clinical, EEG, and pathological findings against outcome of the cases and the testing of various systems of criteria suggested by other groups.

When only apnea was considered as a criterion of the 503 patients accepted into the NIH collaborative study, 459 (91.25%) died within 4 weeks of entry but 44 (8.75%) regained the ability to breathe on their own and apparently survived; 345 of the patients died a cardiac death, 114 were declared brain dead and taken off the respirator, 26 showed complete recovery, 15 showed incomplete recovery, and 3 were lost to follow-up. Of interest is the fact that of the 41 persons who survived for at least 3 months, 28 had some form of drug intoxication, which accounted for the comatose state. In this group, all but one individual had complete recovery. The other patients suffered from intoxications with another disease state or had vascular diseases (cardiac or cerebral) or some other pathology and had varying degrees of recovery. Excluding the drug cases, in 442 of 500 patients that had follow-up, only one individual can be said to have recovered completely. Most deaths occurred within 3 days of being placed on the respirator [135].

When the constraints of the Harvard criteria were applied to the NIH cases, of the 503 admitted, only 19 completely fulfilled these stringent requirements, but all of them died. If the constraints were relaxed to allow a one-period compliance with the Harvard criteria, 102 patients would have been added, all of whom also died. If constraints were relaxed still further to require apnea, unresponsiveness, and only one flat EEG examination, 189 patients would have been selected. In this instance, 187 of these died, and the two survivors both involved drug overdoses. It became clear that the Harvard criteria applied only to a very special and small minority of nonbreathing comatose patients and that by adopting criteria that took into account only higher brain function rather than peripheral nervous activity, and excluding those with hypothermia, drug intoxications, and some cases of metabolic encephalopathy, a system of criteria could be established that would not only be reliable but also have wide applicability [135].

The suggested criteria for brain death that emerged from the NIH Collaborative Study [141] are as follows:

1. As a prerequisite, all appropriate diagnostic and therapeutic procedures should have been performed.
2. The following should have been observed for 30 minutes at least 6 hours after onset of coma and apnea:
   a. Coma with cerebral unresponsiveness
   b. Apnea
   c. Dilated pupils
   d. Absent cephalic reflexes
   e. Electrocerebral silence (flat EEG)
3. As a confirmatory test, absence of CBF.

Because there is some degree of overlap between some of the criteria, and because it is implied that drug intoxications and hypothermia have been ruled out, when these conditions are present to some degree, it was suggested that some measure of CBF be made as a discriminator for the diagnosis and to also serve where early organ donation is an issue [120,135].

Although the collaborative study effectively answered many questions about adequate criteria for judgment on declaring death, many issues remain, including the following [124,135,140,141]:

1. Legal considerations, wherein some states do not recognize death of the brain as a basis for death declaration
2. The latitude physicians have in declaring death under legal statutes
3. Liabilities arising out of death declarations
4. The issue of intervening cause when, for example, injuries occur to the brain as a result of criminal action and brain death is declared
5. Authority and responsibility in terminating life support systems in individuals who do or do not meet established criteria

6. Arguments over necessary and sufficient conditions for declaring brain death, the NIH and other criteria notwithstanding
7. Religious and ethical questions and considerations apart from death criteria
8. Issues about pathological confirmation of clinical findings
9. Various methods that can be employed to reliably diagnose brain death

Mechanisms of Brain Death

From numerous clinical, pathological, and experimental studies, the primary disease processes that lead to brain death are mostly common entities, as follows in decreasing order of commonness according to the NIH Collaborative Study [141]: cardiac failure (infarction, standstill, valve dysfunction) leading to insufficient, cerebral perfusion; head trauma; stroke (in all its forms); CNS infectious diseases; intoxications and metabolic coma; tumors involving the brain; and miscellaneous conditions that include aspiration, drowning, asphyxia and strangulation, chest trauma, exsanguination, status epilepticus, hypoxia and anesthetic accidents, disseminated intravascular coagulation, decompression sickness, air embolism, and a host of other uncommon events. What all these conditions have in common is some disruption of the BBB or interference with the brain's supply of oxygen or glucose, directly or indirectly, which leads to a major and sustained increase in intracranial pressure that exceeds first venous and then arterial perfusion pressure [119,120,142], leading to loss of perfusion of the brain. To be sure, this circulatory arrest is not always uniform, and some areas of the brain may retain some perfusion, or total brain perfusion may wax and wane as intracranial pressures vacillate in response to treatment and physiological factors. Once sufficient brain has been damaged, the resulting edema usually recruits other previously unaffected regions until the process becomes generalized.

Once CBF ceases and is not restored, irreversible damage results not only to the capillary bed of the brain but also to nerve cells in sequence of their relative vulnerability to ischemia and hypoxia. When the capillary bed is irreversibly damaged, the no-reflow phenomenon occurs such that no matter what is done, reperfusion of the brain cannot take place [43]. It is this aspect of the phenomenon of brain death that is measured by CBF studies. Within very few seconds of total brain ischemia, electrical activity of the brain disappears, which correlates with previous cerebral metabolic studies [143]. To be sure, when there is fractional perfusion of the brain, islands of cortex and other nuclear masses may contribute some elements to an EEG, resulting in a distorted and severely depressed EEG tracing but not electrocerebral silence (ECS). For this reason, persistent low-voltage activity in a deeply comatose patient may delay declaration of death and confound clinicians [144]. The process of brain death need not occur in immediate association with the comatose state and the necessity for the respirator, and it is not inevitably encountered in individuals who are in prolonged and deep coma, as the famous Karen Quinlan case clearly illustrates [145]. In such cases, not all elements of even the most liberal of brain death protocols are satisfied, and declaration of brain death becomes a legally as well as ethically hazardous undertaking. One of the most recent notorious cases is that of Terri Schiavo, who did not meet the established criteria for brain death; rather, other considerations supervened and resulted in the removal of her feeding tube and eventual death [146]. In these cases, there may be severe and multifocal brain damage, but not a respirator brain, such that the individual would never have been able to function in a normal manner but was capable of surviving for an undetermined period even without ventilator support. Neither the law nor the medical profession has yet adequately defined the limits of responsibility and privilege in such situations, and neither has allowed wide latitude in dealing with them.

Respirator Brain

Most neuropathologists agree [122] that the respirator brain has a number of general characteristics that set it apart from virtually any other condition. The typical criteria for gross diagnosis include the following: the patient must have been comatose and on a respirator; the brain should be dusky gray and congested; there should be generalized brain swelling with evidence of uncal, tonsillar, or other herniation, but there may be focal swelling as well; the brain generally does not fix well, even after long immersion in formalin; the brain is soft, often mushy, or nearly liquid; the cerebellum and brain stem are often macerated, and fragments of the cerebellar tonsils may have sloughed into the spinal canal [147,148]; and the pituitary may be similarly soft and grayish. The typical respirator brain is illustrated in Figures 5.28 and 5.29. The changes may be minimal, with good preservation of the normal landmarks, or very advanced, with little preservation of anything but the external anatomy. In some respirator brain cases, the necrotizing process is not uniform and may result in near-total necrosis of the brain stem and cerebellum but varying degrees of preservation of the cerebrum, as in Figure 5.30. Such cases may show persistent but highly abnormal brain electrical activity although the victim is in deep coma and cannot survive because of the necrosis of the posterior fossa structures. In the fresh state, a respirator brain is not odoriferous unless the etiology of the fatal process was infectious.

At times, the upper cord and lower medulla may also participate in the respirator brain phenomenon. This most likely occurs because the blood supply from the vertebrobasilar system via the anterior spinal artery is compromised, and, depending on the degree of collateral circulation from below via the external carotid system, aortic arch, and segmental or radicular arteries, there may be a watershed zone that suffers ischemia (Figure 5.31) [149,150]. This may result in focal hemorrhage mimicking a high spinal cord injury and

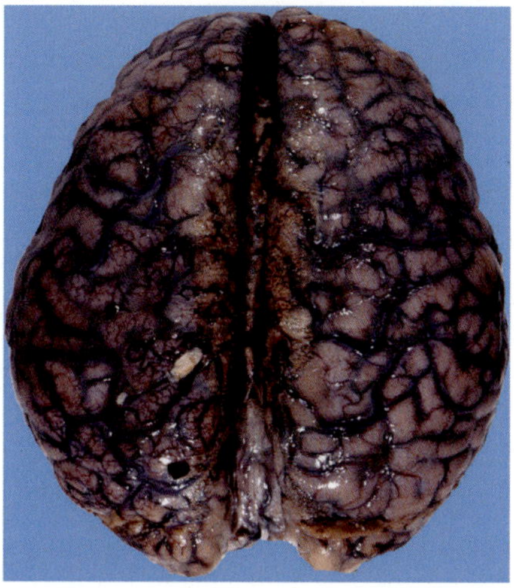

Figure 5.28 This view of the vertex of the cerebral hemispheres of "respirator" brain illustrates the dusky, dark, and congested appearance. This appearance generally takes more than 12 hours of circulatory arrest in a life-supported victim to develop.

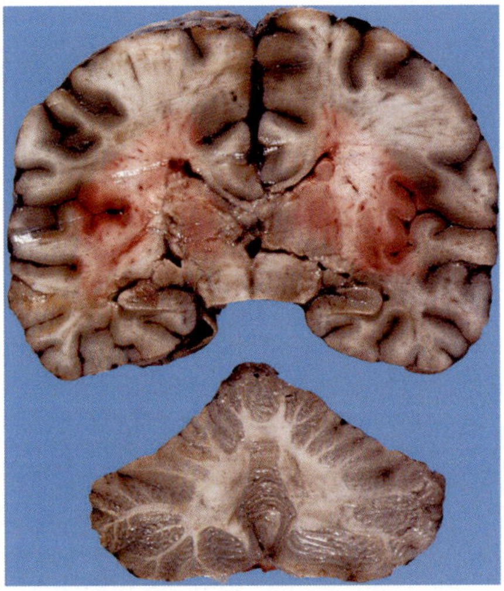

Figure 5.29 This figure shows a coronal section of the cerebrum and a vertical section of the cerebellum of a typical "respirator" brain. Areas of hemorrhage, usually localized or microscopic, are often seen. This hemorrhage may result from partial circulation to the brain as the process developed.

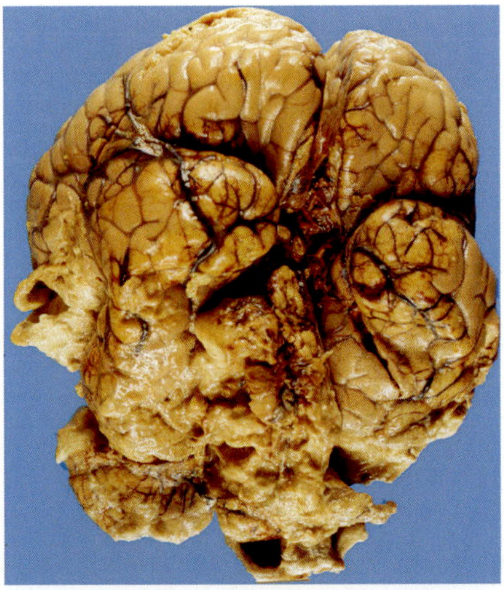

Figure 5.30 This photograph illustrates a "respirator" brain in which the changes are not uniform and are more advanced in the brain stem and cerebellum than in the cerebrum. In cases such as this, it is not uncommon for electroencephalograms to show persistent electrical activity, although the brain stem reflexes are absent and isotope blood flow studies may show some circulation in the cerebrum. (Courtesy of Dr. Y. Konakci and the Cook County Medical Examiner, Chicago, IL.)

giving the erroneous impression of cervical trauma, especially in pediatric cases. An excellent example of spinal respirator brain pathology can be found in Oehmichen's recent text, *Forensic Neuropathology and Neurology* [147]. There is forensic importance to appreciating that the respirator brain phenomenon can involve the cord, especially in alleged child abuse cases where evidence of spinal cord necrosis (even in the absence of demonstrable spinal soft tissue or skeletal trauma) suggests to some that shaking trauma has occurred.

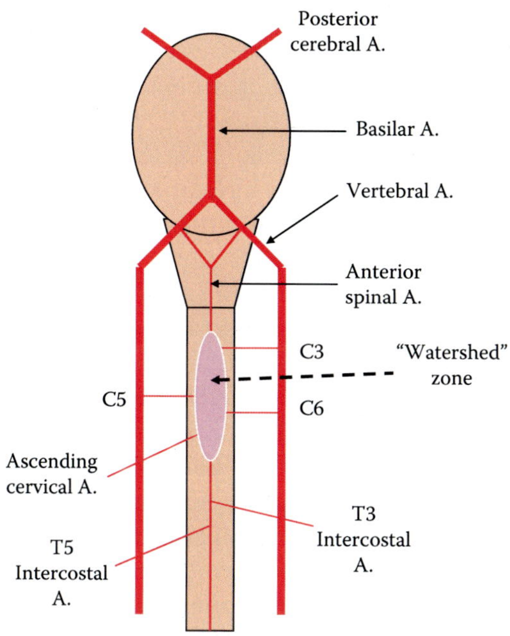

Figure 5.31 This diagrammatic representation of the arterial circulation of the spinal cord illustrates anastamosis with and contributions to the anterior spinal arterial system. From above, arterial blood comes from branches of the vertebral artery that join to form the rostral anterior spinal artery. From below, "radicular" or segmental arterial branches come from the vertebral, ascending cervical and intercostal arteries, forming a "watershed" in the cervical cord (shaded region). When the rostral circulation stops because intracranial pressure is too high (brain death), a potential ischemic zone develops where the lower circulation, unaffected by intracranial dynamics, joins the anterior spinal system. Hemorrhages and necrosis can occur here in some cases of the "respirator" brain. (Adapted from Strong OS, Elwyn A, Truex RC. *Strong and Elwyn's Human Neuroanatomy*. Baltimore: Williams & Wilkins, 1959; Uflacker R, Feldman CJ. *Atlas of Vascular Anatomy: An Angiographic Approach*. Philadelphia: Lippincott Williams & Wilkins, 2007.)

Such an erroneous conclusion may produce a similarly erroneous interpretation of the case, with enormous consequences for an accused individual.

In the fixed state, coronal sections of the hemispheres may be difficult to cut but reveal the same dusky gray appearance as seen externally. The cerebral cortex may fall away from the underlying white matter, as may the basal ganglia. The cerebellum and brain stem may have separated from the brain and be very difficult to cut. It is possible to discern intracerebral or extracerebral hemorrhages that were part of the primary pathology even after long periods on the respirator without cerebral circulation, and an adequate examination of the specimen in spite of its poor state should always be attempted. As a general rule, rather than cutting such brain in the fresh state, cutting after fixation helps facilitate critical examination when required. The best means of diagnosing a respirator brain is by gross examination. Microscopic pathological changes do not offer an unequivocal diagnosis by themselves, and is absolute positive confirmation of the gross findings is not reliable by this means.

The microscopic features of respirator brain are not constant or specific, even though they are consistent with the process that gives rise to the phenomenon. There is less agreement among pathologists on microscopic correlative findings than for gross pathologic impressions. An attempt has been made to correlate gross impressions and specific gross criteria of respirator brains with the microscopic features; however, little reliable correlation could be obtained by statistical analysis [121]. The difficulty lies with the fact that pure postmortem autolysis due to delay in fixation of the specimen often cannot always be differentiated from the changes observed in a respirator brain. The spectrum of autolytic changes includes tissue vacuolation, excessive cutting artifacts (cracks and splits in the tissue, knife marks, etc.), washed-out staining reactions, and dissolution of cells. What may be present in simple autolysis or fixation failure but is generally not present in respirator brains is bacterial growth in the tissue and preservation of peripheral portions of the brain, but liquefaction in the deeper areas. In classic infarctions, there is cellular reaction to the necrotizing process heralded by astroglial proliferation and inflammatory and macrophage responses. In general, these are absent in the classic respirator brain unless the process of ischemia was uneven. It therefore appears that the microscopic examination alone is not a reliable confirmatory tool in establishing the existence of respirator brain changes and that the most reliable confirmation is the gross appearance of the brain. Some have applied immunochemical stains such as β-APP (β-amyloid precursor protein) to brains that have respirator changes in hopes of demonstrating axonal balloons and other supposed signs of traumatic axonal injury. In such cases, the interpretation of any accumulations found in any brain that has suffered global hypoxia/ischemia is unreliable [151].

It is reasonable to ask if delays in refrigeration of the body after death has been declared, as well as delays in performing an autopsy in the brain-dead individual, influence the appearance of the brain so as to confuse the interpretation of respirator brain changes. It appears from an analysis of some 32 cases of brain death in which the temporal sequence of events was carefully noted that such delays are not important in modifying the process under way, and it is apparent that the respirator brain is not produced by such delays [121].

Evolution of Respirator Brain

Once cerebral perfusion has ceased, the brain begins to undergo necrosis. The time pattern of necrosis is dependent on the selective vulnerability of various areas to pressure, ischemia, and hypoxia, yet eventually the whole brain will reflect the necrotizing process. Several factors appear to influence the rapidity with which typical respirator brain changes evolve. These include the acuteness of the illness and probably, to some degree, the amount and duration of brain hypoxia before circulatory arrest. Such factors have been discussed by Lindenberg to influence the process of postmortem autolysis and certainly apply to the respirator brain phenomenon [152,153]. It appears that if there has been some preparative hypoxia or systemic metabolic illness, the brain undergoes retrogressive changes more slowly than if it had been completely healthy before the final insult. This process probably has something to do with lysosomal activation and alterations in intracellular metabolism in the dying state. In any case, the respirator brain process does not occur immediately but takes many hours to develop, subject to inherent and probably indefinable individual variations. It is important to realize that the length of time an individual is on the respirator is not a factor in the development of a respirator brain, but it is the nature of the intracranial environment that determines whether these changes will occur. The most important event that signals the beginning of the process of respirator brain changes (RBCs) is the moment when intracerebral circulation ceases. This may occur hours, days, or weeks after the onset of the apneic comatose state. This moment, however, probably coincides with the onset of ECS, intoxications excluded. From the data in the NIH study, it is concluded that once brain circulation ceases, about 12 hours is required for typical RBCs to be evident grossly. In another study [121], some variation was noted in which some individuals seemed to develop RBCs in as little as 6 hours after circulatory arrest or ECS, whereas others took 24 hours or longer, with the average case showing typical RBCs in 12–16 hours. In the cases that developed RBC rapidly, the individual was almost always stricken acutely, as in severe accidental head trauma, acute intracerebral hemorrhages, or sudden cardiac arrest with delayed resuscitation [121]. The cases that showed delays in development of RBCs were almost always chronically ill persons, such as those with brain tumors, metabolic problems, or infarctions. These observations lend support to the observations of Lindenberg, cited above.

Forensic Considerations in Brain Death

The forensic pathologist generally sees cases in which brain death has been declared only when the manner of death (homicide, suicide, accident, natural, undetermined) is in doubt or involves a cause that is not considered owing to a natural disease process [154]. In many, if not most, of these cases, the brain will show changes typical for a respirator brain. It is incumbent on the forensic pathologist to determine, given the resources at his or her command, the medical cause and manner of death. Invariably, the anatomic basis for the death lies inside the head and reflects the trauma the victim suffered, the vascular disease, or other process that gave rise to the brain-dead state. A common source of consternation on forensic pathology services is the interpretation of the underlying pathology in a severely distorted, if not liquefied, respirator brain and a common notion that such interpretations are impossible. Such a nihilistic view is unfounded because many basic pre-RBC processes do not disappear but may merely be overshadowed by later events. It is important in a case such as a fatal head injury caused by an alleged homicidal beating to conduct a complete neuropathological examination. This usually requires careful removal of the brain followed by formalin fixation. In addition, the entire cerebral dura should be removed and preserved and the cranial vault carefully inspected for fractures. The scalp and galea should be carefully examined for hemorrhages and healing lesions and their locations noted and photographed. Histological sections should be made of all lesions external to the brain, including the meninges, scalp, and skin. This precaution will permit estimates of the time of occurrence of the lesions and their age. In this context, it must be remembered that even though the brain may not have received vascular perfusion, the meninges and other cranial structures probably have received perfusion from extracranial vessels, uninterrupted by events occurring in the brain. Vital reactions will therefore be present and can be evaluated. These baselines can be helpful in correlating the estimated age of lesions in the brain and meninges, such as hemorrhages, contusions, and hematomas. One must remember that the middle meningeal arterial system that nourishes the dura is fed from the external carotid arterial system and is thus not susceptible to the circulatory arrest of the interior vessels of the brain; thus, vital reactions may proceed unhampered in the dura and sometimes for a short distance beneath it.

The interpretation of lesions in the respirator brain is not easy because many antemortem processes do not follow the normal course of events as they would in the presence of circulation. Hemorrhages tend to appear frozen in time, having a dark appearance, little altered by time in the now-inert brain. The process of organization and clot dissolution ceases once circulation has stopped but evolves up to the point of circulatory arrest. An awareness of this phenomenon can permit analysis and bolster confidence in interpretations delivered in court. These situations may arise in cases where a child, the victim of a fatal beating, is maintained for a long period on a respirator far in excess of legal requirements, perhaps because of the hope (on the part of attorneys and the perpetrators) that the evidence will be obscured. Similar situations may arise in adult homicidal beatings where it might be assumed that lesions caused by the beating will have been obscured by the RBCs. Often the outcome of such cases rests on the assurance that underlying lesions do not disappear but may be preserved beneath the artifacts of the respirator brain.

When attempting to examine a respirator brain, it is important not to attempt too fine an examination. It will be impossible to execute the usual 1-cm coronal slices; 2- and 3-cm slices are perfectly acceptable. Handling of the brain should be kept to a minimum, and the handy presence of a pancake turner or broad spatula may assist in moving the fragile slices of the brain to photography for further examination. Although the respirator brain may show hemorrhage or congestion mimicking hemorrhage, true traumatic hemorrhages and contusions can usually be identified and photographed. Tissue blocks for microscopic examination may be taken in spite of an initial prejudice that they will be useless and will probably surprise the skeptical pathologist when examined later.

The pathologist should not be drawn into a conflict that rests on the microscopic confirmation of brain death, for the reasons mentioned above. Gross appearances are quite reliable, as already mentioned. At times, death may have occurred (with absence of CBF or flat EEG tracings) before obvious RBCs had developed. This lack of RBCs does not negate the declaration of brain death, and an explanation of the evolution and mechanism of the process to interested parties can forestall precipitous and pejorative judgments.

Occasionally, especially when brain death has been declared without fulfilling what may be alleged established criteria, the pathologist may find himself or herself at the center of a legal conflict in determining the cause of death. Such situations require great care in analyzing available data and the pathological specimen. When the responsible pathologist feels unprepared for such a judgment, it is essential that the specimen be photographed and preserved so that a consultative opinion can be sought.

References

1. Pardridge WM. Blood–brain barrier delivery. *Drug Discov Today* 2007;12:54–61.
2. Silva GA. Nanotechnology approaches for drug and small molecule delivery across the blood brain barrier. *Surg Neurol* 2007;67:113–6.
3. Muldoon LL, Soussain C, Jahnke K, Johanson C, Siegal T, Smith QR, Hall WA, Hynynen K, Senter PD, Peereboom DM, Neuwelt EA. Chemotherapy delivery issues in central nervous system malignancy: A reality check. *J Clin Oncol* 2007;25:2295–305.
4. Brightman MW, Klatzo I, Olsson Y, Reese TS. The blood–brain barrier to proteins under normal and pathological conditions. *J Neurol Sci* 1970;10:215–39.
5. Begley DJ, Brightman MW. Structural and functional aspects of the blood–brain barrier. *Prog Drug Res* 2003;61:39–78.
6. Hartmann C, Zozulya A, Wegener J, Galla HJ. The impact of glia-derived extracellular matrices on the barrier function of cerebral endothelial cells: An *in vitro* study. *Exp Cell Res* 2007;313:1318–25.

7. Dougherty DD, Rauch SL, Rosenbaum JF, eds. *Essentials of Neuroimaging for Clinical Practice.* Washington, DC: American Psychiatric Publishing, 2004.
8. Klatzo I. Presidential address: Neuropathological aspects of brain edema. *J Neuropathol Exp* 1967;26:1–14.
9. Manz HJ. The pathology of cerebral edema. *Hum Pathol* 1974;5:291–313.
10. Crone C. The permeability of brain capillaries to non-electrolytes. *Acta Physiol Scand* 1965;64:407–17.
11. Milhorat RH. *Cerebrospinal Fluid and the Brain Edemas.* New York: Neuroscience Society of New York, 1987.
12. Hoff JT. Brain edema XIII. In Hoff JT, ed., *The XIII International Symposium on Brain Edema and Tissue Injury.* Ann Arbor, MI: Springer, 2005.
13. Raichle ME, Eichling JO, Grubb RL Jr. Brain permeability of water. *Arch Neurol* 1974;30:319–21.
14. Rabinstein AA. Treatment of cerebral edema. *Neurologist* 2006;12:59–73.
15. Reese TS, Feder N, Brightman MW. Electron microscopic study of the blood–brain and blood–cerebrospinal fluid barriers with microperoxidase. *J Neuropathol Exp Neurol* 1971;30:137–8.
16. Huang S. Regulation of metastases by signal transducer and activator of transcription 3 signaling pathway: Clinical implications. *Clin Cancer Res* 2007;13:1362–6.
17. Dorsam RT, Gutkind JS. G-protein-coupled receptors and cancer. *Nat Rev Cancer* 2007;7:79–94.
18. Brower V. Researchers tackle metastasis, cancer's last frontier. *J Natl Cancer Inst* 2007;99:109–11.
19. Raine CS. Neurocellular anatomy. In Siegel GJ, Albers RW, Brady ST, Price DL, eds., *Basic Neurochemistry: Molecular and Medical Aspects.* Amsterdam: Academic Press/Elsevier, 2006, pp. 3–19.
20. Graham DI. Neuropathology of head injury. In Narayan RK, Wilberger JE Jr, Porlishock JT, eds., *Neurotrauma.* New York: McGraw-Hill, 1995, pp. 43–59.
21. Barkovich AJ. *Pediatric Neuroimaging.* Philadelphia: Lippincott Williams & Wilkins, 2000.
22. Shapiro K, Fried A. Pressure–volume relationships in shunt-dependent childhood hydrocephalus: The zone of pressure instability in children with acute deterioration. *J Neurosurg* 1986;64:390–6.
23. Hoff JT, Xi G. Brain edema from intracerebral hemorrhage. *Acta Neurochir Suppl* 2003;86:11–5.
24. Lee KR, Betz AL, Kim S, Keep RF, Hoff JT. The role of the coagulation cascade in brain edema formation after intracerebral hemorrhage. *Acta Neurochir* (Wien) 1996;138:396–400; discussion, 400.
25. Xi G, Fewel ME, Hua Y, Thompson BG Jr, Hoff JT, Keep RF. Intracerebral hemorrhage: Pathophysiology and therapy. *Neurocrit Care* 2004;1:5–18.
26. Bruce DA, Alavi A, Bilaniuk L, Dolinskas C, Obrist W, Uzzell B. Diffuse cerebral swelling following head injuries in children: The syndrome of "malignant brain edema." *J Neurosurg* 1981;54:170–8.
27. Humphreys RP, Hendrick EB, Hoffman HJ. The head-injured child who "talks and dies": A report of 4 cases. *Childs Nerv Syst* 1990;6:139–42.
28. Snoek JW, Minderhoud JM, Wilmink JT. Delayed deterioration following mild head injury in children. *Brain* 1984;107:15–36.
29. Lobato RD, Sarabia R, Cordobes F, Rivas JJ, Adrados A, Cabrera A, Gomez P, Madera A, Lamas E. Posttraumatic cerebral hemispheric swelling: Analysis of 55 cases studied with computerized tomography. *J Neurosurg* 1988;68:417–23.
30. Ostrowski RP, Colohan AR, Zhang JH. Molecular mechanisms of early brain injury after subarachnoid hemorrhage. *Neurol Res* 2006;28:399–414.
31. Kusaka G, Ishikawa M, Nanda A, Granger DN, Zhang JH. Signaling pathways for early brain injury after subarachnoid hemorrhage. *J Cereb Blood Flow Metab* 2004;24:916–25.
32. Provencio JJ, Vora N. Subarachnoid hemorrhage and inflammation: Bench to bedside and back. *Semin Neurol* 2005;25:435–44.
33. Hinshaw LB. *Pathophysiology of Endotoxin*, Vol. 2. Amsterdam: Elsevier, 1985.

34. Baumgartner JD, Calandra T, Carlet J. *Endotoxin: From Pathophysiology to Therapeutic Approaches*, Vol. XIV. Paris: Flammarion, 1990.
35. Butler KM. Meningococcal meningitis prevention programs for college students: A review of the literature. *Worldviews Evid Based Nurs* 2006;3:185–93.
36. Neuman HB, Wald ER. Bacterial meningitis in childhood at the Children's Hospital of Pittsburgh: 1988–1998. *Clin Pediatr* (Phila) 2001;40:595–600.
37. Thurtell MJ, Keed AB, Yan M, Gottlieb T, Spies JM, Halmagyi GM. Tuberculous cranial pachymeningitis. *Neurology* 2007;68:298–300.
38. Leestma JE. Viral infections of the nervous system. In Davis R, Robertson DM, eds., *Textbook of Neuropathology*. Baltimore: Williams & Wilkins, 1991, pp. 804–903.
39. Shin RK, Balcer LJ. Idiopathic intracranial hypertension. *Curr Treat Options Neurol* 2002;4:297–305.
40. Cinciripini GS, Donahue S, Borchert MS. Idiopathic intracranial hypertension in prepubertal pediatric patients: Characteristics, treatment, and outcome. *Am J Ophthalmol* 1999;127:178–82.
41. Huna-Baron R, Kupersmith MJ. Idiopathic intracranial hypertension in pregnancy. *J Neurol* 2002;249:1078–81.
42. Lin A, Foroozan R, Danesh-Meyer HV, De Salvo G, Savino PJ, Sergott RC. Occurrence of cerebral venous sinus thrombosis in patients with presumed idiopathic intracranial hypertension. *Ophthalmology* 2006;113:2281–4.
43. Ames IA, Wright RL, Kowada M, Thurston JM, Majno G. The no-reflow phenomenon. *Am J Pathol* 1968;52:437–53.
44. Mohr JP. Natural history and pathophysiology of brain infarction. *Circulation* 1991;83(Suppl): I172–75.
45. Spencer PS, Schaumburg HH, Ludolph AC. *Experimental and Clinical Neurotoxicology*. New York: Oxford University Press, 2000.
46. Torack RM, Terry RD, Zimmerman H. The fine structure of cerebral fluid accumulation: II. Swelling produced by triethyl tin poisoning and its comparison with that in the human brain. *Am J Pathol* 1960;36:273–87.
47. Farrar HC, Chande VT, Fitzpatrick DF, Shema SJ. Hyponatremia as the cause of seizures in infants: A retrospective analysis of incidence, severity, and clinical predictors. *Ann Emerg Med* 1995;26:42–8.
48. Tien R, Arieff AI, Kucharczyk W, Wasik A, Kucharczyk J. Hyponatremic encephalopathy: Is central pontine myelinolysis a component? *Am J Med* 1992;92:513–22.
49. Schulman H, Laufer L, Berginer J, Hershkowitz E, Berenstein T, Sofer S, Maor E, Hertzanu Y. CT findings in neonatal hypothermia. *Pediatr Radiol* 1998;28:414–7.
50. Murakami K, Kondo T, Sato S, Li Y, Chan PH. Occurrence of apoptosis following cold injury-induced brain edema in mice. *Neuroscience* 1997;81:231–7.
51. Blinkov S, Glezer IP. *The Human Brain in Figures and Tables: A Quantitative Handbook*. New York: Basic Books, Plenum Press, 1968.
52. Wilmes F, Hossmann KA. A specific immunofluorescence technique for the demonstration of vasogenic brain edema in paraffin embedded material. *Acta Neuropathol* (Berl) 1979;45:47–51.
53. Feigin I, Budzilovich G, Weinberg S, Ogata J. Degeneration of white matter in hypoxia, acidosis and edema. *J Neuropathol Exp Neurol* 1973;32:125–43.
54. Feigin I, Budzilovich GN. Laminar scars in cerebral white matter: A perinatal injury due to edema. *J Neuropathol Exp Neurol* 1978;37:314–25.
55. Miller JD, Piper WR, Statham PFX. ICP monitoring: Indications and techniques. In Narayan RK, Wilberger JE, Polishock JT, eds., *Neurotrauma*. New York: McGraw-Hill, 1995, pp. 429–44.
56. Kelly DF, Doberstein C, Becker DP. General principles of the head injury management. In Narayan RK, Wilberger JE, Povlishock JR, eds., *Neurotrauma*. New York: McGraw-Hill, 1996, pp. 71–101.
57. Miller JD, Piper IR, Jones P. Pathophysiology of head injury. In Narayan RK, Wilberger JE, Povlishock JT, eds., *Neurotrauma*. New York: McGraw-Hill, 1995, pp. 61–9.

58. Chesnut RM. Treating raised intracranial pressure in head injury. In Narayan RK, Wilberger JE, Povlishock JT, eds., *Neurotrauma*. New York: McGraw-Hill, 1995, pp. 445–69.
59. Rosner MJ, Daughton S. Cerebral perfusion pressure management in head injury. *J Trauma* 1990;30:933–40; discussion, 940–1.
60. Muizelaar JP, Marmarou A, DeSalles AA, Ward JD, Zimmerman RS, Li Z, Choi SC, Young HF. Cerebral blood flow and metabolism in severely head-injured children: Part 1. Relationship with GCS score, outcome, ICP, and PVI. *J Neurosurg* 1989;71:63–71.
61. Young JS, Blow O, Turrentine F, Claridge JA, Schulman A. Is there an upper limit of intracranial pressure in patients with severe head injury if cerebral perfusion pressure is maintained? *Neurosurg Focus* 2003;15(6):E2.
62. Lehmenkuhler A, Sykova E, Svoboda J, Zilles K, Nicholson C. Extracellular space parameters in the rat neocortex and subcortical white matter during postnatal development determined by diffusion analysis. *Neuroscience* 1993;55:339–51.
63. Davison AN, Dobbing J. *Applied Neurochemistry*. Philadelphia: F.A. Davis, 1968.
64. Sykova E, Roitbak T, Mazel T, Simonova Z, Harvey AR. Astrocytes, oligodendroglia, extracellular space volume and geometry in rat fetal brain grafts. *Neuroscience* 1999;91:783–98.
65. Hrabetova S. Extracellular diffusion is fast and isotropic in the stratum radiatum of hippocampal CA1 region in rat brain slices. *Hippocampus* 2005;15:441–50.
66. Tao A, Tao L, Nicholson C. Cell cavities increase tortuosity in brain extracellular space. *J Theor Biol* 2005;234:525–36.
67. Shapiro K, Marmarou A, Shulman K. Characterization of clinical CSF dynamics and neural axis compliance using the pressure–volume index: I. The normal pressure-volume index. *Ann Neurol* 1980;7:508–14.
68. Pickard JD, Czosnyka M, Higgins N, Owler B, Momjian S, Pena A. Clinical aspects of disorders of the choroid plexus and the CSF production. In Zheng W, Chodobski A, eds., *The Blood–Cerebrospinal Fluid Barrier*. Boca Raton, FL: Taylor & Francis, 2005, pp. 497–517.
69. Wallach J. *Interpretation of Diagnostic Tests: A Handbook Synopsis of Laboratory Medicine*. Boston: Little Brown, 1974.
70. Zhu DC, Xenos M, Linninger AA, Penn RD. Dynamics of lateral ventricle and cerebrospinal fluid in normal and hydrocephalic brains. *J Magn Reson Imaging* 2006;24:756–70.
71. Aronyk KE. The history and classification of hydrocephalus. In Butler AB, McLone DG, eds., *Neurosurgery Clinics of North America*, Vol. 4. Philadelphia: W.B. Saunders, 1993, pp. 599–609.
72. Greitz D. Cerebrospinal fluid circulation and associated intracranial dynamics: A radiologic investigation using MR imaging and radionuclide cisternography. *Acta Radiol Suppl* 1993;386:1–23.
73. Greitz D, Greitz T, Hindmarsh T. A new view on the CSF-circulation with the potential for pharmacological treatment of childhood hydrocephalus. *Acta Paediatr* 1997;86:125–32.
74. Egnor M, Zheng L, Rosiello A, Gutman F, Davis R. A model of pulsations in communicating hydrocephalus. *Pediatr Neurosurg* 2002;36:281–303.
75. Bergsneider M, Alwan AA, Falkson L, Rubinstein EH. The relationship of pulsatile cerebrospinal fluid flow to cerebral blood flow and intracranial pressure: A new theoretical model. *Acta Neurochir* 1998;71(Suppl):266–8.
76. Bradbury MW, Cole DF. The role of the lymphatic system in drainage of cerebrospinal fluid and aqueous humour. *J Physiol* 1980;299:353–65.
77. Shapiro K, Marmarou A, Portnoy H, eds. *Hydrocephalus*. New York: Raven Press, 1984.
78. Milhorat TH. The third circulation revisited. *J Neurosurg* 1975;42:628–45.
79. Johnston IH, Rowan JO. Raised intracranial pressure and cerebral blood flow. 3. Venous outflow tract pressures and vascular resistances in experimental intracranial hypertension. *J Neurol Neurosurg Psychiatry* 1974;37:392–402.
80. Marmarou A. Pathophysiology of intracranial pressure. In Narayan RK, Wilberger JE, Povlishock JT, eds., *Neurotrauma*. New York: McGraw-Hill, 1995, pp. 413–28.
81. Friden HG, Ekstedt J. Volume/pressure relationship of the cerebrospinal space in humans. *Neurosurgery* 1983;13:351–66.

82. Friden H, Ekstedt J. CSF dynamics modeling in man. In Nagai H, Kamiya K, Ishii S, eds., *Intracranial Pressure IX*. Tokyo: Springer, 1994, pp. 502–3.
83. Schwab S, Erbguth F, Aschoff A, Orberk E, Spranger M, Hacke W. "Paradoxical" herniation after decompressive trephining. *Nervenarzt* 1998;69:896–900.
84. Avezaat CJ, van Eijndhoven JH. Clinical observations on the relationship between cerebrospinal fluid pulse pressure and intracranial pressure. *Acta Neurochir* (Wien) 1986;79:13–29.
85. Papasian N, Frim DM. A theoretical model of benign external hydrocephalus that predicts a predisposition towards extra-axial hemorrhage after minor head trauma. *Pediatr Neurosurg* 2000;33:188–93.
86. Hyreh SS. Orbital vascular anatomy. *Eye* 2006;20:1130–44.
87. Muller PJ, Deck JH. Intraocular and optic nerve sheath hemorrhage in cases of sudden intracranial hypertension. *J Neurosurg* 1974;41:160–6.
88. Ballantyne AJ. The ocular manifestations of spontaneous subarachnoid hemorrhage. *Br J Ophthal* 1943;27:383–414.
89. Walsh FB, Hedges TR Jr. Optic nerve sheath hemorrhage: The Jackson Memorial lecture. *Am J Ophthalmol* 1951;34:509–27.
90. Smith DC, Kearns TP, Sayre GP. Preretinal and optic nerve-sheath hemorrhage: Pathologic and experimental aspects in subarachnoid hemorrhage. *Trans Am Ophthalmol Otolaryn Soc* 1957;61:201–11.
91. Luedemann W, von Rautenfeld DB, Samii M, Brinker T. Ultrastructure of the cerebrospinal fluid outflow along the optic nerve into the lymphatic system. *Childs Nerv Syst* 2005;21:96–103.
92. Killer HE, Laeng HR, Flammer J, Groscurth P. Architecture of arachnoid trabeculae, pillars, and septa in the subarachnoid space of the human optic nerve: Anatomy and clinical considerations. *Br J Ophthalmol* 2003;87:777–81.
93. Ommaya AK, Goldsmith W, Thibault L. Biomechanics and neuropathology of adult and paediatric head injury. *Br J Neurosurg* 2002;16:220–42.
94. Smith SL, Andrus PK, Gleason DD, Hall ED. Infant rat model of the shaken baby syndrome: Preliminary characterization and evidence for the role of free radicals in cortical hemorrhaging and progressive neuronal degeneration. *J Neurotrauma* 1998;15:693–705.
95. Smith SL, Hall ED. Tirilazad widens the therapeutic window for riluzole-induced attenuation of progressive cortical degeneration in an infant rat model of the shaken baby syndrome. *J Neurotrauma* 1998;15:707–19.
96. Lantz PE, Adams GG. Postmortem monocular indirect ophthalmoscopy. *J Foren Sci* 2005; 50:1450–2.
97. Lantz P. Postmortem detection and evaluation of retinal hemorrhages. In *American Academy of Forensic Sciences*, Seattle, 2006, abstract G-14, p. 271.
98. Levin AV. Ocular complications of head trauma in children. *Pediatr Emerg Care* 1991;7:129–30.
99. Matshes E. Retinal and optic nerve sheath hemorrhages are not pathognomonic of abusive head injury. In *American Academy of Forensic Science Annual Meeting*, 2010, Abstract G-1, p. 272.
100. Selhorst JB, Gudeman SK, Butterworth JF 4th, Harbison JW, Miller JD, Becker DP. Papilledema after acute head injury. *Neurosurgery* 1985;16:357–63.
101. Steffen H, Eifert B, Aschoff A, Kolling GH, Volcker HE. The diagnostic value of optic disc evaluation in acute elevated intracranial pressure. *Ophthalmology* 1996;103:1229–32.
102. Hayreh SS. Optic disc edema in raised intracranial pressure: V. Pathogenesis. *Arch Ophthalmol* 1977;95:1553–65.
103. Hayreh SS, Hayreh MS. Optic disc edema in raised intracranial pressure: II. Early detection with fluorescein fundus angiography and stereoscopic color photography. *Arch Ophthalmol* 1977;95:1245–54.
104. Black PM. Normal-pressure hydrocephalus: Current understanding of diagnostic tests and shunting. *Postgrad Med* 1982;71:57–61, 65–7.
105. Greitz D. Paradigm shift in hydrocephalus research in legacy of Dandy's pioneering work: Rationale for third ventriculostomy in communicating hydrocephalus. *Childs Nerv Syst* 2007;23:487–9.

106. Widenka DC, Wolf S, Schurer L, Plev DV, Lumenta CB. Factors leading to hydrocephalus after aneurysmal subarachnoid hemorrhage. *Neurol Neurochir Pol* 2000;34(Suppl):56–60.
107. Massicotte EM, Del Bigio MR. Human arachnoid villi response to subarachnoid hemorrhage: Possible relationship to chronic hydrocephalus. *J Neurosurg* 1999;91:80–4.
108. Suzuki H, Muramatsu M, Tanaka K, Fujiwara H, Kojima T, Taki W. Cerebrospinal fluid ferritin in chronic hydrocephalus after aneurysmal subarachnoid hemorrhage. *J Neurol* 2006;253:1170–6.
109. Watanabe K. Long-term observation of arachnoid villi after subarachnoid hemorrhage: An electron microscopic study in dogs. *Tohoku J Exp Med* 1979;128:161–73.
110. Shaw C, Alvord ECJ. Hydrocephalus. In Duckett S, ed., *Pediatric Neuropathology*. Baltimore: Williams & Wilkins, 1995.
111. Kahlon B, Sjunnesson J, Rehncrona S. Long-term outcome in patients with suspected normal pressure hydrocephalus. *Neurosurgery* 2007;60:327–32; discussion, 332.
112. Tsakanikas D, Relkin N. Normal pressure hydrocephalus. *Semin Neurol* 2007;27:58–65.
113. Modic MT, Kaufman B, Bonstelle CT, Tomsick TA, Weinstein MA. Megalocephaly and hypodense extracerebral fluid collections. *Radiology* 1981;141:93–100.
114. Kapila A, Trice J, Spies WG, Siegel BA, Gado MH. Enlarged cerebrospinal fluid spaces in infants with subdural hematomas. *Radiology* 1982;142:669–72.
115. Handique SK, Das RR, Barua N, Medhi N, Saharia B. External hydrocephalus in children. *Ind J Radiol Imag* 2002;12:197–200.
116. Azais M, Echenne B. Idiopathic pericerebral swelling (external hydrocephalus) of infants. *Ann Pediatr* (Paris) 1992;39:550–8.
117. Piatt JH Jr. A pitfall in the diagnosis of child abuse: External hydrocephalus, subdural hematoma, and retinal hemorrhages [Electronic resource]. *Neurosurg Focus* 1999;7(4):E4.
118. Kanev PM, Park TS. The treatment of hydrocephalus. In Butler B, McLone DG, eds., *Hydrocephalus (Neurosurgical Clinics of North America)*, Vol. 4. Philadelphia: W.B. Saunders, 1993, pp. 611–9.
119. Korein J, Braunstein P, George A, Wichter M, Kricheff I, Lieberman A, Pearson J. Brain death: I. Angiographic correlation with the radioisotopic bolus technique for evaluation of critical deficit of cerebral blood flow. *Ann Neurol* 1977;2:195–205.
120. Korein J, Braunstein P, Kricheff I, Lieberman A, Chase N. Radioisotopic bolus technique as a test to detect circulatory deficit associated with cerebral death: 142 studies on 80 patients demonstrating the bedside use of an innocuous IV procedure as an adjunct in the diagnosis of cerebral death. *Circulation* 1975;51:924–39.
121. Leestma JE, Hughes JR, Diamond ER. Temporal correlates in brain death: EEG and clinical relationships to the respirator brain. *Arch Neurol* 1984;41:147–52.
122. Moseley JI, Molinari GF, Walker AE. Respirator brain. Report of a survey and review of current concepts. *Arch Pathol Lab Med* 1976;100:61–4.
123. Walker AE, Diamond EL, Moseley J. The neuropathological findings in irreversible coma: A critique of the "respirator." *J Neuropathol Exp Neurol* 1975;34:295–323.
124. Wijdicks EFM, ed. *Brain Death*. Philadelphia: Lippincott Williams & Wilkins, 2001.
125. Plum F, Posner JB. *The Diagnosis of Stupor and Coma*. Philadelphia: F.A. Davis, 1982.
126. Cuneo RA, Caronna JJ, Pitts L, Townsend J, Winestock DP. Upward transtentorial herniation: Seven cases and a literature review. *Arch Neurol* 1979;36:618–23.
127. Miller NR, Newman N, Biousse V, Kerrison JB, eds. *Walsh and Hoyt's Clinical Neuro-Ophthalomology*. Philadelphia: Lippincott Williams & Wilkins, 2004.
128. Pearce JM. Kernohan's notch. *Eur Neurol* 2006;55:230–2.
129. Oster JM Jr, Hildenbrand P, Tronic B, Cosgrove GR. Reversible Kernohan notch. *Neurology* 2007;68:368.
130. Makino A, Soga T, Obayashi M, Seo Y, Ebisutani D, Horie S, Ueda S, Matsumoto K. Cortical blindness caused by acute general cerebral swelling. *Surg Neurol* 1988;29:393–400.
131. Parizel PM, Makkat S, Jorens PG, Ozsarlak O, Cras P, Van Goethem JW, van den Hauwe L, Verlooy J, De Schepper AM. Brain stem hemorrhage in descending transtentorial herniation (Duret hemorrhage). *Intensive Care Med* 2002;28:85–8.

132. Alexander E Jr, Kushner J, Six EG. Brain stem hemorrhages and increased intracranial pressure: From Duret to computed tomography. *Surg Neurol* 1982;17:107–10.
133. Heiskanen O. Cyst of the septum pellucidum causing increased intracranial pressure and hydrocephalus: Case report. *J Neurosurg* 1973;38:771–3.
134. Hakim S, Venegas JG, Burton JD. The physics of the cranial cavity, hydrocephalus and normal pressure hydrocephalus: Mechanical interpretation and mathematical model. *Surg Neurol* 1976;5:187–210.
135. Walker AE. *Cerebral Death*. Baltimore: Uban & Schwarzenberg, 1981.
136. Cushing H. Some experimental and clinical observations concerning states of increased intracranial tension. *Am J Med Sci* 1902;124:375–400.
137. Hughes JR. Limitations of the EEG in coma and brain death. *Ann NY Acad Sci* 1978;315:121–36.
138. Riishede J, Ethelberg S. Angiographic changes in sudden and severe herniation of brain stem through tentorial incisure: Report of five cases. *Arch Neurol Psychiatr* 1953;70:399–409.
139. Youngner SJ, Bartlett ET. Human death and high technology: The failure of the whole-brain formulations. *Ann Intern Med* 1983;99:252–8.
140. School AH. A definition of irreversible coma: Report of the Ad Hoc Committee of the Harvard Medical School to examine the definition of brain death. *JAMA* 1968;205:337–40.
141. Collaborative Study. An appraisal of the criteria of cerebral death: A summary statement. *JAMA* 1977;237:982–6.
142. Balslev-Jorgensen P, Heilbrun MP, Boysen G, Rosenklint A, Jorgensen EO. Cerebral perfusion pressure correlated with regional cerebral blood flow, EEG and aortocervical arteriography in patients with severe brain disorders progressing to brain death. *Eur Neurol* 1972;8:207–12.
143. Brierley JB, Graham DI, Adams JH, Simpsom JA. Neocortical death after cardiac arrest: A clinical, neurophysiological, and neuropathological report of two cases. *Lancet* 1971;2:560–5.
144. Bennett DR, Hughes JR, Korein J, Merlis J, Suter C. *Atlas of Electroencephalography in Coma and Cerebral Death*. New York: Raven Press, 1976.
145. Kinney HC, Korein J, Panigrahy A, Dikkes P, Goode R. Neuropathological findings in the brain of Karen Ann Quinlan: The role of the thalamus in the persistent vegetative state. *N Engl J Med* 1994;330:1469–75.
146. Wijdicks EF. Minimally conscious state vs. persistent vegetative state: The case of Terry (Wallis) vs. the case of Terri (Schiavo). *Mayo Clin Proc* 2006;81:1155–8.
147. Oehmichen M, Auer RN, König HG. *Forensic Neuropathology and Neurology*. Berlin: Springer-Verlag, 2006, pp. 319–29.
148. Herrick MK, Agamanolis DP. Displacement of cerebellar tissue into spinal canal: A component of the respirator brain syndrome. *Arch Pathol* 1975;99:565–71.
149. Strong OS, Elwyn A, Truex RC. *Strong and Elwyn's Human Neuroanatomy*. Baltimore: Williams & Wilkins, 1959.
150. Uflacker R, Feldman CJ. *Atlas of Vascular Anatomy: An Angiographic Approach*. Philadelphia: Lippincott Williams & Wilkins, 2007.
151. Oehmichen M, Meissner C, Schmidt V, Pedal I, König HG, Saternus KS. Axonal injury—A diagnostic tool in forensic neuropathology? A review. *Foren Sci Int* 1998;95:67–83.
152. Lindenberg R. Systemic oxygen deficiencies. In Minckler J, ed., *Pathology of the Nervous System*, Vol. 2. New York: McGraw-Hill, 1971, pp. 1583–617.
153. Lindenberg R. Anoxia does not produce brain damage. *Jpn J Legal Med* (Nihon Hoigaku Zasshi) 1982;36:38–57.
154. Gerber P. Brain death, murder and the law. *Med J Aust* 1984;140:536–7.

Physical Injury to the Nervous System

6

JAN E. LEESTMA
KIRK L. THIBAULT

Contents

Introduction

Probably the most common neuropathologic condition that confronts the forensic pathologist, and that is thought of as the most typical of forensic problems by the neuropathologist, is some form of head–brain or spinal trauma. The spectrum of traumatic injuries that is observed on any reasonably active forensic service is truly impressive in its diversity. The injuries seen at the autopsy table are a function of many distinct, although interactive, phenomena that need to be considered before a proper and informed interpretation of the case can be made. Obviously, available historical and clinical information needs to be reviewed, along with witness accounts of an incident of what purportedly occurred and scene or witness investigation reports. The age of the individual is very important because neural trauma often shows different faces at different age groups. As with any forensic examination, autopsy or not, documentation and notation of all external injuries should be made and preserved in photographs. The highly advanced and inexpensive digital photographic methods are preferred, and equipment now available provides excellent results, with the added advantage of the ability to transmit copies electronically and via the Internet. Digital images are now accepted by the courts in most jurisdictions.

The autopsy examination and analysis of neurotrauma cases should be firmly rooted in an appreciation of injury biomechanics because mechanisms of injury are often the central focus of the forensic exercise. To permit even a cursory injury biomechanics analysis, the forensic pathologist and his or her investigators must collect and preserve information about the traumatic event and the scene (the "loading" environment, which is discussed below). To do this, one must have an appreciation of the kinds of information that might be required.

The kind of information that should be collected and documented when possible, on any trauma case, neural included, may be invaluable to a mechanistic understanding of the case and, if properly done, may permit a detailed, science-based analysis by a biomechanics professional. Included in this body of information should be accurate weight and measurements of the body (especially true in infant and childhood cases). It should also include accurate and photographically preserved information about the scene of the death or occurrence with some sort of scale in the photographs from which distances can be easily observed or calculated. Characteristics of the environment (indoor, outdoor, temperature, weather conditions, etc.) should be noted or researched. If the victim may have fallen, characteristics of the apparent takeoff point should be noted, as should intervening objects and protuberances. The actual or candidate impact surface(s) should be examined and, if possible, sampled and photographed. In the case of a floor with a covering, samples of the covering should be taken. If there are objects that might be candidates for causing injuries, these, too, should be carefully examined, not only for trace evidence but also for their physical characteristics and surfaces as well as weight. Surface characteristics may be quite valuable in linking an object with so-called pattern injuries in the skin of the victim. If possible, the objects of interest should be preserved as evidence for later examination if this should prove necessary. It may be possible that DNA evidence can be recovered from objects of interest to link the victim not only with the object but also possibly with a candidate perpetrator.

Other important information, especially when head injuries are being evaluated, is whether the head was moving at the time of impact or still relative to the impacting force, the location of the impact site, the dimensions (area) of the impact site, and whether or not the scalp or skull was intact. Although simple observations will generally not yield dynamic aspects of the event, it may be possible to estimate the mass, velocity, and direction of the impacting object, the time characteristics of the impacting event (pulse height and width), the nature and extent of other injuries, and the physiological state of the individual at the time of the impact.

Also important are a host of postimpact events, such as vital function status over time; the degree of hypoxemia or cerebral ischemia; changes in intracranial pressure; the presence or absence of subarachnoid, intraventricular, or intracerebral hemorrhage; whether attempts at resuscitation were made and their effectiveness; whether operative intervention occurred; and the duration of the postinjury clinical course before death, with some appreciation of how many ancillary or medical personnel "had their hands on" the victim and how many institutions treated the individual. Because many external variables can affect the type and extent of posttraumatic neural lesions, it is little wonder that, except in the most typical and routine cases, there is often great difficulty in interpreting, correlating, and understanding them. Fortunately, the greater number of forensic brain trauma cases have sufficient accompanying information that a reasonably accurate interpretation can be made by the experienced forensic pathologist, who has probably seen hundreds or thousands of head trauma cases, but there is still a sufficiently large number of examples in which interpretation is not only difficult but perhaps also vital to disposition of a case.

When neuropathological expertise is available to the forensic pathologist, it is often unfortunate that the neuropathologist may not be able to offer a great deal of help in interpretation because of lack of experience with brain trauma in his or her usual hospital neuropathologic material. This deficiency often results from head trauma cases not being autopsied in the hospital because many of them are medical examiner's cases, because the neurosurgeons in a particular institution are not inclined or able to treat neurotrauma, or because in nonforensic cases autopsy permits are not obtained. This lack of exposure to brain trauma, not only in practice but also during the training period, may leave most neuropathologists with a minimal practical knowledge of the subject, even though they may have read extensively on the issues involved at one time or other.

An additional factor that affects all interested parties is the comparative lack of textual material in works on forensic pathology and neuropathology relating to the pathology of brain trauma and injury biomechanics, although this deficiency has to some extent been remedied in recent years by increasing attention to the broader area of neurotrauma by researchers and clinicians, with a corresponding increase in original articles and monographs on the subject. The amount of literature on brain injury, however scattered, is extensive, going back to antiquity, typified by *The Edwin Smith Papyrus* [1], with much of it still worth reading. By the same token, it now behooves the neuropathologist and forensic pathologist to incorporate at least some injury biomechanics into their training and lifelong learning process. An increasing number of highly qualified biomechanicians are available for consultation and opinion, although the literature that is directly accessible to the pathologist is often sparse because biomechanicians often publish in specialty journals not normally part of a medical institution's library. In part, the authors hope to remedy some of this difficulty and prompt the reader to become more familiar with the theory (physics), practice, and methods of injury biomechanics. Pursuant to this task, relevant basic background material will be presented to provide a context for at least an appreciation of this branch of science in the evaluation and analysis of neural trauma cases. It is natural to try to think about highly complex phenomena in a simplistic way and dynamic phenomena in terms of static processes as part of the learning process, but to cling to these intellectual devices rather than to replace them with more enlightened and dynamic concepts may result in errors of clinical or pathological interpretation.

In the case of neurotrauma, there is a tendency to think of injuries as occurring at the moment of trauma and the traumatic process as having been essentially completed within moments of its occurrence. This concept is not only incomplete but also wrong. By the same token, to think of brain injuries following one localized impact or event as being similarly localized, involving only one structure or producing one apparent injury, is also naive.

As a general principle, when the head or any other part of the body is subjected to an accelerative force, this is generally referred to as an inertial force by most physicists and engineers. Such a force results in a change of the motion status of the object (head). An impact would be an example of such an inertial event. In such an event, there may appear to be no localized injury in the scalp, skull, brain, or its covering in some instances, but there is increasingly compelling evidence to show that the *whole* brain is subject to inertial forces, no matter how apparently insignificant the obvious injury appears. It is important to note, however, that the amount and extent of injury is related to the amount of force involved.

It might be convenient to think of trauma as a virus and the brain to which it is exposed as being totally infected but showing focal rather than obvious diffuse lesions. Nevertheless, the virus is everywhere, perhaps causing subtle changes, not grossly obvious but potentially functionally significant. Clinical evidence for this notion can be found in several recent longitudinal studies in which a whole range of meningeal or brain injuries appeared in the course of recovery, not to mention a whole range of derangements in neural function that also appeared. For example, psychometric testing of victims of even minor head injury reveals quantifiable dysfunction that may persist after long periods or show enhancement of these abnormalities if trauma is repeated, however minor [2–7]. It appears that repeatedly brain-injured persons, especially those with certain apolipoprotein E-4 genotypes, may be especially vulnerable and show Alzheimer-like changes in their brains later in life [8,9]. The issue of sports-related repetitive brain trauma is currently having considerable impact on the continuing discussion over the advisability of banning professional boxing in the United States and other countries because of the high degree of risk for brain damage in its participants [10–16]. Hard contact sports such as various forms of football, lacrosse, and hockey also appear to inflict on their players long-term neural, behavioral, as well as physical consequences. Pathological support for the clinical studies is more difficult to come by, but enough studies have been completed based on human postmortem, longitudinal clinical studies, as well as experimental animal material, to support the concepts outlined above [17–23]. These areas of neurotrauma are currently topics of great interest and study and will be discussed in detail below.

The following discussion will first deal with the basics that one must understand to properly explore basic injury biomechanics of neurotrauma, and then each anatomic component of the cranium will be dealt with in turn with respect to the anatomy of the structure, its relationship to other structures, and its characteristics that relate to physical injuries of that structure and their interpretation.

The focus of the following biomechanical discussion of central nervous system (CNS) trauma will incorporate the experimental data developed in the areas of subdural hematoma and diffuse axonal injury, two related intracranial pathologies in terms of the underlying loading mechanism. During the discussion, specific attention will also be focused on the differences between the mechanisms of these pathologies as they relate to the age-dependent properties of the developing pediatric CNS and constitutive tissues (skull, suture, brain, neurovasculature), an area of research that is currently gaining greater and much-deserved attention. The discussion will cover the overarching concepts of inertial versus contact loading of the head (applied load), the dependence of injury mechanism on the various physics of the applied load (direction, magnitude, duration), the kinematics of the head and the intracranial contents during the applied loading event, and the tissue and cellular level consequences of these kinematics. If this terminology is not somewhat familiar to you, please consult the beginning of this chapter for a brief introduction to physics and mechanics.

In general, the intracranial contents may be affected by external loading to the head in two ways: through the direct interaction between the displacing (e.g., ridges, prominences of the bony architecture) or deforming skull (in-bending, penetration, displaced fractures) or the intracranial partitions (falx, tentorium, etc.); and via relative motion created between the skull/dura and the intracranial contents by virtue of those contents' lagging behind the motion of the skull during acceleration of the head. The former case describes direct contact trauma, often associated with injuries such as contusion, laceration, and epidural hematoma, whereas the latter describes impulsive, inertially induced trauma, often associated with subdural hematoma (SDH), subarachnoid hemorrhage (SAH), and diffuse axonal injury (DAI/TAI). To clarify, when we refer to diffuse axonal injury in this context, we are referring to traumatic, stretch-induced injury to the axons resulting from external loading to the head versus hypoxic/ischemic injury.

Biomechanics

Biomechanics is a subspecialty within the field of bioengineering. Bioengineering is the application of traditional engineering principles (mechanical, electrical, chemical, structural, etc.) to living systems. Injury biomechanics extends the emphasis of this subspecialty to understanding the way in which living systems become injured when exposed to a traumatic mechanical environment. In other words, human injury biomechanics is a field of engineering dedicated to understanding how living things get injured. Injury biomechanics combines extensive background and training in physics, mathematics, and mechanical engineering with the life sciences and medical background specific to a particular living system, be it human, animal, or otherwise. Applying the principles of injury biomechanics to understanding how a particular portrait of trauma occurred complements the approach traditionally used in the fields of forensic pathology and neuropathology. Often, when a particularly detailed understanding of an injury-causing event is required, the clinician and engineer work together to develop a highly sophisticated and rigorous, evidence-based analysis of the injuries and the injury-causing event itself.

An engineer studying injury biomechanics is studying *failure*, that is, how a particular structure, when exposed to a particular loading environment or loading event, ceases to be able to perform or behave as physiologically "normal." In the traditional engineering sense, failure usually means that the structure of something has been compromised and can no longer perform as intended. Consider the example of an I-beam that is part of the support structure for a bridge; due to various influences, the I-beam may become weakened and unable to carry its required load as part of the bridge's support. Ultimately, the I-beam may fail completely (the I-beam may break), often with disastrous consequences not only for that I-beam but also for the entire system of which it was a part (the entire bridge). Following such a failure, forensic experts are brought in to try to understand how and why that failure occurred, what sequence of events led to that failure, what defects or changes in the structure contributed to its failure, and how that failure may be prevented in the future. The engineers and scientists studying the failure rely on their understanding of the physics that define the loading environment in which the I-beam performed its day-to-day task of carrying a load within the bridge's structure (was the load normal, or did factors such as wind or heavy traffic change the normal load?). They rely on their understanding of the material, shape, and configuration of the I-beam to determine how the forces generated within that loading environment, when applied to the specific I-beam, created stresses and strains within the I-beam and how the I-beam responded to those mechanical forces. They study how the I-beam's ability to withstand the loading environment to which it was exposed changed over time, either through long-term chronic changes, due to environmental factors (e.g., corrosion), or through short-term acute changes that may have instantaneously caused the I-beam to become compromised (e.g., a car accident on the bridge during which the I-beam was damaged and weakened). They compare the loads acting on the I-beam to its known load-carrying ability and its failure threshold to determine if the I-beam's ability to withstand the loading environment was exceeded. Once the engineers and scientists studying the failure have characterized the loading environment of the I-beam, the mechanical properties of the I-beam, and the failure thresholds of the I-beam, they are able to determine a failure mechanism, that is, a specific explanation of how and why the I-beam, and the bridge, failed.

This analogy serves as an intuitive scaffold upon which to build an explanation of injury biomechanics. Understanding injury from a biomechanical perspective may be divided into three general areas of exploration: (1) defining the loading environment in which injury occurs; (2) characterizing the mechanical properties of the cells, tissues, organs, and systems that may potentially fail in a given loading environment, and determining how the loading environment may cause failure in those constituent elements; and (3) defining in quantitative terms the injury tolerance of the cell, tissue, organ, or system—that is, the threshold levels of the various engineering parameters (force, stress, strain, energy, etc.) at which failure occurs. The following discussion will elaborate on each of the three areas as they pertain to biomechanical analysis of injury and the determination of injury mechanism.

Loading Environment

Loading environment is a descriptive term that refers to the forces acting on a particular living system to cause injury. *Load* is a generic term for external influence acting on a person, organ, or other structure—a load may be a force (*stress*) expressed as force per unit area. This *stress* results in deformation of a structure from its original configuration, expressed in change in length or other dimension per unit of original length or dimension (*strain*). The physical parameters that are used to characterize a loading environment will be discussed in detail later in this chapter. Examples of a loading environment in which head injury may occur include a motor vehicle collision, a fall onto a cement floor, or a gunshot to the head. A biomechanical analysis of injury begins with a quantitative characterization of the loading environment to which an injured person was exposed. A familiar example is a motor vehicle collision in which the loading environment of the collision is studied by performing a crash test, that is, recreating the collision in the laboratory setting and using various instruments and techniques to measure the crash forces acting on the vehicle and the vehicle occupants. This type of analysis is performed by crashing a vehicle in a controlled manner, similar to the collision being investigated, and using anthropomorphic test devices (ATDs, or crash dummies) to measure the loads acting on the head, neck, torso, spine, etc., of the vehicle occupants. This methodology allows the engineer to quantify the crash loads generated by the collision and determine how those crash loads get applied to the various anatomical regions of the vehicle occupants.

Injury is a dynamic process that occurs over time, whether it is a period of milliseconds or minutes. One should appreciate, however, that the injury process is not over at the end of the loading event(s), rather can continue in the form of a cascade of reactions that may extend beyond the even for hours, days, weeks, and longer. From a biomechanical perspective, the time over which a loading event takes place is crucial to understanding injury mechanism; many biological tissues and systems are not only sensitive to how much load they receive but also sensitive to the rate, rate of change, and duration of loading. Take, for example, the loading environment of someone hopping off a step onto the floor versus the loading environment experienced by a high-performance fighter pilot executing a high-g maneuver. In both loading environments, the body of an individual may experience similar forces acting in the vertical (superior–inferior) direction (approximately 8–10g, or 8–10 times the force exerted on the person by the earth's gravity; more on this later). The landing following a hop off a step may expose the individual's body to that 8g load for a fraction of a second, with no physiologic or traumatic consequences; however, a high-g maneuver in a high-performance aircraft that exposes the pilot to a sustained 8g load for several seconds may cause physiologic compromise to the point where the pilot blacks out due to altered cerebral perfusion. Injury biomechanics typically concentrates on understanding the acute loading phase of an injury that occurs over milliseconds during a traumatic insult, versus the secondary, reactionary sequelae and chronic physiologic changes that take place following the primary insult.

There are complex loading circumstances that should be appreciated. Most falls are mediated by the force of gravity that results in a uniform rate of acceleration (rate of change of velocity or dv/dt). The loading circumstances of a roller-coaster ride, for example, results in rates of acceleration (inertial loading) that are variable (da/dt) and may be likened to a "jerking" scenario. This type of loading circumstance may introduce complexity to injury analysis.

Mechanical Properties of Cells, Tissues, Organs, and Systems

To understand the consequences of the loading environment on the body, one must be able to relate the external loads acting on the body to some measure of compromise or failure of the body, system, organ, tissue, or cell of interest [24]. To this end, the biomechanical engineer seeks to determine the mechanical properties of the cells, tissues, organs, and systems that make up the human body. *Mechanical property* is an intrinsic characteristic of a particular material or structure and is defined broadly as a description of how the particular material or structure behaves in response to mechanical loading. For example, the mechanical properties of the various bones that constitute the skull have been studied in depth in an attempt to characterize the various loading levels and loading types required to produce fracture. Various experimental techniques, taken from traditional materials testing methods, are employed to measure the bone's resistance to tension, compression, and bending. These experiments provide data about the bone's resistance to its various loading conditions and the bone's failure characteristics once the loading conditions begin to exceed the normal range of the bone's mechanical environment. Similar testing has been conducted on the various tissues and elements of the head, neck, and intracranial contents to provide a quantitative tool for relating how external loads affect the tissues during a traumatic event.

Mechanical characterization of the constituents of the head, neck, and CNS has been performed from the whole-body gross anatomical level (e.g., human volunteers, human surrogates, animal models) through the organ and tissue level (e.g., whole brain, skull, spine and spinal cord) through the individual constitutive tissues (e.g., blood vessels, skull bones and sutures, brain tissue sections, dura) to the cellular level (e.g., isolated axons, neural cells, endothelial cells). Understanding how the loading environment affects, and potentially disrupts, the structure and function of the biological systems and their underlying physiology on all of these levels is a critical component of predicting how a particular loading environment results in injury.

As is apparent with almost every biological material and structure, the mechanical properties of a particular element may change in response to the loading environment, inherent physiological processes, or natural growth and development. The unique ability of a bone, for example, to rearrange its configuration in response to its loading environment is an important factor to consider when characterizing the mechanical properties of a biological system. Likewise, the constraints placed on, and the rapid growth and development of, the newborn and infant braincase to accommodate brain growth result in a dynamically changing mechanical structure with respect to how the structure may respond to external loads (intrauterine pressure, birthing forces, impact loading, etc.). These considerations are of particular importance in the context of injury when one considers failure and trauma of the rapidly and dynamically developing tissues of the head, neck, and CNS of the developing newborn, infant, and young child.

Injury Tolerance

Of particular importance in the study of injury biomechanics is the determination of *injury tolerance criteria*. Injury tolerance criteria are broadly defined as the levels, or ranges, of a particular physical parameter (e.g., force, acceleration, stress, strain, impact velocity, energy) above which failure (injury) of a particular element, tissue, organ, or system may occur. Recall that failure may be structural or functional and may manifest itself in many different ways specific to the particular system. For example, consider the neuropathological entity traumatic or diffuse axonal injury (TAI-DAI), injury to the central white matter of the brain that manifests itself clinically as loss of consciousness. Biomechanical studies of this entity, from the gross anatomical level to the cellular level, have been performed to elucidate the underlying mechanism responsible for producing TAI-DAI. These studies demonstrate that TAI-DAI is actually a continuous spectrum of pathology, from the mildest clinical expression of confusion, stupor, and brief loss of consciousness (concussion) to severe, permanent loss of consciousness (coma). The corresponding mechanical spectrum ranges from transient mild stretch of the axon, with near-instantaneous recovery (functional failure with recovery), to permanent, irreversible damage to the structure of the axon itself (frank structural failure). The loading conditions that the head must experience throughout this range of axonal failure have been defined biomechanically through the use of real-world accident reconstruction; human surrogate and ATD testing; animal, physical, and mathematical models of the brain; and cellular models of the neural cell, the axon, and the constituents of neural tissue affected by TAI-DAI. These models have yielded the graded spectrum and corresponding threshold levels of critical strains within the axon and neural cell required to disrupt normal electrophysiology and neural activity, gross strains within the central white matter resulting from angular acceleration of the head, and the threshold levels of angular acceleration of the head required to produce the continuous spectrum of TAI-DAI observed clinically. These thresholds, as well as others associated with various traumas to the head and neck, will be covered in detail later in this chapter.

Injury tolerance criteria are essential to our understanding of how and why injury occurs. In the context of forensic investigation of injury, one often performs a biomechanical analysis to determine if a particular loading environment provides the requisite loading conditions to exceed the thresholds for the observed trauma. If it is possible to reconstruct an injurious event and determine how a victim was exposed to a particular loading environment, then it is often possible to compare the loads experienced within that reconstructed environment to the loads known to result in trauma. Methodical determination of the loading environment, utilization of the mechanical properties of the head and neck, and application of the threshold levels of load at which injury to the head and neck occurs permit the biomechanical engineer to determine the biomechanical fingerprint of the injury mechanism that links a particular event history (loading environment) with the corresponding set of observed evidence.

Consider the example of a forensic investigation involving the death of a child from head injuries. By history, the child was said to have fallen and impacted his or her head on the floor; however, the nature of the head injuries that the child sustained necessitates an objective determination of the potential for those injuries resulting from the described fall versus another, differential explanation. A biomechanical analysis of scene evidence aids in the definition of the loading environment. Knowledge of the mechanical properties of the child's scalp, skull, brain, and blood vessels permits the engineer to determine, in quantitative terms, the consequences of that loading environment on the head and neck and its constituents. Comparison of the loads applied to the head and neck within the reconstructed loading environment and the injury tolerance criteria for the observed injuries permits the engineer to evaluate objectively and quantitatively the potential for the observed injures in the context of the loading environment described by history and physical evidence. This type of analysis complements the investigation conducted by the forensic pathologist in making a determination of injury mechanism and cause of death.

Introduction to Biomechanics: A Primer

The previous section introduced the conceptual framework upon which the field of biomechanics is built. As can be appreciated, biomechanical engineering, like its clinical counterparts, requires specialized knowledge. Biomechanics relies on concepts, conventions, and terminology that may be foreign or vaguely familiar to a nonengineer. The following discussion will serve as a brief introduction to some of the underlying physical, mathematical, and scientific concepts essential to the study of biomechanics. The reader is directed to several excellent and thorough texts, listed in the references, for further detail and discussion. Where possible, the concepts covered in this section will be reinforced with contextual examples in an effort to make somewhat abstract concepts more easily appreciated.

No discussion of biomechanics can start without a basic understanding of the laws of physics. For purposes of discussion, we will assume that we are not dealing with structures on the atomic level or with phenomena approaching the speed of light; we are therefore dealing with the area of physics known as *classical mechanics*.

The relationships that govern the inherent properties of objects and the way in which objects move and interact with other objects and the environment were elegantly solved and summarized by Englishman Sir Isaac Newton (1642–1727). Newton first presented his laws of motion in 1686, in his work *Philosophiae Naturalis Principia Mathematica*, or simply *Principia* (published by S. Pepys, London, 1686). In the context of injury, Newton's laws of motion apply to the way our bodies interact with our environment and the forces governing these interactions, and they play a crucial role in evaluating injury mechanism. These laws bear repeating, for they form the context of the remaining discussion.

Newton's Laws of Motion

Newton's First Law of Motion

> *Every body persists in its state of rest or of uniform motion in a straight line unless it is compelled to change that state by forces impressed upon it.*

This law is often referred to as the law of *inertia*, a property inherent in matter that defines its ability to continue in its natural state of motion in the absence of external forces acting on it. A key concept inherent in this law is the *reference frame* in which the object is characterized. A reference frame is a contrivance used to establish the point of view from which an object or system of objects is observed. Motion is not an absolute property but is, rather, a property relative to a particular point of view, or reference frame. Take, for example, the driver of a car moving down the road. If the reference frame for the system we define is anchored to the ground, then we observe the driver moving by the fixed ground reference at some speed; however, if the same system is characterized relative to a reference frame anchored to the car, then the driver is not moving, or has zero velocity, relative to that car-mounted reference frame. The first law makes no distinction between a body at rest and a body in motion, due to the relative nature of the observer's reference frame. It states that the body, due to its inertia, will maintain its uniform motion until acted upon by a force. A force applied to that body could change that body's motion, a fact that necessitates a working definition of force.

Force

> *Force is an action or agency that causes a body of mass, m, to accelerate. It may be experienced as a lift, a push, or a pull. The acceleration of the body is proportional to the vector sum of all forces acting on it (known as net force or resultant force).*

This definition introduces several terms and concepts that will be discussed in detail later in this chapter. However, in a general sense, a force is simply an action that causes a body to change its motion. We experience forces every day when we interact with other people, objects, and our environment. Our muscles develop forces within them that, when applied to our skeleton, permit us to lift objects, stand up, and walk. Wind blowing against us exerts a force on our body. Riding a bicycle results from our exertion of forces on the bicycle's components and reacting to the forces exerted on us by the terrain over which we ride. Force is not a foreign concept in everyday experience but, when treated in the mathematical sense, requires a concise and quantitative definition. We will define force explicitly and discuss how we go about accounting for force in a system of objects and their environment.

Newton's Second Law of Motion

The mathematically concise definition of

$$\vec{F} = m\vec{a}$$

states that the acceleration, a, of an object is proportional to the sum (net) of all of the forces, F, acting on that object. Notice that the F and a have arrows placed over them; this denotes that they are *vector* quantities (possessing both magnitude and direction), a concept that will be discussed shortly. m denotes the *mass* of the object of interest. Mass is a measure of the amount of matter that constitutes an object and is an intrinsic property of that object. The more massive an object, the lower the resulting acceleration of that object for a specific degree of applied force.

Mass is not to be confused with the common concept of weight; our weight, W, when we step on a bathroom scale, is the measure of the force that our body mass, m_{body}, exerts on the scale under the influence of the constant force of gravity upon it. Numerically, g incorporates all the elements that go into the establishment of the magnitude of the earth's gravitational field. In equation form, our weight, W, can be expressed as

$$W = m_{body}g$$

The force of the earth's gravity causes objects that are not constrained within the proximity of the earth to accelerate (fall) toward the earth's center at the constant rate of 32.2 feet per second each second (ft/s^2), or 9.81 meters per second per second (m/s^2). When we step on a bathroom scale, the scale is indicating the force that our body mass is applying to the scale as a result of our mass being attracted toward the earth (and the scale that is between us and the earth's surface). The force that the earth's gravitational field creates is proportional to the earth's mass, shape, and some other variables; the moon, for example, is less massive than the earth, and its gravitational field is proportionally smaller, resulting in a smaller force due to the lunar gravitational field (approximately one-sixth that of the earth). Thus, if we weighed ourselves on Earth and then went to the moon and repeated the measurement, we would weigh one-sixth of what we would on Earth. However, we did not lose any of our mass; we were simply applying less force to the scale because of the decreased force of gravity on the moon.

Shortly, we will expand our definition of force and explore the relationship between motion and the forces that result in motion.

Newton's Third Law of Motion

To every action there is always an opposed and equal reaction; or, the mutual actions of two bodies upon each other are always equal, and directed to contrary parts.

If body A exerts a force on body B, body B simultaneously exerts an equal force back in the opposite direction on body A. These forces lie along the same line of action, namely, the line joining the two bodies. An analogy is that if one pushes a stalled car, the car in effect pushes back at one with the same force. From this simple example, we can appreciate the significance of the third law as it relates to the study of injury biomechanics.

Newton's laws of motion result in a powerful and elegant expression of the nature of interaction between objects and the environment. As the previous discussion has demonstrated, there are some mathematical concepts, conventions, and terminology that require further explanation. The following discussion will focus on a brief explanation of some of the more important concepts that form the framework for a quantitative approach to understanding how we interact with other objects and our environment and how these interactions pose the potential for injury.

Kinematics and Kinetics

There are two general concepts to explore first: *kinematics* (the motion of an object) and *kinetics* (the forces associated with causing motion of the object). In the previous discussion of Newton's laws of motion, we touched upon the foundation of these concepts. Kinematics terms that may be familiar to the reader include *displacement*, *velocity*, and *acceleration*; kinetics terms that may be familiar include *force*, *momentum*, and *impulse*. In combination, the laws governing our understanding of kinematics and kinetics form the foundation of classical mechanics.

Kinematics

Kinematics can be defined as the study of motion without regard to the forces required to produce that motion. Consider the act of driving your car. You can change the location of your car by driving it a certain distance in a certain direction (25 feet northwest). You can drive your car at a certain rate of speed (velocity), in a certain direction (55 miles per hour, heading south). You can change the direction or rate of speed (velocity) of your car over some time by steering or by speeding up or slowing down (negotiating the entrance ramp to the interstate and going from 25 to 55 miles per hour in 10 seconds). All of these familiar terms are actually explicitly defined concepts in the study of kinematics, or motion. When you move your car a certain distance in a certain direction, your car experiences a displacement, often represented by the letter *S*.

Displacement is expressed in units of distance, such as feet or meters. As your car experiences a displacement over some period of time, the car achieves a velocity, *V*. Velocity is expressed in units of distance per unit time, such as feet per second, miles per hour, meters per second, or kilometers per hour. Finally, as your vehicle changes its speed in a straight line over some period of time, it is said to undergo linear acceleration often depicted as *a*, expressed in units of velocity per unit time over time such as feet per second per second, or kilometers per hour per hour; often this expression of acceleration is shortened to feet per second squared (ft/s^2).

Used throughout this chapter are notations that describe features of motion and their relationship to the quantities noted above [25]. A convention that is often employed makes use of notations used in calculus. For example, $dS/dT = V$ represents how speed is calculated using d*S*, which is the span of distance through which an object moves over the time interval of interest (d*T*). To repeat, an automobile may move 1 mile (d*S*) in 1 minute (d*T*) or 88 feet per second or 60 miles per hour for its *V* at the completion of its path of measurement. Terminology that may be used to label the relationship between distance and time is called *velocity*, the first derivative of distance traveled with respect to time (d*S*/d*T*), or the rate of change of distance with respect to time.

Another important relationship, noted above, is embodied when an object such as ball is dropped to the earth (accelerates). The ball starts out with zero velocity but ends up with another velocity when it strikes the ground (terminal velocity). The acceleration, α, from the resting state to terminal velocity proceeds at about 32.2 feet per second each second (32.2 ft/s^2). What this motion represents is the rate of change of the velocity of the object (ball). It can be expressed as noted before as

$$dV/dT = \alpha$$

Not all accelerations are constant or regular in comparison with gravity, which accelerates every object at the same rate. An example of this difference might be a slingshot and a stone, a roller coaster (as mentioned above), or a hot rod at a local drag strip. In these circumstances, the object to be accelerated starts out at zero velocity and attains some terminal velocity; however, its rate of acceleration will not be determined by gravity but, rather, by the nature of the propelling force and its capabilities. The nonconstancy of such accelerations can be measured and graphed to illustrate their motion. The calculations for such nonlinear accelerations require more advanced mathematics than simple differential calculus, as will become apparent later on and relates to head impacts; thus, by extension, the relation, dα/d*T*, to represent the rate of change of acceleration, α, would represent a special case that would apply to a gravity acceleration, where the answer to the rate of change of acceleration (due to gravity) would be graphed as a straight line, whereas if acceleration were variable it would be represented in a graph as a curved or wavy line to describe all aspects of the acceleration, including the peak acceleration. Using a function, discussed below in connection with impulse, it is possible to obtain an average acceleration measure, which is often reported in biomechanical studies such as those of Duhaime et al. [26] and Prange et al. [27].

It is important to note that displacement, velocity, and acceleration are *vector* quantities. That is, they have associated with them a *magnitude* and a *direction*. For example, velocity is a vector that possesses both a magnitude (commonly called "speed," e.g., 55 miles per hour) and a direction (e.g., north). If the car is traveling at a constant velocity, this means that its speed and direction remain constant. However, the velocity of a vehicle can change over time (experience acceleration) simply by altering the direction of travel or speed. Changing either one of the components of the vector (magnitude or direction) constitutes a change in the vector quantity itself. It should also be noted that there may be several vectors of velocity and acceleration acting upon a body at any one time independent of one another. Without belaboring the point, this distinction is important to understand and consider because injury is often dependent on not only the magnitude of simultaneous specific loads but also the directions of those loads.

The nature of motion can be described in two general ways: translation and rotation. *Translation* occurs when every point of a body travels along identical parallel paths but may take place in one, two, or three dimensions (along a line, in a plane, or through space, respectively).

Rotation, on the other hand, takes place when every point, at every instant of time, executes circular motion about some axis; such an axis may change position in space. The corresponding quantity defining this motion is the angular displacement (Θ, Theta), which is not a vector quantity. Elements along a radial line at different distances from the axis of rotation will have identical rotational motion but different translational motion. A simple example of the relation between angular motion (rotation) and linear motion (translation) is the rotating bicycle wheel.

If one spins a bicycle wheel about its center of rotation, the axle, the hub (closer to the center of rotation) will appear to be moving slowly relative to the tire (farther from the center of rotation). The hub and tire both complete one revolution in the same amount of time (i.e., they have the same angular velocity), but a point on the tire (far from the center of rotation) has a greater linear velocity at any instant than a point on the hub. Angular velocity, $\omega = d\Theta/dt$, and angular acceleration, $\alpha = d\omega/dt = d^2\Theta/dt^2$, are vector quantities in general but are scalar (arithmetically additive) parameters when motion is restricted to a plane. Angular velocity produces linear velocity of any point on the object, $v = r\Theta$, and the angular acceleration produces two components of linear acceleration, a component tangential to the path, $a_t = r\omega$, and a normal component directed from the point in question toward the axis of rotation, $a_n = r\omega^2$, where r is the distance from the point under consideration to the axis of rotation.

A measure often employed for angular or rotational motions and accelerations related to these is radians per second (rad/s) or radians per second per second (rad/s^2), respectively. There are 360 degrees in the circumference of a circle. This circumference may also be expressed in radians, or how many lengths of the radius of the circle define the circumference of a circle. Because the formula for the circumference (C) of a circle is $C = \pi D$, and D (diameter) is $2R$ (radii), $C = 2\pi R$. This means that there are 6.28 rad in a circle circumference; thus, a radian is equivalent to 57.32 degrees. If one knows the radius, then angular motion such as velocity and acceleration can be expressed in linear terms, such as feet/s or feet/s^2, respectively.

Most motion is a combination of translation and rotation, and the relationships between translation and rotation are important concepts to understand when applying biomechanical approaches elucidating injury mechanism. We will discuss this concept in detail when examining the biomechanics of brain injury.

Kinetics

Kinetics can be defined as the study of the forces that create or affect motion. In the previous example of driving a car, we demonstrated the physical parameters associated with the kinematics, or motion, of the car without regard for how that motion was produced. In distinction, understanding the kinetics of that motion requires knowledge of how the forces generated during driving affect the motion of the car. Forces that act on the car during driving include the torque generated by the engine, drive train, and wheels; the friction acting at the tires to propel and stop the car and to accommodate steering and cornering; the suspension forces acting on the sprung mass of the vehicle; and other factors. By understanding the relationship between the forces acting on the car to create motion (kinetics) and the motion of the car itself (kinematics), one may change those forces in an educated way to influence the motion of the car and, for example, reach a destination safely or increase the car's performance. Extending the analogy to the human body, by understanding the relationship between the kinetics and kinematics of the head and neck and its constituent systems, we can measure, model, and predict the influence of external forces acting on the body and its systems. This is especially important as external forces approach levels known to cause injury.

Momentum and Energy

As we discussed previously, if the motion of a body can be characterized, then we can begin to explore and quantify the nature of the forces acting on that body to create its motion. Some additional physical concepts that are important in the analysis of the motion and forces resulting in injury include momentum and energy. Like the previous relations defining kinematics and kinetics, these physical quantities are governed by clearly definable physical laws and form a useful framework upon which to analyze the interaction of objects and their environment. Because injury is typically the consequence of a body interacting with other objects or elements of the surrounding environment, the importance of understanding the nature of momentum and energy in the context of understanding trauma is evident.

Momentum is defined as the product of an object's mass and velocity. An object's momentum, $\boldsymbol{p}(\vec{p})$, is defined physically as the product of its mass, m, and its velocity, $\boldsymbol{v}(\vec{v})$, remembering that momentum and velocity are vector quantities and are represented in bold type here rather than employing the overhead arrow. In equation form, this becomes

$$\boldsymbol{p} = m\boldsymbol{v}$$

Momentum is expressed in corresponding units, such as lbmft/s or kgm/s, where lbm denotes pounds mass or slug. The phenomenon of momentum will be discussed in practical terms below with respect to impulse and the physics of the falling head.

In a closed system of objects that are not acted on by some force outside the system, momentum is conserved—this means that the sum of all of the momentum in the closed system remains constant, although it can be redistributed, or exchanged, among the various objects in the system. Because velocity is a vector quantity, as discussed previously, momentum is also a vector quantity; that is, momentum has associated with it a magnitude and a direction.

Newton's second law of motion, commonly written as $F = ma$, was actually expressed by Newton in terms of momentum. Specifically, "the rate of change of momentum of a body is proportional to the resultant force acting on the body and is in the direction of that force." These relations can be expressed by

$$F = \frac{\mathrm{d}}{\mathrm{d}t}(mv)$$

where mass times velocity (mv) is momentum (p). Another way of expressing the relation is

$$F = m\frac{\mathrm{d}v}{\mathrm{d}t} \text{ where } \frac{\mathrm{d}v}{\mathrm{d}t}$$

is the time rate of change of velocity or acceleration (α), which reduces to $F = ma$, the most commonly used expression of Newton's second law [25,28].

That is, the force acting on an object is proportional to the time rate of change of the momentum of that object. Different types of objects can have the same momentum, as long as the product of their mass and velocity are equal; however, the properties of the object itself often govern how that object may exchange momentum with other objects and the environment during interaction. Take, for example, a BB shot from a BB gun and a baseball being pitched by a professional pitcher. The mass of the BB is small compared to the baseball, but the muzzle velocity of a BB may be many times greater than the fastball pitcher's pitch speed. If the product of mass and velocity for each object is equal, and both objects strike a person in the head with that same momentum, the outcome for the victim can be very different, however. The inherent properties of the BB and the baseball, when compared to each other and to the head of the victim, will, in part, dictate how momentum is exchanged over time, and force is imparted, to the victim's head during impact. This is a function of the area of contact, with the BB likely penetrating the scalp or even the skull, and the baseball accelerating the head and bruising the scalp.

In the context of studying injury, the concepts of *impulse* and *momentum* are useful in determining the nature of the forces acting on a body during a brief application of an external force, where other external forces such as the earth's gravitational field are negligible. For example, consider the instant in time when a falling person strikes his or her head on a tile floor. During the brief period over which the contact between the head and the floor takes place, other forces in the environment may be neglected, as the contact force developed between the head and the floor will dominate the outcome of the event. The force acting on the head during this type of loading is called an impulse, which in a sense implies a nonuniform acceleration as opposed to the force of gravity that exists. Impulse, J, is a physical quantity that is related to the change in the momentum of an object during the brief application of the impulsive force, and is written mathematically as

$$J = \int F(t)\mathrm{d}t = m(\Delta V)$$

where F is the impulsive force acting over some interval of time, dt. The "s"-shaped symbol ($\int$) represents the mathematical operation of integration: the impulse, J, is the *integral* of the force acting over the interval of time dt and is equal to the change in momentum of the object upon which that force is acting. The integral of the force–time impulse can loosely be thought of as a summation, or average, of force over the time interval of interest (or essentially the area under the plot of the curve of the event).

Carrying the example of the head impacting the floor further, if we know something about the pre- and postimpact velocity of the head and we assume a reasonable approximation of the time over which the impulsive force acted during the impact, we can estimate the impulsive force acting on the head during the impact. If we can estimate that impulsive force through analysis, then we can make comparisons of that estimated force to values of force required to produce injury—skull fracture tolerance criteria, for example—to determine the feasibility of a particular impact scenario as it relates to the clinically or pathologically observed outcome. Because injury typically takes place over very brief periods of time, when external forces other than the impulsive forces acting on the victim can be effectively neglected, the relationship of impulse and momentum is a useful tool in the study of injury biomechanics, particularly as it relates to impact. These principles are illustrated in Figures 6.1 and 6.2. Figure 6.3 illustrates the convention of orientation of planes of motion for the head.

Energy is an inherent property in the physical world that is *conserved*, meaning it is neither created nor destroyed but, rather, exchanged and transformed into other states. Like momentum, if we characterize the energy in a closed system at some state, we can track how that energy is exchanged and altered into other forms as objects within the system interact. In general, there are two forms of energy to be aware of in the context of characterizing a loading environment: potential energy and kinetic energy. *Potential energy* is generally defined as the stored energy an object possesses by virtue of its position

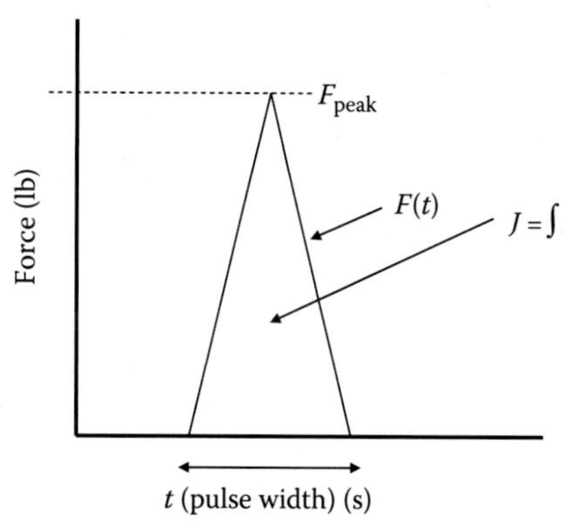

Figure 6.1 This diagram illustrates an idealized impact event of an object such as a head striking the floor. The impact event, once contact is made with the floor, results in deceleration of the head from a terminal velocity to a resting velocity of zero over an interval of time and the dissipation of momentum of the head over time. It is possible to calculate the average acceleration of this event by determining, according to the integral above, the area under the "curve," which in this case is idealized into an isosceles triangle, the formula for the area of which is 1/2 base times height (base = pulse width or time and height is the peak force attained). In practice with dummies such as the CRABI series, the shape of the force "curve" more often resembles that of a sine wave, making calculations somewhat more difficult. The curve results from complexities during the impact event such as changing elasticity of the head, deformation, and other factors [298]. These factors make a simple calculation of α = dv/dt, alluded to above, inappropriate.

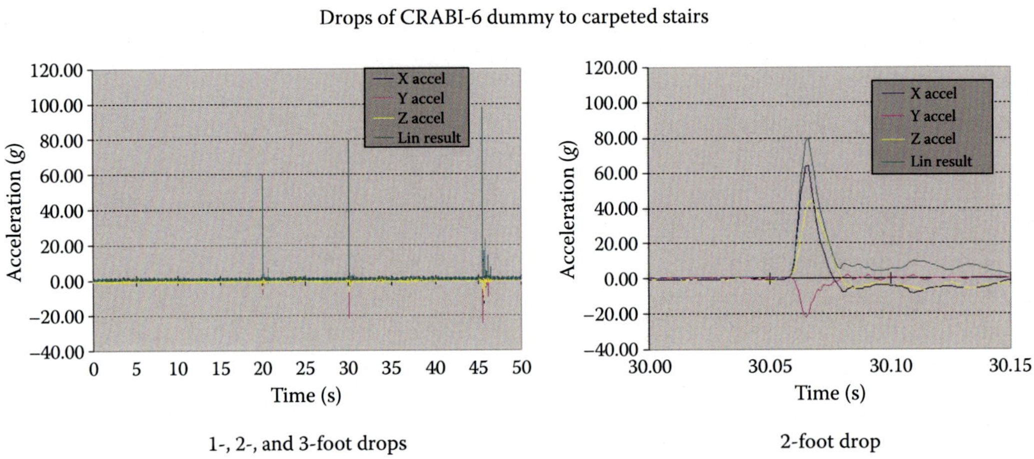

Figure 6.2 These panels illustrate pulses of deceleration in horizontal test drops of a CRABI-6 (model of 6-month-old baby) dummy on carpeted hard wood stairs from heights of 1, 2, and 3 ft (left panel) (about 60*g*, 80*g*, and 100*g*, respectively). The right panel shows the acceleration pulse shapes of the head (*X*, *Y*, *Z* planes and the linear result of all three axes) for a 2-ft drop. It should be noted that in a drop like that modeled, accelerations of the head occur in all three planes. It is this complexity that results in rotational accelerations in the mass of the head. (Courtesy of Chris Van Ee, PhD, Design Research Engineering, Novi, Missouri.)

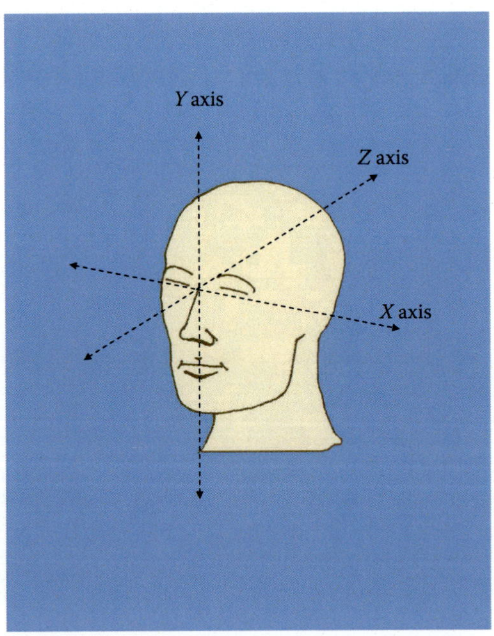

Figure 6.3 This diagram illustrates the Cartesian convention for anatomical axes [89]. Side-to-side movements are along the *X*-axis, up and down movements are along the *Y*-axis, and front-to-back movements are along the *Z*-axis. The transverse or tangential plane is defined by the *X* and *Z* axes. The coronal plane is defined by the *X* and *Y* axes, and the sagittal plane by the *Y* and *Z* axes.

or location within a *conservative field*—typically the gravitational field of the earth. A conservative field is one in which the work done in moving an object of unit mass around a closed loop within that field is zero. *Kinetic energy* is often defined as the energy of motion and is proportional to the square of the velocity of an object. These definitions are abstract and could use a little simplification and elaboration, so an example is helpful.

In the earth's gravitational field, when we raise an object off the ground, we do work to change the object's elevation from ground level to some height, h, above the ground. *Work* is a term that refers to the energy required to exert a force through a distance and is a measure of energy expended to perform that work. Mathematically, work, W, is the product of a force, F, exerted over a distance, d:

$$W = Fd$$

In keeping with our simple example, we use the metabolic energy available to our muscles to raise the ball from ground level to a height h above the ground. In this sense, when we do work, we are adding energy to the system. The ball's potential energy (stored energy) changes when we do work as a result of its change in position within the earth's (conservative) gravitational field. In doing so, we have transferred the energy involved in performing that work from our muscles to the potential, or stored, energy possessed by the ball.

Tracking the transformation of energy within a conservative system is an accounting exercise, in that we can define the energy in a system at some state (often known as the initial state) and then define the energy at some other state (often known as the final state). By virtue of the conservative nature of energy, the initial and final energy states must be equal—recall that energy can neither be created nor destroyed but, rather, simply changes form. This powerful concept leads to the conclusion that if we can account for all of the energy in each state, we can sum, or add up, the energy terms in the initial and final states and balance them. Symbolically, we can account for the total amount of energy in the system:

$$\sum \text{Energy}_{\text{initial}} = \sum \text{Energy}_{\text{final}}$$

The sum of energy in the initial state equals the sum of the energy in the final state. Why is this useful? Returning to our example, we define the initial and final states of energy for our simple action of lifting a ball from the ground to a height h above the ground. The ground is an important concept in physics because it provides a *reference point* for assessing the amount of potential energy an object possesses within the earth's gravitational field. By definition, if an object is located on the ground, it possesses no potential energy. When the ball is raised above ground, it acquires potential energy as a result of its elevation above the ground. Mathematically, the energy the ball possesses at a particular elevation, h, above the ground is defined as

$$U = mgh$$

In our example, we can define the initial and final states of energy, U_i and U_f, respectively, for the ball:

$$U_{\text{initial}} + U_{\text{added}} = U_{\text{final}}$$

where $U_i = 0$ and $U_f = mgh$:

$$U_{added} = U_f - U_i = mgh$$

and set these two states equal. This permits us to determine, for example, the amount of energy that was required of our muscles to perform the work of elevating the ball. In the English system of units, energy is expressed in pound-feet (lbft); in the SI system, energy is expressed in Nm (newton-meters) or joules (J).

More often, we do not necessarily want to find the amount of energy transformed for a specific action but, rather, we use the concept of conservation of energy to estimate other physical parameters helpful in determining injury potential. For example, what happens if we let the ball in our previous example fall from the height *h* above the ground back to the ground and let the ball strike the ground? Here, the initial state of the ball is at the height *h* above the ground, and the final state of the ball is at the instant it strikes the ground, with the height above the ground returning to zero. In the process of allowing the ball to fall from its stationary position at height *h* to its position at height 0, the ball acquires a velocity by virtue of gravity's accelerating the ball toward the ground. In the process of falling toward the ground, the ball's energy is transformed from potential energy (stored energy resulting from its elevation above the ground) to kinetic energy (energy of motion). Kinetic energy is defined mathematically as

$$\text{KE} = 1/2\, mv^2$$

We can account for the transformation of energy by defining the initial and final states of energy for the ball as before; however, we will cast the summation of the energies in a slightly different form. We will sum the potential and kinetic energies for each state and set those sums equal:

$$U_i = \sum \text{PE}_i + \text{KE}_i = U_f = \sum \text{PE}_f + \text{KE}_f$$

where PE represents potential energy and KE represents kinetic energy. This equation means that the sum of the potential and kinetic energies that the ball possesses in each state must be equal. In equation form:

$$U_i = mgh + 0 = U_f = 0 + 1/2\, mv^2$$

To apply this equation, we must define the variables *h* and *v* with values specific to our environment, so let us extend the example: a ball sits at rest on a table whose surface is 36 in above the floor. The ball falls from the table and strikes the floor. What is the impact velocity of the ball at the instant it strikes the floor?

To solve this problem, we must define the initial and final states of energy for the ball and set those states equal:

$$U_i = \sum \text{PE}_i + \text{KE}_i = U_f = \sum \text{PE}_f + \text{KE}_f$$

Rewriting our accounting in terms of the energies, we get

$$U_i = mgh_i + 1/2\, mv_i^2 = U_f = mgh_f + 1/2\, mv_f^2$$

Let us examine the specific definitions of our environment in the context of the variables h and v. The ball is initially at rest, located 36 in above the ground. In mathematical terms, this means that the initial height, h_i, is 36 in (3 ft) and the initial velocity, v_i, is zero for the ball's initial state. In the final state, the ball is just at the instant where it is striking the ground; the final height, h_f, is zero, and we want to find the final velocity, v_f, which is the ball's velocity at impact.

If we insert these quantities into the energy balance we performed above, we get

$$mgh_i + 0 = 0 + 1/2\ mv_f^2$$

As can be appreciated, some of the terms in the energy balance drop out because of the physical values assigned as zero. When we rearrange the energy balance equation with our values inserted, we get the following result for the final velocity:

$$v_f^2 = 2gh_i \text{ or } v_f = \sqrt{2gh_i}$$

This approach permits us to calculate the final velocity of the ball in terms of its initial height above the ground; we do not need to know the mass of the ball to do so. We compute the impact velocity to be 13.9 ft/s. Note that the mass, m, of the object is not included in the result. As an aside, this brings to mind the mythologized experiment of Galileo Galilei, often regarded as the father of modern science. The story goes that Galileo demonstrated that objects achieve uniform acceleration toward the earth independent of their mass by simultaneously dropping objects of different masses off the "Leaning Tower" of Pisa and having them strike the ground at the same time. Although the actual event apparently never occurred, and other individuals had demonstrated the concept before Galileo, the physical principle is nonetheless born out by the above application of the conservation of energy, a concept that Galileo appreciated through his study of pendulums.

To summarize this brief physics primer, there are several fundamental laws and concepts within physics that can be applied to understand injury with a scientific, quantitative approach. Specifically, through the application of concepts such as kinematics, kinetics, and conservation of momentum and energy, the loading environment for a particular injury-producing event may be analyzed and characterized in a quantitative manner to explore the potential for injury within that environment. The accelerations, forces, velocities, and energies generated within those environments, when applied to the human body, may result in injury; finding the levels of these physical quantities at which injury occurs, the thresholds for injury, is a major area of research in the field of human injury biomechanics.

To appreciate the effect of the laws of physics on the human body, we will briefly introduce the concept of injury in terms of the mechanical consequences of applying a loading environment to the human body and its systems, organs, tissues, and cells. In the next discussion, some basic concepts will be discussed to provide a foundation for understanding injury and failure in terms of engineering mechanics.

Engineering Mechanics

Previously, we discussed Newtonian mechanics in terms of the physical concepts of kinematics and kinetics, or the motions of objects and the forces required to produce those motions. In distinction, the mechanics of materials and structures, or engineering mechanics, focuses on the effects that those forces have on the structure of an object: does a particular force stretch or compress an object? Bend or twist an object? Change the object's shape, size, or volume? Thus, in addition to understanding the forces acting on an object, one must consider the inherent properties of the object and how those properties influence the response of the object to applied forces. In this regard, the study of injury biomechanics relies on a branch of engineering known as continuum mechanics.

Continuum mechanics may be defined as the study of the mechanical properties of a body that can be continually subdivided into infinitesimally small elements, with properties being those of the bulk material. In a *continuum*, one assumes that an object is composed of a material that is uniform in structure and behaves mechanically the same throughout its entire volume. One can appreciate that biological tissues are often composed of several different structures and elements; however, the continuum approach may be utilized if one chooses an appropriate scale with which to assume continuum behavior. Thus, if we treat bone or skin as a continuum, we are assuming that its gross mechanical properties are the same throughout a particular sample, recognizing that the scale of the piece of tissue is large compared with the microscopic elements that constitute the gross material. This is analogous to characterizing a piece of steel as a continuum, acknowledging that steel is made up of a lattice of atoms at the atomic level but treating the gross material as a uniform continuum. Obviously, as we explore injury mechanisms on various levels, from the gross macroscopic whole-body level through the organ and tissue level and down to the microscopic cellular level, the definition of our continuum changes with the appropriate scale of the structures being studied.

So what happens when a force is applied to an object with particular mechanical properties? From our previous discussion of physics, the object's motion may change (it may be accelerated), and it may interact with other objects and the surrounding environment. When studying injury biomechanics, these interactions are of particular importance because, in addition to external forces acting to accelerate an object, these forces may also *deform* an object. Injury, recall, is the point at which a particular biological structure is loaded such that the structure fails. The crux of injury biomechanics is in understanding how a particular external applied force results in deformation and failure of a biological structure.

Deformation

In the most general sense, deformation is defined as the change in conformation, shape, or size of an object. In engineering parlance, there are two basic types of deformation: a change in shape with preservation of the original volume of the object (deviatoric deformation) and a change in volume of an object with a preservation of the original shape (dilatational deformation). Real-world deformations are often a combination of both.

Deformations of an object may result in many ways, but there are specific descriptive terms in engineering parlance that describe the fundamental modes of deformation. These include *tension, compression, shear, bending,* and *torsion. Tension* is a mode of deformation that results from pulling on something and causing it to elongate. *Compression* is a mode of deformation that results from pushing an object and causing it to shorten. Tension and compression may be visualized by pulling or pushing on the ends of a spring and causing the spring to become longer or shorter, respectively, than the spring's original length. An example of tensile failure in injury is stretching and rupture of a blood vessel, ligament, or axon. An example of compressive failure in injury is the fracture of a long bone or vertebral body due to axial compression.

Shear

Shear is a mode of deformation that causes adjacent planes of an object to slide past each other in a direction parallel to the direction of the applied load. This may be visualized by setting a deck of playing cards on a table and pushing on an edge of the cards on the top half of the deck, causing the top cards to slide across the bottom cards in the direction of the applied load and parallel to the plane of the table. Brain tissue sustains shear loading during high-magnitude angular accelerations of the head, a loading condition associated with clinical entities such as traumatic or diffuse axonal injury (TAI-DAI).

Bending

Bending is a mode of deformation that is specific to objects that are substantially longer than they are wide or deep, like an I-beam or a femur. When a *bending moment* is applied to the ends of a beam-like object, the object will bend. Bending can be visualized by grasping a pencil with your hands on either end and placing your thumbs on the underside of the pencil in the middle of the pencil's length—pushing upward on the middle, or mid-span, of the pencil with your thumbs while constraining the ends of the pencil with your hands will cause the pencil to bend upward in the middle. Application of a bending moment to the pencil will result in deflection, or upward displacement, of the pencil at mid-span; this deflection will be proportional to the properties of the wood that constitutes the pencil's body (i.e., the material properties of the wood) as well as the way in which the cross section of the pencil is configured (i.e., the pencil's structural properties). Long bone fractures with "butterfly fragments" and linear skull fractures from in-bending of the skull during head impact with a flat surface are examples of failure during bending.

The dependence of the bending response on the material properties of the pencil wood and the way in which that material is arranged highlight the distinction between an object's material properties (i.e., mechanical properties inherent to the actual material of which the object is composed) and the object's structural properties (i.e., the mechanical properties related to the way in which the material is arranged). We will explore the distinction between material and structural properties later in this summary of continuum mechanics, as it plays an important role in understanding how the human body adapts and responds to its mechanical loading environment.

Torsion

Torsion is a mode of deformation associated with the twisting of an object. Torsion may be visualized by grasping a cylindrical object at each end, such as a cardboard tube from a roll of paper towels, and twisting one end relative to the other. Applying a twist, or torque, to one end of the tube while constraining the other end causes the tube to twist and deform along its length. Spiral fractures of long bones are classic examples of injurious torsional loading to failure.

Force, Displacement, Stress, and Strain

Objects may be subject to external forces and deform in response to those applied loads. From an engineering point of view, it is important to be able to quantify the deformation as well as the object's resistance to deformation under a particular load. Take, for example, a long bone such as a tibia. We would like to be able to characterize the response of that tibia to various types of external forces resulting in deformation (e.g., tensile, compressive, shear, bending, and torsion loading) to understand the various types of fractures that are observed clinically in the tibia. We can mount that tibia in a *material testing machine*, a device that permits the engineer to carefully apply a specific load or deformation to a *test specimen* in a controlled manner and measure the response of the test specimen (the tibia). We can apply a tensile or compressive load to the tibia by pulling or pushing on the ends of the specimen (distraction or oblique fracture); apply a shear load by fixing the middle of the specimen in two separate grips and moving the grips in opposite directions perpendicular to the long axis of the tibia (transverse fracture); apply a bending load by positioning the tibia horizontally, supporting the ends on "knife edge" blocks and pushing downward on the middle of the bone (bending fracture with butterfly fragment); or apply a torsional load by twisting the ends of the tibia in opposite rotation (spiral fracture). In each loading mode, we can measure the force, F, developed within the specimen and the displacement, δ, or deformation of the specimen during the loading process. The resulting test data are typically plotted on a force–displacement curve, a plot of the displacement and the corresponding force at that displacement. These are physical quantities specific to the test specimen's shape, size, and conformation and will vary for different-size specimens. We can normalize the force and deflection values by introducing two new parameters that account for the geometric properties of a test specimen, allowing comparison of the force–deflection response of a particular specimen to similar, different-sized or different-shaped specimens. These two parameters are called stress and strain.

Stress, σ, is defined generally as force divided by the area over which that force acts. Mathematically,

$$\sigma = \frac{F}{A}$$

In the context of a tensile test on our example tibia, the stress developed within the shaft of the tibia may be computed by dividing the measured force by the tibia's cross-sectional area at a specific location along the length of the tibia. The introduction of the geometry of the tibia (its cross-sectional area) essentially normalizes the force response and permits the force response of one tibia to be compared with another larger or smaller tibia in a direct way. Examples of the units of stress are pounds per square inch (psi) or newtons per square meter—the pascal (Pa).

Strain, ε, is generally defined as a change in length of an object divided by the original length of that object. Mathematically,

$$\varepsilon = \frac{\delta}{L_0}$$

where δ represents the change in length and L_0 represents the original length. This relation is the displacement analog of the relation between force and stress; that is, the geometry of an object is used to normalize the displacement, or deformation, of that object so that displacements in one object may be compared directly to displacements in a similar but smaller or larger object. In the context of our tibia example, if we mount the specimen in the test machine in preparation for a tensile test, we can appoint the middle section of the tibia's length (i.e., the diaphysis) as the "gauge length" of the test specimen. The gauge length of a tensile test specimen is the gauge or reference length of the undeformed specimen and is the original length used in the computation of strain. We assume that most of the specimen's deformation occurs in the gauge length during a test. As the tensile test proceeds, the gauge length region will elongate. This elongation, or change in length, is measured and divided by the original gauge length to compute strain. Units of strain include inch per inch (in/in), millimeter per millimeter (mm/mm), etc.—that is, length per length, which is essentially a dimensionless quantity. Strain can be thought of as a deformation that is a percentage of the original length. Tensile strain can also be expressed in terms of a stretch ratio, λ, where an elongation is represented by a value greater than unity (e.g., an elongation of 20% greater than the original length is expressed as a stretch ratio of 1.2) and compression is represented by a value less than 1. Sometimes a strain can be expressed explicitly as a positive or negative value, representing a tensile or compressive strain, respectively (e.g., +0.1 represents a 10% elongation and −0.2 represents a 20% compressive strain).

Why are these mechanical parameters important? First, they permit the engineer to characterize an object's response to an external load in a meaningful way, taking into account the object's geometry. Second, if stress and strain can be related to each other mathematically, a quantifiable, descriptive characterization of a material's behavior can be derived.

The simplest relation between stress and strain was developed by Robert Hooke in 1660. Among his many contributions to science, Hooke realized that certain materials deformed in a predictable way, and he published this observation in the form of an anagram: *ceiiinosssttuu*, which, when rearranged, reveals the Latin phrase *Ut tensio, sic vis*, or "As the extension, so the force." What Hooke observed was that the force developed within an object was directly proportional to the displacement applied to the object. Consider the example of a scale used to weigh fish—the scale is essentially a spring with a hook on the end and a pointer that, when the device is loaded with a fish, points to the weight of the fish on a printed scale on the face of the device. This device relies on Hooke's observation that the displacement of the spring inside the scale is in direct proportion to the applied load. Mathematically,

$$F = kx$$

where F is the applied force, x is the resulting deflection (elongation) of the spring, and k is a constant representing the stiffness, or spring constant, of the spring. The spring constant is expressed in terms of the force required to deflect the end of the spring a given amount, for example, 50 lb/in. If the fish we attach to the scale weighs 50 lb, the pointer on the end of the spring will move downward 1 in in response, as the spring stretches the predicted length. When the spring constant is known, a rule indicating weight can be printed on the scale so that the distance the pointer on the end of the spring moves points to the corresponding weight of the fish on the printed rule.

Hooke's observation is applicable to certain materials as well, expressed mathematically as

$$\sigma = E\varepsilon$$

where σ is stress, ε is strain, and E is a constant. Materials that obey this relation are known as linear elastic materials owing to the linear relationship between stress and strain. When a Hookean material deforms in response to an external load, it deforms in a predictable way that is related to the properties of the material. This constant, E, is called the *modulus of elasticity* of a material (sometimes referred to as the material's *Young's modulus*) and is a measure of the material's *stiffness*, in the same way that a spring constant is a measure of the stiffness of a spring. Casting Hooke's law in terms of stress and strain permits the determination of a property inherent to the material (stiffness) and independent of the configuration of the material.

For example, bone is a biological material that essentially behaves like a Hookean material. When we perform a tensile test on our tibia from the previous example, the force–deflection data that are measured can be converted to stress–strain data, as discussed previously. The resulting *stress–strain* curve will have an initial linear region that typifies a Hookean, linear elastic material. The slope of this linear portion of the stress–strain curve is equal to the modulus of elasticity, E. Thus, the stiffness of a material can be determined experimentally and is a useful parameter in characterizing the mechanical behavior of a material and predicting the response of that material to loading.

When such a material is loaded and deformed within its range of linear elastic behavior, the removal of the applied load will result in the material's returning to its original, undeformed state. That is, all of the deformation is elastic and not permanent, persisting only while the applied load is present. If a spring is stretched to a length within its linear elastic range, removal of the load stretching the spring will cause the spring to return to its original length. Structural injury typically begins to occur outside the region of linear elastic behavior and requires additional consideration of the stress–strain response of an object beyond the linear elastic region.

The example stress–strain curve for bone has some other notable features that are critical to understanding failure and injury. As we stretch the tibia further and further, the force developed within the test specimen begins to deviate from typical linear elastic behavior. In general, the point at which the deviation from linear elastic behavior occurs is known as the material's *yield point*. The stress and strain at which yield occurs are known as the *yield stress* and *yield strain*. Qualitatively, the material is beginning to "give way," and this point represents the precursor to material failure. Unlike elastic deformation within the range of linear elastic behavior, deformation beyond a material's yield point will result in some permanent, residual deformation. Although the elastic portion of the deformation will be recovered upon removal of the applied load, the residual deformation will persist. This residual deformation is known as plastic deformation.

As deformation proceeds through the yield point of a material, the shape of the stress–strain curve usually changes such that subsequent increases in strain within the material result in smaller increases in stress when compared to linear elastic behavior. Eventually the deformation of the material reaches a point where failure of the material occurs and the stress within the material decreases dramatically to zero—the material can no longer support the applied load. The peak value of stress preceding this precipitous decrease is the material's *failure point*. Stress and strain at this point are known as the material's *ultimate stress* and *ultimate strain*.

Recall that failure and injury in living systems may be structural (as discussed above) or functional. Structural failure usually involves behavior of biological materials in the region between their yield and failure points. However, it is important to consider that functional failure may occur at lower levels of deformation, such that normal physiologic function is interrupted but structural integrity (in the continuum sense) is not compromised.

Finally in this engineering primer is a brief discussion of some mechanical concepts to consider when approaching injury from a biomechanical engineering perspective. First is the distinction between material properties and structural properties. A material possesses inherent properties such as its stiffness (modulus of elasticity). These properties can be measured or computed with various testing techniques and permit quantitative characterization of the material's response to loading independent of how the material is shaped or configured. However, the way in which a material is arranged to form a structure will also affect the way that structure responds to an applied load. For example, consider the material properties of steel. A specimen of solid steel can be configured into a typical test specimen and tested in a material testing machine to measure its stress–strain response and compute E, its modulus of elasticity. Now consider various steel objects and their individual responses to bending, for example. A tubular member, an I-beam, and a solid bar made of identical steel may all have different responses to an identical applied load due to the way in which the steel is shaped and configured for each structure. The shape, size, and configuration of each member may be optimized in a way that uses the appropriate amount of steel to satisfy loading requirements, weight, shape, or conformational requirements as well as constraints of cost and fabrication methods and other factors.

Imagine an I-beam in a bridge that could constantly sense the applied load (a load that may vary with traffic, wind, temperature, etc.) and then change its structural properties to optimize its load-carrying capacity to the current, prevailing applied loads. The human body performs these same optimizations in an amazing variety of ways. The skull, for example, needs to deform to accommodate vaginal delivery, remain compliant to accommodate brain growth, and then become essentially rigid to provide protection and a stable environment for its contents. It also needs to be lightweight and accommodate internal vasculature. The optimization of the skull bones and sutures is an elegant solution that combines the lightweight and strong sandwich construction (inner table, diploë, outer table) typically employed in the lightweight panel design of aircraft wings with the energy-absorbing and growth-accommodating elements of the sutures. These design elements grow and develop over the requisite period to permit maturation. The femur is another example of the body's ability to reconfigure itself in response to its loading environment—the cross section of the femur changes through absorption and redeposition of bone to optimize the stress distribution along the femur's length. These changes occur in response to changes in the load sensed by the bone, and knowledge of this mechanism is essential in promoting healthy bone healing after a fracture. Thus, although we treat biological materials with standard engineering techniques, we tacitly acknowledge the limitations of our ability to abstract and characterize the material and structural behavior of these highly complex systems.

It is also important to recognize that most biological tissues are sensitive to not only the magnitude of an applied load but also the rate at which that load is applied. For example, the response to compression of the newborn head and the intracranial contents during vaginal birth (quasi-static or very slow rate loading) may be entirely different than the response under the same compressive loads applied at high rates (i.e., impact). This phenomenon is known as strain-rate sensitivity and is an important concept to consider in the context of the high-loading-rate environment of mechanical injury. This effect is common in biological tissues owing to the nature of the constituents that make up those tissues. Most biological tissues are mixtures of solids and fluids, mixtures that give those tissues a correspondingly complex mechanical response to an applied load. *Viscoelastic* materials are a specialized class of materials exhibiting such behavior, and the field of rheology, for example, is one scientific discipline that combines the application of the principles of elasticity of solids and fluid mechanics to study such materials. Many biological materials that are studied in the context of injury exhibit viscoelastic behavior, and thus an understanding of their response to high-strain-rate loading is essential when attempting to determine how those materials fail in the dynamic environment of trauma. Strain rate is expressed in terms of the amount of strain applied over a specific interval of time—for example, 0.1 in/in/s—and is expressed in units of reciprocal seconds; thus, 0.1 in/in/s is written as 0.1 s^{-1}. From a biomechanical perspective, traumatic injury typically occurs at strain rates greater than 1 reciprocal second (i.e., 1 s^{-1}).

Although this primer has covered a vast amount of physics and engineering ground and is by no means a complete discussion of the underpinnings of the biomechanics of injury, it will hopefully equip the reader with background to appreciate the basic biomechanical aspects of injury and injury mechanism as a complement to the explanations articulated by standard clinical, forensic pathological description. There are several textbooks that the reader may wish to consult for further discussions of physics, continuum mechanics, and applications of these concepts to biological structures. Some specific examples include the following: physics—Halliday et al. [28]; statics and dynamics—Beer et al. [29]; material properties—den Hartog [30]; and continuum mechanics—Fung [31].

Scalp

The scalp [32] is composed of five layers, from superficial to deep, as illustrated in Figure 6.4.

The thickness of the scalp in the adult is highly variable, ranging from a few millimeters to about a centimeter, depending on the location on the head and the age and sex of the individual. In the infant, the thickness of the scalp may be less than 3 mm but is highly elastic. In the child it increases in thickness with age, so that by puberty it approaches the thickness of the adult scalp. Its resiliency depends on the location on the head and the age of the individual. The biomechanical properties of skin, including several regions of the scalp, have been studied using standardized penetrometers [33]. The penetrability using a 1/16-in-diameter rod requires static force of between 15 and 20 lb to penetrate the skin of the face, arm, or knee but only 5–7 lb at the thinnest part of the face, near the eye sockets. Other parameters of scalp injury for the above penetrator or edged devices have also been reported, as have tensile and compressive strengths for scalp that indicate that scalp tissue is the most resistant to crushing of all the skin specimens tested [33]. Like most soft tissues of the body, the scalp displays viscoelasticity; that is, it responds to stresses in a nonlinear manner with respect to time and loads. With respect to tensile strength of skin, the percentage elongation (strain) varies with age, from 1.0 between ages 10 and 29 years to 0.57 in the 70- to 79-year age group, meaning stretch ability diminishes with age [33].

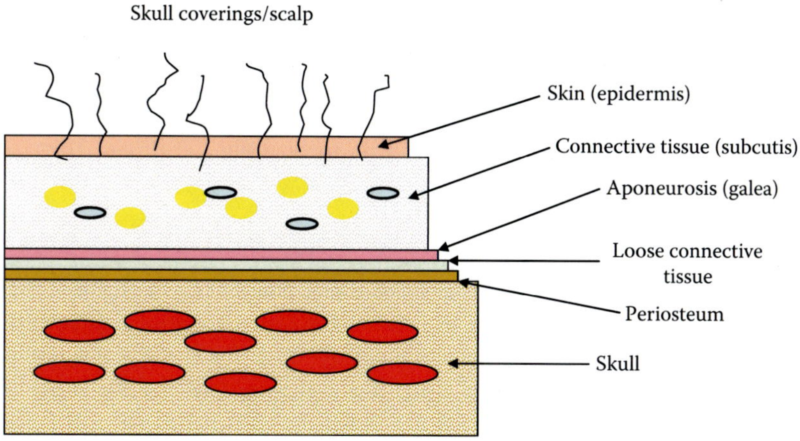

Figure 6.4 This diagram illustrates the composition and layers of the scalp above the skull: (1) the skin with its hair; (2) the subcutaneous connective tissue; (3) an aponeurotic layer, which is composed of epicranial muscle such as the temporalis and the galea aponeurotica; (4) loose connective tissue; and (5) the periosteal connective tissues that overlie and are bound tightly to the skull. The periosteum is responsible for making bone and generating the connective tissue cells that can repair fractures and other injuries to the skull.

The scalp is highly vascular and will bleed briskly when lacerated. From a traumatologic standpoint, the scalp is the first barrier to impact, providing a significant degree of protection to underlying structures by absorbing and damping the effects of impacts. Like most other areas of skin, there are natural lines of cleavage (so-called Langer's lines or creases) that on the head tend to run circumferentially and are thought to represent longitudinally running parallel collagen fibers in the dermis. The skin has been subjected to biomechanical analysis, and many of its mechanical properties are known, including variations in males and females for most age groups. For example, the tensile modulus along the lines of Langer is about four times that across the lines, which may explain why lacerations from blunt force impacts or punctures course as they do, tending to run parallel to the Langer lines [34].

The scalp serves to widen and lower the peaks of transient impacts and may absorb 35% or more of the energy of an impact, according to Gurdjian [35], but Melvin reported that less than 13% of the impact energy is absorbed by the scalp [30]. The intact scalp over the skull increases the resistance to skull fracture in experimental models by nearly 10 times compared to conditions when it is absent. Similarly, when there is a mat of hair over the impact site, a significant but less impressive protection is also afforded the victim.

Injuries of the Scalp and Skin

When performing a forensic autopsy, it is vital that the scalp be reflected and the locations of any subgaleal hemorrhages be noted, diagrammed, and photographed. This observation provides valuable collateral information that will aid in interpretation and correlation of underlying brain pathology by allowing identification of the sites of impact. In the forensic setting, the practical importance of the scalp is that it provides information to the pathologist regarding the location and character of impacts. Various impacting instruments may leave patterns in the scalp, which provide insight into the type of weapon or object involved. These may take the form of abrasions (scrapes), bruises (contusions), lacerations (cuts), tears, avulsions, or imprints of some distinctive surface. Such pattern injuries are well described in detail in many of the standard works on forensic pathology [36–40] and only a brief review will be attempted here. Scalp injuries for the neuropathologist must be taken against the greater context of neurotrauma to provide a complete picture of a traumatic event and perhaps its meaning.

Abrasions

Abrasions, or scraping injuries to the scalp or other skin surfaces, occur because of tangential applications of force producing friction between the surface of contact and the skin, damaging the superficial layers of the skin or scalp. The degree of damage is dependent on the nature of the contacting surface and its roughness, how much force and in what direction the forces are applied, as well as a number of factors operating in the victim. In the immediate period of the abrasion injury, the skin may show little other than blanching or erythema, which, depending on the depth of the injury, will give way to bleeding, generally of an oozing capillary character. With the passage of time, serous oozing and scab formation may form, and if there has been an accompanying deeper dermal capillary injury, a bruise formed by dissecting capillary hemorrhage may involve the injury area. This process may continue even though vital signs have been lost for a time. If abrasions of the skin have occurred postmortem, bleeding can occur from puddling of blood by gravity and may give the impression of a premortem injury. Furthermore, as the skin dries postmortem and is subject to autolysis, abrasions may take on a brownish discoloration that may confuse estimates of aging and dating of the lesions, which should be approached cautiously in any case.

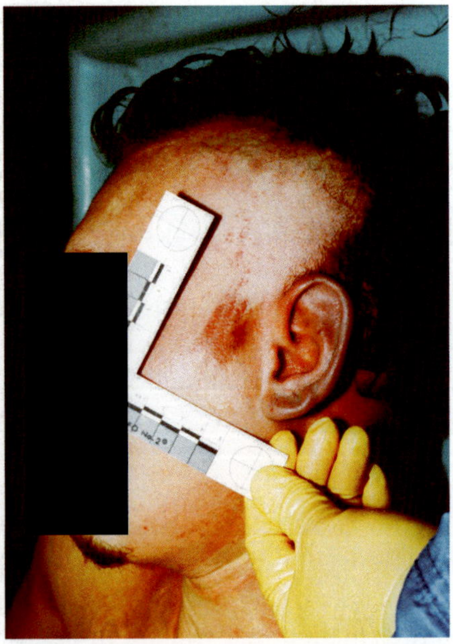

Figure 6.5 This photograph of the left side of the face of a victim of a "bar fight" illustrates an abrasion with ill-defined margins extending from the zygomatic region upward to the temporal scalp likely due to a fist blow. This victim died as a result of a posterior impact with the floor that caused a large basilar skull fracture.

Because abrasions tend to have features that often suggest a direction from a frictional surface, inferences can be made concerning the body position and the contacting surface, especially if macrophotographs are taken to reveal tags of epidermis that are elevated during the contact event and tend to elevate portions of the epidermis along the axis of the contacting surface. An example of a typical facial abrasion is shown in Figure 6.5.

Contusions

Contusions, which often accompany abrasions, are capillary hemorrhages within the deep subcutaneous regions of the skin even though they appear to be surface phenomena. Over time these hemorrhages tend to diffuse away from the impact site and may dissect into fascial planes that may cause the hemorrhages to appear some distance away from the original injury. This is illustrated by the phenomenon of black eyes ("raccoon" eyes), as illustrated in Figure 6.6. Black eyes can result from several things, artifactual and real. If the eyes are removed at autopsy before the body is opened and venous blood has had a chance to flow away, postmortem bleeding may occur and dissect into the orbital tissues and then to eyelids and face. Such a circumstance at first glance might lead to the impression of head trauma, and may lead to a civil law suit for damaging the body and making it unsightly. True pathological processes such as cavernous sinus thrombosis and basilar skull fracture that courses through orbital bones or nearby paranasal sinuses may also produce black eyes. The forensic importance of treating this observation carefully should be obvious. Other circumstances in which apparent subcutaneous hemorrhage may occur at some distance from a possible injury include hemorrhage into mastoid skin (so-called Battle's sign), which may occur from a basilar skull fracture, and hemorrhage into the scrotum resulting from intravenous access in the groin.

The visual aging and dating of skin bruises is notoriously inaccurate and imprecise, as has been pointed out many times in the literature [41–44]. Histological aging and dating is not much better, showing wide variations in tissue reactions over time. Red blood cells generally hold their tinctorial characteristics for about 48 hours after extravasation but then over the succeeding 2 or 3 days become paler and more lavender colored with the hematoxylin and eosin (H&E) stain. By 5–7 days after extravasation, red cells become indistinct

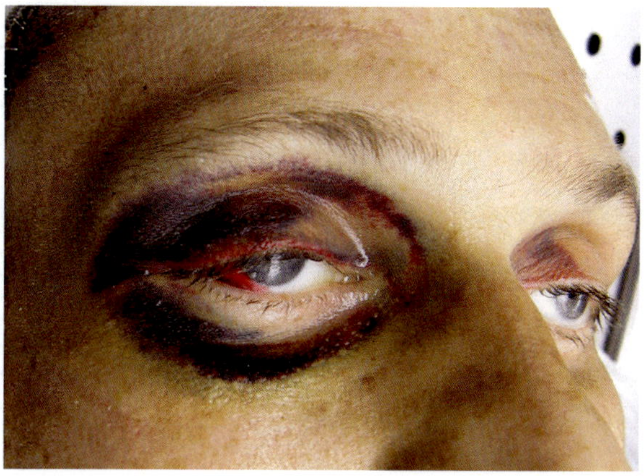

Figure 6.6 This photograph illustrates typical "raccoon eyes" in an individual involved in an altercation who apparently suffered a blow from a fist to the face and fell backward to pavement, sustaining a "hinge"-type basilar skull fracture that extended into the orbital bones.

and often empty at about the time the first detectable hemosiderin by the Prussian blue reaction is possible and macrophages are in evidence. Fibroblastic proliferation and capillary proliferation are usually evident after about a week, and sometimes before, from time of injury [45–48]. Beyond this time, accurate aging and dating may be problematic [49].

One of the most important forensic aspects of contusions and contusion/abrasions is the possibility of distinctive patterns caused by the impacting contact object or surface. Flat surfaces with some degree of texture with tangential contacts tend to leave linear tracks. If contact is more perpendicular, the textures, if pronounced enough, may imprint themselves onto the skin surface. Typical examples are textured fabrics, carpeting, furniture coverings, checkered or knurled surfaces of tools, weapons, belts, or shoe soles, as shown in Figure 6.7. Often these injuries can be matched dramatically with items or objects at the scene or seized from an alleged perpetrator and thus constitute valuable physical evidence to the authorities.

When the scalp or skin has been struck with linear objects not possessing sharp edges, characteristic imprints may also be made. One of the most typical is the pattern left on the skin (commonly on the thorax but also on the scalp) by a pipe, rod, belt, whip, or other more or less linear object. In these instances, the primary contact region is blanched by compression of the weapon, and the peripheral edges are hemorrhagic and dark; a phenomenon often referred to as railroad tracking or tramline bruising is illustrated in Figure 6.8. Sometimes the relative position of the assailant and the victim can be inferred from the patterns of the blows from the linear object (see Figure 6.9).

Ligatures and similar objects can leave imprints on the skin of the neck as well and can often also provide linkage to physical evidence that might be available (see Figure 6.10). The imprints of fingers in the form of bruises or abrasions made by the

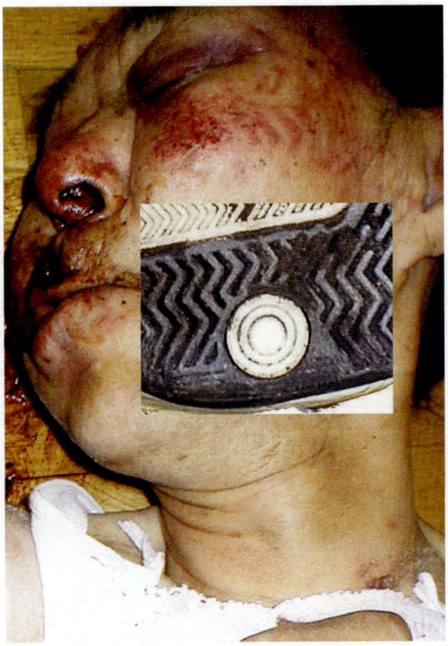

Figure 6.7 This composite photograph illustrates patterned contusions/abrasions on the face of a victim of a homicidal attack that matched to the sole pattern of an athletic shoe from a suspect in the attack.

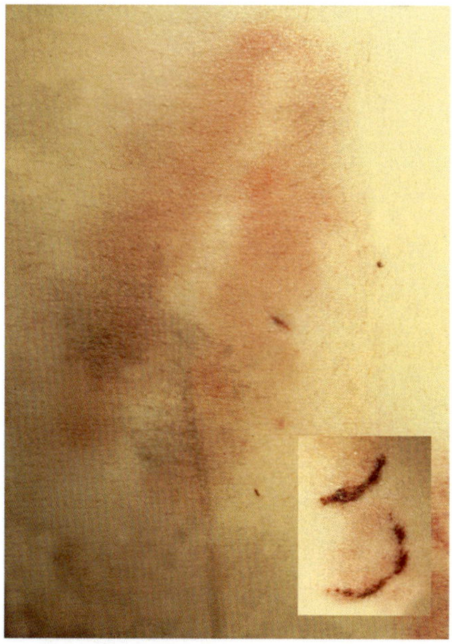

Figure 6.8 This composite photograph of the skin of the back or a victim of a homicidal beating involving a metal pipe, possibly conduit pipe, which left a linear blanched track bordered by erythema ("tramline" pattern). The inset shows two wounds elsewhere on the body that likely represent an "end-on" impact with the pipe. (Courtesy of Dr. Lee F. Beamer, Office of the Medical Examiner, Cook County, IL.)

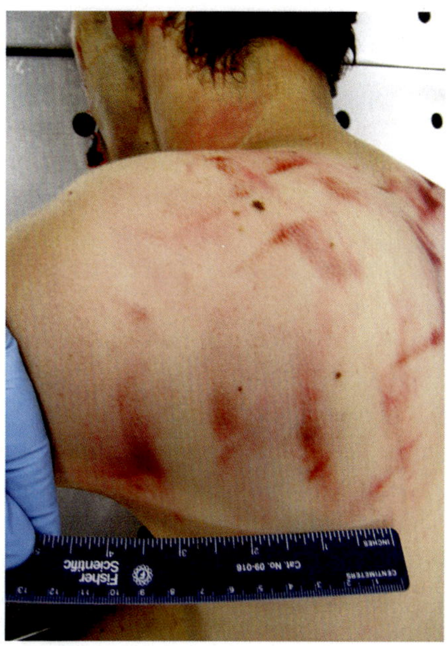

Figure 6.9 This photograph of the left shoulder/back area of a victim of a homicidal beating by multiple assailants illustrates numerous "tramline" imprints from a linear weapon that appear at different angles to one another, strongly suggesting blows from different directions and possibly from more than one assailant. The victim died of a head injury with extensive basilar skull fracture.

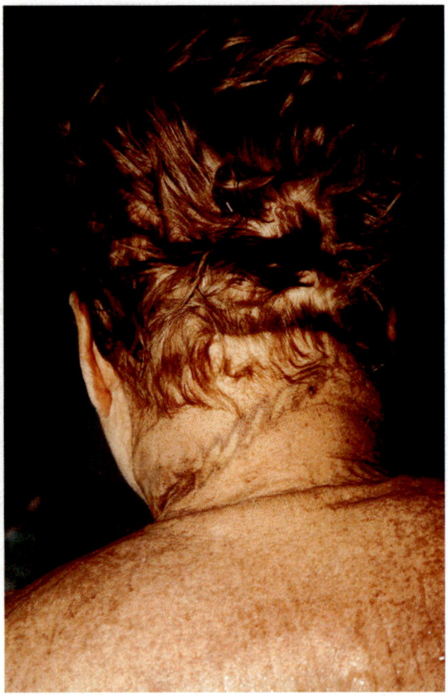

Figure 6.10 This photograph of the posterior neck in an exhumation autopsy of a man who had hanged himself 2 years before illustrates the imprint of the ligature that was used.

fingernails on the skin is another example of imprint evidence; however, care must be exercised in interpretation of such marks and their possible correlation with a perpetrator. In these instances, it is vital that accurate photographs with a scale in the picture frame be made for later comparison with the hands of a potential perpetrator, again with scales in the photograph. The marks made by knuckles may be discernable on the skin of a victim, but because of distortions on the struck surface, accurate comparisons may be difficult or impossible. Fist blows may or may not leave discernable pattern bruises, but in most cases bruising is rather diffuse on the face and scalp, rendering correlation imprecise and probably unreliable.

In vehicular/pedestrian impacts, all manner of imprint contusions and abrasion contusions are possible. A classic event is a pedestrian being struck from behind by an oncoming automobile where the bumper contacts the back of the legs, often leaving an imprint of the bumper on the victim and fracturing the lower extremities at the impact site. Following the impact, the struck victim is often propelled upward and backward to strike the hood and windshield of the vehicle, where further injuries, some of them possibly causing imprints, may occur. The grille on the front of the automobile may likewise leave imprints on the contacted skin. Protruding objects and surface of vehicles may also afford an opportunity for leaving patterned imprints on the skin. The possibilities for these are endless. When victims are overrun by a vehicle, imprints of the tire treads may be left on the skin and offer linkage comparisons. Surfaces on the undercarriage of the vehicle may also leave patterned injuries, but often these are so widespread or complex, mixing contusions with extensive abrasions ("road rash"), that precise interpretations are impossible (see Figure 6.11).

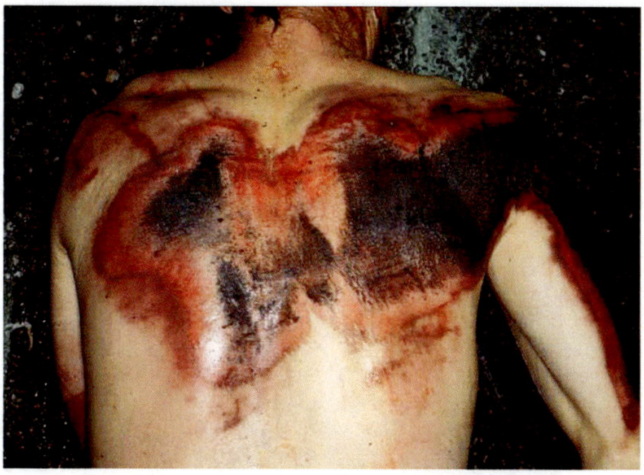

Figure 6.11 This photograph of a vehicle–pedestrian accident in which the victim was dragged beneath the vehicle on pavement illustrates the extensive abrasions and other injuries often referred to as "road rash." (Courtesy of Dr. Andreas Buettner, Munich, Germany.)

Lacerations

Lacerations or cuts occur most often when an edged surface impacts the skin, the scalp being no exception. There are many forms of lacerating injuries that are governed by the impacting surface and its mass, the force of the impact (momentum), the portion of the scalp or skin that is struck, and the direction of the impact and relationship to Langer's dermal lines [34]. Lacerations may be caused by pointed objects such as knives, ice picks, pencils or pens, fabricated weapons ("shivs" or "shanks"), pointed fragments of wood, wire, metal fragments, or debris. When the point of contact is broader, more linear lacerations may occur. When sharp-edge surfaces such as those of knives, swords, axes, broken bottles, glass shards, and metallic fragments strike the skin, relatively clean-edge lacerations commonly occur. Such cuts will not have strings of tissue or vessels crossing the incisions. These lacerations may occur perpendicular to the skin surface or occur at angles and undercut the skin surface. The determinant of how deeply the wounds affect the underlying tissues is a function of the force (momentum) of the impacting cutting surface, as determined by its mass and velocity, its sharpness (concentration of force), and the resistance of the tissues encountered. If the cutting surface is irregular, irregular lacerations will result. Penetration of bone (skull or other bones) and entrance into the brain or spinal canal may occur, as a function of the impacting sharp object. Stab wounds by sharp-pointed weapons have many identifying and confounding characteristics that often pose forensic challenges. These are well discussed in standard works on forensic pathology [37,39,40] and will not be covered here.

When impacting objects or surfaces are not sharp but still cause failure of the skin, these lacerations have many complex features that include shapes that may not match the impacting edge as well as crushing or incomplete disruption of the skin and underlying tissues, leaving strands of tissue, vessels, and nerves across the laceration (see Figure 6.12). Because the laceration is not sharp, forces may be dissipated into the surrounding tissues, causing, in addition to a laceration, variable bruising that can diffuse away from the immediate region with time and extend into the postmortem period. Objects like a tire iron, metal bar, conduit, gas or water pipe, baseball or cricket bat, piece of lumber, or other relatively heavy material can produce a variety of injuries to the skin or scalp. If there is

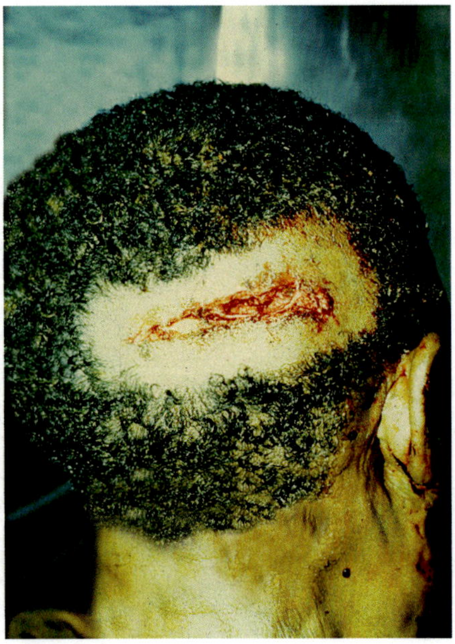

Figure 6.12 This photograph of the posterior scalp of a victim of a homicidal beating illustrates a linear tearing laceration apparently caused by a blow with a baseball bat. Beneath the laceration was an extensive skull fracture and a large subdural hematoma. (Courtesy of the Office of the Medical Examiner, Cook County, IL.)

a rigid structure such as the skull or other cranial bone immediately beneath the skin, a laceration is more likely to result from blows with these objects than if there is more soft tissue or muscle beneath the impact site. On the scalp especially, blows with more or less massive linear instruments may produce a curious laceration that may have a double-Y appearance, in which there is a linear laceration with tissue bridges across it, and at either end the skin has split into a Y pattern owing to the shape of the underlying skull surface and the unevenness of the forces at the end of the impact site, causing splitting of the scalp (see Figures 6.13 and 6.14). Such lacerations usually require a nearly perpendicular impact with the cranium. If the angle of impact is other than perpendicular, the scalp may be torn away from the underlying cranium, often producing an irregular laceration rather than a linear one. When heavy objects are wielded, there is almost always an underlying skull fracture or some form of intracranial injury associated, such as epidural hematoma, subdural hematoma, or brain contusion. When there is not such an injury, it is likely that the object was of relatively low mass, such as a hollow tube or some other configuration other than a solid mass.

Impacts (blows) with tools such as hammers, wrenches, flashlights, and other implements may leave characteristic imprints of the striking surface. Typical are the imprints made by hammers (see Figure 6.15). The typical carpenter's hammer often leaves crescent-shaped lacerations with some element of crushing of tissues, with tissue bridges in the cut. If the claw of the hammer is the striking surface, it may cause double sharp-edged penetrations, usually with underlying similar fractures, or if somewhat tangentially impacting, it may tear and rip the skin or scalp. By the same token, a ball peen hammer may produce punctate crushing lacerations typical for its rounded conical shape. Hatchets and axes characteristically produce extensive deep cuts and underlying skeletal and brain injuries.

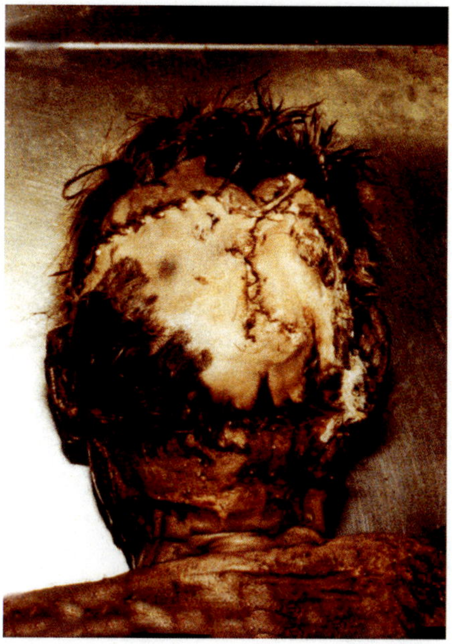

Figure 6.13 This photograph of the posterior scalp in an exhumation autopsy of a victim of a homicidal beating with a large iron pipe illustrates a "double Y" laceration sutured in the original autopsy below the lateral incision (sutured) through which the brain was removed. The body had been interred 10 years previously.

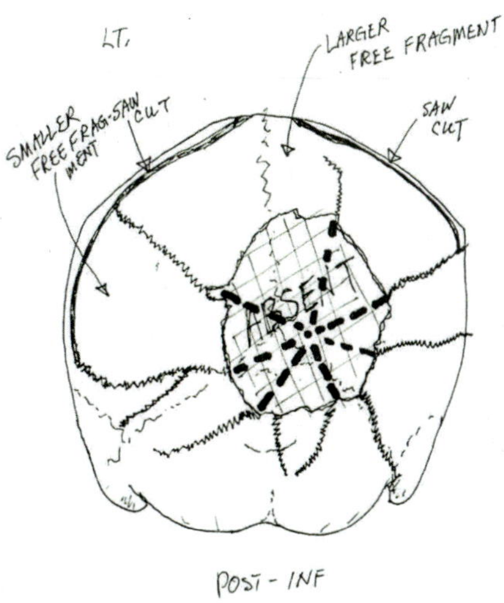

Figure 6.14 This drawing of the posterior skull of the victim in Figure 6.13. illustrates the massive stellate-complex skull fracture that resulted from the blow. The central part of the fracture apparently had been removed and not replaced at the original autopsy.

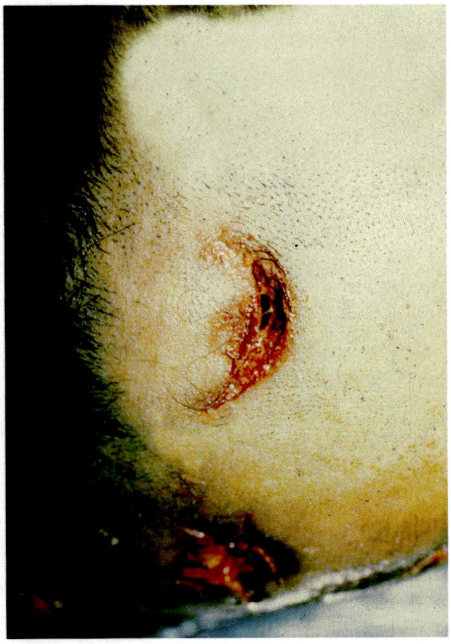

Figure 6.15 This photograph of the scalp of a victim of a homicidal attack with a hammer illustrates the typical crescent-shaped laceration of this type of weapon. There was an underlying skull fracture and brain injury. (Courtesy of Dr. Shaku Teas, Office of the Medical Examiner, Cook County, IL.)

Other objects cause their own variations of scalp wounds. Such objects are often found at the death scene and can be matched with wounds (see Figure 6.16).

Impacts during falls, accidental or suicidal, upon edged objects or elements of a building may produce massive lacerations and usually also cause devastating underlying cranial injuries, as illustrated in Figure 6.17. Impacts on solid, relatively flat surfaces by the head in fall scenarios can produce a spectrum of lacerations that can appear to have been caused by blows with an edged object. In these cases, even though the lacerations are spectacular and sometimes apparently multiple and unconnected, and there is no skull fracture or internal

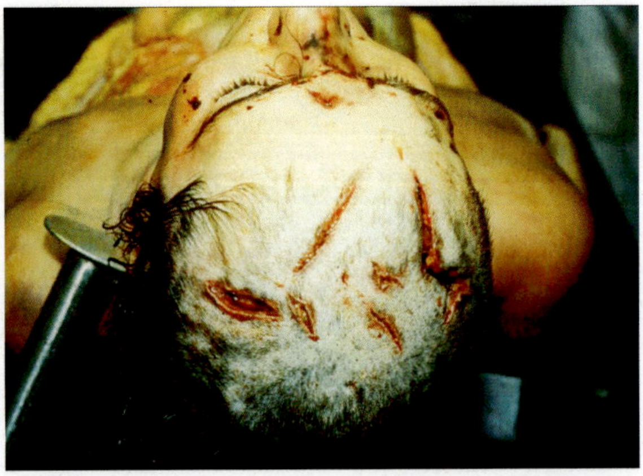

Figure 6.16 This photograph illustrates the wounds produced by a dumbbell found at the scene in a beating homicide. (Courtesy of Dr. Andreas Buettner, Munich, Germany.)

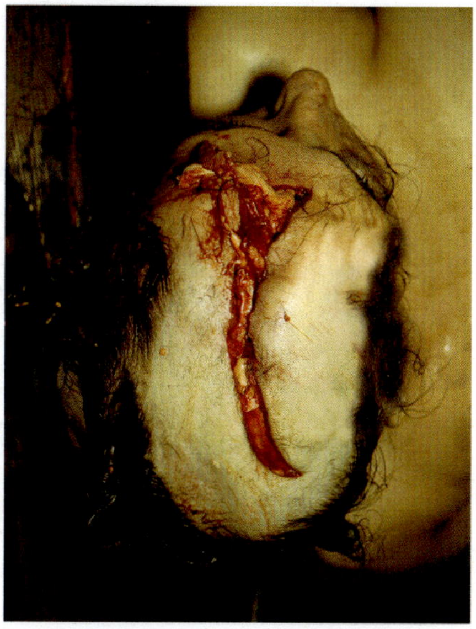

Figure 6.17 This photograph of the top of the head of a victim who apparently jumped from a road overpass and may have struck a traffic barrier below illustrates an extensive scalp laceration and open cranial wound. There was a continuation of the vertex fracture to the skull base but no neck injury was found. (Courtesy of Dr. Y. Konakci, Office of the Medical Examiner, Cook County, IL.)

cranial or brain injury, the splitting of the skin is caused by local forces that overcome the resistance of the scalp (see Figure 6.18). The flat surface impact may produce a stellate complex laceration or linear or curved lacerations with tissue bridges and a penumbra of dermal bruising. If there are irregularities in the impact surface, such as moldings or points or textures, these may affect their own additions to the injuries observed and may correlate their injury patterns with the impact surfaces. Scalp lacerations, because the scalp is so vascular, can lead to exsanguination upon occasion. Determination of the precise cause of death in such cases may be difficult and confusing.

Other Injuries to the Scalp

Often, the injuries to the scalp do not provide a true indication of the severity of the underlying trauma, which may come to light only when the scalp is reflected during the autopsy. This is especially true in infants [50]. The locations and extent of subgaleal hemorrhages as well as the exposure of fracture lines in the skull are far more important in this regard. The importance of nonimpact scalp injuries is well known in the analysis of stabbing and missile injuries to the head and is covered in this chapter and in many texts on forensic pathology [37,38,40]. Other forms of scalp injury include avulsion of the scalp [39], subgaleal and other hemorrhages due to hair pulling [51] (see Figure 6.19), and cephalohematomas that occur in connection with birth. When there has been a surgical procedure involving the scalp such as placement of an intracranial pressure monitor, ventricular drain, burr hole or craniotomy, the deep scalp will invariably become involved in a spreading dissection of hemorrhage at its deepest levels. Many craniotomies employ head positioning devices to firmly affix the head to the operating table. These devices make use of pointed pins that often penetrate the scalp and reach the skull. The same can be said for stereotactic frames.

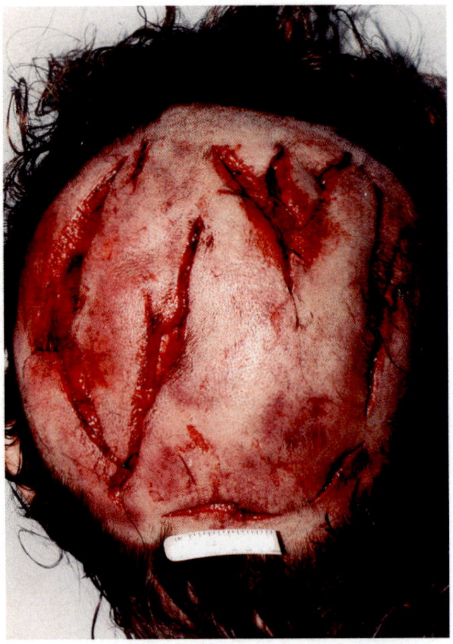

Figure 6.18 This photograph of the scalp of the back of the head of a victim who apparently sustained multiple falls in a narrow stairwell illustrates a complex pattern of large scalp lacerations without underlying skull fracture, subdural hematoma, or brain injury. These lacerations were likely caused by impacts against a wall. Death was caused by exsanguination over a period of an hour or more. Note the tearing quality of the lacerations and the bruising that surrounds them that is consistent with a nonedged impact surface.

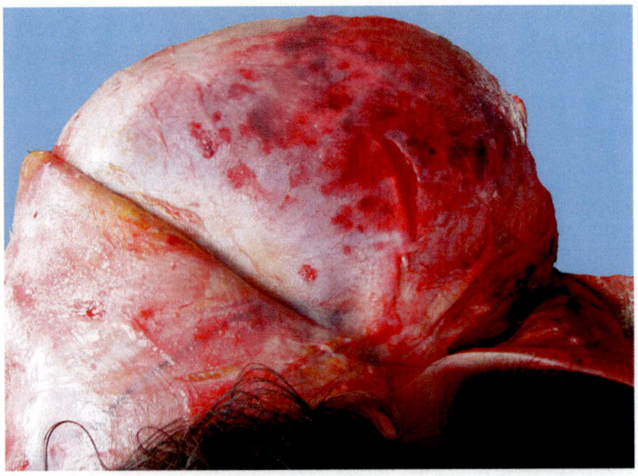

Figure 6.19 This photograph of the left lateral deep scalp illustrates multiple focal and sometimes confluent deep galeal hemorrhages in a young female who was the victim of an assault that likely involved hair pulling. There was no external evidence of impact in this location and the finding only appeared when the scalp was peeled back at autopsy.

These devices may cause hemorrhage in the deep scalp that spread in the galeal tissues and may be confused with impact points. The forensic importance of this phenomenon is that these iatrogenic processes will likely obliterate or overshadow any preexisting galeal hemorrhage from an impact; thus, an interpretation of deep scalp hemorrhages in these kinds of cases probably should not be attempted. It may be possible to differentiate true traumatic impacts from iatrogenic ones by histological examination, and suspected pretreatment hemorrhages should always be sampled histologically to search for chronic inflammation, macrophages, siderophages, etc.

The aging and dating of scalp lesions are far from a simple problem, although most pathologists have a reasonable knowledge of the stages of repair and resolution of hemorrhagic lesions that can be applied to lesions of the scalp; however, there are a number of issues that must be borne in mind when attempting to date them. Every individual probably has a slightly different capacity for tissue repair and reaction to injury. The infant may be able to repair and resolve injuries more rapidly than can an elderly individual, just as the healthy person's response to injury is likely to be more rapid than the chronically ill person's. The nature of underlying medical conditions, likewise, is also a factor, but by how much cannot be predicted. For example, an individual who has a hematological or bleeding disorder, diabetes, or a neoplastic disease or is immunosuppressed will likely offer a different response to injury than other individuals. Additionally, environmental circumstances may complicate wound interpretation. Such circumstances include whether the wound was clean or contaminated and whether burning, electrical, or chemical injury was involved; the environmental temperature may also be important [38]. There is literature based on human and animal wound healing, but precision and accuracy leave a good deal to be desired for every circumstance. It should be stressed that hard-fast and reliable rules for aging and dating skin lesions do not exist [36,47,49]; thus, a healthy respect for what is not known should temper attempts to age and date cutaneous injuries.

Postmortem Skin Injuries

Differentiation of antemortem and postmortem injuries to the scalp and skin may sometimes be an issue. As above, there are general principles that can usually be applied. These include the principle that the absence of a vital reaction (inflammatory response, repair reactions) connotes postmortem injury or injury proximate to the time of death. It is commonly supposed, also, that bleeding cannot occur after vital signs have ceased. This latter notion is not always true, and it must be borne in mind that postmortem bleeding can occur and simulate antemortem hemorrhaging [36,39,40]. This phenomenon can occur when there is considerable venous congestion before death and later injury or when a dependent portion of the body (including the head) is injured after death. Pooled blood may leak profusely out of a postmortem wound or, more importantly, dissect and suffuse into the vicinity of a postmortem cut or injury, giving the impression of a true vital injury. This phenomenon can be observed when, shortly after death, eyes are removed for corneal transplantation before performance of the general autopsy or embalming. The act of dissecting the orbital tissues in the presence of a distended venous system may cause considerable orbital hemorrhage with dissection into the fascial planes of the face, producing what appear to be massive black eyes as has been mentioned above.

Skull and Periosteum

Anatomy

The cranium is a composite of 11 bones (frontal, ethmoid, lacrimal, nasal, maxilla, mandible, zygoma, sphenoid, temporal, parietal, and occipital). Sometimes where the sutures meet, supernumerary interosseous (Wormian) bones may occur (see Figure 6.20). These bones are sometimes referred to as *os incae* [52]. Such bones are particularly common at the lambdoidal (junction of the two parietal bones with the occipital bone) suture [53–55]. Occasional sutures may also be found in the frontal bone, where its two embryonic plates have joined (metopic suture), and also in the occipital bone (mendosal suture) [56]. Generally, these latter sutures are invisible by the time the infant is a year old. Occasionally, these sutures may persist into adulthood. The forensic significance of these anatomic variants is that they may be misinterpreted radiologically as fractures [57].

In the fetus, the skull bones are separate, lying within plates of cartilage, and gradually fill in so that at birth the skull is essentially complete; however, there are junctions that have not fully fused, represented by the anterior fontanel and posterior fontanel. The pattern of suture closure is highly variable, and they are expandable well into childhood. The largest fontanel, the anterior fontanel, generally has closed by 12–18 months of age, with the others usually closing before. At the point at which all the sutures are closed, the skull has fully ossified and, for all intents and purposes, biomechanically functions as would the adult skull—a rigid encasement for the brain.

The skull bones vary in thickness, depending on the location, with some of the thickest and densest bone in the brow ridges and near the occiput, with the thinnest and most delicate in the temporal region and orbits, and with the parietal bone somewhat intermediate between them. The skull in the adult is a diploë with an outer and inner continuous smooth layer of bone, but the center is punctuated with many marrow spaces, vessels, and fat. In the infant, the diploic character of the skull is not declared until about a year of age or older. On the surface of the skull, at the junction with the scalp, is the external periosteum. Attached rather firmly to the undersurface of the skull is the dura, which also acts as an inner periosteum of the skull. The periosteum is capable of making bone, and when fractures or other injuries to the skull have occurred, repair and ossification are accomplished first by the periosteum and later by proliferating osteogenic cells that

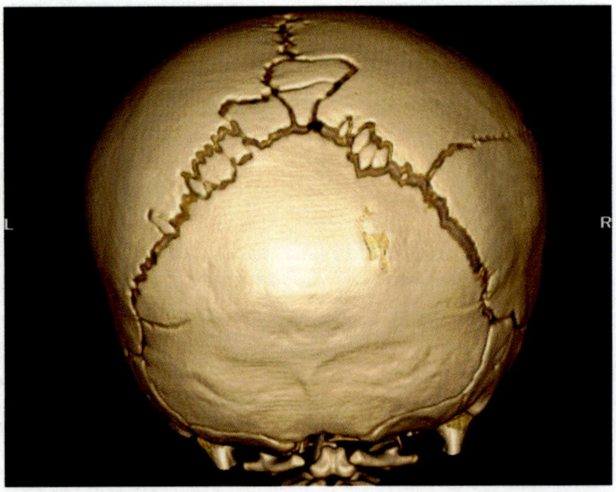

Figure 6.20 This three-dimensional computerized reconstruction of an MRI study in a young infant shows the posterior skull with sagittal and occipital sutures that contain many interosseous (Wormian) bones. There is a linear bony defect in the right parietal region that probably represents an aberrant suture. Autopsy did not show any soft tissue damage or hemorrhage in this region.

eventually bridge the gap of injury. Coursing within and above the dura, sometimes within the lower surface of the skull, and certainly indenting it, are branches of the middle meningeal arterial system that is derived from the external carotid system. This vascular system provides arterial blood to the dura and skull bones. Venous drainage occurs via vessels that drain externally in the facial system of veins and also internally via valveless emissary veins that empty into the deep venous plexuses of the skull base and ultimately into the jugular system.

The immature skull is equipped to undergo potentially large deformations associated with vaginal childbirth and thus possesses flexible cartilaginous bones and hinge-like membranous joints between the bones formed by the periosteum. The mechanical properties of the bones and sutures vary greatly over the first few years of life as the infant brain grows and develops. With growth and development, the bones of the skull increase in thickness and differentiate into their sandwich construction of the dense inner and outer tables surrounding the diploë.

The parietal bone, for example, increases in thickness from approximately 1–2 mm at birth to approximately 10 mm at maturity. The prominences of the parietal bones (parietal eminences) are the growth centers, from which the bone growth emanates radially, forming a mechanical structure whose properties vary according to the anatomical loading direction (loading oriented parallel to the radial fibers vs. across the radial fibers). This mechanical behavior is analogous to the behavior of corrugated cardboard, a structure that carries bending loads more effectively along the direction of the corrugations than in the direction across the corrugations. Other biomechanical features of the infant skull have been provided by studies on infant cadaver heads and by other means [58–63].

Mechanical Characteristics of the Skull

In contrast, the sandwich composite into which the bones typically develop at maturity provides a stiff, lightweight structure that is capable of carrying external (e.g., impact, crush) loads effectively in bending and shear. The cortical inner and outer tables of the bones provide bending and shear strength to the structure, whereas the diploë core provides space for intracranial channels as well as a lightweight, energy-absorbing cancellous bone core, much like engineered sandwich structures as in aircraft wing panels, architectural building "skins", etc. The skull bones are a structural composite that achieves an optimum balance of weight, stiffness, and energy-absorbing ability.

The curved sandwich structure of the adult skull acts like an architectural dome, receiving an external load at a point along the curvature and distributing that load across the bone. The load is carried by the bone to its margins, where the load is shared and transmitted to the other skull bones via the sutures. In the immature skull, the membranous sutures are incapable of supporting a bending load and possess little ability to absorb energy (e.g., from an impact). As the skull matures, the joints between the bony plates of the skull begin to achieve their typical interdigitated conformation, with the joint between bones possessing a network of collagenous connective tissue. The interdigitation of the sutures provides a large surface area over which the joints form, and the connective tissue network present in the joint, in concert with the increased surface area, forms an effective means of absorbing energy transmitted between bones during impact loading of the skull, for example.

Adult human cranial bone and its individual components have been tested in tension [33,64–66], bending [67,68], compression [64,65], and with simple shear [66] to characterize the mechanical response of the skull to traumatic loads. Wood [66] tested human cortical cranial bone in tension and reported rate-dependent increases in the elastic modulus and the ultimate stress, decreases in the ultimate strain, and no significant rate dependence of energy absorbed to failure. Sutures have been tested in bending [68,69] and in pendulum impact tests [69] to determine the mechanical properties of the sutures in the skull. Using the frontoparietal sutures of the mature goat skull, Jaslow [69] has shown that sutures absorb more energy during impact than adjacent cranial bone, and the ability of the suture to absorb energy increases with the amount of interdigitation. The presence of collagen within the suture and the highly irregular surface created during failure are thought to provide the suture with its energy-absorbing capabilities. Collagen has been shown to absorb at least 100 times more energy than bone per unit volume of tissue, and the amount of collagen within the suture is thought to increase with the degree of sutural interdigitation [69]. Examination of fracture surfaces of cranial bone and suture shows that much more surface area is created at the irregular fracture surface of the suture than at the planar fracture surface of the bone, suggesting that more energy is released from suture at failure than from bone [69]. Thus, the sutures in the adult skull are thought to act as shock absorbers during impact loading of the skull.

The elastic modulus of human cranial bone in bending increases from ≤1000 MPa (quasi-static) to 1370 MPa (dynamic) at birth [27] to ≈8000 MPa at maturity [67]. The quasi-static ultimate stress of cranial bone in tension increases from 10 MPa (porcine) at birth to 43–70 MPa at maturity [64,69]. The quasi-static ultimate strain in tension decreases from 0.034 mm/mm (porcine) at birth to ≈0.0052 mm/mm [67] at maturity. Mature sutures have properties similar to those of adult cranial bone [68]. The elastic modulus and ultimate stress of sutures increase from ≈200 MPa (porcine) and 7 MPa (porcine) [27], respectively, at birth to the values for adult cranial bone, as previously stated.

As a functional unit, the cranial bones and sutures serve to protect the brain from impact injury and focal penetrating trauma. In this capacity, bone is thought to carry and spread load (e.g., in-bending), whereas the sutures are thought to act as shock absorbers; this differentiation in roles is described in the literature [67–69] for quasi-static and impact loading conditions. Whole-head quasi-static compression testing of human surrogates has been performed and discussed in the literature, with the force-deflection curves for newborns and adults published as a function of the loading direction (anterior–posterior loading and lateral loading). It has been reported that whole-head stiffness in infants is about 10% of that of adults [27,58,63,70] and that there is a progressive increase in stiffness from birth to age 6 months [27,58]. Although impact accelerations from dropped infant cadaver heads showed differences between impacts at the forehead (about 40*g*) compared with impacts at other sites (about 60*g*), A–P and lateral loading experiments showed little difference in skull stiffness, whereas in adults A–P stiffness has been reported to be about 50% greater than in side-to-side loading [27,71]. While the compliance of the immature skull makes it capable of large deformations to accommodate vaginal childbirth, this property also makes the developing infant head highly susceptible to high-rate deformation from impact loading, a particularly interesting topic that will be explored in detail from a biomechanical perspective.

Fractures of the Skull

Fractures of the skull can be conveniently classified according to many schemes, all of which are very similar [72–74]. Evans [2] divided them as follows:

I. Closed fractures
   A. Simple linear fractures
   B. Simple comminuted or "egg shell" fractures
   C. Complicated linear or comminuted fractures
II. Fractures that transect the middle meningeal artery or venous channels, producing epidural hematoma
   A. Fractures that cross major venous sinuses and produce massive venous bleeding
   B. Fractures that cross cranial nerves, causing them damage
   C. Depressed skull fractures
III. Open skull fractures
   A. Simple
   B. Comminuted
   C. Depressed
   D. Fractures that traverse paranasal sinuses or the petrous portion of the temporal bone

A more morphological classification, which does not in any way conflict with the above, is the scheme of Gurdjian [35]:

1. Linear fracture of calvarium or base
2. Basilar skull fracture
3. Depressed skull fracture
4. Comminuted fracture of calvarium or base
5. Diastatic skull fracture
6. Expressed skull fracture
7. Stellate skull fracture
8. Multiple fractures
9. Combinations of above

General Skull Fracture Mechanics

The potential for skull fracturing depends on the location of the applied load, the magnitude of the load, and the nature of the surface applying the load to the head. The types of fracture, mechanisms, and parameters influence fracture type. With respect to linear and remote linear fractures, there is usually an impact against a flat surface. In-bending failure occurs first on the tensile surface (inner table) under the point of load, with fracture lines that can course across regions of high stress (thin stress concentrations, defects, etc.). Example surfaces are floors and broad flat surfaces (automotive interiors, tables, etc.).

With respect to comminuted or comminuted depressed fractures, there may be focal loading or more than one focal surface, such as edges, corners, or shaped objects. As the surface becomes more focal, the mechanism goes from bending to shear, which yields punch-type fractures. These fragments can lacerate the dura and brain, causing further problems. Example surfaces are steering wheel rims, pipes, hammers, and edges of furniture.

Various skull bones have different tolerances to fracture, as the experimental literature demonstrates [33,65,75,76]. A measure of the differences by age of skull bone is the elastic modulus (stress/strain). Studies have shown that for neonatal skulls, the elastic modulus is less than 1000 MPa (mega-pascals), but from 6 to 20 months of age it has risen to 3000 to nearly 4000 MPa. In the adult, the elastic modulus may approach 10,000 MPa [58,67,77–79]. The concept of skull buttresses, developed by Le Count and Apfelbach [73] and extended by Gurdjian et al. [80], is that there are strips of skull arranged vertically from the skull base to the vertex that have greater structural integrity than other areas and thus will tend to, when loaded, duct energy upward and allow fractures to follow buttresses and generally not to cross them. The main buttresses run from the orbital rim upward, from the junction of the zygomatic arch and temporal sphenoid bone upward, from the mastoid bone upward, and from the occiput upward [74]. Thus, impacts to the frontal region tend to run vertically, as do impacts to the occiput. Lateral impacts tend to produce horizontal fractures, and crushing forces tend to produce bilateral vertical fractures.

Attempts to study skull fracture mechanics include whole-head impact and isolated bone testing using tensile, bending, compression, and other approaches [81–85]. Recent studies have increased the knowledge base, especially in infantile skull fracture mechanics [70,86]. These various techniques have resulted in a compilation of skull fracture tolerance data for the various bones and various types of impact surfaces (Table 6.1), expressed through various physical parameters, including acceleration, force, and energy.

It is not uncommon for fractures of the facial bones to occur along with fractures of the skull. These fractures have also received study and have been classified in a number of ways, one of the more popular of which is the system of Le Fort [33,87–89]. The Le Fort I fracture horizontally separates the maxilla from the central facial skeleton. The Le Fort II fracture separates the central facial triangular unit from the skull, including the nasal bones and central maxilla but sparing the zygomatic bones. The Le Fort III fracture separates the entire central facial skeleton, including the maxilla, zygomatic bones, and inferior orbital bones, from the rest of the skull. The mechanics of these fractures is beyond the

Table 6.1 Work of Several Studies as Shown in Which Significant Numbers of Cadaver Specimens Were Studied

Bone	Range (N)	Mean (N)	Number of Cases	Reference
Frontal	2670–8850	4930	18	[83]
	4140–9880	5780	13	[84]
	2200–8600	4780	13	[85]
Temporal–parietal	2215–5930	3490	18	[83]
	2110–5200	3630	14	[84]
	2500–10,000	5200	20	[85]
Parietal	5800–17,000	12,500	11	[85]

Source: Derived from Allsop DL. Skull and facial bone trauma: Experimental aspects. In Nahum AM, Melvin EC, eds., *Accidental Injury: Biomechanics and Prevention.* New York: Springer-Verlag, 1993, pp. 247–67.

Note: It is obvious that the ranges of force required to produce fractures was wide, but the means tend to be quite similar and provide at least some context for the fractures of different cranial bones. N = Newton.

scope of this work and will not be discussed here. An excellent compilation and discussion of facial bone fracture tolerance literature and fractures of the facial skeleton can be found in Nahum and Melvin's text [89] and Galloway's text [74].

Linear Skull Fracture

As the name implies, linear skull fractures are usually rather simple, straight-line fractures occurring over the convexity of the skull or the base, and they constitute nearly 70% of all skull fractures and mostly affect the parietal bone. These fractures generally radiate away from the site of impact, where out-bending of the skull in response to impact has occurred, and follow a course determined by the strength of the bone in its path and, to some degree, the direction of the impacting force (see Figure 6.21). The fracture line will tend to run in the direction of the impact toward areas of weakness, including foramina, and may cross them. Lines may extend for only a few centimeters and be confined to the vertex or base or involve both with full or partial thickness of the diploë. Quite often there is more than one fracture line, not all of which necessarily intersect at the point of impact, but generally they do [2,72,73].

The clinical effect of a simple linear skull fracture is usually minimal by itself, but if the fracture line passes over a branch of the middle meningeal artery, it can lead to epidural hematoma (discussed below), lacerate a cranial nerve or damage a vessel if it passes through a foramen, or open a sinus cavity, which can result in cerebrospinal fluid (CSF) rhinorrhea or otorrhea and possibly infection. If none of the above complications occurs and there is no injury or only minimal injury to the brain from contusions or hemorrhage, there are frequently no obvious symptoms or neurological sequelae, and the fracture may be difficult to visualize radiographically [90,91]. This fact often causes issues for forensic interpretations, especially when clinicians discount the possibility for minimal symptoms in association with skull fractures and imply that their lack somehow casts suspicion upon another person.

Simple linear fractures, especially if they do not fully involve both the inner and outer tables of the skull, may be difficult to observe at autopsy unless the calvarial surface is carefully inspected, the skull cap percussed when removed (for a "cracked pot" sound),

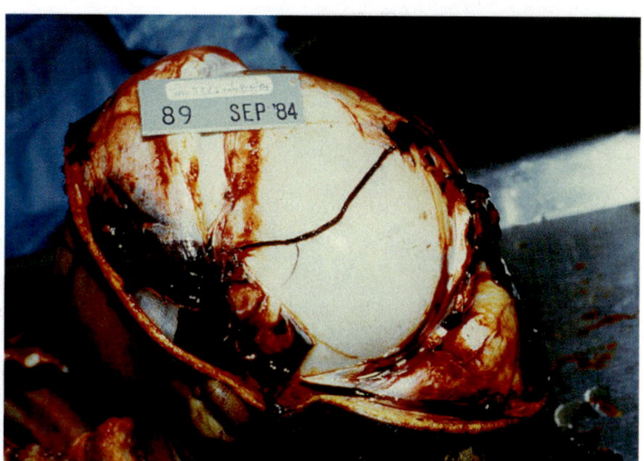

Figure 6.21 This photograph of lateral mostly linear skull fracture from a homicidal blow to the side of the head with a heavy object illustrates an accompanying large subgaleal hemorrhage and a secondary fracture line. Note the sharp edges on the fracture line and blood within. (Courtesy of Dr. Shaku Teas, Office of the Medical Examiner, Cook County, IL.)

and if the dura on both the vertex and the base is not stripped away. Postmortem radiography may or may not reveal some fractures, but most will be visualized if care is taken in technique. In child abuse cases, fractures that are found are usually widely spaced, in contradistinction to the narrow linear fractures seen in adults. The factor that most influences fracture spreading is intracranial pressure, which in turn is governed by evolving mass effects of subdural hematomas, brain hemorrhage, and edema that may be present.

The healing process in the skull fracture does not result in a callus as would be seen in a rib or long bone fracture, rather it causes an elevation of tissue at the edge of the skull fracture, producing a lip or rounded edge along the fracture line that is visible grossly and microscopically within about 2 weeks after occurrence [92–95]. Examples of this finding can be seen in Figure 6.22. At this point, the fracture may or may not have much tissue bridging the fracture line, but as time passes the tissue bridge becomes more and more evident and significant structurally, and at autopsy the skull bones of a fracture may require some force to separate them, which should not be done by the prosector.

Linear and other skull fractures heal at variable rates and may be visible radiographically for many months after occurrence. Pathologically, healing occurs from the periosteum of the external surface of the skull and perhaps more robustly from the periosteal activity of the dura [92]. The calvarial fracture eventually leads to deposition of first fibroblastic tissue, then osteoid, and then bone within the fracture line associated with reactive cells (see Figure 6.23). There are no good and reliable histological or radiological criteria for accurately aging and dating skull fractures; thus, fracture age can only be estimated.

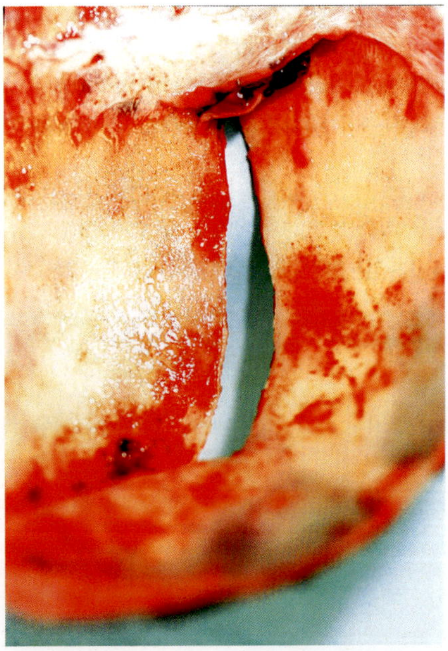

Figure 6.22 This photograph shows a parietal skull fracture in a 1-month-old female who was born 3 weeks premature. The baby had been apparently overlain in bed by the father and was found to be unresponsive. Autopsy did not reveal any bruising on the head. There was an acute upon chronic subdural hematoma, which had a neomembrane consistent with about 1 month duration. The child's body weight was in the 50th percentile but the head was in the 90th percentile. Note the somewhat rounded or lipped (nonsharp) edges of the fracture line, which connotes healing, in this case probably birth-related 1 month before.

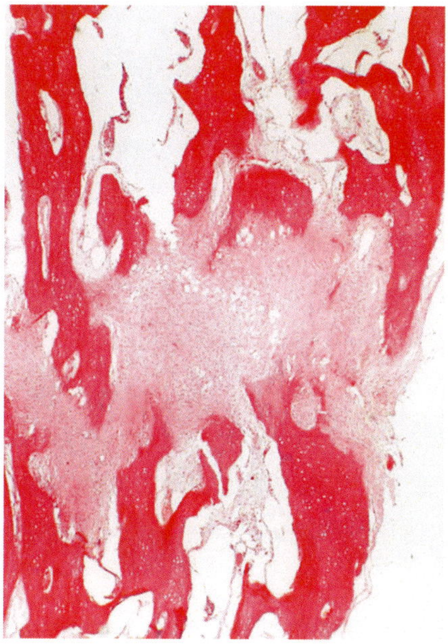

Figure 6.23 This low-power photomicrograph of a decalcified portion of a healing skull fracture in a 5 1/2-month-old baby shows connection of the fracture line with fibrous connective tissue. The fracture is probably several weeks or more old, in keeping with a chronic subdural hematoma on the opposite side of the head. Grossly the fracture line was barely visible and was accompanied by a thickened and discolored region in the subgaleal connective tissues overlying it.

Correlative histological changes in pericranial soft tissues, such as degree and extent of hemosiderin/hematoidin, the inflammatory reaction both grossly and microscopically, as well as the estimated age of a coexistent subdural hematoma, may aid in estimating the ages of the processes.

Upon occasion, a skull fracture may grow and not heal. The phenomenon is often referred to as a "growing" skull fracture, which almost always is seen in children. The phenomenon leads to an expanding fracture line that may never heal and may or may not be associated with cystic fluid accumulation (leptomeningeal cyst) beneath the fracture. Why this complication of skull fracture occurs is not entirely clear [96–98].

Basilar Skull Fracture

Fractures of the base of the skull can take several forms, from relatively simple linear basal fractures to more complex and structurally discontinuous fractures that may cross from side to side, often along the petrous ridges, or arc around the posterior fossa, or extend into the orbital roofs (see Figure 6.24). Fractures of the vertex from impacts there can, and often do, extend into the base, but most basilar fractures result from impacts to the occiput, sides of the head, or front of the head (hat band), although this is not absolute. As with other fractures, deformation of the skull after loading from an impact creates in- and out-bending and stress lines that may exceed the structural tolerance for the skull. The pattern of basilar fractures generally follows the direction of the impact; for example, lateral impacts produce side-to-side fractures, and axial impacts produce axial fractures. This is not to say that patterns may not be complex, but these general rules are said to commonly

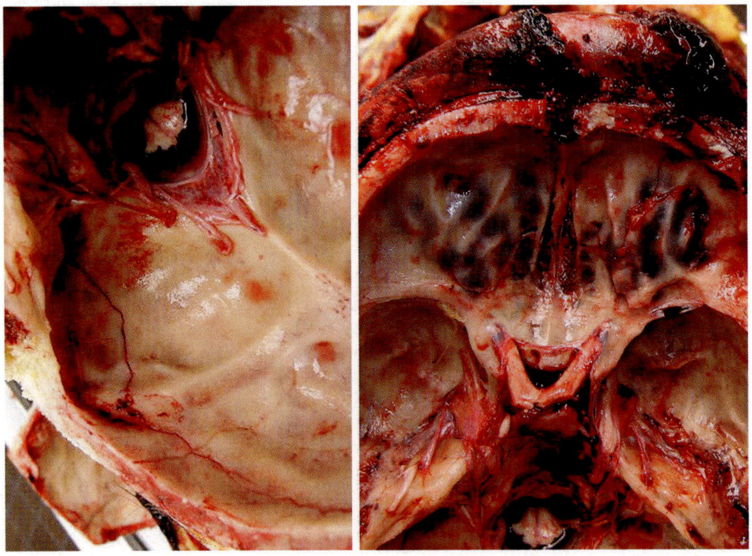

Figure 6.24 This composite photograph of the open cranium of an individual who fell backward, striking his occiput on pavement after an apparent punch to the central face during a brawl, illustrates a complex basilar skull fracture. On the right panel, many fracture lines criss-cross the orbital plates and apparently do not join with a jagged fracture of the posterior fossa on the left side as shown in the left panel. Here a fracture line passes from the floor of the posterior fossa forward to the petrous bone, crosses it, and appears to arc into the clivus. There was also a longitudinal fracture in the midline of the frontal bone that became diastatic at the vertex. An issue in this case was whether these fractures were the result of one event or two.

apply [35,72–74,99,100]. Experience has shown, however, that the intuitive interpretation of the mechanisms of basilar skull fractures is fraught with error. Harvey and Jones [101] reported the diversity of impact sites and character, all of which produced predominantly side-to-side (hinge) fractures of the skull base (see Figure 6.25), not infrequently with unconnected orbital fractures or sometimes separate fractures that often were diastatic to the sagittal suture. Some of these impacts were blows delivered by a fist to the apex of the mandible [100]. The knowledge of the biomechanics of basilar skull fractures is incomplete, owing to the complexities of these fractures and the difficulty in studying and modeling them.

The issue of contracoup fractures primarily of the orbital plates in association with basilar fractures has been the subject of controversy over the years regarding the mechanisms for this [102,103]. Suffice it to say that the thin bone of the orbital roof contributes to such fractures by either in–out forces or out–in forces that can occur with occipital impacts and the pressure waves of the contracoup phenomenon (discussed below). An example of an out–in orbital fracture is illustrated in Figure 6.26.

There are several major complications that can arise with basilar skull fractures. These include the following: laceration or trauma to cranial nerves in their foramina, damage to arteries or venous sinuses at the base with potential for both extracranial and intracranial fatal hemorrhage [104], opening a paranasal sinus with CSF leakage and risk of infection [105], laceration of pituitary stalk, fracture through inner ear structures, explosion or implosion of the orbital contents [102,103], and contusions of the inferior surface of the brain and cerebellum. Generally, the more forceful the impact and severe the injury, the

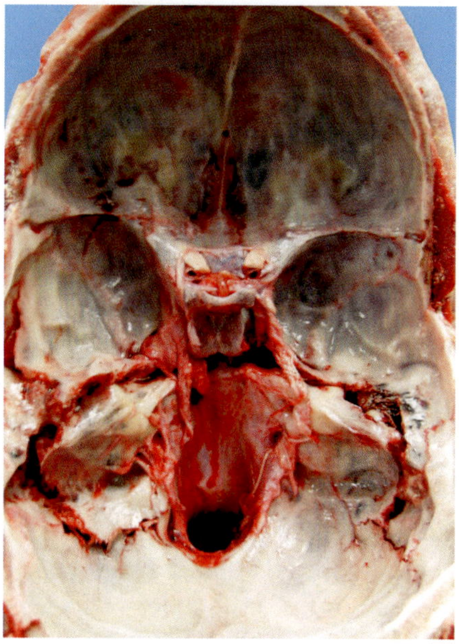

Figure 6.25 This photograph of the skull base from a victim of a beating in which he fell backward striking his head on pavement illustrates a so-called hinge basilar skull fracture. Note the fracture line passing across the clivus from side to side and arcing on the left side forward into the middle fossa and posterior on both sides into the posterior fossa.

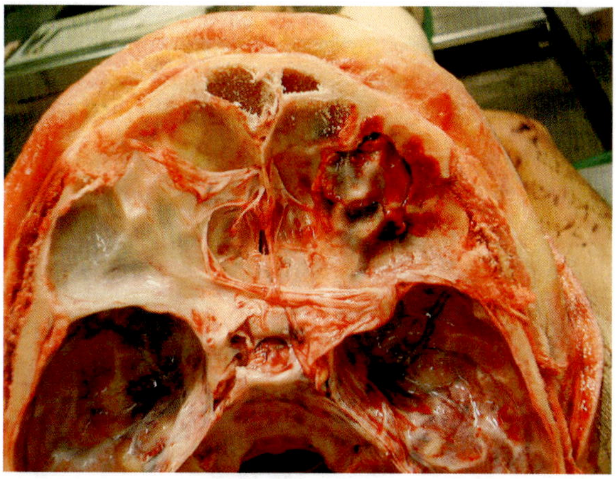

Figure 6.26 This photograph of the skull base of a man who had sustained a very forceful blow to the right eye in a fight and later died in a roll-over automobile accident (involving a high blood alcohol level) of neck injuries illustrates what is likely a "blow-out" fracture of the orbital roof from the blow. A small laceration of the orbital lobe was found, which was not considered to be the cause of death. (Courtesy of Dr. David Taylor, Rotorua, New Zealand.)

more of these complications are to be expected. Basilar skull fractures commonly produce raccoon eyes; bleeding from the ears, nose, or mouth; as well as CSF leaks from ears or nose.

With respect to the kinds of forces that are required to produce significant basilar skull fracture in man, it is very common to observe such fractures when an individual experiences an occipital fall against a hard surface, as on the ice in winter time; when falling down stairs and striking the head; or when falling backward, even a short distance, to a hard floor, as from a bar stool. Homicidal blows to the head with objects like baseball bats, iron pipes, bricks, and "two-by-four" routinely produce basilar fractures, as do impacts sustained in accidental and suicidal falls from heights. Pedestrian and vehicular accidents are also prominent etiologies for such fractures. In these latter instances, ring fractures of the posterior fossa and often associated pontomedullary avulsion injuries are seen [106–109].

Trauma that frequently leads to basilar skull fractures also causes epidural as well as subdural hematomas and almost always causes some degree of cerebral contusion and inner cerebral trauma (traumatic axonal injury—TAI) (discussed below). Therefore, basilar fracture is a much more significant lesion clinically and pathologically than a simple linear fracture of the convexity. Demonstration of these fractures at autopsy is best accomplished by stripping the basal dura away to expose the basal calvarium. When fractures are discovered, they should at the very least be described anatomically in the autopsy report, but they are better diagrammed or photographed so that at a later time their course and extent can be correlated with other information in the case. It is also appropriate to open the orbits, paranasal sinuses, and petrous bones to document injuries. Histological sampling for possible aging and dating processes is recommended.

Depressed Skull Fracture

One of the most serious forms of skull fracture is the depressed skull fracture, which can occur when pointed objects or objects that are massive and moving slowly impact the skull [35,110]. In such an instance, a circle or plate of calvarium may be punched out, or pushed into the intracranial space, and may not move outward again. Sometimes such fractures have a stellate appearance with several radiating fracture lines within the punched-out portion of bone. Typical situations producing depressed fractures are blows with very heavy objects, such as a baseball bat, brick, or hammer, or falls, such as a head-first plunge into shallow water in a swimming pool. The effect of such a fracture is often to deform the brain and deeper structures so as to lacerate the dura and sometimes the superior sagittal sinus, to produce subdural or epidural bleeding, lacerate or contuse the underlying brain, and most certainly exert pressure on underlying brain and decrease intracranial volume. The morbidity and mortality with such a fracture are much greater in the short term than almost any other type.

It may be possible to observe depressed skull fractures at autopsy, and, as expected, the affected area is caved in. However, more likely, some surgical procedure will have been performed to elevate the fracture, so that only the evidence of the procedure remains and the description of the fracture must be obtained from preoperative radiographs or medical records.

Comminuted and Multiple Fractures

Comminuted fractures may be relatively simple but are frequently multiple and are those in which shattering or fragmentation of the skull occurs and in which the fragments are separated and often override each other. Such fractures are produced in much the same manner as depressed skull fractures, by huge impacts (high momentum), usually of relatively low velocity [35]. The fractures usually occur at the site of impact but may show wide areas of fragmentation, often with fragments that do not rebound. This is commonly seen

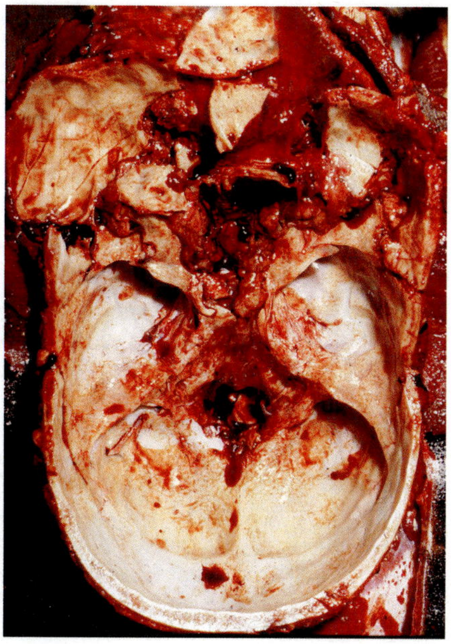

Figure 6.27 This photograph of the skull base in a victim of a violent beating with a hammer illustrates the degree of skull fragmentation that can occur from blows by heavy objects.

in repeated blows to the head with a weapon such as a hammer (illustrated in Figure 6.27), which not only shatters the skull but also results in an open cranial wound. Associated brain injuries are very common, and the morbidity and mortality rates of such fractures are high.

Another circumstance in which complex fractures of the skull occur is in static head injuries (static loading) with a nonmoving or stationary head. A typical circumstance is that of a prone or supine victim who may be beaten about the head with a weighted flashlight, pipe, heavy night stick, rock, fire extinguisher, or two-by-four, or stomped or otherwise, so that the head is crushed. Here the skull may be shattered or crushed with sometimes surprisingly little damage to the brain. Brain damage, if it occurs, can occur with in-driven fragments of the skull fracture or severe deformation of the brain by the impacting object once the skull has been broken. In these circumstances, there are often unconnected bilateral split-type fractures observed [111–113]. Crushing injury often involves the facial skeleton in addition to the skull, and severe injuries typically include CSF rhinorrhea or otorrhea, open cranial injury, and orbital or oral injury. Occasionally, a surprisingly mild injury may occur to the brain, especially in infants who may or may not display immediate neurological symptoms.

Diastatic Fracture

Diastatic fractures are those in which the fracture line involves separation of one or more cranial bone sutures. These fractures are most often seen in children and are commonly associated with epidural hematoma formation, laceration of the dura by the sharp edges of the fracture, and severe brain injury. They often occur as a result of large impacts to the head with blows, falls, or industrial accidents, or under circumstances where the individual, usually a child, is bodily swung against a wall or other immovable object by the legs, as in fatal child abuse or falls from height [114–116]. Sometimes fall-type impacts,

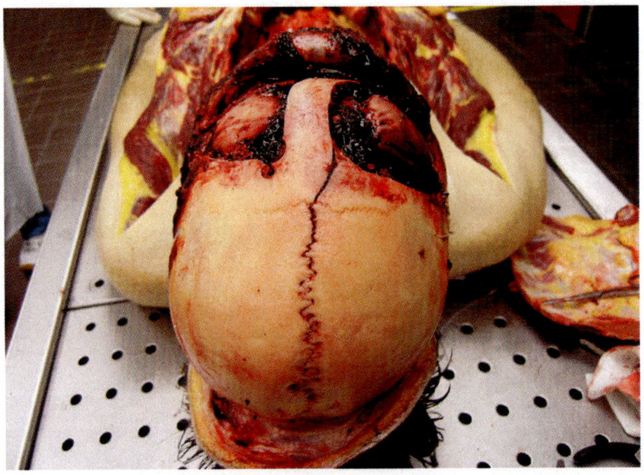

Figure 6.28 This photograph illustrates a frontal diastatic fracture in the individual also shown in Figure 6.24, who apparently sustained a blow from a fist to the right orbital region and then fell backward, striking his head on pavement and sustaining a complex basilar skull fracture. The two frontal openings are due to an attempted cranial decompression. Here the fracture line emanates from the right orbital rim and courses upward and backward along the sagittal suture. Diastatic fractures are more commonly seen in infants than adults. The forensic question in this case concerned whether the frontal fracture was caused by a fist blow or was part of the complex basilar skull fracture caused by the occipital impact site.

if they occur near sutures, will permit extension of a linear fracture into the suture and split it, especially if there is significantly raised intracranial pressure from edema or subdural hematoma. Instances of basilar skull fractures can have a diastatic component, as can other forms of fractures (see Figure 6.28).

Expressed Skull Fracture

These rather uncommon, usually massive fractures involve fragmentation or shattering of the skull in which pieces of the skull come to lie outside the normal curvature of the calvarium in the pericranial tissues, in the orbit or sinuses, or physically outside the head. Such horrible fractures usually result from massive head trauma, often involving missiles or blasts. Such injuries are not always fatal because of special circumstances in which the skull is crushed but the head was not accelerated, and thus significant kinetic energy was not transmitted or dissipated within the brain but rather was dissipated externally. However, in most cases, brain and other trauma are so severe that death results most likely from brainstem destruction [35].

Forensic Aspects of Skull Fractures

There are several relevant forensic issues involving fractures of the skull, few of which involve skull fractures in isolation, but most of which involve other aspects of head trauma. One of these issues involves fracture of the skull in children, discussed below and in Chapter 7, in which there is a question of child abuse as a cause for the skull fracture and other brain injuries that may be present. Another circumstance that sometimes arises is the issue of skull fractures that occur in connection with physical altercations or assaults. In these circumstances, it may become an issue of whether a punch with a fist produced a skull fracture or whether some other or a secondary impact may have been involved that may have caused a basilar fracture.

Infantile Skull Fractures

Considerable insight into infant skull fracture has resulted from several radiological and clinical studies on skull fractures in children and on the injuries that occur when children and infants fall accidentally [114,115,117]. These studies report that accidental drops and falls in infants and young children only occasionally produce skull fractures and then usually, but not exclusively, simple linear ones without any neurological complications or sequelae. When fractures of the skull in young children are more extensive or complex and involve brain injury (subdural, epidural, subarachnoid hemorrhage, or brain hemorrhage) and neurological symptoms and sequelae, many authors have expressed the opinion that these instances should be considered evidence of willful injury (child abuse) [116,118,119]. The problem with this assertion is that there is extensive literature in which simple, relatively short-distance falls have resulted in simple as well as complex skull fractures in infants, with and without a spectrum of injuries ranging from apparently occult cranial and brain injuries seen in imaging studies but not evident clinically, to fatal outcomes.

Many reports often cited to support the claim that short falls do not injure children [116,117,119] are based on incident reports and similar situations where abuse is unlikely and infants were accidentally dropped. In these studies, only occasional skull fractures were reported along with humerus and clavicular fractures and essentially no sequelae. These studies were reported in the pre–computerized tomography (CT) or magnetic resonance imaging (MRI) era; thus, it can never be known if there were occult but potentially significant cranial injuries, as Greenes and Schutzman [90] and Fickenscher et al. [91] reported. Further, except for the occasional skull fracture cases, it cannot be known how the infant impacted the floor; thus, it is inappropriate to infer that impacts to the head during short falls do not cause injury, because most of the children likely did not hit their heads. In other studies in which head-first fall impacts occurred, a very different picture of injury potential emerges. In these studies [90,120] a variety of short-fall scenarios on young infants produced skull fractures, subdural hematomas, and other injuries. These injuries were not always apparent immediately after their occurrence, but when symptoms appeared, they did so over many hours, days, or even weeks. In relation to skull fractures, among the most important reports are those by Weber [121–123]. Weber did a series of experiments employing horizontal drops on 50 infant cadavers, dropping them from about 32 in to a variety of flooring surfaces, padded and unpadded. These drops resulted in a 100% incidence of a variety of simple and complex skull fractures, with drops to hard flooring surfaces from newborns to age 8 months. Because the infants were dead, it was obviously impossible to assess any associated neural or meningeal injury. Regardless, the observation of the skull fractures is real. Perhaps it is worth noting that in young infants, most of the skull has not yet taken on the adult diploic form [70] and is quite thin compared with the skull of the adult. Weber [122] noted that most of the fractures occurred in bone that was 0.1–0.4 mm in thickness without a diploë.

The observations of Weber have been extended using unembalmed human heads from 1-, 3-, and 11-day-old infants by Prange and associates [124] and subjecting them to a number of quasi-static and dynamic compression tests and were dropped on to rigid surfaces from 15 and 30 cm so that impacts occurred at five different locations (vertex, occiput, forehead, right and left parietal regions) with instrumentation that recorded peak accelerations, stiffness of the heads in the different locations of impact, and other parameters of impact. The results were compared with comparable maneuvers employing the instrumented Child Restraint and Airbag Interactions (CRABI) 6-month-old dummy device. It is impressive that with a 15 cm drop height (about 6 in), peak accelerations to the center of mass of the head ranged between about 25g and 65g, with the vertex drop having the highest acceleration and the forehead drop having the lowest. For the 30 cm drop (about 1 ft), accelerations ranged from about 40g to nearly 120g, with the same variations in acceleration by impact site as with the 15 cm drop. Comparisons with the CRABI-6 dummy drops showed the dummy experienced somewhat greater accelerations than did the human heads for lateral head impacts. These data indicate that even in what most would regard as very short falls, the potential for serious injury exists in infants.

An important parameter that distinguishes infant head impacts from those of adults is that the infant head experiences much more compression and deformation at impact than the adult, which will affect how forces affect the impact response. A number of analyses of these differences have resulted in scaling methods [124,125] that permit comparisons between adult head and infant head impact responses.

Most recently, Lloyd [86], in his doctoral thesis at Duke University Department of Biomedical Engineering, studied the heads of 14 infants, 8 adults, and 6 dummy heads under various impact and other biomechanical experimental conditions and reviewed what is known about impact parameters for the human head. This study, much too detailed to be specifically discussed here, provides a great deal of information about the infant head not available before and clearly shows that sufficient information is known to rebut the common assertion that "nothing" is known about infant head impacts.

It should be stated again that clearly more information on the biomechanical parameters is desirable, but the gaps in knowledge are gradually being filled in [52,54,62,63,70,86,125].

Skull Fractures from Blows

Skull fractures often occur from blows with wielded objects such as clubs, stones, bricks, and baseball bats but can occur from blows with a fist unaided by any object. When some additional object besides a clenched fist is employed in an altercation, skin lacerations often result that reflect the surface characteristics of the object. Such candidate objects may include rings or jewelry that may leave a characteristic and correlatable pattern of injury. Lacerations can also occur with a fist blow without any additional object, but these tend to be tearing-type lacerations rather than sharp-edged ones, and often only a bruise occurs. Biomechanical analysis of punches has been undertaken, usually employing professional boxers and volunteers. Atha et al. [126] studied a series of punches by a professional fighter as he punched a padded target mass suspended as a pendulum. Within 100 ms of the start of a punch, the fist had traversed 0.49 m and had attained a velocity of 8.9 m/s. The peak force upon impact (after 14 ms of contact) was 4096 N (0.4 ton), which the authors calculated to represent a blow to a human head of 6320 N (0.63 ton) with an acceleration of 53g. This was judged equivalent to a blow delivered by a padded wooden mallet with a mass of 6 kg swung at 20 mph. Another study by Whiting et al. [127] examined the kinematics of punches by four professional boxers and found that average contact velocities ranged from 5.9 to 8.2 m/s, with peak velocities of 6.6–12.5 m/s within 8–21 ms before contact with the test surface. These authors noted few significant differences in these figures, whether a gloved or naked fist was employed. Viano et al. [100] performed similar studies using Olympic boxers of different weights who threw punches at a Hybrid

III dummy. The resultant impacts were studied using high-speed video recording and instrumentation of the dummy. They found that a sweeping punch (hook) produced the greatest change in fist velocity (11.0 ± 3.4 m/s and force of 4405 ± 2318 N to the head and a loading of the neck of 855 ± 537 N, which resulted in accelerations of 71.1 ± 32.2*g* or 9306 ± 4485 rad/s). Several other studies have yielded similar results [128]. The forces attained by punches are well within the failure parameters of human skulls, which in the frontal region for adults have been reported to be between 1000 and about 1400 lb (4448 and 6200 N) [33].

Contracoup Fractures

The concept of so-called contracoup fracture is a controversial one in the literature and has been so for many years, but it appears to be a bona fide phenomenon [102,103]. Fractures that are generally accepted as contracoup are mostly seen in the orbital portions of the frontal bones as simple linear fractures or more complex, even stellate, fractures [129,130]. Bilateral orbital contrecoup fractures are uncommon but not rare and exist as separate, nonjoined fractures. These fractures presumably arise out of pressure differentials between the intracranial orbital surface and the intraorbital space during conditions that would be expected to produce typical contrecoup contusions of the frontal lobes, as in occipital falls or heavy blows or in gunshot wounds. In these circumstances, discussed below, negative pressure (suction forces) within the frontal region, because of differential movements of brain versus skull with occipital impacts, causes implosion of the relatively thin and weak orbital roof. It is unlikely that sufficient forces can exist in other areas of the skull to allow implosion fractures in the event of head injury, but pathological conditions and certain very special circumstances may permit contrecoup fractures to occur elsewhere.

Under rare circumstances, the base of the skull may become fractured by blows to the mandible. In such circumstances, the mandibular condyles may rupture upward through the temporal–mandibular joint and be driven into the middle cranial fossa and produce brain injury. Such impacts can also produce extensive basilar skull fractures and all the complications that can occur with them [101].

Meninges

Anatomy

Classically, the meninges are composed of the dura (pachymenix), the arachnoid, and the pia (leptomeninges). The meninges invest the brain and spinal cord and provide a complex and vital interface between the cranial cavity and spinal canal and the brain and spinal cord. The dura is sometimes thought of as melding with or joining a thin, translucent membrane called the arachnoid. Despite confusion of this relationship, the dura and arachnoid are one membrane normally that some have divided into two or three layers (see Figures 6.29 and 6.30). At the junction with the skull, the dura acts as a periosteum and is able to generate collagen, osteoid, and bone. The dura, on the whole, is relatively tough, having the appearance of thick parchment, and contains abundant collagen that interlaces extensively in its outer layers that lie close to the skull [131,132]. The character of the dura changes about halfway through its thickness, with somewhat less collagen and different intercellular specializations between the fibroblastic and other cells [132]. The

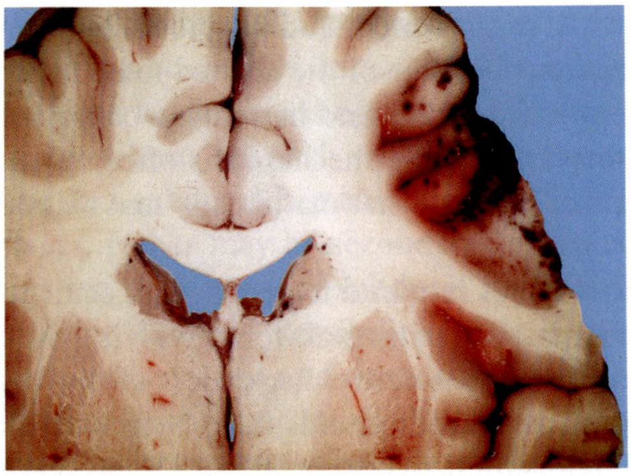

Figure 6.39 This photograph is of a coronal section of the brain of an individual that died of an acute subdural hematoma on the right side that has fallen away, revealing underlying hemorrhagic infarction in the cortex. This lesion was not due to traumatic contusion but rather to a pressure effect on cortical vessels of the overlying subdural hematoma.

shift of the brain, such as uncal grooving, tonsillar herniation, herniation of the cingulate gyrus on the side of the hematoma beneath the falx to the opposite side, and herniation of the orbital lobe into the middle fossa or portions of the temporal lobe into the frontal fossa. In case of a posterior fossa subdural hematoma [166], there may be tonsillar as well as upward transtentorial herniation of the cerebellum with brain stem distortion. If herniation has been extreme, usually associated with surgical extraction, branches of the posterior cerebral artery on the side of the hematoma may have been compressed against the edge of the tentorium. The capillaries served by these vessels, damaged by low or absent blood flow, may bleed when pressure is released and blood flow reestablished, causing a hemorrhagic infarction in the inferior temporal and medial posterior occipital lobes or other locations (herniation infarction). Hemorrhagic infarction of the medial occipital lobe, including area 17, the visual cortex, may occur (see Chapter 5). Furthermore, the rapid unilateral herniation caused by an acute subdural hematoma may produce a secondary Duret hemorrhage in the midline or tegmentum of the pons or midbrain (see Chapters 3 and 5).

The maximal complication of acute subdural hemorrhage includes all of the above but also includes development of the respirator brain as a consequence of raising the intracranial pressure to a point beyond which adequate cerebral perfusion could occur [194] (see Chapter 5). Other traumatic lesions may also be present in the brain, including various types of contusions and intracerebral and intraventricular hemorrhages. The characteristics and pathogenesis of these lesions are discussed individually below.

Forensic Issues

Many of the aspects of subdural hemorrhages from the forensic point of view center about interpretations about the age and speed of evolution of the lesion(s), the kinds of trauma (force, direction, circumstances) that could have produced them, the causal relationship to the death, the relation to symptoms described or observed, and the utility or ability to diagnose and treat the lesion by clinicians. Clearly, these issues involve determination of not only the cause but also the manner of death as well as implications to possible criminal or civil legal actions in relation to the case. It thus behooves the pathologist or neuropathologist to carefully document at autopsy, by description, sketch, or photograph, the lesions seen, the volume of the hematoma, and the relationship to other lesions (internal and external). Histological sampling of several portions of the subdural hematoma and any other visible lesions of the dura is essential in providing the best possible forensic information.

It is often reported in operative notes that a given subdural hematoma was acute. Such observations are based on visual inspection by an operating surgeon who, in all likelihood, has little or no interest in the nuances of aging a subdural hematoma. Most hospitals require that any tissue removed at surgery be submitted to a pathologist for examination. It is to be desired that all such specimens be examined histologically, because within apparently acute clots older reactive processes may be present that have vital importance forensically but little importance medically. The forensic pathologist or neuropathologist, when evaluating a case in which aging and dating of a subdural hematoma is an issue, when there has been a surgical procedure requests not only the pathology report but also the microscopic slides of the specimen. A relatively uncommon situation may occur in which a chemical analysis of the subdural clot may be undertaken to determine blood alcohol and drug levels and their relation to the inciting events or circumstances. A number of studies have been made of these types of determinations, and many have concluded that valuable forensic evidence may be obtainable by these means [195–197].

Subacute Subdural Hematoma

Subdural hematomas that have remained undetected or unoperated on for at least 3 days to as many as 14 days after inception are usually arbitrarily referred to as subacute subdural hemorrhages. Some authors may narrow or extend these time limits or may further subdivide subdural hematomas into acute, early subacute, subacute, late subacute, and chronic varieties [179,198] based on clinical parameters. Nevertheless, from a pathological standpoint, every subdural hemorrhage would appear to have been acute in the beginning and may or may not evolve or be allowed to evolve through the succeeding clinically significant steps. Regardless of the subdivisions of the middle group of hematomas, they are clearly able to persist this long because of the ability of the victim to tolerate them or because of their inherently more slowly evolving mass effect by whatever mechanism [182]. This more benign character is reflected in the mortality rate of this group of lesions, about 22%, as compared with a 60% or greater mortality rate in acute lesions [179].

Subacute hematomas present their own set of challenges and risks to the patient compared with acute hematomas, one of which is the increased risk of misdiagnosis and failure to treat them. This may be due to the less striking onset of symptoms, which may be rather nonspecific, and their lesser tendency to be associated with severe head trauma, especially in older individuals. The fundamental pathophysiological issue is the rate of accumulation of the hematoma, the ability of the brain to compensate for its increasing mass effect, and the coexistence of other lesions, which can modify this compensatory mechanism. These would include the extent and severity of cortical and deep brain trauma and how much edema may be developing in these lesions in a delayed fashion. The degree of systemic trauma and the cardiovascular status of the patient may also intervene at some point (e.g., cerebral ischemia due to blood loss) to produce cerebral edema and magnify the mass effect of the hematoma. Nevertheless, at some critical point, the mass effect of the hematoma may reach a level at which decompensation occurs and intracranial pressure rise leads to herniation, brain stem compression, or cerebral circulatory embarrassment, with fatal or long-lasting effect on brain function, as discussed in Chapter 5.

Pathology of Subacute Subdural Hematoma

The pathological appearance of subacute subdural hematomas depends on the age of the hematoma and on other factors, which include other conditions that may be present, such as bleeding tendencies, other blood dyscrasias, the presence of infection and the nature of the inflammatory response in the individual, and other environmental factors [199]. Clot liquefaction occurs as a result of the normal process of fibrinolysis and repair mediated by enzymatic activity within the clot due to both intrinsic and extrinsic factors [200–202]. Red blood cells begin to fade, lyse, and leak their contents into the clot, and macrophages and fibroblasts begin to migrate into the clot to engulf and digest the products of degeneration [203]. At this point, the clot has begun to lose its dark red or black appearance and begins to take on a more brownish color, with more degenerated portions showing a tan, orange, or even yellow appearance due to the metabolism of blood pigments. Hemosiderin-laden macrophages become more and more prominent at the edges of the clot initially, then all through it, until by 14–21 days after inception the clot is completely liquefied but not necessarily replaced by straw-colored or clear fluid. The histology of the aging subdural

Table 6.2 Verbal Data on Histological Aging of Subdural Hematomas of Known Age in Surgical Specimens from 105 Adult Patients

Interval	Clot	Dural Side	Arachnoid Side
24 hours	Intact RBCs	Thin layer fibrin	Thin layer fibrin
36 hours	Intact RBCs	Early fibroblastic activity	Thin layer fibrin
4 days	Loss of RBC sharp contour and variability of staining	2–4 layers of fibroblasts	Thin layer fibrin
5 days	Loss of RBC sharp contour and variability of staining	3–5 layers of fibroblasts. First siderophages appear at edges	Thin layer fibrin
7–8 days	Laked RBCs, clot liquefies, fibroblasts enter clot	12–14 layers of fibroblasts; neomembrane visible grossly when clot scraped away	Thin layer fibrin
11 days	Broken up into islands by capillaries and fibroblasts and thick strands of fibrin	Fibroblasts migrate around the edges of the clot	Siderophages are visible on arachnoid side
15–17 days	Most original RBCs lysed. Capillary formation obvious	Membrane 1/3 to 1/2 dural thickness	Variably thin, earliest complete neomembrane. Clot may be completely enveloped
18–26 days	Clot completely liquefied. Larger vessels permeate	Membrane same thickness as dura. Siderophages in membranes	Membrane up to dural thickness. Siderophages in membranes
27–36 days	Large capillaries	Well-formed membrane	Well-formed membrane
1–3 months	Giant capillaries secondary bleeding and fresh RBCs	Hyalinization of membranes, less cellular, more collagen	Hyalinization of membranes, less cellular, more collagen. Nearly thickness of dura
3–6 months	No original RBCs and only focal rebleeding	Hyalinized neomembrane	Hyalinized neomembrane
>1 year	No RBCs	Resembles dura	Resembles dura

Source: Data from Munro D, Merritt HH, *Arch Neurol Psychiatr* 35, 64–78, 1936.

Note: This schema, in one form or another, has been relied upon by pathologists for many years.

hematomas can best be analyzed according to the scheme of Munro and Merritt [204], as depicted in Table 6.2 [205].

The microscopic appearances of subdural hematomas of differing ages are shown in Figures 6.40 through 6.48. As is clear from these figures and from the material from many forensic services that involve infants and children, it is not at all uncommon to find with a

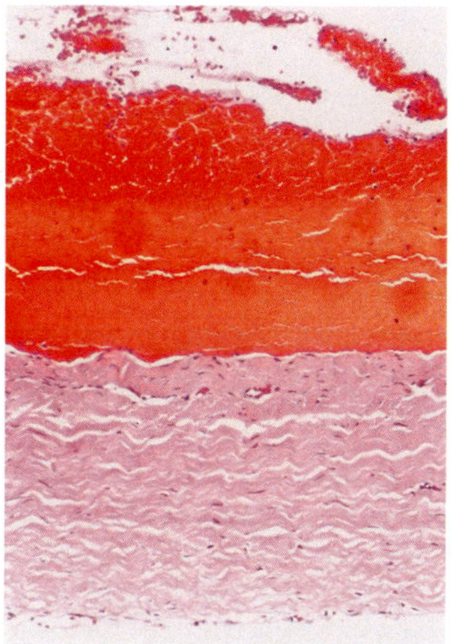

Figure 6.40 This is a lower-power photomicrograph of an H&E-stained section of dura with attached acute subdural hematoma in a child. The child died within 24 hours of having suffered a major cranial impact that was probably inflicted. Note the preservation of erythrocytes in the clot, little or no cellular reaction in the clot, and no reaction or fibrin deposition at the dura–clot interface.

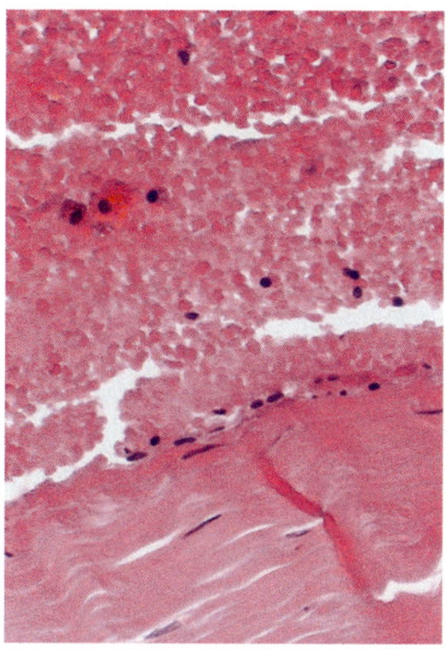

Figure 6.41 This is a higher-power photomicrograph of an H&E-stained subdural hematoma in a child who died about 5 days after an apparent fall, but the parent was accused of abusing the child. Note the variable staining characteristics of the erythrocytes in the clot and the development of macrophages that are phagocytosing red cells and some appear to have processed the hemoglobin into hemosiderin. At the interface between the clot and dura, there is only a minimal reaction in flat cells, which are probably fibroblasts, and some fibrin deposition. Elsewhere these changes are more evident but still early.

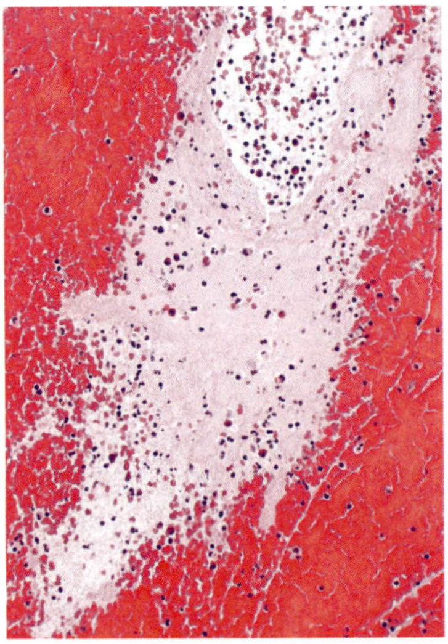

Figure 6.42 This medium-power H&E-stained photomicrograph of the central portion of a subdural hematoma, not including the dura, reveals islands of fibrin and lymphoid cells separating the clot that appears mostly composed of intact and fully staining red cells. Some macrophages contain pigment. Enmeshed in the mass of fibrin are erythrocytes that have a faded, lavender color. In other sections not shown, a neomembrane appears to be 5–7 days old (Table 6.2). This clot clearly represents recent clot (0–2–3 days old) mixed with an older clot in the process of aging.

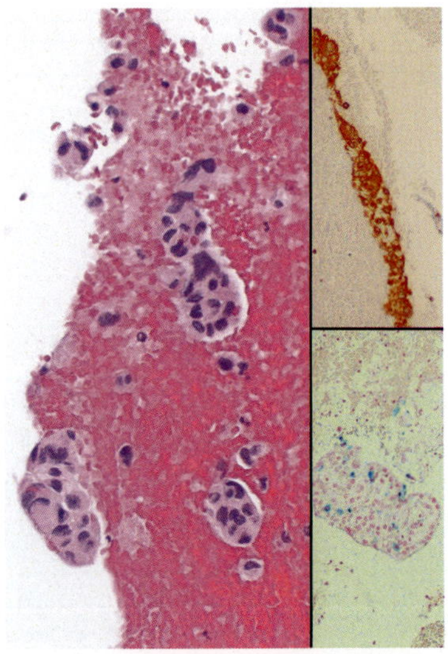

Figure 6.43 This high-power photomicrograph (left panel) of a portion of a subdural hematoma clot removed at surgery from an apparent victim of child abuse illustrates clumps of proliferated arachnoid cells enmeshed in a clot that has preserved but also variably stained erythrocytes. The neurosurgeon had reported no neomembrane and the clot to be "acute" but sent it for pathological examination. The CT scan had suggested a "mixed density" subdural hematoma. The appearance of erythrocytes and the appearance of reacting arachnoidal cells clearly indicate this hematoma is recent, not acute in the strict sense of the word, and possibly 3–5 days or more old. In the upper right panel is a vimentin immunostain that labels these cells as being of arachnoidal origin. In the right lower panel is an iron stain that illustrates that at least some of the cells have taken up iron. A CD-68 stain (not shown) shows a few cells within the arachnoid cell clumps are positive. It is not known if arachnoid cells possess phagocytic properties.

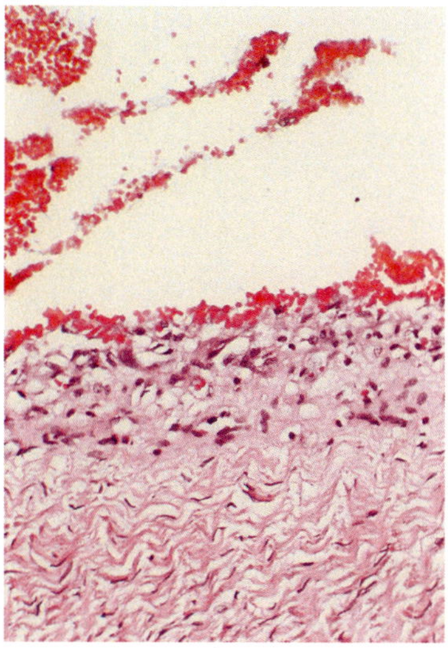

Figure 6.44 This higher-power photomicrograph of an H&E-stained section of a subdural hematoma includes a portion of the dura. This hematoma was from a 14-month-old child. There is an inexact history of the child having fallen about a week before, and possibly other times before the child decompensated and was hospitalized. A caregiver was charged with child abuse. Autopsy revealed a subdural hematoma adherent to the dura and thought to be acute. Microscopic examination, however, revealed a developing neomembrane of about 10 layers of cells and some small capillaries. A few pigmented cells were noted. It is estimated that this neomembrane was about 7 days old.

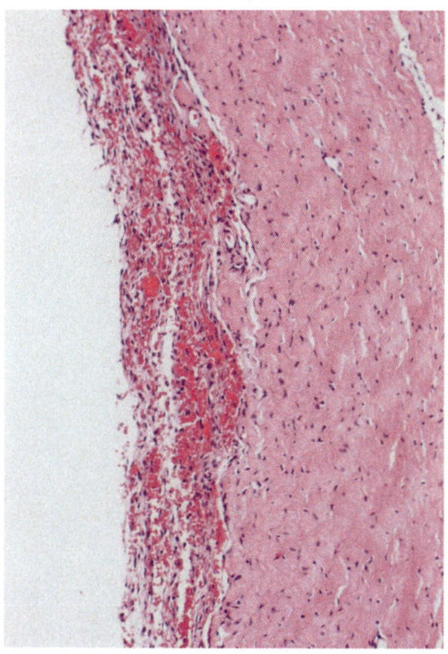

Figure 6.45 This medium-power photomicrograph of an H&E-stained section of a subdural hematoma attached to the dura from a 2-year-old child that was thought to have been the victim of abuse. The membrane is composed of about 15 or more layers of reactive cells and capillaries that are evident at the dural interface. Collagen is clearly being laid down and there is also recent hemorrhage within the membrane composed of intact erythrocytes. Other portions of the clot have fallen away during sampling or processing. It is estimated that this membrane is about 10 days old.

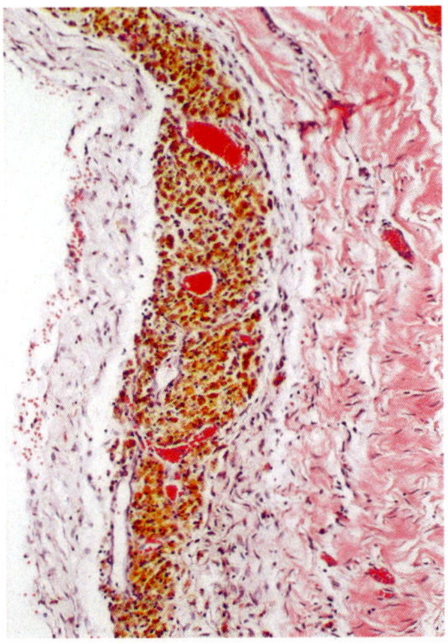

Figure 6.46 This photomicrograph is of an H&E-stained section from a subdural hematoma in a young child. There had been a more acute clot on the surface that was carried away. The circumstances in this case were unclear, and one of the caregivers was charged with child abuse. This hematoma membrane is complex, possibly being composed of two layers separated by a dense band of hemosiderin and hematoidin-containing macrophages. Well-developed capillaries are noted and in some places the thickness of this membrane is well over one-half of thickness of the dura. It is difficult to estimate the age of this hematoma but it appears that the oldest components are "weeks" old or older.

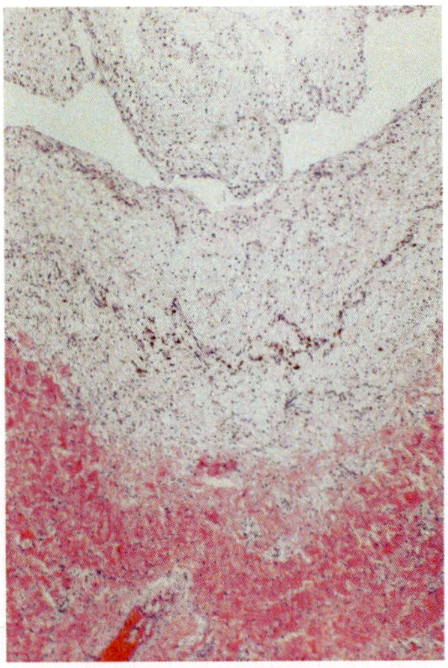

Figure 6.47 This lower-power photomicrograph is of an H&E-stained section of a chronic subdural hematoma in a 3 1/2-month-old child that had an active medical history that included difficult birth and prematurity, numerous physicians' visits before experiencing an acute decompensation (ALTE), and was essentially dead on admission to hospital. Thick subdural hematoma membranes, some with recent bleeding on them, were discovered. Here the neomembrane is nearly as thick as the dura, and composed of several lamellae each having siderophages and a capillary network. There is extensive delicate collagen within all the membranes. It is likely that this hematoma emanated from birth and may have had several episodes of bleeding. With hematomas this old, it is exceedingly difficult to precisely age them histologically. It may be best to regard these lesions simply as "old" chronic subdural hematomas.

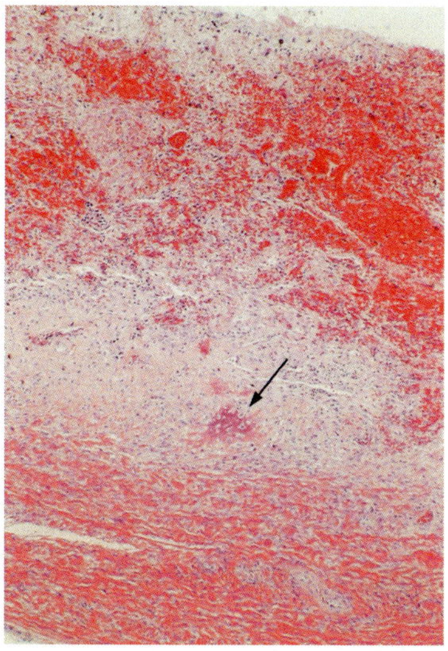

Figure 6.48 This photomicrograph illustrates a chronic subdural hematoma in an infant with a thick neomembrane that contains recent hemorrhage as well as a focus bone formation (arrow) and collagen.

subdural hematoma blood and reactions of several ages, reflecting the possible continued addition of new blood to the clot by periodic repeat bleeding. This bleeding need not imply repeated trauma but is an inherent part of the character of this lesion [206]. The transition from subacute hematoma to chronic hematoma is subtle but is generally conceded to coincide with the development of cellular organization of the clot by formation of a neomembrane that surrounds it. Radiologically, the hematoma is usually of mixed density at this point.

Chronic Subdural Hematoma

Chronic subdural hematoma is a somewhat broadly defined, commonly encountered, clinically and pathologically important group of subdural hemorrhages of at least 2 weeks of age. They blur pathologically and clinically with subacute subdural hematomas of older age but, from a pathological standpoint, form a distinct phase when a cellular organizing membrane, however tenuous, has formed over the undersurface of the hematoma (Figures 6.48 and 6.49). There are many controversial aspects to subdural hematomas, including their etiology, clinical diagnosis, and pathogenesis, which will be discussed below.

Pathogenesis and Pathology

In some series, up to half of all chronic subdural hematomas do not have a clear-cut traumatic historical etiology, at least in older individuals in whom the majority of such lesions occur. The reason for this age disparity, and for other aspects of the chronic lesion, is probably the increasing subarachnoid space that occurs with diminution of brain size after age 55. This increased CSF space and corresponding decrease in brain size allow greater movement of the brain inside the cranial vault, even with incidental accelerations. In addition, the bridging veins leaving the cortical surface to enter the venous sinuses are longer and likely to be under strain, as well as weaker in the elderly, and thus more susceptible to tearing. Another factor is that with an increased CSF space in the cranium, there is more potential space that can be occupied by a space-taking hematoma before symptoms appear. Aronson and Okazaki [207] computed threshold volumes for hematomas at various ages and noted that with the average expected loss of brain weight (and volume) of about 5% in individuals between 55 and 75 years, an additional potential space of about 65 ml may exist. This space may be utilized by an enlarging subdural hematoma by gradually driving out CSF by pressure-induced reabsorption and may thus forestall the development of symptoms [180].

The origin of subdural hematoma neomembranes has been studied for many years [203] and appears to be a product of proliferation of boundary layer cells at the upper boundary of the hematoma within the dura and not to a significant degree from the lower surface of the boundary layer. Perhaps more important is what influences how neomembranes form [208]. Animal models of chronic subdural hematomas have considerable limitations to this understanding, owing in no small part to the difficulty in producing them. It is possible to produce truly chronic enlarging subdural hematomas experimentally in animals by injecting blood only into the subdural compartment, however [182]. In these and other experiments, hematomas produced all resolved and were reabsorbed, eventually failing to produce a typical chronic lesion [209]. In 1972, Watanabe and coworkers [210] were able to report a model that seemed to overcome these difficulties by mixing blood with CSF. They found that when freshly collected, canine whole venous blood and human or canine CSF were mixed (in ratios from 20:1 to 5:1) and held at 37°C in test tubes, a clot was formed that seemed to possess a surface membrane composed of a dense fibrin mat. Other experimental models have also been studied [211].

As mentioned above, one of the most distinctive features of chronic subdural hematomas (Figures 6.40 through 6.47) is the formation of an organizing membrane over their surfaces and the process of potential enlargement of the hematoma with time. In most adults, the formation of completely enveloping neomembranes about the hematoma requires between 15 and 21 days to accomplish, probably depending on several variables, including the size of the original clot, possibly the age of the victim, and underlying disease states. In infants and children, less time may be required, although a systematic study in this age group has not been accomplished.

Why subacute–chronic subdural hematomas enlarge has been the subject of much speculation and experimentation over the years [212]. Gardner and others proposed that the liquefying blood within a dural clot was hyperosmolar and thus drew in water to make it enlarge [182]. Weir and Gordon [201] showed that this hypothesis was not tenable and, with others [200], postulated that capillary rebleeding and fibrinolytic factors in the neomembrane wall caused incremental bleeding, adding to the volume of the clot [213], an interesting and compelling study. Another impressive study was accomplished by Ito et al. [214] who injected radioactive chromium-labeled red blood cells from the patients' own blood, back into patients with known chronic subdural hematomas who were about to undergo surgery for their removal. These workers found that during the period of time that elapsed between injection and removal of the hematoma, with analysis of the fluid within 6–14 hours, radiolabeled blood was demonstrated within the hematoma, indicating an active and ongoing hemorrhage into the clot. Thus, the best evidence to date suggests that the probable mechanism behind the formation of chronic subdural hematomas is persistent bleeding from capillary vessels in the neomembrane. This bleeding may be incremental but occasionally may occur rapidly for unknown reasons or related to coagulopathy to produce catastrophic decompensation that may lead to death, apparently without any significant new traumatic event [206]. How frequently this occurs is not known because few studies have concentrated on this issue and controlled for the many variables in these cases.

There is a group of expanding, chronic subdural lesions referred to as subdural hygromas that would support the nontraumatic etiology of at least some of these lesions. Hygromas, usually seen in infants and children, are rather enigmatic lesions that have all the features of a chronic subdural hematoma, except that trauma may not have been recorded and the amount of blood in the lesion may be minimal. Such hygromas can develop as a complication of meningitis, hydrocephalus with or without shunting intervention, or minimal or significant head trauma with or without skull fracture in children or adults [215–218], or may occur spontaneously. They may expand to cause symptoms or may be discovered incidentally in a manner that is very similar or identical to that of subdural hematomas. The etiology of these hematoma-like expanding lesions that possess neomembranes is presumably due to some injury, by inflammation, trauma, or unknown causes, to the boundary zone between the dura and arachnoid. The dural border cells begin proliferating, and capillaries join the process but, because of their fragility, leak blood or plasma into the space created, which creates a vicious cycle.

The implications of the pathogenesis of both subdural hygroma and chronic subdural hematoma for treatment are that to perform a large craniotomy with resection of the neomembranes may cause the process to recur, whereas if the hematoma–hygroma cavity is opened, drained, and irrigated until the effluent fluid is clear, this may allow collapse of the cavity with apposition of the membrane surfaces and their subsequent healing with cessation of the process. Sometimes the cavity is shunted with success. These approaches seem to be effective and now form the treatment of choice for these lesions.

As previously mentioned, a clear-cut history of head trauma is obtained in cases of chronic subdural hematoma in only about 50% of cases of all age groups. Where it is obtained, the trauma may not be major but might include a simple bump on the head or a minor fall (on the ice in winter, missing a chair, and falling to the floor without head impact). Sometimes the history obtained includes an episode of sneezing, coughing (in connection with a cold or bronchitis), constipation (straining at stool), or vomiting or retching where some Valsalva-like action occurred in an elderly person [219]. The symptoms observed once a subdural hematoma has begun under these circumstances (usually in the elderly) are often vague. There may be headache associated with ill-defined loss of function in an aged person, such as slowing of intellect, loss of memory, development of personality changes, lethargy or apathy, loss of concentration and attention span, confusion, failure or blurring of vision, loss of hearing, weakness, stumbling or loss of coordination, or a host of other symptoms that might be passed off as signs of old age or a mild stroke. The important features of these symptoms are that they have evolved over a relatively short period of time (weeks or months) and that they increase in severity over the long run but may show fluctuation from day to day. In cases in which an episode of head trauma is taken as the starting point, the development of symptoms has often been shown to occur 5–6 weeks later, making causal connections in many cases difficult [181,182,198]. Although chronic subdural hematomas may persist and be discovered after having been present for months or even years, most are diagnosed by some means within 3 or 4 months of inception.

Early chronic subdural hematomas, as previously defined, are those that possess a recognizable neomembrane over their entire surface and are usually between 2 and 3 weeks of age (Table 6.2). In the autopsy specimen, such hematomas range in size from only a few millimeters thick and a few square centimeters in area to a centimeter or more in thickness and an area that covers the entire lateral dural surface (Figures 6.49 and 6.50). They may be homogeneous, tan-brown, or variable with dark brown areas, depending on the extent of recent bleeding. The inner (arachnoidal) side of the hematoma should be covered with a thin, glistening membrane that is delicate and can be scraped away easily with a knife tip but nevertheless prevents the clot from falling away. On cut section, the hematoma will be completely or partially liquefied, containing a grumous liquid that may have the appearance of motor oil. The microscopic appearances of early membranes are described below.

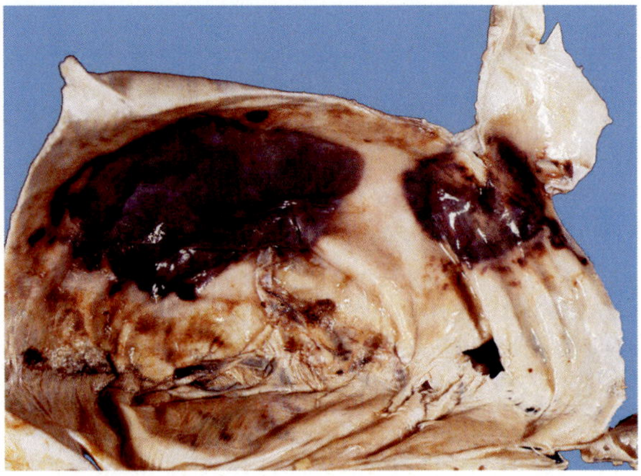

Figure 6.49 This photograph illustrates a typical chronic subdural hematoma, in this case from an adult. There appear to be two separate hematomas enclosed by a thin, translucent neomembrane but there is actually a neomembrane between the two lesions that may have separated them. Like most chronic subdural hematomas, recent blood is evident within the cavities. The origin of this bleeding is probably spontaneous, arising from capillaries in the neomembrane (see text). It was estimated that this hematoma was a month or more old.

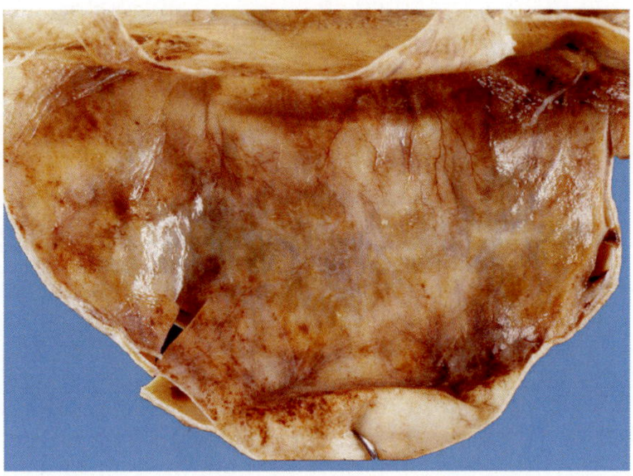

Figure 6.50 This photograph of an old chronic subdural hematoma in an elderly man reveals mostly a flat thick pigmented patch on the hemidura. It is likely that a few small fluid-filled cavities remained but were opened in taking the specimen. Bleeding is minimal. Such a hematoma may be many months or even years old.

Older, more well-developed chronic subdural hematomas will have a gross appearance that resembles a pancake or rubber sac containing a bluish or brownish liquid (Figure 6.51). The neomembranes will be opalescent or completely opaque, depending on their age, owing to the deposition of collagen. Hematomas of this age may be single, multiple, or multiloculated, each with its own character (Figure 6.52). The contents of the sac may range from

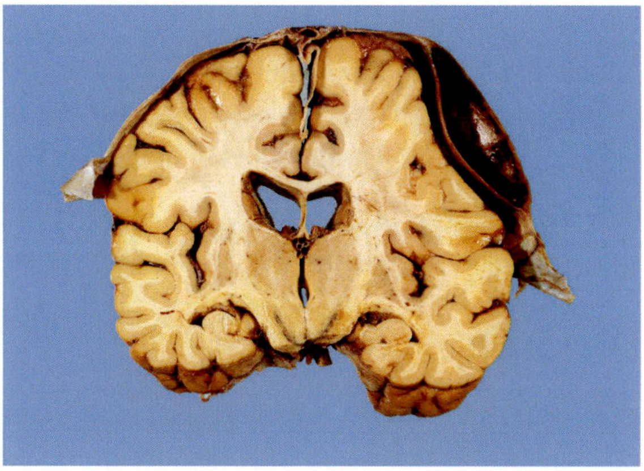

Figure 6.51 This photograph of a coronal section of brain and dura shows a chronic subdural hematoma with blood within the cavity. Note that the hematoma has effaced the right hemisphere and has produced some midline shift. Such lesions are commonly found at autopsy in elderly individuals who have been dwindling functionally before death. Often a traumatic history is elusive or nonexistent.

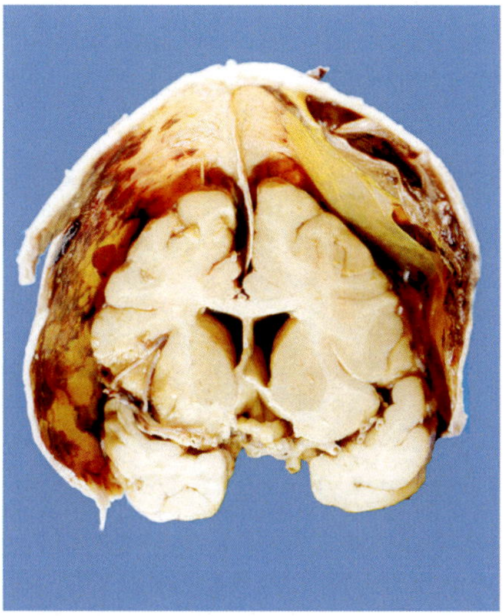

Figure 6.52 This photograph of a coronal brain section with cerebral dura intact illustrates the truly enormous dimensions that chronic subdural hematomas may reach on occasion in a minimally symptomatic individual. This individual was a 65-year-old man found unresponsive on his driveway in the morning. He had a history of alcohol abuse for many years. He appeared to have fallen while intoxicated. He had complained of headaches recently, apparently had seen a physician, and was being medicated for hypertension. (Courtesy Dr. Edmund Donoghue, Office of the Medical Examiner, Cook County, IL.)

bloody brown fluid to nearly clear, straw-colored fluid. The gross pathological appearance of the brain that underlies a chronic subdural hematoma may show discoloration and thickening of the arachnoid and adhesion of the arachnoid to the underlying cortex, usually with associated old cortical contusion or softening. Such an area will usually be tan, orange, or yellow in color [220], even many years after the hematoma has been resolved one way or another. At times, careful examination of the exposed surface of the arachnoid under the hematoma will reveal a scarred cord, which may have been the scarred vessel from which the hemorrhage originated. From time to time, one will encounter what appears to be a completely resolved, plaque-like, old subdural hematoma, shown in Figure 6.53.

The appearance of the brain is often striking with respect to the indentation and deformation that is caused by a chronic hematoma. Figure 6.54 illustrates this phenomenon.

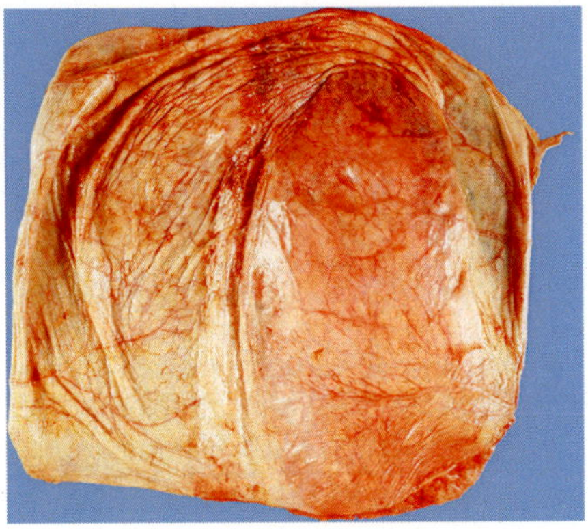

Figure 6.53 This photograph shows the vertex cerebral dura with an ovoid very old, apparently resolved, subdural hematoma found incidentally in the case of an elderly man found dead at home. Such lesions may occasionally contain bone (as is illustrated in another case in Figure 6.48). The age of the lesion is not known. (Courtesy of Dr. Mitra Kalelkar, Office of the Medical Examiner, Cook County, IL.)

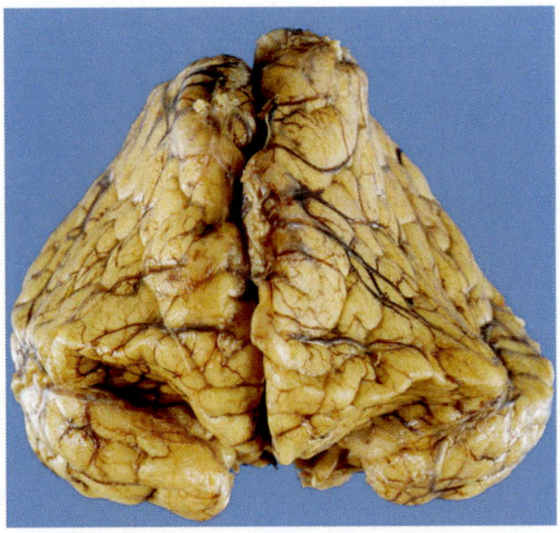

Figure 6.54 This photograph of the frontal aspect of the brain illustrates the effect on the brain of bilateral chronic subdural hematomas. In this case, the victim was an elderly man who was a nursing home resident in a demented state and was found dead in his bed. The dementia has evolved over a 6-month period after an unconfirmed report that the man had fallen on an icy sidewalk about 6 months previously. Plain skull films had been made but no CT scan was done. (Courtesy of the Office of the Medical Examiner, Cook County, IL.)

Deformations such as those illustrated generally do not reexpand if the hematoma is removed or drained, for reasons that are not clear, even though some resolution of neurological symptoms may occur upon removal. Shifts of midline structures are common, and occasionally midline shifts may cause sufficient distortion of the inner brain structures so that obstruction of the foramina of Monro may impede CSF flow and produce unilateral hydrocephalus, brain shift with herniation, decompensation, and death.

Histologically, the dating and aging of subdural hematoma membranes is not simple, owing to the dynamic character of the lesion, and is dependent to a large degree on the sampling of the membrane for examination. As alluded to before, a general guideline published more than 70 years ago by Munro and Merritt [204], which is still useful today, described the stages of evolution of the subdural hematoma membrane and provided specific criteria to aid in aging of the lesions. The information is summarized and presented in Table 6.2.

From an examination of the table, it can be seen that beyond about 6 months of aging, it is not reliable to affix an age to dural hematoma membranes, but that reasonable estimates may be made on their age before that time. As has been cautioned before, in reference to attempting to precisely age hemorrhages, there may be some variation in the evolution of changes from individual to individual, and histological sampling may be another variable factor; thus, rigid precision is not justified, although reasonable estimates can be made that have evidentiary and forensic value. It is indeed unfortunate that more recent and extensive data on hematoma aging are not available, especially in reference to subdural hematomas in infants and children, but from personal experience, the Munro–Merritt paradigm can be reasonably applied to infants and children.

In older individuals, especially those who have suffered many episodes of head trauma, such as chronic alcoholics, epileptics, ataxic individuals, and stroke victims, it is not uncommon to find chronic subdural hematomas with multiple layers in them. Sometimes there may be three or four layers of collagenized membranes totaling 1 cm or more in thickness with or without a persistent cavity. These lesions no doubt arose from separate episodes of fresh bleeding beneath a prior hematoma with or without an accompanying trauma. In other individuals, hematoma membranes may be found frequently in which there is no longer a cavity present and there is no activity whatsoever within what remains of the original lesion. Such findings underscore the fact that probably many subdural hematomas, even some that reach the chronic phase and may have enlarged at one time or another, resolve by themselves without any intervention. The prevalence of this phenomenon is nearly impossible to determine.

Forensic Issues

Chronic subdural hematomas provide a fertile field in forensic pathology, in neuropathology, and for the legal profession because of the special character of these lesions. They frequently occur without known trauma or other historical cause; often evolve silently and with great subtlety; mimic a number of other conditions; are easily missed clinically, even by the most adept and competent clinicians; and may cause permanent disability or death if untreated or treated too late. The lesion is the central focus for medical malpractice suits, often for failure to diagnose/treat; for product liability and insurance claims; and in criminal cases. Such cases often involve the judgment of forensic pathologists and neuropathologists regarding linkage of the hematoma with a temporal event, the relation between the lesion and symptoms observed, and possible causal variables. The presence of a chronic subdural hematoma does not necessarily imply that there has been recent trauma—an issue that is commonly raised regarding intervening cause, fixation of liability, or responsibility during litigation. It is part of the natural history of such lesions that they bleed of their own accord [173,206,214]. It often becomes difficult, if not impossible, to determine if additional trauma has caused recent bleeding, and the application of common sense is usually required to resolve such issues. In such cases, it is important to determine if there are any other signs of recent traumatic lesions in the brain, such as contusions or new hematomas, which might bolster an argument that recent trauma aggravated an underlying condition or caused death.

When confronted with a case in which a chronic subdural hematoma is found, it behooves the pathologist to carefully document the location and extent as well as the appearance of the lesion by descriptions, notes, drawings, and photographs. Measurements of the thickness of membranes are important, as is histological examination of a strip of all hematomas encountered. Taking of such sections represents an important bit of neuropathological evidence, without which considerable embarrassment and frustration may result at a later time, should the matter of age and duration of the hematoma become an issue.

Central Nervous System

Brain as a Whole

Physically, the brain mass is composed of neurons, glial cells, vessels, and extracellular space and is covered in meningeal membranes. The number of neurons has been estimated to be between 10 billion and 18 billion and astrocytes at least 5–10 times this number. Gray matter composition is quite variable from region to region, but in the neocortex the ratio of gray matter as a whole to the volume of neuron somas has been reported as 27:1 [221]; thus, for every neuron volume, there are 27 times the volumes of other structures, such as glial cells, vessels, and extracellular space. The extracellular space, a subject of considerable controversy in measurement technologies over the years, appears now to be about 25% of brain volume [222]. As for the glial cells, it has been reported that every cubic millimeter of brain matter contains about 100,000 glial cells and that the brain contains between 100 billion and 130 billion of them, accounting for perhaps 50% of the brain's mass. In the gray matter, each cubic millimeter has been reported to contain 500–800 mm of capillaries, and for white matter, there are about 200 mm of capillaries per cubic millimeter [221]. The total volume of capillaries in the whole brain is said to be about 3% of brain volume. The shear volume density of brain vessels can be appreciated from arteriovenous injection/corrosion studies and other preparations. In terms of proximity between capillaries and neurons, every neuron is only a short distance, from three to five capillaries, and is essentially covered by astrocytic foot processes. The bed of astroglia covers the body of the neuron and surrounds synapses and may territories whose functions are still poorly understood.

The brain is normally supplied by four arterial vessels in the normal state, the two internal carotid arteries and the two vertebral arteries. Anatomic variants in these vessels are not uncommon, and about 25% of adults have only one functioning vertebral artery. The internal carotid arteries arise from the common carotid arteries and traverse the cavernous sinus upward into the cranial cavity, giving off the ophthalmic artery, then forming the circle of Willis, and continuing on to form the middle cerebral and anterior cerebral arterial trees. The vertebral arteries arise from the subclavian arteries and ascend within the costotransverse foramina of the cervical spine to penetrate the dura at the foramen magnum, where they course upward to form the basilar artery. The vertebrobasilar system gives rise to the anterior spinal artery and the cerebellar arteries and joins with the circle of Willis to form the posterior cerebral arteries and posterior communicating vessels.

Axon

Each neuron possesses a single axon that may terminate in a short distance upon another neuron or form a recurrent collateral fiber that terminates on the same neuron soma, but a large number of axons in the brain may reach 20 or more centimeters in length, and some, like those emanating from large pyramidal neurons in the motor cortex, may journey more than a meter before synapsing in the anterior horn motor neuron of the spinal cord. Such comparatively vast lengths of an axon for a neuron that may be 100 or more microns at its greatest dimension, and the realities for its survival and maintenance of its terminal, are impressive, considering that most protein synthesis occurs in the neuron cell soma, virtually all materials destined for the nerve cell terminus must be transported to the axon terminus, and depleted materials must be transported back to the cell body by axoplasmic transport mechanisms [222].

Axonal Transport cytoplasmic streaming, or the movement of cytoplasm within the cell, has been known since the invention of the microscope. In the nervous system, this process has special significance since vital neuroplasmic components must be transported from the neuron body to the periphery via the axon. This process was defined by the work of Weiss [223] who ligated peripheral nerves and charted the build-up of axoplasm proximal and distal to the ligation. A large body of literature regarding the processes involved in axonal transport exists. A classical view has been that protein synthesis can occur only in the neuron cell body; however, recently, this concept has been questioned by the demonstration of axonal synthesis of proteins and other components [224–226]. By the same token, products of catabolism and vital neuron-bound signaling molecules from the periphery, which inform the neuron of the status of its neural terminus and axon, must be, and are, transported back to the soma [227]. When an axon is injured or severed, a sequence of changes occurs in the neuron, its axon, and in the distal damaged axon. This process is often referred to as Wallerian or anterograde degeneration. Within a few days after a peripheral axon has been damaged, the axoplasm undergoes degeneration with lysis of the cytoskeleton with vesicle and bleb formation. This is followed by profound changes in the neuron cell body with dissolution of Nissl bodies (chromatolysis) and swelling, among other changes. Protein synthesis increases and if the cell survives, a new axon grows into the myelin sheath. Meanwhile the myelin sheath of the distal damaged axon deteriorates. Eventually the sprouted new axon may find its way into the distal residual sheath and may reach the normal nerve terminus, but this is far from guaranteed [228,229]. The process of nerve degeneration and regeneration depends heavily on the complex process of axonal transport.

Transport of materials from neuron soma to the periphery is referred to as anterograde or orthograde transport, and transport from periphery back to the soma as retrograde transport. These processes occur in the central and peripheral nervous systems. Anterograde transport can occur at a spectrum of rates, ranging from fractions of a millimeter to 8–10 mm per day ("slow" transport) and involves the transport of hundreds of proteins and other molecules by association with the microtubular cytoskeleton and microtubule-associated proteins of the axon [230]. "Fast" anterograde transport of vesicular profiles and mitochondria can occur much faster at speeds ranging from 50 to hundreds of millimeters per day and generally occurs in an irregular ("stop and go") pattern [231–234]. Retrograde transport, is most easily observable optically using Nomarski® differential interference contrast microscopy or other new optical methods in living axons in the form of vesicles moving toward the neuron. The movement of particles is robust and reveals that some proceed in the same "stop and go" pattern as for anterograde transport and ranges between 100 and 200 mm/day [234]. It appears that retrograde transport makes use of actin and other motor proteins [230]. Retrograde axonal transport is important in maintaining communication of the peripheral nerve ending with the neuron cell body and to ensure that the neuron continues anterograde transport of supplies to the periphery. It is also important in the pathogenesis of rabies, herpes simplex, and other viral diseases by transporting the viruses from the periphery to the cell body and thence to the CNS [235–237]. Soluble macromolecules from the periphery that may have a toxic effect on the neuron, such as chemotherapeutic agents like Adriamycin [238,239], or tracer substances like horseradish peroxidase and various lectins [239], are also transported.

Both anterograde and retrograde axonal transport are energy dependent, meaning that the same things the brain as whole requires moment to moment (oxygen, glucose, and blood flow, and thus ATP), the axons do also [240]. Thus disruption of these vital elements will result in dysfunction or breakdown in axonal transport, although thresholds and exact parameters have not been established.

When axons are subjected to physical stress, a number of processes become involved in upsetting axonal transport. These involve damage to the neural membrane that may cause calcium fluxes to active proteases that can focally affect the cytoskeleton and disrupt transport in the affected portion. Physical forces may actually fracture or break the cytoskeleton but not necessarily the axon itself so that transport cannot occur past a certain point, forward or backward. Thus transport proceeds along the axon until the zone of dysfunction is approached where vesicles and other materials then build up, much like a multicar traffic accident on an expressway. It is this problem that can cause the blebs, spheroids, and swellings that are demonstrated by β-app staining. It should be obvious that anything that disrupts the axonal microenvironment (chemical or physical) can produce axonal pathology. Here lies an important forensic issue: the differentiation of true traumatic axonal injury from the effects of the immediate axonal environment (hypoxia, etc.) [241].

Brain

The brain is suspended in CSF, the properties of which have been discussed in Chapter 5. The brain is tethered to the cranium by pial-arachnoid trabeculae (see Figures 6.29 and 6.32), by bridging veins that run from the cortical surface to the arachnoid and dura (see Figure 6.32), by the supplying arteries of the circle of Willis at the base of the brain, by the cranial nerves at the base of the brain and along the brain stem, and by the spinal cord. Further support for the mass of the brain occurs because of the compartmentalization by the dura. The falx cerebri provides midline structural support. The tentorium provides inferior support between the brain and the cerebellum.

Pathobiology of Neurotrauma

Although it might appear obvious at first that an impact to the head would produce disruption and hemorrhage in some part of the brain or its covering or some other form of injury, it is not at all obvious precisely how an impact produces a lesion when it does not directly or immediately physically tear or disrupt the tissue. When one observes the autopsy specimen of the brain of a trauma victim some days after the traumatic event, one might suppose that all injury occurred at the time of trauma, but this is not so. The process of reaction evolves over many hours, days, weeks, or even months or years to produce what is observed clinically and pathologically [242]. This dynamic process of the evolving lesion has been best studied in connection with experimental spinal cord trauma [243,244], in which a calibrated weight is dropped onto the exposed cord and the time sequence of events followed in serial experiments. Allowing for differences between brain and spinal cord and the experimental model, for purposes of this illustration, there are probably few differences at the tissue level of the evolution of the traumatic lesion. However, some general principles can be extracted from these observations [245].

At the instant of trauma, if the site of ultimate injury in the cerebral cortex or spinal cord, for example, were to be examined grossly, little would be revealed. This is not to say that the neural function would be normal. Very early, possibly instantly, after a physical impact, a phenomenon known as neural shock occurs. In the case of spinal cord trauma, this takes the form of immediate paralysis and blockage of all forms of neural transmission. In the cerebral cortex, a neurophysiological counterpart, spreading depression, occurs. The process by which this develops is poorly understood [244,246] but involves rapid shutdown of membrane ion channel function.

Even if obvious physical disruption of the tissue did not occur, the first visible events tend to be vascular [245,247]. Within the vessels of the area, congestion, perivascular edema, and eventual capillary hemorrhages occur, but perhaps not for an hour or more, depending on the severity of the impact. Eventually, edema (blood–brain barrier breakdown) and hemorrhage are expected to spread with time, until the margins of the lesion are clearly outlined. It would only be after the vascular and edema components of the injury are well established that structural integrity of the neuropil is lost and necrosis occurs. Once the necrotizing process is under way, in which axons, dendrites, neurons, and other tissue components become irreversibly damaged, repair reactions will occur with activation and migration of macrophages, phagocytosis, glial swelling, and capillary growth. When enough time has elapsed to allow for complete removal of necrotic tissue elements, glial scarring will develop and restore the blood–brain barrier. This pattern of tissue reaction is remarkably nonspecific and occurs in almost any ischemic, infective, or other destructive process. Comparatively little neural regrowth occurs in a traumatic lesion in the brain, although rewiring and some functional restoration are possible although unpredictable. The same is likely true for the cord. The peripheral nervous system, on the other hand, is capable of regrowth of axons and remyelination, although this is often incomplete and sometimes abortive and nonproductive, as in the case of a traumatic neuroma, in which aberrant connections may produce pain and curious but troublesome symptoms, such as phantom limb phenomena [248].

Perhaps of greatest interest is not the grossly obvious or even the early minor microscopic events in the traumatic lesion but, rather, the subcellular and functional processes that are occurring in response to the trauma. Work using organized tissue CNS culture preparations indicates that perhaps the earliest lesions occur in the cytoskeleton (microtubules) of neuritic processes without any physical disruption of the cell membrane [249]. In spite of no obvious early cell membrane damage visible by electron microscopy, membrane channel function is altered. This alteration may take the form of damaged ion channels, which could account for the phenomenon of neural shock. Another effect of altered membrane permeability is the influx of calcium ions into the cells from the extracellular space or from structures within the cell and so-called glutamate-induced excitotoxicity [250]. Increased calcium and other ions also enter the extracellular space from a subtly compromised capillary bed in the region. Such an influx of calcium ions activates proteases in the tissue, which ultimately leads to necrosis. These issues have been more thoroughly studied in experimental spinal cord injury than in brain injury.

It is therefore quite clear that the traumatic lesion, whether in the meninges or neural parenchyma of the brain or cord, develops through several phases, each with its own pathophysiology and outcome, which may or may not lead to the next phase, depending on the severity of the injury and the efficiency of repair. Grcevič [251], Adams et al. [252], Ommaya et al. [253], and many others [254] have described a concept of this process in the brain now known by many names, such as diffuse axonal injury (DAI), traumatic axonal injury (TAI), inner brain trauma, and intermediary coup injury [130]. Some of these terms imply that inner brain injury is an axonal phenomenon, which it certainly is, but the injury process involves vessels and the dynamic processes that operate in the inner brain environment. Grcevič [251] has made the observation that the neurotraumatic process is composed of those lesions that are directly related to the primary traumatic event (membrane dysfunction and organelle dysfunction), followed by a sequence of those that are secondary (lesions caused by edema, inflammatory mediator release, hemorrhage in adjacent normal tissue, etc.) and those tertiary or quaternary lesions that occur as a result of associated injuries or clinically important systemic and thus global dysfunctions, such as hypoxia, acidosis, alteration in the clotting mechanism, embolization, disorder of pressure/volume equilibria, hydrocephalus, infection, surgical intervention, and underlying medical conditions such as diabetes, hypertension, and alcoholism [255]. Each of these processes has a life cycle of its own that, nevertheless, may become superimposed on or altered by another coexisting process in evolution. One might also consider such processes not as separate events but, rather, as a cascading phenomenon. In any case, the traumatic process is anything but static, stereotyped, and inherently predictable.

Within the context of this dynamic process, it is appropriate to consider the nature of clinical observations and studies performed on the head trauma victim [2]. On the clinical front, the Glasgow group [252,256,257] has developed a method of grading and monitoring the progress of head trauma victims, from which predictions of outcomes are possible. This method and its various modifications take into account the changing character of brain trauma. Radiographic studies and other imaging methods, most notably the CT and MRI scans, provide very valuable concrete information on the lesions that are present at the time the study is made [258]. Herein lies a conceptual trap into which many clinicians and pathologists fall. Such studies are static observations, one frame of a longer movie, and unless repeated or done in a serial fashion, they provide little clue to the possible course of the lesions in the future or its dynamic character. It is often assumed, because a CT, ultrasound, or MRI study is negative, that no significant process is occurring intracranially, and it often comes as a shocking surprise when a repeat study or autopsy reveals massive lesions where none were suspected or documented in life. These common occurrences of the hospital or forensic autopsy service constantly underscore the highly dynamic nature of traumatic processes within the CNS. This phenomenon of temporal development of traumatic lesions is sometimes useful in aging and dating intracranial traumatic lesions in relation to external events, such as beating or altercation, a homicide by gunshot, or fire, or the allegation that observed brain lesions are postmortem processes rather than premortem. Such questions may arise in connection with criminal prosecutions and may involve expert testimony by a neuropathologist.

Injury Mechanisms in Central Nervous System Trauma

From a biomechanical perspective, trauma to the CNS and its neural and vascular elements has been studied extensively in the adult, from the gross anatomical level to the cellular level, through the use of human surrogates, animal models, analytical and mathematical models, isolated tissue models, and cellular models, as discussed above [33,35]. The multilevel approach to understanding injury mechanism permits the researcher to correlate real-world loads that may be applied to the head with the pathophysiological consequences of those loads on the system, tissue, and cellular constituents that constitute the CNS and its vasculature. This approach has been used to study well-known clinical phenomena such as acute subdural hematoma and diffuse axonal injury, for example, with the goal of defining the specific injury mechanism and injury tolerance criteria for these clinical entities in the hopes of applying the findings to the development of prevention through proper aircraft, vehicle, and restraint systems designs; therapeutic intervention; and rehabilitation strategies [35,192,254,259–261].

The focus of the following biomechanical discussion of CNS trauma will emphasize the experimental research performed in the areas of subdural hematoma and diffuse axonal injury, two related intracranial pathologies in terms of the underlying loading mechanism. During the discussion, specific attention will also be focused on the differences between the mechanisms of these pathologies as they relate to the age-dependent properties of the developing pediatric CNS and constitutive tissues (skull, suture, brain, neurovasculature), an area of research that is currently gaining greater and much-deserved attention. The discussion will cover the overarching concepts of inertial versus contact loading of the head (applied load), the dependence of injury mechanism on the various physics of the applied load (direction, magnitude, duration), the kinematics of the head and the intracranial contents during the applied loading event, and the tissue and cellular level consequences of these kinematics. If this terminology is not somewhat familiar to you, please consult the beginning of this chapter for a brief introduction to physics and mechanics.

In general, the intracranial contents may be affected by external loading to the head in two ways: through the direct interaction between the displacing (e.g., ridges, prominences of the bony architecture) or deforming skull (in-bending, penetration, displaced fractures) or the intracranial partitions (falx, tentorium, etc.); and via the relative motion created between the skull/dura and the intracranial contents by virtue of those contents' lagging behind the motion of the skull during acceleration of the head. The former case describes direct contact trauma, often associated with injuries such as contusion, laceration, and epidural hematoma, whereas the latter describes impulsive, inertially induced trauma, often associated with SDH, SAH, and DAI/TAI. To clarify, when we refer to DAI in this context, we are referring to traumatic, stretch-induced injury to the axons resulting from external loading to the head versus hypoxic/ischemic injury. The importance of context of this process deserves a brief review, below.

Head Injury Mechanisms

Often, head injury mechanisms are not purely contact related or inertially induced but, rather, are combinations of contact and impulsive loading. This is often a point of confusion as one attempts to separate the contact (blunt force) injuries from the inertially induced (acceleration–deceleration) injuries. As a matter of course, the terminology of *blunt force* and *acceleration–deceleration* serves as convenient shorthand for forensic descriptions of injury mechanism but is arbitrary in the biomechanical sense, and these terms are rarely used by biomechanicians. In this discussion, we will abandon those terms and use *contact* to mean the physical interaction between objects, the head and the ground or a baseball bat and the head, for example, and we will use the term *inertial* or *impulsive* to mean the loading of the head generated by virtue of the head's acceleration. We will use the term *acceleration* to mean the head's change in velocity over time (dV/dT), whether it is speeding up or slowing down or merely changing direction at a constant speed (recall that displacement, velocity, and acceleration are vector quantities that possess both a magnitude and a direction). Thus, we can have a pure contact event with no resulting inertial event (e.g., a person is lying with his or her head on the ground and someone hits that person's constrained head with a baseball bat), a purely inertial event involving no contact (e.g., the occupant of an automobile sustains whiplash of the head on the neck without contacting the seat, head rest, etc.), or a combination of the two (e.g., a person in a bar room brawl is punched in the side of the face, sustaining fractures, and is also knocked unconscious by the resulting inertial load to the head). It is important to be able to understand and appreciate the differences between these loading conditions as they relate to CNS injury biomechanics because, as stated previously, the goal of establishing a particular CNS injury mechanism is to relate the gross anatomical loading condition applied to the head to the resulting neural and vascular trauma.

Another important concept to appreciate is the difference between translation and rotation of the head during a particular loading event. Translation is simply a linear, or straight-line, motion in three dimensions; rotation is defined as the pivoting, or angular motion, of a body about its geometric or inertial center, typically. Most motion in the real world is a combination of these two basic types and is referred to as curvilinear motion; that is, any complex motion can be characterized as a combination of translation of the center of mass of an object and a rotation about that center. The head is coupled to the torso by the neck, and this kinematic constraint typically results in both translation and rotation of the head for most loading events applied to the freely moving head. In reality, the rotation of the head is usually not about its center of mass but may be a rotation about a point outside the head itself (e.g., the upper, mid-, or lower cervical spine), a condition that is generally termed angular motion of the head. One exception is pure axial translation of the head such that the head moves coincident to the superior–inferior (often referred to as the Y-axis) of the head (see Figure 6.3), resulting in axial compression or extension of the cervical spine. However, in most cases, the unconstrained head will be free to rotate on the neck during a loading event, even if the loading event itself is applied in pure translation.

For example, if a person is standing upright and is struck on the occiput by a baseball bat traveling in a straight line parallel to the ground, the head will experience a contact event. By virtue of the impulsive loading imparted to the head by the baseball bat, momentum will be transferred from the moving baseball bat to the head, and the head will experience a subsequent acceleration. During the sagittal plane (Z-axis) acceleration of the head, the head will displace forward from the impulsive loading applied by the baseball bat; however, the head will experience forward flexion and rotation as the neck constrains the pure linear motion of the head. During this curvilinear motion, the head will sustain a change in angular velocity over a short period, resulting in angular acceleration of the head. Thus, the pure linear motion of the baseball bat results in curvilinear motion of the head by virtue of the head's connection to the neck. If the head is struck on the side, an X-axis movement as well as other movements will occur. Remember, then, that the motion of the head is not dictated simply by the loading applied to it from any one direction, but also by factors such as the kinematical constraints imposed upon it by its mass and physical connections to the rest of the body.

Why is this distinction between translation and rotation important? As with other physical parameters governing injury mechanism, certain types of CNS trauma are dependent on the nature of the kinematics of the head; that is, certain types of CNS trauma occur during a loading event as a result of the linear component of head motion, whereas others occur as a result of the angular component of the head motion. For example, the biomechanics and forensic correlation of inertially induced injuries, such as SDH and DAI, are attributed to rotation of the head and concomitant intracranial consequences of the head's angular motion. The consequences of a head translation versus a rotation in terms of CNS injury and injury mechanism are distinctly related to the mechanical and structural properties of the neural and vascular elements and structures, a significant concept that we will explore in detail in the remaining discussion. It should be remembered that while the head may experience angular or rotational movements during a traumatic event, in most instances, the movements before impact have little or no effect on the injuries sustained, most of which occur from rotational forces at and after impact (postimpact phenomena). The preimpact movements are generally of a low rate of change compared to the much more substantial forces of impact that can be complex and multiplanar.

Central nervous system (CNS) trauma in general and brain injury in particular have been the subjects of intensive biomechanics investigation for the past five decades. Therefore, CNS trauma is the example that is used to demonstrate the concepts of transition from the macroscopic to the microscopic level of biomechanics research. Some of the earliest studies [4,35,192,261–267] suggested that the translational and rotational accelerations of the head serve as a macroscopic descriptor and predictive index with regard to the incidence of brain injury. Subsequent investigations, including human volunteer experiments and animal model studies [192,254–268], confirmed that the inertial loading, its direction, duration, and magnitude relative to the anatomy, can produce a broad spectrum of the neuropathological findings. These various forms of injury to the brain include the following: cerebral concussion, cortical contusion, focal intracerebral hematoma, subdural hematoma, and diffuse axonal injury with prolonged coma. Each of these pathologic entities is distinctive and represents the structural or functional failure of the discrete elements within the brain. Each of these forms of CNS trauma has specific failure criteria, mechanisms of injury, and tolerance levels. This may be further confounded by the age of the patient.

With the exception of crush injury, the mechanical forces that lead to CNS trauma are applied dynamically with a characteristic time course of 50 ms or less. The injury models in the biomechanics literature are designed to investigate the underlying mechanisms of injury, determine the threshold of mechanical stimuli that produce injury, and explore the time course of the pathophysiological events to define windows of opportunity and strategies for therapeutic intervention. The macroscopic analysis of CNS injury is complicated by the fact that the tissue or organ responses are dictated by the cellular responses, all of which may be confounded by factors that alter these mechanical and physiologic responses, such as age. To this end, researchers have attempted to develop a multilevel approach to understanding CNS injury mechanisms, correlating gross head-loading events to the corresponding mechanical and pathophysiological effects at the organ, tissue, and cellular levels. Several different injury models and techniques have been employed in this regard, including real-world injury databases, human surrogates, anthropomorphic test devices (ATDs, or crash test dummies) [269], animal models, isolated organ and tissue studies, and cellular models of injury.

This discussion will focus on the biomechanical approach to elucidating the injury mechanisms related to diffuse axonal injury (DAI) and acute subdural hematoma (ASDH), two clinical entities that epidemiological data indicate are responsible for significant mortality and morbidity associated with CNS injury. From a biomechanical standpoint, DAI and acute SDH have a similar causative mechanism in that they are both found to occur as the result of angular acceleration (inertial loading) of the head, resulting in differential motion between the skull/dura and the brain/pia–arachnoid. This differential motion is the result of the inertia of the brain: when an external load is applied to the head (e.g., an impact), the scalp, skull, and adherent dura accelerate as a result of the impulsive loading and transfer of momentum to the head. By virtue of its mass, the brain and its intimate membranes lag the motion of the skull and dura, resulting in relative motion between the two anatomical elements. This differential motion results in strain within the brain (parenchymal neural and vascular elements) or the vasculature on the surface of the brain (e.g., the bridging vessels). Although the common element linking the mechanisms of DAI and SDH is angular acceleration of the head, the actual outcome of that acceleration is dependent on loading direction, duration, and magnitude. Diagrams and cartoons are often employed in legal proceedings by experts to illustrate supposed movements of the brain in some injury scenarios (such as manual shaking). Often these demonstrative aids mislead because of no attention being paid to magnitude and duration of the accelerative forces involved and the thresholds that must be attained or exceeded for meaningful differential brain movement to occur.

The major factor contributing to the directional dependence of DAI and SDH is the intracranial anatomy and compartmentalization of the intracranial contents by the falx and the tentorium. Experimental studies of DAI and acute, traumatically induced SDH in subhuman primate and physical model studies have demonstrated the directional dependence of these clinical entities. For example, DAI is associated with coronal plane (i.e., lateral movement of the head in an arc) and, to a lesser extent, axial plane angular acceleration of the head [192,268]. During this loading condition, the falx constrains motion of the contralateral cerebral hemisphere, while the ipsilateral hemisphere continues to move in the direction of the angular motion. This constrained differential motion of the brain results in stretch of the axonal tracts within the deep central white matter, correlating anatomically with the corpus callosum, rostral brain stem, and basal ganglia. For example, consider the driver of an automobile whose vehicle is impacted on the driver's side (T-boned). The driver will appear to move toward the driver's side interior door panel as his or her vehicle is pushed out from under him or her toward its passenger's side. Real-world incidents like this have demonstrated contact between the left side of the driver's head and the buckling and deforming engine cover of the incoming, colliding vehicle. In this example, the head of the driver moves laterally in an arc from right to left and then comes to an abrupt halt when its left side impacts the intruding engine cover of the striking vehicle. The skull and dura stop moving during contact, but the brain continues to rotate in its original direction until arrested by some force. In this case, the ipsilateral (left) hemisphere continues to move within the cranial vault while the contralateral (right) hemisphere's movement is arrested by the falx. At high enough levels of load, this condition results in strain (stretch) within the left corpus callosum, rostral brain stem, and basal ganglia areas, classic locations for DAI lesions. Similar impact scenarios include professional American football players who sustain helmet-to-helmet contact on the ear hole of their helmet, the optimum lateral impact load that will result in coronal plane angular acceleration of the head.

In contrast, the gross head movement associated with SDH is sagittal plane angular acceleration of the head, with occipital impacts creating the most conducive loading for stretching of bridging vessels [193]. During an occipital impact, for example, a backward fall with an occipital impact on the ground, the head is abruptly brought to a stop while the brain continues to rotate rearward. In this case, the motion of the cerebral hemispheres is parallel to the falx and is constrained by the tentorium. As the cerebral hemispheres move rearward relative to the skull, the cortical insertion end moves relative to the dural insertion end and the vessel elongates. Additionally, the anatomical orientation of the bridging vessels, exiting from the cerebrum and sweeping forward as they insert into the dural sinus, enhances the stretch of the vessels during an occipital impact. Conversely, during a frontal impact, the cerebral hemispheres move forward relative to the dura; however, the forward-swept orientation of the vessels causes them to buckle, protecting them from stretch. Unilateral versus bilateral subdural injuries are typically the result of an asymmetric impulsive load acting on the head, such that the head is not subject to a pure sagittal plane rotation but to a combination of sagittal, coronal, and axial rotation. The compartmentalization of the brain by the falx and the tentorium, as discussed previously, will arrest the motion of parts of the brain while others are free to continue rotating, resulting in nonuniform distribution of strain within the various bridging vessels and unilateral or asymmetric pathology.

Further distinguishing the mechanism of DAI and SDH is the duration of the impulse that results in the injurious angular acceleration of the head. SDH is associated with short, spiked loading pulses (e.g., 5–10 ms typically), whereas DAI is associated with longer, attenuated pulses (e.g., 30–50 ms). This behavior is consistent with the frequency-dependent depth of propagation of strain through viscoelastic media, such as the brain, where higher-frequency (shorter-duration) loads result in shallow disturbances of the underlying viscoelastic medium and lower-frequency (longer-duration) loads result in deeper propagation of the disturbance.

Finally, the magnitude of the applied load has a direct result on the outcome of the nature and severity of CNS injury. In gross anatomical terms, the load applied to the head is traditionally expressed in terms of the force, linear acceleration, or angular acceleration. These physical parameters are easily measured in the laboratory setting, and instrumentation permitting the measurement of these parameters as a function of time is installed in the current state-of-the-art anthropomorphic test devices to capture, for example, the acceleration–time history of a loading event. Of particular biomechanical importance is the level of loading above which injury occurs—this level of load is called the injury threshold, and determination of these threshold values of head acceleration, for example, leads to injury tolerance criteria, quantitative values of a particular physical parameter that describes the likelihood or risk of injury. Thus, the ability to correlate traumatic levels of head acceleration with a specific CNS injury is a particularly useful relationship to establish, as it leads not only to a better forensic understanding of the forces involved in causing injury but also to targeting of design criteria for safety engineers who develop protective strategies for injury mitigation and prevention. For example, protective safety devices (helmets, air bags, seat belt systems, etc.) can be configured so that the head accelerations generated during typical loading events in which these protective devices are used fall below the applicable and acceptable injury tolerance criteria for specific forms of head injury. These injury tolerance criteria come in several forms, including general indicators of injury risk (i.e., injury assessment reference values) and explicit physical parameters related to specific CNS pathologies (i.e., angular acceleration thresholds for SDH and DAI).

Injury assessment reference values (IARVs) are expressions developed to relate the loads measured with the on-board instrumentation of an ATD to the risk of injury for a particular anatomic structure. IARVs were first proposed for the adult midsized (50th percentile) male ATD by biomechanical engineers at General Motors [269]. These IARVs evolved into a set of values for the entire family of Hybrid III ATDs and utilize injury risk curves to establish the threshold value of loading for each parameter, each threshold representing a 5% risk of significant injury predicted for the specific anatomy [269]. The IARV is not injury specific, though; that is, it does not discriminate among the various forms of trauma for the specified anatomic region. For example, the IARVs for head acceleration represent the threshold for brain injury of AIS = 4. AIS represents the injury classification of the Abbreviated Injury Scale, a system developed to quantify injury based on anatomical region and severity; the scale ranges from 1 (minor) to 6 (currently untreatable). The AIS system was developed through collaboration between the Association for the Advancement of Automotive Medicine (AAAM) and the Society of Automotive Engineers (SAE) as a tool for investigating automotive crash epidemiology. The AIS was originally developed for impact injury assessment. Examples of AIS for brain injuries include subdural hematoma AIS 4 = 50 cc for adult, AIS 5 >50 cc for adult; and AIS 5 diffuse axonal injury (white matter shearing). The IARVs for peak linear acceleration of the head for the range of adult ATDs are 193g (small female), 180g (midsize male), and 175g (large male) [89].

The IARVs for the adult Hybrid III ATDs were adapted to form the corresponding IARVs for child Hybrid III ATDs and infant and toddler CRABI (Child Restraint Air Bag Interaction) ATDs. These pediatric IARVs were developed by scaling adult IARVs, the scale factors developed for the head, including consideration of the head size and failure properties of the skull. The brain's mechanical properties were assumed to be similar in variation with age to those of the calcaneal tendon, a tissue whose age-dependent properties exhibit the typical biphasic change in stiffness as a function of development [269,270]. Discussion of the scaling relation for each IARV is beyond the scope of this chapter, but a detailed discussion of the relations may be found in the published literature [33,79,270–273]. The IARVs for peak linear head acceleration for the range of pediatric ATDs are 50*g* (6-month-old), 51*g* (12-month-old), 52*g* (18-month-old), 175*g* (3-year-old), and 189*g* (6-year-old) [269]. For a more detailed discussion of IARVs, please consult the excellent review of the subject by Mertz [269].

Other approaches sought to develop reliable measures for human brain injury thresholds. Gurdjian and coworkers, working at Wayne State University in Detroit, developed one such scale, the Wayne State Tolerance Curve (WSTC) [263]. This curve showed that durations of acceleration that were longer than 5 ms but below 75–100*g* would likely not exceed the brain's tolerances. For pulse durations shorter than 5 ms, higher *g* forces could be tolerated. Many shortcomings of this scale were pointed out, and a number of other tolerance scales were developed [274]. These include the head protection criteria (HPC), the generalized acceleration model for brain injury threshold (GAMBIT), and the so-called 3 ms criterion [274], each of which either has sufficient scientific issues or lacks universal acceptance. Currently, the most widely employed head injury tolerance function adopted by the National Highway Safety Administration (U.S. federal government) is the so-called Head Injury Criterion (HIC) [274,275].

The HIC can be calculated using the following formula:

$$\mathrm{HIC} = \max(t_1,t_2)\left[\frac{1}{t_2-t_1}\int_{t_1}^{t_2} a(t)\,\mathrm{d}t\right]^{2.5}(t_2-t_1)$$

where a is the head acceleration in multiples of the force of gravity (g), as would be determined by averages of three accelerometers (X, Y, Z axes) placed at the center of gravity of the head. This complicated relation can be expressed in another way if one ignores some specifics of the relationship between translational and rotational motions and yields the value for HIC by

$$\mathrm{HIC} = (\mathrm{d}V^{2.5}/\mathrm{d}T^{1.5}) \text{ or } (\mathrm{d}V^{2}/\mathrm{d}T)(\mathrm{d}V/\mathrm{d}T)^{0.5}$$

where $\mathrm{d}V^2$ is the change in kinetic energy of the head during the acceleration. HIC is inversely proportional to the rate of change of the kinetic energy, $\mathrm{d}T$, and is proportional to the square root of the rate of change of the specific *momentum*, $\mathrm{d}V/\mathrm{d}T$ [275]. The HIC may be calculated over various time intervals, and one of the most frequently employed is for 36 ms, sometimes referred to as the HIC_{36}. With these parameters, if the HIC does not exceed the value of 1000, the likelihood for head injury in a 50th percentile male is low, and above this value the chance of injury rapidly increases, such that at HIC values of 3000, almost all such victims would experience serious head/brain injuries. Experimentally, HIC values for likelihood of skull fractures have correlated with the incidence of skull fractures in cadavers [274,275]. Nevertheless, there are many limitations for applications of the HIC, although in injury correlations in real-life situations and simulations and application, such as automobile crashes, air bag deployment, and helmet design, the HIC has proven useful. Other threshold HIC values have been estimated for infants and children.

Angular acceleration injury tolerance criteria were developed from experimental research, including animal and physical models of injury, isolated tissue failure models, cellular injury models, and analysis of real-world injury data [193,276–280]. Recall the mechanism of subdural hematoma (SDH), which many regard as resulting from bridging vessel stretch failure: a rapid change in velocity of the head results in relative motion between the brain and the skull/dura, causing displacement of the insertion points of the cortical bridging vessels and stretch of the vessel itself. If the stretch is great enough (typically 50% increase in the resting length of the vessel), failure of the vessel may occur and hemorrhage into the subdural potential space will result [152,279–282]. The analogous condition relating angular acceleration of the head to axonal injury has been elucidated in the literature as well, demonstrating a graded pathophysiologic response of the axon to axial stretch developed during deformation of the brain during angular acceleration. The onset of clinically observable disruption of function coincides with axonal elongation of approximately 5%, with greater levels of impairment corresponding to greater levels of stretch. The impairment ceases to be spontaneously reversible at approximately 15% stretch, with primary axotomy occurring at about 25% stretch. These elemental threshold levels of tissue failure for DAI and SDH correspond to approximately 4500 rad/s^2 angular acceleration in the coronal plane for the onset of DAI (i.e., 5% axonal stretch) and 4500–7500 rad/s^2 sagittal plane angular acceleration for acute SDH.

Holbourn [264,265] observed the importance of rotation in the production of certain intracranial pathologies and suggested that it is rotation that is responsible for creating injurious deformations of the brain. This concept is consistent with the mechanical properties of brain tissue, whose bulk modulus (resistance to change in volume) exceeds its shear modulus (resistance to shear loading) by several orders of magnitude (300,000 psi vs. 10 psi) [30]. The physical consequence of these mechanical properties is that the brain can resist linear acceleration but deforms easily during angular acceleration (think of a spreadable solid like mayonnaise).

The pediatric population presents interesting variations on the adult mechanism of injury. As discussed previously, the infant head develops rapidly during the first 2 years of growth, evolving from a compliant, deformable structure into the relatively rigid adult braincase. In the adult, the braincase is relatively rigid, and an impact to the skull will result in diffuse relative motion between the brain and the skull, as discussed previously (impulsive loading). This is in contrast to an impact in the younger child and infant, in which the compliance of the braincase may also lead to gross deformation of the skull and concomitant deformation of the underlying neural and vascular tissues. During the transition from the compliant infant braincase into the fully mature rigid braincase, the mechanism of trauma of the underlying neural and vascular elements may shift from a primarily deformation-mediated mechanism in the infant to a primarily inertially mediated mechanism in the mature system.

In the case of inertially induced injuries in the immature brain, the driving physical variable affecting the relationship between head loading and the resulting axon or vessel stretch is the mass of the brain itself. That is, the critical strain developed within the brain is dependent on the mass of the brain (its inertial properties)—this concept assumes that the material properties of the brain are identical in the infant and adult, an assumption that is not entirely valid and will be addressed subsequently. Scaling methods based on the work of Holbourn and Ommaya have been derived and developed to relate the thresholds from one system (the model system, e.g., the adult) to another system (the prototype system, e.g., the infant). The scaling relationship takes the adult threshold and scales it to a corresponding infant threshold based on the brain masses of the two subjects of interest [283]. The scaling relationship (see Figure 6.55) has also been used to scale primate data to humans, again based on brain mass, and is derived from physical law [264,265,279]. It has been proposed by Ommaya et al. [283] that for angular accelerations, concussion tolerance is related to

$$R = \frac{C}{m^{2/3}}$$

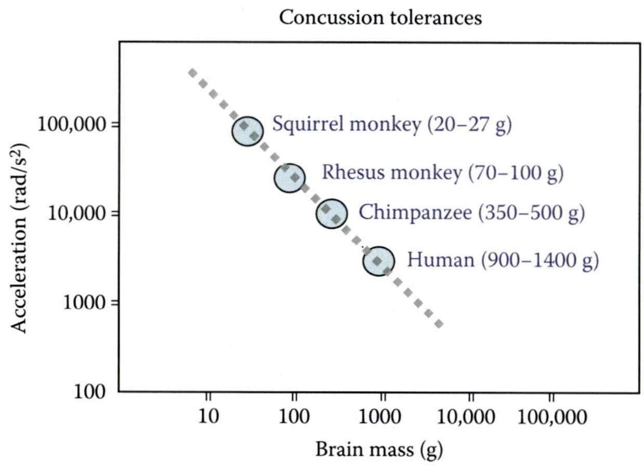

Figure 6.55 This graph, created by Ommaya et al. based on theoretical work of Holbourn [267,283], depicts the relationship between brain mass and injury thresholds. It should be pointed out that the only experimentally derived value was that for the rhesus monkey brain and that the others were theoretically predicted, based on other experimental work in various species. This is not to say that there is no merit in this "curve" since many experiments done since this work was published have shown that smaller brains clearly require more acceleration to produce brain injury than larger ones, and human studies approximate the observations and hypotheses of Ommaya et al. [267]; however, caution should be applied when using this "curve." (From Ommaya A et al. *Proceedings of the 11th Stapp Car Crash Conference*, Society of Automotive Engineers (SAE), 1967, pp. 47–52.)

where C is an empirically derived constant, m is the mass of the brain in question, and R is rotational acceleration in rad/s^2. Ommaya et al. [283] also pointed out that for translational accelerations, the relation is

$$A = \frac{C}{m^{1/3}}$$

in an example to estimate the concussion injury threshold for a 3-year-old child, based on the known threshold of the adult. The brain masses associated with each system are 1400 g for the adult and 1000 g for the 3-year-old. In this example, we will use a conservatively high estimate of the adult SDH threshold of 7500 rad/s^2 [165], scaling to 9300 rad/s^2 for the 1000-g brain prototype; Löwenhielm's [152] criterion for vessel rupture is published as 4500 rad/s^2, which would scale to 5600 rad/s^2 for the 1000-g brain mass. The somewhat counterintuitive result is that in order for the smaller-mass brain to achieve a similar level of stretch as the large-mass brain, the small-mass brain must be subjected to a larger angular acceleration. The deformations predicted within the brain based on these scaling results have been explored computationally [284] and through physical model studies of idealized geometries (cylinders) as well as primate and human skull models [63]. Introduction of the mechanical properties of the brain (e.g., the complex shear modulus) into the scaling relationship has demonstrated that the higher-scaled angular acceleration values predicted for the infant brain are decreased slightly with the consideration of the lower stiffness of the infant brain tissue when compared with the adult tissue [77].

The driving force behind the biomechanical research into the mechanism of these injuries is the quest to link the gross head-loading conditions (loading magnitude, loading direction, pulse duration) to the associated neuropathological entities observed clinically. As an example of the multilevel approach to understanding the relationship between gross head loading and the effects of that loading in terms of injury, consider the development of the biomechanical model of DAI. From mild episodes of concussion, with only momentary loss of consciousness, up to and including the prolonged vegetative state represents the spectrum of the clinical manifestations that constitute the biomechanical entity called diffuse axonal injury. Mechanically induced loss of consciousness for varying periods of time is the direct result of the dynamic strains experienced by the axons in the central white matter of the brain. Physiologically, the degree to which the axons stretch determines the changes in axolemma permeability through the transient development of mechanical defects within the membrane. In response to this alteration in membrane permeability, calcium moves rapidly into the cytosol and causes the membrane to depolarize. The amount of calcium that enters the cell is in direct proportion to the magnitude of the membrane strain and the persistence of the defects. The cell quickly handles small amounts of calcium quite easily through clearance or sequestration; however, as the strain increases, the net calcium flux increases and the cell can be overwhelmed. As cytosolic free calcium concentrations reach approximately 50 μM, enzymes are activated that cause disruption (depolymerization) of the microtubules and neurofilaments. The osmotic pressure increases in response to this newly generated protein solution and the cell begins to swell. Hydrostatic pressure then leads to quasi-static axolemma strain and ultimately secondary axotomy.

This injury mechanism has been studied with a multilevel approach by

1. Producing varying degrees of traumatic unconsciousness in an animal model
2. Examining the pathology at the electron microscope level
3. Using physical models of the skull and surrogate brain material to estimate the magnitude and topographic distribution of the strain field within the brain under loading conditions identical to those of the subhuman primate model
4. Stretching axons (squid giant axon, sciatic nerve of the frog single-axon prep, and NT2 cells in culture) to measure the electrophysiological response and the changes in cytosolic free calcium
5. Mathematical models of the deformation response of the brain to inertial loading
6. Mathematical models of the membrane strain-induced alterations in the two-phase flow through pores or slits in the membrane
7. Comparing the estimated tolerance levels for the spectrum of DAI with medical records and biomechanical data of human events (e.g., football, boxing, hockey, auto accidents, workplace injuries, and accidents in the home)

In the past, primate models of CNS were used to replicate specific forms of injury. By subjecting physical models or surrogates of the skull–brain structure to loading conditions that produced these discrete forms of brain injury in the primate model, researchers were able to estimate the magnitude and temporal nature of the deformations that were experienced by the various neural and neurovascular elements in association with these injuries. With this information, strategies were developed to investigate the biomechanics of injury at the isolated tissue and cellular levels to begin to simplify this complex analysis. Accordingly, researchers designed instrumentation that permitted the study of isolated axons, blood vessels, and cells in culture under conditions of controlled mechanical deformation. Utilizing these technologies, they demonstrated that high-strain-rate deformation of the axolemma led to an elevated level of intracellular calcium. They showed that membrane ionic permeability is directly affected by high-strain-rate deformation of the axon, which in turn leads to an immediate elevation in cytosolic free calcium ion concentration. Neural tissue can respond by sequestering calcium or pumping it from the cytoplasm, but at some point, these coping mechanisms become overwhelmed. This traumatic rise in cytosolic free calcium in neurons has been implicated in cytoskeletal disruption, functional impairment, cell swelling, and, ultimately, cell death.

The relationships between the energies associated with various events (an auto collision environment, falls, assaults, and impact by moving objects) and the forces applied to the individual are sometimes difficult to determine. With respect to the CNS, impact to the head and the associated inertial loads produce deformation of the neural and neurovascular components that constitute the more macroscopic structures of the brain. The complex pathophysiological process, which accompanies the mechanical distortion to the CNS, can be studied by investigating the response of isolated tissue elements and single cells to mechanical stimuli. By developing failure criteria for the components that constitute the brain, we can begin to simplify this otherwise arduous task and, in the process, provide a scientific basis for the development of improved head injury tolerance criteria. In other words, researchers have related the gross impulsive head loads measured in the real world to the effects of those loads at the microscopic level, attempting to move biomechanics and injury research toward the areas of membrane mechanics, cytomechanics, and transport process analysis at the cellular level [285].

Based on the previous discussion, the neural elements of the CNS experience deformations that can result in a continuum of injury response in the sense that there are levels of strain that produce no response, spontaneously reversible forms of trauma, and irreversible injury and cell death. If the physical and mathematical models can help estimate the deformations experienced by the components of the CNS, then it is reasonable to explore methods of subjecting isolated tissue elements or single cells to controlled mechanical stimulation. Researchers have examined the role of mechanical forces in the etiology of head injury by observing the response of an isolated unmyelinated axon to rapid elongation [286]. A graded depolarization in response to increasing levels of strain and strain rate in the squid giant axon has been observed. This graded response suggests a spectrum of injury severity for individual axons, ranging from mild, reversible injury for stretch ratios less than or equal to 1.10 to permanent deficit at 1.20 and structural failure at 1.25, which will be discussed later.

Diffuse axonal injury (DAI) observed in a subhuman primate model appears morphologically as microscopic abnormalities distributed throughout the white matter, independent of any focal injury. One feature of the axonal damage observed is abnormally shaped nodes of Ranvier, structures unique to myelinated nerves. In addition, the variation in the mechanical structure between the node and internode suggests that strains may not be distributed uniformly along the myelinated fiber, as is assumed for the unmyelinated axon.

Biomechanical data do exist for peripheral nerves. Okamoto, as quoted by McElhaney et al. [33], noted that the human sciatic and median nerves could elongate about 18% under load, and could sustain static loads of 54 and 20 kg, respectively. To assess physiological responses to tension, Thibault et al. [287] dynamically stretched frog sciatic nerve bundles, a myelinated nerve preparation, and measured the compound action potential as an indicator of functional viability. Response to injury varied from a transient alteration in the signal with small stretch to an irreversible change in the compound action potential following a large stretch. Gray and Ritchie [288] demonstrated functional changes, including reversible conduction block and altered action current, in a single myelinated frog axon due to static stretch. Another preparation utilizing the giant axon of the squid, *Loligo pealei*, was subjected to uniaxial extension at high strain rates to examine the pathophysiological response of the axon to stretch. The test preparation included membrane potential electrodes and custom-designed calcium ion-selective electrodes, all of which were mounted on the stage of a microscope. Recordings of the membrane potential and the cytosolic free calcium ion concentrations as a function of the strain and the tensile forces developed within the axon were made, enabling the researchers to study the response of the isolated tissue to mechanical stimulation. The intention of these experiments was to attempt to elucidate the thresholds for the tissue response to a well-controlled mechanical insult.

The degree to which the membrane depolarizes is a reasonable measure of the severity of the injury; however, the recovery of the resting membrane potential to a point where it is once again excitable is an important consideration from a purely functional point of view. This observation is not unlike the clinical aspects of brain injury with regard to the duration of the neurological changes that accompany a head injury. To investigate the mechanisms of injury to the isolated axon and to further explore the functional relationships between mechanical deformation and neuropathophysiology, researchers have measured the changes in intracellular calcium following various levels of stretch-induced axonal injury (see Figure 6.56).

The response of the isolated axon to mechanical stimulation appears to exhibit an injury pattern that is continuous in the sense that the severity level is graded and dependent on the level of insult in an exponential manner. The thresholds for specific forms of injury are reasonably well defined at the single-cell level when one measures the membrane potential and the intracellular free calcium ion concentration. A plateau region of the previous curve indicates that the calcium ion concentration will rise to external levels once one reaches region D (in Figure 6.56). This region must therefore be considered fatal for the single cell.

The isolated tissue studies afford the opportunity to investigate the issue of whether there is a direct correlation between the gross mechanical stimulation and the resulting

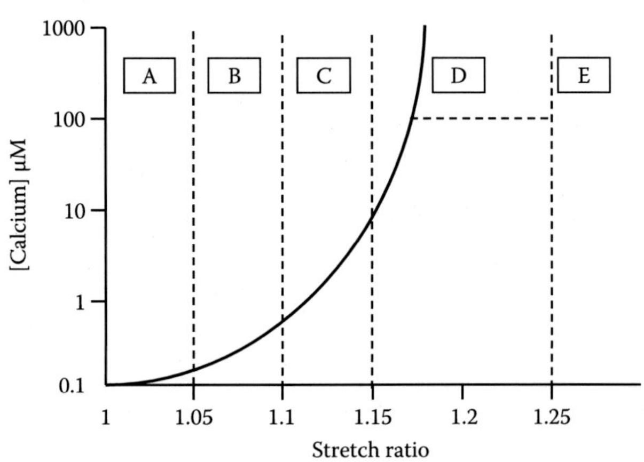

Figure 6.56 This graph demonstrates the functional relationship between the magnitude of the mechanical strain, expressed as the stretch ratio, and the peak values of the intracellular calcium changes that delineate the physiological changes associated with the ultimate outcome of the experiment. (Courtesy of L.E. Thibault, PhD.)

pathophysiological manifestations at the level of the axon. If such a correlation exists, then the injury tolerance criterion may be assigned on the basis of this correlation, provided we have the ability to relate the field variables within the brain to the loads that are applied to the head. One must consider the evidence base for the application and utilization of injury tolerance criteria when attempting to analyze an injury-producing event.

Hopefully, the reader can appreciate the level of understanding and analysis that forms the basis for the biomechanical model of DAI as an example of the laboratory and field techniques used by the biomechanical engineer to quantify and characterize the loading environment, injury mechanism, and injury tolerance criteria for a specific pathological entity.

Brain Contusions

Bruising injuries (focal microvascular injuries) of the brain (Figure 6.57), or contusions, have been observed for centuries, and the mechanisms by which they are produced have been speculated on for nearly as long. For several centuries at least, it was noted that when blows to the head occurred, contusions tended to be observed directly beneath the impact site if there were any immediate brain injuries; whereas in injuries sustained in falls in which the head struck the ground, for instance, there was a notable lack of injury in the brain at the site of impact but often a massive pattern of contusions in the brain at a location exactly opposite the point of impact (contrecoup). The most common instance of the latter phenomenon is a backward fall in which the occiput strikes the ground or pavement, with or without skull fracture, and produces massive contusions in the frontal and temporal lobe tips. To explain contusions that occur directly beneath the impact of a blow to the head (coup contusions) would appear far easier than to explain the counterintuitive finding of contusions in an opposite part of the brain to the impact site when the impact has been due to a fall (contrecoup contusions), but in actuality any theory of brain contusion must hold an explanation not only for both classic forms of contusion but also for all other forms of impact injury to the brain. This conundrum was well known more than 200 years ago, when one of the first public debates was held in Paris in 1766 on the mechanisms involved in the production of cerebral contusions, especially contrecoup contusions. In the two centuries that have elapsed since the so-called contusion contest of Paris, the

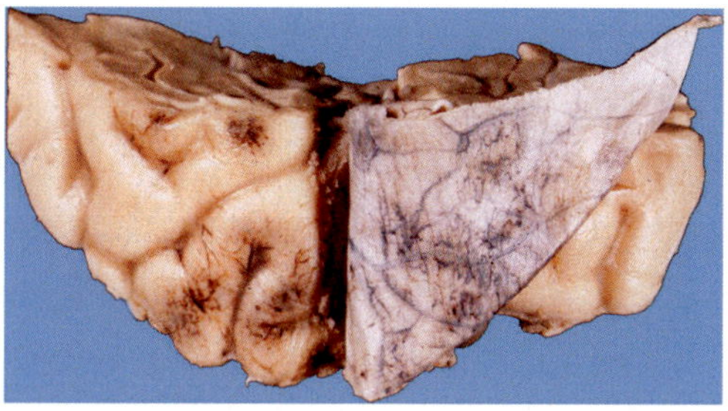

Figure 6.57 This photograph of the frontal lobes with a portion of the overlying dura illustrates recent areas of focal brain contusion. Note the capillary character of the contusion and that the dura is also involved. In time, these contusions will give way to a necrotic surface lesion with a cavitary and brown–yellow appearance.

issues raised have still not been completely resolved or universally agreed on [289,290]. The various theories on the formation of contusions are presented and discussed below.

Vibration Theory of Contusions

Although this particular theory was favored by members of the Paris Academy of Surgeons of 1766 after hearing all the arguments at the time, few subscribe to this notion today. Basically, this theory proposed that impacts to the skull create vibrations that pass through it and arrive at a site opposite the impact where the vibrational energies of the impact are focused and thus have their greatest effect in perhaps fracturing the skull but certainly damaging the brain [291]. Some experimental evidence was offered in support of this proposition in 1835 by Gama, who suspended thin threads in flasks filled with a viscous liquid; when he struck the threads, they seemed to vibrate with the force of the impact. Although a few subsequent workers supported this theory, the emergence of other, more elegant models gradually eclipsed it.

Transmitted Force Waves Theories

Somewhat more attractive hypotheses based on model experiments and experiments that utilized human skulls emerged in the later 1800s. An important observation was made by Felizet as quoted by Goggio [291,292] in a series of experiments in which he dropped skulls and proved that in spite of apparent rigidity, the skull was capable of measurable deformation of the impact point. This observation was incorporated by Duret [293] into a theory that gave rise to a school of thought in the next century that persists today—the cavitation theory. However, the crux of Duret's theory rested with the fact that he felt that impacts to the skull caused not only deformation at the site of impact (in-bending) and expanding lines of force that resulted in deformation at the site opposite (out-bending), which produced a vacuum at that point, but also a wave of force transmitted through the brain that focused at the site opposite the impact point and ruptured blood vessels in the brain, producing the typical contrecoup phenomenon. A number of experiments at the time and later seemed to support this attractive idea. Courville [289,294] retained large portions of this theory and concluded that lesions in the brain produced by impacts were caused by waves of force reacting to the various structures encountered in passage, such as cortical–subcortical anatomy, penetrating blood vessels, bony prominences, and barriers such as the falx. In support of this view, Courville felt that he could demonstrate damage along the paths of the lines of force within the brain and between coup and contracoup contusions.

Brain Displacement Theory

The leading proponent of this concept, W.R. Russell, incorporated his observations that the brain was capable of movement inside the skull during impacts into a theory that included some aspects of the vibrational theory. He felt that the contrecoup phenomenon was due to the sudden arrest of the portion of the brain that lay opposite the impact site, tearing itself away from its superficial attachments by its own momentum. Later, experiments done in collaboration with Denny-Brown [4] and those of others supported the vacuum theory of Duret and were thought to explain intermediary lesions also on the basis of altered intracerebral pressures. This basic theory still enjoys considerable support today.

Skull Deformation Theory

By extension or modification of the vibrational hypothesis of Felizet and some of the ideas of Duret, Monro and others suggested that contrecoup contusions arose out of a combination of displacement of the brain on impact (lag of the brain behind the skull) and deformation of the skull, which resulted in the skull's slapping the brain at the side opposite the impact site and producing a contusion. This model has been criticized by many, including Goggio [292], but supported by others, such as Unterharnscheidt and Sellier [246], and has been used as an explanation for other forms of brain injury, namely, inner cerebral trauma, by Grcevič [295].

Pressure Gradient Theory

Taking the ideas of Duret and others, Goggio [292] in 1940 showed, using simple mathematics dealing with hydrodynamic phenomena, that greatly lowered pressures exist at sites opposite the impact point in vessels filled with fluids. These lowered pressures, he reasoned, could distend and even rupture small blood vessels if the model were applied to the brain. These ideas were further explored by Gross [296], who created several models for demonstrating the phenomenon using glass vessels that he photographed under impact conditions, which showed cavities at locations opposite the impact locus. Using high-speed cinematography during various impact situations, other workers have shown cavitation to occur in model situations using artificial brains in sectioned calvaria or transparent or sectioned calvaria containing actual brain matter [35]. Pressure transducers placed in the skulls of experimental animals have documented zones of negative pressure at sites opposite impact locations that were of sufficient duration and magnitude that cavitation could occur [35].

Cavitation arises out of tension failure in a fluid when it is exposed to focal, nonuniform pressures or shear forces, such as in the water surrounding a spinning propeller. In a region where pressures are greatly lowered, perhaps for only an instant, the ambient pressure is less than the vapor pressures of water or of dissolved gases, so that vaporization occurs. The implications of such an event occurring in brain matter, or within vessels in the region of lowered pressure, are apparent. As was the case with the brain displacement theory, from which this differs only slightly, many feel that at least part of the actual mechanism for both coup and contrecoup contusions lies here.

Rotational Shear Force Theory

This theory, most notably proposed by Holbourn [264,265] in 1943, grew out of experiments performed in the 1800s with skulls and other containers that were filled with gelatin and subjected to impacts. These studies clearly showed that movement of the intracranial contents relative to the skull was possible and that shearing strains could develop in the brain as a result of rotational movements. Holbourn contrasted rotational and translational impacts with respect to injuries incurred in each and concluded that accelerations with a rotational component were more likely to produce brain injuries than purely translational ones. He then went on to develop several models that predicted likely sites of brain injury with various impact patterns. These analyses indicated that shear strains were more likely to occur over the frontal/temporal regions, regardless of impact site, than elsewhere and in locations where the underlying skull was less smooth than other places. Shear strains can tear cerebral tissue or blood vessels, resulting in focal hemorrhagic injuries. With comparatively few additions, deletions, or criticisms, Holbourn's theories now represent the most universally accepted theory on deep brain traumatic lesions and to some explain the contrecoup phenomenon as well. Many elements of this basic theory have been substantiated in recent animal studies [2,193,253,254,297].

It should be stated that a good deal of confusion and misuse of the terminology regarding rotational brain injuries has arisen. Many have misinterpreted preimpact events such as motions of the head, as in shaking or whiplash scenarios, as having some influence on the neural injury that results after impact loading. The use of the term *rotation* applies to what is happening inside the brain after impact, not what happens before, which has little or no influence on neural injury in most circumstances. Rotational movements are imparted to the brain if the forces are large enough upon impact and are related to the geometry of the cranium against the impacting surface, the vectors' directions of movements of the head at impact, the composition of the encasement, and the mechanical properties of neural tissue involved in a complex interaction [298]. Another aspect of confusion has resulted from a misinterpretation of certain experimental neurotrauma models in which very high-acceleration rotational movements were imparted by a device to experimental animals, chiefly various species of monkeys [253,254], and produced all manner of meningeal and neural injuries. The loading durations in these experiments centered about 15–20 ms at thousands of radians per second per second. These numbers clearly fall within the dynamics of fall-impact scenarios and cannot remotely be attained by manual shaking by a human being [26,27]. Thus, although some would refer to these experiments as being nonimpact, in a sense they are, but in a physical sense they are not, because the interaction of the head with an impacting surface is minimized or eliminated by the encasement of the animal's head; the kinetics of the event on the brain, absent the impact phenomena such as deformation, is essentially the same as an impact. Other issues that surround this phenomenon are discussed in detail in Chapter 7.

Mechanisms Overview

In recent years, there has been a resurgence of interest in neurotrauma, with extensive and important animal research that has permitted considerable testing of old hypotheses regarding brain injuries. The results of this work indicate that there is no doubt that the skull is not a completely rigid structure and is capable of considerable deformation during impacts. Deformation can occur locally with significant in-bending and rebound, especially when the head is fixed during the impact. In-bending of the skull upon a fall-type impact may cause the head to bounce, perhaps several times. These secondary impacts are not trivial and may significantly contribute to the final cranial injury that is observed clinically and pathologically.

With respect to the contrecoup phenomenon, it is likely that some elements of most of the foregoing theories are probably valid but that one single unified theory has not yet been established. Although a discussion of theories might have educational or, at the very least, entertainment value for the forensic pathologist or neuropathologist, the issue of somehow explaining the phenomenon of contrecoup contusion, and the difference between injuries typical for blows and falls, becomes a vital task when the pathologist attempts to communicate with lawyers, law enforcement officials, and especially judges and juries. The very concept of contrecoup contusion is counterintuitive and, if not adequately explained, can give the impression that the expert "doesn't know what he is talking about." A proper approach in beginning to explain this phenomenon to a skeptical lay jury is to confess that the notion does not appear logical at first but that it has been observed for more than 200 years and that animal experiments have given some clues about how it occurs. Even though a complete theoretical explanation may not be possible, the vacuum or cavitation theory of contusions seems fairly easy for laypersons to grasp when, for the sake of simplicity and at the expense of exactitude, the brain can be likened to a sphere suspended in a fluid container. When the container is accelerated, the brain lags behind the container and at impact continues to move relative to the container, producing a vacuum at the site opposite the point of impact. This vacuum can damage vessels and brain substance, giving rise to the bruise at this point. It can also be pointed out that, for some reason, brain tissue can withstand positive pressures more effectively than negative pressures, again supporting the vacuum hypothesis of contracoup contusion.

Sometimes it is necessary to explain various other traumatic lesions in the brain on the basis of shear force injury. Again, the notion of the movable brain can be invoked, but this time it is appropriate to point out that the brain, being jelly-like, can move relative to itself and often in opposite directions. This occurrence can literally act to tear the brain apart in some locations. Although this explanation is not altogether correct or complete, it captures enough of the truth to communicate the basic problem to laypersons. A vital point here is that brain movement in response to acceleration has a threshold and that any motion of the head does not necessarily set the brain moving within the cranial cavity or cause brain damage. For example, simple manual shaking of a baby cannot exceed this threshold and thus cannot damage the brain, but an impact, even one due to a relatively short fall with head impact, can [299,300].

Brain Contusions due to Blows

A blow, in this context, can be defined as an impact to the head that is delivered usually by a discrete object that either is held by someone or otherwise strikes the head, willfully or not, of a nonfalling victim. That is, in most applicable scenarios the head is at rest when an impact load is applied to it. It should be obvious from this rather inexact definition, which depends to some degree on common sense and common usage of the term, that strict definitions might pose problems. In any case, for purposes of this discussion, it might be useful to differentiate blows into several classes, in which they are separated on the basis of their kinetic energy compared with the inertia of the head. Thus, there is a class of blows that would tend to dissipate their energy locally in the scalp and skull, with comparatively little dissipation of energy in accelerating the head. Examples of these would be impacts by objects of low mass with low velocity, such as sticks, small stones, and empty lightweight bottles or cans. Such impacts, if they did not produce substantial deformation of the skull, would be expected to produce only an abrasion or laceration of the scalp, with or without a subgaleal hemorrhage, with no fracture, and with no underlying brain injury. Scalp injuries were discussed earlier in the chapter.

A second class of blows might be those that are produced by larger, more massive objects, moving at the same or higher velocities when striking the head and thus possessing much more kinetic energy and momentum. This energy, as before, would have to be dissipated in some manner. Considerable amounts of energy are absorbed by the scalp and by the skull during its in-bending, and some may be spent into the brain by generating movements within it. If the energy of such a blow is such that it does not significantly accelerate the head but does indent the skull, injuries may be seen in the brain immediately underlying the impact site, the impact site being identified by superficial lacerations or abrasions and by the presence of subgaleal hematomas. Precisely how the underlying brain is injured is still subject to controversy but may be the result of shear strains, in-bending the skull, or vibration of the deformed skull, which may cause alternating positive and negative pressures locally with or without cavitation. Mechanisms aside, the classically observed lesion in such an impact is a single or multiple, more or less cone-shaped lesion with its base facing the skull and its apex facing into the brain, as illustrated in Figure 6.58. Recognizing that time is required to develop such a lesion and that there are definite phases of evolution, as discussed above, the classic blow lesion lies along the perpendicular axis of the blow. It may be confined to the cortex and appear as only a slight contusion with little other than capillary bleeding or as a much larger, deeper lesion with extensive hemorrhage and necrosis, extending into the subcortical white matter. In infants, whose skulls are malleable, some of these generalizations do not apply.

Generally, there is good empirical correlation between the degree of injury sustained and the mass/velocity relationship (momentum) of the impacting object. Objects that produce injuries as described may include conduit or steel pipe of 1 in diameter or less, a policeman's night stick, a soft drink or beer bottle, a tightly clenched fist or hand edge in a karate blow, a pistol barrel or butt, or any other instruments. These include some of the most common weapons employed for the purpose of striking the head in fights and confrontations. Owing to the diversity of the objects and the variability of force and velocity applied to such a blow, the injuries are highly variable.

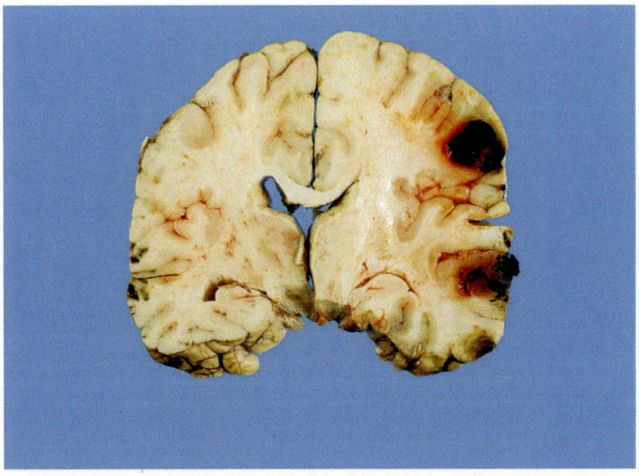

Figure 6.58 This photograph of a coronal section of brain from a victim of a beating with a heavy object, quite possibly a baseball bat, illustrates two lateral hemorrhagic lesions on the right side. The upper one appears to be a "ball" hemorrhage beneath the cortex that may be a coup lesion, and the lower one more superficial. There was a lateral skull fracture that may have caused the lower lesion (fracture contusion). Near the inferior lateral portion of the right temporal lobe is another contusion, which may represent a "gliding" contusion from the blow. On the left para-Sylvian region are a group of small contracoup contusions. (Courtesy of Dr. Carol Haller, Office of the Medical Examiner, Cook County, IL.)

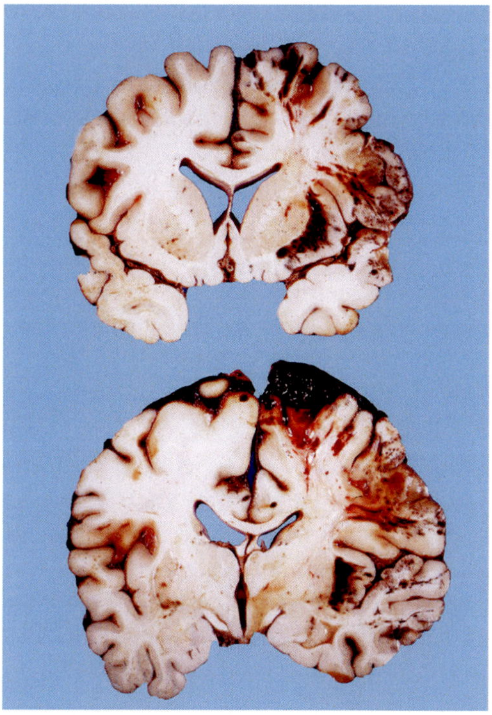

Figure 6.59 These coronal sections of the brain of an individual who was struck on the right side of the head with a "2 × 4" board illustrates extensive coup-type contusions as well as an adherent acute subdural hematoma at the vertex and a number of subcortical contusion hemorrhages. A much less obvious pattern of contracoup contusions is seen on the left side of the brain. Survival was about 24 hours. (Courtesy of Dr. Richard Lindenberg, Office of the Medical Examiner, Baltimore, MD.)

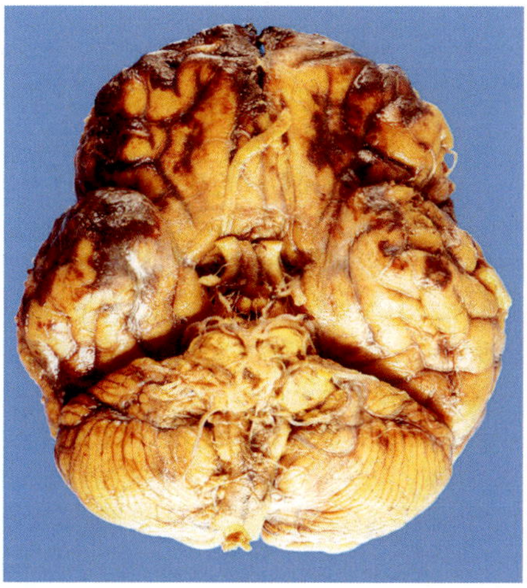

Figure 6.60 This photograph of the base of the brain from a man assaulted by multiple blows to the back of the head with a steel crow bar illustrates the pattern of contrecoup and probably gliding contusions of the frontal and temporal lobes of the brain without much evidence of injury to the posterior cerebellum or occipital lobes. Such "fall-like" blows approximate the kind of injury expected from an occipital fall on a rigid surface. (Courtesy of the Cook County Medical Examiner's Office, Cook County, IL.)

It sometimes happens that in the course of a fall, the head may strike the sharp edge of a nearby object, such as a table edge, a bookshelf, or a sharp object on the ground, such as a bit of broken brick or stone. In this event, even though the injury is the result of a fall, some of the injuries may appear as though they were produced by a blow, but they are interval events. These injuries may show a scalp abrasion or laceration, a subgaleal hematoma at the site of impact, and contusional lesions immediately in the underlying brain with no sign of contrecoup contusion, with or without skull fracture. In isolation, with no historical or circumstantial information, these injuries may be very difficult to interpret with certainty, and often one can say no more than that the injuries appear consistent with a blow or at least an impact with an edged object by an unknown means. Associated injuries, toxicology, and witness accounts, however developed, are very useful in resolving such troublesome interpretations. By the same token, when witness accounts provide information that seems at variance with the injuries observed, this information, when fed back to law enforcement officers and investigators, can yield the truth from witnesses or suspects who are confronted with evidence at variance with their "story."

A third class of blow-type impact might involve objects whose momentum overcomes the inertia of the head and accelerates it (Figures 6.60 and 6.61). Impacts of this type include blows with baseball bats, cricket bats, weighted or lead-filled pipes or homemade saps, bits of lumber (a two-by-four), a club, a metallic baton such as an "ASP," a crow bar, or a heavy multicell flashlight, which is commonly carried by law enforcement personnel. When violently swung against the head, these objects are capable of delivering enough force to the head to deform the skull and accelerate the head in such a manner that the forces involved approximate those encountered in falls. These types of impacts, even though they are blows and are supposed to produce only coup contusions (at the site of impact), may produce both coup and contrecoup contusions, or contrecoup contusions only, with or without skull fractures. In general, when the skull is fractured, there is a tendency for a lesser degree of contusion of both coup and contrecoup types, although fracture contusions may be produced (discussed below).

These fall-like blows, like the paradoxical blow-like falls mentioned above, can be troublesome to interpret or explain to laypersons. Such cases may involve very different outcomes, depending on how they are described in the final report or on the death certificate, and might be classified as accidental, suicidal, or, more likely, homicidal manners of death. Additional information, such as witness accounts, observations of the scene, associated injuries, and toxicological data, as well as circumstantial evidence of the victim and his or her surroundings, may be vital in resolving such difficult interpretations. Examples of difficult situations in which these issues arise are altercations where no appropriate weapon is found, but the victim may have been pushed or fallen against a protruding object and not willfully struck; situations in which a large vehicle with a protruding external rearview mirror or other object may possibly have struck the victim in passing; and events on a construction site when a swinging or dropped object of sufficient mass and velocity may have accidentally struck the victim. In these cases, inspection of the scene and careful questioning of witnesses may provide information that allows a solution to the interpretation.

A fourth form of blow-type impact injury involves two circumstances: when the velocity and mass of the object are very large compared with the inertia of the head and when the head is struck with an object whose momentum is equal to or larger than the inertia of the head but the head is fixed (by resting against a firm surface) or otherwise immobilized at the time of impact, producing what amounts to an almost-static loading or crush scenario. These situations may result in what might seem paradoxical injuries: shattering of the skull with comparatively little bruising, coup or contrecoup, of the brain; and perhaps no loss of consciousness due to the impact. In this case, the skull is broken very early in the event to such a degree that forces are likely to be centrifugal rather than centripetal, and shear forces or negative pressures never have a chance to develop and produce brain injury. Some very strange and rare examples of this extreme form of injury may even cause the brain to be thrown completely clear of the cranium in a remarkably intact state.

Other unusual circumstances in which blows may bring about brain injuries other than typical surface coup contusions may be seen when a heavy object such as a board or a heavy book is used to strike the top of the head, when an impact strikes the head tangentially, or when an impact occurs at the lower jaw such that the mandibular condyles are driven upward through the base of the skull and directly injure the brain. Such instances are rare and are only fleetingly mentioned in the literature [35]. In the former instances, no surface contusion may be seen but, rather, a spectrum of lesions that resemble those of so-called inner cerebral trauma [295] or contrecoup lesions most commonly associated with fall-type impacts. These lesions often involve inner cerebral contusions or shearing injuries to the corpus callosum, subcortical white matter hemorrhages, avulsions of the choroid plexus, hemorrhages into the tela choroidea, and even basal contrecoup contusions [239]. Most of these lesions are illustrated in figures to follow. The importance of these unusual forms of impact injury is that they may cause the forensic pathologist confusion in interpretation. Furthermore, especially in choroid plexus avulsions and tela choroidea hemorrhages, there may only be intraventricular and subarachnoid hemorrhage and no obvious contusion. In such a case, the fatal event may be intraventricular hemorrhage. A careful dissection of the brain will usually show some small intraparenchymal hemorrhage at the root of the plexus where the avulsion took place or may include laceration of the septum pellucidum with rupture of septal veins. These lesions have only occasionally been mentioned in the literature in spite of the fact that they occur with regularity on any active forensic pathology service. In such injuries, there has probably been significant in-bending or distortion of the skull such that shear forces and other mechanisms produce the lesions. Unfortunately, no experimental models of these types of impacts have been reported, and thus any suggested mechanism must remain hypothetical.

Pathological Appearances of Blow-Type Lesions

The classic coup contusion is found over the exposed cerebral or cerebellar hemispheres and not at the base of the brain or in the midline because it is produced by direct action of the force of the blow, probably by in-bending of the skull at the point of impact and its associated effects. The earliest and most subtle contusion (short interval between injury and death) is a microvascular or capillary hemorrhage, which may appear as a focal discoloration or bruise on the surface of the cortex, usually at the crown of a gyrus. The contusions from such a blow may extend only a short distance into the brain, with the broad base of the cone of contusion lying in the gray matter and fading into the white matter, or may be somewhat diffuse on one side, with or without accompanying subcortical hemorrhages (Figures 6.58 and 6.60). It must be borne in mind that the evolution, and thus the appearance, of a coup contusion at autopsy is dependent on the length of survival. With the passage of time, coup contusions, like contracoup contusions, undergo necrotizing changes and then repair reactions, which have been studied by many investigators using

This mode of neural injury has a long history. Many observers, primarily neurosurgeons, recognized that victims of closed head trauma often remained unconscious for prolonged periods after nonmissile head injuries. In the period before artificial ventilation, if the victim was not able to breathe on his or her own, survival was limited; however, with the advent of life support methods, there were comparatively few impediments to sustaining head-injured comatose patients indefinitely. This permitted many investigations, both clinical and pathological, into why these persons remained unconscious and, when or if they awakened, what caused the often-profound neurological and cognitive deficits they experienced. Another population of patients were those who did not suffer a major brain injury but who, in effect, suffered many smaller brain injuries in the course of their amateur or professional careers as prizefighters. The studies of Strich [321–323] of the brains of such individuals led to the observation that often-profound loss of deep white matter axons and other pathologies that sometimes resembled Alzheimer's disease pathology might be responsible for the "punch drunk" state of these people. It was perhaps the rather profound axonal loss and related demyelination of the deep white matter that gave rise to the rather unfortunate term *diffuse axonal injury* (DAI), which has evolved considerably since it was first popularized by Adams and his coworkers [256]. The term diffuse implies lesions everywhere. It would perhaps have been more appropriate to use the term disseminated or multifocal to describe the axonal pathology observed.

A number of systematic studies of human pathological material relevant to inner brain trauma have been made, the most notable of which are the studies by Adams et al. [252–256] in Scotland and the very careful analysis of 66 cases of fatal human brain trauma conducted by Grcevič [251] in Yugoslavia. In Grcevič's study, all cases were victims of closed head trauma, whose span of survival after trauma (mostly traffic or pedestrian accidents) varied from essentially 0 to 846 days. The brains of these victims were studied with large windowpane paraffin sections, and the lesions seen were correlated with the sites of presumed impact (frontal, vertex, occipital, or lateral) and the types of forces that acted on the brain (linear translation or rotational) as judged by external injuries, observations by police or other witnesses, and the period of survival. If these cases are grouped into those whose brains suffered an anterior–posterior form of acceleration (so-called centroaxial trauma) and those who did not, the majority of victims (more than 90%) had the former. The survival spans were divided into the following groups: 0–1 hours, 1–24 hours, 1–4 days, 5–14 days, 15–29 days, 30–89 days, and those who survived 90 days or more. In general, the distribution of cases was nearly similar, with about 12% of the case population in each group. The only exception was a larger number of persons who died 5–14 days postinjury (about 25%).

The locations of macroscopic and microscopic lesions, as discerned from whole-brain microscopic sections, showed the following. Frontal, vertex, and occipital (centroaxial) impacts had the most extensive distribution of lesions, whereas lateral impacts appeared to be more selective, and virtually all centroaxial traumas showed midline or paramedian pathology. The most frequently affected areas were the corpus callosum, septum pellucidum, fornix, tela choroidea, paraventricular areas (paraventricular complex), and hippocampal area (hippocampal complex) [251,301]. In the early deaths, the lesions reported by Grcevič [251] took the form of hemorrhagic lesions (streak, petechial, or ball hemorrhages), but in later deaths they were lytic, cavitated, rarified, gliotic, or demyelinated. Many affected areas contained siderophages. With the pattern of inner cerebral trauma, Grcevič [251,295] also includes the diffuse paraventricular lesions of the white matter described originally by Strich [321,323]. The spectrum of inner cerebral trauma is illustrated in Figures 6.64 and 6.65.

From whole subserially examined brains with varying survival times, Grcevič interpreted the diffuse white matter changes as an extension of the paraventricular complex of lesions, which are due to deformation of the ventricular system and laterolateral stretching of the brain when the impacting forces acted along the longest diameter of the skull (fronto-occipital or occipitofrontal) and caused bulging outward of the lateral aspects of the skull according to the concept of Lindenberg [129,130] and Unterharnscheidt and Sellier [246]. According to Grcevič, these diffuse changes are the ultimate sequelae of pathological processes that occurred acutely at a specific focus (epicenter) and radiated outward as a sort of traumatic penumbra, forming a zone in which damage had greater and greater potential for reversibility the farther away from the epicenter that it appeared. The studies of Grcevič give evidence that within the epicenter zone of primary injury, many of the irreversible lesions of inner cerebral trauma (disruptions of axons, synapses, capillaries, and other vessels) are limited to this zone and that in periepicentric areas recovery of integrity of structure and function may take place. This vasocentric theory has been largely ignored by proponents of the primary axonal injury aspects of inner cerebral injury, although there is much to merit its inclusion in the collective of this complex form of neurotrauma.

Secondary factors, such as edema, hypoxia, microvascular ischemia, and probably a host of other phenomena acting within this zone, influence the reversibility of any of the injuries sustained and may lead to the perception of diffuse white matter damage, when in reality the basis of such apparently diffuse lesions is actually focal and secondary factors to which the brain was exposed during the posttraumatic period caused expansion of the lesions. In chronic cases—those that survive more than 90 days—the process of demyelination and sclerosis of the white matter shows a clear image of fanning out from the most affected periventricular regions toward the subcortical until eventually normal tissue prevails (see Figure 6.67). In the areas of the brain that contain long tracts or long commissures, as in the brain stem, corpus callosum, or internal capsule, the axonal swellings and

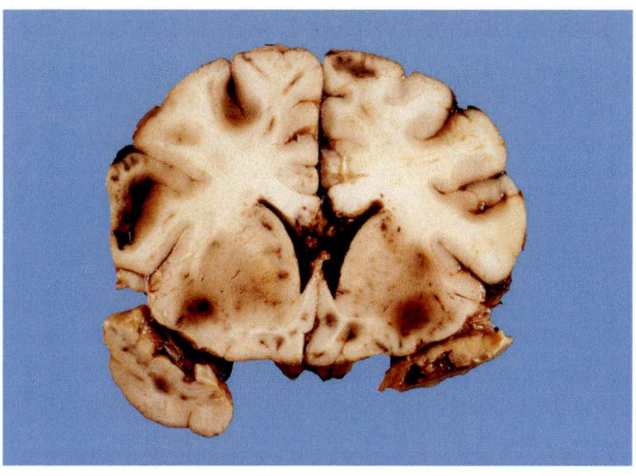

Figure 6.67 This coronal section of the brain of the victim of closed head injury from a vehicular accident illustrates the multifocal character of the lesions in inner cerebral trauma ranging from streak and ball hemorrhages in cortex and subcortex and smaller lesions throughout the basal ganglia as well as the lesion of the corpus callosum that included a septum tear and intraventricular hemorrhage. (Courtesy of Dr. Carol Haller, Office of the Medical Examiner, Cook County, IL.)

retraction bulbs may be encountered long distances away from the traumatic epicenter, as demonstrated by silver stains and now by immunochemical methods such as β-app [316,329]. It appears that such lesions are due to stretching rather than shearing forces, as envisioned in laterolateral stretching of the corpus callosum in frontal or occipital impacts of the head and in long tracts of the brain stem in centroaxial injuries, as described by Lindenberg [129,130].

To place these reactions in a proper perspective, it is appropriate to recall briefly the physiological processes involved in axonal transport, which is where the pathology of axonal injury is played out (earlier in the chapter). These pathologies all involve the cytoskeleton [330,331]. Axonal ballooning may be observed, according to some, within 90 minutes [332], within a few hours of injury [315] to between 24 and 48 hours postinjury [317], and they may persist by silver staining methods for many years. Most workers now have abandoned the many silver staining methods for axons in favor of immunochemical preparation that detects β-app and other proteins carried by axonal transport [318,319]. Other molecular tags have also been employed such as neuron-specific enolase (NSE) [332], anti-neurofilament [333], anti-ubiquitin [334] and other immunostaining methods. To repeat an element of an earlier discussion of the diagnosis of axonal injury, there are many confounding variables to the interpretation of axonal stains that must include the almost inevitable hypoxia/ischemia and increased intracranial pressure that attends virtually every head injury case. These secondary phenomena can mimic true traumatic axonal injury as Oehmichen et al. [241] have pointed out. A great deal of controversy has found its way into the courts with regard to the interpretation of β-app staining [318,335–340]. The controversies center about the specificity of β-app staining for its mechanism (physical forces vs. hypoxia/ischemia and other chemical factors); what the time window for the development of the changes is; are there "diagnostic" patterns or distributions of β-app staining that can offer specificity and differentiate between physical force injury and something else? Another issue about alleged axonal injury is what are the minimal forces or kinematics that can produce axonal pathology? Can axonal pathology be present in someone who was not unconscious or perhaps even symptomatic? Can axonal injury be diagnosed using CT or MRI technologies in the early postinjury period?

With regard to specificity and differentiation issues for β-app staining, virtually all authors of papers on the subject issue cautionary statements about interpretations and the confounding effects of parallel processes such as hypoxia/ischemia, cerebral edema, etc., which are all encountered in the head-injured patient [317,342–345]. Perhaps the most complete and careful study regarding the interpretations of axonal injury using β-app staining was the essentially double-blinded study of Oehmichen et al. [241]. In this study, 252 brain specimens were examined systematically using 119 fatal nonmissile closed head injury cases, 30 gunshot fatalities, 51 cases of fatal hypoxia/ischemia, 14 cases with brain death due to mechanical trauma and 18 with nonmechanical injury, and 20 with hemorrhagic shock. They found that 65%–100% of all cases of closed head injury, fatal brain hypoxia/ischemia, and brain death with a survival of more than 3 hours had axonal pathology. The hemorrhagic shock cases did not show axonal injury. Further, a statistically significant difference between traumatic and non-trauma-induced brain injury could not be demonstrated. Also there was no correlation between axonal injury and the different types of external forces involved. The authors concluded: "...biomechanical inferences for reconstruction purposes are not possible." These authors also pointed out that β-app positivity was an indicator of vitality apparently requiring at least 3 hours of vital signs, however altered, to be expressed.

Oehmichen and his colleagues conducted another study [316], examining the pons in another series of head-injured victims compared with a similar group with hypoxic/ischemic brain damage using β-app. Again it was concluded that "...beta-APP expression in the pons is a reliable indicator of AI (axonal injury) but does not discriminate between injuries caused by traumatic strain or shearing mechanisms and secondary damage due to cerebral hypoxia–ischemia or edema."

These two studies of Oehmichen et al. challenge assertions made by others [337–342,346,347] in print as well as in court testimony that not only can traumatic axonal injury be discriminated from hypoxia/ischemia and edema, but that a specific mechanism for the supposed axonal injury could be inferred. It seems clear that these issues are far from settled; thus, the applications of the technologies to assess axonal injury in the forensic situation leave much to be desired.

It appears the window in time during which physical forces acting on axons separate from hypoxia/ischemia may be very small (no earlier than 30 minutes after injury and possibly no longer than a few hours post injury). Further, if 90 minutes or perhaps less is needed after injury to develop axonal swellings, and "fast" axonal anterograde transport proceeds at 200 mm/day or 8.33 mm/h, the locus of pathology at 90 minutes postinjury will be possibly about 12 mm in extent, perhaps less. The geometry of the physical lesion cannot be known or predicted, thus the chances of finding a highly focal lesion, perhaps in the corpus callosum, may be small. Further, the specific regional blood flow and oxygen tension in the same region after trauma cannot be known, nor can it be easily known when secondary phenomena are operating, such as cerebral blood flow dysfunctions, hypoxia, etc. Potentially, these complex phenomena could be tested and analyzed, but at present, there are too many scientific issues hovering over so-called DAI/TAI so that forensic interpretations must be very conservative and measured or not employed at all.

Many victims of head trauma, young or old, suffer from increased intracranial pressure sufficient to overwhelm vascular autoregulation and eventually give rise to the "respirator brain" phenomenon (see Chapter 5). This phenomenon results from insufficient perfusion pressure and eventual cessation of meaningful cerebral perfusion leading to necrosis of the brain and possibly the upper to middle cervical spinal cord. This process of circulatory embarrassment is not uniform topographically or temporally, which means that possibly "watershed" regions of the brain (junctions of perfusion territories) may be deprived of effective sustaining perfusion ahead of other regions. These uneven deficits may result in persistent, although dysfunctional, electrical activity rather than an electrically silent brain, which can observed in the EEG [348,349] in deeply comatose and nonbreathing patients. This means also that some territories in the brain may suffer ischemic/hypoxic damage while others are functional as the "respirator" brain phenomenon evolves. This also means that axons within those territories most likely have disruptions in their axonal transport process, which can be manifested by focal accumulation of proteins such as β-app. These focal disruptions can occur at several places along an axon of long passage such as an axon passing from one cortical area across the corpus callosum to a cortical or other area in the opposite hemisphere until the entire axoplasmic transport process stops. Any axon of long passage may be similarly affected (axons from motor areas in the cortex to the brain stem or below or axons from one cerebellar hemisphere to the other). The importance of this is that what may appear to be axonal injury due to physical forces may in fact be due to local metabolic disturbances.

With respect to the threshold for axonal injury due to physical forces, the work of Ommaya et al. in several publications [192,253,266,267] established a number of parameters using higher primates. This work was continued at the University of Pennsylvania by Gennarelli, Thibault, and their colleagues [193,254,268,277,287]. Basically, these and other workers found that 60-degree sagittal accelerations were tolerated better than 60-degree lateral (side-to-side) accelerations produced by a mechanical device that did not employ percussion–impact from clinical–neurological as well as neuropathological perspectives. It was found that in the rhesus monkey, angular accelerations of 40,000 rad/s^2 yielded >99% chance of concussion. Using a mass-scaling paradigm, it was determined that in an adult human male, about 7500 rad/s^2 was required to yield the same >99% chance of concussion. For a 50% chance of concussion, about 10,000 rad/s^2 was required for rhesus monkeys and was imputed to be about 1200 rad/s^2 for an adult human [253,261] and somewhat less than 10,000 rad/s^2 for a human infant [283]. Experiments determined that acceleration times (pulse duration) in the monkey were generally in the range of 7–12 ms [283] and using observations for adult humans, a somewhat longer pulse duration (about 20 ms). When physical impacts against unyielding surfaces were modeled, accelerations were much more pronounced, reaching 170,000 rad/s^2 with pulse durations of about 5 ms [300].

To put these observations in perspective, a number of model injury scenarios have been studied. Manual human shaking of instrumented models for infant human head accelerations, by Duhaime et al. [26] and Prange et al. [27], found that accelerations of 1100–2600 rad/s^2 and pulse durations of 100–200 ms were attainable, making the shaking action unlikely to cause axonal injury. Other potential injury scenarios have been modeled, including drops to a typical crib mattress and other typical mattress surfaces [300,350]. These studies have shown that acceleration at impact, associated pulse duration, and *g* forces are well below those that would be expected to cause brain damage; thus, the determinants of injury are velocity at impact, the impact surface rigidity, the acceleration in three planes at impact, and mass and other characteristics of the head.

The question of whether axonal injury can occur in an individual who has apparently suffered a head injury yet experienced no loss of consciousness is a thorny question, especially in view of the recent attention being paid to professional athletes (boxers, football players, hockey players, etc.) that suffer repeated apparent concussion [13,22,23,351–355]. It seems abundantly clear that such scenarios do damage the brain and result in cognitive decline, behavioral alterations, and other higher-order neurological dysfunction in the victims, often many years after the incidents. Precisely what the tolerance limits for repeated concussive events are have yet to be determined, nor have the specific physical injuries that have occurred with each event.

Pathology of Brain Stem Injury

In the extensive study of human brain and brain stem trauma by Grcevič and his coworkers [251,295], it is abundantly clear that, just as in the cerebrum [356], in the brain stem there are many favored sites for small traumatic epicenters, many of which can be recognized on CT scans retrospectively, and include punctate lesions in the superior colliculi, in the brachium conjunctivum, about the cerebral aqueduct and edges of the upper fourth

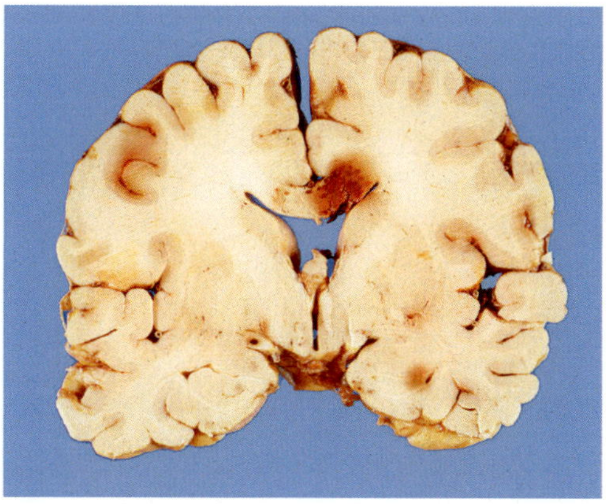

Figure 6.68 This photograph of a coronal section of the brain from a 40-year-old woman, a victim of an apparent hit-and-run vehicular accident, illustrates another example of inner cerebral trauma with a prominent hemorrhagic lesion in the corpus callosum. The victim apparently suffered an impact to the right side of the head, causing a mandibular fracture and relatively small bilateral subdural hemorrhages but no skull fracture. The victim was on ventilation support for 12 days before she died. (Courtesy of Dr. Shaku Teas, Office of the Medical Examiner, Cook County, IL.)

ventricle, in the midline reticular formation, and at the junctions of the cerebral peduncles with the midbrain. Pontine lesions are also common, as in Figure 6.69. In early deaths, the lesions take the form of small hemorrhagic lesions (streak, petechial, or ball hemorrhages), which may be visualized in CT and MRI scans if the viewer appreciates that such lesions exist. In more chronic cases, where death occurs later, brain stem lesions are lytic, cavitated–rarified, gliotic, or demyelinated, many of which contain siderophages. The traumatic penumbra effect seen clearly in the cerebral injuries is less evident in the brain stem, but probably the same principles apply. These patterns of injuries have been seen in other human neuropathological studies and in higher animal models of brain trauma [193,252,254,259,357,358].

The mechanisms for brain stem lesions appear more related to downward displacement, as described by Lindenberg and Freytag [359], than lateral displacement in the cerebrum. Some correlation and support for this notion can be found when the types of impacts are related to the severity of brain stem injuries. For instance, lesser stem injury was sustained in lateral cranial impacts and resulted in longer survivals than in the centroaxial types of trauma. Brain stem lesions may be missed or neglected because they are not as large or obvious as lesions in the cortex, but their importance is much greater functionally than that of cerebral lesions. In terms of clinical symptomatology, it goes without saying that lesions in this region, and especially those involving the reticular formation, would have profound impact on the state of consciousness of a head trauma victim and logically account for the prolonged deep coma that many such victims suffer [181,252,259,360]. Precisely how the brain stem receives perhaps a disproportionate degree of trauma as compared with other areas is not clear, but because it is the point at which all neural structures impinge before exit from the cranium, it must represent a focus for stretching, torsional, and oscillatory movements. Similarly, as the brain moves with an impact, the upper brain stem may be driven into the tentorial notch or otherwise vibrate against it, causing flexion or stretching. These movements probably exert strains on axons and vessels that will ultimately produce

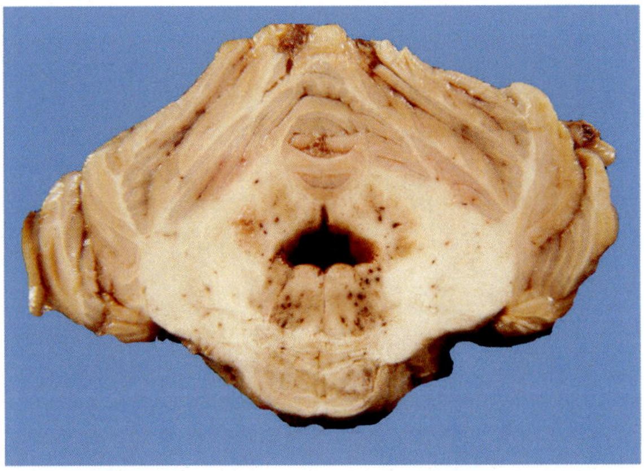

Figure 6.69 This section of the cerebellum and pons from the case in Figure 6.65 illustrates multiple punctate hemorrhages and general congestion about the fourth ventricle and pontine tegmentum. The damage to the reticular formation explains why such individuals are deeply comatose and will likely remain that way until they die. (Courtesy of Dr. Carol Haller, Office of the Medical Examiner, Cook County, IL.)

lesions or in some extreme hyperextension (whiplash) or rotatory movements of the neck may actually avulse the pons from the midbrain, the pons from the medulla, or the medulla from the upper cervical cord (see Figures 6.72 and 6.73) [108,359].

As with any traumatic lesion in the brain, the gross appearance changes with time and the period in which vital signs are present. If survival lasted several hours or days, petechial hemorrhages in the tectum and tegmentum are often the most typical (Figure 6.69). At times, the lesions will be more severe and widespread [358]. These lesions age or are modified by the effects of herniation due to expanding lesions (edema, subdural or epidural hematoma, intracerebral hematoma) in the brain, which may cause Duret hemorrhages

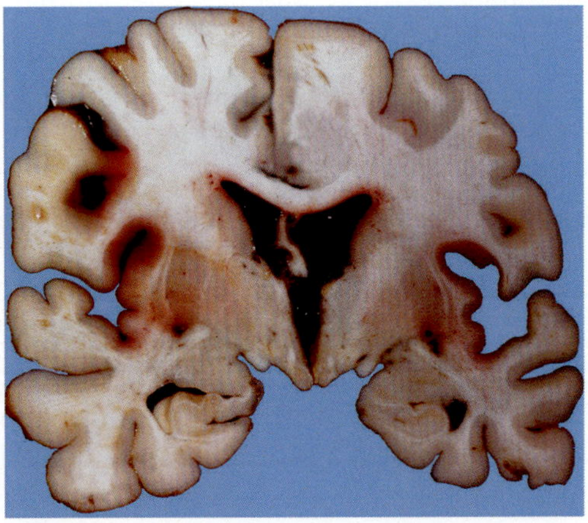

Figure 6.70 This coronal section of the brain of a vehicle–pedestrian accident illustrates an intraventricular hemorrhage due to avulsion of the choroid plexus–tela choroidea. In many such cases, the impact appeared to involve, at least in part, a tangential impact (side-swipe) of the vehicle with the victim. There was no skull fracture and no subdural hematoma present. The individual died within a few hours in hospital while in deep coma. (Courtesy of the Office of the Medical Examiner, Cook County, IL.)

that overshadow the underlying primary traumatic pathology. If Duret hemorrhages are not present, the petechial lesions may fade and become less apparent grossly and may eventually in time become very difficult, if not impossible, to observe grossly. However, microscopically there are often many lesions visible [35,360,361]. These are especially well illustrated in myelin-stained preparations (Figure 6.71) or preparations that highlight gliosis, such as the Holzer stain, the immunochemical stain GFAP, and the various axon stains (Bodian, β-app, etc.). Typical examples of challenging cases are those who have remained in a comatose state long after their injury yet seem to have little pathology to account for the prolonged coma. Studies in these individuals will usually show neuronal loss and gliosis, glial stars (inflammatory nodules), and evidence of axonal damage (ballooning or retraction balls) in the reticular formation of the midbrain and upper pons [251,295,310,316,322].

Traumatic Pontomedullary and Cervicomedullary Avulsion

In the course of the practice of forensic neuropathology, especially in cases of trauma, one will occasionally observe that the pons and medulla have become partially or completely separated or that the cervicomedullary junction may show the same lesion (see Figures 6.72 and 6.73). Such lesions have been described in the literature for many years [108,359,362,363] but still somehow are often rejected as artifacts of brain removal by many pathologists and neuropathologists. A careful analysis of many cases reveals several important observations that characterize the lesions and the circumstances under which they occur. In Lindenberg and Freytag's series [359], most victims were automobile drivers or passengers. In the author's unpublished series from the Cook County Medical Examiner in Chicago, although there were a number of automobile drivers and passengers who were victims of this lesion, most were pedestrians struck by vehicles. An analysis of the accidents in both instances indicates that most victims were struck from the rear or in such a

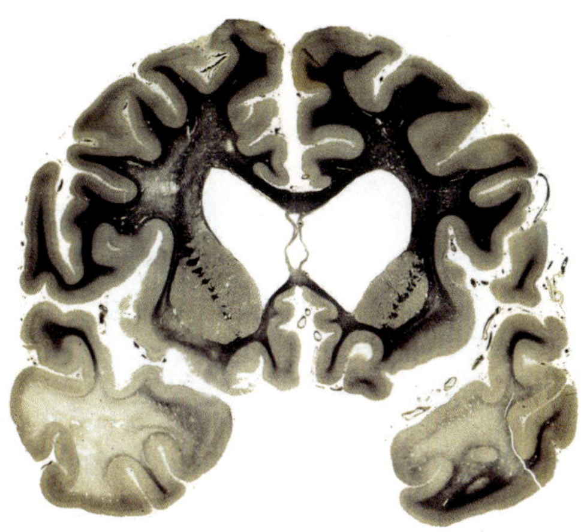

Figure 6.71 This "window pane" celloidin section stained with the Woelcke myelin stain illustrates myelin pallor most pronounced in the temporal lobes and to a lesser extent in the centrum ovale and other regions. There is also hydrocephalus *ex vacuo*. This man, a truck driver, apparently fell asleep and crashed into a bridge viaduct. There was no skull fracture or subdural hematoma. The victim was deeply comatose but eventually recovered to some degree but remained neurologically incapacitated for 2 years, finally dying of pneumonia. (Courtesy of Ms. Dolores Janis and the Departments of Pathology and Neurology, Veterans Administration Hospital, North Chicago, Illinois.)

with other signs of brain trauma such as satellite streak or ball hemorrhages or surface contusions. Collateral evidence in the general autopsy of hypertensive disease or the lack thereof may also be helpful. On rare occasions, unequivocal interpretations are not possible.

Delayed Posttraumatic Apoplexy

Sometimes referred to as *Spät Apoplexie* in the German literature, or more recently as delayed traumatic intracerebral hemorrhage (DTICH), and first described by Bollinger in 1891 [364], the syndrome refers to the sudden, often fatal, intracerebral hemorrhage in an individual who has sustained head trauma, even minor in character, after a symptom-free interval of a few days, weeks, or even months. The usual interval in suspected cases is within 1–2 weeks of the injury [365]. There should be no evidence of underlying vascular disease to explain the bleeding, and the site of hemorrhage may be in the deep white matter anywhere in the brain, in the brain stem, or even involving the subarachnoid space. Two possibilities are said classically to exist for the origin of the hemorrhage: that an intracerebral vessel was injured on impact and was weakened or surrounded by a small, clinically silent ischemic or hemorrhagic lesion; or that a vessel of the circle of Willis or other surface portion of the brain was injured by shearing forces, producing an intimal/medial tear that subsequently dissected and formed a pseudoaneurysm, or ruptures [366,367]. The latter phenomenon has been extensively reviewed by Krauland and Maxeiner [368,369]. Another very reasonable etiology is unsuspected underlying cerebral vascular amyloid disease [370–372] that resulted in a weakened vessel bed that trauma might have affected; however, one can never know if a traumatic event interacted in any way with this natural disease process.

The issue of delayed brain hemorrhage in the context of trauma regularly occurs in the forensic arena and is often the subject of personal injury litigation. A practical means of evaluating such cases has been suggested by Lindenberg and Freytag [129] and includes a very careful review of the history of the victim, including any history of hypertension, vascular disease, diabetes, and the like. Attention should be paid to anything that may have happened to the victim during the symptom-free interval, and the circumstances of the alleged injury must be investigated with care. A careful neuropathological examination must involve a search for evidence of or lack of vascular disease and the location of the hemorrhage compared with any traumatic lesions that may be present. Because the stress of an injury may lead to fat embolization or thromboembolism from preexisting atheroma in the neck of great vessels or the heart, these sites must be examined as part of a careful and thorough systemic autopsy. Sometimes trauma to a neck vessel or the heart may cause an intimal tear that subsequently thromboses or embolizes to the brain and can be mistaken for *in situ* posttraumatic apoplexy. Potential cases should also be stained for amyloid. DTICH remains a controversial entity.

Traumatic Injury to Cerebral Vessels

As has been previously mentioned, injuries to the neck and head can result in damage to arteries or veins. The consequences of this damage may be immediate and due to avulsion, tearing with bleeding, or injury that leads to thrombosis, dissection, or obstruction, with the potential for pseudoaneurysm formation, which is uncommon or delayed, as discussed above. Beyond the context of dural and subdural hemorrhages, intracranial arterial injuries are more common than venous ones. Krauland [369] has explored this subject intensively and demonstrated, via painstaking dissections, the spectrum of arterial injuries. Several circumstances involving primary vascular injury not infrequently have forensic importance. These are traumatic arteriovenous fistulas, injuries to neck vessels in connection with chiropractic manipulation [373–376], and traumatic avulsion of branches of the circle of Willis with massive subarachnoid hemorrhage.

Arteriovenous fistulas may form after penetrating injuries of the neck or head, or complex basilar fractures may occur in which both an artery and vein, usually in proximity, are injured and a fistula forms. This can occur within the cavernous sinus, in the dura, or in the spine [377–379]. Many of these lesions can be treated endovascularly by embolization or insertion of coils. The consequence of fistulas may be hemorrhage or some element of heart failure due to the high flow character of the lesion.

Injuries to the Circle of Willis and Basal Vessels

Issues over injuries caused by inexpert chiropractic manipulation, chiefly of the neck, have been noted over many years [373,375,376]. These injuries may result in vertebral arterial damage or direct injury to the cord. Vascular damage can occur by causing an intimal tear that either dissects or thromboses the vessel, perhaps leading to a stroke or embolization.

Avulsions or tear of circle of Willis vessels are not particularly common, but when they occur, they will almost always end up on a forensic pathology service with an individual dead of a massive subarachnoid hemorrhage that may at first glance be interpreted as a ruptured aneurysm. Krauland [369,380] reported 37 cases of his and others of individuals who generally sustained a single or multiple blows or impacts to the chin or side of the face. This author collected 28 additional cases from the literature [381–389] and from his own case files. Of the 67 victims reviewed, only 5 were females. The average age was 36 years and the range in ages was 15–76 years. The circumstances of the traumatic events most commonly involved a physical altercation, most commonly involving one or more blows with a fist, and sometimes kicks to the face or side of the head. The victims usually became unconscious immediately or rapidly. Most did not respond to resuscitative efforts either at the scene or during transport to a medical facility. Some victims survived in a comatose state for a day or two before dying. Autopsy usually revealed bruises and sometimes lacerations of the face, often on one side, with or without fractures of the zygoma, jaw, or base of the skull. The presence of alcohol in the blood was very common. All had basal subarachnoid hemorrhage, and many also showed intraventricular hemorrhage. The patterns of arterial injuries are displayed graphically in Figure 6.74. Precise localization of arterial tears, splits, and avulsions was often not reported, although most reports stated that no aneurysms were found.

While most of the cases reviewed reported that the injurious incident was witnessed, actual recording by video or photography of the traumatic event has not been reported. The following two case examples appear to be unique, in that in one a video was made with a phone camera and in the other, a surveillance camera captured the fatal attack [390].

Case 1: A 25-year-old man at a party challenged several of the women there to hit him, maintaining they could not "knock him out." A young woman accepted the challenge and struck the man on the left side of the face with her balled right fist. The phone-cam video taken by one of the party attendees and collected by the police clearly shows the blow to

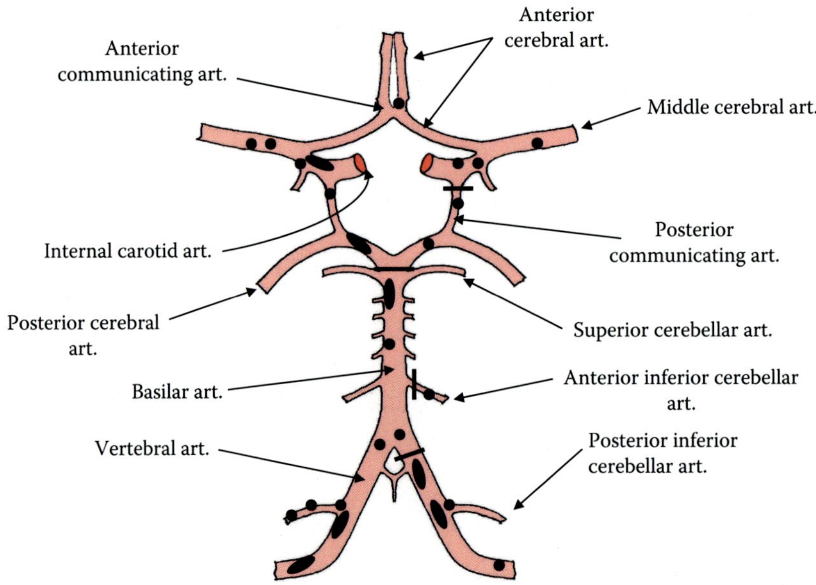

Figure 6.74 This diagrammatic representation of the basal arteries of the brain (circle of Willis) illustrate locations and types of reported injuries to the arteries in 67 reported cases that usually involved one or two impacts to the head, usually blows with a fist. In virtually all of these cases, the victim collapsed quickly and generally was dead before they reached hospital. All had basal subarachnoid hemorrhages. Round dark circles indicate the approximate location of an unspecified injury. Dashed lines indicate where a total avulsion of a vessel occurred. Dark ovals indicate where a longitudinal tear in the wall of the vessel occurred. Data were collected from Krauland [369,380] and from other authors' reports [381–389].

have twisted the victim's head to the right. The victim appeared stunned but remained upright for about a minute then collapsed. It was determined that he had ceased breathing shortly thereafter. Resuscitative attempts at the scene were begun and continued by emergency personnel, and upon arrival at hospital, but were abandoned when the victim did not respond. Autopsy revealed the victim to weigh 140 lb and to be 68 in. tall. The lungs weighed 790 and 1110 g and the heart was 370 g with no underlying pathology. Blood alcohol was 15 mg/dl, and there were cannabis metabolites detected. There was no subdural hemorrhage or skull fracture. The base of the brain is shown in Figure 6.75. The site of arterial injury was probably on the left side of the medulla consistent with vertebral or posterior inferior cerebellar artery avulsion–tear [390].

Case 2: A 44-year-old man who was walking on a railroad station platform in the north of Germany was struck on the right side of his face–neck in an unprovoked attack by an intoxicated assailant who was unknown to him. The victim fell to the pavement and died in hospital 10 hours later without regaining consciousness. The events of the attack were recorded on a surveillance camera. Autopsy revealed only a basal subarachnoid hemorrhage and intraventricular hemorrhage. No subdural hemorrhage or skull fracture was noted. No other significant pathology was reported. The site of arterial injury was at the dural entrance of the left internal carotid artery shown in Figure 6.76 [390].

Regarding the mechanisms for the observed arterial injuries in the typical cases, several possibilities have been suggested [380,391–394]: the force of the blow(s) rotated the head on the neck and/or hyperextended the neck, resulting in torsion of the basal vessels,

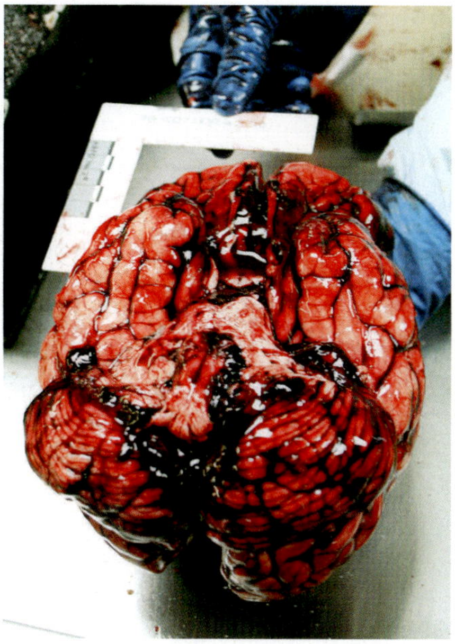

Figure 6.75 This photograph is of the unfixed base of the brain of a young man struck with one forceful blow to the side of his face by a young woman, as described in text. It appears the basilar and vertebral arteries have been torn away (artifactually), but there appears to be more concentration of blood where the left PICA would have been.

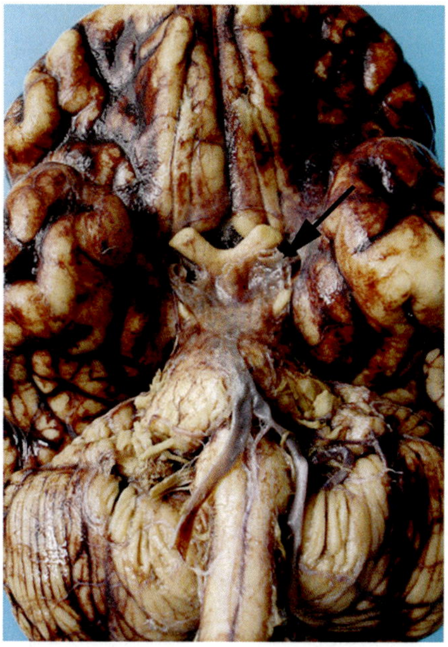

Figure 6.76 The basal surface of the brain in this victim of a single blow to his face while walking on a train platform, as described in the accompanying case example, shows extensive basal subarachnoid hemorrhage. A rent (black arrow) was discovered at the entrance of the left internal carotid artery into the cranial cavity. Microscopic examination showed extensive hemorrhage within the dural sheath at the skull base. (Courtesy of Dr. Andreas Buettner, Rostock, Germany.)

particularly in the vertebro-basilar complex, with tearing or avulsion. Another possible scenario is that the force of the blow(s) involved the lateral neck, which could compress the internal carotid artery possibly sending a pulse of high pressure upward that may rupture a vessel intracranially. Such a mechanism might explain the arterial injuries in the anterior circle of Willis near the carotid entrance. It is also possible that inherent weakness due to inadequacies of the internal elastic lamina in portions of the circle of Willis might render that area vulnerable to not only pressure pulses but also physical forces.

Another aspect of these cases that deserves examination is why the victims die so quickly. In another situation, rupture of an aneurysm, victims may become unconscious rapidly but very often survive to reach hospital and benefit from treatment. Many of these victims also display intraventricular hemorrhage, not from tissue damage but from extension of subarachnoid blood upward via the cerebello–pontine angle foramina. The mechanisms of unconsciousness in acute subarachnoid hemorrhages is thought to involve a rapid rise in intracranial pressure due to arterial hemorrhage into the subarachnoid space and possibly into the ventricles, and the direct toxic effect of blood on the brain and/or ependymal surface or vessels that may go into spasm. In the case of traumatic arterial rupture, the greater percentage of victims have bleeding that involved the lower circle of Willis where blood supply may have been compromised to vital medullary centers of respiratory control (see Chapter 9). Such deprivation could relatively quickly shut down the respiratory drive, leading to a rapid cessation of vital functions.

Only a few experiments regarding the possible injury biomechanics of these arterial injuries have been investigated [391,393]. Another important but separate mechanism might be the posterior head impact on pavement that often accompanies a blow to the face. Such secondary impacts often involve extensive basilar skull fractures ("hinge" fractures) [101]. In backward undefended falls with basilar fractures, it is comparatively uncommon but not unknown to observe vessel avulsions or tears [369].

When one encounters a basal subarachnoid hemorrhage with evidence by witnesses or findings, that an impact occurred on the face, chin, or neck, the autopsy is vital to a proper interpretation of the case. Care must be taken in removing the brain so as not to artifactually tear basal vessels or leave behind those that might have been avulsed or transected by the traumatic event. The brain should be photographed, especially the base of the brain, and then the arachnoid over the base should be carefully stripped away. A gentle stream of water should then be splayed on the vessels to wash away the blood, to hopefully reveal tears or rents in the circle of Willis vessels. If this is not done before fixation, the blood may harden, making dissection later almost impossible. If possible, the tear or rent should be studied histologically with elastic connective tissue stains to reveal elastic lamina injury or deficiencies.

Traumatic Cerebral Edema

Whenever there has been physical cerebral or spinal cord injury, some degree of edema will inevitably occur in the vicinity of the lesion. If one subscribes to the classification of vasogenic and cytotoxic forms of edema (discussed in greater detail in Chapter 5), some disruption of the blood–brain barrier quite early will result in vasogenic or extracellular edema. If this edema is not compensable, its mass and pressure effects may affect vascular perfusion in the region, resulting in secondary ischemia of the region, which will alter metabolism in nearby cells, resulting in cytotoxic or intracellular edema. This form of edema may also be produced by release of neurotoxic products of inflammation or cell injury (cytokines) that alter cell membrane function and may irreversibly damage affected cells, usually neurons. Regardless of which form of edema exists in response to trauma, it may spread well outside the traumatized region and involve the whole hemisphere or the whole brain. In this instance, there is a grave risk of excessive and irreversible increases in intracranial pressure, herniation, and perfusion failure, which may lead to brain death.

Traumatically induced edema, from whatever cause, is always capable of expanding the intrinsic mass effects of any lesion present in the adult; however, in the child who has suffered head trauma, cerebral edema may occur in connection with even apparently mild injury and may lead to death [395,396]. A typical example of this phenomenon may be seen in the child who falls from a window to the pavement or is struck by a vehicle, who may or may not suffer a skull fracture and may or may not suffer loss of consciousness, but within hours of the traumatic episode may become stuporous and drift into coma from elevated intracranial pressure. This phenomenon has been observed for many years by emergency room physicians and neurosurgeons but has not been satisfactorily explained. A possible explanation may lie in the fact that cerebral blood flow in response to injury differs with age. In children under the age of 5 years, impacts to the head may result in increased cerebral blood flow, whereas in the adult the response may be just the opposite [397–400]. With increased blood flow into a possibly damaged vascular bed, the blood–brain barrier may be more likely to open, giving rise to massive edema, which may or may not be fatal. The importance to the pathologist of this phenomenon is when attempting to develop a mechanism for death with the confusing and seemingly inconsistent finding of little evidence of brain trauma in the face of massive edema, with no obvious anatomic cause. Suffice it to say that even though the explanations are not satisfactory, this phenomenon has been observed on a regular basis in forensic pathology practice, and one should not hesitate to assign a traumatic cause to such deaths, even though a lucid interval may have occurred.

In the adult, cerebral edema of a traumatic origin, if long standing, may have deleterious effects on myelin that may lead to demyelination [304]. Altered metabolic states such as prolonged acidosis, or associated conditions such as fat embolism, and the basic nature of shearing forces that might have injured long axons of passage can also be satisfactory explanations for apparent demyelination about contusions or deeper brain lesions; however, some workers feel that at least some of the demyelination observed (discussed above) in some cases is due to edema alone. This contention is difficult to prove or disprove.

Pulmonary Edema in Connection with Head Trauma

In some cases of head trauma, usually severe, the victim may suddenly appear to suffer cardiac failure as evidenced by severe massive pulmonary edema [401]. The basis for this edema appears to have at least some neurogenic component but may interact with other factors, such as disseminated intravascular coagulation, fat embolism, hypovolemic shock, electrolyte disturbances, and thoracic injuries that may also affect myocardial function [402–404]. The mechanisms of so-called neurogenic pulmonary edema are not yet understood, but trauma may not be the only underlying condition giving rise to the phenomenon. An association with epilepsy and the sudden unexpected death in connection with seizures has also been reported [403–407] and is discussed in Chapter 9 [408].

Posttraumatic Demyelination

After any destructive lesion of the cerebral cortex, it is inevitable that there will be some reflection of loss of axonal input to the white matter by pallor of myelin beneath the lesion. This myelin pallor is usually lost as sections are examined at greater and greater distance from the lesion. Often this pattern of pallor is greatest about the ventricles, as described by Grcevič and many others [251], and in other instances the loss is apparently quite diffuse, involving much of the centrum ovale or temporal lobe white matter (see Figure 6.71), and is quite independent of the degree of cortical pathology [181,304,323]. In such cases, the degree of demyelination is so evident that the appearance closely resembles myelin loss as seen in one of the leukodystrophies, with sparing of the subcortical "U" fibers. The basis for this pathological appearance is probably locally extensive axonal injury from shear or stretching forces (traumatic epicenter), as well as by myelin loss caused by secondary factors such as edema, inflammation, microvascular ischemia, and a host of other factors that produce the traumatic penumbra previously discussed. The loss of axons can usually be demonstrated by silver or other axonal stains. Focal glial scarring (glial or inflammatory nodules) may be scattered throughout the devastated white matter and may also appear in transitionally damaged regions. In any case, a protracted period of survival after injury is usually required to allow the development of this lesion, although the functional consequences of the lesion are apparent early on in the form of protracted coma, severe frontal lobe dysfunction, and dementia.

Posttraumatic Hydrocephalus

Whenever there is a cerebral contusion or another form of significant brain trauma such as inner cerebral trauma, including subdural hematoma, there is almost always some degree of subarachnoid hemorrhage in connection with the event. In the case of closed head trauma, which produces the pattern of inner cerebral trauma as described by Grcevič and others [251,254,256,295], hemorrhage may result quite frequently from tears in the tela choroidea [301] of the lateral third ventricle in connection with centroaxial trauma (along the long axis of the skull) and need not occur only with major episodes of injury.

The amount of hemorrhage is highly variable and virtually unpredictable; nevertheless, any blood in the subarachnoid space is irritating and may cause a cellular reaction in the arachnoid and subarachnoid space [303]. This may lead to altered CSF absorption by mechanisms that are probably not related to fibrosis of the arachnoid villi, but through more complex mechanisms, discussed in detail in Chapter 5. Disturbed CSF absorption or transport can lead to an acute rise in intracranial pressure and hydrocephalus. Probably more commonly, subtle subarachnoid bleeding may set into motion a prolonged scarring reaction, which may result in not only decreased absorption of CSF but also a rising impedance to flow, both of which can give rise to sustained or periodic rises in intracranial pressure and hydrocephalus. This latter form of hydrocephalus is often discovered incidentally at autopsy in a victim of remote head trauma who has died of some other cause or who has died of complications of the trauma. Some individuals will have shown some symptomatology of their acquired hydrocephalus and may have been classified as suffering from so-called low-pressure or normal-pressure hydrocephalus, which is also discussed in Chapter 5. Typical symptoms of this condition are dementia, ataxia, and bladder and bowel control problems. In other old head trauma cases, especially those in which there has been a good deal of inner cerebral (TAI) trauma, volume loss of cerebral matter may produce hydrocephalus ex vacuo, also shown in Figure 6.71.

The pathological picture of these phenomena is that of a moderate dilatation of the ventricles in a symmetrical pattern, usually patency of the basal cerebellar foramina (Luschka and Magendie), but fibrosis, opalescence, and sometimes tan or brown discoloration of the leptomeninges. Frequently the septum pellucidum will be thin or fenestrated and the fornices reduced to thin threads, giving evidence of the chronic distention of the ventricles that was present. In some cases, dramatic improvement of neurological and mental status results from shunting CSF surgically. Occasionally, some individuals will have effectively shunted themselves by so distending their ventricular chambers that a blowout between ventricle and subarachnoid space may occur in the floor of the third ventricle, in the anterior tips of the temporal horns, in the base of the occipital horns, or through a dilated ventricle beneath a traumatic contusion where the overlying brain is thinned.

Postconcussive Syndrome—Cerebral Concussion

Much confusion abounds regarding the relationship between cerebral contusion (a bruise of the brain) and cerebral concussion. Both have a pathology [409] and occur together, but concussion is usually considered a clinical entity that is regularly observed in head-injured patients in one degree or another and usually consists of posttrauma headache, dizziness, fatigue, some degree of memory difficulty (including amnesia), irritability, depression, episodic disorientation, blurring of vision, tinnitus and deafness, and difficulty in concentration. These symptoms wax and wane; may persist for days, weeks, months, or even years following head injury; and have been extensively described [410,411]. Neuropsychological testing of such individuals, who may be otherwise neurologically normal, shows clear-cut differences in performance from controls and even in the same patient over time as healing occurs [411]. In some individuals, behavioral symptoms may take the form of personality change, antisocial behavior, or frank psychosis. For many years, no structural basis for these symptoms was appreciated, but careful examinations of the brains of recovered posttrauma victims have shown a panoply of lesions in their brains that include evidence of axonal damage in the cerebral and brain stem white matter (axonal balloons seen in silver-stained preparation and more recently using immunohistochemical reactions such as for β app) [241,409], focal astroglial scars (so-called glial nodules or inflammatory nodules) [251,310,321], deep white matter pallor, and sometimes hydrocephalus. These lesions are found in addition to any contusions or other obvious injuries that may have occurred but cannot be separated from them. As mentioned in other portions of this chapter, there is increasing evidence that even minor head trauma results in some damage to the brain, visible or not, which forms the basis for the functional and symptomatic difficulties in most people who have suffered a head injury [410]. The magnitude of the symptoms of the postconcussive state correlates with the degree of severity of the injury, the presence or absence of unconsciousness, and the duration of coma, if any.

In victims who have sustained, in connection with head trauma, a period of coma, there may be severe postconcussive symptomatology, including prolonged anterograde or retrograde amnesia, disorientation, behavioral dysfunctions including psychosis, and dementia. These conditions may clear in time or persist. There is a rather poor specific correlation of the lesions found in the brains of such victims with their clinical state, which reflects in part our lack of precise knowledge with respect to the loci in the brain of the processes of mentation, memory, and behavior.

Posttraumatic Dementia and Neurodegenerative Disease

A demented state following head trauma, related or not to some disturbance of consciousness (semicoma), has been recognized for many years [294,321,409,412] and has gained prominence before the public most recently [22,23]. A more subtle, yet perhaps more widely recognized, syndrome associated with chronic and repeated head trauma is the so-called punch drunk syndrome or dementia pugilistica. In both of these conditions, which are perhaps only ends of the spectrum, the pathological substrate appears to be due to damage in portions of the limbic, rhinencephalic, and mesial diencephalic regions, such as the hippocampal formations, fornices, cingulum, substantia nigra, and ventral tegmentum of the midbrain [251,295,322,323]. Lesions in these regions are a consistent part of the pattern of inner cerebral trauma and, with the exception of the hippocampal and cingular lesions, have little to do with cortical injuries. Extensive axonal damage of such areas as well as deep periventricular white matter damage can contribute to this clinical syndrome. All these injuries can be caused by blows (single or repeated) but most commonly follow falls or complex injuries such as those sustained in traffic accidents or open head injuries such as gunshot wounds.

In the case of the chronically traumatized brains of prizefighters or other athletes who repeatedly suffer head trauma, for example, a number of pathological studies have been performed that indicate that, in addition to some of the lesions listed above, reflective of diffuse axonal injury, a reaction in the cerebral cortex may occur that produces neurofibrillary tangles indistinguishable from Alzheimer's disease [413]. It is not at all certain whether the Alzheimer changes can be brought about by repeated trauma or are merely coincidental, but a possibility exists that Alzheimer-like changes can be caused by lesions that undercut the cortex, suggested by studies in animals. Nevertheless, the association of trauma and Alzheimer's disease must remain conjectural.

An association of trauma and other neurological degenerative diseases has also been suggested, which include possibly posttraumatic Pick's disease, posttraumatic Parkinson's disease, and posttraumatic motor neuron disease. In the case of trauma-associated Parkinson's disease, an anatomic basis is not unreasonable in that in inner cerebral trauma there is a profusion of focal midbrain pathology that could directly injure the substantia nigra and the locus coeruleus but could also interrupt the nigral–striatal pathways [360], indirectly resulting in decreased dopaminergic supply to the striatum. The case for an anatomic connection between adult motor neuron disease (amyotrophic lateral sclerosis) and repeated trauma is unclear at best, but a statistical correlation has been established between the two conditions [414]. Perhaps to complete the spectrum of neurological diseases ascribed to repeated head trauma, an association has even been drawn between trauma and Creutzfeldt–Jakob disease, although it is difficult to explain conceptually how a transmissible unconventional agent (prions) might be activated or inoculated in the course of closed head trauma.

Posttraumatic Epilepsy

Epileptic seizures associated with head trauma should be separated into those that occur early (in the immediate posttrauma period) and those that develop late (long after the injury), as their pathogenesis is probably quite different. In the immediate posttrauma period, only a minority of head trauma victims display seizure activity. The percentages reported by various authors run between 2% and 5% of cases more than 15 years of age and somewhat higher (up to 9%) in those younger than 15 years [415]. Most cases (nearly 85%)

of early posttraumatic epilepsy show their seizures in the first few days after the injury, and the remaining 15% will show their seizures over an extended period of a month or two after injury. In most cases, those showing these forms of seizures are severely brain injured and almost always have some form of intracranial hemorrhagic process in evolution or a depressed skull fracture or a penetrating injury to the brain. The seriousness of the injuries that show secondary seizures is also reflected in an increased mortality rate (see Chapter 9) in such victims. In those who survive their injuries, there is a four times greater chance of their developing late posttraumatic epilepsy than those who do not have a seizure immediately connected with their head trauma [181]. The types of seizures observed may be focal or generalized, although focal motor fits are the most common and are probably related to the highly focal nature of the inciting lesion.

The prevalence of late posttraumatic seizures is subject to considerable variation, given the variability of the degree and severity of head injuries suffered, and ranges from as little as 3% for minor injuries to as much as 100%, in which penetrating injuries of the brain have occurred. In general, late seizures develop a few months after the initial trauma, with about 67% of cases developing within the first year, 89% within the first 2 years, and virtually all patients who are going to develop seizures due to their trauma having done so by 5 years postinjury [2,181]. The type of seizure observed has a focal quality often with generalization in about 40% of cases, with about 20% of cases said to have temporal lobe seizures [181,416]. Of those who show late development of seizures, 80% will continue to have seizures for the remainder of their lives. The risk of late posttraumatic seizures is increased (four times) if there were early seizures, if there was a depressed skull fracture (about 60% incidence), and if there was an intracranial hematoma (about 35%), and if no depressed skull fracture or no intracranial hematoma existed, the incidence may be as low as 2% of cases [181]. If one compares statistics for the incidence of epilepsy in brain-injured patients in the various major wars of the last century, there is remarkable congruency [177]. If injuries did not result in a torn dura, the incidence of epilepsy was 35%; if the dura was torn, the incidence was 41%–43%, regardless of in which war the injury occurred. It is also apparent that figures for civilian brain injuries follow a very similar pattern and are not markedly different from those of the military.

Acknowledging the significant possibility of developing posttrauma epilepsy in serious head injuries, there is considerable difference of opinion and practice among neurosurgeons and neurologists in prophylactically treating posttraumatic epilepsy. Possibly as a consequence of a laissez-faire attitude on the part of some clinicians and a similar attitude on the part of patients, it appears that those individuals who have epilepsy as a result of traumatic injury, who do not take anticonvulsant medication on a regular basis or at all, and who abuse alcohol may have a significant risk of developing sudden unexpected death, presumably in connection with a seizure [417]. The phenomenon of sudden unexpected seizure-associated death is discussed in detail in Chapter 9.

Posttraumatic Blindness

Apart from intraocular and intraorbital causes of blindness after head trauma due to retinal separation, laceration, and direct trauma to the globe, perhaps by missiles, foreign bodies, or bone fragments, or transsection or trauma to the optic nerve or chiasm as a consequence of basal skull or central facial fractures, impairment of vision or blindness may result from damage to the retrogeniculate optic pathway. This can occur with massive coup, contrecoup, fracture, or gliding contusions involving the posterior inferior temporal lobe, in which damage may occur to portions of the optic radiations. This is particularly true for the inferiorly running Meyer's loop, which passes forward from the lateral geniculate body, around and under the temporal horn of the lateral ventricle, and then posteriorly and medially toward the primary optic cortex (Brodmann area 17) in the calcarine gyri of the mesial occipital lobes (illustrated in Chapter 5). If the traumatic process, primary or secondary, is deep enough, portions of this pathway may become interrupted, resulting in quadrantic or hemianoptic field defects [418].

A more common condition, hemorrhagic infarction of the calcarine and neighboring gyri in the occipital lobe, occurs in connection with brain swelling and herniation. In this instance, owing to edema from contusions or mass effects from subdural, epidural, or intracerebral hematomas, the mesial temporal lobe may herniate through the tentorial opening to such an extent that in its most posterior portion the temporal lobe compresses one or more branches of the posterior cerebral artery against the tentorium, resulting in obstruction of blood flow. These branches of the artery are usually those that supply the mesial occipital lobe cortex, including the calcarine gyri. Because the obstruction is often transitory, as a result of therapeutic intervention, the supplied vascular bed is damaged and bleeds upon restoration of circulation, when intracranial pressure is diminished, producing a hemorrhagic infarction with loss of function in the ischemic and necrotic cortex. This complication is usually unilateral but may be bilateral. When this latter condition exists, the victim may become cortically blind. This and other complications of herniation and brain swelling are discussed in more detail in Chapter 5.

Posttraumatic Brain Tumors

At first consideration, to imply an association between cerebral trauma and development of a neoplasm would seem unwarranted; however, this issue is regularly raised in medical–legal circles in connection with workers' compensation hearings, veterans benefit hearings, and insurance or personal injury cases. What is more, there is considerable medical literature on the subject in which several cases appear to clearly represent bona fide instances of trauma–tumor linkage. The usual tumor encountered is a meningioma seen years after an open head injury in which foreign materials have been embedded in the brain. Criteria that may be applied to the evaluation of possible cases are discussed in detail in Chapter 2.

Infectious Complications of Head Trauma

Although intracerebral infection (brain abscess, subdural empyema, meningitis) most typically is recognized as a complication of skull fracture, all of these conditions may occur in the absence of known fractures of the skull. The possible mechanisms for this infection are the following: subtle fracture of the base of the skull, perhaps involving a paranasal sinus that is not recognized clinically, pathologically, or even radiologically; disruption of the cribriform plate with or without CSF rhinorrhea; transient alteration of blood flow in the emissary venous system toward the intracranial circulation from the face and scalp, where laceration and contamination may have occurred; a transient bacteremia in connection with abdominal, thoracic, skeletal, or other secondary trauma; and iatrogenic contamination during surgical or other medical procedures. The pathology of the various intracranial infectious processes is discussed in detail in Chapter 2.

Neuropathology of Repetitive Head Injury

As mentioned above, in recent years the debate on the legitimacy of prizefighting as a sport has intensified, and the banning of this activity has been called for in the public press. No doubt, as a result of increasing medical scrutiny and scientific studies of boxers and the kinds of lesions and neurological and psychological deficits they acquire, the public has responded. A recent monograph on the subject by Unterharnscheidt and Unterharnscheidt [419] discusses the issues and history of the problem in detail. In several of the preceding sections of this chapter, reference has been made to several lesions regularly observed in professional fighters and, in some cases, of prizefight fatality. To recapitulate, the following have been reported [3,10,413,419–422]: organic brain syndromes that include dementia, slurring of speech, apathy, incoordination, amnesia, and seizures; parkinsonism associated with interruption of the nigral–striatal pathways and depigmentation of the substantia nigra; Alzheimer's neurofibrillary tangles; focal gray and white matter scars and gliosis; cortical atrophy; hydrocephalus; cava of the septum pellucidum; lacerations and alterations in the fornices; and subdural hematomas. In spite of this long list of the reported effects of prizefighting, there are those that maintain it is harmless [423]. It is interesting to note that most, if not all, lesions declared by various authors to have resulted from a career in boxing belong to the pattern of inner cerebral trauma, which may mean that even relatively mild forces of acceleration bring about lesions in the same areas that more severe and violent forces do. The implication here is that the biomechanical structure of the brain, more than anything else, is the predictor of the pattern of injuries observed rather than the traumatizing force. To be sure, most brain lesions ascribed to boxing are found in persons who have had a long career in the ring, but recent evidence indicates that the significant percentage of fighters who would otherwise appear to be normal have physical evidence of brain damage by CT or MRI scans of the brain and by sophisticated psychometric examination [421] and that there may be no such thing as an episode of head trauma that does not leave evidence of its occurrence if sensitive enough studies are made.

Spine and Spinal Cord Injury

Anatomical Considerations

The spinal cord, the continuation of the medulla into the spinal canal, is on average about 30 g in weight and is said to be about 2% of brain weight, with quite a bit of variability. The volume of the cord is about 28 cc, with the gray matter forming about 5 cc of this. The specific gravity of the cord is about 1.034 [221]. The cord is tethered within the spinal canal by the nerve roots that exit and enter the meninges, the segmental arteries and veins, and the denticulate ligaments, all of which serve to limit lateral movements of the cord but which permit a small degree of axial movements that correspond with normal movement of the spinal skeleton. The vascular supply to the cord rostrally arises from the anterior spinal artery (vertebrobasilar system) and anastomoses, with a number of contributing arteries that are quite anatomically variable that come from segmental arteries and so-called radicular arteries (see Figure 6.77). There are a number of real and potential watersheds in a zone of shared perfusion that can have pathological and clinical significance. The venous drainage is complex and often plexiform.

The spinal canal is invested with meninges in continuity with those in the intracranial compartment with similar, if not identical, structures. Some data exist regarding the

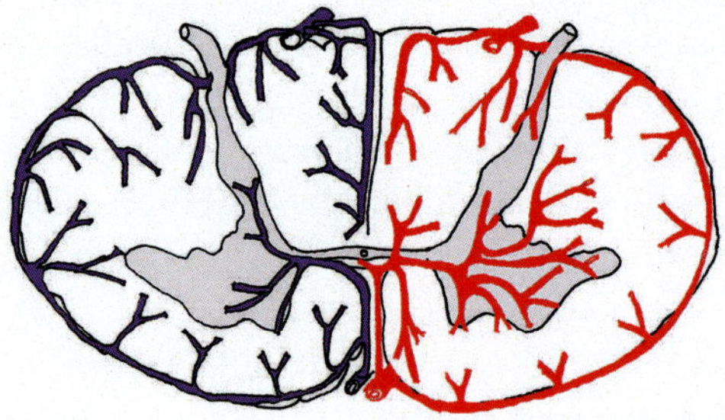

Figure 6.77 This diagram illustrates arterial (red) and venous (blue) vascular supply and drainage to the cervical cord. The anterior spinal artery (lower midline of the cord) arborizes and supplies the anterior (ventral) mid portion of the cord, while the posterior spinal arterial system supplies the posterior and some of the circumferential areas. A "watershed" of sorts exists between the territories of the anterior and posterior spinal fields in the white matter of the cord.

biomechanical properties of spinal dura that indicate that the dura is more capable of elongation in persons younger than 60 years than those who are older. There are sex differences in mechanical properties as well [33].

The spinal skeleton is composed of 7 cervical, 12 thoracic, and 5 lumbar vertebrae, which are individual bones separated by intervertebral discs and stabilized by a system of ligaments and facet articulations with each other. The first cervical vertebra (atlas) articulates with the skull base, forming the atlanto-occipital articulation. The fifth lumbar vertebra articulates with the fused mass of the sacrum, which is without intervertebral discs. It joins with a vestigial coccyx. The spine normally has an S shape, with obvious curves in the cervical and lumbar regions. The vertebrae at each anatomic level (cervical, thoracic, and lumbar) have typical characteristics. Posterior (sensory) rootlets leave the cord and form the dorsal root ganglia, which then meet the anterior (motor) rootlets to form the spinal roots, which then exit via the intervertebral foramina and differentiate into nerve plexuses and their branches and the sympathetic trunks.

The cervical spine is capable of greater mobility and complexity of mobility than other parts of the spine, being capable of flexion, extension, lateral movements, and rotation. The degree of movement is a function of individual characteristics of interspinal ligaments, facets, paraspinal muscles, age, disease states, and extent of prior injury or surgery. The biomechanics and kinematics of the spine make up a complex body of information, much too extensive to be covered in detail here. The interested reader is referred to texts and monographs devoted to these matters [125,424–428]. Only selected spinal injuries that have relatively common forensic importance will be covered here.

Biomechanical Aspects of the Spine

The biomechanical properties of the cervical spinal skeleton have been the subject of extensive study using animals, human cadavers, human volunteers, and various test dummies [274,424,428–431]. With respect to the different loading parameters, Table 6.3 illustrates various thresholds for the cervical spine using volunteers and in cadavers. As might be

Table 6.3 Injury Tolerances to Cervical Spine

Response	Test Source	Threshold	Threshold Value	Source
Extension	Volunteers	No injury	23.7 Nm	314
	Volunteers	Pain	47.3 Nm	315
	Cadavers	Ligamentous injury	56.7 Nm	314
Flexion	Volunteers	Pain	59.4 Nm	314, 315
	Volunteers	Pain—maximum tolerance	87.8 Nm	315, 314
	Cadavers	Ligamentous injury	189–190 Nm	315, 314
Compression	Cadavers	Facet dislocation	1.72 kN	317
		Compression Fx	4.8–5.9 kN	316
Tension	Volunteers	No injury	1.1 kN	315
	Cadavers	Failure	3.1 kN	318
Anterior–posterior shear	Volunteers	No injury	845 N	315
	Cadavers	Failure	2 kN	314

Note: This table displays injury tolerances to the cervical spine based on the work of Goldsmith and Ommaya [430], Mertz and Patrick [431], and others [429,433,443,446]. Nm, newton-meters; kN, kilo-newtons; N, newtons.

expected, tolerance levels will vary between adults and infants and between males and females under the various testing parameters [274,428].

Just as injury criteria have been developed for cranial injury, attempts have been made to apply some of the methodology to the neck, which obviously is a much more mechanically complex structure than the cranium. A number of assumptions have been made out of necessity, and specific injury scenarios must be employed, for example, anterior–posterior (whiplash) loading, frontal and posterior and lateral impacts, and

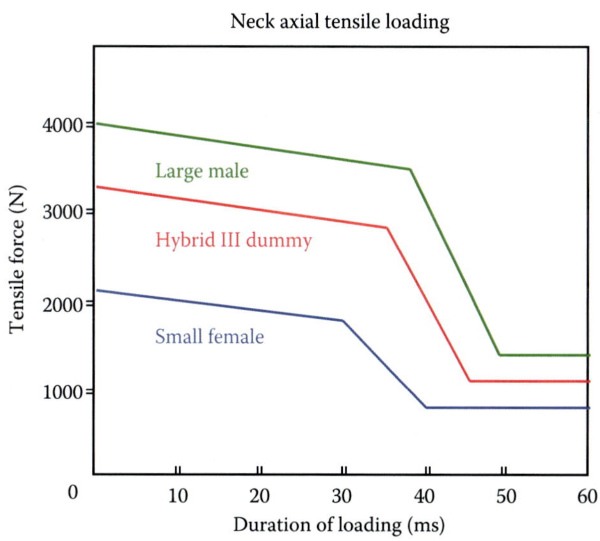

Figure 6.78 This graph illustrates the dynamics of tensile loading to the neck in three systems. With loading above each of the "curves," there is the potential of "significant" neck injury and presumably below these "curves" such loading can be tolerated. The studies of Mertz [269] show that for relatively short-duration loads, the tolerance of the neck is relatively constant until load durations >30 ms occur at which load tolerance levels precipitously decline and the potential for injury increases but remains relatively constant to the limits of the experiments.

compressive loading [274]. The differences in various parameters of loading are illustrated in Figures 6.78 through 6.80. These graphs provide a general perspective for neck injury scenarios and their likelihood of occurring with respect to sex and stature. These figures can be compared with those values obtained from volunteers, as illustrated in Table 6.3.

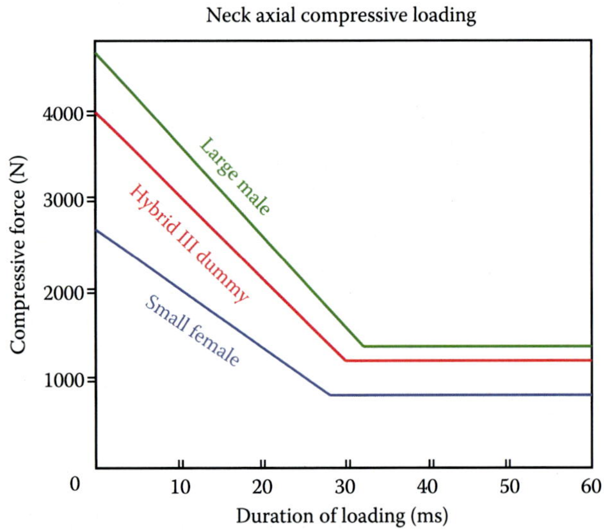

Figure 6.79 Here it appears that the tolerance of the neck for compressive loading diminishes rapidly for loads of durations longer than 30 ms and then remains relatively constant over the duration of the experiment from 30 to 60 ms at a much lower level of tolerance. Note the differences in response as compared with tensile loading (Figure 6.78). (From Mertz HJ. Anthropomorphic test devices. In Nahum AM, Melvin JW, eds., *Accidental Injury: Biomechanics and Prevention*. New York: Springer-Verlag, 1993, pp. 66–80.)

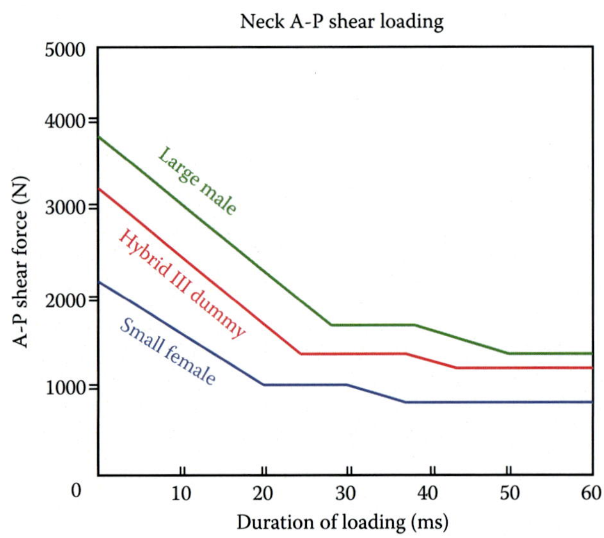

Figure 6.80 This graph illustrates the responses of the neck to shear loading (side to side). These "curves" resemble those for compressive loading (Figure 6.79) and indicate that tolerance rapidly diminishes for loading durations longer than about 20 ms.

Epidemiologic and Clinical Aspects of Spinal and Spinal Cord Injury

Spinal injuries constitute an important and complex group of cases that have a major personal and economic impact on individuals as well as society. In a 1985 review, it was noted that more than 70 million people required medical attention or restriction of activity because of spinal injuries of all causes [432]. This resulted in 144 million bed-days of disability and 433 million days of restricted activity. Approximately 10%–20% of all hospital admissions for nervous system trauma are due to injuries of the spinal cord. Worldwide, spinal cord injuries occur at annual rates of between 13 and 50 cases per million people. The United States, in general, reports relatively higher rates of occurrence. Spinal cord injuries occur most frequently among older adolescents and young adults, with males being at greater risk than females. There are no precise epidemiological figures for spinal skeletal injuries, with or without spinal cord injury, because many of these injuries are occult but not without eventual consequence [433]. The most common immediate causes of injuries are [428] motor vehicular accidents, including cycle accidents (36.7%); falls (15.9%); injuries due to firearms (11.7%); injuries associated with sporting and recreational activities (especially diving and football) (about 16%); and others (about 20%). With respect specifically to sporting activities, diving accidents account for 21% of spinal injuries, and snowmobiling, parachuting/sky diving, motorcycles and ATVs, and equestrian activities account for about 10% of spinal injuries each.

With respect to spinal cord injuries in connection with motor vehicle accidents, in the United States the highest incidence of traumatic paraplegia is found in individuals involved in head-on collisions or those ejected from the vehicle during the crash. It is remarkable that 50% of spinal cord injuries result from single-vehicle crashes, which raises the issue of alcohol intoxication, an important contributing factor in these cases. Drivers or occupants of sports utility vehicles, trucks, or larger vehicles seem especially vulnerable to spinal injuries, and they suffer nearly twice the expected rate of this complication than occupants of automobiles, bicycles, or other motorized vehicles [432,434,435].

Although general correlations mentioned above for motor vehicle accidents and spinal cord injuries have been made, the specific details that might relate to patterns of injury are not commonly analyzed. This seems to apply also to analyses of other etiologies of spinal trauma, such as victims of falls and injuries due to suicide attempts. It is of interest that falls in suicide attempts result in more severe injury than accidental falls [436,437]. Diving accidents are an important cause of spinal injuries and tend to affect young males between the ages of 15 and 25 more commonly than other groups. These injuries usually involve damage between the fourth and sixth cervical spinal cord levels, sustained when the diver's head strikes the bottom of a pool, lake, or other body of water, causing compression or burst fractures of the spinal column [438,439]. Spinal injuries sustained during American football games occur at a rate of approximately 2–14 cases per 100,000 population [440]. Rugby and trampoline accidents are also highly represented in the sport-associated spinal injuries, as are water skiing and snow skiing, ski jumping, competitive motorcycle racing, and a host of vigorous body-contact sports or sports where falls are common.

Injury to the Upper Cervical Spine

Pathology

To fully appreciate the mechanisms of high spinal injury, one must appreciate the unique anatomy of this region. The first cervical vertebra (the atlas) supports the occiput and is held in place by a number of ligaments. The transverse ligament of the atlas encloses and restricts motion of the odontoid process of the second cervical vertebra (the axis), which might otherwise indent the pontine base. There are 24 pairs of paraspinal muscles that are attached to the cervical spine [429]. A careful analysis of these anatomic structures has yielded a number of models that lend themselves of finite element analysis during various injury scenarios [441,442].

A variety of loading scenarios alone or in combination may cause injury to the spinal skeleton, chiefly the cervical region, and may also lead to spinal cord injury. These basic mechanisms include compression (vertical loading), compression/flexion, compression/extension, tension, tension/extension, tension/flexion, torsion, horizontal shear, and lateral bending [428]. Disruption of the transverse ligament of the atlas may occur in anterior–posterior shear or rotational injuries of the spine, resulting in atlantoaxial subluxation with or without odontoid fracture. Compressive loading such as might occur with vertex impacts (by fall or blow) may cause compression fracture (Jefferson's fracture—illustrated in Figure 6.81) of the anterior and posterior arches of the atlas (C-1) with lateral displacement of the lateral masses onto the axis (C-2) [74,443]. Like atlantoaxial subluxation, this injury usually does not injure the cord because there is ample space about the cord to accommodate encroachment on the spinal canal. Another common fracture, the so-called hangman's fracture, illustrated in Figure 6.80, consists of fracture of the pedicles of the axis (C-2), resulting in anterior dislocation of C-2 or C-3 with or without odontoid process fracture. This injury is typically seen in judicial hangings [444,445] and automobile accidents in which the neck is forcibly hyperextended and rotated; however, in many accident cases, the spinal cord may not be injured, due to considerable space surrounding the cord in the region. Of course, in judicial hangings, damage is extensive, involving the cord and brain stem as well as fractures of other cervical vertebrae, the hyoid bone, and other neck structures.

When the head is hyperextended, as with loading to the face and jaw, more or less in the midline, a variety of cervical spinal injuries can occur. A common circumstance occurs when unrestrained automobile passengers strike the dashboard. Of course, many of these types of impacts have now been obviated by the preventive actions of vehicular air bags. The frontal loading often causes facet dislocations, which may become locked by overriding of vertebrae or not. Fractures of the hangman's type of C-2 may also occur, along with other injuries to the neck. A special circumstance of hyperextension may occur when a pedestrian is struck from behind. The force of this scenario may be so great that a so-called ring fracture of the skull base may occur [428,446]. In this instance, basically the skull base is

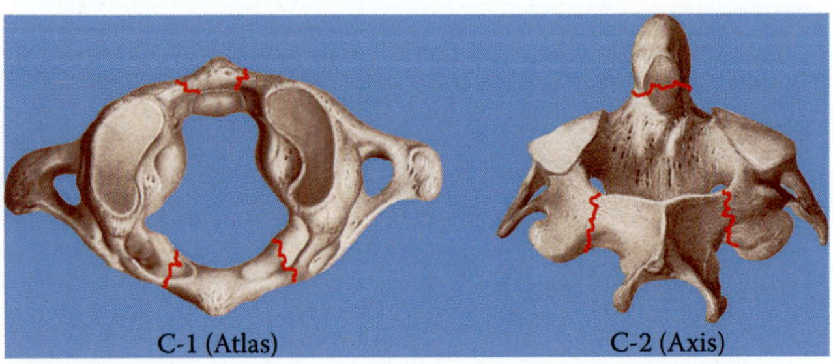

Figure 6.81 This illustration depicts on the left (C-1) a typical Jefferson's fracture and on the right (C-2) a typical pattern of "hangman's" fractures.

avulsed by the tensile forces of the articulating spine. In the course of this injury, it is very common that a pontomedullary or cervicomedullary avulsion may occur [108].

Middle and Lower Cervical Injuries

Injuries to the cervical spine and cord between spinal segments C-4 and C-8 occur with great regularity and form the most common type of immediately nonfatal spinal injury [89]. Cord lesions may occur with or without spinal fracture, but spinal ligamentous injury is almost always present, resulting in dislocation or subluxation. The motions responsible are one or more of the following: hyperflexion, hyperextension, hyperrotation, or compression of the spinal column. Hyperflexion injuries may occur with blows to the back of the neck, in a shallow-water diving injury, when motorcyclists are flipped forward from their cycles, in automobile crashes with distortion of the passenger compartment, or in rollover automobile situations when the victim is unbelted. Fractures observed in hyperflexion injuries may involve pinching off of the anterior part of the vertebral body, with the posterior parts being displaced backward into the spinal canal, producing so-called teardrop fracture. Hyperextension, as mentioned above, occurs sometimes in wrestling matches or fights where a forceful hammerlock is used and in posterior impacts, as in rear-end collisions. A variety of injuries to the spine and cord may result, which can include injury to the pontomedullary junction, as noted above. Rotational forces (and complex combinations of movements), common in automobile accidents, may produce subluxation with facet interlocking (unilateral or bilateral) and other forms of dislocation with impingement of the spinal canal. When the middle cervical spine is fractured, dislocated, or subluxated, spinal cord injury is usually more severe than similar injuries sustained to the upper cervical region, and there is a higher incidence of complete rather than incomplete lesions associated.

Clinical Aspects

Clinically, the most critical period for survival is the first 3 months after spinal cord injury. Factors influencing survival include the level of the spinal injury, degree of respiratory control remaining, degree of sensory and motor disabilities, age of the patient, and degree of associated neurological or systemic injuries or diseases. The most immediate problem is one of respiratory control. In cases where the level of injury is at the fourth cervical level or higher, diaphragmatic control via the phrenic nerve may be minimal or lost, resulting in dependence on the accessory muscles of the respiration subserved by the eleventh (spinal accessory) nerve, which is rarely damaged. If other conditions exist during the acute phase of the injury, which may include aspiration, pulmonary contusional injury, or secondary insults associated with the traumatic episode, such as shock lung, multiple organ failure, fat or air embolism, pneumothorax, hemothorax, rib fractures, cardiac injury, or pulmonary edema, the already compromised pulmonary function may be overwhelmed, resulting in death.

In individuals whose injuries are below the fourth cervical level, or in those who have stabilized and respiration may be less of an issue, disability of bladder and bowel function becomes a more immediate concern but soon translates into long-term problems of management. Stasis of urine or feces in an uncontrollable bladder or bowel is a ready nidus for infection. Chronic cystitis and pyelonephritis are the nemeses that continually stalk the spinal-cord-injured patient but can be managed with a careful medical and surgical regimen. The personal impact of spinal cord injury on a victim may far outweigh the physical injuries, and the victim's own response to his or her injury plays a significant role in the outcome. Depression and suicide are common complications of spinal injury and must be considered carefully by the forensic pathologist who has occasion to autopsy a spinal-cord-injured individual. An important legal and ethical controversy surrounds the right to live and die in spinal-cord-injured patients and has been the subject of a popular play and movie, authored by Brian Clark in 1972 (*Whose Life Is It Anyway?*), and a number of lawsuits over the right to die and assisted suicide in the quadriplegic or paraplegic spinal cord injured.

An important forensic issue that commonly arises in litigation for damages and medical costs in connection with a spinal cord injury is the question of mortality, morbidity, quality of life, and survival potential. With modern techniques for immediate treatments after injury and a comprehensive program of rehabilitation and maintaining nutritional support, bladder and bowel function, as well as respiratory support and pulmonary toilet, long-term survivals for such victims are now expected, compared with lesser outcomes only 10 years ago [447–449]. The excitement over the potential of stem cell research in the treatment of spinal cord injury has yet to be realized.

Other circumstances in which the spine and spinal cord may be injured and in which there may be forensic considerations include spinal injury after chiropractic manipulation [374,450–452], in connection with child abuse, due to alleged product failure, as a complication of spinal surgery for disc or other spinal skeletal disease, in connection with gymnastic or other exercise regimens, and in the martial arts training or demonstrations [453–455]. A host of other special situations may be encountered, but each demands, for proper analysis and interpretation, a careful pathological approach and an appreciation of the complex issue involved.

Spinal injury may result in fractures, dislocations, or subluxations of the spine with or without spinal cord injury. In one study [456], it was reported that in only 14% of spinal fractures did injury to the cord occur. Of interest is the phenomenon of SCIWORA (spinal cord injury without radiological abnormality), which has been reported to occur in 17% of cases [456,457]. When the spinal cord is injured, the clinical state of quadriplegia or paraplegia may occur. Quadriplegia (or tetraplegia) is the paralysis of all four limbs and usually indicates an injury above the level of emergence of the roots serving the brachial plexus (fourth cervical). It is possible that some function may be preserved but may allow only movement of the shoulders and preclude movement of the arms and hands. Paraplegia is paralysis of the lower extremities and variable portions of the trunk due to injury of the spinal cord below the emergence of the brachial plexus (first or second thoracic segment).

Spinal-cord-injured individuals may suffer either complete or partial (incomplete) loss of function below the level of injury after spinal shock dissipates. In the latter, in which some motor or sensory function is preserved, the prognosis is generally better. Some individuals use the terms *paraparesis* and *quadriparesis* to describe incomplete paralysis while reserving *paraplegic* and *quadriplegic* for complete motor paralysis. Others use the latter terms to describe the general level of injury for both complete and incomplete lesions [425]. According to Green et al. [458], complete and incomplete injuries are represented about equally in the population. There appears to be a relative increase in the incidence of quadriplegia (50%–70%) versus paraplegia (30%–50%) in recent years due to more traffic accidents and more reporting of such accidents [459]. Despite the phenomenon of spinal shock, immediate neurological assessment can predict the long-term outcome relatively accurately [458]. Ducker and Walleck [460] indicated that 85% of those who show an immediate complete injury will tend to retain a complete symptomatology at the end of 1 year, whereas those with immediate incomplete signs and symptoms have a greater tendency to experience at least some additional neurological recovery by the end of a year.

Spinal cord injuries are often classified according to the neurological deficits observed [425]. Incomplete lesions have been subclassified into various syndromes: posterior cord, anterior cord, central cord, hemicord, or Brown-Séquard syndromes. However, Green et al. [458] indicate that most patients with incomplete lesions do not fall into any clear-cut syndrome. An excellent overall review of the clinical and radiological aspects of human spinal cord trauma, covering many of the following subtopics, is provided by Braakman and Penning [459].

Concurrence of Craniocerebral and Spinal Injuries

Many spinal cord injuries occur in conjunction with vehicular accidents where multiple and complex patterns of trauma are typical, involving both head and spinal trauma—so-called trauma in continuity [459,461,462]. Davis et al. [463] reviewed a series of 50 acute fatal cases of craniocerebral trauma, most of which occurred as a result of vehicular accidents, in which 33 of 50 victims died instantly. Concurrent brain and spinal cord lesions were found in 61% of the cases. This is illustrated in the circumstance in which high cervical spinal cord trauma coexists with pontomedullary or other brain stem injury [108,459], which may produce sudden death or, in cases that survive for some period, the so-called Déjérine onion skin pattern of sensory loss.

Thoracic and Lumbar Spinal Injuries

The upper thoracic spine from T-1 to T-10 enjoys considerably more resistance to injury than does the cervical spine because of added stability of the thoracic rib cage and costovertebral ligaments [89]. Fracture dislocations and rotational injuries require great force and consequently are comparatively uncommon. In contrast to the stability of the upper thoracic spinal column, the lower thoracic and lumbar spine is more vulnerable to injury because of increased flexibility in this region and the lack of lateral stability of the ribs. Fractures and dislocations can occur here with or without spinal cord injury. Rotational and flexion forces rather than extension forces seem to be more important in the pathogenesis of spine and cord injuries in this region, and compression injuries are uncommon. In the lower lumbar and lumbosacral region, compression injuries with bursting fractures of vertebral bodies are the most common but do not necessarily involve injury to the cord. These types of injuries are common in military pilots who survive airplane crashes (in which the craft "bellies" in) and in individuals who sustain sitting-position injuries. Pathological and incidental fractures in this region are common in connection with osteoporosis, disorders of calcium–phosphorus metabolism, and metastatic disease, although cord lesions in these conditions are uncommon.

Pathology of Spinal Cord Injury

The usual types of pathological changes seen with impact injury of the spinal cord are remarkably consistent, regardless of the particular mechanisms of the injury. Even in clinically complete traumatic spinal cord injury with total loss of function below the level of the injury, the cord is functionally but not usually physically transected. Actual physical transsection only occurs in extreme situations where massive fracturing and distortion of the spine, penetrating injuries, crush, or other devastating injuries have occurred. The foregoing clinical section has emphasized the more commonly encountered combinations of spinal cord lesions in association with fracture or dislocation of spinal bones. However, it is recognized that the spinal cord may be traumatically injured in the absence of the latter [464], and the converse is also obviously true. In recent years, the acronym SCIWORA (spinal cord injury without radiological abnormality) has been applied to this not-uncommon situation [457,465], especially in the pediatric age group. In patients who live long enough to reveal the effects of irreversibly induced traumatic injury of the cord, distinct patterns of necrosis or nerve fiber alterations are observed in the traumatized segment of the spinal cord. This, along with other features of pathology, is discussed below. Birth-related spinal and spinal cord injuries are discussed in Chapter 4.

Acutely Fatal Spinal Injury

In examining patients dying of or with acute spinal cord injuries, one may be struck with a paucity of change, especially in the spinal cord tissue itself, especially if death has occurred within an hour or so of the incident, usually from collateral injuries. Therefore, it becomes all the more imperative to examine the spinal column by postmortem radiography using plain films, CT, or MRI methods [461,462], and to dissect and examine soft tissues and the spinal bones and canal carefully at autopsy [463,466]. In this regard, it is important to know the relationships between the level of the spinal bones (vertebrae) and the spinal cord. These arrangements are described in many standard anatomy texts.

As has been indicated by Davis et al. [463], soft tissue disruption and hemorrhage, especially of neck musculature, are frequently observed at the site of bone fracture (or dislocation) or ligamentous tears. Although hemorrhages in relationship to the spinal meninges are not consistently found, perivascular petechial intramedullary hemorrhages of the spinal cord, diffusely involving segments at as well as above and below the level of osseous or ligamentous disruption, are to be expected in acute fatal cases of craniospinal trauma. Other than petechial hemorrhage, the spinal cord in early lesions is characteristically normal in appearance [466], except, of course, in those minority of cases in which it is lacerated or completely disrupted. The latter usually occurs only in the most violent cases, in which there is severe spinal column disruption or penetrating (bullet, knife) wounds, which are discussed in Chapter 8.

Traumatic Myelopathy Associated with Delayed Death

Under well-controlled experimental conditions, the progression of pathological changes in the cord following an impact injury has been well defined in a variety of animals, such as rats, cats, and monkeys, with spinal cords traumatized by direct impact injury with a calibrated weight and application of balloons, heat, cold, and radiofrequency lesioning [467–470]. The endpoint of severe injury leading to complete loss of function is the development of a cone of necrosis (Figure 6.82) involving all or most of the entire area of subpial spinal cord tissue at the level of maximal change and tapering above and below this region beyond the point of impact. In principle, this progression to a necrotic zone is essentially what happens in humans in the usual type of spinal column–cord traumatic injury. It is very important to note that in the delayed time period, after the acute hemorrhages in

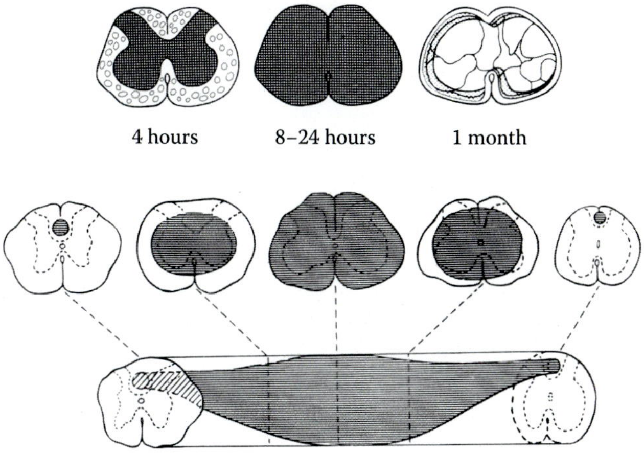

Figure 6.82 This diagram illustrates the time and injury course that is typical for a "complete" spinal cord injury in man or in experimental animals. Before an hour, comparatively little is seen grossly or microscopically, but usually by 4 hours postinjury the central cord will bear the brunt of the reaction, expanding to involve more or less the whole cord at the most injured segment by 8–24 hours. By about a month, postinjury the damaged cord is cystic. (Courtesy of Dr. J.D. Balentine.)

soft tissue and near the meninges have subsided, the cord, unlike the injured (contused) brain, often looks relatively normal exteriorly. At autopsy, it is imperative to expose it at the appropriate levels relative to the trauma history and clinical findings and to identify the necrotic zone (Figure 6.83) by touch and visually. When the cord is cross-sectioned segmentally, typical appearances are as shown in Figure 6.84. Eventually, a more cystic lesion is noted (Figure 6.85). Such cystic changes can be easily identified by transillumination

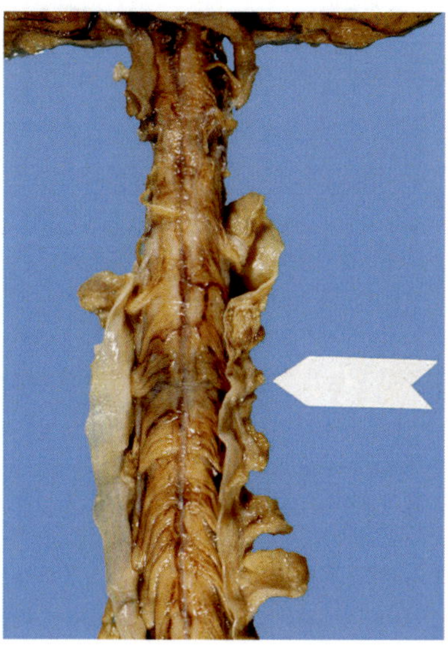

Figure 6.83 This photograph illustrates the external appearance of a traumatized cervical cord segment (arrow) in which the victim, of a traffic accident, died within a few hours of other injuries. Note the congestion at one segment.

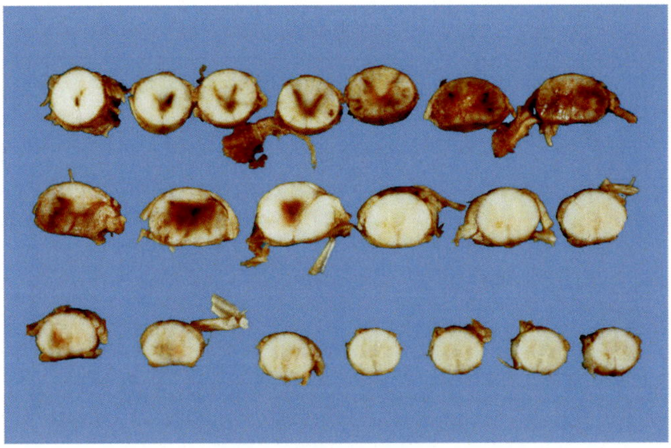

Figure 6.84 This photograph shows segmental cross sections of the cord from a victim of spinal cord injury who died several days after being injured. The typical central cord (gray matter) congestion and hemorrhagic necrosis is seen, in this case mostly above the main lesion and blends into the most injured segments that are totally hemorrhagic and necrotic. The lesion then tapers to a central lesion below the lesion.

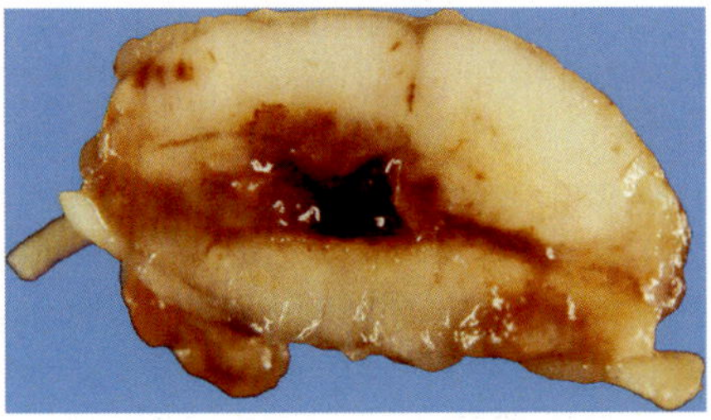

Figure 6.85 This photograph of a single cross section of an injured spinal cord illustrates the cavitary nature of the central cord lesion (above or below the most injured segment) as it usually appears within about 2 weeks after injury.

before the cord is sectioned. It is apparent from considering the experimental model of spinal cord injury that it is important to assess many levels of the spinal cord to find the level of maximum change, which should correspond to the clinical level of neurological impairment. This is more easily identified after necrosis has developed. Under experimental conditions, this point is reached within 8–24 hours postinjury [471]. A similar latent period has been found in humans where macroscopic changes, independent of acute hemorrhages, require 6–24 hours to develop [472]. The progressive changes in the development of irreversible injury, and hence necrosis, involve the evolution of vascular alterations, hemorrhage, edema, and necrotic cellular changes [471,473].

Resolution of Necrotic Events

The necrotic phase of cord injury is followed by a phase of resolution in which phagocytosis by polymorphonuclear leukocytes (within 24 hours) and macrophages (1–3 days, progressing until 2–4 weeks) leaves a residual empty (cystic) area. The latter is surrounded by a variable amount of neovascularization and astrocytic gliosis. Gliosis following traumatic spinal cord injury in humans is quite often relatively sparse in comparison to its emphasis in research on spinal cord transsection and the glial barrier to regeneration hypothesis [474]. The cystic changes in traumatized spinal cord may take many months to years to fully develop, and they may have clinical significance as a syndrome of posttraumatic syringomyelia [475].

Incomplete Lesion

The above discussion has focused on the complete spinal cord lesion in which there is a functional transsection clinically and a zone of complete or near-complete cross-sectional necrosis, despite the intact meninges and often-small amounts of subpial neuropil. The incomplete lesion is more difficult to describe because it is less commonly encountered at autopsy, despite its clinical frequency. In such cases, the evolution of necrotic events is limited to various regions of the spinal cord, with sparing of other zones. The posterior or anterior part of the cord may be affected predominantly. Often the peripheral white matter is spared, giving the appearance of central cord necrosis. Human autopsy material and animal tissue in experimental spinal cord injury have clearly shown that the center of the spinal cord is especially vulnerable to traumatic forces and that many of the resulting myelopathies begin in this zone and spread circumferentially. However, analysis of reviews of the neuropathology of spinal cord trauma [462,466,472] reveals a great deal of variability in the topography of incomplete lesions, and it is not wise to oversimplify their anatomic dimensions.

Nontraumatic Myelopathies

Compressive Myelopathies In addition to the general category of impact injury of the spinal cord and traumatic impact myelopathy, which may be a combination of acute compression with sudden forceful impaction and distortion, impressive myelopathies develop without an associated impact injury but in connection with relatively prolonged intrinsic mechanical compression of the cord by impingement of the canal or by protruding intervertebral discs. Spinal stenosis [476,477] or compression may be congenital, as in achondroplasia; developmental, as in various defects of neural closure; neoplastic or metabolic, as in osteoporosis; or iatrogenic, inflammatory, or degenerative, as in the case of spondylitis, which is widespread and the most common form. Of course, any of these conditions may be compounded by an incident of trauma, which further compromises the integrity of the spinal cord.

Spondylitis [425,476] is a disease of unknown etiology, which affects men more than women, beginning often in the third decade and affecting the cervical spine, usually between the C-2 and C-7 levels, and the lumbar region from L-3 downward more than other regions. The disease results in proliferation of bone such that the spine becomes essentially fused in the affected areas and the spinal canal becomes narrowed, often with nodular growths of bone that may indent and individually compress the cord (osteophytes) or may compress and narrow the passageway for the vertebral arteries [478,479]. In an already narrowed spinal canal, trauma is an added risk in the affected portions of the spine. The two most common forms of spondylitic myelopathy occur in the mid- to lower cervical region and in the lower lumbar and cauda equina region of the cord. When the cord specimen from a victim of spondylitis is examined pathologically, the cord appears almost beaded at times, with obvious indentations, usually in the anterior surface but in other portions as well [480]. The cord may be softened and necrotic in these regions, perhaps as a result of infarction due to compression of the anterior spinal arteries, although this point is controversial. The cut section and microscopic examination of the cord often reveal small patchy or larger areas of white and gray matter necrosis and long tract degeneration. In sections above the lesion, ascending degeneration of tracts (primarily recognizable in the dorsal columns) can be demonstrated with myelin staining. Below the lesion, descending degeneration can be demonstrated easily in the lateral corticospinal tracts (pyramidal tracts) and sometimes in the ventral medial (uncrossed) pyramidal tract.

Disc disease [476,478] is due primarily to aging of the intervertebral discs with liquefaction and herniation of the nucleus pulposus, with or without weakening or fragmentation of the posterior annulus and its attachment to the longitudinal ligament. There is an alteration in the water and nuclear composition of the nucleus pulposus, resulting in a net decrease in disc volume and elasticity. The net effect of these changes is vulnerability to compression and likelihood of rupture. This can occur in some individuals during early adult years but most commonly occurs in middle age, usually in the lumbosacral regions but also possible in the cervical spine. The thoracic spine is relatively spared by this disease process. After age 60, disc rupture is less likely, but some degree of spondylosis with osteophyte formation is more frequent and may produce identical symptoms. Typical symptoms involve radicular pain (due to lateral rupture of the disc), loss of muscular reflexes, and paraspinal muscular spasm, but only rarely actual spinal cord compression due to midline rupture and herniation. In the cervical region, the C-5 to C-7 discs and in the lumbar region the L-4 to S1 discs are the most commonly affected.

One of the more usual causes of spinal-cord-producing myelopathic changes is encountered in patients suffering from primary or metastatic neoplastic diseases of the spine. This can occur in two ways: neoplastic erosion and destruction of vertebral bodies (pathologic fractures) with collapse and compression of the cord, and by extramedullary primary or metastatic masses compressing the cord. The most common primary tumors that may impinge on the cord are schwannomas and meningiomas. The most common secondary tumors are carcinomas of the lung, breast, kidney, and prostate; lymphomas; myelomas; and malignant melanomas. In the case of pathological fracture of the spine due to metastatic disease or osteoporosis, damage to the cord is less common than injury to the roots, which may cause considerable pain, but when cord damage is sustained, it often occurs in the lower thoracic and upper lumbar regions, producing weakness in the legs, neurological dysfunction of the bladder and bowel, or both. When primary or secondary tumors within the spinal canal compress the cord, there may be associated softening and necrosis of the cord in a circumferential manner, leaving only a thin rim of viable tissue, similar to that seen in severe cases of impact injury. However, the less severe incomplete lesion tends to affect the more peripheral white matter and not the central or paracentral areas of the cord. This is probably related to selective compression of the vessels of the pial arterial plexuses on the cord's surface.

Ischemic Myelopathies Spinal vascular disease is much less common than cerebrovascular disease. The same pathogenetic factors (atherosclerosis, thrombi, emboli) have been responsible for the extremely rare occurrence of spinal cord infarction due to intrinsic occlusive vascular disease [481] and in connection with decompression sickness (the bends) in divers [482]. The clinical manifestations have presented as syndromes of anterior spinal or posterior spinal artery occlusions or complete transverse myelopathies. The anterior spinal artery syndrome is the most common and often is related to infarction of the anterior two-thirds of the spinal cord, a lesion topographically distinct from most traumatic myelopathies. Some studies have indicated that the cervical and lumbosacral enlargements are the most common levels of spinal cord affected [481]. Transient ischemic attacks involving the spinal cord have been described.

Occlusion of spinal veins resulting in central hemorrhage and necrosis of the cord have been reported, although rarely [483]. As with hemorrhagic cerebral infarcts, such cases have revealed more hemorrhage than ischemic necrosis, and in the cord the lesions resemble traumatic hematomyelia more than the usual lesions of spinal cord trauma. However, Kim et al. [484] have reported a case of no hemorrhagic spinal cord infarction attributed to venous obstruction.

In contrast to the focal nature of spinal cord infarction secondary to intrinsic spinovascular or aortic disease, prolonged hypotension may result in central gray matter necrosis of the entire spinal cord. In such cases, often related to prolonged terminal hypotension in critically ill patients, the pericentral zone of white matter may also be involved rather impressively [485]. The topography of this lesion is similar to that of the region considered by many to be the primary area of cord vulnerability to trauma.

Spinal cord necrosis at upper cervical levels (C-2 to C-3) is frequently observed in the brain-dead patient [314,486,487] with irreversible coma on prolonged mechanical ventilation (respirator brain). Usually, the remainder of the spinal cord is structurally viable. In fact, necrotic brain (especially cerebellum) passing down into the subarachnoid space of the cord region may be mistaken for meningitis but can also provoke a meningitis with meningeal vasculitis and secondary vascular lesions in the spinal cord. The problem of spinal cord involvement in the respirator brain is discussed in Chapter 5.

Major Vascular Injury Complicating Trauma

The paramount role of ischemia in the pathogenesis of traumatically induced spinal cord injury and necrosis has been reviewed above. Fundamentally, it is impossible to exclude secondary vascular events as a contributing factor in any form of human trauma, because blood vessels, at most levels down to the capillary, are among the first and major tissue components to react. There are, however, cases in which patients with histories of trauma develop lesions that appear to be primarily vascular in origin. In such cases, it is sometimes difficult to identify the tissue reactions to trauma, suggesting that the sole effect of the latter was on a major blood vessel. This subject is reviewed in depth by Jellinger [488], along with those cases of spinal cord trauma that present primarily as hematomas in meningeal compartments (epidural, subdural, subarachnoid) in the cord proper (hematomyelia).

Consideration of Vascular Anatomy in Lesions of Spinal Cord Trauma and Vascular Disease

In analyzing whether a given case may be primarily traumatic or vascular [489], it is useful to review the anatomy of the human spinal cord and its vascular supply [490–492]. A composite of the arterial and venous blood supply of the upper cord appears in Figure 6.77 and in Figure 5.31 from Chapter 5. In the territory between the circulation of the anterior spinal artery and that of the posterior spinal artery is a border, or watershed, zone of the human cervical spinal cord following the nomenclature and modified selected diagrams of Turnbull [493]. In reviewing the composite, it is worth recalling that most pure ischemic lesions involve primarily the central and anterior gray matter (aortic lesions) or a particular vascular zone (anterior spinal artery). Spinal cord trauma in its most severe form causes segmented death and necrosis of all but a thin rim of subpial parenchyma in and around the region of trauma, with the lesion tapering off for several segments above and below. Prolonged severe hypotension provokes necrosis in the entire center of the spinal cord, including appreciable amounts of pericentral white matter. This is the lesion that most mimics the idealized central cord necrosis of incomplete traumatic lesions. However, prolonged hypotension involves the entire spinal cord; that is, it is not segmental like the myelopathy of trauma.

Glossary of Terms and Units of Measurement

Units of Length

Inch (in) = 2.54 centimeters (cm)	Centimeter (cm) = 0.39 inch (in)
Foot (ft) = 0.3048 meter (m)	Meter (m) = 3.28 feet (ft) = 39.37 inches (in)
Yard (yd) = 0.9144 meter (m)	Meter (m) = 1.09 yards (yd)

Units of Force

Pound-foot (lbf) = 4.448 newtons (N)	Newton (N) = 0.22 pound-foot (lbf)
Kilogram force (kgf) = 9.807 newtons (N)	Newton (N) = 0.10 kilogram force (kgf)

Units of Work

Newton-meter (Nm) = 1 kg-m^2/s^2 = joule (J)

Units of Pressure

Pascal (Pa) = 1 N/m^2 = 0.0001 pound/square inch (psi)
Pound/square inch (psi) = 6896 pascals (Pa)

Angular Measure

Circumference of a circle (C) = πD or $2\pi r$
Circumference of a circle in radians = 2π radians (6.28 rad), where 1 rad = 57.32 degrees

References

1. Breasted JH. *The Edwin Smith Papyrus*, Vol. I. Chicago: University of Chicago Press, 1930.
2. Caveness WF, Walker AE, eds. *Head Injury Conference Proceedings*. Philadelphia: Lippincott, 1966.
3. Critchley M. Medical aspects of boxing particularly from a neurological standpoint. *Br Med J* 1957;1:357–62.
4. Denny-Brown D. Cerebral concussion. *Physiol Rev* 1945;25:296–325.
5. Levin HS, Grossman RG, Rose JE, Teasdale G. Long-term neuropsychological outcome of closed head injury. *J Neurosurg* 1979;50:412–22.
6. Wilson JT, Pettigrew LE, Teasdale GM. Emotional and cognitive consequences of head injury in relation to the Glasgow Outcome Scale. *J Neurol Neurosurg Psychiatry* 2000;69:204–9.
7. Whitnall L, McMillan TM, Murray GD, Teasdale GM. Disability in young people and adults after head injury: 5–7 year follow up of a prospective cohort study. *J Neurol Neurosurg Psychiatry* 2006;77:640–5.
8. Millar K, Nicoll JA, Thornhill S, Murray GD, Teasdale GM. Long term neuropsychological outcome after head injury: Relation to APOE genotype. *J Neurol Neurosurg Psychiatry* 2003;74:1047–52.
9. Teasdale GM, Murray GD, Nicoll JA. The association between APOE epsilon 4, age and outcome after head injury: A prospective cohort study. *Brain* 2005;128:2556–61.
10. Casson IR, Siegel O, Sham R, Campbell EA, Tarlau M, DiDomenico A. Brain damage in modern boxers. *JAMA* 1984;251:2663–7.
11. Kaste M, Kuurne T, Vilkki J, Katevuo K, Sainio K, Meurala H. Is chronic brain damage in boxing a hazard of the past? *Lancet* 1982;2:1186–8.
12. Ryan AJ. Intracranial injuries resulting from boxing: A review (1918–1985). *Clin Sports Med* 1987;6:31–40.
13. Clausen H, McCrory P, Anderson V. The risk of chronic traumatic brain injury in professional boxing: Change in exposure variables over the past century. *Br J Sports Med* 2005;39:661–4; discussion, 664.
14. Ross RJ, Casson IR, Siegel O, Cole M. Boxing injuries: Neurologic, radiologic, and neuropsychologic evaluation. *Clin Sports Med* 1987;6:41–51.
15. Bazarian JJ, Zhu T, Blyth B, Borrino A, Zhong J. Subject-specific changes in brain white matter on diffusion tensor imaging after sports-related concussion. *Magn Reson Imaging* 2012;30(2):171–80.
16. Forstl H, Haass C, Hemmer B, Meyer B, Halle M. Boxing-acute complications and late sequelae: From concussion to dementia. *Dtsch Arztebl Int* 2010;107(47):835–9.
17. Viano DC, Casson IR, Pellman EJ. Concussion in professional football: Biomechanics of the struck player—Part 14. *Neurosurgery* 2007;61:313–27; discussion, 327–8.
18. Pellman EJ, Viano DC; National Football League's Committee on Mild Traumatic Brain Injury. Concussion in professional football: Summary of the research conducted by the National Football League's Committee on Mild Traumatic Brain Injury. *Neurosurg Focus* 2006;21(4):E12.
19. Cantu RC. Chronic traumatic encephalopathy in the National Football League. *Neurosurgery* 2007;61:223–5.
20. Omalu BI, DeKosky ST, Hamilton RL, Minster RL, Kamboh MI, Shakir AM, Wecht CH. Chronic traumatic encephalopathy in a National Football League player: Part II. *Neurosurgery* 2006;59:1086–92; discussion, 1092.
21. Weber JT. Experimental models of repetitive brain injuries. *Prog Brain Res* 2007;161:253–61.
22. Guskiewicz KM, Marshall SW, Bailes J, McCrea M, Cantu RC, Randolph C, Jordan BD. Association between recurrent concussion and late-life cognitive impairment in retired professional football players. *Neurosurgery* 2005;57:719–26; discussion, 719–2.
23. Guskiewicz KM, Marshall SW, Bailes J, McCrea M, Harding HP Jr, Matthews A, Mihalik JR, Cantu RC. Recurrent concussion and risk of depression in retired professional football players. *Med Sci Sports Exerc* 2007;39:903–9.

24. Ethier CR, Simmons CA. *Introductory Biomechanics: From Cells to Organisms*. New York: Cambridge University Press, 2007.
25. Özkaya N, Nordin M. *Fundamentals of Biomechanics Equilibrium, Motion, and Deformation*, 2nd ed. New York: Springer, 1999.
26. Duhaime AC, Gennarelli TA, Thibault LE, Bruce DA, Margulies SS, Wiser R. The shaken baby syndrome: A clinical, pathological, and biomechanical study. *J Neurosurg* 1987;66(3):409–15.
27. Prange MT, Luck JF, Dibb A, Van Ee CA, Nightingale RW, Myers BS. Mechanical properties and anthropometry of the human infant head. *Stapp Car Crash J* 2004;48:279–99.
28. Halliday D, Resnick R, Walker J. *Fundamentals of Physics*. Hoboken, NJ: Wiley, 2005.
29. Beer F Jr, Johnston ER, Clausen WE, Staab GH. *Vector Mechanics for Engineers: Statics and Dynamics*. New York: McGraw-Hill, 2004.
30. den Hartog JP. *Strength of Materials*. Mineola, NY: Dover, 1986.
31. Fung YC. *First Course in Continuum Mechanics*. New York: Prentice-Hall, 1994.
32. Woodbourne RT. *Essentials of Human Anatomy*. New York: Oxford University Press, 1957.
33. McElhaney JH, Roberts VL, Hilyard JF. *Handbook of Human Tolerance*. Tokyo: Japan Automobile Research Institute, 1976.
34. Haut RC. Biomechanics of soft tissues. In Nahum AM, Melvin JW, eds., *Accidental Injury*. 1993, pp. 224–46.
35. Gurdjian E. *Impact Head Injury: Mechanics, Clinical and Preventive Correlations*. Springfield, IL: Charles C. Thomas, 1975.
36. Gonzales TA, Vance M, Helpern M, Umberger CJ. *Legal Medicine: Pathology and Toxicology*. New York: Appleton-Century-Crofts, 1954.
37. DiMaio VJ, DiMaio D. *Forensic Pathology*. Boca Raton, FL: CRC Press, 2001.
38. Camps FE, Robinson AE, Lucas BGB, eds. *Gradwohl's Legal Medicine*. Bristol: A. John Wright, 1976.
39. Spitz WU, Spitz DJ, Fisher RS, eds. *Spitz and Fisher's Medicolegal Investigation of Death: Guidelines for the Application of Pathology to Crime Investigation*. Springfield, IL: Charles C. Thomas, 2006.
40. Knight B. *Forensic Pathology*, 2nd ed. London: Arnold, 1996.
41. Bariciak ED, Plint AC, Gaboury I, Bennett S. Dating of bruises in children: An assessment of physician accuracy. *Pediatrics* 2003;112:804–7.
42. Bohnert M, Baumgartner R, Pollak S. Spectrophotometric evaluation of the colour of intra- and subcutaneous bruises. *Int J Legal Med* 2000;113:343–8.
43. Langlois NE, Gresham GA. The ageing of bruises: A review and study of the colour changes with time. *Foren Sci Int* 1991;50:227–38.
44. Maguire S, Mann MK, Sibert J, Kemp A. Can you age bruises accurately in children? A systematic review. *Arch Dis Child* 2005;90:187–9.
45. Grossman SE, Johnston A, Vanezis P, Perrett D. Can we assess the age of bruises? An attempt to develop an objective technique. *Med Sci Law* 2011;51(3):170–6.
46. Vanezis P. Interpreting bruises at necropsy. *J Clin Pathol* 2001;54(5):348–55.
47. Cummings PM, Trelka D, Springer K. *Atlas of Forensic Histology*. New York: Cambridge University Press, 2011.
48. Raekallio J. Timing of wounds—An introductory review. *Ann Acad Med Singapore* 1984; 13(1):77–84.
49. Janssen W. *Forensic Histopathology*. Berlin: Springer-Verlag, 1984.
50. Wilson EF. Estimation of the age of cutaneous contusions in child abuse. *Pediatrics* 1977; 60:750–2.
51. Hamlin H. Subgaleal hematoma caused by hair-pull. *JAMA* 1968;204:339.
52. Hanihara T, Ishida H. Os incae: Variation in frequency in major human population groups. *J Anat* 2001;198:137–52.
53. Calori L. De' wormiani occipitali ed interparietali posteriori dei cranii nostrali e de quelli delle fontanelle laterali ne' cranii di negro. *Mem R Accad Sci Istituto di Bologna* 1867;7:303–21.

54. Calori L. Wormian occipital and interparietal bones. In Bergman RA, Afifi AK, Miyauchi R, eds., *Illustrated Encyclopedia of Human Anatomic Variation: Opus V: Skeletal System*, Vol. 2007. Iowa City: Univ. Iowa, 2006.
55. Rubini M. Size correlation in Wormian bones. *Anthropol Anz* 1998;56:145–9.
56. Urzi F, Iannello A, Torrisi A, Foti P, Mortellaro NF, Cavallaro M. Morphological variability of pterion in the human skull. *Ital J Anat Embryol* 2003;108:83–117.
57. Roach A. Neuroradiological evaluation. In Coleman M, ed., *Neonatal Neurology*. Baltimore: University Park Press, 1981, pp. 81–153.
58. McPherson GK, Kriewall TJ. The elastic modulus of fetal cranial bone: A first step towards an understanding of the biomechanics of fetal head molding. *J Biomech* 1980;13:9–16.
59. McPherson GK, Kriewall TJ. Fetal head molding: An investigation utilizing a finite element model of the fetal parietal bone. *J Biomech* 1980;13:17–26.
60. Kriewall TJ, McPherson GK, Tsai AC. Bending properties and ash content of fetal cranial bone. *J Biomech* 1981;14:73–9.
61. Kriewall TJ. Structural, mechanical, and material properties of fetal cranial bone. *Am J Obstet Gynecol* 1982;143:707–14.
62. Luck JF, Nightingale RW, Song Y, Kait JR, Loyd AM, Myers BS, Bass CR. Tensile failure properties of the perinatal, neonatal and pediatric cadaveric cervical spine. *Spine* (Philadelphia, PA 1976) 2012;38:E1–12.
63. Margulies SS, Thibault KL. Infant skull and suture properties: Measurements and implications for mechanisms of pediatric brain injury. *J Biomech Eng* 2000;122:364–71.
64. Evans FG. *Stress and Strain in Bones*. Springfield, IL: Charles C. Thomas, 1957.
65. McElhaney JH, Fogle JL, Melvin JW, Haynes RR, Roberts VL, Alem NM. Mechanical properties on cranial bone. *J Biomech* 1970;3:495–511.
66. Wood JL. Dynamic response of human cranial bone. *J Biomech* 1971;4(1):1–12.
67. Hubbard RP. Flexure of layered cranial bone. *J Biomech* 1971;4:251–63.
68. Hubbard RP, Melvin JW, Barodawala IT. Flexure of cranial sutures. *J Biomech* 1971;4:491–6.
69. Jaslow CR. Mechanical properties of cranial sutures. *J Biomech* 1990;23:313–21.
70. Davis MT, Loyd AM, Shen HY, Mulroy MH, Nightingale RW, Myers BS, Bass CD. The mechanical and morphological properties of a 6 year-old cranial bone. *J Biomech* 2012;45:2493–2498.
71. Hodgson V, Gurdjian ES, Thomas L. Development of a model for the study of head injury. In *11th Stapp Car Crash Conference*, Warrendale, PA, Society of Automotive Engineers (SAE), 1967, pp. 432–43.
72. Hooper R. *Patterns of Acute Head Injury*. Baltimore: Williams & Wilkins, 1969.
73. Le Count ER, Apfelbach CW. Pathologic anatomy of traumatic fractures of the cranial bones and concomitant brain injuries. *JAMA* 1920;74:501–11.
74. Galloway A. The biomechanics of fracture production. In Galloway A, ed., *Broken Bones: Anthropological Analysis of Blunt Force Trauma*. Springfield, IL: C.C. Thomas, 1999, pp. 35–62.
75. Travis LW, Stalnaker RL, Melvin JW. Impact trauma of the human temporal bone. *J Trauma* 1977;17:761–6.
76. Melvin JW, Evans FG. A strain energy approach to the mechanics of skull fracture. In *Proceedings of the 15th Stapp Car Crash Conference*, 1971, pp. 666–85.
77. Thibault KL. Pediatric head injuries: The influence of brain and skull properties. Thesis, University of Pennsylvania, 1997.
78. Runge CF, Youssef A, Thibault KL, Kurtz SM, Magram E, Thibault LE. Material properties of human infant skull and suture: Experiments and numerical analysis. In *CDC 8th Injury Prevention through Biomechanics Symposium*, 1998.
79. Irwin A, Mertz HJ. Biomechanical basis for the CRABI and Hybrid III child dummies. In *38th Stapp Car Crash Conference*, 1997.
80. Gurdjian ES, Webster JE, Lissner HR. Observation on prediction of fracture site. Head injury. *Radiology* 1953;60:226–35.
81. Melvin JW. Fracture mechanics of bone. *J Biomech Eng* 1993;115:549–54.

82. Allsop DL. Skull and facial bone trauma: Experimental aspects. In Nahum AM, Melvin EC, eds., *Accidental Injury: Biomechanics and Prevention*. New York: Springer-Verlag, 1993, pp. 247–67.
83. Nahum AM, Gatts JD, Gadd CW, Danforth JP. Impact tolerance of the skull and face. In *12th Stapp Car Crash Conference*, Society Automotive Engineers (SAE), 1968, p. 302.
84. Schneider DC, Nahum AM. Impact studies of facial bones and skull. In *16th Stapp Car Crash Conference*, Society Automotive Engineers (SAE), 1972, p. 186.
85. Alsop D, Warner CY, Wille MG, Schneider DC, Nahum AM. Facial impact response—A comparison of the Hybrid III dummy and human cadaver. In *32nd Stapp Car Crash Conference*, Society Automotive Engineers (SAE), 1988, p. 139.
86. Lloyd A. Studies of the human head from neonate to adult: An inertial, geometrical and structural analysis with comparisons to the ATD head. Thesis, Durham, NC: Duke University, 2011.
87. Le Fort R. Etude experimentale sur les fractures de la machiore superiieure. *Rev Chir* 1901;208:360–479.
88. Hodgson VR, Lange WA, Talwalker RK. Injury to the facial bones. In *9th Stapp Car Crash Conference*, Society Automotive Engineers (SAE), 1965, p. 144.
89. Nahum AM, Melvin JW, eds. *Accidental Injury: Biomechanics and Prevention*. New York: Springer-Verlag, 1993.
90. Greenes DS, Schutzman SA. Occult intracranial injury in infants. *Ann Emerg Med* 1998;32:680–6.
91. Fickenscher KA, Dean JS, Mena DC, Green BA, Lowe LH. Occult cranial injuries found with neuroimaging in clinically asymptomatic young children due to abusive compared to accidental head trauma. *South Med J* 2010;103(2):121–5.
92. Gosain AK, Santoro TD, Song LS, Capel CC, Sudhakar PV, Matloub HS. Osteogenesis in calvarial defects: Contribution of the dura, the pericranium, and the surrounding bone in adult versus infant animals. *Plast Reconstr Surg* 2003;112:515–27.
93. Hammerle CH, Schmid J, Lang NP, Olah AJ. Temporal dynamics of healing in rabbit cranial defects using guided bone regeneration. *J Oral Maxillofac Surg* 1995;53:167–74.
94. Kantorova VI. Inductive role of the edges of the bony defect in the process of regeneration of the bones of the cranial vault in adult rabbits. *Ontogenez* 1978;9:333–44.
95. Osipenkova TK. Histomorphology of healing of fractures, splits, and defects in the cranial bones. *Sud Med Ekspert* 2004;47:3–4.
96. Roy S, Sarkar C, Tandon PN, Banerji AK. Cranio-cerebral erosion (growing fracture of the skull in children): Part I. Pathology. *Acta Neurochir* (Wien) 1987;87:112–8.
97. Drapkin AJ. Growing skull fracture: A posttraumatic neosuture. *Childs Nerv Syst* 2006; 22:394–7.
98. Kingsley D, Till K, Hoare R. Growing fractures of the skull. *J Neurol Neurosurg Psychiatry* 1978;41:312–8.
99. McElhaney JH, Hopper RH Jr, Nightingale RW, Myers BS. Mechanisms of basilar skull fracture. *J Neurotrauma* 1995;12(4):669–78.
100. Viano DC, Bir C, Walilko T, Sherman D. Ballistic impact to the forehead, zygoma, and mandible: Comparison of human and frangible dummy face biomechanics. *J Trauma* 2004;56(6):1305–11.
101. Harvey FH, Jones AM. "Typical" basal skull fracture of both petrous bones: An unreliable indicator of head impact site. *J Foren Sci* 1980;25:280–6.
102. Hein PM, Schulz E. Contrecoup fractures of the anterior cranial fossae as a consequence of blunt force caused by a fall. *Acta Neurochir* (Wien) 1990;105:24–9.
103. Hirsch CS, Kaufman B. Contrecoup skull fractures. *J Neurosurg* 1975;42:530–4.
104. Pollanen MS, Deck JH, Blenkinsop B, Farkas EM. Fracture of temporal bone with exsanguination: Pathology and mechanism. *Can J Neurol Sci* 1992;19:196–200.
105. Contostavlos DL. Exsanguination from impact head trauma: The explanation for the "empty heart" sign. *Foren Sci Int* 1998;95:201–12.

106. Ezzat W, Ang LC, Nyssen J. Pontomedullary rent. A specific type of primary brain stem traumatic injury. *Am J Foren Med Pathol* 1995;16:336–9.
107. Britt RH, Herrick MK, Mason RT, Dorfman LJ. Traumatic lesions of pontomedullary junction. *Neurosurgery* 1980;6:623–31.
108. Leestma JE, Kalelkar MB, Teas S. Ponto-medullary avulsion associated with cervical hyperextension. *Acta Neurochir Suppl* (Wien) 1983;32:69–73.
109. Schulz E, Jahn R. Ring fractures of the base of the skull. *Z Rechtsmed* 1983;90:137–45.
110. Oh S. Clinical and experimental morphological study of depressed skull fracture. *Acta Neurochir* (Wien) 1983;68:111–21.
111. Duhaime AC, Eppley M, Margulies S, Heher KL, Bartlett SP. Crush injuries to the head in children. *Neurosurgery* 1995;37:401–6; discussion, 407.
112. Gonzalez Tortosa J, Martinez-Lage JF, Poza M. Bitemporal head crush injuries: Clinical and radiological features of a distinctive type of head injury. *J Neurosurg* 2004;100:645–51.
113. Takeshi M, Okuchi K, Nishiguchi T, Seki T, Watanahe T, Ito S, Murao Y. Clinical analysis of seven patients of crushing head injury. *J Trauma* 2006;60:1245–9.
114. Barlow B, Niemirska M, Gandhi RP, Leblanc W. Ten years of experience with falls from a height in children. *J Pediatr Surg* 1983;18:509–11.
115. Hahn YS, Raimondi AJ, McLone DG, Yamanouchi Y. Traumatic mechanisms of head injury in child abuse. *Childs Brain* 1983;10:229–41.
116. Hobbs CJ. Skull fracture and the diagnosis of abuse. *Arch Dis Child* 1984;59:246–52.
117. Helfer RE, Slovis TL, Black M. Injuries resulting when small children fall out of bed. *Pediatrics* 1977;60:533–5.
118. Merten DF, Osborne DR. Craniocerebral trauma in the child abuse syndrome. *Pediatr Ann* 1983;12:882–7.
119. Kravitz H, Driessen G, Gomberg R, Korach A. Accidental falls from elevated surfaces in infants from birth to one year of age. *Pediatrics* 1969;44(Suppl):869–76.
120. Howard MA, Bell BA, Uttley D. The pathophysiology of infant subdural haematomas. *Br J Neurosurg* 1993;7:355–65.
121. Weber W. Experimental studies of skull fractures in infants. *Z Rechtsmed* 1984;92:87–94.
122. Weber W. Biomechanical fragility of the infant skull. *Z Rechtsmed* 1985;94:93–101.
123. Weber W. Predilection sites of infantile skull fractures following blunt force. *Z Rechtsmed* 1987;98:81–93.
124. Prange M, Newberry W, Moore T, Peterson D, Smyth B, Corrigan C; Society of Automotive Engineers. Inertial neck injuries in children involved in frontal collisions. In *51st Stapp Car Crash Conference*, Soc Auto Eng (SAE), 2007.
125. Melvin JW. Injury assessment reference values for the CRABI-6 month infant dummy in a rear-facing infant restraint with airbag deployment. In *36th Stapp Car Crash Conference*, Society Automotive Engineers (SAE), 1995, pp. 1553–64.
126. Atha J, Yeadon MR, Sandover J, Parsons KC. The damaging punch. *Br Med J (Clin Res Ed)* 1985;291:1756–7.
127. Whiting WC, Gregor RJ, Finerman GA. Kinematic analysis of human upper extremity movements in boxing. *Am J Sports Med* 1988;16:130–6.
128. Walilko TJ, Viano DC, Bir CA. Biomechanics of the head for Olympic boxer punches to the face. *Br J Sports Med* 2005;39:710–9.
129. Lindenberg R, Freytag E. Trauma of the meninges and brain. In Minckler J, ed., *Pathology of the Nervous System*, Vol. 2. New York: McGraw-Hill, 1971, pp. 1705–65.
130. Lindenberg R. Mechanical injuries of brain and meninges. In Spitz WU, Fisher RS, eds., *Medicolegal Investigation of Death: Guidelines for Application of Pathology to Crime Investigation*. Springfield, IL: Charles C. Thomas, 1973, pp. 420–69.
131. Haines DE, Harkey HL, al-Mefty O. The "subdural" space: A new look at an outdated concept. *Neurosurgery* 1993;32:111–20.

132. Peters A, Palay SL, Webster H DeF. *The Fine Structure of the Nervous System: The Neurons, and Supporting Cells*. Philadelphia: W.B. Saunders, 1976.
133. Mack J, Squier W, Eastman JT. Anatomy and development of the meninges: Implications for subdural collections and CSF circulation. *Pediatr Radiol* 2009;39(3):200–10.
134. Kerber CW, Newton TH. The macro and microvasculature of the dura mater. *Neuroradiology* 1973;6(4):175–9.
135. Roland J, Bernard C, Bracard S, Czorny A, Floquet J, Race JM, Forlodou P, Picard L. Microvascularization of the intracranial dura mater. *Surg Radiol Anat* 1987;9(1):43–9.
136. Shukla V, Hayman LA, Ly C, Fuller G, Taber KH. Adult cranial dura I: Intrinsic vessels. *J Comput Assist Tomogr* 2002;26(6):1069–74.
137. Shukla V, Hayman LA, Taber KH. Adult cranial dura II: Venous sinuses and their extrameningeal contributions. *J Comput Assist Tomogr* 2003;27(1):98–102.
138. Merland JJ, Bories J, Djindjian R. The blood supply of the falx cerebri, the falx cerebelli and the tentorium cerebelli. *J Neuroradiol* 1977;4(2):175–202.
139. Lang J. Zur Vascularisation der Dura mater cerebri. *Z Anat Entwickl-Gesch* 1971;135:20–34.
140. Fox RJ, Walji AH, Mielke R, Petruk KC, Aronyk KE. Anatomic details of intradural channels in the parasagittal dura: Possible pathway for flow of cerebrospinal fluid. Anatomic report. *Neurosurgery* 1996;39:84–91.
141. Browder J, Kaplan HA, Krieger AJ. Venous lakes in the suboccipital dura mater and falx cerebelli of infants: Surgical significance. *Surg Neurol* 1975;4(1):53–5.
142. Browder J, Kaplan HA, Krieger AJ. Venous channels in the tentorium cerebelli: Surgical significance. *Surg Neurol* 1975;3(1):37–9.
143. Maxeiner H. Demonstration and interpretation of bridging vein ruptures in cases of infantile subdural bleedings. *J Foren Sci* 2001;46:85–93.
144. Ehrlich E. Postmortem radiological investigation of bridging vein ruptures. *Legal Med* 2003; 5:225–7.
145. Andrews BT, Dujovny M, Mirchandani HG, Ausman JI. Microsurgical anatomy of the venous drainage into the superior sagittal sinus. *Neurosurgery* 1989;24:514–20.
146. Sharifi M, Kunicki J, Krajewski P, Ciszek B. Endoscopic anatomy of the chordae Willisii in the superior sagittal sinus. *J Neurosurg* 2004;101:832–5.
147. Oka K, Rhoton AL Jr, Barry M, Rodriguez R. Microsurgical anatomy of the superficial veins of the cerebrum. *Neurosurgery* 1985;17:711–48.
148. Meder JF, Chiras J, Roland J, Guinet P, Bracard S, Bargy F. Venous territories of the brain. *J Neuroradiol* 1994;21:118–33.
149. Yamashima T, Friede RL. Why do bridging veins rupture into the virtual subdural space? *J Neurol Neurosurg Psychiatry* 1984;47:121–7.
150. Friede RL. *Developmental Neuropathology*. Berlin: Springer-Verlag, 1989.
151. Löwenhielm P. Biomechanics—Material properties and "tissue damage." *Acta Neurochir Suppl* (Wien) 1986;36:28–30.
152. Löwenhielm P. Dynamic properties of the parasagittal bridging veins. *Z Rechtsmed* 1874;74:55–62.
153. Christensen E. Studies on chronic subdural hematoma. *Acta Psychiat Neurol Scand* 1944; 19:69–148.
154. Haines DE. On the question of a subdural space. *Anat Rec* 1991;230:3–21.
155. Allen DJ, Low FN. Scanning electron microscopy of the subarachnoid space in the dog: III. Cranial levels. *J Comp Neurol* 1975;161:515–39.
156. Nabeshima S, Reese TS, Landis DM, Brightman MW. Junctions in the meninges and marginal glia. *J Comp Neurol* 1975;164:127–69.
157. Fishpool SJ, Suren N, Roncaroli F, Ellis H. Middle meningeal artery hemorrhage: An incorrect name. *Clin Anat* 2007;20:371–5.
158. Yilmazlar S, Kocaeli H, Dogan S, Abas F, Aksoy K, Korfali E, Doygun M. Traumatic epidural haematomas of nonarterial origin: Analysis of 30 consecutive cases. *Acta Neurochir* (Wien) 2005;147:1241–8; discussion, 1248.

159. Mealey J. Acute extradural hematomas without demonstrable skull fractures. *J Neurosurg* 1960;17:27–34.
160. Freytag E. Autopsy findings in head injuries from blunt forces. *Arch Pathol* 1963;75:402–13.
161. Choux M, Lena G, Genitori L. Intracranial hematomas. In Raimondi AJ, Choux M, DiRocco C, eds., *Head Injuries in the Newborn and Infant*, Berlin: Springer-Verlag, 1986, pp. 203–16.
162. Le Roux AA, Nadvi SS. Acute extradural haematoma in the elderly. *Br J Neurosurg* 2007;21:16–20.
163. Edna TH. Acute traumatic intracranial haematoma and skull fracture. *Acta Chir Scand* 1983;149:449–51.
164. Ravi D, Dwarakanath S, Satish R, Gopal S, Venkataramana NK. Spontaneous spinal extradural hematomas. *J Clin Neurosci* 2006;13:269–72.
165. Jamieson KG, Yelland JD. Traumatic intracerebral hematoma: Report of 63 surgically treated cases. *J Neurosurg* 1972;37:528–32.
166. Wang EC, Lim AY, Yeo TT. Traumatic posterior fossa extradural haematomas (PFEDH). *Singapore Med J* 1998;39:107–11.
167. Cheung PS, Lam JM, Yeung JH, Graham CA, Rainer TH. Outcome of traumatic extradural haematoma in Hong Kong. *Injury* 2007;38:76–80.
168. Teasdale GM, Galbraith S. Acute traumatic intracranial hematomas. In Krayenbuhl H, Maspes PE, Sweet WH, eds., *Progress in Neurological Surgery*, Vol. 10. Basel: Karger, 1981, pp. 252–90.
169. Radulovic D, Janosevic V, Djurovic B, Slavik E. Traumatic delayed epidural hematoma. *Zentralbl Neurochir* 2006;67:76–80.
170. Riesgo P, Piquer J, Botella C, Orozco M, Navarro J, Cabanes J. Delayed extradural hematoma after mild head injury: Report of three cases. *Surg Neurol* 1997;48:226–31.
171. Parmar CD, Sinha AK, Hayhurst C, May PL, O'Brien DF. Epidural hematoma formation following trivial head trauma in a child with osteogenesis imperfecta. Case report. *J Neurosurg* 2007;106(Suppl):57–60.
172. Chase W. An anatomic study of subdural haemorrhage associated with tentorial splitting in the newborn. *Surg Gynecol Obstet* 1930;51:31–41.
173. Sherwood D. Chronic subdural hematoma in infants. *Am J Dis Child* 1930;39:980–1021.
174. Wintzen AR. The clinical course of subdural haematoma: A retrospective study of aetiological, chronological and pathological features in 212 patients and a proposed classification. *Brain* 1980;103:855–67.
175. Kotwica Z, Brzezinski J. Acute subdural haematoma in adults: An analysis of outcome in comatose patients. *Acta Neurochir* (Wien) 1993;121:95–9.
176. Fell DA, Fitzgerald S, Moiel RH, Caram P. Acute subdural hematomas: Review of 144 cases. *J Neurosurg* 1975;42:37–42.
177. Jennett B, Teasdale G, Galbraith S, Pickard J, Grant H, Braakman R, Avezaat C, Maas A, Minderhoud J, Vecht CJ et al. Severe head injuries in three countries. *J Neurol Neurosurg Psychiatry* 1977;40:291–8.
178. Jones NR, Blumbergs PC, North JB. Acute subdural haematomas: Aetiology, pathology and outcome. *Aust N Z J Surg* 1986;56:907–13.
179. Stone JL, Rifai MH, Sugar O, Lang RG, Oldershaw JB, Moody RA. Subdural hematomas. I. Acute subdural hematoma: Progress in definition, clinical pathology, and therapy. *Surg Neurol* 1983;19:216–31.
180. Yamaki T, Hirakawa K, Ueguchi T, Tenjin H, Kuboyama T, Nakagawa Y. Chronological evaluation of acute traumatic intracerebral haematoma. *Acta Neurochir* (Wien) 1990;103:112–5.
181. Jennett B, Teasdale G. *Management of Head Injuries*. Philadelphia: F.A. Davis, 1982.
182. Gardner WJ. Traumatic subdural hematoma with particular reference to the latent interval. *Arch Neurol Psychiatr* 1932;27:847–55.
183. Goldschlager T, Rosenfeld JV, Winter CD. "Talk and die" patients presenting to a major trauma centre over a 10 year period: A critical review. *J Clin Neurosci* 2007;14:618–23; discussion, 624.
184. Krauland W. *Ueber die Quellen des akuten und chronischen subduralen haematomas*. Stuttgart: Thieme, 1961.

185. Hannah JA. The aetiology of subdural hematomas. An anatomical and pathological study. *J Nerv Ment Dis* 1936;84:169–86.
186. Maxeiner H. Detection of ruptured cerebral bridging veins at autopsy. *Foren Sci Int* 1997;89:103–10.
187. Cohen MC, Scheimberg I. Evidence of occurrence of intradural and subdural hemorrhage in the perinatal and neonatal period in the context of hypoxic ischemic encephalopathy: An observational study from two referral institutions in the United Kingdom. *Pediatr Dev Pathol* 2009:12;169–76.
188. Geddes JF, Tasker RC, Hackshaw AK, Nickols CD, Adams GG, Whitwell HL, Scheimberg I. Dural haemorrhage in non-traumatic infant deaths: Does it explain the bleeding in 'shaken baby syndrome'? *Neuropathol Appl Neurobiol* 2003;29(1):14–22.
189. Maxeiner H, Spies C, Irnich B, Brock M. Rupture of several parasagittal bridging veins without subdural bleeding. *J Trauma* 1999;47(3):606–10.
190. Speth CP. Personal communication, 2008 and 2013.
191. Barnes PD. Imaging of nonaccidental injury and the mimics: Issues and controversies in the era of evidence-based medicine. *Radiol Clin North Am* 2011;49(1):205–29.
192. Ommaya AK. Head injury mechanisms and the concept of preventive management: A review and critical synthesis. *J Neurotrauma* 1995;12:527–46.
193. Gennarelli TA, Thibault LE. Biomechanics of acute subdural hematoma. *J Trauma* 1982; 22:680–6.
194. Walker AE, Diamond EL, Moseley J. The neuropathological findings in irreversible coma. A critique of the "respirator." *J Neuropathol Exp Neurol* 1975;34:295–323.
195. Hirsch CS, Adelson L. Ethanol in sequestered hematomas. *Am J Clin Pathol* 1973;59:429–33.
196. Moriya F, Hashimoto Y. Medicolegal implications of drugs and chemicals detected in intracranial hematomas. *J Foren Sci* 1998;43:980–4.
197. Smialek JE, Spitz WU, Wolfe JA. Ethanol in intracerebral clot: Report of two homicidal cases with prolonged survival after injury. *Am J Foren Med Pathol* 1980;1:149–50.
198. Cameron MM. Chronic subdural haematoma: A review of 114 cases. *J Neurol Neurosurg Psychiatry* 1978;41:834–9.
199. Zollinger R, Gross RE. Traumatic subdural hematoma: An explanation of the late onset of pressure symptoms. *JAMA* 1934;103:245–9.
200. Ito H, Komai T, Yamamoto S. Fibrinolytic enzyme in the lining walls of chronic subdural hematoma. *J Neurosurg* 1978;48:197–200.
201. Weir B, Gordon P. Factors affecting coagulation: Fibrinolysis in chronic subdural fluid collections. *J Neurosurg* 1983;58:242–5.
202. Fujisawa H, Ito H, Saito K, Ikeda K, Nitta H, Yamashita J. Immunohistochemical localization of tissue-type plasminogen activator in the lining wall of chronic subdural hematoma. *Surg Neurol* 1991;35:441–5.
203. Schachenmayr W, Friede RL. The origin of subdural neomembranes: I. Fine structure of the dura–arachnoid interface in man. *Am J Pathol* 1978;92:53–68.
204. Munro D, Merritt HH. Surgical pathology of subdural hematoma: Based on a study of one hundred and five cases. *Arch Neurol Psychiatr* 1936;35:64–78.
205. Leestma JE, Grcevič N. Impact injuries to the brain and head. In Leestma JE, ed., *Forensic Neuropathology*. New York: Raven Press, 1988, pp. 184–253.
206. Hymel KP, Jenny C, Block RW. Intracranial hemorrhage and rebleeding in suspected victims of abusive head trauma: Addressing the forensic controversies. *J Foren Sci* 2002;7:329–48.
207. Aronson SM, Okazaki H. A study of some factors modifying response of cerebral tissue to subdural hematomata. *J Neurosurg* 1963;20:89–93.
208. Fogelholm R, Heiskanen O, Waltimo O. Chronic subdural hematoma in adults: Influence of patient's age on symptoms, signs, and thickness of hematoma. *J Neurosurg* 1975;42:43–6.
209. Goodell CL, Mealey J Jr. Pathogenesis of chronic subdural hematoma. Experimental studies. *Arch Neurol* 1963;8:429–37.
210. Watanabe S, Shimada H, Ishii S. Production of clinical form of chronic subdural hematoma in experimental animals. *J Neurosurg* 1972;37:552–61.

211. Aikawa H, Suzuki K. Experimental chronic subdural hematoma in mice: Gross morphology and light microscopic observations. *J Neurosurg* 1987;67:710–6.
212. Putnam TJ, Putnam IK. The experimental study of pachymeningitis hemorrhagica. *J Nerv Ment Dis* 1927;65:260–72.
213. Murakami H, Hirose Y, Sagoh M, Shimizu K, Kojima M, Gotoh K, Mine Y, Hayashi T, Kawase T. Why do chronic subdural hematomas continue to grow slowly and not coagulate? Role of thrombomodulin in the mechanism. *J Neurosurg* 2002;96:877–84.
214. Ito H, Yamamoto S, Saito K, Ikeda K, Hisada K. Quantitative estimation of hemorrhage in chronic subdural hematoma using the ^{51}Cr erythrocyte labeling method. *J Neurosurg* 1987; 66:862–4.
215. Stone JL, Lang RG, Sugar O, Moody RA. Traumatic subdural hygroma. *Neurosurgery* 1981; 8:542–50.
216. Wetterling T, Demierre B, Rama B, Spoerri O. The clinical course of surgically treated post-traumatic subdural hygromas. *Acta Neurochir* (Wien) 1986;83:99–104.
217. Wetterling T, Demierre B, Rama B, Nekic M. Protein analysis of subdural hygroma fluid. *Acta Neurochir* (Wien) 1988;91:79–82.
218. Lee KS, Bae WK, Park YT, Yun IG. The pathogenesis and fate of traumatic subdural hygroma. *Br J Neurosurg* 1994;8:551–8.
219. Geddes JF, Talbert DG. Paroxysmal coughing, subdural and retinal bleeding: A computer modelling approach. *Neuropathol Appl Neurobiol* 2006;32:625–34.
220. Strassmann G. Formation of hemosiderin and hematoidin after traumatic and spontaneous cerebral hemorrhages. *Arch Pathol* 1949;47:205–10.
221. Blinkov S, Glezer IP. *The Human Brain in Figures and Tables: A Quantitative Handbook.* New York: Basic Books, Plenum Press, 1968.
222. Siegel GJ, Albers RW, Brady ST, Price DL, eds. *Basic Neurochemistry: Molecular, Cellular and Medical Aspects.* Amsterdam: Elsevier Academic Press, 2006.
223. Weiss A, Hiscoe H. Experiments on the mechanism of nerve growth. *J Exp Zool* 1948; 107(3):315–95.
224. Alvarez J, Torres JC. Slow axoplasmic transport: A fiction? *J Theor Biol* 1985;112(3):627–51.
225. Court FA, Alvarez J. Slow axoplasmic transport under scrutiny. *Biol Res* 2011;44(4):311–21.
226. Serani-Merlo A. Jaime Alvarez and the case against slow axoplasmic transport: Some epistemological reflections. *Biol Res* 2001;34(2):111–5.
227. Lubinska L. On axoplasmic flow. *Int Rev Neurobiol* 1975;17:241–96.
228. Lampert PW, Cressman MR. Fine-structural changes of myelin sheaths after axonal degeneration in the spinal cord of rats. *Am J Pathol* 1966;49(6):1139–55.
229. Vaughn J, Hinds P, Skoff RP. Electron microscopic studies of Wallerian degeneration in rat optic nerves: I. The multipotential glia. *J Comp Neurol* 1970;140:175–206.
230. Roy S, Winton MJ, Black MM, Trojanowski JQ, Lee VM. Cytoskeletal requirements in axonal transport of slow component-b. *J Neurosci* 2008;28(20):5248–56.
231. Brown A. Slow axonal transport: Stop and go traffic in the axon. *Nat Rev Mol Cell Biol* 2000;1(2):153–6.
232. Brown A. Axonal transport of membranous and nonmembranous cargoes: A unified perspective. *J Cell Biol* 2003;160(6):817–21.
233. Leestma JE. Velocity measurements of particulate neuroplasmic flow in organized mammalian CNS tissue cultures. *J Neurobiol* 1976;7(2):173–83.
234. Leestma JE, Freeman SS. Computer-assisted analysis of particulate axoplasmic flow in organized CNS tissue cultures. *J Neurobiol* 1977;8(5):453–67.
235. Gillet JP, Derer P, Tsiang H. Axonal transport of rabies virus in the central nervous system of the rat. *J Neuropathol Exp Neurol* 1986;45(6):619–34.
236. Iwasaki Y, Yamamoto T, Konno H, Iizuka H, Kudo H. Eradication of herpes simplex virus persistence in rat trigeminal ganglia by retrograde axoplasmic transport. *J Virol* 1986;59(2):242–8.

237. Openshaw H, Stampalia L, Asher LS. Retrograde axoplasmic transport of herpes simplex virus. *Trans Am Neurol Assoc* 1978;103:238–9.
238. Yamamoto T, Iwasaki Y, Konno H. Retrograde axoplasmic transport of adriamycin: An experimental form of motor neuron disease? *Neurology* 1984;34(10):1299–304.
239. Yamamoto T, Iwasaki Y, Konno H. Retrograde axoplasmic transport of toxic lectins is useful for transganglionic tracings of the peripheral nerve. *Brain Res* 1983;274(2):325–8.
240. Koenig H. Acute axonal dystrophy caused by fluorocitrate: The role of mitochondrial swelling. *Science* 1969;164(3877):310–2.
241. Oehmichen M, Meissner C, Schmidt V, Pedal I, Konig HG, Saternus KS. Axonal injury—A diagnostic tool in forensic neuropathology? A review. *Forensic Sci Int* 1998;95(1):67–83.
242. Oehmichen M, Eisenmenger W, Raff G, Berghaus G. Brain macrophages in human cortical contusions as indicator of survival period. *Foren Sci Int* 1986;30:281–301.
243. Wagner FC Jr, VanGilder JC, Dohrmann GJ. Pathological changes from acute to chronic in experimental spinal cord trauma. *J Neurosurg* 1978;48:92–8.
244. White RJ, Albin MS, Harris LS, Yashon D. Spinal cord injury: Sequential morphology and hypothermic stabilization. *Surg Forum* 1969;20:432–4.
245. Oehmichen M, Walter T, Meissner C, Friedrich HJ. Time course of cortical hemorrhages after closed traumatic brain injury: Statistical analysis of posttraumatic histomorphological alterations. *J Neurotrauma* 2003;20:87–103.
246. Unterharnscheidt F, Sellier K. Mechanics and pathomorphology of closed brain injuries. In Caveness WF, Walker AE, ed., *Head Injury*. Lippincott, Philadelphia, 1966, pp. 321–41.
247. Oehmichen M, Raff G. Zeitabhaengige histomorphologische Veraenderungern von Rindenprellungsherden nach Contusio cerebri. *Beitr Gerichtl Med* 1978;36:291–4.
248. Reilly KT, Sirigu A. The motor cortex and its role in phantom limb phenomena. *Neuroscientist* 2007;14:195–202.
249. Balentine JD, Greene WB, Bornstein M. In vitro spinal cord trauma. *Lab Invest* 1988;58:93–9.
250. Liu XY, Li CY, Bu H, Li Z, Li B, Sun MM, Guo YS, Zhang L, Ren WB, Fan ZL et al. The neuroprotective potential of phase II enzyme inducer on motor neuron survival in traumatic spinal cord injury *in vitro*. *Cell Mol Neurobiol* 2008;28:769–79.
251. Grcevič N. Topography and pathogenic mechanisms of lesions in "inner cerebral trauma." *Rod Yug Acad Sci* 1982;402:265–331.
252. Adams H, Mitchell DE, Graham DI, Doyle D. Diffuse brain damage of immediate impact type. Its relationship to "primary brain-stem damage" in head injury. *Brain* 1977;100:489–502.
253. Ommaya AK, Goldsmith W, Thibault L. Biomechanics and neuropathology of adult and paediatric head injury. *Br J Neurosurg* 2002;16:220–42.
254. Gennarelli TA. Head injury in man and experimental animals: Clinical aspects. *Acta Neurochir Suppl* (Wien) 1983;32:1–13.
255. Torvik A. Brain lesions in alcoholics: Neuropathological observations. *Acta Med Scand Suppl* 1987;717:47–54.
256. Adams JH, Graham DI, Murray LS, Scott G. Diffuse axonal injury due to nonmissile head injury in humans: An analysis of 45 cases. *Ann Neurol* 1982;12:557–63.
257. Adams JH, Doyle D, Graham DI, Lawrence AE, McLellan DR, Gennarelli TA, Pastuszko M, Sakamoto T. The contusion index: A reappraisal in human and experimental non-missile head injury. *Neuropathol Appl Neurobiol* 1985;11:299–308.
258. Gean AD. *Imaging of Head Trauma*. New York: Raven Press, 1994.
259. Adams JH, Graham DI, Gennarelli TA. Head injury in man and experimental animals: Neuropathology. *Acta Neurochir Suppl* (Wien) 1983;32:15–30.
260. Melvin JW, Lighthall JW, Ueno K. Brain injury biomechanics. In Nahum AM, Melvin JW, eds., *Accidental Injury: Biomechanics and Prevention*. New York: Springer-Verlag, 1993, pp. 268–91.
261. Goldsmith W. The state of head injury biomechanics: Past, present, and future. Part 1. *Crit Rev Biomed Eng* 2001;29:441–600.
262. Scott WW. Physiology of concussion. *Arch Neurol Psychiatr* 1940;43:270–83.

263. Gurdjian ES, Lissner H, Latimer R, Haddad B, Webster J. Quantitative determination of acceleration and intracranial pressure in experimental head injury. *Neurology* 1953;3:417–23.
264. Holbourn AHS. Mechanics of head injuries. *Lancet* 1943;2:438–41.
265. Holbourn AHS. The mechanics of brain injuries. *Br Med Bull* 1945;3:147–9.
266. Ommaya AK, Hirsch AE, Flamm ES, Mahone RH. Cerebral concussion in the monkey: An experimental model. *Science* 1966;153:211–2.
267. Ommaya AK, Hirsch AE. Tolerances for cerebral concussion from head impact and whiplash in primates. *J Biomech* 1971;4:13–31.
268. Gennarelli TA, Thibault LE, Tomei G, Wiser R, Graham D, Adams JH. Directional dependence of axonal brain injury due to centroidal and non-centroidal acceleration. In *31st Stapp Car Crash Conference*, Vol. 31, Warrendale, PA, 1987, pp. 49–53.
269. Mertz HJ. Anthropomorphic test devices. In Nahum AM, Melvin JW, eds., *Accidental Injury: Biomechanics and Prevention*. New York: Springer-Verlag, 1993, pp. 66–80.
270. Chancey VC, Nightingale RW, Van Ee CA, Knaub KE, Myers BS. Improved estimation of human neck tensile tolerance: Reducing the range of reported tolerance using anthromorphically correct muscles and optimized physiologic initial conditions. *Stapp Car Crash J* 2003;47:135–153.
271. Dejammes M, Tarriere C, Thomas C, Kallieris D. Exploration of biomechanical data towards a better evaluation of tolerance for children involved in automotive accidents. In *SAE 28th Stapp Car Crash Conference*, 1984, pp. 427–40.
272. Klinich KD, Hulbert GM, Schneider LW. Estimating infant head injury criteria and impact response using crash reconstruction and finite element modeling. *Stapp Car Crash J* 2002; 46:1–30.
273. Sturtz G. Biomechanical data of children. In *SAE 24th Stapp Car Crash Conference*, 1980, pp. 525–9.
274. Schmitt KU, Niederer P, Walz F. *Trauma Biomechanics: Introduction to Accidental Injury*. Berlin: Springer-Verlag, 2004.
275. Eppinger RH. A prospective view of head injury research. In Bandak FA, Eppinger RH, Ommaya AK, eds., *Traumatic Brain Injury: Bioscience and Mechanics*. Larchmont, NY: Mary Ann Liebert, 1996, pp. 39–43.
276. Boock RJ, Thibault LE. Cerebral vascular deformations in high strain rate loading. Paper presented at the *First World Congress of Biomechanics*, LaJolla, 1990.
277. Gennarelli TA. The spectrum of traumatic axonal injury. *Neuropathol Appl Neurobiol* 1996;22:509–13.
278. Margulies SS, Thibault LE. A proposed tolerance criterion for diffuse axonal injury in man. *J Biomech* 1992;25:917–23.
279. Monson KL, Goldsmith W, Barbaro NM, Manley GT. Axial mechanical properties of fresh human cerebral blood vessels. *J Biomech Eng* 2003;125:288–94.
280. Monson KL, Goldsmith W, Barbaro NM, Manley GT. Significance of source and size in the mechanical response of human cerebral blood vessels. *J Biomech* 2005;38:737–44.
281. Lee MC, Haut RC. Insensitivity of tensile failure properties of human bridging veins to strain rate: Implications in biomechanics of subdural hematoma. *J Biomech* 1989;22:537–42.
282. Meaney DF. Biomechanics of acute subdural hematoma in the subhuman primate and man. Thesis, University of Pennsylvania, 1991.
283. Ommaya A, Yarnell P, Hirsch AE, Harris Z. Scaling of experimental data for cerebral concussion in subhuman primates to concussive threshold for man. In *Proceedings of the 11th Stapp Car Crash Conference*, Society of Automotive Engineers (SAE), 1967, pp. 47–52.
284. Prange MT, Meaney DF, Margulies SS. Defining brain mechanical properties: Effects of region, direction, and species. *Stapp Car Crash J* 2000;44:205–13.
285. Prange MT, Margulies SS. Regional, directional, and age-dependent properties of the brain undergoing large deformation. *J Biomech Eng* 2000;124:244–52.
286. Galbraith JA, Thibault LE, Matteson DR. Mechanical and electrical responses of the squid giant axon to simple elongation. *J Biomech Eng* 1993;115:13–22.

287. Thibault LE, Gennarelli TA, Tipton HW, Carpenter DO. The physiologic response of isolated nerve tissue to dynamic mechanical loads. *Proc Ann Conf Eng Med Biol* 1974;16:176.
288. Gray JAB, Ritchie JM. Effects of stretch on single myelinated nerve fibers. *J Physiol* 1954; 124:84–99.
289. Courville CB. Coup–contrecoup mechanism of craniocerebral injuries. Some observations. *Arch Surg* 1942;45:19–43.
290. Gurdjian ES. Cerebral contusions: Re-evaluation of the mechanism of their development. *J Trauma* 1976;16:35–51.
291. Pudenz RH, Shelden CH. The Lucite calvarium—A method for direct observation of the brain. *J Neurosurg* 1946;3:487–505.
292. Goggio AI. The mechanism of contre coup injury. *Pediatrics* 1941;16:11–22.
293. Duret H. Commotions graves, mortelles, sans lesions (commotions pures) et lesions cerebrales stendues sans commotion dans les tratismes craio cerebraux. *Rev Neurol* 1920;36:888–900.
294. Courville CB. *Forensic Neuropathology: Lesions of the Brain and Spinal Cord of Medicolegal Importance.* Mundelein, IL: Callaghan, 1964.
295. Grcevič N. The concept of inner cerebral trauma. *Scand J Rehabil Med Suppl* 1988;17:25–31.
296. Gross AG. A new theory on the dynamics of brain concussion and brain injury. *J Neurosurg* 1958;15:548–61.
297. Ommaya AK, Grubb RL Jr, Naumann RA. Coup and contre-coup injury: Observations on the mechanics of visible brain injuries in the rhesus monkey. *J Neurosurg* 1971;35:503–16.
298. Goldsmith W. *Impact: The Theory and Physical Behavior of Colliding Solids.* Mineola, NY: Dover Publications, 2001.
299. Reiber GD. Fatal falls in childhood. How far must children fall to sustain head injury? Report of cases and review of literature. *Am J Foren Med Pathol* 1993;14:201–207.
300. Prange MT, Coats B, Duhaime AC, Margulies SS. Anthropomorphic simulations of falls, shakes, and inflicted impacts in infants. *J Neurosurg* 2003;99:143–50.
301. Grcevič N. Traumatic tears of the tela chorioidea: A hitherto unrecognized cause of post-traumatic hydrocephalus. *Acta Neurochir Suppl* (Wien) 1983;32:79–85.
302. Oehmichen M. Vitality and time course of wounds. *Foren Sci Int* 2004;144:221–31.
303. Kennady JC. Investigations of the early fate and removal of subarachnoid blood. *Pac Med Surg* 1967;75:163–8.
304. Nevin NC. Neuropathologic change in the white matter following head injury. *Arch Neurol Psychiatr* 967;35:77–84.
305. Voigt GE, Löwenhielm CG, Ljung CB. Rotational cerebral injuries near the superior margin of the brain. *Acta Neuropathol* 1977;39:201–9.
306. Lindenberg R, Freytag E. The mechanism of cerebral contusions: A pathological anatomic study. *Arch Pathol* 1960;69:440–69.
307. Keiper MD, Ng SE, Atlas SW, Grossman RI. Subcortical hemorrhage: Marker for radiographically occult cerebral vein thrombosis on CT. *J Comput Assist Tomogr* 1995;19(4):527–31.
308. Squier W. The "shaken baby" syndrome: Pathology and mechanisms. *Acta Neuropathol* 2011; 122(5):519–42.
309. Baggenstoss AH, Kernohan JW, Drapeiwski JF. The healing process in wounds of the brain. *Am J Clin Pathol* 1943;13:333–48.
310. Clark JM. Distribution of microglial clusters in the brain after head injury. *J Neurol Neurosurg Psychiatry* 1974;37:463–74.
311. Oppenheimer D. Microscopic lesions in the brain following head injury. *J Neurol Neurosurg Psychiatry* 1968;31:503–16.
312. Freytag E, Lindenberg R. Morphology of cortical contusions. *AMA Arch Pathol* 1957;63:23–42.
313. Oehmichen M. Timing of cortical contusion: Correlation between histomorphologic alterations and post-traumatic interval. *Z Rechtsmed* 1980;84:79–94.
314. Oehmichen M, Auer RN, Koenig HG. *Forensic Neuropathology and Neurology.* Berlin: Springer-Verlag, 2006.

315. Itabashi H, Andrews JM, Tomiyasu U, Erlich SS, Sathyavagisawaran L. *Forensic Neuropathology: A Practical Review of the Fundamentals*. New York: Academic Press, 2007.
316. Oehmichen M, Meissner C, Schmidt V, Pedal I, Konig HG. Pontine axonal injury after brain trauma and nontraumatic hypoxic–ischemic brain damage. *Int J Legal Med* 1999;112:261–7.
317. Sherriff FE, Bridges LR, Sivaloganathan S. Early detection of axonal injury after human head trauma using immunocytochemistry for beta-amyloid precursor protein. *Acta Neuropathol* 1994;87:55–62.
318. Geddes JF, Whitwell HL, Graham DI. Traumatic axonal injury: Practical issues for diagnosis in medicolegal cases. *Neuropathol Appl Neurobiol* 2000;26:105–16.
319. Gultekin SH, Smith TW. Diffuse axonal injury in craniocerebral trauma: A comparative histologic and immunohistochemical study. *Arch Pathol Lab Med* 1994;118:168–71.
320. Peerless SJ, Rewcastle NB. Shear injuries of the brain. *Can Med Assoc J* 1967;96:577–82.
321. Strich SJ. Lesions in the cerebral hemispheres after blunt head injury. *J Clin Pathol Suppl (R Coll Pathol)* 1970;4:166–71.
322. Strich S. Shearing of nerve fibers as a cause of brain damage due to head injury. *Lancet* 1961;2:443–8.
323. Strich SJ. Diffuse degeneration of the cerebral white matter in severe dementia following head injury. *J Neurol Neurosurg Psychiatry* 1956;19:163–85.
324. Kasahara K, Hashimoto K, Abo M, Senoo A. Voxel- and atlas-based analysis of diffusion tensor imaging may reveal focal axonal injuries in mild traumatic brain injury—Comparison with diffuse axonal injury. *Magn Reson Imaging* 2012;30(4):496–505.
325. Lucciichenti G, Giugni E, Peran P, Cherubini A, Barba C, Bivona U, Formisano R, Sabatini U. 3 Tesla is twice as sensitive as 1.5 Tesla magnetic resonance imaging in the assessment of diffuse axonal injury in traumatic brain injury patients. *Funct Neurol* 2010;25(2):109–14.
326. Scheid R, Preul C, Gruber O, Wiggins C, von Cramon DY. Diffuse axonal injury associated with chronic traumatic brain injury: Evidence from T2*-weighted gradient-echo imaging at 3 T. *Am J Neuroradiol* 2003;24(6):1049–56.
327. Takaoka M, Tabuse H, Kumura E, Nakajima S, Tsuzuki T, Nakamura K, Okada A, Sugimoto H. Semiquantitative analysis of corpus callosum injury using magnetic resonance imaging indicates clinical severity in patients with diffuse axonal injury. *J Neurol Neurosurg Psychiatry* 2002;73(3):289–93.
328. Schrader H, Mickeviciene D, Gleizniene R, Jakstiene S, Surkiene D, Stovner LJ, Obelieniene D. Magnetic resonance imaging after most common form of concussion. *BMC Med Imaging* 2009;9:11.
329. Gleckman AM, Bell MD, Evans RJ, Smith TW. Diffuse axonal injury in infants with nonaccidental craniocerebral trauma: Enhanced detection by beta-amyloid precursor protein immunohistochemical staining. *Arch Pathol Lab Med* 1999;123(2):146–51.
330. Povlishock JT. Pathobiology of traumatically induced axonal injury in animals and man. *Ann Emerg Med* 1993;22(6):980–6.
331. Tang-Schomer MD, Johnson VE, Baas PW, Stewart W, Smith DH. Partial interruption of axonal transport due to microtubule breakage accounts for the formation of periodic varicosities after traumatic axonal injury. *Exp Neurol* 2012;233(1):364–72.
332. Ogata M, Tsuganezawa O. Neuron-specific enolase as an effective immunohistochemical marker for injured axons after fatal brain injury. *Int J Legal Med* 1999;113(1):19–25.
333. Christman CW, Grady MS, Walker SA, Holloway KL, Povlishock JT. Ultrastructural studies of diffuse axonal injury in humans. *J Neurotrauma* 1994;11(2):173–86.
334. Staal JA, Dickson TC, Chung RS, Vickers JC. Disruption of the ubiquitin proteasome system following axonal stretch injury accelerates progression to secondary axotomy. *J Neurotrauma* 2009;26(5):781–8.
335. Reichard RR, White CL 3rd, Hogan RN, Hladik CL, Dolinak D. Beta-amyloid precursor protein immunohistochemistry in the evaluation of pediatric traumatic optic nerve injury. *Ophthalmology* 2004;111(4):822–7.

382. Boström K, Helander CG, Lindgren SO. Blunt basal head trauma: Rupture of posterior inferior cerebellar artery. *Forensic Sci Int* 1992;53(1):61–8.
383. Dolman CL. Rupture of posterior inferior cerebellar artery by single blow to head. *Arch Pathol Lab Med* 1986;110(6):494–6.
384. Bunai Y, Nagai A, Nakamura I, Ohya I. Traumatic rupture of the basilar artery: Report of two cases and review of the literature. *Am J Forensic Med Pathol* 2000;21(4):343–8.
385. Dowling G, Curry B. Traumatic basal subarachnoid hemorrhage. Report of six cases and review of the literature. *Am J Forensic Med Pathol* 1988;9(1):23–31.
386. Plant JR, Butt JC. Laceration of vertebral artery: An historic boxing death. *Am J Forensic Med Pathol* 1993;14(1):61–4.
387. Pollanen MS, Deck JH, Blenkinsop B. Injury of the tunica media in fatal rupture of the vertebral artery. *Am J Forensic Med Pathol* 1996;17(3):197–201.
388. Filter ER, Fernandes JR. Fatal traumatic subarachnoid hemorrhage due to assault-related tear of the basilar artery. *J Forensic Leg Med* 2009;16(7):414–6.
389. Miyazaki T, Kojima T, Chikasue F, Yashiki M, Ito H. Traumatic rupture of intracranial vertebral artery due to hyperextension of the head: Reports on three cases. *Forensic Sci Int* 1990;47(1):91–8.
390. Leestma JE, Buettner A. "One punch" fatalities. In *American Academy of Forensic Sciences*, Atlanta, 2012, p. 312.
391. Krauland W, Maxeiner H, Siekmann H. Longitudinal tears of the vertebral arteries. Calculations and experimental findings concerning the conditions (author's transl). *Z Rechtsmed* 1981; 87(1–2):19–26.
392. Simonsen J. Fatal subarachnoid haemorrhages in relation to minor injuries in Denmark from 1967 to 1981. *Forensic Sci Int* 1984;24(1):57–63.
393. Farag AM, Franks A, Gee DJ. Simple laboratory experiments to replicate some of the stresses on vertebro-basilar arterial walls: An investigation of possible mechanisms of traumatic subarachnoid haemorrhage. *Forensic Sci Int* 1988;38(3–4):275–84.
394. Tatsuno Y, Lindenberg R. Basal subarachnoid hematomas as sole intracranial traumatic lesions. *Arch Pathol* 1974;97(4):211–5.
395. Snoek JW, Minderhoud JM, Wilmink JT. Delayed deterioration following mild head injury in children. *Brain* 1984;107:15–36.
396. Bruce DA, Alavi A, Bilaniuk L, Dolinskas C, Obrist W, Uzzell B. Diffuse cerebral swelling following head injuries in children: The syndrome of "malignant brain edema." *J Neurosurg* 1981;54:170–8.
397. Overgaard J, Tweed WA. Cerebral circulation after head injury: 1. Cerebral blood flow and its regulation after closed head injury with emphasis on clinical correlations. *J Neurosurg* 1974;41:531–41.
398. Overgaard J, Tweed WA. Cerebral circulation after head injury: Part 2. The effects of traumatic brain edema. *J Neurosurg* 1976;45:292–300.
399. Overgaard J, Mosdal C, Tweed WA. Cerebral circulation after head injury: Part 3. Does reduced regional cerebral blood flow determine recovery of brain function after blunt head injury? *J Neurosurg* 1981;55:63–74.
400. Overgaard J, Tweed WA. Cerebral circulation after head injury: Part 4. Functional anatomy and boundary-zone flow deprivation in the first week of traumatic coma. *J Neurosurg* 1983;59:439–46.
401. Refines HD, Dill L, Saad S, Hungerford GD. Neurogenic pulmonary edema and missile emboli. *J Trauma* 1980;20:698–701.
402. Sedy J, Zicha J, Kunes J, Jendelova P, Sykova E. Mechanisms of neurogenic pulmonary edema development. *Physiol Res* 2008;57:499–506.
403. Simon RP. Neurogenic pulmonary edema. *Neurol Clin* 1993;11(2):309–23.
404. Bayne LL, Simon RP. Systemic and pulmonary vascular pressures during generalized seizures in sheep. *Ann Neurol* 1981;10(6):566–9.

405. Johnston SC, Darragh TM, Simon RP. Postictal pulmonary edema requires pulmonary vascular pressure increases. *Epilepsia* 1996;37:428–32.
406. Young YR, Lee CC, Sheu BF, Chang SS. Neurogenic cardiopulmonary complications associated with spontaneous cerebellar hemorrhage. *Neurocrit Care* 2007;7:238–40.
407. Mayer SA, Fink ME, Homma S, Sherman D, LiMandri G, Lennihan L, Solomon RA, Klebanoff LM, Beckford A, Raps EC. Cardiac injury associated with neurogenic pulmonary edema following subarachnoid hemorrhage. *Neurology* 1994;44:815–20.
408. Leestma JE, Hughes JR, Teas SS, Kalelkar MB. Sudden epilepsy deaths and the forensic pathologist. *Am J Foren Med Pathol* 1985;6:215–8.
409. Povlishock JT, Becker DP, Miller JD, Jenkins LW, Dietrich WD. The morphopathologic substrates of concussion? *Acta Neuropathol* 1979;47:1–11.
410. Rizzo M, Tranel DD, eds. *Head Injury and Postconcussive Syndrome*. New York: Churchill Livingstone, 1996.
411. McCrea MA. *Mild Traumatic Brain Injury and Postconsussion Syndrome: The New Evidence Base for Diagnosis and Treatment*. New York: Oxford University Press, 2008.
412. Aronson SM. Pathologic considerations in head injury. In Feiring H, ed., *Brock's Injuries of the Brain and Spinal Cord and Their Coverings*. New York: Springer-Verlag, 1974, pp. 42–72.
413. Corsellis JA, Brierley JB. Observations on the pathology of insidious dementia following head injury. *J Ment Sci* 1959;105:714–20.
414. Kurland LT, Mulder DW. Epidemiologic investigations of amyotrophic lateral sclerosis: I. Preliminary report on geographic distribution, with special reference to the Mariana Islands, including clinical and pathologic observations. *Neurology* 1954;4:355–78.
415. Annegers JF, Grabow JD, Groover RV, Laws ER Jr, Elveback LR, Kurland LT. Seizures after head trauma: A population study. *Neurology* 1980;30:683–9.
416. Laidlaw J, Richens A. *A Textbook of Epilepsy*. Edinburgh: Churchill-Livingstone, 1982.
417. Lathers CM, Schraeder PL, eds. *Epilepsy and Sudden Death*. New York: Marcel Dekker, 1990.
418. Lindenberg R, Walsh FB, Sacks JG. *Neuropathology of Vision: An Atlas*. Philadelphia: Lea & Febiger, 1973.
419. Unterharnscheidt F, Unterharnscheidt JT. *Boxing: Medical Aspects*. London: Academic Press, 2003.
420. Thomassen A, Juul-Jensen P, de Fine Olivarius B, Braemer J, Christensen AL. Neurological, electroencephalographic and neuropsychological examination of 53 former amateur boxers. *Acta Neurol Scand* 1979;60:352–62.
421. Hahnel S, Stippich C, Weber I, Darm H, Schill T, Jost J, Friedmann B, Heiland S, Blatow M, Meyding-Lamade U. Prevalence of cerebral microhemorrhages in amateur boxers as detected by 3T MR imaging. *Am J Neuroradiol* 2007;29:388–91.
422. Zetterberg H, Hietala MA, Jonsson M, Andreasen N, Styrud E, Karlsson I, Edman A, Popa C, Rasulzada A, Wahlund LO et al. Neurochemical aftermath of amateur boxing. *Arch Neurol* 2006;63:1277–80.
423. Loosemore M, Knowles CH, Whyte GP. Amateur boxing and risk of chronic traumatic brain injury: Systematic review of observational studies. *BMJ* 2007;335:809.
424. Backaitis SH, ed. *Biomechanics of Impact Injuries and Injury Tolerances of the Abdomen, Lumbar Spine, and Pelvis Complex*. Warrendale, PA: Society of Automotive Engineers, 1995.
425. Bridwell KH, DeWald RL, eds. *The Textbook of Spinal Surgery*. Philadelphia: Lippincott-Raven, 1997.
426. Benzel E. *Biomechanics of Spine Stabilization*. Rolling Meadows, IL: American Association of Neurological Surgeons, 2001.
427. Adams MA, Burton K, Dolan P, Bogduk N. *The Biomechanics of Back Pain*. Edinburgh: Churchill Livingstone Elsevier, 2006.
428. McElhaney JH, Meyers BS. Biomechanical aspects of cervical trauma. In Nahum AM, Melvin JW, eds., *Accidental Injury: Biomechanics and Prevention*. New York: Springer-Verlag, 1993, pp. 311–61.

429. Van Ee CA, Nightingale RW, Camacho DL, Chancey VC, Knaub KE, Sun EA, Myers BS. Tensile properties of the human muscular and ligamentous cervical spine. *Stapp Car Crash J* 2000;44:85–102.
430. Goldsmith W, Ommaya AK. Head and neck injury criteria and tolerance level. In Aldman B, Chapon A, eds., *The Biomechanics of Impact Trauma*. Amsterdam: Elsevier, 1984, pp. 149–87.
431. Mertz H, Patrick L. Strength and response of the human neck. *Stapp Car Crash Conf Proc* 1971;710855:207–55.
432. Kraus JF. Epidemiological aspects of acute spinal cord injury. A review of incidence, prevalence, causes and outcome. In Becker DP, Pavlishock JT, eds., *Central Nervous System Trauma Status Report*. Bethesda, MD: National Institute of Neurological and Communicative Disorders and Stroke (NINCDS), 1985, pp. 313–22.
433. Lentle BC, Brown JP, Khan A, Leslie WD, Levesque J, Lyons DJ, Siminoski K, Tarulli G, Josse RG, Hodsman A; Scientific Advisory Council of Osteoporosis Canada, Canadian Association of Radiologists. Recognizing and reporting vertebral fractures: Reducing the risk of future osteoporotic fractures. *Can Assoc Radiol J* 2007;58:27–36.
434. Peek-Asa C, Kraus JF. Estimates of injury impairment after acute traumatic injury in motorcycle crashes before and after passage of a mandatory helmet use law. *Ann Emerg Med* 1997;29:630–6.
435. Kraus JF, Franti CE, Riggins RS. Neurologic outcome and vehicle and crash factors in motor vehicle related spinal cord injury. *Neuroepidemiology* 1982;1:223–38.
436. Girard R, Minaire P, Castanier M, Berard E, Perrineriche B. Spinal cord injury by falls: Comparison between suicidal and accidental cases. *Paraplegia* 1980;18:381–5.
437. Kennedy P, Rogers B, Speer S, Frankel H. Spinal cord injuries and attempted suicide: A retrospective review. *Spinal Cord* 1999;37:847–52.
438. Aito S, D'Andrea M, Werhagen L. Spinal cord injuries due to diving accidents. *Spinal Cord* 2005;43:109–16.
439. Korres DS, Benetos IS, Themistocleous GS, Mavrogenis AF, Nikolakakos L, Liantis PT. Diving injuries of the cervical spine in amateur divers. *Spine J* 2006;6:44–9.
440. Brown RL, Brunn MA, Garcia VF. Cervical spine injuries in children: A review of 103 patients treated consecutively at a level 1 pediatric trauma center. *J Pediatr Surg* 2001;36:1107–14.
441. Camacho DL, Hopper RH, Lin GM, Myers BS. An improved method for finite element mesh generation of geometrically complex structures with application to the skullbase. *J Biomech* 1997;30(10):1067–70.
442. Camacho DL, Nightingale RW, Ronbinette JJ, Vanguri SK, Coates DJ, Myers BS. Experimental flexibility measurements for the development of a computational head-neck model validated for near-vertex head impact. In *41st Stapp Car Crash Conference*, Soc Auto Eng (SAE), 1997.
443. Beckner MA, Heggeness MH, Doherty BJ. A biomechanical study of Jefferson fractures. *Spine* 1998;23:1832–6.
444. Reay DT, Cohen W, Ames S. Injuries produced by judicial hanging: A case report. *Am J Foren Med Pathol* 1994;15:183–6.
445. Spence MW, Shkrum MJ, Ariss A, Regan J. Craniocervical injuries in judicial hangings: An anthropologic analysis of six cases. *Am J Foren Med Pathol* 1999;20:309–22.
446. Myers BS, McElhaney JH, Doherty BJ, Paver JG, Gray L. The role of torsion in cervical spine trauma. *Spine* 1991;16:870–4.
447. Branco F, Cardenas DD, Svircev JN. Spinal cord injury: A comprehensive review. *Phys Med Rehabil Clin N Am* 2007;18:651–79.
448. Bracken MB, Holford TR. Neurological and functional status 1 year after acute spinal cord injury: Estimates of functional recovery in National Acute Spinal Cord Injury Study II from results modeled in National Acute Spinal Cord Injury Study III. *J Neurosurg* 2002; 96(Suppl):259–66.
449. Vogel LC, Klaas SJ, Lubicky JP, Anderson CJ. Long-term outcomes and life satisfaction of adults who had pediatric spinal cord injuries. *Arch Phys Med Rehabil* 1998;79:1496–503.

450. Schmitz A, Lutterbey G, von Engelhardt L, von Falkenhausen M, Stoffel M. Pathological cervical fracture after spinal manipulation in a pregnant patient. *J Manipulative Physiol Ther* 2005;28:633–6.
451. Dupeyron A, Vautravers P, Lecocq J, Isner-Horobeti ME. Complications following vertebral manipulation—A survey of French region physicians. *Ann Readapt Med Phys* 2003;46:33–40.
452. Stevinson C, Honan W, Cooke B, Ernst E. Neurological complications of cervical spine manipulation. *J R Soc Med* 2001;94:107–10.
453. Oler M, Tomson W, Pepe H, Yoon D, Branoff R, Branch J. Morbidity and mortality in the martial arts: A warning. *J Trauma* 1991;31:251–3.
454. Cecil KM, Hills, EC, Sandel ME, Smith DH, McIntosh TK, Mannon LJ, Sinson GP, Bagley LJ, Grossman RI, Lenkinski RE. Proton magnetic resonance spectroscopy for detection of axonal injury in the splenium of the corpus callosum of brain-injured patients. *J Neurosurg* 1998;88:795–801.
455. Pieter W. Martial arts injuries. *Med Sport Sci* 2005;48:59–73.
456. Riggins RS, Kraus JF. The risk of neurologic damage with fractures of the vertebrae. *J Trauma* 1977;17:126–33.
457. Bosch PP, Vogt MT, Ward WT. Pediatric spinal cord injury without radiographic abnormality (SCIWORA): The absence of occult instability and lack of indication for bracing. *Spine* 2002;27:2788–800.
458. Green BA, Klose KJ, Goldberg M. Clinical and research considerations in spinal cord injury. In Becker DP, Pavlishock JT, eds., *Central Nervous System Trauma Status Report*. Bethesda, MD: National Institute of Neurological and Communicative Disorders and Stroke (NINCDS), 1985, pp. 341–68.
459. Braakman R, Penning L. Injuries of the cervical spine. In Vinken PJ, Bruyn GW, eds., *Handbook of Clinical Neurology*, Vol. 25. New York: Elsevier North Holland, 1976, pp. 227–376.
460. Ducker TB, Walleck CA. Recovery from spinal cord injury. In Becker DP, Pavlishock JT, eds., *Central Nervous System Trauma Status Report*. Bethesda, MD: National Institute of Neurological and Communicative Disorders and Stroke (NINCDS), 1985, pp. 369–75.
461. Braakman R. Traumatic lesions of the spine. In Rosenberg R, ed., *The Clinical Neurosciences*, Vol. 2. New York: Churchill Livingstone, 1983, pp. 1467–90.
462. Schneider RG. Trauma to the spine and spinal cord. In Kahn E, Crosby EC, Schneider RG, Taren JA, eds., *Correlative Neurosurgery*. Springfield, IL: Charles C. Thomas, 1969, pp. 597–648.
463. Davis D, Bohlman H, Walker AE, Fisher R, Robinson R. The pathological findings in fatal craniospinal injuries. *J Neurosurg* 1971;34:603–13.
464. Perna E, Petrone G, Liguiori R, Serino D, DeRosa G, Calabro A. Tetraplegia from trauma of the cervical spine in the absence of fractures and luxations. *J Neurol Sci* 1975;3:170–5.
465. Liao CC, Lui TN, Chen LR, Chuang CC, Huang YC. Spinal cord injury without radiological abnormality in preschool-aged children: Correlation of magnetic resonance imaging findings with neurological outcomes. *J Neurosurg* 2005;103(Suppl):17–23.
466. Kakulas BA, Bedbrook GM. A correlative clinico-pathologic study of spinal cord injury. *Proc Aust Assoc Neurol* 1969;6:123–32.
467. Baydin A, Cokluk C, Aydin K. A new minimally invasive experimental spinal cord injury model in rabbits. *Minim Invasive Neurosurg* 2007;50:170–2.
468. Basso DM, Beattie MS, Bresnahan JC. Graded histological and locomotor outcomes after spinal cord contusion using the NYU weight-drop device versus transection. *Exp Neurol* 1996;139:244–56.
469. Haghighi SS, Perez-Espejo MA, Rodriguez F, Clapper A. Radiofrequency as a lesioning model in experimental spinal cord injury. *Spinal Cord* 1996;34:214–9.
470. Metz GA, Curt A, van de Meent H, Klusman I, Schwab ME, Dietz V. Validation of the weight-drop contusion model in rats: A comparative study of human spinal cord injury. *J Neurotrauma* 2000;17:1–17.

471. Balentine JD. Pathology of experimental spinal cord trauma: I. The necrotic lesion as a function of vascular injury. *Lab Invest* 1978;39:236–53.
472. Jellinger K. Neuropathology of cord injuries. In Vinken PJ, Bruyn GW, eds., *Handbook of Clinical Neurology*, Vol. 25. New York: Elsevier North Holland, 1976, pp. 43–121.
473. Balentine JD, Dean DL Jr. Calcium-induced spongiform and necrotizing myelopathy. *Lab Invest* 1982;47:286–95.
474. Kao CC, Bunge RP, Reier PJ, eds. *Spinal Cord Reconstruction*. New York: Raven Press, 1983.
475. Barnett HJM, Jousse AT. Post-traumatic syringomyelia (cystic myelopathy). In Vinken PJ, Bruyn GW, eds., *Handbook of Clinical Neurology*, Vol. 26. New York: Elsevier North Holland, 1976, pp. 113–57.
476. Rothman RH, Simeone FA, eds. *The Spine*. Philadelphia: Saunders, 1982.
477. Gunzberg R, Szpalski M, eds. *Lumbar Spinal Stenosis*. Philadelphia: Lippincott Williams & Wilkins, 2000.
478. van Royen BJ, Dijkmans BAC, eds. *Ankylosing Spondylitis: Diagnosis and Management*. New York: Taylor & Francis, 2006.
479. Calin A, Taurog JD, eds. *The Spondylarthritides*. New York: Oxford University Press, 1998.
480. Hughes J. *Pathology of the Spinal Cord*. London: Lloyd-Luke, 1966.
481. Garland H, Greenberg J, Harriman DG. Infarction of the spinal cord. *Brain* 1966;89:645–61.
482. Yoshiyama M, Asamoto S, Kobayashi N, Sugiyama H, Doi H, Sakagawa H, Ida M. Spinal cord decompression sickness associated with scuba diving: Correlation of immediate and delayed magnetic resonance imaging findings with severity of neurologic impairment—A report on 3 cases. *Surg Neurol* 2007;67:283–7.
483. Hughes JT. Venous infarction of the spinal cord. *Neurology* 1971;21:794–800.
484. Kim RC, Smith HR, Henbest ML, Choi BH. Nonhemorrhagic venous infarction of the spinal cord. *Ann Neurol* 1984;15:379–85.
485. Young W. Blood flow, metabolic and neurophysiological mechanisms in spinal cord injury. In Becker DP, Pavlishock JT, eds., *Central Nervous System Trauma Status Report*. Bethesda, MD: National Institute of Neurological and Communicative Disorders and Stroke (NINCDS), 1985, pp. 463–73.
486. Schneider H, Matakas F. Pathological changes of the spinal cord after brain death. *Acta Neuropathol* 1971;18:234–47.
487. Leestma JE. Neuropathology of brain death. In Eelco FM, ed., *Brain Death*. Philadelphia: Lippincott Williams & Wilkins, 2001, pp. 45–60.
488. Jellinger K. Traumatic vascular disease of the spinal cord. In Vinken PJ, Bruyn GW, eds., *Handbook of Clinical Neurology*, Vol. 12. New York: Elsevier North Holland, 1972, pp. 556–630.
489. Tator CH, Koyanagi I. Vascular mechanisms in the pathophysiology of human spinal cord injury. *J Neurosurg* 1997;86:483–92.
490. Gillilan LA. The arterial blood supply of the human spinal cord. *J Comp Neurol* 1958;110:75–103.
491. Gillilan LA. Veins of the spinal cord. Anatomic details; suggested clinical applications. *Neurology* 1970;20:860–8.
492. Brockstein B, Johns L, Gewertz BL. Blood supply to the spinal cord: Anatomic and physiologic correlations. *Ann Vasc Surg* 1994;8:394–9.
493. Turnbull IM. Blood supply of the spinal cord. In Vinken PJ, Bruyn GW, eds., *Handbook of Clinical Neurology*, Vol. 12. New York: Elsevier North Holland, 1972, pp. 478–91.

Child Abuse
Neuropathology Perspectives

7

JAN E. LEESTMA

Contents

Introduction and Historical Background

Throughout history, most societies have exhibited ambivalent and often inconsistent behaviors toward children: on the one hand, espousing the value and sanctity of the child and, on the other, condoning if not codifying various modes of maltreatment. In some countries, such as Sweden, rigorous and sweeping laws protect all aspects of the child's life, whereas in others, maltreatment, slavery, sexual exploitation, infanticide, and mutilation are tolerated. In most advanced societies, a well-defined system of law exists for children to grant to them the same degree of protection under the law afforded to adults, but even in ancient times laws existed that proscribed the killing of babies and children, and various punishments were stipulated for individuals found guilty of this activity [1]. However, it was well recognized that it was often not possible to determine if the death of a child was due to natural causes or the actions of another. Autopsies, after a fashion, even in medieval times, were often sought to resolve this issue, and the legal quandaries posed by difficulties in obtaining reliable medical information were well known. The discovery by Swammerdam in 1667 [2–4] that the lungs of infants who had breathed floated in water whereas those of stillborns did not constitute a valuable advance in pathological knowledge that went a long way toward proving infanticide at the time. Further reports corroborated this early observation; however, like many historic observations and the conclusions that arose from them, experience and research have developed exceptions. It is now recognized that lungs of stillborn infants can sometimes float, for which there may be several reasons. Among them are bacterial contamination with gas formation, manipulation after stillbirth, attempted resuscitation, possibly elastic expansion of the thorax in precipitous deliveries of the stillborn infant, and probably others [5].

Very early on, there were observations regarding fatal head trauma in infants and children, which led many writers of the late seventeenth and eighteenth centuries to advise against striking the heads of infants or children for fear of producing bleeding inside the skull or "water on the brain." In 1860 Ambroise Tardieu, published probably the earliest learned treatise on the syndrome of the battered child based largely on autopsy study [6]. This work is said to contain virtually all the elements of injury that were later "rediscovered" and brought to the attention of the medical world under the term *battered child syndrome* by the publications and pioneering work of C. Henry Kempe and his colleagues during the early 1960s [7,8]. The body of literature has now expanded to more than 25,000 citations [9]. The efforts of Kempe and other efforts led to research studies, one of which, conducted by the American Humane Society, revealed that in a single year in the United States, there were 662 reported cases of child abuse, 27% of which had resulted in death of the child [10]. Furthermore, a review of papers on subdural hematomas in infancy that date from the late 1800s into the early 1900s clearly implies in some case reports the strong likelihood of abusive injury as a basis for the injuries [11,12]. It is interesting to note that in some of these case reports, fundoscopic examinations revealed retinal hemorrhages, a finding that, again, was rediscovered many years later and about which there is considerable interpretive controversy. There have been a number of reports on the magnitude of fatal child abuse in given populations, but out of necessity for the methods employed and many basic uncertainties that underlie the cases, these figures are estimates only [13,14].

An outgrowth of the evolving public awareness that child abuse exists and is probably widespread has given rise to a host of local and national organizations whose purpose is education, prevention, advocacy, and direct service in the field of child abuse. Through the influence of these groups, most states now have some official organization to which reports of abuse and neglect must be made and which can mandate actions to be taken to protect the injured child [1,15]. In most states, any individual, layperson, or physician who observes abuse or neglect of a child by anyone is obligated to report his or her observations or suspicions to a state or local agency [16–18]. In the state of Illinois, this agency is the Department of Children and Family Services, which maintains 24-hour-a-day telephone operators to receive calls. Anyone who reports suspected or observed child abuse is protected by the law and is never asked to confront an accused person. All reports are investigated by presumably competent professional personnel of the department before any action is taken relative to the alleged abuser or the child. In some communities, computer data banks exist that allow hospital emergency rooms to coordinate information on possible previous emergency room visits to other hospitals by an injured child in order to develop an awareness of repeated injury and take corrective action. This and other information on file at child welfare agencies may be an exploitable resource to law enforcement agencies and to the medical examiner/coroner when he or she is called on to determine if a death occurred within the context of potential abuse. An outgrowth of reporting laws and the increasing coordination and power of child welfare agencies has been abuse of the system and an unintended extension of power and influence over persons suspected or accused of abusing their children. In many jurisdictions in the United States, child protective services, regardless of judicial processes regarding criminal proceedings against alleged perpetrators or their outcome, can pursue an independent course of action that may deprive parents of their children and force them to incur disabling financial burdens to essentially prove their innocence. The lack of uniform standards or criteria for removal of children from a home may inappropriately empower vindictive and zealous social workers to exact their own perception of justice in cases that may or may not actually be adjudicated in a court of law.

The problem of child abuse, over the past 40 years, has led to a number of phenomena within the medical community. Many pediatrics residency programs and teaching hospitals have now established child abuse response teams, interdisciplinary child abuse teams, child abuse training programs, and fellowships in child abuse. Recently, board certification in child abuse has become available for pediatricians [19]. The role of the clinician in determining the cause and manner of injury (before death) is problematic, but has nevertheless been adopted widely. Two issues arise with the clinician's involvement. First, contrary to what may be communicated to potentially accused persons, is that if the potentially accused tells the clinician what she or he did, then the child's life might be saved. This line of questioning is disingenuous at best and deceptive at worst. The treatment of a head injury, which is the physician's role, does not depend on this sort of information. Second, despite alleged training in child abuse, there is no or almost no input into the educational training exercise by qualified forensic scientists and pathologists whose disciplines are cause of injury and manner of death determinations using science and hopefully not dogma.

Many of the above organizations have become politically and legally active largely within the context of providing counsel, primarily to police authorities and prosecutors, and in some cases to assume a nearly prosecutorial or adjudicative position. As a consequence of increasing vigor in seeking prosecutions of possible abusers, a body of law has developed that has elevated child abuse to special status, often demanding very harsh penalties not only for the death of a child but also for child endangerment or condoning abuse. Many of these offenses carry with them mandated long prison terms with very little legal leeway for judges. Various aspects of this issue are discussed in Chapter 2. Against the background of difficult forensic case analysis, a dead child, high interest in the community and media, and the severe punishment for anyone accused of harming a child make for a very high-stakes endeavor on the part of the pathologist.

The involvement of the general pathologist, forensic pathologist, or neuropathologist in the phenomenon of child abuse is multifaceted [20]. On the one hand, as concerned citizens, there is an important role that such health-care professionals can play in raising public and professional awareness to the problem; however, there is also an important professional and statutory responsibility to report suspected cases and to assist in legal processes that come into play when a child dies out of neglect or overt action on the part of another. This role is often very difficult because there is frequently conflicting information regarding a fatal event. The child cannot speak for himself or herself, and in the case of nonfatal abuse, if the child is old enough to communicate, he or she may not be believed. Furthermore, there is often a high degree of concern and anxiety on the part of physicians that if an accusation is made, it will or cannot be proved, and libel or damage actions may follow. Comparatively few physicians consider themselves experts on the problem of child abuse, and even many forensic pathologists are uncomfortable with such cases [21,22]. The issue first realized in the seventeenth century still remains: how can it be determined if a fatality was the result of accident or willful action? A further complication in the analysis of fatalities in children is the fact that they may not be due to willful abuse; some children are purposefully killed under circumstances that do not constitute child abuse in the usual sense [23,24]. A study conducted by Copeland [24] on case material collected over nearly 30 years in Miami-Dade County, Florida, indicates that about 45% of homicides in children under the age of 12 years occurred within the context of child abuse, but about 42% did not, and in 14% the circumstances were either unknown or undetermined. The perpetrators of these crimes are similar in characteristics to those who fatally injure children by abusing them (about 70% are parents). The neuropathological characteristics in this total group differ little from those series involving abuse only, in that more than 50% suffer some form of serious skull or brain injury.

Pathology of Child Abuse

Current texts and references on forensic pathology all contain important information on the typical forms of child abuse that lead to death. These references should be consulted for more details and illustrations [2,15,25]; however, the following represents a condensed survey of information for purposes of orientation or review. Discussions of head injury in children in relation to possible child abuse are found in Chapter 6, and discussions on cerebral edema, hydrocephalus, and intracranial pressure/volume issues are found in Chapter 5. Some reiteration of these issues will appear below.

The analysis of potential or alleged child abuse fatalities by the forensic pathologist poses one of the most difficult challenges possible. Child abuse fatalities rarely involve identification problems of the body, DNA trace evidence is rarely involved, witnesses who can or will provide information are only rarely encountered, confessions are often suspect, trace evidence is rarely germane, and the case almost always hinges on circumstantial evidence and medical opinion that may be ill-informed, prejudiced, or based on dogma. Almost every alleged child abuse case, especially involving young infants, includes the possibility of some preexisting brain injury or other condition, possibly emanating from birth, or the possibility of inherited or acquired disorders of bleeding/coagulation or some other process that can mimic traumatic lesions. At least some service should be paid by the pathologist to the long list of differential and confounding conditions that may be present before reaching a decision concerning both the cause and manner of death.

The elements of the battered child syndrome that are commonly reported include [5,15,25–27] the following:

- An infant usually less than 1 year of age who displays evidence of multiple episodes of injury, consisting of many healing dermal injuries, including burns, cuts, and scars
- Multiple skeletal fractures, skull fractures, subdural or epidural hematomas, spine or neck injuries
- Retinal and optic nerve sheath hemorrhages, and other retinal pathologies
- Malnourished and poorly cared for
- Smaller than normal for the age
- Usually will have been reported to have died or collapsed at home
- Found dead in bed [assumed or purported sudden infant death syndrome (SIDS)]
- Usually reported to have been injured following a fall or falls (while changing diapers, bathing, etc.)
- Reported to have suddenly stopped breathing or choked—acute life-threatening event (ALTE)
- Had a seizure with subsequent coma
- Reported to have pulled hot liquids on themselves
- Reported to have become entangled in bedclothes

Evidence may surface that the child had been seen repeatedly in emergency rooms for similar injuries over a period of time, often at different institutions. Not infrequently the child may appear normal and well fed with no obvious outward signs of injury. There may be a history of similar injuries in other children in the family or previous fatalities in infants. The family may be from any socioeconomic class, well or poorly educated, but careful inquiry may reveal that one or both parents had themselves been victims of abuse or neglect as children [28]. The account given to explain the injuries in the child by the parent or caregiver may change on questioning or when the parent or caregiver is confronted with suspicions or evidence of abuse [29]. One must be ever mindful that circumstances under which admissions or confessions are obtained may be coercive or otherwise suspect, and information thus obtained may be tainted. Furthermore, admissions and confessions may or may not be factual, complete, or true at all for reasons that are the subject of a robust literature [30–32].

Older children who are victims of abuse may be suffering from cerebral palsy or mental retardation [7,33] and sometimes have been abused and injured by many members of the family, including siblings [34,35]. In some families where more than one baby has died suddenly and unexpectedly and may have been signed out as SIDS, there is always the suspicion, often justified, that these deaths were not natural; however, there are familial diseases, such as "ion-channel-opathies" that cause the so-called long Q-T syndrome, and others that result in multiple unexpected and apparently unexplained deaths of infants [36, 37]. Such cases have often only come to light through the untiring and diligent efforts of counselors or attorneys to uncover family histories. This is especially true of the Cannings case in the United Kingdom [38], where a mother who lost three children and nearly a fourth due to sudden unexpected death was convicted of murder but whose life sentence was overturned on appeal.

Occasionally, caregivers or parents will confess to smothering a child who was considered a SIDS victim; thus, the SIDS problem is a constant source of concern for forensic pathologists [39–41]. In recent years, a newly appreciated form of child abuse that may involve suffocation of the infant by a caregiver, so-called Munchausen-by-proxy, poses yet another challenge for the forensic pathologist [42,43]. A number of aspects of the SIDS phenomenon are discussed in Chapter 4.

Before Autopsy in Suspected Child Abuse

Autopsies on possible victims of child abuse may well be the most complex and challenging of any forensic case, even though perhaps at the outset a given case may appear simple. The interaction of inherited disorders, accident scenarios, medical treatment effects, and inflicted injuries demands careful attention to detail and an appreciation for possibilities that include many rare conditions of which the average forensic pathologist may be unaware; however, ignorance of such conditions cannot be an excuse for an erroneous conclusion that may have serious consequences for persons who may be accused of injuring the child victim. Although it is unsatisfying professionally, there is often plenty of justification for the forensic pathologist to use the "undetermined" manner of death in many cases.

Upon beginning an analysis of a possible abuse fatality, information that should be available to the forensic pathologist charged with determination of cause and manner of death before an examination of the body of a suspected victim of child abuse is vital in the interpretation and correlation of subsequent anatomic findings of the body surface, in the viscera, or in the central nervous system [44]. This information should include as detailed a history as possible of the events leading up to the death. This information may be in the form of a police report; ambulance, emergency room, or hospital records (including birth records); radiographs or radiographic reports; or notes made by one or more investigative officers, perhaps of a child welfare agency. This information should include a narrative account by the adults present or any witness of the events that occurred, as well as an account of what, if any, medical treatment had been rendered recently, including prescription drugs and proximate immunizations and why they were administered.

It is also important, at some point before sign-out, to have a report available, including photographs of the scene (or to have made a personal visit), which include the state of repair and cleanliness of the surroundings and proximity of beds to windows, radiators, and other objects. The composition of the floor and its covering is also important to later interpretation of head injuries and possible pattern injuries that might be observed on the skin. If falls from cribs or other furniture or surfaces are alleged to have occurred, measurements and photographs of these surfaces should be taken with scales in the photographs. Any stains should be sampled and appropriately collected for analysis. The presence of pets, other children, and adults and their relationship to the child may also be important. Attention should be paid to the state of repair and cleanliness of the clothing the victim is wearing or was wearing at the time of death or injury. If there are soiled towels or papers on the scene, they should be preserved for later analysis. Further considerations on proper scene analysis are beyond the scope of this discussion and are within the ken of the burgeoning field of scene forensics and trace evidence analysis.

General Autopsy

The general state of nutrition of the body must be noted, and measurements of body length, crown–rump length, head circumference, and weight must be recorded and compared with values from "well baby" records. The external examination of the body obviously can reveal important clues about the nature and extent of injuries and evidence of past injuries [44]. Such external appearances may include multiple lacerations in various stages of healing or pattern injuries as would be caused by a belt buckle, switch, whip, or ligature. There may be few, if any, external signs of bruising, yet there may be extensive subcutaneous injuries, including fractures of the limbs, ribs, and skull, that are only visible when the internal examination is conducted. Burns of various forms may be seen, which may suggest the cause of these injuries as being a cigarette, a hot iron, a scalding liquid, etc. Bites and puncture wounds and bruises may also be visible. The presence of any lesion, including a diaper rash, scars, hyperpigmentation or hypopigmentation, or keloids, should be noted and photographed [2,25,27]. Examination of the body orifices may reveal signs of injury, but care should be exercised in premature interpretation of any dermal or mucosal injury because there may be many causes, including medical treatment or examinations, that may give an ominous impression of inflicted injury, including sexual abuse. Smears of the orifices may also be useful in determining the presence of semen and establishing valuable DNA evidence. The patterns of external injuries seen in child abuse cases have been described in detail in many texts and monographs cited above. It is common to discover tears or other injuries to the interior of the mouth and frenulum that may attributed to forceful feeding or some other abusive action; however, intubation and resuscitation may also cause such lesions. Bruises of the pinnae of the ears, often viewed with extreme suspicion, may also be iatrogenic, caused by straps from a respirator mask or adhesive tape. Likewise, injuries to the penis, vulva, and anus may not be due to abuse but, rather, insertion of catheters, thermometers, or other instruments. Nevertheless, these lesions, when found, should be photographed and possibly sampled histologically.

The internal examination should include whole-body radiography to document any recent or healed fractures of long bones, ribs, pelvis, and skull [45–47]. Tissue samples of any external lesion should be taken to establish the nature of the lesion and its age. Fractures that are observed should also be sampled histologically for documentation and age determination and to determine if they are indeed fractures. Very often radiology reports may indicate fractures of the skull or metaphyses of long bones or ribs that, at autopsy, prove not to be fractures but, rather, anatomic variants of bone formation, aberrant vascular channels, or variant sutures in the case of the skull (Wormian–interosseous bones). It is vital that these "lesions" be documented and sampled histologically.

A careful examination of the viscera may reveal old and recent traumatic lesions that may include lacerations of viscera, tears in the mesentery, and puncture or other injuries of the viscera. If intravascular catheters were employed, they should be left *in situ* so that if there is possible puncture of a viscus from a misplaced catheter, its relationship to the hemorrhage or injury can be ascertained. It is vital that histological sampling of visceral hemorrhages or other lesions be made in order to provide aging/dating information on the injuries, which may permit correlation with historical events or facts in evidence.

Neuropathological Autopsy Examination

Because head injury is such a common component of alleged and known child abuse fatalities, it is essential that a proper examination be conducted and appropriate documentation of injuries and other conditions be effected. This latter can be accomplished by making diagrams of any lesions found and photographing them with reasonable quality media, as well as collecting appropriate tissue samples for storage and histological preparations.

As a part of the general external examination, bruises, abrasions, lacerations, and any other potential lesion of the scalp, neck, and back should be identified, described, measured, and memorialized. Any lesions in the scalp should be clearly visualized after having been photographed by shaving the area and repeating the process of photography. Histological sampling may be dictated by needs to preserve the face for showing at a funeral service; however, subcutaneous tissues, which are where most hemorrhages occur, can be sampled without disfigurement if care is taken. The scalp should be reflected according to standard procedures that reveal the skull and its periosteum. The deep scalp tissues should be carefully examined for hemorrhage, which may represent impact points, taking care to differentiate from possible surgical interventions such as placement of intracranial pressure monitors, burr holes, or surgical sites. Generally when such procedures have been performed, interpretation of subgaleal hemorrhage is made very difficult, if not impossible, owing to the often extensive diffusing hemorrhage that results from the procedure. Nevertheless, any lesions should be photographed.

The skull should be sawed or cut to allow atraumatic exposure of the dura and brain; however, before sawing, care should be taken to determine if there may be a skull fracture by percussing with the finger for a "cracked pot" sound. If fractures are found, they should be photographed and the fracture edges sampled for histological examination. Once the skull cap is removed, the dura can be inspected for lesions. If it has not been torn during removal of the skull cap, a careful incision should be made around the circumference of the head using curved scissors such as Mayo scissors to avoid damaging the brain beneath. The falx can be cut carefully to allow the dura to be reflected over the brain's surface to reveal hemorrhage if present. Posteriorly, the dura just above the tentorium can be cut. If care is taken, the dura can be reflected upward so that the near midline can be examined to see if bridging vein injury has occurred and, if so, to attempt to locate such an injury and photograph it. When this examination has been completed, the dura can be separated from or left with the brain as it is removed. By the same token, basal dural sinuses should be opened in search for thrombosis. Paranasal sinuses should also be opened for signs of infection. Wherever hemorrhages are found, iron stains should be performed in addition to the usual hematoxylin and eosin (H&E) stains.

There are a number of monographs and books that provide instructions for brain removal and many of the above-mentioned dissections [5,27,44,47,48]. The brain should be removed carefully to avoid creating disruptions. Generally, a good method involves gently elevating the frontal lobes and cutting the optic nerve, carotid arteries, and other cranial nerves after the tentorium has been cut circumferentially with the curved scissors. With the brain gently tilted backwards and supported, the cervical–medullary junction can be severed with a long-handled scalpel and the brain can then be removed, carefully examined, weighed, and then placed in fixative for later examination. This can be effected by suspending the brain in a volume of 10% formalin that is buffered that exceeds the volume of the brain by at least three times. The brain can be suspended by a length of string passed beneath the basilar artery and tied around the opening of the brain crock or container. If this is not done, the brain may sink and become distorted during fixation. If possible, formalin should be changed after a few days. Fixation of the brain under these circumstances is usually complete within a week or two, at which time it can be washed and dissected.

The basal dura of the skull should be stripped and placed along with the vertex dura in the brain container. If appropriate, the eyes may be removed via sawing of the orbital roofs. Paranasal sinuses can be entered and examined if appropriate (in possible cases of meningitis), and the petrous portions of the temporal bones can likewise be sawed and examined or removed and fixed. The exposed cranial base should be examined and photographed if any fractures or other lesions are present. Histological sampling of any lesions should be done as well.

In general practice, the spinal cord can be examined via the open thorax and abdomen by sawing away the vertebral bodies; however, in cases of alleged or suspected child abuse, the spinal cord should be removed by a posterior approach with an incision from the occiput downward. The soft tissues can be elevated away from the spine, and any areas of hemorrhage can be exposed and documented. The cord can be exposed by sawing the posterior vertebral arches. Inspection of the spinal dura can then proceed, again with photographs being taken of any lesions. The entire spinal cord should be carefully removed, avoiding too much pulling and tugging to avoid artifacts of removal. The spinal roots can be individually cut and the spinal cord with its dura to the lumbosacral region (cauda equina) removed. The spinal cord with its dura can then be placed in the brain container and fixed. Like the brain, sectioning of the cord in the fresh state in possible abuse autopsies should be avoided. The cord can be examined at the time of brain cutting.

It may be appropriate to obtain samples of peripheral nerve and muscle if there is any suspicion of diseases of these systems. Samples of the lumbar and brachial plexuses are easily reached from the normal autopsy incisions. Samples of the deltoid, intercostal, psoas, and other muscles can also be easily obtained if needed.

After the brain, cord, and dural specimens are fixed, they should be washed with running water until much of the formalin odor is gone. The dura should be examined for any staining or discontinuity, and such areas should be sampled for histological examination. The superior sagittal sinus should be opened and inspected for thromboses. If suspected, these should be sampled histologically. The brain can be sectioned in any plane if required for a particular anatomic correlation, such as with the plane of an imaging study; however, generally, coronal sections no more than 1 cm thick should be made and laid out on a tray in an orderly manner after the brain stem–cerebellum has been separated by a single sweep of a scalpel at the midbrain level. These structures can then be sectioned in a number of ways [49]. Often it is convenient to make a section through the cerebellar rostral vermis parallel to the brain stem and then place the cerebellum–brain stem flat and make cross sections from top to bottom, to display the entire brain stem. It may be required to angulate the crosscut to maintain cross sections of the brain stem. These sections can then be laid out with the brain.

Inspection of the sections can then proceed, noting the locations and distributions of lesions and taking representative sections for photography and histological sampling. An appropriate routine sampling should include several areas of the cortex and underlying white matter (frontal, parietal, occipital, temporal). It may be appropriate to sample the corpus callosum. An effective section that will show the insular cortex and underlying basal ganglia, including the ependyma, is made via the insula to the ventricle, and this is then divided into two pieces to permit embedding. A section of the hippocampus should be made. A section should be made of each level of the brain stem, with one section of the cerebellum. As for the spinal cord, the dura should be opened and the crosscut made at 1-cm levels throughout its extent, sampling for histological study each major division with the dura. If lesions are found, more extensive sampling should be made.

If nerves and muscle are to be studied, both cross- and longitudinal sections should be prepared. If the eyes have been taken, they can be fixed and sectioned with a razor blade on each side of the limbus, providing two culottes and a central cylinder of the eye. A section can be made through this cylinder to include the optic nerve for embedding. Other specimens can be decalcified if needed and prepared.

Neuropathological and Forensic Issues in Child Abuse Cases

The specific traumatic conditions such as epidural and subdural hematomas, skull fractures, brain injuries, and neck and spinal cord injuries are dealt with from several perspectives in other chapters, but some repetition is required here to facilitate communication. The following are common issues in the forensic neuropathology of child abuse fatalities. Some of these are technical, physiological, mechanistic, clinical, and pathological, but many are professional, in that often profound disagreement exists over many aspects of the abuse scenario and its effects. An effort will be made to discuss these, giving the various positions on the issues and their basis.

Dermal and Scalp Injuries

As has been discussed earlier in Chapter 6, the scalp is a layered structure that can be injured in many ways from so-called blunt impacts (blows or falls) that cause bruising; by splitting, incision, and cutting (laceration) by wielded objects or from contact with various surfaces during falling (accidental or inflicted); and by being punctured with pointed objects (medical treatments or other occurrences). Other forms of dermal injury can occur from thermal effects, such as heating or cold. Various mechanisms include immersion, splashing, and exposure to heat or cold air or surfaces. Injuries can occur from vermin, animals (pets or wild), biting by another person, and injury from ligatures, constricting materials, or objects making impressions on the skin. Gunshot, missile, and fragmentation injuries may also be seen, although not usually in the abuse situation [5,24]. These conditions are discussed in Chapter 8.

Several important aspects of dermal injury in potential abuse scenarios should be kept in mind when making a case analysis. One is that in infants and young children, the extent of external evidence of injury may not correlate with the severity of underlying injury to the skull or brain; it is possible to have virtually no visible external injury yet have massive injuries in deeper structures. The reason for this is that an impacting object or surface may cause in-bending of the malleable skull such that the skin is not compressed between the object and the softer and deformable skull. Thus, a full appreciation of deeper injuries may not be achievable unless proper imaging is done or an autopsy is performed. Another important issue is the estimation of the age of a skin lesion by external inspection. Although many profess to be able to accomplish such aging, objective investigation of the problem has shown that at best, visual inspection is an estimate and may be able only to differentiate between recent, resolving, and older dermal injuries, with no sharp lines between these arbitrary and vague designations [50,51]. If there is a point of agreement, it appears that when a bruise is yellow, it is generally older than 18 hours [52]. Attempts have been made using instrumentation such as photometers to age dermal injuries, but with only measured success [53,54]. Among the many confusional factors in skin injury aging are the variabilities of dermal pigmentation and individual characteristics, observer consistency with color perceptions and descriptions, and the depth at which hemorrhage in the skin has occurred. The more superficial bleeds tend to appear more red than the deeper bleeds, which appear more blue, but beyond this little or no reliable other conclusions can be drawn.

Another area that requires caution in interpreting skin lesions involves differentiation of inflicted injuries from those that might have occurred in connection with medical treatment and hospitalization or other reasons having nothing to do with abusive injury. Typical examples are often-unrecorded instances in which venous access had been attempted via a scalp vein in an infant, electrode damage to the skin (EEG or other recording electrodes), injuries caused by head restraint devices during neurosurgical procedures, and lesions caused by tape, elastic straps, or other surfaces such as ventilation pipes, nasogastric tubes, and tracheal catheters that may have impressed the skin and caused pressure injury. Often photographs of the victim in an intensive care unit before death can provide correlations of dermal injuries that the pathologist might not suspect because these objects are no longer in evidence. Quite often, infants or children will be positioned unconscious in a bed or crib in a manner that puts pressure on the occiput and may cause pressure injury, which may pose confusion as the lesion is being an impact point during inflicted injury. Still other examples are bruises to the face, chin, lips, and neck that can occur in the course of intubation and cardiopulmonary resuscitation (CPR). Differentiation of these from truly inflicted injuries may be difficult to impossible but can be aided by careful reading of emergency room and CPR notes that may describe preexisting injuries before resuscitation.

The role of histology in aging bruises leaves a lot to be desired if using only H&E staining and paraffin sections. Generally, bruises do not involve the upper layers of the skin but, rather, occur in the subdermis and present with highly variable vital reactions, including inflammation [55]. Iron staining generally will not stain siderophages from 3 days to about 7 days after injury, and later aging using this method is imprecise [56]. A number of aging and dating schemes have appeared in recent texts, to which the reader is referred [57,58]. Enzyme histochemical staining of skin bruises and other injuries has been employed by some workers, with mixed success [55]. Newer methods than can probe for induction of the apoptosis pathway and collagen synthesis in response to injury show duration-dependent alterations; however, precision is problematic, as is the availability of what are essentially research techniques to the forensic pathologist in most circumstances [59–61].

Interpretation of possible pattern injuries to the face, skin, and scalp may be highly correlated with some object surfaces present at a scene on occasion; however, in most instances, vague patterns on a victim offer little chance of correlation. A common perception is that punctate bruises may or do indicate fingertip impressions due to gripping. Of course, sometimes crescent-shaped fingernail impressions can be demonstrated and even correlated with DNA of the victim under the nails of an offender, but vagueness of impressions often frustrates such an analysis. It is vital that if there appear to be patterned impressions or bruises, good photographs with scale rulers in the field be taken so that size comparisons may be made with candidate surface or objects at the scene.

The correlation of various other forms of skin wounds with objects is a science in and of itself and will not be reviewed here. The interested reader can find ample discussion of these matters in standard forensic pathology texts [2,5,26,27] and in Chapter 6.

Skull Fractures and Abuse

The types and characteristics of skull fractures in children as well as adults have been discussed in Chapter 6 in detail, especially with respect to the injury biomechanics of fracturing. The following discussion may repeat to some degree that which appears elsewhere in this volume. An infant skull obviously has different physical properties than does the skull of the older child or adult. In the infant, the skull bones are thin and as yet unfused to make a solid cranium. This means that the skull is malleable and, when impacted or compressed, will bend inward with or without fracturing to deform the brain and possibly tear intracranial vessels, venous channels, tentorium or other parts of the dura, and possibly the brain itself. This also means, as mentioned above, that even with significant deep injuries the scalp may show little or nothing. Generally, if the skull is fractured by an impact, it will tend to be a linear parietal fracture with highly variable deeper injuries. If fractures are more complex (depressed, expressed, multiple, diastatic, widely spaced, or growing) and have associated brain injury, a number of workers have expressed the opinion that such fractures strongly suggest an abusive etiology, but this is not necessarily so [62,63]. An example of a complex or stellate skull fracture from a case of alleged child abuse is illustrated in Figure 7.1.

A number of studies approaching the issue of accidental versus inflicted head injuries have reported that accidental falls only occasionally or rarely cause skull fractures or brain injury [14,15]. One of the earliest of these studies is that of Helfer et al. [64], who

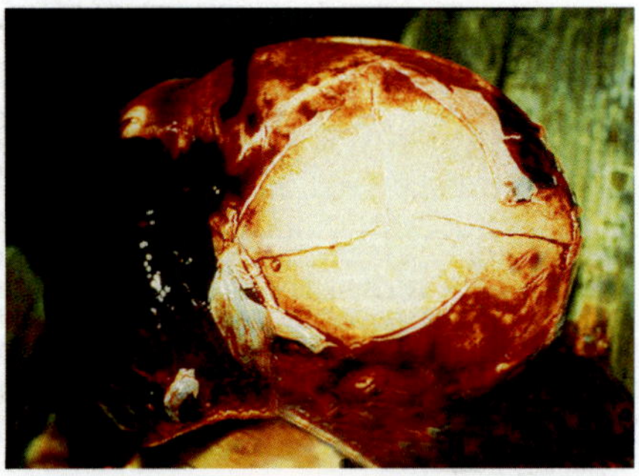

Figure 7.1 Lateral view of an abusive skull fracture in a 4-month-old child. The mother was reported to have repeatedly beaten the baby practically from birth until the child's death. Note the extensive subgaleal and scalp hemorrhage that covers most of the scalp tissues on the left side of the head. If there has been surgery or insertion of a pressure monitor, these procedures can produce a similar extensive hemorrhage pattern and can overshadow underlying hemorrhage or make interpretations of what is iatrogenic and what is a preexisting lesion difficult. (Courtesy of the Office of the Medical Examiner, Cook County, IL.)

collected information on 161 children brought to an urban hospital between 1969 and 1975 after having had falls as reported. A total of 176 incidents were investigated. Of these, 169 were reported to have been a fall from beds or sofas of 90 cm or less, 5 were from heights of 120 cm, and 2 were from 150-cm heights. Most of the children suffered no injury at all. However, in 37 of them, injuries were discovered that were considered nonserious and included assorted bruises, bumps, and scratches. In only six were there injuries that were more serious: three clavicular fractures, two skull fractures (unilateral with 1 mm or less fracture line width), and one humerus fracture. The two children with skull fractures experienced no neurological complications and no subdural or epidural hematomas. All cases of fracture were apparently uncomplicated. A further 85 children were studied in connection with incidents occurring while hospitalized for other problems. These children were also 5 years of age and younger and were reported to have fallen in most cases about 90 cm from a hospital bed. Of these children, 57 showed no apparent injury, 17 showed minor abrasions or cuts or bloody noses, 20 children had a bruise, and only one, who fell off an emergency room cart, was shown to have a skull fracture with no complications. A total, then, of 246 cases were reviewed by these workers, who found only four instances of skull fracture, none of which was accompanied by neurological signs; all of which were unilateral, nondiastatic fractures; all of which showed a fracture line of 1 mm or less; and none of which had any evidence of subdural or epidural hematoma. Other reports noted a low incidence of serious head injuries from accidental falls and concluded that serious injuries occurring with reported falls spoke loudly for an abusive rather than an accidental cause [29,63,65–67].

Unfortunately, there are issues of significance with the interpretation of these reports. Most of the early studies, like those of Helfer et al. [64], occurred in the era before computed tomography (CT) and magnetic resonance imaging (MRI) scanning, so that the possibility of occult injuries in a child that appeared not to have been injured might have been overlooked, a situation that has been since appreciated [68,69] as a common issue in pediatric emergency room practice. Another is the implied assumption that the children had struck their heads yet mostly were not injured. In fact, the points of impact were not specified in the reports, except that nonhead impacts can be inferred from those children who injured their arms, shoulders, or other body parts and not their heads. Ignoring these criticisms, the studies basically confirmed what is generally known—that children fall a lot and mostly do not hurt themselves seriously when doing so, and when they fall, they do not necessarily fall on their heads. A number of other observers have noted this and clearly indicate that even low-height falls in which the head strikes the floor or ground can cause serious injuries, some of which can be fatal [70–74]. It cannot be accurately estimated what percentage of children who fall hit their heads, but in studies that report more complete accident statistics, when injuries occur, those that involve the head make up about half of the injuries and body injuries make up the other half [72,75].

A series of important studies involving infant cadavers that were dropped on various surfaces from table height (82 cm) has been reported by Weber [76–78]. These studies, which employed 50 infant and child cadavers from neonates to infants up to about 8 months of age, as well as examined 82 cases from the literature, showed that "in special cases, fractures cannot be avoided even after falls onto softly cushioned ground" [78]. These studies clearly indicate that when the head strikes a largely unyielding surface after a fall from less than 3 ft, skull fractures can occur, sometimes nonsimple ones. This study cannot address, of course, the consequences of the skull fractures because the children were already dead. To assess or estimate possible consequences, one must look to clinical studies such as those of Greenes and Schutzman [68] and of Fickenscher et al. [69], where there may be an incidence of 20% to about 50% of occult head injury in those infants who apparently were clinically uninjured but had imaging evidence of a spectrum of cranial and intracranial injuries. Precisely how many of these children might have developed subsequent symptomatology is not known, but it has been estimated that more than 25% of them will return to the hospital or clinic with symptoms that may or may not have to be treated [68]. The conclusion from this information is that infants and children can and do suffer serious injuries even from short falls with head impacts against hard surfaces, and it cannot be said unequivocally that injuries sustained provide reliable information concerning what happened before the impact.

Generally, the higher the fall height, the more serious the injuries that can occur, which is logical because the energetics of falls are largely determined by the terminal velocity the body reaches at time of impact on a firm surface by Newtonian physics. The terminal velocity of a free fall for any object is

$$V = \sqrt{2GS}$$

where V is the velocity in feet/second at the impact with the floor or ground surface, S is the distance in feet of the fall, and G is 32.2 ft/s/s—the force of gravity. Once contact of the head with the impact surface occurs, a series of events occur that determine the amount of acceleration (or deceleration) that will occur to the mass of the head. These events are not totally predictable, although their effect on acceleration can be estimated. If the characteristic of the impact surface, scalp (thickness, stiffness, etc.), and skull (stiffness and other properties) are known or can be estimated, estimates may be made for the so-called stopping distance (the distance that it takes for the head to decelerate from the terminal velocity to a resting state). The stopping time (the time it takes for the head to decelerate from the terminal velocity to a resting state) may also be estimated. Depending on many factors, a stopping distance for a hard surface is on the order of 1/4 in. to about 1/2 in., and the stopping time may be about 4–10 ms. As the head would be decelerating during the impact, the rate of deceleration (in several planes) is likely not to be linear but will change during the short time of the impact event due to deformation and other dynamic events in the impact with a head (real or modeled). This deceleration event may have a pulse shape that is complex but most commonly approximates a sine wave. Owing to the complexities involved, precise calculations of g forces during a head fall are not easily made, but they can be compared to modeled data using instrumented dummies, as shown in Figure 6.2 in Chapter 6.

It is common for nonphysicists or nonengineers to fail to appreciate how impressive the force of gravity is and how high the velocity any body, including the head, can attain in comparatively short distances of falling. Table 7.1 illustrates this principle using the velocity formula cited above using the English units of measurement.

Examples of such falls in which a CRABI-6 dummy head (model of a 6-month-old baby) struck carpeted wooden stairs indicate that a 1-ft fall attained 50–60g. A 2-ft fall attained 80–87g, and a 3-ft fall attained 98–116g (data provided by C. Van Ee, PhD, Design Research Engineering of Novi, Michigan). These values would be different for different ages and conditions, but some points of reference can be gleaned from these data.

Table 7.1 Peak Terminal Velocities Any Body Will Attain in Falling to Floor or Other Flat Surface from a Horizontal Position

Distance of Fall (ft)	Peak Velocity (ft/s)	Peak Velocity (mi/h)
1	8.02	5.47
2	11.35	7.74
3	13.9	9.48
4	16.04	10.94
5	17.94	12.23
6	19.66	13.40
10	25.38	17.30
20	35.89	24.47
30	43.95	34.61

Note: This table displays peak terminal velocities reached by any object falling from a distance in feet to a floor surface under the influence of gravity only. For each foot of drop, the velocities are displayed in feet/second, and in miles/hour. The velocity reached is independent of the mass of the object. Calculations are based on Newtonian physics for a falling body: $V = \sqrt{2GS}$ (V in ft/s; G = 32.2 ft/s^2; distance in ft).

From a practical point of view, the notion that infants cannot suffer serious injuries from short falls is illogical. If one were to imagine a baby being propelled into a wall at 5–10 miles per hour (equivalent of a 1- to 3-ft fall), as if being thrown forward into a wall, would one seriously maintain that they would not be injured? The nature and extent of injuries would, of course, be determined by what body part struck the wall first and what clothing or protective devices might dampen the forces of the impact, but the facts remain, sustained by our own everyday experiences, that no one in his or her right mind would assume that walking into a wall at several miles per hour or more would not be injurious to an adult, much less to an infant.

With respect to skull fractures, there are circumstances, also discussed in Chapter 6, in which an infant suffers more than one skull fracture, often on opposite sides of the head and often with significant intracranial injury that may or may not become immediately evident [79–81]. It should be kept in mind that a mechanism for this type of fracture may be profound distortion of the head by compression (more or less static loading), as from a heavy object such as a piece of furniture or television set [82], someone who has fallen on the child, or vehicular accidents, essentially crushing the head [83]. In such circumstances, sufficient deformation of the head has occurred that the skull splits, not necessarily along suture lines, usually with extension into the skull base. Curiously, although the injuries may prove fatal, recovery, often with limited neurological deficits, is possible [80,89].

Spinal Injury in Child Abuse

By all rights, cervical and other spinal injuries in infancy and childhood are uncommon or rare [84–86] and, when observed, often have an obvious explanation, such as in a vehicular accident or air bag deployment [90,91]. The importance of spinal cord injuries in child abuse is difficult to ascertain [84]. There are very few reports of abuse-related spinal cord injury [85–89]; the most prominent of these is that of Hadley et al. [92]. In this report, 13 cases are presented that were alleged to have been victims of shaking, although certain ambiguities in the basis for this within the article are confusing: eight children died, but only six were autopsied, the details of which were only vaguely reported. In a study by Leestma [93] that spanned 30 years of literature, among the 54 cases from among 324 analyzed, there were only 4 in which some form of spinal injury was reported, but this number should be viewed against the fact that only 6 cases had information relating to the spine or cord in the case reports. In any case, it appears justified to regard spinal injury in child abuse to be uncommon or rare. The significance of this observation is in the context of the alleged shaken baby syndrome (SBS; discussed in detail below). Injury thresholds for the infantile neck, incomplete as they are, appear to be in a range that if shaking of a violent nature occurred in a young infant, the spinal column and cord would be injured well before intracranial injuries could occur [94]. The context of tensile loading/failure parameters for the neck employed by Bandak [94] is in keeping with those illustrated in Figure 6.75 in Chapter 6. Given the allegation of many that shaking deaths are common in child abuse, it is troublesome to the concept that so few cases of spinal injury have been observed. What appears to be a relative paucity of spinal cord injury due to abuse may be due to the clinical difficulties in appreciating spinal injury in a comatose baby or the lack of proper radiological study that may or may not show structural injury in spite of neurological injury (so-called SCIWORA) [90,95]. Sometimes an apparent false diagnosis of spinal injury in abuse cases is made because the respirator brain process extends into the upper cord, producing lesions that may resemble trauma [96]. This issue is discussed in Chapter 5.

Epidural Hematoma and Child Abuse

Epidural hematomas, although they may occur in conjunction with impact trauma that may be abusive or accidental, are usually not forensic issues unless there are delays in appearance of symptoms from such a lesion, which can occur very commonly [97–99]. After a traumatic event that usually involves a skull fracture and laceration of a branch of the middle meningeal arterial tree, there may be a period of unconsciousness that may clear to a lucid state. Although epidural hematomas have classically been thought to occur by arterial rupture, some workers have questioned this assertion by noting that venous channels follow the middle meningeal artery and may be the source of bleeding [100,101]. Consciousness may not be lost at all until the mass effect of the epidural hematoma reaches a critical mass, and then consciousness may be lost slowly or rapidly [97]. With prompt surgical intervention, survivability may reach 90% [98]. Varying degrees of neurological deficits may, of course, follow.

In the infant, epidural hemorrhages are virtually always caused by a traumatic event, very often the result of child abuse, but they can occur in connection with difficult births, misplacement of catheters, craniotomies near or remote from the hematomas, and with osteogenesis imperfecta [102–104]. These hemorrhages are every bit as serious in the young as they are in older individuals but probably occur less frequently on aggregate (about 2% of cases in the series of Hahn et al. [29]). This may be because the branches of the middle meningeal arteries are generally intradiploic until the skull becomes firmly ossified and the fontanels are firmly closed. Owing to the plasticity of the infant skull, which will tend to give with force rather than break, it is correspondingly less likely that dural arteries will be disrupted unless major dislocation and distortion or major fracture occurs. However, this same plasticity may allow avulsion of branches of the middle meningeal artery or accompanying veins from the undersurface of the skull in response to distorting trauma and thus may cause epidural hemorrhages in the absence of skull fracture [100,105]. Epidural hemorrhages can occur anywhere over the brain, including in the posterior fossa, the most dangerous location [106]. Early recognition and surgical treatment of these lesions are vital if the child's life is to be preserved, because intracranial pressure may rise very rapidly, leading to midline shifts, herniation, brain stem compression, respiratory embarrassment, coma, and death. Occasionally, posterior fossa epidural hemorrhages evolve slowly, in a manner not normally envisioned for such a lesion in this location; therefore, the finding of a delayed fatal outcome with such a lesion should not cause confusion.

Subdural Hematomas and Child Abuse

Subdural hematomas are a common injury in the allegedly abused child, but they are by no means always caused by intentional actions. The biomechanics and mechanisms for occurrence of subdural hematomas in infancy, childhood, and adulthood are discussed fully in Chapter 6 but in the context of child abuse will be discussed here with some inevitable repetitions.

The classic view of subdural hematoma is that physical forces in most instances cause tearing or rupture of cortical veins as they pass into the so-called border zone between the arachnoidal membrane and the dura, eventually entering the superior sagittal sinus. When bleeding occurs by whatever mechanism, it accumulates in the potential space between dura and arachnoid, often referred to as the subdural space. Other possible mechanisms for subdural hemorrhages, especially in infants, include hypoxia [107,108]. Controversy exists about many aspects of subdural hematomas (acute or chronic) and subdural fluid collections (hygromas) and how these lesions progress [109]. These issues are discussed in detail in Chapter 6 and will not be repeated here.

In the context of possible child abuse, the finding of a subdural hematoma has many forensic issues:

1. What is required to produce a subdural hematoma in an infant or child?
2. What symptoms attend the occurrence of a subdural hematoma and when do they appear?
3. What happens over time to a subdural hematoma?
4. What is the relationship between subdural hematomas and retinal hemorrhages?
5. What is the relationship between skull fracture and subdural hematomas?
6. Can mechanisms of injury or injury scenarios be inferred from the findings of a subdural hematoma?

What Is Required to Produce a Subdural Hematoma in an Infant or Child?

Most subdural hematomas in infancy and childhood are caused by physical forces that act on cerebral veins or other vessels in the dura or dura–arachnoid interface (border zone), causing them to become injured and bleed at some point after injury. That is not to say that all subdural hematomas have a physical force basis [107,109,110]. Examples include disorders of bleeding/clotting that may be inherited, such as one or more clotting factor deficiencies, or acquired deficiencies, such as vitamin K deficiency. Other inherited conditions include sickle cell and other hemoglobinopathies (including combinations), glutaric acidemia, and other disorders of amino acid metabolism. Many of these conditions are discussed in Chapter 4. Cerebral venous or sagittal sinus thrombosis of known or unknown causes may produce subdural hematomas and other forms of intracranial hemorrhage. On rare occasions, vascular anomalies may also produce subdural hemorrhages. Birth-related injuries, known or unknown, may produce subdural hematomas that may later declare themselves. These and other causes and their mechanisms are discussed in other chapters.

Physical forces that deform the cranium, such as in blow or fall impacts or crushing/compression events, may bring about injury to the cerebral "bridging" veins wherever they are coursing or other venous channels. Thus, loading scenarios include both static and dynamic-impulse loading events that may affect the vessel by straining forces or by hydrostatic loading forces. With the exception of static loading events, subdural hematomas due to physical events all involve impacts of the head with a nonyielding surface. The parameters of such impacts have been studied in a variety of animal and model systems and yield peak accelerations from 25,000 to more than 100,000 rad/s^2 and peak angular velocities from 200 to about 1000 rad/s, with pulse durations from 17.13 to 22.8 ms. Accelerative forces (based on axis of rotation of the head structure) have been measured or calculated to reach between 380*g* and 436*g*, depending on impact surfaces and model design [110]. When these parameters are compared with a large series of primate animal studies that were seeking to correlate force levels and occurrence of dural and brain injuries, the injury threshold for subdural hematoma occurred above about 35,000 rad/s^2 and above about 100 rad/s velocity, and brain injury thresholds were above about 40,000 rad/s^2. Similar results have been reported by Prange et al. [111].

During unassisted or unaugmented fall scenarios, where instrumented dummies such as the CRABI-12 and Hybrid III were allowed to fall to a dense carpeted surface from 3- to 4-ft heights, in which the head struck the surface, peak *g* forces of 121–189*g* were recorded in the CRABI-12 dummy (with angular accelerations from 7600 to 21,700 rad/s/s and velocities of 25–49 rad/s), and with the Hybrid III dummy (simulating a 3-year-old baby) impact forces of 287–349*g* were recorded (with angular acceleration of 16,000–79,000 rad/s/s and velocities of 16–65 rad/s). It is clear that in these experimental short-fall scenarios, injury thresholds may be exceeded. If one examines the case literature regarding short falls in young infants of various ages, subdural hematomas can clearly occur, as has been shown by Howard et al. [112] and others [68,113,114]. It is not known what the lowest injury threshold for infantile subdural hematoma might be, but it appears that forces near or greater than 100*g* can cause subdural hemorrhages in apparently normal infants. Force levels of 100*g* can occur by simple Newtonian physics calculations for 3- to 4-ft falls to a variety of common floor coverings. The occurrence of subdural hemorrhages in an infant does not rule out accidental falls but, of course, does not exclude an inflicted scenario [112].

A major controversy exists regarding whether apparent nonimpact events such as shaking can produce subdural hematomas. This position is vigorously propounded by many clinicians and child abuse experts [115–118] and organizations [119]. The same studies cited above [110,112] have examined the force parameters produced by shaking dummies that mimic the physics of purported shaking events. These studies have conclusively shown that with manual shaking of a baby dummy, regardless of whatever effort is expended, the acceleration duration time for one pulse is about 10 times longer than that occurring in a fall-type impact (250 ms vs. 20 ms), and peak accelerations for shakes are on average no larger than average 10–12*g*. These parameters place such scenarios well outside the known injury thresholds for both subdural hematomas and brain injury [111,120]. Thus, shaking (so-called acceleration/deceleration forces) accomplished without impact by an individual simply cannot physically attain sufficient force to produce intracranial pathology by this means. This is not to say that injuries cannot occur, for they clearly can, but that they involve upper spinal skeletal/soft tissue and spinal cord injuries, as has been shown by Bandak [94], although in practicality such injuries appear to be rare [93].

What Symptoms Attend the Occurrence of a Subdural Hematoma in an Infant, and When Do They Appear?

Acute subdural hematomas can evolve over minutes, hours, days, or longer and may or may not produce symptoms proximate to the injurious event. This lag period, often referred to as a lucid interval by some, is highly variable due to several physiological bases but occurs. It is impossible to know what percentage of infants who have a subdural hematoma will experience some sort of lag period, because unless the infant is subjected to imaging studies or subdural hematoma is suspected or diagnosed, it may never come to light; however, this phenomenon is probably not uncommon, as has been suggested by studies such as that of Howard et al. [112]. Infants who appear neurologically normal after a reported short-fall event have been found to have subdural hematomas [68,69], and infants who have known subdural hematomas but for whom clinical interventions have been postponed for various reasons may declare their injuries at a later time [68,112,121]. In spite of this literature, some maintain that lucid intervals in subdural hematomas of infancy rarely occur and, if present, mean that a false history was provided [121]. The time course for appearance of symptoms after a head injury is governed by many factors, such as the ability of the victim to compensate for the evolving mass lesion using pressure/volume equilibrium processes (see Chapter 5). In this environment, the rate of accumulation and the ability rate possible of the brain to mobilize space to accommodate the hematoma by absorption and transport of cerebrospinal fluid (CSF) are vital. By the same token, the presence of other mass lesions that may or may not be mobilizable, such as arachnoid cysts, subdural hygromas, or other fluid collections, may degrade the compensation mechanism (see Chapter 5) and permit decompensation. If there are complicating processes, such as brain injury (traumatic axonal injury) or hypoxia/ischemia, that produce cerebral edema, which is a mass effect that must be taken into account against the pressure/volume mechanisms, these may degrade the response mechanism and cause symptoms to appear sooner than otherwise. Similarly, if there is an intracranial hemorrhage or blockage to CSF flow, or compression of the brain by a depressed skull fracture, these, too, will degrade the ability to compensate and hasten symptom appearance.

Commonly, symptoms related to a subdural hematoma result mostly from increased intracranial pressure due to its mass and collateral mass-making process, outlined above. These symptoms, before total decompensation, may be relatively nonspecific, such as lethargy, irritability, vomiting, poor feeding, and choking. These symptoms may wax and wane sometimes for days. They may progress to deeper disorders of consciousness, leading to deep coma and apnea, which, unless corrected, will lead to irreversible brain damage and death in a relatively short time. In the course of rising intracranial pressure, unilateral and eventually bilateral pupillary changes may be observed owing to pressure on the third cranial nerve (see Chapter 5). Once intracranial pressure rises significantly above 20 mm Hg, cerebral circulation will be imperiled, and it is likely that serious and permanent brain damage or brain death will occur regardless of therapy.

What Happens over Time to a Subdural Hematoma?

The true natural history of acute subdural hematoma is not known, because it is not possible to study a representative population of those who acquire a subdural hematoma and follow them long enough. Nevertheless, with respect to the population that is diagnosed with subdural hematomas in infancy, it appears that the incidence at least on one population was 12.8 of every 100,000 children/year, with 85% of these in children younger than 1 year [122,123]. It is clear that some infants acquire a subdural hematoma and never show symptoms or apparent ill effects from it [12]. What the percentage of the true population is for these kinds of cases is not known. It appears that in cases of head trauma, little or no subdural bleeding occurs, but apparently a rent develops allowing CSF to flow into the border zone between the dura and arachnoid, producing a hygroma that may enlarge over time. In other circumstances, it appears that only bleeding from a torn or injured bridging vein or other structure may occur into the border zone. Such lesions may be absorbed in time, and others continue to progress into a chronic process (chronic subdural hematoma). Many have suggested that the progressive hematomas result from a mixing of CSF and venous blood. These concepts are discussed in detail in Chapter 6. An example of a vertex acute subdural hematoma is illustrated in Figure 7.2.

Regardless of the theories behind subdural hematoma natural history, it has been known for more than 100 years that some subdural hematomas become chronic and enlarge, with varying consequences [123,124], and that chronic subdural hematomas regularly are shown to contain recent bleeding, or rebleeding, as some prefer. The mechanisms for chronic subdural hematoma enlargement have been studied for many years (see Chapter 6) and are thought to be due to leakage from capillaries in the neomembrane. This bleeding is usually incremental over weeks or longer and may or may not escalate into a

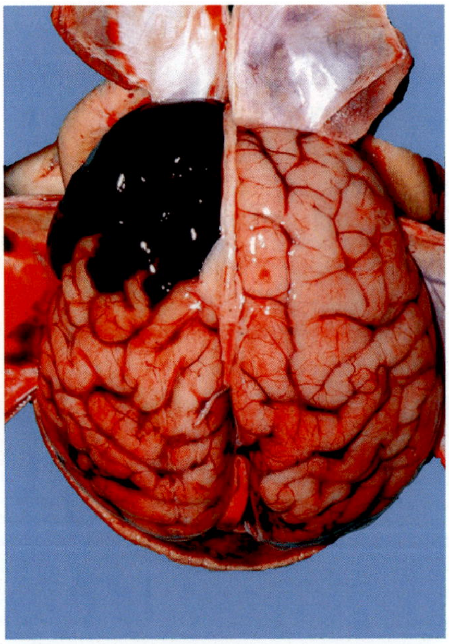

Figure 7.2 Vertex of the brain with its dura in an older child, illustrating a dark clot easily separated from the dura. Typically, cortical veins are often distended beneath the clot. Some portions of clot appear to be adherent to the dura, which suggests some days of aging on the process. This can only be assessed by microscopic examination. This issue often more properly calls for the designation for such hematomas as *recent*, avoiding the use of the term *acute*, which may imply or impose a restrictive aging measure. (Courtesy of the Office of the Medical Examiner, Cook County, IL.)

sudden major bleed that can cause decompensation, but this does occur [123,125] and does not necessarily mean that a new episode of trauma (or abuse) occurred. Chronic subdural hematomas all have a neomembrane composed of proliferating fibroblasts, capillaries, macrophages, and other inflammatory cells that evolves over the course of about 2 weeks [126,127]. The character of these components and their extent can be used for forensic purposes in terms of aging and dating the subdural hematoma [128]. See also Table 6.2 in Chapter 6.

An important amount of forensic information can be developed from the CT or MRI scans of the head obtained on admission to the hospital of a child with subdural hematoma [129]; however, often from simply examining the radiology report only, one may get little helpful information or even confusing information because of the brevity or aridness of the report. To overcome this common problem, one may have to view the studies themselves or do so with a radiologist while making it clear what one is looking for if it is present. It will be important to properly characterize any fluid collections or apparent bloody collections in the subdural compartment and to attempt to differentiate between subdural and subarachnoid hemorrhages. Subdural hemorrhages in CT images may be homogeneous or not. When they are not, as in mixed-density hematomas, significant diagnostic challenges present themselves. It may be impossible using CT imaging to differentiate between so-called hyperacute subdural hematomas and subacute or more chronic subdural hematomas with some element of recent hemorrhage within them [130–132]. The different densities within a subdural hematoma may be due to clotted versus unclotted components or mixing of the clot with CSF [133]. MRI scanning methods appear to be more sensitive and discriminating than CT scans for determining the age of subdural hematomas. One must be aware and critical of radiological opinions that venture too far into mechanisms based on the studies and the tendency for some radiologists to feel that they can assign culpability for or causality to the lesions they see, for such opinions may not have a scientific basis and have profound impact on a legal action that may involve the case [134,135].

Chronic subdural hematomas may reach spectacular proportions, especially if many weeks or months have elapsed between injury (which may or may not be known) and declaration of symptoms. The hematoma may be largely composed of straw-colored or dusky fluid with varying degrees of hemosiderin visible pathologically or in MRI studies. From time to time, the neomembrane will have many layers within it, strongly supporting the fact that several episodes of bleeding, often one on top of another, have occurred. An example of an extraordinary chronic subdural in infancy is illustrated in Figure 7.3. In such cases, when the information has been charted, head circumference has accelerated well beyond the norm, whether it was appreciated or not. In imaging studies, the hematoma may be shown to stretch bridging veins around or over the hematoma. It is not illogical to expect that such elongated vessels might rupture by themselves or in response to what would ordinarily have been an inconsequential physical force causing rapid increase in mass and its consequences. This problem and the potential for sudden decompensation in infants with chronic subdural hematomas and fluid collections have been addressed by Papasian and others [135,136]. An example of an allegedly abused child's CT scan on admission for a head injury is illustrated in Figure 7.4.

A problem that seems to have been underappreciated clinically and pathologically is the effect that a subdural hematoma, almost regardless of its mass, has on the underlying brain. It is very common in imaging studies to observe dark (underperfused) brain beneath a subdural hematoma [129,137]. In time, this brain, if the child survives, will

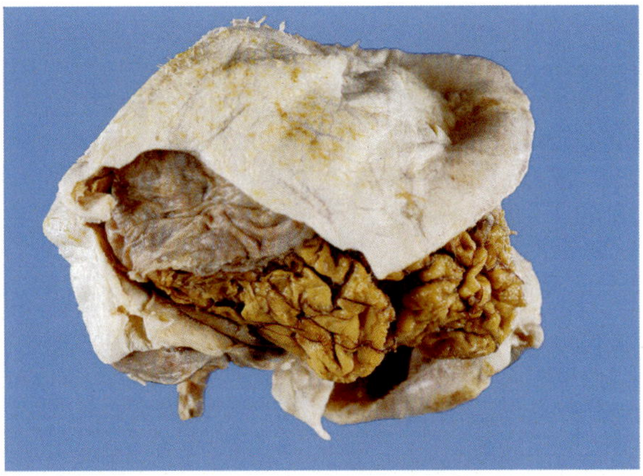

Figure 7.3 Coronal section of dura and brain from which the dura was not stripped at autopsy but, rather, fixed along with the brain, illustrating a huge bilateral chronic subdural hematoma with multiple neomembranes and obvious aging discoloration of its components. Head circumference was well over the 99th percentile in this toddler, who decompensated and died shortly after admission to hospital. The brain, however, was shrunken due to hypoxic–ischemic tissue loss. (Courtesy of Dr. Carol Haller, Office of the Medical Examiner, Cook County, IL.)

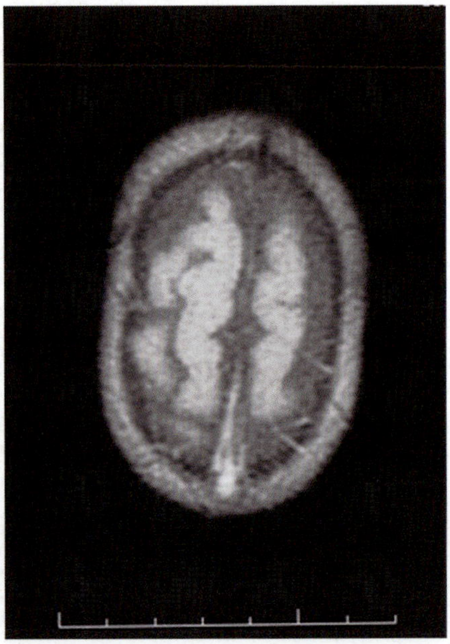

Figure 7.4 CT image near the vertex of 7-month-old male, born at 26 5/7 weeks' gestation, who was reported to have fallen from a car seat on a couch to the concrete floor, demonstrating bilateral large vertex fluid collections with an acute component in the midline falx. There was associated ventricular enlargement as well. The skull is clearly scaphycephalic, and the fluid collection is bridged by elongated veins. The child had retinal hemorrhages. The child had surgical drainage of the fluid collections and survived. The history of the child was that after birth he had respiratory distress syndrome, sepsis, a patent ductus arteriosus, a ventricular septal defect, and anemia and showed a grade II germinal matrix hemorrhage with intraventricular extension. The child had a number of apneic episodes while at home. The father was charged with abuse and convicted. Cases such as this, with so many complexities and processes, challenge interpretation and are not atypical for many cases alleged to be abuse.

become degenerate and show atrophy and sometimes cystic degeneration of the cortex and underlying white matter. Often larger areas of dark brain occur outside the dimensions of the subdural hematoma. These areas of the brain will also deteriorate and become atrophic, sometimes leading to a "walnut" brain in the affected areas, as illustrated in Figures 7.5 and 7.6. The mechanism behind these processes is probably multifactorial. A subdural hematoma will compress the subarachnoid space beneath it, even if the actual hematoma pressure is not great. If the theories of Greitz are correct, that there is a complex process of microcirculation in the arachnoid and brain surface that is dependent on subtle blood flow regulation [129,138] (see also Chapter 5), normal function of the capillary bed is likely to be affected, resulting in a local disruption in cerebrovascular autoregulation that could lead to ischemia. Clinically, many infants have superimposed hypoxia from immediate respiratory failure or difficulty of or delays in intubation that exacerbate any circulatory difficulties.

Of course, if the subdural hematoma has significant mass effect and increased local pressure, local ischemia is very likely and can be exacerbated by any global alterations in cerebral blood flow due to increased intracranial pressure or peripheral hypoxia. Often, the dark areas of brain are said to result from physical forces of an impact on the brain, which may not be true. If the skull is malleable enough and has indented and deformed the underlying brain sufficiently, this explanation is tenable, but so-called traumatic axonal injury is generally manifested by deeper lesions in the white matter in critical locations having no direct relationship to the site of impact. Thus, the dark brain beneath a subdural

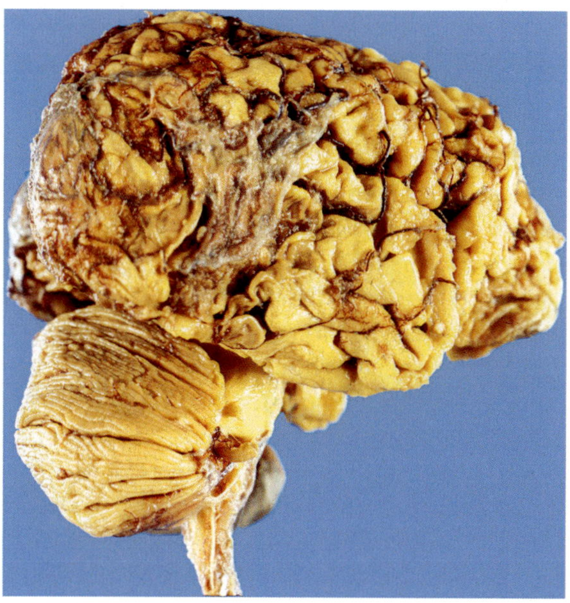

Figure 7.5 Left side of the brain of a 2-year-old infant at death. At age 1 month, the child was said to have fallen from a crib to the floor, striking his head. The child survived a lengthy hospitalization but had severe neurological deficits that included little neuromuscular development, seizures, and blindness. The child was tube fed and died with pneumonia. Abuse was alleged. This brain shows extensive cortical atrophy and meningeal thickening typical of a "walnut brain." (Courtesy of Dr. Robert Kirschner, Office of the Medical Examiner, Cook County, IL.)

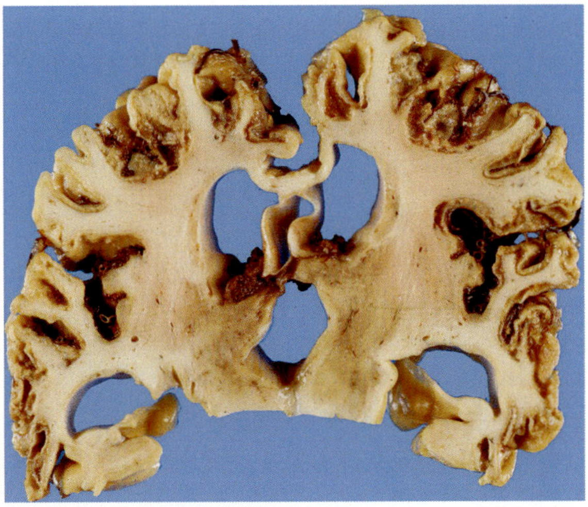

Figure 7.6 Coronal section of the brain shown in Figure 7.3 illustrating the profound cortical loss from global hypoxia–ischemia at the time of the injury. There is hydrocephalus *ex vacuo*. The white matter and deep nuclei were hard and rubbery, reflecting gliosis. (Courtesy of Dr. Robert Kirschner, Office of the Medical Examiner, Cook County, IL.)

hematoma may have a physiological explanation and not be part of any measure of the degree of forces involved in alleged trauma. It should also be remembered that until the infant skull is mostly ossified, surface contusions are probably not possible in response to falls or blows.

What Is the Relationship between Subdural Hematomas and Retinal Hemorrhages?

When subdural hematomas and retinal hemorrhages or retinal folds are found in a pediatric patient, as they often are, to many these findings are tantamount to a diagnosis of abuse and are said to rarely occur outside the context of abuse. This position is unjustified and prejudicial, especially when the mechanism for the coexistent lesions is said to be due to shaking [12,139]. Retinal hemorrhages in conjunction with both acute and chronic subdural hemorrhages have been described for more than 100 years [12]. The causal mechanisms for subdural hematoma-associated retinal hemorrhages and retinal folds in infancy have been sought for many years, and it appears that such hemorrhages, even large ones, can be seen in a variety of conditions with and without subdural hematomas and in nonabuse situations [140–142]. When there is a subdural hematoma that is symptomatic with or without additional mass effects from cerebral edema, increased intracranial pressure will likely result. Ommaya and others [137] have suggested that cerebral venous spasm or venous hypertension and possibly hypoxia may produce retinal hemorrhages. Other workers have developed evidence for and have refined this mechanism [144–146]. The work of Muller and Deck [146] summarized 40–50 years of prior work and has provided compelling evidence that increased intracranial pressure exerts a tourniquet-like action on the optic nerve sheath, through which the central retinal vein courses and compresses it, causing backup of blood into the eye and retina that can rupture, causing retinal and optic nerve sheath hemorrhages (see also Chapter 5). It would appear that this mechanism is the unifying process in head injury and other kinds of conditions that show retinal hemorrhages but does not explain why some cases of increased intracranial pressure in infants have a high incidence of retinal hemorrhages whereas others apparently do not. Lantz and colleagues [141] have examined more than 1000 eyes in a general and forensic autopsy service using both indirect ophthalmoscopy and pathological examinations, and have found about 25% of both adult and infant cases has a spectrum of retinal hemorrhages, often to the ora serrata, and retinal folds in conditions that were clearly not abuse. Matshes has reported similar findings [147]. If one does not take into account a control group, any statement of the exclusivity and specificity for retinal hemorrhages for abuse scenarios can have no meaning.

There are instances in which chest compressions raise intrathoracic pressure and therefore central venous pressure, such as in some cases of CPR, crushing injuries, Valsalva maneuvers, prolonged and forceful coughing, and vomiting, that may cause retinal hemorrhages [147–152]. How commonly resuscitation retinal hemorrhages occur is open to debate, with some maintaining that this is rare [153,154]. It is not clear why there is such disparity in the supposed frequency of CPR-related retinal hemorrhages; however, factors other than CPR might be involved that have not been controlled for in the studies, such as coagulopathy. The general phenomena of thoracic pressure from a variety of causes and in various circumstances and retinal hemorrhages have often been lumped under the term *Purtscher's retinopathy* [155,156]. The basis for such hemorrhages is said to result from increased thoracic pressure with impairment of venous transport to the heart (Valsalva maneuver), causing backup in the peripheral venous system, including the eye. Another condition, known as Terson's syndrome, also involves retinal and vitreous hemorrhages sometimes with retinal folds, usually in individuals who have a significant subarachnoid hemorrhage, commonly a ruptured aneurysm [157,158]. It appears that underlying the syndrome is increased intracranial pressure and not some other property of subarachnoid hemorrhage.

What Are the Relationships among Head Injury, Skull Fracture, and Subdural Hematomas?

Subdural hematomas can occur with or without skull fractures in infants, but few occur without apparent head impacts in the study of Leestma [93]. The basis for the very small number of infants who apparently did not suffer impact injury to the head yet had subdural hematomas is not known, and it cannot be known because most of these children did not have autopsies because they survived. It is possible that impacts, abusive or not, occurred but produced no external signs of injury; that these children had unknown coexistent contributory conditions such as chronic subdural hematomas/hygromas, bleeding, or clotting abnormalities; or that some other mechanism was operating. Unfortunately, insufficient data are available on these comparatively few published cases to permit a robust analysis. As it stands, the case database is insufficient to draw the conclusion that nonimpact subdural hematoma cases occurred because of shaking forces.

Can Mechanisms of Injury or Injury Scenarios Be Inferred from the Findings of a Subdural Hematoma?

This question can only be answered partially. Most subdural hematomas in infants appear to have a physical traumatic basis, whether due to falls, drops, blows, or some other head impact scenario. There are conditions other than trauma that can cause subdural hematomas, however. Many of these are discussed in Chapter 4. Precisely what impact scenarios occurred cannot be inferred with precision or accuracy from any characteristic of the subdural hematoma itself, but they can be put into an injury context on the basis of other findings, such as skull fractures, external injuries, and accompanying skeletal or body injuries. It may be possible, by analyzing the accompanying injuries, to develop some gradation of injury forces or mechanics that may or may not have forensic significance or reliability; thus, caution is advised. The occurrence of retinal pathology with a subdural hematoma, dealt with above and in Chapter 6, probably cannot be used to determine with accuracy the injury severity or forces that may have been involved, except to infer that some element of increased intracranial pressure and possibly some element of hypoxemia occurred in the injury scenario, with these things often attending more severe head injuries and those that appear to involve inflicted injury than occur in accidental scenarios.

Brain Injury in Child Abuse

Injury to the brain in abuse scenarios is common and may or may not be due to physical forces acting on the brain to produce intracranial vascular injury, axonal injury, hemorrhage, or other pathologies. Physical forces acting on the brain may damage it on the basis of deformation of the brain by an impact to an unossified or unfused skull (usually infants less than 6 months of age), by deformation of the brain and direct damage to the brain by a skull fracture in an ossified or unossified skull, or by inner brain injury (variously referred to as diffuse axonal or traumatic axonal injury [DAI/TAI]) caused by forces acting on the brain itself.

In the infant younger than 6 months, deformation injury, however it occurs, usually will not produce classic cortical contusions, either coup or contrecoup. These lesions require a rigid, ossified, and fused skull to occur by various proposed mechanisms (see Chapter 6). In young infants, deformation injury may produce what is known as contusional tears [159]. These lesions appear as necrotizing and often hemorrhagic slits at the gray–white matter junction in various places but commonly beneath the superior frontal convolution at the vertex, in the temporal lobes, and sometimes in the insular cortex (see Figure 7.7). The mechanism of these lesions may be due to differential mechanical properties of cortex and white matter that in deformations of the infant brain result in separation of the two structures, probably at points of greatest strain. These lesions can be visible in imaging studies, although they may not be recognized for what they are by radiologists who may be unfamiliar with the lesion. These lesions are rarely, if ever, seen in older children or adults who suffer impact injuries to the head.

Other brain injuries that may be the outcome of abuse result in direct brain injury by virtue of a special form of impact that may cause penetrating or disruptive injury to the brain, such as a blow with an object like a hammer, pipe, knife, or hatchet. Certain fall scenarios with impact against an edged surface or protruding surfaces may also penetrate the cranium and directly injure the brain or perhaps vital structures such as the superior sagittal sinus, from which hemorrhage may enter the brain (see Figure 7.8). These scenarios are comparatively uncommon and may represent homicidal actions and not necessarily actions of abuse in the accepted meaning of the term.

Impacts of the head, whether by accidental or inflicted falls, as discussed in Chapter 6, are "moving head" injuries in which the head is accelerated by gravitational forces to some terminal velocity governed by the distance the head has fallen. After contact with a floor or other nonyielding surface from which the head decelerates (negatively accelerates) to

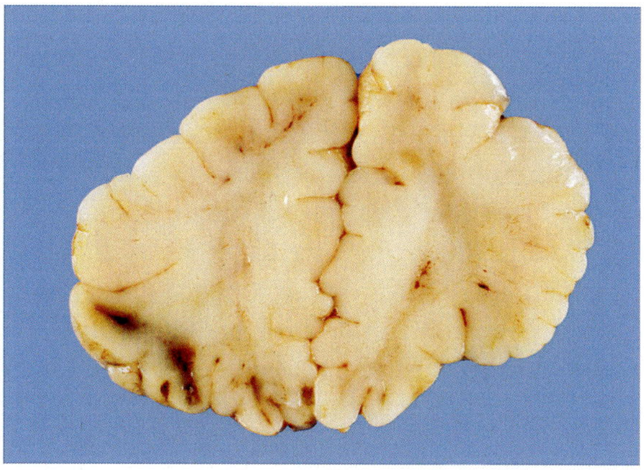

Figure 7.7 Coronal section of the frontal lobes of a 1-month-old infant who was reported to have been dropped, striking its head. The baby survived in the hospital for a few days and had retinal hemorrhages and a left-sided skull fracture. Abuse was alleged. This photograph illustrates subcortical hemorrhagic lesions beneath several gyri. These lesions are thought to represent contusional tears due to distortion of the brain, permitted by the malleable skull and the force of the impact. It is not possible to determine, from this illustration, if the impact was inflicted or accidental. Such contusions should not be regarded as contrecoup since the skull of such a child is not ossified and rigid. (Courtesy of Dr. Carol Haller, Office of the Medical Examiner, Cook County, IL.)

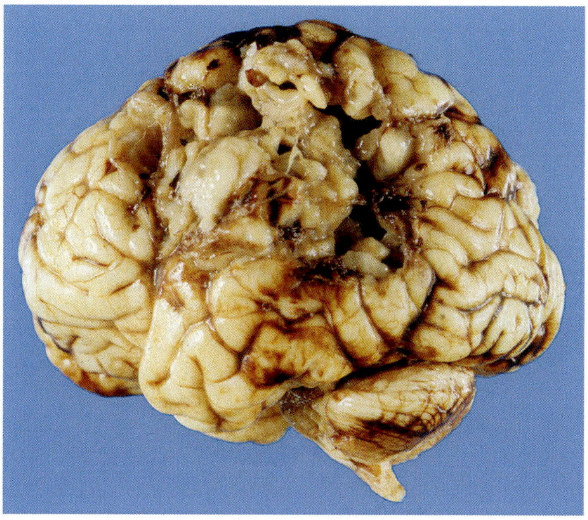

Figure 7.8 Left side of the brain of a 4-week-old male, who was said to have been dropped to the floor by the father and survived 4–5 hours. There was a complex stellate fracture on the left with bilateral subdural hematoma and basilar skull fracture. Autopsy revealed a large contusion on the left scalp and face. The child was operated on for the subdural hematomas but did not survive. Found also at autopsy were lesions deeper in the brain that suggested birth-related injuries. Here the cortex of the brain is lacerated, most likely by the inward movement of the fracture and distortion forces (fracture contusion), which was judged to be abusive. (Courtesy of Dr. H. Wayne Carver, Office of the Medical Examiner, Cook County, IL.)

a resting or zero velocity, various vector forces act on the head and brain that are dependent on the type of impacting surface, velocity of the head at impact, and position of the head at impact. These factors may introduce angular accelerations (rotational forces) in the postimpact interval into the brain that may produce brain injury. The nature, extent, and distribution of such brain injuries are determined by many factors, discussed in detail in Chapter 6. An important aspect of this is what forces [160] are involved in the coronal or sagittal plane of the head, because there are different injury thresholds depending on the planes of force. In general, extensive research has shown that coronal plane angular accelerations tend to produce more DAI/TAI than sagittal vectors. Regardless of the plane of force, it must be borne in mind that at angular accelerative forces below about 10,000 rad/s^2, the likelihood of function or morphologically discoverable lesions is low, but the likelihood of injury increases with higher levels of accelerative force, above about 25,000 rad/s^2 [143]. The mere fact that some degree of rotational forces before impact is acting on the brain does not mean that meningeal or brain injuries will result because the degree of forces is insufficient. It is another fact that in inflicted injuries that involve throwing of the body of an infant, comparatively little additive force over and above gravity occurs and probably does not significantly alter the injury profile. In situations where a body is swung against a vertical object, gravity will play a minor role, and the energetics of such a scenario can be estimated by biomechanical analysis and evaluated against this body of information. There is no evidence that shaking or some other force that precedes a fall-type scenario has any effect on the ultimate forces and injuries that may occur.

Traumatic axonal injury to the brain, however it occurs, is a dynamic process, discussed in detail in Chapter 6, beginning at a subcellular level in axons involving the neural membrane, cytoskeleton, and cellular organelles. These alterations are not visible radiologically, grossly, or microscopically in the early phases (many minutes) of the postinjury period. About 20 minutes or longer after injury, alterations in the axon and its function, as well as in the immediate vascular environment, evolve. These, too, are probably not visible grossly or radiologically but may be visible microscopically. Over the next hour to two, these changes may evolve to include vascular permeability, alterations in axoplasmic transport that may still not be visible grossly by CT scanning but possibly by MRI scanning and likely by microscopic examination, which may make use of histological methods that highlight the axonal cytoskeleton, such as β-app immunostaining in selected areas of the brain [161–164]. A problem with interpretation of axonal changes in alleged child abuse cases involves confounding processes that are very frequently present and which may introduce identical axonal changes that are not the result of direct physical forces acting on the cytoskeleton of the axon, such as hypoxia, ischemia, hemorrhage, and edema involving the brain, which are almost all present in a severely brain-injured baby from secondary and tertiary phenomena, not the primary insult [165–167]. During the first few hours after brain injury, axonal pathology can develop, and if death occurs during this time and other confounding causes of axonal injury mentioned above are minimal or absent, it may be possible that the axonal changes are due purely to physical phenomena. After this period, it is difficult to conceive of cases in which some degree of edema, hypoxia/ischemia, or other circulatory alterations, as well as hemorrhage, has not occurred and can overshadow the apparently purely traumatic axonal injury. Thus, in practical terms, it is questionable for any axonal pathology to have significant forensic value with respect to causal mechanism. To fully study the potential value for axonal injury from a mechanistic standpoint, it would be necessary to prospectively collect a large number of cases, controlling for any known confounding variable relating to axonal pathology in human cases, a near-impossible task. If there were a reliable animal model, the same care in experimental design would have to be exercised, again a Herculean task. Thus, it would appear prudent to regard axonal pathology and its forensic importance with great caution [168–170].

Rib Fractures and Alleged Child Abuse

The radiological or pathological discovery of rib fractures in infants is regarded by many as a strong indication of abuse, particularly if the fractures are multiple, posterior, and of different ages, as evidenced by healing calluses [45,167]. Such fractures are often found in head-injured children who were likely abused [15,167,171], the implication being that the fractures are part of the abuse scenario. As mentioned above, abuse-related rib fractures tend to be posterior (within 5–10 cm of the vertebral column) [172]. Typical older rib fractures are shown in Figure 7.9. Precisely how these presumably abuse-related fractures occur is not clear, but they appear to involve compression of the thorax, which causes torsional strain on the rib near its most rigid anchor point, at the vertebral column (see Figure 7.10) [173]. Other fractures that may be related to CPR or other chest trauma, as in vehicular accidents, falls, or crushing injuries, may occur laterally or at the costochondral junction [26,174,175] and may be accompanied by intra-abdominal injuries. It appears that although CPR-related rib fractures in children do occur, they are considered rather uncommon [176], if not rare [177–180]. It should be kept in mind that comparative rarity of

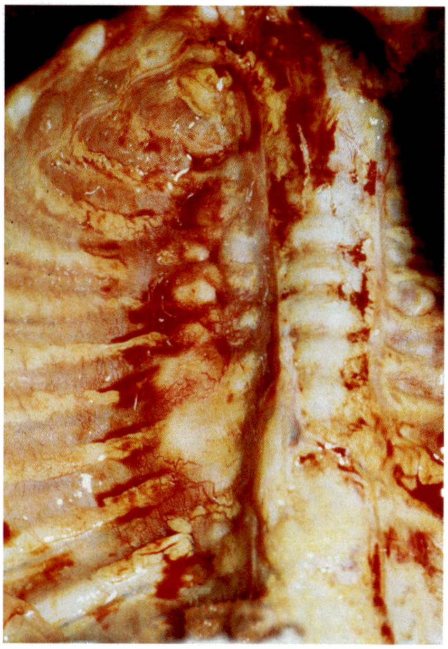

Figure 7.9 Open thorax showing numerous healing bulbous posterior rib fractures on both sides in this 2-month-old female, found unresponsive in bed. The child was dead on arrival at hospital. Autopsy revealed numerous old rib fractures, several long bone fractures, and a skull fracture that were deemed to be abusive. (Courtesy of Dr. Shaku Teas, Office of the Medical Examiner, Cook County, IL.)

obvious and add additional complexity in the analysis of infants suspected of having been abused who have multiple fractures of differing ages. Even in the face of OI or perhaps temporary brittle bone disease, such children may be victims of abuse, but differentiation of abuse from nonabuse may be impossible.

It is increasingly being appreciated that hypovitaminosis in infants and newborns is common. This may be due to insufficient maternal vitamin D consumption or supplementation, or diminished levels of vitamin D in breast milk and in some formulas. In such infants, fractures can occur apparently during incidental handling of the baby and as strange as it may seem, seem to be relatively asymptomatic as compared with true trauma-associated skeletal fractures. It would be wise to regard a baby with literally dozens of fractures to have been suffering from some form of metabolic bone disease [194].

Fractures of the Long Bones and Child Abuse

Caffey [195] is often credited with pointing out the association of head injuries in infants with fractures of the long bones to raise the probability that child abuse was involved. In his original publication, he reported six cases in which there were a total of 27 fractures in all portions of the arm and leg bones (14 metaphyseal and 9 diaphyseal locations). The association of chronic subdural hematoma and long bone fractures had been noted in some cases by Sherwood in 1930 [12]. The differential diagnosis of such fractures apart from abuse and accidents includes rickets, OI, scurvy, and other conditions [196]. While rickets is commonly thought of as a disease in developing and poor countries, it is probably more common in the United States than one might think and can be a source of unexplained long bone fractures. A variety of terms have been applied to long bone fractures, but those involving the epiphyseal region have been classified by Salter and Harris [197,198]. Fractures in this region appear to have a high probability of being due to abuse according to Silverman [199] and Kleinman [200].

The Salter–Harris classification of epiphyseal fractures [197,198] is illustrated diagrammatically in the proximal tibia in Figure 7.13. Type I fracture involves complete separation of the epiphyseal plate from the metaphysis through the cartilaginous interface but does

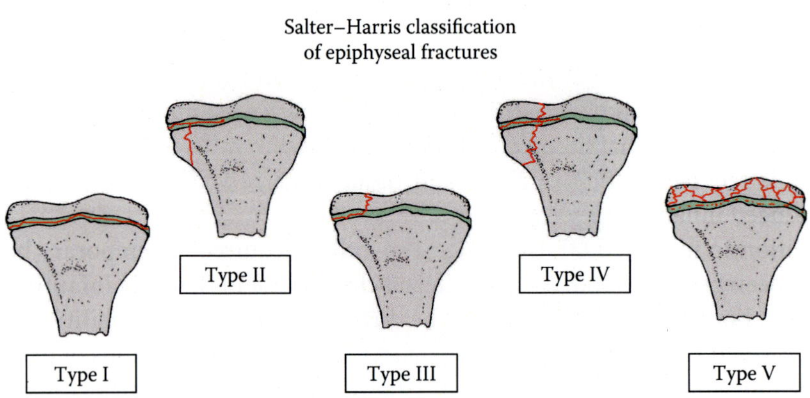

Figure 7.13 Various forms of metaphyseal fractures commonly observed in infancy according to the Salter–Harris classification [185]. There are obviously many more variations in end-bone fractures that are more severe and extensive, but this classification is often employed in cases of suspected child abuse.

not involve bony fracture. Type II, or typical "corner" type fracture, involves basically a chip fracture of the metaphysis, probably with some cartilaginous separation as well. Type III involves a segmental fracture of the epiphyseal plate but not the metaphysis. Type IV involves a combination of types II and III with segmental fracture of the epiphyseal plate, cartilage, and metaphysis. Type V involves basically a crushing of the epiphysis. The red lines illustrate pattern of fracture injury.

Over time, the corner or "bucket handle" fractures (type II) primarily of the proximal tibia and to some extent epiphyseal separations of humerus and other bones, as well as periosteal elevations, became popularly accepted as occurring frequently in abusive situations and less commonly in accidental situations [198,200]. The cause of many of these injuries was thought due to vigorous pulling and handling of the extremities by an adult. The mechanisms of type I and type II fractures are thought to be due to shearing (tangential) or avulsive (tensile) forces. Type III and type IV fractures appear to be mostly due to shearing (tangential) forces, whereas type V fractures are due to compressive loading. Whether, or how many, such lesions are actually due to abusive actions such as shaking is open to question and apparently has never been extensively studied biomechanically.

An almost-infinite variety of supracondylar, condylar, and distal epiphyseal fractures can occur, but with the exception of distal epiphyseal fractures, they usually affect adults because most of these fractures appear to occur with rotational forces on the extremity when it is loaded, which would not be the case with infants. Certain high-energy scenarios can also affect children [201].

An issue that exists in the analysis of any alleged fracture is the reliability of the radiological diagnosis of the alleged fracture and correlations with autopsy examinations. Errors can, of course, be those of a missed lesion or an incorrectly diagnosed lesion. Radiological examination accuracy and reliability are predicated on the use of proper techniques, whether the study involves plain films, CT scans, or other radiological methods. Fractures may be present but missed radiologically for many reasons, including poor technique; rotation of the injured bone so that the fracture is obscured; structures within the bone that may mimic a fracture line (vascular structures, aberrant sutures, anomalous structures); the location of the fracture below the level of resolution of the technique; superimposition of other structures obscuring the fracture or producing artifacts that may mimic a fracture; "volume averaging" in CT or MRI, or other artifacts of such techniques, obscuring a fracture; and the level of expertise of the radiologist [133,167,202]. It behooves both radiologists and those using their interpretations to be aware of the potential for error and the temptation to imply mechanisms to static images [203]. Another issue is the aging and dating of fractures in infancy by radiography or pathology examinations. Such estimations are approximate at best [55,200,203].

Other types of fractures of long bones may be described as transverse (a straight lateral break), oblique, spiral, comminuted (multiple fragments that may penetrate the skin), or segmental, in which a section of the long bone is separated from the proximal and distal diaphysis. The probable mechanisms of these fractures differ from type to type. A simple transverse diaphyseal fracture may result from forces like those that break a stick (three-point loading) and can occur from manual forces of blow-type impacts that strike the bone laterally, whether by intent or not. Oblique fractures usually involve an approximate 45-degree-angle fracture line with respect to the longitudinal axis of the bone. These fractures appear to result from relatively greater compressive forces than bending (lateral) forces or from bending and torsional forces also. Spiral fractures are thought to result from a combination of tensile (pulling) and rotational (twisting) forces of relatively low velocity

[198]. Comminuted or complex fragmented fractures of long bones vary considerably in extent and are generally due to high levels of external force in a weight-bearing attitude, usually in the lower extremity. Often, complex forces, as in vehicular or pedestrian accidents, are responsible and difficult to reconstruct or model. Segmental fractures may result from a localized application of forces by a broad-based surface. The mechanics of these and many other fractures are dealt with in great detail elsewhere [204–206].

Nontraumatic Forms of Child Abuse

Although most cases of child abuse involve physical, traumatic injuries to the infant or child, there is a spectrum of injuries to the nervous system that can result as a consequence of parental action or inaction. These include all manner of actions, such as neglect scenarios, for example, deprivation of food or water [207–209], and placing children in environments that are too hot, for example, closed automobiles in summer [210,211], or in unheated environments [212]. There is also a broad spectrum of intentional or unintentional circumstances that include feeding children with salt [213,214], excessive amounts of water [215], alcohol [216], and various therapeutic drugs [217,218] and drugs of abuse [43]. It may be difficult to differentiate between accidental and deliberate poisoning in an infant or young child, but the functional capabilities of young children must be kept in mind, and the fact that a child is not physically capable of having drunk from a sealed bottle may elicit the true story from the abuser.

Intentional smothering or suffocation or other parental mistreatment of infants may produce seizures or be reported as apneic episodes or SIDS phenomena during repeated visits to emergency rooms and clinics (an unusual form of the Munchausen syndrome) [42,218]. In some instances, such maltreatment may result in death; in others, it has some lingering effect on the child that hinders brain development and represents an often-hidden cause of child morbidity and mental subnormality.

Malnutrition

Although there are undeniable maturational and psychological effects of malnutrition in the young as well as the adult, the central nervous system appears morphologically remarkably resistant to nutritional deprivation. Studies made in several notorious famines from World War II to the present famines in Africa and elsewhere have provided a significant body of information concerning the impact on structure and function of the nervous system by severe malnutrition [219–221].

When starvation occurs in the first few months, and probably within the first few years of life, there are permanent residua with respect to neurological and psychological development, which have been observed in humans as well as in experimental animals. Such studies [222,223] indicate that, at least in the very young, there is a lowering of brain weight below that expected for age-matched controls, which may or may not resolve when proper nutrition is provided. In some instances, there is a decrease in the quantity of white matter associated with enlargement of the ventricles. The functional impact of poor nutrition even in adults is a notable and sometimes severe depression of intellectual functioning, with observable neurological dysfunction including tremors, weakness, and ataxia, and psychological abnormalities [224]. These deficits may persist if starvation occurs during the first few years of life and are more severe when it occurs in the first few months of life. The histological reflections of this deprivation are not always obvious by normal methods but may require highly specialized methods such as Golgi impregnations and electron microscopic methods. Such studies show retarded dendritic and synaptic development in large populations of neurons that may be permanent. In general, such methods do not readily lend themselves to the forensic situation and, furthermore, relatively few pathologists or neuropathologists are skilled in their use or interpretation. Nevertheless, evidence may exist if it is important enough to make the effort to secure it.

Failure to Thrive—Marasmic Death

The issue of marasmic death was first recognized by Rene Spitz in his pioneering work on infants confined to orphanages and foundling homes in the early 1900s [224]. At that time, it was a well-known phenomenon that many abandoned babies and young children failed to develop in spite of apparently adequate nutrition and care. This syndrome has been referred to as hospitalism, marasmus, or, more recently, failure to thrive [224,225]. After studying these children and their circumstances for many years, Spitz and coworkers [224] found that infants, and later other investigators found that even young animals, when deprived of a reasonably consistent "mother figure," failed to develop properly and often lacked the will to survive. When nursing routines were changed to provide for consistency in the group of caretakers to the infant, and when the infant was handled and physically stimulated by the mother figure, survivability improved dramatically.

In many homes where the infant is not wanted, or the mother is very young and unable or unwilling to care for the child, a situation not unlike the foundling home syndrome develops, and failure to thrive may result. When neglect is coupled with physical abuse or failure to adequately feed the infant, the risks of death increase dramatically. The actual cause of death in such infants has never been discovered, although many physicians clearly recognize the importance of the will to live and implicate the lack of it in such deaths. An analogous situation presents itself much more commonly on every autopsy service when cases of terminal cancer of the very elderly are autopsied. In a significant number of such cases, no clear-cut anatomic cause of death is ever found, in spite of careful gross and microscopic examinations. To be sure, many of the terminal cases show cachexia and disseminated tumor, but no actual terminal event can be identified [226]. The enigma of such cases is a source of frustration to every pathology resident who discovers this phenomenon and eventually develops some gentle subterfuge in signing such cases out. One might ask: is this phenomenon any different than that of infant failure to thrive? Possibly not.

A particular challenge to the forensic pathologist, and sometimes to the neuropathologist, arises when one or both are called on to testify in a legal setting regarding the cause and manner of death of an infant who has been neglected, possibly in combination with overt abuse and some element of starvation. In such cases, there may or may not be a history of admission to a hospital for malnutrition or, euphemistically, failure to thrive, and there may or may not be evidence of physical abuse at the time of autopsy. When obvious abuse is absent, probably very few of these cases are labeled homicide for lack of evidence deemed sufficient to merit prosecution. Even when there is evidence of physical abuse, but there is no obvious anatomic cause of death, many of these cases are never correctly labeled as homicides (death at the hands of another). In the latter case, it is quite understandable that forensic pathologists would be hard-pressed to communicate the cause of death to a state's attorney, judge, or jury; nevertheless, there are circumstances in which surprisingly strong testimony from a pathologist can be presented in such difficult cases.

It is by employing the analogy of the lack of an obvious anatomic cause of death in terminal neoplasia or in the aged that a strategy may lie for presenting medical evidence in abuse–failure to thrive cases. Everyone recognizes that terminally ill and elderly people may die suddenly and apparently without cause [227], perhaps out of a failure of some vital force known as the will to live [228]. Why should the impotent and helpless infant, faced with an impossible situation in which there is no care or constant harassment or abuse, not simply give up? The following case illustrates such a phenomenon.

A 9-month-old child was left in the care of his biological father, who had not been living with the child's mother, while the mother was at the hospital delivering another child of uncertain parentage. While in the father's care, the child cried a great deal and constantly wet his diapers. Ostensibly to prevent the diaper wetting, the father deprived the child of food and water over a period of a week. During that time, he apparently repeatedly beat and cut the child and probably also burned him with cigarette butts. He locked the child in a closet most of the time. The child was found dead. The autopsy revealed an emaciated and dehydrated youngster with ample evidence of child abuse, but no clear-cut anatomic cause of death was found. Such cases have been reported by others [116].

The father in this case was placed on trial for homicide, and the defense was based largely on the fact that the pathologist could not specify an anatomic cause of death, and because the cause of death could not be determined, the father could somehow not be blamed for the death. At the trial, a consultant pathologist presented the findings at the autopsy and the extent of the injuries and freely admitted that no one specific injury was responsible for the death but that the aggregate of all the injuries, including starvation, dehydration, and psychological state of the child, were the cause of the death. A conviction resulted that was sustained on appeal.

So-Called Shaken Baby Syndrome

Historical Background

In the course of the evolving field of child abuse, a concept about which there are many controversies is that children are commonly injured by shaking. This concept has developed to such an extent that the so-called shaken baby syndrome has become a generic term often used to describe any abused child with head injuries [117,229]. Deep professional disagreements have arisen over a number of complex issues embedded in the syndrome and continue to be the subject of strong arguments both inside and outside the courtroom. The "nanny" case (*Commonwealth of Massachusetts v. Woodward*, 1997) in Cambridge, Massachusetts, brought the highly contentious nature of SBS cases to the public via *Court TV* and subsequently in a continuing saga of print and television reexaminations of the case and its issues [229]. In a sense, since this celebrated case, the adjudication of alleged child abuse, and particularly SBS cases, has never been the same, and strong polarization between advocates of SBS and those who question its very existence continues. The following traces the evolution of the concept of SBS and the published basis for it as well as the problems with the concept and mechanisms of SBS.

Caffey is usually given credit for defining the so-called shaken baby syndrome [195,230,231]. Apparently, his conception of this phenomenon arose out of the anecdotal case histories provided by a child care nurse who apparently habitually shook infants in her charge in an attempt to quiet their crying. This nurse allegedly caused the death of three infants and "maimed two others," apparently by shaking them. Caffey recounted clinical and autopsy findings in two of the fatal cases [231]. He obtained his data by personal communication with a pediatrician who had apparently been involved in the cases and obtained autopsy reports of these babies. It should be noted that these cases were never published in full or reported elsewhere than in the popular print media. Attempts made to locate the autopsy reports by the author have been fruitless.

In Caffey's case "H", a 12-day-old female infant had been apparently well until admission to the hospital after having awakened crying as if in pain. There were no external signs of injury, but respiration was gasping and the anterior fontanel was bulging. Ophthalmologic examination revealed diffuse fundal hemorrhages. The baby died 3 hours after admission. Autopsy revealed no skull fracture, pulmonary edema, and a small subcapsular hemorrhagic laceration of the liver. The brain showed bilateral subdural hematomas and subarachnoid hemorrhage as well as subpial bleeding and lacerations of the cerebral parenchyma, perivascular intracerebral hemorrhages, and apparently hypoxic changes in neurons. The optic nerves were congested and edematous with sheath hemorrhages and numerous hemorrhages in the retina. This case occurred in 1948. It is not clear if an admission of shaking was ever obtained by the nurse or if this was the case in which she was alleged to have said that "one of her babies died after she had pounded it on the back to get a bubble up."

In Caffey's case "K", an 11-week-old female infant was found to have a bulging anterior fontanel and had awakened crying and lethargic but became semicomatose and cyanotic on admission to the hospital. Caffey reported that the ocular fundi were invisible. The CSF was bloody. The child died 2 hours after admission. No signs of trauma were visible other than a small abrasion on the left knee and abdominal wall. No fractures were noted. Autopsy data were limited to the brain, which was reported as showing bilateral subdural hematomas (near bridging veins) with subarachnoid hemorrhages on both sides. Microscopic examination revealed subarachnoid hemorrhage but no intracerebral bleeding. The eyes were not examined. This case occurred in 1956. Apparently, the nurse who had cared for this baby confessed during a coroner's inquest that she had "seized her by both arms and shook her until her head bobbed and she became faint." The nurse in question was incarcerated for many years and at this writing is still alive but has declined requests for an interview.

Much of the so-called shaken baby literature is linked with the alleged connection between supposed shaking trauma and hemorrhages and other pathologies of the retina and with the coexistent presence of subdural hematomas and no clear history of an obvious accidental fall from height, vehicular accident, or other out-of-the-home situation. In a review of infantile subdural hematomas, Sherwood, in a 1930 publication [12], cited a number of previous case studies in which the authors had reported hemorrhages in the eye grounds in young infants with acute or chronic subdural hematomas. Many of his case presentations have a distressingly familiar tone; for example

> A 4 1/2-month-old female was admitted to the hospital in 1928 because of irritability and convulsions, followed by unconsciousness. When the child awakened, she showed no symptomatology, but physical examination revealed bilateral large hemorrhages in the eye grounds. Although the mother suffered from syphilis, the baby apparently did not. Subdural tap yielded blood and xanthochromic fluid. The hospital course was 4 weeks long. The child gained weight and continued to do well with no recurrence of seizures [12].

It is clear from Sherwood's case descriptions and his subtle suggestions that he was likely reporting instances of abusive trauma in young infants, in case studies that mirror many of those reported over the next 70 years. It is interesting that in almost none of the literature that has appeared in the explosion of reports on abusive head injury in infants and alleged syndrome has any cognizance been taken of a large body of relevant case material from the past that addresses important issues relative to allegedly abusive head trauma that are often controversial and described as new.

In 1958, Hollenhorst and Stein [232] reported 47 cases of infants with subdural hematoma, subdural hygroma, or subarachnoid hemorrhage and who had had eye ground examinations. Positive or possible histories of trauma were noted in 23 of 47 cases. About half of the traumatized patients had evidence of retinal hemorrhages. In general, the incidence of ocular pathology was significantly greater in infants who had been traumatized than in those who had not, and a similar correlation was found with the severity of trauma. Mechanisms of trauma were not reported, and no mention of shaking trauma was made, although the veiled comment "subjected to trauma" strongly suggested but did not identify child abuse as the cause.

Other literature often cited in reference to retinal pathology associated with battering or shaking includes the article of Kiffney in 1964 [233], who reported a single case of a battered baby that, in addition to multiple skull fractures and subdural and subarachnoid hemorrhages, had bilateral vitreous hemorrhages and retinal detachment. He stated that "ocular signs have not been common in the reported cases of this (battered baby) syndrome." In a short note, Gilkes and Mann in 1967 [234] noted that the presence of retinal hemorrhages, which "may well be helpful in the diagnosis of the physically abused child." The authors further suggested that the retinal pathology might not be due to direct physical forces or the presence of subdural hemorrhages but might possibly be due to concomitant extreme rises in intracranial and intraocular venous pressures as did Hollenhorst and Stein [232]. The authors mentioned possible correspondence to Purtscher's retinopathy, where compressive injury to the chest might produce retrograde elevated venous pressure or fat emboli that might cause retinal hemorrhages. Harcourt and Hopkins in 1971 [235] reported general observations in 11 apparently abused children and reported case histories in 4 of these infants in greater detail. It appears that all but two children had intraocular hemorrhages in association with a spectrum of intracranial pathology that included mostly subdural hematomas (not every case), four cases of skull fracture, and a high incidence of soft tissue trauma (not otherwise defined). No mechanism of trauma was described. No instance of shaking was reported. The authors cited a number of other papers, including those of Gilkes and Mann [234] and Hollenhorst and Stein [232] and suggested that severe intraocular hemorrhage might indicate that physical abuse had occurred.

In 1971, Mushin [236] reported 12 cases (4 in detail) of battered babies with ocular injuries, including retinal and vitreous hemorrhages, retinal separations, and other intraocular pathology in association with skeletal and cranial fractures, subdural hematomas, and other cranial injuries. The author postulated that intraocular injury might be proportional to the level of force involved in the trauma and that permanent visual damage was more likely in the more severely injured babies. He also pointed out that ocular damage may be a marker for battering. In another paper, Mushin and Morgan [237] apparently re-reported one of their previous cases but added another one in which apparently admitted prolonged and forceful shaking had occurred associated with subdural hemorrhages, intraocular hemorrhages, and extensive external bruising. The authors again suggested that certain ocular conditions in childhood should raise the issue of possible battering as a cause.

Also in 1971, Friendly [238] reported five cases in detail of apparently battered children, four of whom later died, who had a spectrum of ocular pathology (retinal hemorrhages, papilledema, etc.) associated with various other injuries, including skeletal and skull fractures, subdural hematomas, and other intracranial hemorrhages. General findings were reported in 49 others. The author addressed the issue of ocular pathology in raising the suspicion of child abuse in relation to the responsibility for reporting suspected child abuse to relevant agencies as required by law in many states. A very similar article by Jensen et al., also published in 1971, reinforced Friendly's conclusions [239].

Perhaps one of the most often-quoted papers that many regard as the progenitor of the SBS is that of Guthkelch [240], who was apparently the first to invoke the mechanism of repeated acceleration/deceleration forces in infants to explain abusive brain injuries in babies who apparently had no evidence of external injuries but had subdural hematomas. Guthkelch was aware of the work of Caffey, who had not yet invoked the shaking phenomenon, as well as the cases reported by Weston [4], who did include in a history the statement that shaking of the baby was involved. Guthkelch reported two cases, the first of a 6-month-old boy who was admitted to the hospital with seizures and coma. He was found to have bilateral subdural hematomas and died in spite of surgery. Autopsy was reported to show torn bridging veins associated with the subdural hemorrhages. The mother had reported that the child had choked in association with several fits of coughing and that she shook him, whereupon he convulsed. Inartful compression of the chest by the distraught mother was thought responsible. The second case was of a 6-month-old boy, vomiting and convulsions and a possible diagnosis of meningitis. The child had bilateral retinal hemorrhages and was eventually discovered to have a subdural hematoma. Parental violence was not suspected initially, but after this child was treated and discharged, his twin brother was admitted to the hospital with a femoral fracture with no explanation for its cause. The original baby was readmitted with recurrence of the subdural hematoma and showed apparent digital imprints on his forearms that matched an adult digit. The parents denied abuse but admitted they "might have" shaken the baby when he cried at night. Guthkelch concluded his article [240] with the following statement, which seems to have become the watchword for many in years to come: "It follows that since all cases of infantile subdural hematoma are best assumed to be traumatic until proven otherwise it would be unwise to disregard the possibility that one of these has been caused by serious violence…when there are only trivial bruises or indeed no marks of injury at all, and (to) inquire, however guardedly or tactfully, whether perhaps the baby's head could have been shaken." It is interesting that in recent years, Guthkelch has had second thoughts about his statements, since there were no experiments or biomechanical citation in the article, and now regards his original thoughts more as hypotheses than fact, and now urges great caution in implying exact mechanisms of injury from the findings of subdural hemorrhages and retinal hemorrhages.

Several other authors reported cases similar to those of Caffey [230,231] and Guthkelch [240], in which intracranial injuries (subdural hematomas, subarachnoid hemorrhages with and without hemorrhage in the brain) were found without apparently significant external injuries, with and without retinal hemorrhages, sometimes in the context of admissions of shaking, but mostly not. Eisenbrey [241] did not present any case data of his own but summarized the work of others, including Ommaya et al. [242], who had studied experimental so-called whiplash head injuries in animals for several years and had developed a whiplash biomechanical animal model, and came to a number of conclusions that appear to have set the tone for the next 20 years, even though it is quite likely Ommaya's conclusions [242] were misinterpreted (in these "whiplash" experiments, the acceleration produced by a machine that did produce pathology in the primates was vastly different than those produced by manual shaking as Duhaime et al. [110] and Prange et al. [111] have shown). Eisenbrey concluded: "The data presented, we believe, supports the conclusion that the presence of retinal hemorrhage in a child under 4 years old should strongly suggest the possibility of battering (child abuse and WLS [whiplash shaking]). In a traumatized child with multiple injuries and an inconsistent history, the presence of retinal hemorrhage is pathognomonic of battering." These notions have now been criticized as unsupported by science by many authors [243–245].

Retinal Hemorrhages and Other Intraocular Pathology

In the 20 years that followed the report of Caffey of 1974 [231], the subject of retinal hemorrhage and other forms of retinal pathology in apparently traumatized infants, and their association with a specific physical mechanism, received a great deal of attention in the literature. A number of mechanisms for retinal hemorrhages were proposed: direct mechanical effects of shaking by Greenwald et al. [246]; hemodynamic forces in the chest, such as compression [247]; vitreoretinal traction [247]; venous congestion in the retina [137,145, 146]; increased intracranial pressure [146]; or combinations of these. There seems to be no question that intraocular pathology is very common in battered babies for reasons that still remain incompletely unexplained, but it does not appear appropriate to regard retinal hemorrhages as only being caused by abusive trauma [93]. As for the question of shaking in the mechanism of retinal hemorrhages, the causal association is anything but clear [248], even though many feel it is a marker for this mode of injury [154,248].

Retinal hemorrhages by themselves are regarded by many as rather nonspecific for abusive injury, but some others regard extensive retinal hemorrhages that reach the ora serrata or the presence of perimacular retinal folds (retinoschisis) as indicative of abusive injury and shaking trauma. Recent postmortem eye examinations on a large general autopsy population of infants, children, and adults have shown that all forms of retinal hemorrhage and retinal folds are not specific to inflicted head trauma but can be seen in a variety of traumatic as well as nontraumatic circumstances [141,142,147]. Retinal folds have been described in apparent accidental head injuries in infancy as well [249]. Further analysis of case reports of 325 allegedly abusively injured babies, of which 54 carried with them some admission on the part of a caregiver of shaking, indicated that no statistical inference of correlation between mode of injury and the presence of retinal pathology could be demonstrated [93].

Biomechanical Analysis of Shaking

The first attempt to mechanically analyze the phenomenon of shaking a baby was published by Duhaime et al. in 1987 [110]. This study and others [111] are discussed in Chapter 6. In the Duhaime et al. study, models were constructed of 1-month-old infants fitted with accelerometers. Three variants of the model were developed with different neck structures. One of these had as a neck attachment to the model cranium with a simple hinge with no resistance and with a fixed arc of rotation. The other two used rubber attachments with low to moderate resistance and moving centers of rotation. The geometry of the infant model paralleled appropriate head and body measurements and contained a head that corresponded to the 730- to 870-g typical head weight for the age. Instead of a brain, the cranial cavity was filled with wet cotton so that no sloshing about of cranial contents could occur during the experiments. Such movements would have rendered the studies physiologically invalid. The body was similarly modeled for size and weight to a typical 1-month-old baby. The model skull was constructed from a thermoplastic material that was malleable to mimic that of a young infant. The axis of rotation for the center of mass of the head on the neck for this model was 9 cm. Adult male and female volunteers held the models by the thorax and shook them in the anterior–posterior plane many times and, at the end of the free shaking period, impacted the occipital part of the skull against a metal bar or a padded surface. At least 20 trials were conducted on each of the three models, for a total of 69 shaking episodes and 60 shaking episodes with impacts.

These experiments showed that the mean tangential acceleration for all 69 shaking episodes was 9.29*g* (1138 rad/s^2) and that the mean tangential acceleration for impacts was 428.18*g* (52,475 rad/s^2), and a 50 times greater acceleration for impacts than for free shakes. Significantly, the mean time course of a typical shake was 106.6 ms but for impacts was 20.9 ms. The frictionless hinged neck allowed mean accelerations of the head to 13.85*g*, but the rubber necks resulted in mean accelerations of 5.7*g* and 7*g*. The neck design produced no significant difference in accelerations during impacts. Not surprisingly, impacts to padded surfaces resulted in lower *g* forces (380.6*g*), compared with 489.5*g* with an impact to the iron surface. When these levels of acceleration were compared to scaled animal data [143], the levels of acceleration for pure shaking were well below those which produced subdural hemorrhages and diffuse axonal injury in extensive animal studies [110,160]. The authors concluded that, in effect, impact was the defining and causative event in an abusive episode and that shaking, unless the child had some underlying brain disease, did not cause intracranial pathology. The use of models in shaking scenarios has often been criticized because the model was not living. That the model is of course not living, is beside the point. These studies simply measure forces, not their effects. To assess biological effects, one must rely on the huge body of animal work and to some degree work that involved humans in accidents, car crashes, air bag deployments, and other events that have yielded numerical data to which the model data can be compared [113,143].

The Duhaime et al. [110] paper, perhaps more than any other at the time, raised very serious questions about the general view that shaking of an infant caused a group of injuries (subdural hemorrhage, retinal hemorrhages, brain swelling) said to occur in no other scenario. Other experiments have shown that the injury thresholds for rotational forces for a brain are approximately inversely related to the 2/3 power of the brain's mass with reasonable precision using several different animal models [113]. This means that the smaller the brain mass, the greater the forces are required to produce an analogous injury, compared with a larger brain mass, which is more sensitive. These principles have been tested and incorporated into all sorts of brain injury models and scenarios employed by the military, automobile industry, aircraft industry, and government regulators who have determined the design parameters and requirements of various restraint devices, auto air bags, other occupant safety devices, and football and military helmets. Any differences or errors that have come from all the work on human injury tolerance studies are not sufficient to disqualify this body of comparative data from consideration [250]. To suppose that only by testing the end subject, a living baby, can meaningful data be obtained is not only ethically unacceptable but scientifically nihilistic.

In 2003, Prange et al. [111] reported results from a study that essentially repeated Duhaime et al.'s [110] work using a slightly different model and experimental design. This model was constructed to parallel a 1.5-month-old baby with a 1.13-kg head weight. Like Duhaime et al. [110], these workers used a hinge attachment for the head on the trunk with an axis of rotation of 9.2 cm. Accelerometers were installed in the model head. As before, a number of volunteers performed 61 trials of shaking followed by an occipital impact against 4-in foam padding, carpet pad, or bench top. Additionally, the model was dropped from heights of 0.9 and 1.5 m onto the same types of surfaces. Although *g* force measurements of peak acceleration were not reported (but can be calculated easily), the results of the study showed that shaking produced an angular velocity of 28 rad/s and an acceleration of 2640 rad/s^2 (about 24*g*), which was quite similar to the peak acceleration found in the Duhaime experiments. The impact experiments indicated that an angular acceleration into a stone bench top produced a peak acceleration of 173,000 rad/s^2, which translates into a peak acceleration of 1622*g*. The drop scenario onto concrete of 0.9 m (about 3 ft) yielded about half the acceleration of the inflicted impact. Despite some of the differences in the results between the Duhaime et al. [104] and Prange et al. [110] studies, the conclusions were essentially the same; that is, the forces involved in shaking are not sufficient to cause subdural hematomas or primary axonal injury in an infant.

A confusing and perplexing paper by Cory et al. [251] basically contended that the Duhaime et al. [110] work was unreliable and sufficiently so to "warrant the exclusion of such testimony in cases of suspected shaken baby syndrome." The authors cited in support of their conclusion papers by Hadley et al. [92], Alexander et al. [115], and Gilliland and Folberg [252]. The Hadley et al. paper [92] deals with a report of 13 infants, 8 of whom died, who had been abusively injured as determined by a multidisciplinary committee. It was alleged that the 13 infants had been injured because of shaking, but it is unclear from the paper if this was only a suspicion, a determination, or a fact. All of the infants had subdural hemorrhages and retinal hemorrhages. In the six babies who were autopsied, none were said to have a skull fracture, but no comment was made about other evidence of cranial impact. All of the six were reported to have cervical subdural or epidural hemorrhage and proximal spinal cord contusions. It is difficult to interpret this case series in view of the equivocal basis for determining that shaking had occurred, the lack of full information about cranial impact evidence other than the absence of skull fractures, and the true meaning of the spinal subdural and epidural hemorrhage and supposed contusions. Spinal epidural hemorrhage in babies who are brain dead is considered by many to be artifactual [253]. Subdural hematoma in the intracranial compartment can dissect downward into the subdural space in the spinal canal and may not represent traumatic spinal subdural hematoma [253,254]. Hemorrhagic changes in the upper spinal cord in babies who are brain dead may be a function of the respirator brain pathology of circulatory deficits emanating from the arrested anterior spinal arterial supply from the vertebrobasilar system as it meets the contributions to the anterior spinal circular from unaffected supply from the aorta and radicular arteries [255,256].

The Alexander et al. paper [115] reported an analysis of 24 babies initially concluded as victims of SBS, 12 of whom apparently had no evidence of cranial impact. The diagnosis of SBS was arrived at by a multidisciplinary team. The authors employed circular reasoning to defend the diagnosis of SBS and present no individual case data.

The Gilliland and Folberg [252] paper deals with an analysis of 80 deaths in presumably abused babies. Evidence of shaking was derived from the presence of finger marks or rib fractures, subdural or subarachnoid hemorrhage, or a history of vigorous shaking. The probative validity of the first two criteria was not and has never been established. The confession of a caregiver of having shaken a baby does not establish if this action produced the observed injuries or if the confessor did things beyond shaking [31,32,257].

In summary, none of these several papers can be considered to have scientifically established a link between observed pathology and shaking. The deficiencies of such anecdotal reports have been discussed in detail by Donohoe [258] and in general by Greenhalgh [259].

The experimental design in the Cory et al. study involved models similar to those used by Duhaime et al. [110] and Prange et al. [111]. In one of the shaking patterns, the baby model in this study was held horizontal and shaken in a "gravity assisted" position. This positioning was reported to result in greatly increased accelerations, in part caused by the chin of the baby model striking the chest and the occiput striking the back of the baby model, which essentially introduced two impacts to the scenario. The authors employed calculations using the Head Injury Criterion (HIC) paradigm [260] and concluded that shaking under the conditions they employed could produce intracranial injury. The injury scenario created in this study is probably unphysiological in that even though chin/occiput self-impacts have been suggested in the literature, there is good reason to suppose that before cranial injury will occur, even if one accepts that the head can pass through a greater than 180 degree (3 rad) arc, the neck would fail [260].

Recently, many of the aspects of the model testing done by Duhaime et al. [110] and Prange et al. [111] were repeated using a CRABI-12 (equivalent of a 12-month-old baby) dummy fitted with state-of-the-art (as of 2008) instrumentation by Van Ee (see Table 7.2). The results of several horizontal drop tests to linoleum-covered hard flooring from heights of 1–5 ft, and comparisons with manual shaking and various known accidental events such as car crashes, are depicted in Figure 7.14. It is obvious, as shown by others [110, 111], that shaking forces yield *g* forces in the 10*g* range as compared with even a 2-ft drop, which yielded about 100*g*. Once again, sophisticated biomechanical analysis of the shaking

Table 7.2 Forces Involved in Manually Shaking a CRABI-12 Instrumented Dummy

Test Type	Peak *g*	HIC	Peak Angular Acceleration
Shake 1	10	4	2994
Shake 2	10	5	2969
Shake 3	10	4	3039
Shake 4	10	4	3428
Shake 5	9	3	2898

Source: Courtesy of Chris Van Ee, PhD, Design Research Engineering Inc., Novi, Michigan.

Note: This table reports the results of manual shaking of a CRABI-12 dummy, which corresponds to a 12-month-old baby (weight 22 lb). The figures reflect the most powerful of several successive shakes for each trial. The shakes were produced by a 210-lb male holding the dummy by laterally placed hands gripping the thorax and vigorously shaking forward and backward. These maneuvers yielded *g* forces of about 10*g*. Peak accelerations in *g*, HIC (Head Injury Criteria), and peak angular acceleration in rad/s^2.

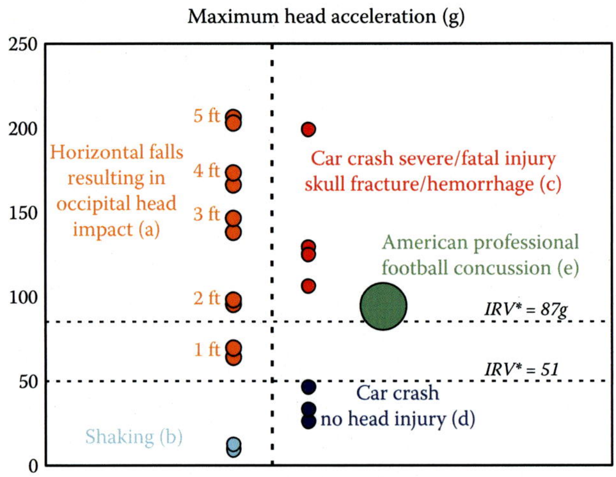

Figure 7.14 Chart displaying data derived from experiments using an instrumented CRABI-12 dummy (equivalent to 12-month-old baby). The shaking results are depicted in Table 7.2. A number of horizontal drops of the dummy were performed from heights of 1, 2, 3, 4, and 5 ft above a linoleum-covered hard floor (a), with impact to the occipital region of the head. The resultant forces are markedly different from shakes and are compared with other known and studied injury scenarios, such as concussive forces suffered by professional football players [261], car crash victims without head injuries [262] as studied with the CRABI-6 (equivalent to 6-month-old baby), and car crash victims with head injuries as studied with the CRABI-6 dummy [262]. Injury reference values (IRVs), in *g*, are derived from the work of Mertz [263] and Klinich et al. [262]. (Courtesy of Chris Van Ee, PhD, Design Research Engineering Inc., Novi, Michigan.)

maneuver, compared with other traumatic events, is well below thresholds in which intracranial injuries would be expected and provides verifiable proof that allegations by some that shaking is equivalent to a multistory fall or a high-speed car crash are false. When these scenarios are modeled or calculated, the forces involved are magnitudes greater than manual shaking can attain [261–263].

A scenario that is not uncommonly related in alleged child abuse cases involves stairway falls or drops and an infant. Sometimes the degree of external injury or even sub-scalp injury appears minimal even though there may be a subdural hemorrhage. This may raise the specter of a theory that shaking occurred rather than an impact.

Stairway falls are often complex with tumbling, sliding, bouncing, and often multiple impacts to the head. Therefore, any such fall must be examined carefully in terms of what the "story" was and what injuries revealed themselves at an autopsy if there was a fatality. It is often proposed by child abuse experts that stairway falls are benign and/or when such a scenario is given by a caregiver or accused individual, it is often stated that the injuries observed were not or could not be consistent with the history. Such a statement may be gratuitous, based on lack of competence to make such a judgment or simple prejudice. Stairway falls have been biomechanically examined. One such study by Van Ee involved a series of drop-falls of a CRABI-12 (12-month surrogate) model down a carpeted staircase. The results of these experiments are depicted in Figures 7.15 and 7.16. In these figures several scenarios and the forces of impact acceleration to the central mass of the model head are depicted. When multiple steps were involved, the model usually tumbled resulting in a

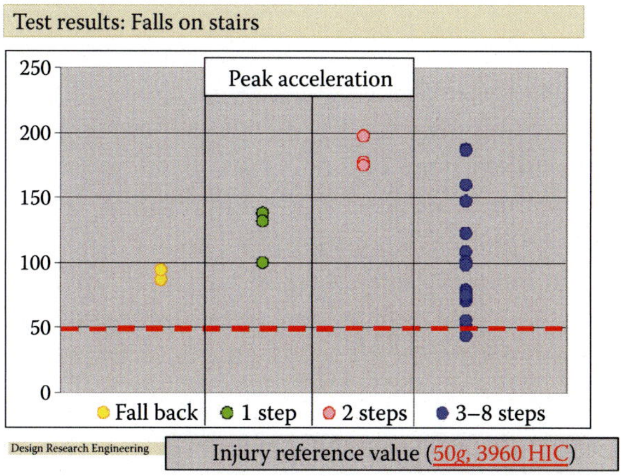

Figure 7.15 This figure depicts peak accelerations in *g*'s for various drop-falls on a carpeted wood stairway using a CRABI-12 instrumented dummy. (Courtesy of Chris Van Ee, PhD, Design Research Engineering Inc., Novi, Michigan.)

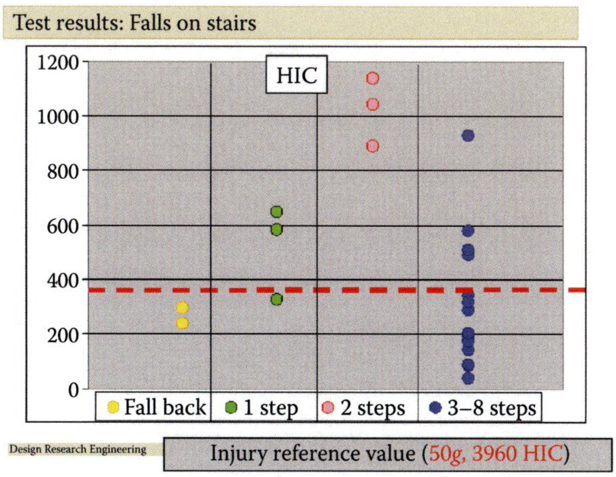

Figure 7.16 This figure depicts HIC (Head Injury Criterion) values for the same scenarios as shown in Figure 7.15. Red dashed line represents threshold for likelihood of serious head injury occurring. (Courtesy of Chris Van Ee, PhD, Design Research Engineering Inc., Novi, Michigan.)

number of greater or lesser impacts, which are illustrated. Suffice it to say, even a more or less free fall onto one step or two can result if there is a head impact first, in accelerations of 100–200*g*, well within the range to produce subdural hemorrhages and potentially brain injury. The accompanying HIC values are shown in Figure 7.16. The HIC is a computed value described and discussed in Chapter 6. It has been used extensively in predicting outcomes from auto crash tests and other accident scenarios using surrogates [262,263].

Other Issues in the Shaken Baby Syndrome

One of the two tenets of SBS by those who espouse the theory is that on shaking, the infant victim is immediately injured and rendered unconscious. The same is held true for abusive injury in which an impact of some sort may have occurred that produced a subdural hematoma, skull fracture, or some other pathology, and therefore the individual present at the time the infant becomes ill and decompensates is the perpetrator [116,117,121]. The other tenet is that the constellation of acute subdural hematoma, retinal hemorrhages, and brain swelling is most likely to have been caused by an inflicted injury, including shaking, and that this collective is uncommonly seen in any other scenario [116–118]. Such blanket pronouncements are not only misleading but also false.

The so-called lucid interval, or perhaps more properly the latent interval, between injury and appearance of symptoms is a well-known phenomenon; it is more common in some types of head injury than others (epidural hematoma vs. subdural hematoma) but is hardly rare, especially among infants. Of course, infants who suffer head injuries that are significant can become immediately unconscious after injury but may not always do so. The more extensive and destructive a head injury is, the more likely that immediate unconsciousness occurs. A number of recent studies have shown that infants who experience some sort of head injury that may bring them to the hospital do not appear particularly ill when examined yet have been shown to have occult head injuries such as skull fractures, subdural and epidural hematomas, and other forms of intracranial brain pathology when they were subjected to CT or MRI scanning [68]. In a particular study of Greenes and Schutzman [68], the aim was to provide criteria for emergency room physicians who were confronted with a history of a head injury situation but the infant appeared normal by physical examination. It was recommended that those infants with a scalp swelling be scanned. In a group of 101 such infants at the Boston Children's Hospital, about 19 of them were found to have occult head injuries. This study followed some of the injured babies, and apart from some of them who were treated with anticonvulsants, apparently none required further treatment. The authors noted that in infants who had been symptomatic, about 33% of them came back at some point for further treatments; thus, a significant percentage of head-injured children have ongoing problems that may or may not have been appreciated initially. It is interesting to note that virtually all of the scenarios of injury included falls of generally 2–4 ft.

Another study, by Howard et al. [112], reported 28 cases of infants brought to the hospital with head injuries and subdural hematomas. All were younger than 2 years. Half of the cases were thought to have been injured in connection with abuse (three cases mentioned some history of shaking, all of which had evidence of scalp impacts), and the other half appeared to have been accidentally injured, mostly in connection with short falls. The intervals between when injury occurred and hospitalization occurred varied from a few hours to 28 days, with nine of these cases being admitted less than 8 hours after injury and the remainder after that. Seven of the cases had mixed-density subdural hematomas, and the remainder had apparently dense homogeneous hematomas, indicating at least some of them may have been evolving into subacute or chronic subdural hematomas. Retinal hemorrhages were common, and eight of the babies had scalp swellings, but the others apparently did not. This report clearly shows that injuries do not immediately declare themselves and that a spectrum of clinical behavior occurs in head-injured, abused or nonabused, babies. Another observation is that the entire alleged discriminating constellation of injuries occurred in apparently accidentally injured babies as well as in the abused group.

A recent review [93] of 325 published cases reported over a 30-year period of infantile head injury presumably due to abuse, including 54 cases in which someone admitted to shaking the infant in some fashion, discovered that in 49 of 325 cases information was provided about the time interval between injury and hospitalization. Twenty-six percent of these cases had more or less immediate appearance of symptoms following injury, but the remainder showed latencies of hours to days to weeks. Eighty-six percent of the 215 cases that provided information about retinal hemorrhages had them, and 85% had acute subdural hematomas. Fifty-eight percent of the 69 cases with information about chronicity had chronic subdural hematomas. There was no statistical correlation between admitted shaking and any clinical or pathological variable in the cases. Thus, it appears that the latent period between injury and symptom appearance is common and that the co-occurrence of subdural hematoma, retinal hemorrhages, and other intracranial pathologies, as well as retinal hemorrhages, has no discriminating power to indicate abuse or a particular mode of injury.

There are many important papers that further cast doubt on the veracity of the proclaimed elements of the SBS. Many physicians maintain that injuries observed in babies do not correspond with the history of an event provided and, thus, such histories are false [14–16,264]. The above-cited reports of Greenes and Schutzman [68] and Howard et al. [112] clearly indicate that short falls can and do cause serious injuries. The report of Plunkett [71] analyzed a case of a 2-year-old girl who fell perhaps 4 ft from a play gym, videotaped serendipitously while doing so, and died with a subdural hematoma and retinal hemorrhages. The report of Piatt [136] illustrates a very short fall in an infant with a subdural fluid collection/external hydrocephalus who suffered retinal hemorrhages and collapse but survived. The as-yet-unpublished study of Lantz [141] indicates that in more than 1000 autopsies on a general and forensic service, when the eyes were examined by a variety of methods, about 20% of the cases (spanning all age groups) had some form of retinal hemorrhage (localized or extensive) under a variety of conditions not related to head trauma. In 116 of these cases who were younger than a year, 20.9% of them had retinal hemorrhages. These infants had died from prematurity-related causes, SIDS, pneumonia, herpes simplex infections, congenital cardiac defects, asphyxia, cerebral venous thrombosis, and other conditions. Thus, in a relatively unselected general population, retinal hemorrhages at autopsy are not uncommon and appear to have no discriminatory potential for signaling abuse, shaking, or any other particular mechanism for occurrence.

Another process that may confound the interpretation of abuse and the occurrence of often-minimal brain pathology in the face of disabling and fatal cerebral edema (often mistakenly called diffuse axonal injury) is the phenomenon of so-called malignant cerebral edema, which may occur after relatively mild head injuries in children [265–267]. This process is discussed in more detail in Chapters 5 and 6 but will be summarized here. There are circumstances in which infants and young children may fall and strike their heads with apparently little immediate consequence, only to appear seriously ill or moribund hours or longer afterward in the hospital. These children appear to suffer from a cascading process of cerebral edema that may have its basis in an immature blood–brain barrier system that is vulnerable [266,267]. Quite often this edema is resistant to therapy, and the child may die from increased intracranial pressure and respirator brain phenomena. It is not known how common this phenomenon is and how often some component of it overlays head trauma, abusive or not, in the pediatric population. From a forensic point of view, it appears that the phenomenon does exist, and may not correlate with fall distance or other standard measures of potential injury severity.

Summary

The problem of analysis of potential or suspected child abuse fatalities, especially in younger children, is a very difficult task, having to deal with a commonly embedded mind-set that holds that certain findings rarely or never occur outside the environment of abuse and have considerable discriminatory potential to rule out accidental injuries, medical conditions, or combinations in favor of abuse. Virtually all the hallowed tenets of SBS have been challenged on the basis of scientific principles and have been found wanting or wrong. Does this criticism mean that there is no such thing as injury in connection with shaking (in the absence of impact)? Not at all. It means that given the best information that is currently available, it appears that shaking forces that a human can achieve, without an impact, do not apparently and predictably cause brain injuries but could cause cervical spinal injuries, which are uncommonly observed. It also means that it is not known if there are some infants who might suffer intracranial injuries from shaking because there is some underlying disease process or condition that lowers the injury threshold for them as compared with normal babies. This latter question has not been addressed in a systematic way and must remain open.

The job of the forensic pathologist of trying to figure out what happened to a dead child is not easy. There are many possibilities of etiology in what is nearly always a multifactorial problem. Given these complexities, like it or not, clear-cut interpretations in a situation where there are no forthcoming witnesses, no independent physical evidence, differences in professional opinions, and meager knowledge about many aspects of the problem are frequently not possible. When an interpretation is given, the answers must be scientifically supportable, not to the standard of "more likely than not" but to a much higher standard, akin to that demanded in the best and most critical scientific disciplines. This standard is required because the results of an analysis may have profound consequences to an individual accused of harming the child, perhaps not very different from the basis for and consequences of the amputation of a limb or embarkation on a highly risky medical treatment. All of these decisions must be based on the best evidence available and not on dogma or prejudice.

Furthermore, it is becoming increasingly apparent that infants may present with what at first impression may appear to be traumatic injuries (subdural hematoma, cerebral edema, retinal hemorrhages, skeletal or skull fractures, coma, and apnea) but which may be caused by or contributed to by previously unsuspected inherited conditions (hemoglobinopathies, disorders of amino acid metabolism, coagulopathies, etc.), vitamin K deficiency, vitamin D deficiency and rickets, brittle bone diseases, unsuspected birth injuries, arachnoid cysts and fluid collections, and many other conditions that may be uncommon to rare. Rarity of a condition in a general population is not a disqualification for the etiological importance of that condition against the context of alleged or possible abuse, because by the selection process that operates, bringing an infant to a hospital emergency room or an autopsy service removes this child from population statistics. Thus, even uncommon and rare conditions become less so in the context of the evaluation of child abuse and should engender caution.

The interested reader is referred to three detailed and scholarly reviews of SBS as seen from the perspective of the law [243–245]. There are many recent celebrated cases in which individuals convicted of harming infants presumably by shaking them were successful in postconviction relief on the basis of flawed science regarding the mechanism(s). Many of these are discussed in detail in these reviews, which are available in full text, online.

References

1. Clark RE, Freeman J, Adamec CA. *The Encyclopedia of Child Abuse*. New York: Facts on File, 2007.
2. Camps FE, Robinson AE, Lucas BGB, eds. *Gradwohl's Legal Medicine*. Bristol: A. John Wright, 1976.

3. Radbill SX. A history of child abuse and infanticide. In Helfer RE, Kempe CH, eds., *The Battered Child*. Chicago: University of Chicago Press, 1974, pp. 3–21.
4. Weston JT. The pathology of child abuse. In Helfer RE, Kempe CH, eds., *The Battered Child*. Chicago: University of Chicago Press, 1968, pp. 77–100.
5. Knight B. *Forensic Pathology*. London: Arnold, 1996.
6. Tardieu A. Etude medico-legale sur les sevices et Mauvais traitments exerces sur des enfants. *Ann Hyg Publ Med Leg* 1860;13:361–98.
7. Kempe CH, Silverman FN, Steele BF, Droegenmueller W, Silver HK. The battered-child syndrome. *JAMA* 1962;181:17–24.
8. Kempe CH. Child abuse—The pediatrician's role in child advocacy and preventive pediatrics. *Am J Dis Child* 1978;132:255–60.
9. Greeley CS. The evolution of the child maltreatment literature. *Pediatrics* 2012;130(2):347–8.
10. Helfer RE. The epidemiology of child abuse and neglect. *Pediatr Ann* 1984;13:745–51.
11. Chase W. An anatomic study of subdural haemorrhage associated with tentorial splitting in the newborn. *Surg Gynec Obstetr* 1930;51:31–41.
12. Sherwood D. Chronic subdural hematoma in infants. *Am J Dis Child* 1930;39:980–1021.
13. Keenan HT, Runyan DK, Marshall SW, Nocera MA, Merten DF, Sinal SH. A population-based study of inflicted traumatic brain injury in young children. *JAMA* 2003;290:621–6.
14. Reece RM, Sege R. Childhood head injuries: Accidental or inflicted? *Arch Pediatr Adolesc Med* 2000;154:11–5.
15. Reece RM, Ludwig S, eds. *Child Abuse: Medical Diagnosis and Management*. Philadelphia: Lippincott Williams & Wilkins, 2001.
16. Levi BH, Brown G. Reasonable suspicion: A study of Pennsylvania pediatricians regarding child abuse. *Pediatrics* 2005;116:e5–12.
17. Webster SW, O'Toole R, O'Toole AW, Lucal B. Overreporting and underreporting of child abuse: Teachers' use of professional discretion. *Child Abuse Negl* 2005;29:1281–96.
18. Van Haeringen AR, Dadds M, Armstrong KL. The child abuse lottery—Will the doctor suspect and report? Physician attitudes towards and reporting of suspected child abuse and neglect. *Child Abuse Negl* 1998;22:159–69.
19. American Board of Pediatrics. Certification in child abuse pediatrics. Available at https://abp.org, 2013.
20. Kanda M, Thomas JN, Lloyd DW. The role of forensic evidence in child abuse and neglect. *Am J Foren Med Pathol* 1985;6:7–15.
21. Gall D, Weil B. Confidentiality and the obligation to report child abuse: Case for discussion. *Prog Clin Biol Res* 1983;139:47–8.
22. Weisberg R, Wald M. Confidentiality laws and state efforts to protect abused or neglected children: The need for statutory reform. *Fam Law Q* 1984;38:143–212.
23. Christoffel KK, Liu K. Homicide death rates in childhood in 23 developed countries: U.S. rates atypically high. *Child Abuse Negl* 1983;7:339–45.
24. Copeland AR. Homicide in childhood. The Metro-Dade County experience from 1956 to 1982. *Am J Foren Med Pathol* 1985;6:21–4.
25. Cameron JM, Rae LJ. *Atlas of the Battered Child*. Edinburgh: Churchill Livingstone, 1975.
26. DiMaio VJ, DiMaio D. *Forensic Pathology*. Boca Raton, FL: CRC Press, 2001.
27. Spitz WU, Spitz DJ, eds. *Spitz and Fisher's Medicolegal Investigation of Death: Guidelines for the Application of Pathology to Crime Investigation*. Springfield, IL: Charles C. Thomas, 2006.
28. Oates RK, Forrest D, Peacock A. Mothers of abused children: A comparison study. *Clin Pediatr (Phila)* 1985;24:9–13.
29. Hahn YS, Raimondi AJ, McLone DG, Yamanouchi Y. Traumatic mechanisms of head injury in child abuse. *Childs Brain* 1983;10:229–41.
30. Conti RP. The psychology of false confessions. *J Credib Assess Witness Psychol* 1999;2:14–36.
31. Leo RA, Ofshe RJ. The consequences of false confessions: Deprivations of liberty and miscarriages of justice in the age of psychological interrogation. *J Crim Law Criminol* 1998;88:429–97.

32. Kassin SM. On the psychology of confessions: Does innocence put innocents at risk? *Am J Psychol* 2005;60:215–26.
33. Diamond LJ, Jandes PK. Child abuse in a cerebral-palsied population. *Dev Med Child Neurol* 1983;25:169–74.
34. Green AH. Child abuse by siblings. *Child Abuse Negl* 1984;8:311–7.
35. Halperin SM. Family perceptions of abused children and their siblings. *Child Abuse Negl* 1983;7:107–15.
36. Arnestad M, Crotti L, Rognum TO, Insolia R, Pedrazzini M, Ferrandi C, Vege A, Wang DW, Rhodes TE, George AL Jr, Schwartz PJ. Prevalence of long-QT syndrome gene variants in sudden infant death syndrome. *Circulation* 2007;115:361–7.
37. Wedekind H, Bajanowski T, Friederich P, Breithardt G, Wulfing T, Siebrands C, Engeland B, Monnig G, Haverkamp W, Brinkmann B, Schulze-Bahr E. Sudden infant death syndrome and long QT syndrome: An epidemiological and genetic study. *Int J Legal Med* 2006;120:129–37.
38. R. v Cannings [2004] EWCA Crim 01, Case No. 200201711 D3. Supreme Court of Judiature, Court of Appeal (Criminal division). Available at http://www.familylawweek.co.uk/site aspx?i=ed1654.
39. Byard R, Krous H, eds. *Sudden Infant Death Syndrome. Problems, Progress and Possibilities.* London: Arnold, 2001.
40. Bajanowski T, Vennemann M, Bohnert M, Rauch E, Brinkmann B, Mitchell EA, GeSID Group. Unnatural causes of sudden unexpected deaths initially thought to be sudden infant death syndrome. *Int J Legal Med* 2005;119:213–6.
41. Cote A, Russo P, Michaud J. Sudden unexpected deaths in infancy: What are the causes? *J Pediatr* 1999;135:437–43.
42. Truman TL, Ayoub CC. Considering suffocatory abuse and Munchausen by proxy in the evaluation of children experiencing apparent life-threatening events and sudden infant death syndrome. *Child Maltreat* 2002;7:138–48.
43. Galvin HK, Newton AW, Vandeven AM. Update on Munchausen syndrome by proxy. *Curr Opin Pediatr* 2005;17:252–7.
44. Norman MG, Smialek JE, Newman DE, Horembala EJ. The postmortem examination on the abused child: Pathological, radiographic, and legal aspects. *Perspect Pediatr Pathol* 1984;8:313–43.
45. Kleinman PK, Marks SC Jr, Richmond JM, Blackbourne BD. Inflicted skeletal injury: A postmortem radiologic-histopathologic study in 31 infants. *AJR Am J Roentgenol* 1995;165:647–50.
46. McGraw EP, Pless JE, Pennington DJ, White SJ. Postmortem radiography after unexpected death in neonates, infants, and children: Should imaging be routine? *AJR Am J Roentgenol* 2002;178:1517–21.
47. Ludwig J. *Handbook of Autopsy Practice*. Totowa, NJ: Humana Press, 2002.
48. Isaacson G. Postmortem examination of infant brains: Techniques for removal, fixation, and sectioning. *Arch Pathol Lab Med* 1984;108:80–1.
49. Earle KM. *Examination of the Brain (Necropsy Technique)*. Washington, DC: American Registry of Pathology.
50. Maguire S, Mann MK, Sibert J, Kemp A. Can you age bruises accurately in children? A systematic review. *Arch Dis Child* 2005;90:187–9.
51. Bariciak ED, Plint AC, Gaboury I, Bennett S. Dating of bruises in children: An assessment of physician accuracy. *Pediatrics* 2003;112:804–7.
52. Langlois NE, Gresham GA. The ageing of bruises: A review and study of the colour changes with time. *Foren Sci Int* 1991;50:227–38.
53. Bohnert M, Baumgartner R, Pollak S. Spectrophotometric evaluation of the colour of intra- and subcutaneous bruises. *Int J Legal Med* 2000;113:343–8.
54. Yajima Y, Funayama M. Spectrophotometric and tristimulus analysis of the colors of subcutaneous bleeding in living persons. *Foren Sci Int* 2006;156:131–7.
55. Janssen W. *Forensic Histopathology*. Berlin: Springer-Verlag, 1984.
56. Betz P, Eisenmenger W. Morphometrical analysis of hemosiderin deposits in relation to wound age. *Int J Legal Med* 1996;108:262–4.

57. Itabashi H, Andrews JM, Tomiyasu U, Erlich SS, Sathyavagiswaran L. *Forensic Neuropathology: A Practical Review of the Fundamentals*. Amsterdam: Academic Press, Elsevier, 2007.
58. Oehmichen M, Auer RN, Koenig HG. *Forensic Neuropathology and Associated Neurology*. Berlin: Springer-Verlag, 2006.
59. Betz P. Immunohistochemical parameters for the age estimation of human skin wounds: A review. *Am J Foren Med Pathol* 1995;16:203–9.
60. Suarez-Penaranda JM, Rodriguez-Calvo MS, Ortiz-Rey JA, Munoz JI, Sanchez-Pintos P, Da Silva EA, De la Fu A, Concheiro-Carro L. Demonstration of apoptosis in human skin injuries as an indicator of vital reaction. *Int J Legal Med* 2002;116:109–12.
61. Sawaguchi T, Jasani B, Kobayashi M, Knight B. Post-mortem analysis of apoptotic changes associated with human skin bruises. *Foren Sci Int* 2000;108:187–203.
62. Hobbs CJ. Skull fracture and the diagnosis of abuse. *Arch Dis Child* 1984;59:246–52.
63. Kravitz H, Driessen G, Gomberg R, Korach A. Accidental falls from elevated surfaces in infants from birth to one year of age. *Pediatrics* 1969;44(Suppl):869–76.
64. Helfer RE, Slovis TL, Black M. Injuries resulting when small children fall out of bed. *Pediatrics* 1977;60:533–5.
65. Nimityongskul P, Anderson LD. The likelihood of injuries when children fall out of bed. *J Pediatr Orthop* 1987;7:184–6.
66. Williams RA. Injuries in infants and small children resulting from witnessed and corroborated free falls. *J Trauma* 1991;31:1350–2.
67. Lyons TJ, Oates RK. Falling out of bed: A relatively benign occurrence. *Pediatrics* 1993;92:125–7.
68. Greenes DS, Schutzman SA. Occult intracranial injury in infants. *Ann Emerg Med* 1998;32: 680–6.
69. Fickenscher KA, Dean JS, Mena DC, Green BA, Lowe LH. Occult cranial injuries found with neuroimaging in clinically asymptomatic young children due to abusive compared to accidental head trauma. *Southern Med J* 2010;103:121–5.
70. Helling TS, Watkins M, Evans LL, Nelson PW, Shook JW, Van Way CW. Low falls: An underappreciated mechanism of injury. *J Trauma* 1999;46:453–6.
71. Plunkett J. Fatal pediatric head injuries caused by short-distance falls. *Am J Foren Med Pathol* 2001;22:1–12.
72. Kim KA, Wang MY, Griffith PM, Summers S, Levy ML. Analysis of pediatric head injury from falls. *Neurosurg Focus* 2000;8(1):e3.
73. Wang MY, Kim KA, Griffith PM, Summers S, McComb JG, Levy ML, Mahour GH. Injuries from falls in the pediatric population: An analysis of 729 cases. *J Pediatr Surg* 2001;36:1528–34.
74. Root I. Head injuries from short distance falls. *Am J Foren Med Pathol* 1992;13:85–7.
75. Lallier M, Bouchard S, St-Vil D, Dupont J, Tucci M. Falls from heights among children: A retrospective review. *J Pediatr Surg* 1999;34:1060–3.
76. Weber W. Experimental studies of skull fractures in infants. *Z Rechtsmed* 1984;92:87–94.
77. Weber W. Biomechanical fragility of the infant skull. *Z Rechtsmed* 1985;94:93–101.
78. Weber W. Predilection sites of infantile skull fractures following blunt force. *Z Rechtsmed* 1987;98:81–93.
79. Takeshi M, Okuchi K, Nishiguchi T, Seki T, Watanabe T, Ito S, Murao Y. Clinical analysis of seven patients of crushing head injury. *J Trauma* 2006;60:1245–9.
80. Gonzalez Tortosa J, Martinez-Lage JF, Poza M. Bitemporal head crush injuries: Clinical and radiological features of a distinctive type of head injury. *J Neurosurg* 2004;100:645–51.
81. Duhaime AC, Eppley M, Margulies S, Heher KL, Bartlett SP. Crush injuries to the head in children. *Neurosurgery* 1995;37:401–6; discussion, 407.
82. Yahya RR, Dirks P, Humphreys R, Rutka JT, Taylor M, Drake JM. Children and television tipovers: A significant and preventable cause of long-term neurological deficits. *J Neurosurg* 2005;103(Suppl):219–22.
83. Prasad MR, Ewing-Cobbs L, Baumgartner J. Crush head injuries in infants and young children: Neurologic and neuropsychologic sequelae. *J Child Neurol* 1999;14:496–501.

84. Brown RL, Brunn MA, Garcia VF. Cervical spine injuries in children: A review of 103 patients treated consecutively at a level 1 pediatric trauma center. *J Pediatr Surg* 2001;36:1107–14.
85. Kokoska ER, Keller MS, Rallo MC, Weber TR. Characteristics of pediatric cervical spine injuries. *J Pediatr Surg* 2001;36:100–5.
86. Platzer P, Jaindl M, Thalhammer G, Dittrich S, Kutscha-Lissberg F, Vecsei V, Gaebler C. Cervical spine injuries in pediatric patients. *J Trauma* 2007;62:389–96; discussion, 394–6.
87. Oral R, Rahhal R, Elshershari H, Menezes AH. Intentional avulsion fracture of the second cervical vertebra in a hypotonic child. *Pediatr Emerg Care* 2006;22:352–4.
88. Rooks VJ, Sisler C, Burton B. Cervical spine injury in child abuse: Report of two cases. *Pediatr Radiol* 1998;28:193–5.
89. Thomas NH, Robinson L, Evans A, Bullock P. The floppy infant: A new manifestation of nonaccidental injury. *Pediatr Neurosurg* 1995;23:188–91.
90. Ghatan S, Ellenbogen RG. Pediatric spine and spinal cord injury after inflicted trauma. *Neurosurg Clin N Am* 2002;13:227–33.
91. Cirak B, Ziegfeld S, Knight VM, Chang D, Avellino AM, Paidas CN. Spinal injuries in children. *J Pediatr Surg* 2004;39:607–12.
92. Hadley MN, Sonntag VK, Rekate HL, Murphy A. The infant whiplash–shake injury syndrome: A clinical and pathological study. *Neurosurgery* 1989;24:536–40.
93. Leestma JE. Case analysis of brain-injured admittedly shaken infants: 54 cases, 1969–2001. *Am J Foren Med Pathol* 2005;26:199–212.
94. Bandak FA. Shaken baby syndrome: A biomechanics analysis of injury mechanisms. *Foren Sci Int* 2005;151:71–9.
95. Bosch PP, Vogt MT, Ward WT. Pediatric spinal cord injury without radiographic abnormality (SCIWORA): The absence of occult instability and lack of indication for bracing. *Spine* 2002;27:2788–800.
96. Oehmichen M. Brain death: Neuropathological findings and forensic implications. *Foren Sci Int* 1994;69:205–19.
97. Ersahin Y, Mutluer S, Guzelbag E. Extradural hematoma: Analysis of 146 cases. *Childs Nerv Syst* 1993;9:96–9.
98. Cheung PS, Lam JM, Yeung JH, Graham CA, Rainer TH. Outcome of traumatic extradural haematoma in Hong Kong. *Injury* 2007;38:76–80.
99. Pillay R, Peter JC. Extradural haematomas in children. *S Afr Med J* 1995;85:672–4.
100. Fishpool SJ, Suren N, Roncaroli F, Ellis H. Middle meningeal artery hemorrhage: An incorrect name. *Clin Anat* 2007;20:371–5.
101. Yilmazlar S, Kocaeli H, Dogan S, Abas F, Aksoy K, Korfali E, Doygun M. Traumatic epidural haematomas of nonarterial origin: Analysis of 30 consecutive cases. *Acta Neurochir* (Wien) 2005;147:1241–8; discussion, 1248.
102. Chaiyasate S, Halewyck S, Van Rompaey K, Clement P. Spontaneous extradural hematoma as a presentation of sinusitis: Case report and literature review. *Int J Pediatr Otorhinolaryngol* 2007;71:827–30.
103. Heyman R, Heckly A, Magagi J, Pladys P, Hamlat A. Intracranial epidural hematoma in newborn infants: Clinical study of 15 cases. *Neurosurgery* 2005;57:924–9.
104. Parmar CD, Sinha AK, Hayhurst C, May PL, O'Brien DF. Epidural hematoma formation following trivial head trauma in a child with osteogenesis imperfecta. Case report. *J Neurosurg* 2007;106(Suppl):57–60.
105. Mori K, Handa H, Munemitsu H, Oda Y, Hashimoto N, Kojima M. Epidural hematomas of the posterior fossa in children. *Childs Brain* 1983;10:130–40.
106. Dirim BV, Oruk C, Erdogan N, Gelal F, Uluc E. Traumatic posterior fossa hematomas. *Diagn Interv Radiol* 2005;11:14–8.
107. Squier W, Mack J. The neuropathology of infant subdural haemorrhage. *Foren Sci Int* 2009;187:6–13.
108. Scheimberg I, Cohen MC, Zapata Vazquez RD, Dilly S, Al-Adnani M, Turner K, Sethuraman C. Non-traumatic intracranial and subdural hemorrhage and hypoxic ischaemic encephalopathny

in fetuses, infants and children up to 3 years of age: Analysis of two audits of 636 cases from two referral centers in the UK. *Pediatr Dev Pathol* 2013;16:149–59.
109. McNeely PD, Atkinson JD, Saigal G, O'Gorman AM, Farmer JP. Subdural hematomas in infants with benign enlargement of the subarachnoid spaces are not pathognomonic for child abuse. *Am J Neuroradiol* 2006;27:1725–8.
110. Duhaime AC, Gennarelli TA, Thibault LE, Bruce DA, Margulies SS, Wiser R. The shaken baby syndrome: A clinical, pathological, and biomechanical study. *J Neurosurg* 1987;66:409–15.
111. Prange MT, Coats B, Duhaime AC, Margulies SS. Anthropomorphic simulations of falls, shakes, and inflicted impacts in infants. *J Neurosurg* 2003;99:143–50.
112. Howard MA, Bell BA, Uttley D. The pathophysiology of infant subdural haematomas. *Br J Neurosurg* 1993;7:355–65.
113. Goldsmith W, Plunkett J. A biomechanical analysis of the causes of traumatic brain injury in infants and children. *Am J Foren Med Pathol* 2004;25:89–100.
114. Fung EL, Sung RY, Nelson EA, Poon WS. Unexplained subdural hematoma in young children: Is it always child abuse? *Pediatr Int* 2002;44:37–42.
115. Alexander R, Crabbe L, Sato Y, Smith W, Bennett T. Serial abuse in children who are shaken. *Am J Dis Child* 1990;144:58–60.
116. Lazoritz S, Palusci VJ, eds. *The Shaken Baby Syndrome: A Multidisciplinary Approach*. New York: Haworth Maltreatment & Trauma Press, 2001.
117. Minns RA, Brown JK, eds. *Shaking and Other Non-accidental Head Injuries in Children*. London: Mac Keith Press, 2005.
118. Case ME, Graham MA, Handy TC, Jentzen JM, Monteleone JA. Position paper on fatal abusive head injuries in infants and young children. *Am J Foren Med Pathol* 2001;22:112–22.
119. American Academy of Pediatrics. American Academy of Pediatrics Committee on Child Abuse and Neglect: Shaken baby syndrome: Inflicted cerebral trauma. *Pediatrics* 1993;92:872–5.
120. Bandak FA. On the mechanics of impact neurotrauma: A review and critical synthesis. *J Neurotrauma* 1995;12:635–49.
121. Willman KY, Bank DE, Senac M, Chadwick DL. Restricting the time of injury in fatal inflicted head injuries. *Child Abuse Negl* 1997;21:929–40.
122. Jayawant S, Rawlinson A, Gibbon F, Price J, Schulte J, Sharples P, Sibert JR, Kemp AM. Subdural haemorrhages in infants: Population based study. *BMJ* 1998;317:1558–61.
123. Hymel KP, Jenny C, Block RW. Intracranial hemorrhage and rebleeding in suspected victims of abusive head trauma: Addressing the forensic controversies. *J Foren Sci* 2002;7:329–48.
124. Parent AD. Pediatric chronic subdural hematoma: A retrospective comparative analysis. *Pediatr Neurosurg* 1992;18:266–71.
125. Hwang SK, Kim SL. Infantile head injury, with special reference to the development of chronic subdural hematoma. *Childs Nerv Syst* 2000;16:590–4.
126. Loh JK, Lin CL, Kwan AL, Howng SL. Acute subdural hematoma in infancy. *Surg Neurol* 2002;58:218–24.
127. Munro D, Merritt HH. Surgical pathology of subdural hematoma: Based on a study of one hundred and five cases. *Arch Neurol Psychiatr* 1936;35:64–78.
128. Feldman KW, Brewer DK, Shaw DW. Evolution of the cranial computed tomography scan in child abuse. *Child Abuse Negl* 1995;19:307–14.
129. Barkovich AJ. *Pediatric Neuroimaging*. Philadelphia: Lippincott Williams & Wilkins, 2000.
130. Sargent S, Kennedy JG, Kaplan JA. "Hyperacute" subdural hematoma: CT mimic of recurrent episodes of bleeding in the setting of child abuse. *J Foren Sci* 1996;41:314–6.
131. Barnes PD, Robson CD. CT findings in hyperacute nonaccidental brain injury. *Pediatr Radiol* 2000;30:74–81.
132. Steinbok P, Singhal A, Poskitt K, Cochrane DD. Early hypodensity on computed tomographic scan of the brain in an accidental pediatric head injury. *Neurosurgery* 2007;60:689–94; discussion, 694–5.
133. Barnes PD. Ethical issues in imaging nonaccidental injury: Child abuse. *Top Magn Reson Imaging* 2002;13:85–93.

134. Barnes PD, Krasnokutsky M. Imaging of the central nervous system in suspected or alleged nonaccidental injury, including the mimics. *Top Magn Reson Imaging* 2007;18:53–74.
135. Papasian NC, Frim DM. A theoretical model of benign external hydrocephalus that predicts a predisposition towards extra-axial hemorrhage after minor head trauma. *Pediatr Neurosurg* 2000;33:188–93.
136. Piatt JH Jr. A pitfall in the diagnosis of child abuse: External hydrocephalus, subdural hematoma, and retinal hemorrhages [Electronic resource]. *Neurosurg Focus* 1999;7(4):e4.
137. Dias MS, Backstrom J, Falk M, Li V. Serial radiography in the infant shaken impact syndrome. *Pediatr Neurosurg* 1998;29:77–85.
138. Greitz D. Paradigm shift in hydrocephalus research in legacy of Dandy's pioneering work: Rationale for third ventriculostomy in communicating hydrocephalus. *Childs Nerv Syst* 2007;23:487–9.
139. Tongue AC. The ophthalmologist's role in diagnosing child abuse. *Ophthalmology* 1991;98: 1009–10.
140. Gardner HB. Retinal folds. *Arch Ophthalmol* 2007;125:1142.
141. Lantz P. Postmortem detection and evaluation of retinal hemorrhages. In *American Academy of Forensic Sciences*. Seattle, 2006, abstract G-14, p. 271.
142. Lueder GT, Turner JW, Paschall R. Perimacular retinal folds simulating nonaccidental injury in an infant. *Arch Ophthalmol* 2006;124:1782–3.
143. Ommaya AK, Goldsmith W, Thibault L. Biomechanics and neuropathology of adult and paediatric head injury. *Br J Neurosurg* 2002;16:220–42.
144. Walsh FB, Hedges TR Jr. Optic nerve sheath hemorrhage: The Jackson Memorial lecture. *Am J Ophthalmol* 1951;34:509–27.
145. Smith DC, Kearns TP, Sayre GP. Preretinal and optic nerve-sheath hemorrhage: Pathologic and experimental aspects in subarachnoid hemorrhage. *Trans Am Ophthalmol Otolaryn Soc* 1957;61:201–11.
146. Muller PJ, Deck JH. Intraocular and optic nerve sheath hemorrhage in cases of sudden intracranial hypertension. *J Neurosurg* 1974;41:160–6.
147. Matshes E. Retinal and optic nerve sheath hemorrhages are not pathognomonic of abusive head injury. Abstract G-1, American Acad Foren Sci Annual Meeting, 2010, p. 272.
148. Odom A, Christ E, Kerr N, Byrd K, Cochran J, Barr F, Bugnitz M, Ring JC, Storgion S, Walling R, Stidham G, Quasney MW. Prevalence of retinal hemorrhages in pediatric patients after in-hospital cardiopulmonary resuscitation: A prospective study. *Pediatrics* 1997;99(6):E3.
149. Weedn VW, Mansour AM, Nichols MM. Retinal hemorrhage in an infant after cardiopulmonary resuscitation. *Am J Foren Med Pathol* 1990;11:79–82.
150. Gayle MO, Kissoon N, Hered RW, Harwood-Nuss A. Retinal hemorrhage in the young child: A review of etiology, predisposed conditions, and clinical implications. *J Emerg Med* 1995;13:233–9.
151. Geddes JF, Talbert DG. Paroxysmal coughing, subdural and retinal bleeding: A computer modelling approach. *Neuropathol Appl Neurobiol* 2006;32:625–34.
152. Kocak N, Kaynak S, Kaynak T, Oner HF, Cingil G. Unilateral Purtscher-like retinopathy after weight-lifting. *Eur J Ophthalmol* 2003;13:395–7.
153. Gilliland MG, Luckenbach MW. Are retinal hemorrhages found after resuscitation attempts? A study of the eyes of 169 children. *Am J Foren Med Pathol* 1993;14:187–92.
154. Gilliland MG, Luckenbach MW, Chenier TC. Systemic and ocular findings in 169 prospectively studied child deaths: Retinal hemorrhages usually mean child abuse. *Foren Sci Int* 1994;68:117–32.
155. Agrawal A, McKibbin M. Purtscher's retinopathy: Epidemiology, clinical features and outcome. *Br J Ophthalmol* 2007.
156. Tomasi LG, Rosman NP. Purtscher retinopathy in the battered child syndrome. *Am J Dis Child* 1975;129:1335–7.
157. Medele RJ, Stummer W, Mueller AJ, Steiger HJ, Reulen HJ. Terson's syndrome in subarachnoid hemorrhage and severe brain injury accompanied by acutely raised intracranial pressure. *J Neurosurg* 1998;88:851–4.

158. Keithahn MA, Bennett SR, Cameron D, Mieler WF. Retinal folds in Terson syndrome. *Ophthalmology* 1993;100:1187–90.
159. Lindenberg RL, Freytag E. Morphology of brain lesions from blunt trauma in early infancy. *Arch Pathol* 1969;87:298–305.
160. Gennarelli TA, Thibault LE, Adams JH, Graham DI, Thompson CJ, Marcincin RP. Diffuse axonal injury and traumatic coma in the primate. *Ann Neurol* 1982;12:564–74.
161. Gleckman AM, Bell MD, Evans RJ, Smith TW. Diffuse axonal injury in infants with nonaccidental craniocerebral trauma: Enhanced detection by beta-amyloid precursor protein immunohistochemical staining. *Arch Pathol Lab Med* 1999;123:146–51.
162. Blumbergs PC, Scott G, Manavis J, Wainwright H, Simpson DA, McLean AJ. Topography of axonal injury as defined by amyloid precursor protein and the sector scoring method in mild and severe closed head injury. *J Neurotrauma* 1995;12:565–72.
163. Oehmichen M, Meissner C, Schmidt V, Pedal I, König HG, Saternus KS. Axonal injury—A diagnostic tool in forensic neuropathology? A review. *Foren Sci Int* 1998;95:67–83.
164. Oehmichen M, Meissner C, Schmidt V, Pedal I, Konig HG. Pontine axonal injury after brain trauma and nontraumatic hypoxic–ischemic brain damage. *Int J Legal Med* 1999;112(4):261–7.
165. Kaur B, Rutty GN, Timperley WR. The possible role of hypoxia in the formation of axonal bulbs. *J Clin Pathol* 1999;52:203–9.
166. Kleinman PK, Marks SC Jr, Nimkin K, Rayder SM, Kessler SC. Rib fractures in 31 abused infants: Postmortem radiologic–histopathologic study. *Radiology* 1996;200:807–10.
167. Kleinman PK, Marks SC, Spevak MR, Richmond JM. Fractures of the rib head in abused infants. *Radiology* 1992;185:119–23.
168. Al-Sarraj S, Fegan-Earl A, Ugbade A, Bodi I, Chapman R, Poole S, Swift B, Jerreat P, Cary N. Focal traumatic brain stem injury is a rare type of head injury resulting from assault: A forensic neuropathological study. *J Forensic Leg Med* 2012;19(3):144–51.
169. Hortobagyi T, Wise S, Hunt N, Cary N, Djurovic V, Fegan-Earl A, Shorrock K, Rouse D, Al-Sarraj S. Traumatic axonal damage in the brain can be detected using beta-APP immunohistochemistry within 35 min after head injury to human adults. *Neuropathol Appl Neurobiol* 2007;33(2):226–37.
170. Reichard RR, Smith C, Graham DI. The significance of beta-APP immunoreactivity in forensic practice. *Neuropathol Appl Neurobiol* 2005;31(3):304–13.
171. Rubin DM, Christian CW, Bilaniuk LT, Zazyczny KA, Durbin DR. Occult head injury in high-risk abused children. *Pediatrics* 2003;111:1382–6.
172. Kleinman PK, Schlesinger AE. Mechanical factors associated with posterior rib fractures: Laboratory and case studies. *Pediatr Radiol* 1997;27:87–91.
173. Ng CS, Hall CM. Costochondral junction fractures and intra-abdominal trauma in non-accidental injury (child abuse). *Pediatr Radiol* 1998;28:671–6.
174. Gunther WM, Symes SA, Berryman HE. Characteristics of child abuse by anteroposterior manual compression versus cardiopulmonary resuscitation: Case reports. *Am J Foren Med Pathol* 2000;21:5–10.
175. Dolinak D. Rib fractures in infants due to cardiopulmonary resuscitation efforts. *Am J Foren Med Pathol* 2007;28:107–10.
176. Feldman KW, Brewer DK. Child abuse, cardiopulmonary resuscitation, and rib fractures. *Pediatrics* 1984;73:339–42.
177. Kemp AM, Butler A, Morris S, Mann M, Kemp KW, Rolfe K, Sibert JR, Maguire S. Which radiological investigations should be performed to identify fractures in suspected child abuse? *Clin Radiol* 2006;61:723–36.
178. Spevak MR, Kleinman PK, Belanger PL, Primack C, Richmond JM. Cardiopulmonary resuscitation and rib fractures in infants: A postmortem radiologic–pathologic study. *JAMA* 1994;272:617–8.
179. Maguire S, Mann M, John N, Ellaway B, Sibert JR, Kemp AM; Welsh Child Protection Systematic Review Group. Does cardiopulmonary resuscitation cause rib fractures in children? A systematic review. *Child Abuse Negl* 2006;30:739–51.

180. Durani Y, DePiero AD. Images in emergency medicine: Fracture of left clavicle and left posterior rib due to birth trauma. *Ann Emerg Med* 2006;47:210.
181. Hartmann RW Jr. Radiological case of the month: Rib fractures produced by birth trauma. *Arch Pediatr Adolesc Med* 1997;151:947–8.
182. Barry PW, Hocking MD. Infant rib fracture—Birth trauma or non-accidental injury. *Arch Dis Child* 1993;68:250.
183. Bulloch B, Schubert CJ, Brophy PD, Johnson N, Reed MH, Shapiro RA. Cause and clinical characteristics of rib fractures in infants. *Pediatrics* 2000;105(4):E48.
184. Rizzolo PJ, Coleman PR. Neonatal rib fracture: Birth trauma or child abuse? *J Fam Pract* 1989;29:561–3.
185. Paterson CR, Burns J, McAllion SJ. Osteogenesis imperfecta: The distinction from child abuse and the recognition of a variant form. *Am J Med Genet* 1993;45:187–92.
186. Paterson CR, McAllion SJ. Classical osteogenesis imperfecta and allegations of nonaccidental injury. *Clin Orthop Relat Res* 2006;452:260–4.
187. Paterson CR, McAllion S, Miller R. Heterogeneity of osteogenesis imperfecta type I. *J Med Genet* 1983;20:203–5.
188. Byers PH. Osteogenesis imperfecta. In Royce PM, Steinmann B, eds., *Connective Tissue and Its Heritable Disorders: Molecular, Genetic and Medical Aspects*. New York: Wiley-Liss, 1993, pp. 317–50.
189. Steiner RD, Pepin M, Byers PH. Studies of collagen synthesis and structure in the differentiation of child abuse from osteogenesis imperfecta. *J Pediatr* 1996;128:542–7.
190. Marlowe A, Pepin MG, Byers PH. Testing for osteogenesis imperfecta in cases of suspected non-accidental injury. *J Med Genet* 2002;39:382–6.
191. Miller ME, Hangartner TN. Temporary brittle bone disease: Association with decreased fetal movement and osteopenia. *Calcif Tissue Int* 1999;64:137–43.
192. Miller ME. Hypothesis: Fetal movement influences fetal and infant bone strength. *Med Hypotheses* 2005;65:880–6.
193. Miller ME, Hangartner TN. Bone density measurements by computed tomography in osteogenesis imperfecta type I. *Osteoporos Int* 1999;9:427–32.
194. Keller KA, Barnes PD. Rickets vs. abuse: A national and international epidemic. *Pediatr Radiol* 2008;38(11):1210–6.
195. Caffey J. Multiple fractures in the long bones of infants suffering from chronic subdural hematoma. *AJR Am J Roentgenol* 1946;56:163–73.
196. Bishop N, Sprigg A, Dalton A. Unexplained fractures in infancy: Looking for fragile bones. *Arch Dis Child* 2007;92:251–6.
197. Salter RB, Harris WR. Injuries involving the epiphyseal plate. *J Bone Joint Surg (Am)* 1963; 45:587–622.
198. Galloway A. The biomechanics of fracture production. In Galloway A, ed., *Broken Bones: Anthropological Analysis of Blunt Force Trauma*. Springfield, IL: C.C. Thomas, 1999, pp. 35–62.
199. Silverman FN. Radiologic and special diagnostic procedures. In Kempe CH, Helfer RE, eds., *The Battered Child*. Chicago: University of Chicago Press, 1980, pp. 215–40.
200. Kleinman PK, Marks SC, Blackbourne B. The metaphyseal lesion in abused infants: A radiologic–histopathologic study. *AJR Am J Roentgenol* 1986;146:895–905.
201. Kleinman PK, Marks SC, Adams VI, Blackbourne BD. Factors affecting visualization of posterior rib fractures in abused infants. *AJR Am J Roentgenol* 1988;150:635–8.
202. Kleinman PK, Marks SCJ. A regional approach to classic metaphyseal lesions in abused infants: The distal tibia. *AJR Am J Roentgenol* 1996;166:1207–12.
203. Chapman S. The radiological dating of injuries. *Arch Dis Child* 1992;67:1063–5.
204. Ethier CR, Simmons CA. *Introductory Biomechanics from Cells to Organisms*. New York: Cambridge University Press, 2007.
205. Dougherty DD, Rauch SL, Rosenbaum JF, eds. *Essentials of Neuroimaging for Clinical Practice*. Washington, DC: American Psychiatric Publishing, 2004.

206. Kellogg ND, Lukefahr JL. Criminally prosecuted cases of child starvation. *Pediatrics* 2005;116: 1309–16.
207. Fieguth A, Gunther D, Kleemann WJ, Troger HD. Lethal child neglect. *Foren Sci Int* 2002; 130:8–12.
208. Whitehead FJ, Couper RT, Moore L, Bourne AJ, Byard RW. Dehydration deaths in infants and young children. *Am J Foren Med Pathol* 1996;17:73–8.
209. McLaren C, Null J, Quinn J. Heat stress from enclosed vehicles: Moderate ambient temperatures cause significant temperature rise in enclosed vehicles. *Pediatrics* 2005;116:e109–12.
210. Centers for Disease Control. Heat-related deaths—United States, 1999–2003. *Morb Mortal Wkly Rep* 2006;55:796–8.
211. Knight LD, Collins KA. A 25-year retrospective review of deaths due to pediatric neglect. *Am J Foren Med Pathol* 2005;26:221–8.
212. Baugh JR, Krug EF, Weir MR. Punishment by salt poisoning. *South Med J* 1983;76:540–1.
213. Meadow R. Non-accidental salt poisoning. *Arch Dis Child* 1993;68:448–52.
214. Lin CY, Tsau YK. Child abuse: Acute water intoxication in a hyperactive child. *Acta Paediatr Taiwan* 2005;46:39–41.
215. Case ME, Short CD, Poklis A. Intoxication by aspirin and alcohol in a child: A case of child abuse by medical neglect. *Am J Foren Med Pathol* 1983;4:149–51.
216. Wagner C, Bowers W. Cardiomyopathy in a child induced by intentional ipecac poisoning. *Air Med J* 2006;25:236–7.
217. Fenton AC, Wailoo MP, Tanner MS. Severe failure to thrive and diarrhoea caused by laxative abuse. *Arch Dis Child* 1988;63:978–9.
218. Maslanka AM, Scott SK. LSD overdose in an eight-month-old boy. *J Emerg Med* 1992;10:481–3.
219. Neugebauer R, Hoek HW, Susser E. Prenatal exposure to wartime famine and development of antisocial personality disorder in early adulthood. *JAMA* 1999;282:455–62.
220. Moynihan N. The effects of famine on brain growth in children. *Trans Med Soc Lond* 1982; 99–100:108–10.
221. Smart JL. Vulnerability of developing brain to undernutrition. *Ups J Med Sci Suppl* 1990;48:21–41.
222. Morgane PJ, Austin-LaFrance R, Bronzino J, Tonkiss J, Diaz-Cintra S, Cintra L, Kemper T, Galler JR. Prenatal malnutrition and development of the brain. *Neurosci Biobehav Rev* 1993;17:91–128.
223. Hulshoff Pol HE, Hoek HW, Susser E, Brown AS, Dingemans A, Schnack HG, van Haren NE, Pereira Ramos LM, Gispen-de Wied CC, Kahn RS. Prenatal exposure to famine and brain morphology in schizophrenia. *Am J Psychiatry* 2000;157:1170–2.
224. Spitz R. *The First Year of Life: A Psychoanalytic Study of Normal and Deviant Development of Object Relations*. New York: International University Press, 1965.
225. Olsen EM, Skovgaard AM, Weile B, Jorgensen T. Risk factors for failure to thrive in infancy depend on the anthropometric definitions used: The Copenhagen County Child Cohort. *Paediatr Perinat Epidemiol* 2007;21:418–31.
226. Maizler JS, Solomon JR, Almquist E. Psychogenic mortality syndrome: Choosing to die by the institutionalized elderly. *Death Educ* 1983;6:353–64.
227. Haynes CF, Cutler C, Gray J, Kempe RS. Hospitalized cases of nonorganic failure to thrive: The scope of the problem and short-term lay health visitor intervention. *Child Abuse Negl* 1984;8:229–42.
228. Koel BS. Failure to thrive and fatal injury as a continuum. *Am J Dis Child* 1969;118:565–7.
229. Plunkett J. Shaken baby syndrome and the death of Matthew Eappen: A forensic pathologist's response. *Am J Foren Med Pathol* 1999;20:17–21.
230. Caffey J. On the theory and practice of shaking infants. Its potential residual effects of permanent brain damage and mental retardation. *Am J Dis Child* 1972;124:161–9.
231. Caffey J. The whiplash shaken infant syndrome: Manual shaking by the extremities with whiplash-induced intracranial and intraocular bleedings, linked with residual permanent brain damage and mental retardation. *Pediatrics* 1974;54:396–403.

232. Hollenhorst RW, Stein H. Ocular signs and prognosis in subdural and subarachniod bleeding in young children. *Arch Ophthalmol* 1958;60:187–92.
233. Kiffney GT. The eye of the "battered child." *Arch Ophthalmol* 1964;72:231–3.
234. Gilkes MJ, Mann TP. Fundi of battered babies. *Lancet* 1967;2:468–9.
235. Harcourt B, Hopkins D. Ophthalmic manifestations of the battered-baby syndrome. *Br Med J* 1971;3:398–401.
236. Mushin AS. Ocular damage in the battered-baby syndrome. *Br Med J* 1971;14:402–4.
237. Mushin AS, Morgan GM. Ocular injury in the battered baby syndrome: Report of 2 cases. *Br J Ophthalmol* 1971;55:343–7.
238. Friendly DS. Ocular manifestations of physical child abuse. *Trans Am Acad Ophthalmol Otolaryngol* 1971;75:318–32.
239. Jensen AD, Smith RE, Olson MI. Ocular clues to child abuse. *J Pediatr* 1971;8:270–2.
240. Guthkelch N. Infantile subdural haematoma and its relationship to whiplash injuries. *Br Med J* 1971;2:430–1.
241. Eisenbrey AB. Retinal hemorrhage in the battered child. *Childs Brain* 1979;5:40–4.
242. Ommaya AK, Faas F, Yarnell P. Whiplash injury and brain damage: An experimental study. *JAMA* 1968;204:285–9.
243. Tuerkheimer D. Science-dependent prosecution and the problem of epistemic contingency: A study of shaken baby syndrome. *Ala Law Rev* 2011;62:513–69.
244. Imwinkelried E. Shaken baby syndrome: A genuine battle of the scientific (and non-scientific) experts. *UC Davis Legal Stud Res Paper Ser* 2009;194:1–44.
245. Findley K. Examining shaken baby syndrome convictions in light of new medical scientific research. *Okla City Univ Law Rev* 2012;37:219–51.
246. Greenwald MJ, Weiss A, Oesterle CS, Friendly DS. Traumatic retinoschisis in battered babies. *Ophthalmology* 1986;93:618–25.
247. Massicotte SJ, Folberg R, Torczynski E, Gilliland MG, Luckenbach MW. Vitreoretinal traction and perimacular retinal folds in the eyes of deliberately traumatized children. *Ophthalmology* 1991;98:1124–7.
248. Buys YM, Levin AV, Enzenauer RW, Elder JE, Letourneau MA, Humphreys RP, Mian M, Morin JD. Retinal findings after head trauma in infants and young children. *Ophthalmology* 1992;99:1718–23.
249. Lantz PE, Sinal SH, Stanton CA, Weaver RG. Perimacular retinal folds from childhood head trauma. *BMJ* 2004;328:754–6.
250. Gennarelli TA, Thibault LE. Biomechanics of acute subdural hematoma. *J Trauma* 1982;22: 680–6.
251. Cory CZ, Jones MD, James DS, Leadbeatter S, Nokes LD. The potential and limitations of utilising head impact injury models to assess the likelihood of significant head injury in infants after a fall. *Foren Sci Int* 2001;123:89–106.
252. Gilliland MG, Folberg R. Shaken babies—Some have no impact injuries. *J Foren Sci* 1996;41: 114–6.
253. Rutty GN, Squier WM, Padfield CJ. Epidural haemorrhage of the cervical spinal cord: A postmortem artifact? *Neuropath Appl Neurobiol* 2005;31:247–57.
254. Duhaime AC, Christian C, Armonda R, Hunter J, Hertle R. Disappearing subdural hematomas in children. *Pediatr Neurosurg* 1996;25:116–22.
255. Oehmichen M, Auer RN, König HG. Permanent global ischemia. In Oehmichen M, Auer RN, König HG, eds., *Forensic Neuropathology and Neurology*. Berlin: Springer Verlag, 2006, pp. 319–29.
256. Wijdicks EFM, ed. *Brain Death*. Philadelphia: Lippincott Williams & Wilkins, 2001.
257. Leestma JE. "Shaken baby syndrome": Do confessions by alleged perpetrators validate the concept? *Am J Phys Surg* 2006;11:14–6.
258. Donohoe M. Evidence-based medicine and the shaken baby syndrome: Part I. Literature review, 1966–1998. *Am J Foren Med Pathol* 2003;29:239–42.

259. Greenhalgh T. *How to Read a Paper: The Basics of Evidence Based Medicine*. London: BMJ Publishing Group, 1997.
260. Schmitt KU, Niederer P, Walz F. *Trauma Biomechanics: Introduction to Accidental Injury*. Berlin: Springer-Verlag, 2004.
261. Pellman EJ, Viano DC, Tucker AM, Casson IR, Waeckerle JF. Concussion in professional football: Reconstruction of game impacts and injuries. *Neurosurgery* 2003;53:799–812.
262. Klinich KD, Hulbert GM, Schneider LW. Estimating infant head injury criteria and impact response using crash reconstruction and finite element modeling. *Stapp Car Crash J* 2002; 46:1–30.
263. Mertz HJ. Anthropomorphic test devices. In Nahum AM, Melvin JW, eds., *Accidental Injury: Biomechanics and Prevention*. New York: Springer-Verlag, 1993, pp. 66–80.
264. Chadwick DL, Chin S, Salerno C, Landsverk J, Kitchen L. Deaths from falls in children: How far is fatal? *J Trauma* 1991;31:1353–5.
265. Bruce DA, Alavi A, Bilaniuk L, Dolinskas C, Obrist W, Uzzell B. Diffuse cerebral swelling following head injuries in children: The syndrome of "malignant brain edema." *J Neurosurg* 1981;54:170–8.
266. Snoek JW, Minderhoud JM, Wilmink JT. Delayed deterioration following mild head injury in children. *Brain* 1984;107:15–36.
267. Humphreys RP, Hendrick EB, Hoffman HJ. The head-injured child who "talks and dies." A report of 4 cases. *Childs Nerv Syst* 1990;6:139–42.

Gunshot, Penetrating, and Blast-Related Injuries to the Nervous System

8

JAN E. LEESTMA
JOEL B. KIRKPATRICK

Contents

Introduction

Penetrating wounds involving the nervous system are very common in a forensic service and mostly involve projectiles fired by firearms, but other forms of penetrating injury to the nervous system include stab wounds; solid fragments from explosions; flying objects and glass in structural collapses, hurricanes, or tornadoes; industrial accidents; and occasionally novel situations, such as vehicular accidents or falls. Recent wars have brought the spectrum and tragedies of missile and fragment injuries to the evening news nearly every day. Explosions and blast injuries have become increasingly common as a part of warfare and urban terrorism, which will bring these cases to the forensic services and, with them, the challenges of interpretation.

Firearms

It is an unfortunate fact of modern life, certainly in the United States but also with increasing frequency elsewhere in the world, that injuries and deaths due to firearms are common and increasingly so, both in civilian life in presumably peaceful societies not at war and in zones of conflict, where firearms and explosive devices wreak a devastating toll on civilians as well as combatants. Much of what will be discussed below is "classical" in the sense that the basics of gunshot wounds have been known for a long time, and excellent chapters on gunshot and missile wounds can be found in most forensic pathology texts, to which the reader is referred [1–6]. There are also a number of focused texts dealing only with gunshot wounds [7,8] or with various aspects of firearms, including ballistics [9,10], that the reader might find useful.

This chapter provides a selective review of the voluminous literature on missile ballistics and wounding and shows how these principles may be applied in examining, recording, and understanding the wounds of the brain and spinal cord created by missiles of various kinds. The flux of human relations is such that new styles of violence appear with each generation, so it is timely to include as well a discussion of blast and explosive fragment wounds encountered during wartime or in terrorist attacks. The particular characteristics of gunshot and stab wounds of the spinal cord are described.

Basic Aspects of Firearms

One may classify firearms in many ways, but Di Maio [8] stratifies them into handguns (single-shot pistols, derringers, revolvers, and autoloading or automatic pistols) and so-called long guns (rifles, shotguns, submachine guns, and machine guns). The basic principle behind any gun is an explosive charge and a projectile that is propelled upon ignition of the charge into a barrel and beyond at a high velocity, with variable accuracy and distance. In times past, the explosive charge usually consisted of a measure of black powder (mixture of saltpeter, charcoal, and sulfur) placed into a blind-ended steel cylinder, packed with wadding to hold the charge in a compacted state, followed by a bullet usually invested with cloth wadding to provide a pressure seal between the bullet and the gun barrel. At the blind end of the cylinder, a small opening of some sort communicated with, in the case of a flintlock musket, a pan containing more powder, which could be struck by a spring-loaded hammer containing a piece of flint that would generate a spark when released to ignite the powder in the pan and then the powder in the cylinder, propelling the projectile outward. At first, the barrels of such guns were smooth, but later, spiral grooving (rifling) of the barrel provided greater accuracy than the smooth-bored rifles. Further advancements in rifle technology included having an openable breech into which a premade cartridge containing powder and bullet could be put. In these and later weapons, ignition was affected by placing a nipple on the breech over which could be placed a percussion cap that, when struck by the weapon's hammer, would ignite the powder charge. Now such weapons are collector's items and curiosities but still occasionally cause injuries, accidental or not.

Modern firearms virtually all now consist of rifled barrels, well-formed and engineered bullets of various compositions and designs, and metallic or plastic cartridges that contain a primer, smokeless powder, which, of course, produces smoke on combustion, but much less than with black powder of a former era. There are various breech or loading designs that hold the cartridges. Methods of firing may include an external hammer or an internal hammer that strikes the primer and causes the cartridge to fire. In the case of pistols, cartridges may be held in a cylinder, like in the case of a revolver (holding five or more shells). In these weapons, the fired cartridges remain in the cylinder and must be manually reloaded. In the case of automatic weapons, pistols, submachine guns, or machine guns, a vertical or other form of clip houses up to a dozen or more cartridges (in many handguns), and hundreds of cartridges (rounds) are loaded into the weapon chamber by various mechanisms in many of the automatic and semiautomatic weapons often referred to as "assault" weapons. In these guns, after the first cartridge is manually loaded into the chamber, after firing, the recoil or the gases of discharge of the weapon activate mechanisms that expel the spent cartridge, cock the firing mechanism, and load a fresh cartridge. This cycle can be unitary, as in typical automatic pistols or semiautomatic rifles, but can cycle in bursts or continuous firing, depending on the design of the weapon, as in some shotguns, submachine guns and machine guns.

There are reference books available that provide information on the dimensions of virtually all bullets of any caliber and the myriad cartridge cases designed to hold them for the various firearms. These books are employed by amateur shooters who reload their own ammunition but provide valuable specialized information and comparisons with so-called factory loads for the reloader [11]. The conventions used to describe ammunition and bullets are sometimes confusing and arbitrary, but generally the bullet diameter is the distance between the grooves in the barrel, with the lands (crests of the rifling grooves) being smaller than the diameter of the bullet, which imparts rifling grooves onto the projectile after exit. These grooves have forensic importance in determining what bullet was likely fired from what gun, if both are available for analysis [8].

There are scores of commercial smokeless powders and bullets, all of which have parameters that will predict the performance of the cartridge within general limits [11]. Such measures of performance rest on the cartridge designation, which usually includes the caliber of the bullet (in America that is usually expressed in hundredths of an inch, e.g., .22, .25, .32, .38, but in other countries it is expressed in metric units, e.g., 7.65 mm), but also on the type and quantity of powder used. There are many formulations and shapes of smokeless powder grains, which can have forensic significance. There are tables in reloading and other reference books that will give estimated muzzle velocity and ballistics information for various combinations of bullets and powder. The final performance of any cartridge is governed by the parameters of the cartridge; individual characteristics of the weapon, such as rifling pattern, chamber and its characteristics, and barrel length and barrel characteristics; and of course, the competence of the shooter and the ambient circumstances.

Once the cartridge is fired, the powder explodes under high pressure, generating gases and combustion products that force the bullet or projectile(s) down the barrel for a variable distance. The composition of this gas plume consists of primer components (often heavy metal residues), burned and unburned powder, carbon and hydrocarbons, in addition to carbon monoxide, carbon dioxide, water vapor, and nitrogen and sulfur compounds, to name a few. The behavior of this gas cloud and its composition with distances from the barrel constitute important forensic information that can estimate the distance of a weapon from its victim and other valuable information, discussed below. Often, test firings of suspect weapons are required to produce soiling patterns that may then be applied to the individual case. The plume of gas, smoke, and combustion products exiting a pistol have been amply illustrated by Di Maio [8] and Spitz et al. [5], who illustrate in many photographs a shower of sparks and debris that virtually envelop the hand of the shooter and weapon. From these high-speed photographs, one can easily appreciate that a great deal of material exits from the muzzle of a gun under high pressure, at thousands of pounds per square inch.

The projectile or bullet spins at a rate determined by the rifling grooves in the gun barrel and the transit time in the barrel (velocity of the bullet). Various firearms have different numbers of spiral rifling grooves in the barrels, from four to six or more per inch, and most often with a right-hand twist [8]. The spinning of the bullet imparts a gyroscopic action to the projectile that lends stability to it, to a point. If the velocity and spin of the bullet are too great and there are inequities in the projectile, it may not run "true" but, rather, precess, yaw, or tumble in flight. Thus, when such a bullet strikes a surface, it may produce not a round hole but a keyhole pattern or some other shape. The characteristics of a bullet in flight are generally those of a rather flat parabola, rising slightly upon exit from the barrel muzzle and gradually succumbing to the force of gravity drawing it downward, away from the aiming point. As strange as it may seem, if one were to poise a bullet at the muzzle of a gun and drop it at the exact moment the fired bullet exited the muzzle, both bullets would strike the ground at the same time if the weapon were fired horizontally and the ground surface was flat, because the vector force of gravity is independent of the horizontal vector forces in the gun. If there are interfering forces, such as wind or rain, the path of the fired bullet may vary. These variations are taken into account by experienced shooters, civilian or military.

An important aspect of ballistics is the kinetic energy of the projectile, which is determined by the relation: $KE = 1/2\ MV^2$, where, depending on the system of units employed, mass is in newtons, pound-feet, or slugs; velocity is in meters/second or feet/second; and KE can be expressed in pound-feet or newton-meters (joules). Kinetic energy is associated with motion; thus, every moving object has kinetic energy. This energy and work are conceptually identical. In a given system, energy must be conserved, and whatever happens, as in a bullet passing into tissue and eventually coming to rest, all of the energy must be accounted for or dissipated. This is done by imparting motion to tissues and fluids, fracturing bones, vaporizing fluids, generating heat, penetrating clothing, etc., as the bullet loses velocity and ultimately comes to rest. This is not to say that one can arithmetically account for or even calculate where all the energy goes in most situations but that the kinetic energy of a moving bullet will be accounted for once a resting state is achieved. The reader is referred to Chapter 6, in which the physics that surround this concept of kinetics and the units employed are discussed.

The importance of these relations is that potential work (which might be thought of as damage that can be done) is a function of mass of the bullet, but much more so of the velocity of the bullet; thus, a slow-moving .45 caliber pistol bullet moving at 800 ft/s will produce far less tissue damage than a .22 caliber bullet moving at 2700 ft/s. The latter's physics is exploited in the design and use of military rifles such as the M-16 or Kalashnikov AK-47, which employ small-caliber bullets but high muzzle velocity and produce impressive amounts of tissue and skeletal damage [12].

Bullets come in many designs. Each has certain exploitable characteristics that can be tailored for its application. Many small-caliber weapons, such as the ubiquitous .22 caliber cartridge, usually contain soft lead alloy projectiles of varying elemental composition. Such projectiles will tend to mushroom and fragment easily when striking tissue, and they may or may not exit the body. Larger-caliber bullets tend to have a copper or other metallic jacket investing the typical lead alloy core, partially or completely. There are other bullets that may appear externally to be typical for the lead-filled projectile but may actually contain no lead, rather they contain copper or copper composite particles [13]. These bullets (see Figures 8.1 and 8.2) are designed to fragment upon entry into tissues and produce devastating local damage, yet do not exit the body. They are primarily designed for "varmint" shooting. The more typical lead-filled bullets or hollow-point or partitioned projectiles will tend to penetrate intact more deeply into tissues than a simple lead alloy bullet. Bullets may have other design features, such as partitions in the bullet and openings or other features of the tip that may cause the bullet to penetrate deeply in tissue or to mushroom while staying intact and causing extensive tissue damage along its path. Such bullets are typical for those employed in game hunting. Such designs are prohibited in warfare by international conventions. There are still other bullet designs that employ a hardened steel or other alloy core that will enable the bullet to penetrate armor [14]. Although sale

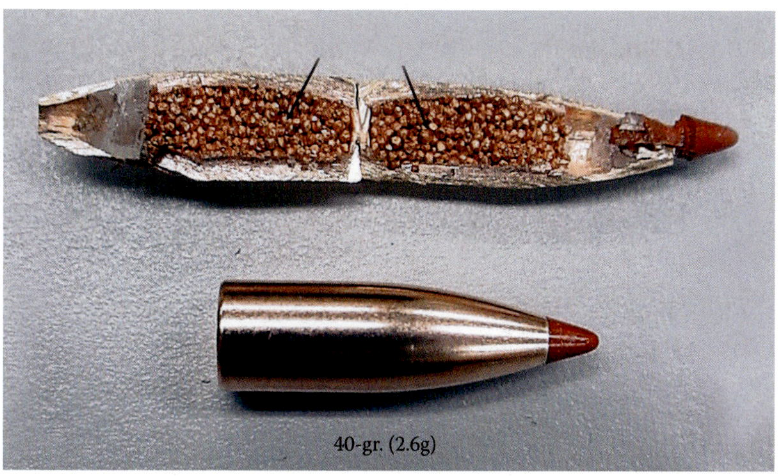

Figure 8.1 Pictured here is a 40-grain Nosler BT-NT® fragmenting rifle bullet that appears like the typical lead-filled projectile, but upon splitting, the composition of the bullet is revealed to be composed of a hollow copper jacket filled with copper granules (arrows) [13]. (Courtesy of L.C. Haag, Forensic Sciences Services, Carefree, Arizona, and with permission of the *Am J Foren Med Pathol* 2013:34;50–5 and Williams & Wilkins.)

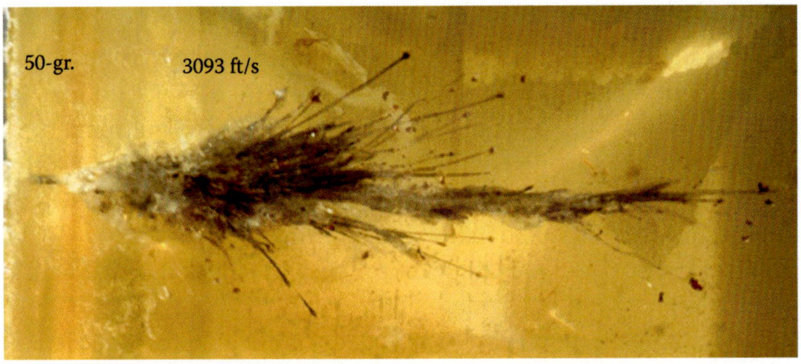

Figure 8.2 Pattern of fragmentation of bullet of a design similar to the Nosler bullet in Figure 8.1 but produced by another manufacturer is seen in a block of Perma-Gel®, a new material comparable to ballistics gelatin. Here the projectile disintegrated into a shower of metallic particles within about 10 in after entering the Perma-Gel block at 3093 ft/s [13]. (Courtesy of L.C. Haag, Forensic Sciences Services, Carefree, Arizona, and with permission of the *Am J Foren Med and Pathol* 2013:34;50–5 and Williams & Wilkins.)

of many such cartridges is regulated and supposedly limited to law enforcement or the military, they find their way illicitly into civilian and often criminal hands and thus may be encountered on a forensic service.

As mentioned above, bullets may or may not follow a true parabolic path from gun to target but may be deflected in transit by building surfaces or may experience deflections at the target. Such deflections or interferences may be caused by clothing, ornaments or jewelry, buttons, zippers, or other items of personal adornment [7,8]. These may cause the bullet to deflect, tumble, or fragment, producing multiple tracks and variable injuries. By the same token, the bullet may strike a bone and be deflected or fragmented. Sometimes bullets may display internal ricochets within the body or cranial cavity, as discussed below. The analysis of such incidents may make forensic interpretation difficult. By the same token, a bullet may strike an object or surface before striking the victim, producing a ricochet, which may further complicate bullet path analysis. A variant of this is an unfortunate accident in which someone fires a gun in the air, perhaps in a celebration or demonstration. The bullet will rise until its velocity is zero and then will turn around and head earthward, ideally terminating in the same velocity it had when it was fired, but this will likely not be the case because of air resistance, tumbling, and other factors. Nevertheless, if someone is in the path of the descending bullet, serious injury or death may result and the shooter will likely never realize that someone has been injured or killed.

When a high-velocity bullet strikes human tissue, the missile causes three dramatic changes in the target or tissue it strikes. First is the shock wave, which moves through the tissue at approximately the speed of sound (in water at body temperature, 4888 ft/s), actually moving ahead of the missile. Although the overpressure of the shock wave may be as much as 60 atm, its duration is extremely brief. There is scant evidence in the ballistics literature that the shock wave by itself is particularly harmful [15]. This position may require reassessment in the light of new experimental observations on trauma from shock waves in blasts and under various circumstances and in various materials [16–20]. The second change is the actual path that the bullet hollows out as it passes through the tissue. There is extensive disruption of tissue as well as total destruction of nerve cells and blood vessels in this permanent track [21–23]. The size of the permanent track is dictated by the effective diameter of the missile, which is its actual diameter increased by any instability or deformation. The last change, and often most important, is the temporary cavity. This follows the missile like the wake of a boat. The temporary cavity expands several times wider than the actual missile, and may contract and expand several times. After several milliseconds, it disappears, leaving the permanent track to mark the passage of the missile. The damage from the temporary cavity consists of stretching of blood vessels and nerve fibers. War experience has established that much of the tissue surrounding the temporary cavity is permanently devitalized and that the extent of damage is deceptive when examining the wound in a more-or-less fresh state.

The size of the temporary cavity is a function of the velocity of the missile and the density of the substance penetrated. High-velocity missiles, such as those from military rifles, create a huge temporary cavity, 10 to 14 times the diameter of the missile [24]. Slower missiles also create a temporary cavity, but a much smaller one. Conventional handguns, for example, make a temporary cavity perhaps five times the diameter of the missile (Figures 8.1 and 8.2). The designation of a missile as high or low velocity is somewhat arbitrary, and each author seems to differ, but the dividing line is conveniently placed at the speed of sound in air, 1100 ft/s. As a useful first approximation, most handguns are considered to be low-velocity weapons.

Wound Profile

Fackler and Malinowski [24] have developed the concept of the wound profile to characterize the wounding potential of a missile. This group has used standardized, large slabs of ordnance gelatin to measure the track and trap the missile (Figures 8.3 and 8.4). This demonstrates the permanent track plainly and, in addition, gives an accurate picture of the temporary cavity from the perpendicular fracture lines that radiate out from the permanent track. This allows visualization of the temporary cavity without the technically arduous task of high-speed cinematography and is preferable to using soap or clay to trap the missile because those media demonstrate only the temporary cavity and not the permanent cavity. Two types of injury occur: crushing injury results from penetration (the full extent of the missile track in the tissue), missile fragmentation (which will produce multiple tracks), and the size of the permanent cavity; stretch injury is caused by the temporary cavity. The potentially injurious effects of stretching depend strongly on the tissue. Owing to the well-recognized damaging effects of stretching and tearing of nerve fibers on electrical conduction, myelin, and nerve cell survival, central nervous system tissue can be assumed to be very sensitive to stretch damage.

As mentioned above, other materials besides the missile are ejected at the muzzle, in particular, gases from the exploding powder, as illustrated by Fatteh [25], Moritz [26] and others [5,8]. These can enter contact wounds, substantially increasing the damage potential of the missile and altering the characteristics of the wound. Other muzzle products are unburned powder, carbon soot, and debris such as wadding. These also can enter the wound and impart special markings to the skin at close range, which can be used as evidence.

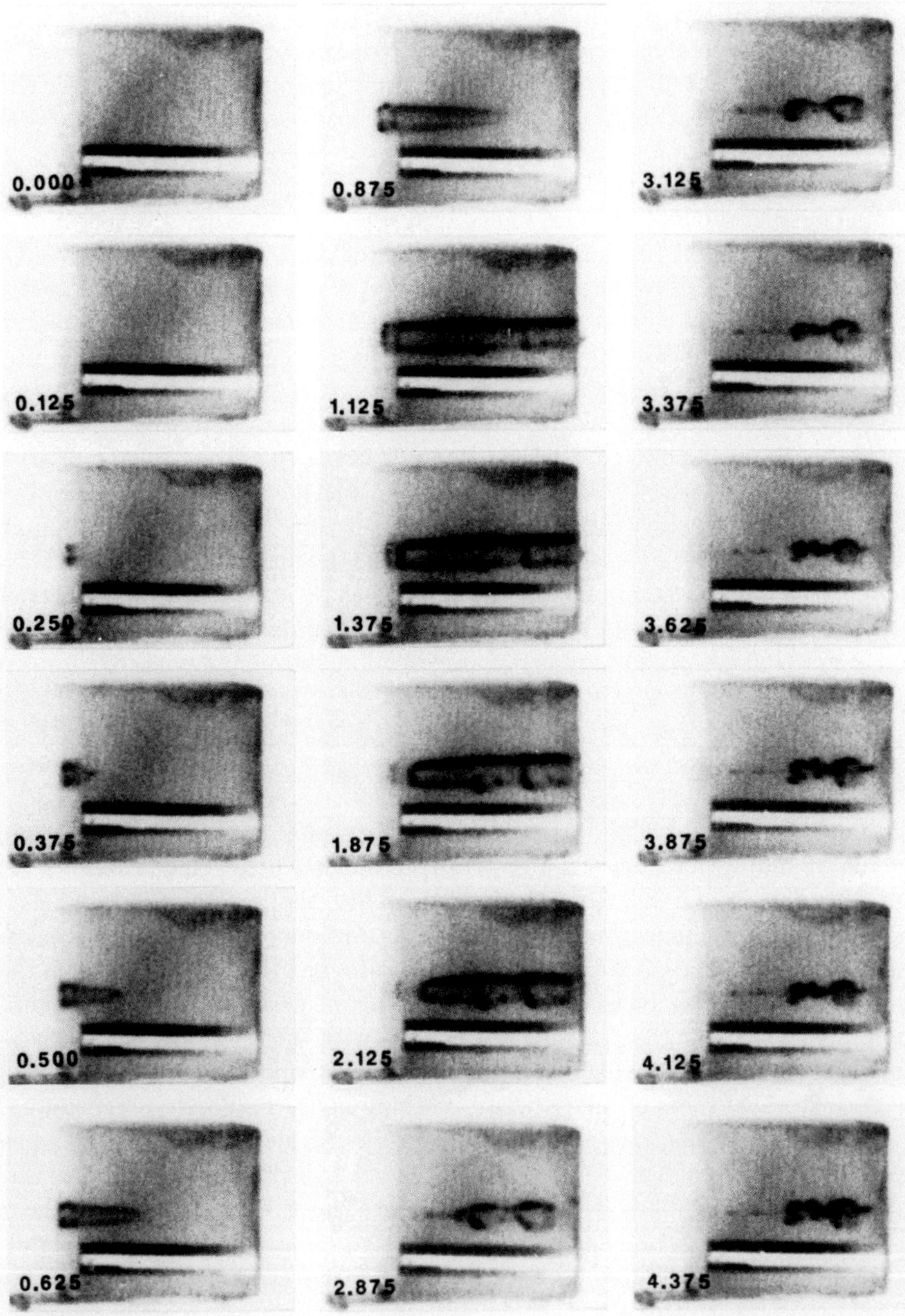

Figure 8.3 Series of photographs of a gelatin block study of temporary cavities caused by a .38 caliber hollow-point bullet. The velocity of the missile at the block surface was 922 ft/s. Gelatin concentration was 13%, similar to soft tissue and cerebral gray matter. The figures in the lower left corners show time in microseconds after the shot, indicated by the arrows, as the bullet approaches the block in the first frame. (Courtesy of the late Mr. Roy Mills, Department of Pathology, University of Texas Southwestern, Dallas, Texas.)

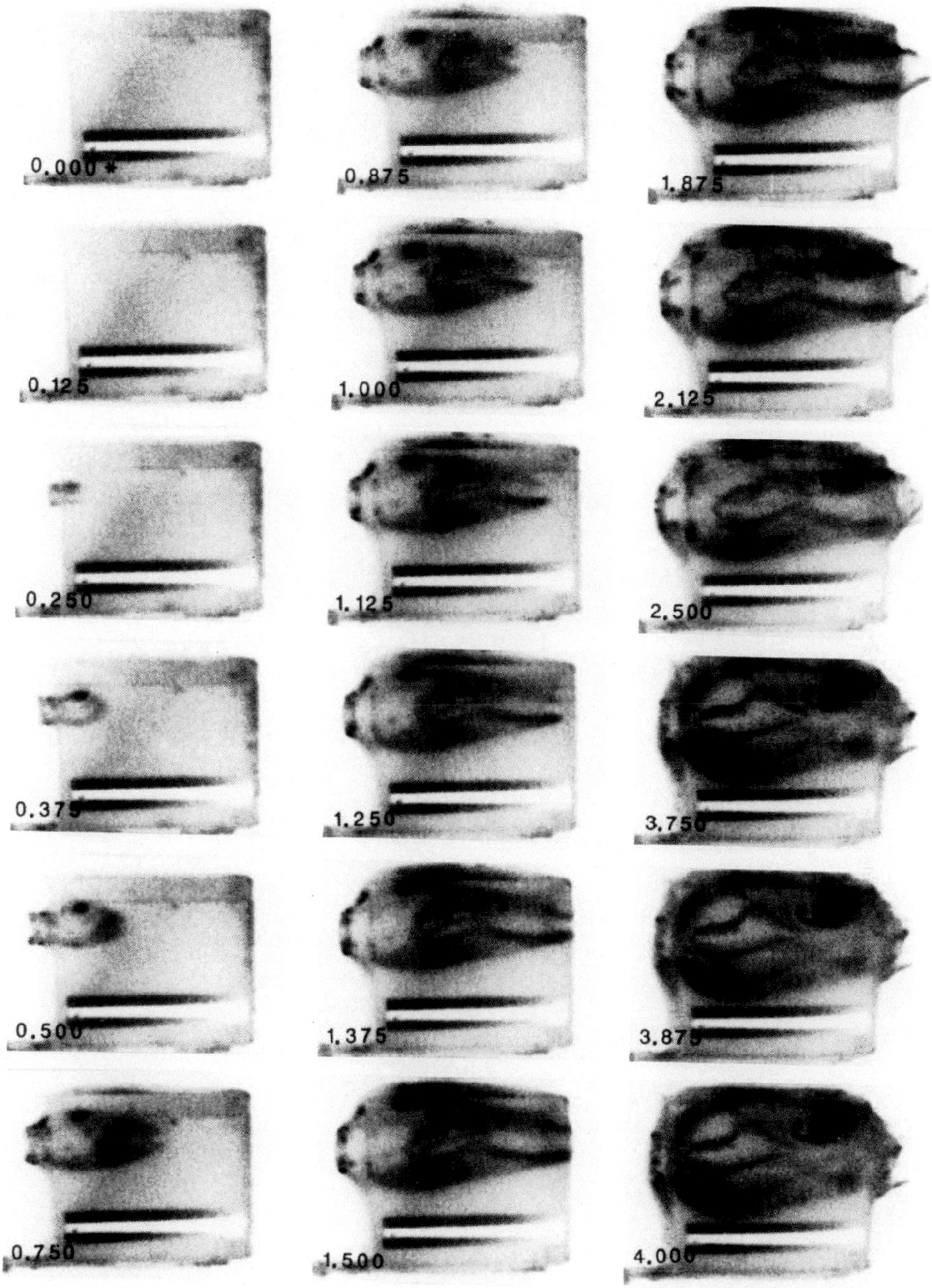

Figure 8.4 This series, like that in Figure 8.3, is of gelatin block shot with a .38 caliber steel-jacketed bullet. The gelatin concentration in this series was 26%, similar to cerebral white matter. The muzzle velocity of the bullet was 1053 ft/s. Note that the temporary cavity expands and then contracts with passage of time. (Courtesy of the late Mr. Roy Mills, Department of Pathology, University of Texas Southwestern, Dallas, Texas.)

Variations in Wounding from Different Weapons

Handguns

The muzzle velocity of most handguns with ammunition available to the civilian population is less than 1000 ft/s, so the great majority of wounds encountered in peacetime are those created by low-velocity missiles [8]. The total damage imparted by a missile is determined by the loss of kinetic energy while the missile passes through the tissue, as noted above. Hence, missiles that perforate and exit a structure may actually do less harm than missiles that expend the last of their kinetic energy and remain in the tissue. This latter circumstance applies in the majority of low-velocity missiles in civilian practice. The forensic pathologist or surgeon can expect to identify part or all of the missile that has come to rest somewhere within the body, as in most cases of head wounds. Although the missile, after passing through the brain, may not have enough energy to penetrate the skull again and exit, it often has enough to bounce off the opposite wall of the cranial bone, running around beneath it or ricocheting within the cranial vault. Freytag [27] observed a 40% frequency of ricochet, and other series have produced similar results [5,8], as illustrated in Figure 8.5.

The second most damaging characteristic of a missile, after velocity, is instability of the projectile. Yaw is the most significant form of instability within the wound track [8,27]. The tumbling motion of the bullet creates asymmetrically varicose patterns in the wound track [23] and prevents accurate prediction of the size and configuration of the permanent track from the size and direction of the missile alone. Bullets with a center of gravity near the front of the missile, such as the .45 caliber bullet of the familiar U.S. military sidearm, tend

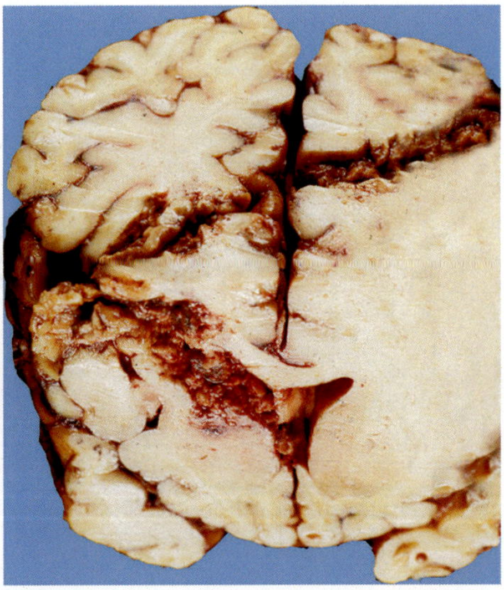

Figure 8.5 Specimen is cut along the axes of the bullet path from a suicidal gunshot wound from a .38 caliber pistol with a 5-in. barrel to the head of a 24-year-old African American woman with a history of epilepsy and depression. The photograph shows the initial bullet path from the left parietal region diagonally across the brain to the opposite side, where it struck the skull and fragmented, sending a shower of lead particles forward and diagonally downward into the right lateral ventricle. A complex basilar skull fracture was also found. The woman was found dead in a chair with the gun on the floor. No suicide note was found. (Courtesy of Dr. H. Wayne Carver II, Office of the Medical Examiner, Cook County, IL.)

not to yaw [8,24]. In contrast, a long, slender bullet, such as that of a military rifle, will inevitably yaw, because its center of gravity is relatively far from the rear of the bullet. This may also account for mushrooming of the base of the bullet, if it is actually traveling backward when it strikes a hard obstruction [8]. Deformation of the missile is another contributing cause of instability. Military ammunition, by international convention, is fully jacketed in metal, preventing very much deformation in tissue, although yaw frequently occurs. Most of the commonly available civilian ammunition is fully jacketed with a copper alloy or only partially jacketed, which allows the soft lead core to mushroom upon striking a hard surface like bone. The appearance of the missile may be much altered by these effects. DeMuth [28] has observed that soft (unjacketed) bullets propelled at greater than 3000 ft/s may break up just after entering tissue, effectively eliminating the permanent wound track and delivering the entirety of the kinetic energy possessed by the missile. This occurs in the civilian setting when some hunting ammunition is used that may not be jacketed, and fragmentation of the bullet within the wound produces a "lead shower." The search for missiles, especially if fragmented, is a tedious but necessary task; here the use of x-ray is a great time saver and may mean the difference between success and failure. In recent years, the development imaging sciences have given rise to the virtual autopsy (virtopsy), in which computerized tomography (CT) and magnetic resonance imaging (MRI) scanning have been used in forensic centers with great success, such that a number of forensic services now employ these advanced methods to analyze gunshot cases and many others [29,30]. The usual forensic service, however, generally lacks such advanced methods, and thus the tried-and-true old-fashioned bullet fragment search still has validity.

Military and Hunting Rifles

The high-velocity missiles usually perforate and may not be found in the body. In these cases, identification of the entry and exit wounds becomes an important indicator of the direction of the shot in relation to the victim. The small entry wound and the larger, sometimes vast, exit wound are well recognized in the literature and relatively easy to identify with certainty, bearing in mind the tendency for inward beveling of the skull at entrance and outward beveling at exit (see below).

There are exceptions to the larger exit wound, such as the close range (2 ft or less) wound from a military rifle (M-16) described by Dimond and Rich [31]. Another exception is the blowback effect of muzzle gases that may be injected into the wound. This has been recognized as a cause of enlargement of the entrance wound in a case of suicide by a closely held magnum pistol [16,32]. Other bizarre and confusing firearm wounds may occur in head wounds in which the entering projectile may actually exit after an internal ricochet from the entrance wound [33].

One effect of expansion of the temporary cavity is a shock-like herniation of the cerebellar tonsils at the foramen magnum. Freytag [26] found herniation contusions in more than 20% of fatal head wounds from low-velocity handguns, and this effect is magnified in high-velocity wounds. The expansion effect can also contuse the inferior surfaces of the frontal lobes. Contraction and reexpansion of the temporary cavity may avulse portions of tissue out of the exit wound and may suck debris into the permanent track. When the temporary cavity occurs within a confined space such as the cranial vault, the expansion may be sufficient to fracture the skull in multiple places, especially the thin orbital plates [5,8], or literally to blow it apart [34]. Butler and coworkers [35] showed that this explosive characteristic of high-velocity missiles was due to the temporary cavity, by experimenting with animal heads with the brain *in situ* and empty skulls. In the whole head, the high-velocity missile caused explosion of the skull. In the empty skull, only the entry and exit holes were made. Experimentally, ring hemorrhages and swelling of astrocyte foot processes have been seen even in sites remote from the high-velocity missile track [21,22,36]. The hypothalamus, brain stem, and cerebellum are most vulnerable to these distant forms of injury.

Tangential wounds may cause significant injuries, especially from high-velocity missiles. These may produce gash-like wounds and form gutter-like depressed fractures in the skull. In such cases, the underlying brain will have extensive superficial contusions adjoining the fracture, even if the dura remains intact, which are caused by the slapping effect of the inbending bone [37]. Contusions of the underlying brain from glancing shots by low-velocity missiles are less likely or smaller.

Shell and Munitions Fragments

In wartime, shell fragments account for more head injuries than do rifles [38]. This is especially true in recent Middle Eastern conflicts, where improvised explosive devices (IEDs) have taken a huge toll. Many of the IEDs have been fabricated to contain nails, ball bearings, and other bits of metal that will be propelled at high velocity away from the bomb. Such fragments may have extremely high initial velocity, sometimes several thousand feet per second, but they may be quickly slowed by air friction due to the irregular shape and unstable motions. In many roadside bomb explosions, fragments of the device penetrate vehicles where secondary fragments may be generated. In the Vietnam War, fatal head injuries from shell fragments occurred at an average range of 3 m from the victim, whereas fatal head wounds from rifle bullets were at an average range of 41 m from the victim. Shell fragment wounds at greater ranges than 3 m tended to permit survival. The steel helmet was effective protection against shell fragments but not against military rifle bullets or, in recent years, from the high-velocity fragments of IEDs [38]. The relevance in this context is to terrorist bomb attacks of civilian facilities, in which these injuries may also be expected [39,40].

Two historical remarks are germane. Cushing [41], during World War I, observed that almost anything on the battlefield—fragments of equipment, jewelry, or clothing—could become airborne secondary missiles when struck by bullets or bombs that impart movement to them (transfer of kinetic energy). Also, these diverse materials could be present in the wound. Conversationally, the term *shrapnel* is sometimes used to refer to shell fragments. Henry Shrapnel in 1784 invented an explosive artillery shell that contained musket balls. In use until World War I, the shrapnel shell was replaced by one that contained higher-velocity steel darts, or flechettes. Thus, shell fragments causing current war injuries are not shrapnel except in a historical sense. Additional aspects of explosions and blast effects are discussed below.

Shotgun Wounds

Shotguns are a special form of rifle or long gun, in which the cartridge is composed of a metallic base and a paper, plastic, or composite cartridge case, as described above. The cartridge then contains shot of various sizes and compositions sometimes along with polyethylene, polypropylene, or other granular plastic material to fill in the air spaces between the shot [42]. The typical shotgun is smooth bored and may be manually operated or automatically loaded for single shots, but multishot and rapid fire as well as automatic shotguns (so-called street sweepers), once available only to law enforcement, have now found their way into the gang and other criminal cultures and thus affect the civilian population.

There are a number of unique aspects to shotgun wounds in comparison to single-projectile rifle or pistol wounds. The typical shotgun shell contains, as mentioned above, various kinds of wadding (paper or plastic) and filler materials that are expelled from the gun along with the shot or other projectiles contained in the shell. In many, if not most, modern shotgun shells, instead of a disk-like paper wad that separates the powder charge from the pellets, a plastic cup-like wad that may partially surround the pellets has been substituted. This cup-wad keeps the pellets in a more tightly packed pattern, which is desired for most hunting applications. Upon exit from the barrel of the shotgun, the cup-wad's "petals" fold outward, releasing the pellets, and then tend to fall away after a few feet [8], but the pellets continue forward. The forensic significance of this is that the cup-wad, if the shot is within 20 ft or more of the victim, will leave an imprint on the skin like the petals of a flower. The pattern may be identifiable with the manufacturer of the ammunition and thus has forensic significance not only for the distance to the victim but also in potentially identifying the shooter, who may be in possession of unfired ammunition when apprehended, to which scene evidence may be compared [8].

As the expelled pellets fly away from the shotgun, they tend to spread with increasing distance. This spreading is influenced by the gauge of the shotgun (.410, 20, 16, 12, etc.), which is a measure of the bore diameter of the gun. The lower the gauge and larger the diameter of the bore, the farther the pellets will be propelled. Other factors influencing range and spread of the pellets are the charge in the shell, the size (and therefore the number) of pellets, whether the shell has a cup-wad, and if the gun barrel at its terminus has a choke. The choke narrows the bore somewhat to tend to keep the pellets together. Some special forms of chokes may shape the pellet pattern from a circular one to a rectangular or other pattern for special uses [8]. A variation on the theme is a shotgun that by manufacture or improvisation has a much shorter barrel than normal ("sawed off" shotgun). Such weapons will scatter their pellets in a broad pattern, generally if the barrel length is less than 12 in. [8], but lack range. There are handguns (Derringers, or pocket pistols) that can accept a .410 shotgun shell, and there are bird-shot cartridges for other handguns that can produce wounds like those of a shotgun.

Pellet size varies from bird shot, which are rather small pellets in the range of 3–4 mm, to buckshot (20+ pellets), in which the pellets may be 8 mm in diameter (four or five pellets). There are specialized forms of shotgun loads in which there are no pellets but, rather, a single projectile, which may take the form of a thimble-shaped lead slug with rifling grooves impressed on its surface to allow it to spin on exit even though there is no rifling in the gun (rifled slugs). Other single-projectile shotgun ammunition may contain various designs of a sabot, a heavier projectile. These types of ammunition are often employed by hunters, by choice or by law, for big-game hunting, especially in populated areas.

As with other firearms, wound characteristics for shotguns vary with the distance they are at discharge from the victim. At relatively close range, the mass of pellets may not have spread and do not produce anything but a round wound hole. If the gun is close enough, stippling and sooting of the skin may be seen or, if in contact with the skin, a stellate torn wound edge pattern may be seen. The damage inflicted by shotgun wounds can be horrific and, in the case of head wounds inflicted accidentally or by suicide, the gunshot may destroy the skull, face, head, and brain and scatter blood and tissue widely about the death scene. Typical examples of these kinds of wounds are illustrated in every forensic pathology text [1–5]. In less devastating wounds, there may be multiple entrance wounds from the multiple pellets, making the use of x-ray technologies almost mandatory to enable the pathologist to recover the projectiles at autopsy, or, for that matter, the neuropathologist at a brain cutting.

Not all shotgun injuries occur from being struck by the missiles in the gun. Excessively charged home-loaded shotgun shells can cause a characteristic injury in which the breech of the shotgun is destroyed and the shell casing, following Newton's third law, is ejected backward from the barrel. The casing may be driven into the orbit and frontal or temporal lobes. Similar injuries have been caused by improvised firearms like "zip" guns.

Unusual or Nonweapon Firearms

Slaughter Guns and Stud Guns

Slaughter pistols and stud guns are sometimes chosen for suicide, particularly in Europe, or may occasionally cause serious or fatal wounds in accidental circumstances. The device for stunning large animals at slaughter ejects a plunger by an explosive charge or pneumatic release. Because the plunger is captive but does penetrate the brain, the injuries are those of a very low-velocity missile. Nevertheless, such an injury is often fatal [43–45]. Stud guns or bolt guns are used for construction applications. For safety precautions, the device must have the muzzle firmly depressed against the target or it will not fire. The charge, often a blank .22 of .38 caliber cartridge especially designed for this application, propels a nail or other construction material into the work surface, be it wood, metal, or sometimes concrete. Sometimes the nail projectile will penetrate the board or wall and injure another worker or bystander some distance away, or the tool may be used with suicidal intent [45,46]. An example of a nail stud gun suicidal injury is illustrated in Figures 8.6 and 8.7.

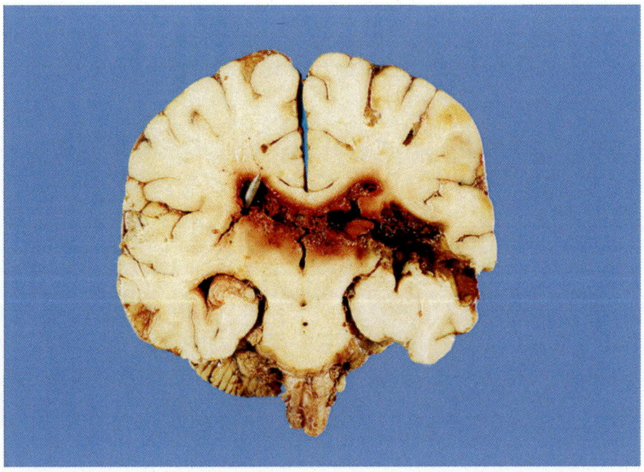

Figure 8.6 Section of the brain of a 25-year-old construction worker who committed suicide with a nail stud gun pressed against the left temple. The nail projectile traversed the brain, lodging in the right lateral ventricle. The nail apparently tumbled upon entrance into the brain. Such suicides are uncommon but well known in the forensic community. (Courtesy of Dr. Mitra Kalelkar, Office of the Medical Examiner, Cook County, IL.)

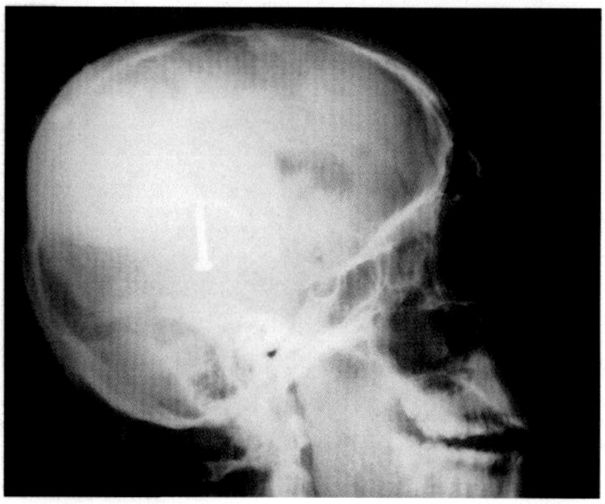

Figure 8.7 Plain lateral postmortem radiograph of the case in Figure 8.6. It illustrates the position of the nail projectile. (Courtesy of Dr. Mitra Kalelkar, Office of the Medical Examiner, Cook County, IL.)

Riot Control Weapons

Rubber and plastic bullets have been used by military and police personnel during riots and in other circumstances where nonlethal forces are required since they were introduced in 1973 [47]. There are a number of designs for the firearms used to propel rubber or plastic projectiles at relatively low velocity that expand in flight or on impact to increase the contact surface area and prevent penetration of the body. In spite of good intentions, numerous fatalities with the supposedly nonlethal projectiles have resulted in well-known areas of past conflict, such as South Africa, Israel and Palestine, and Northern Ireland. Injuries and their severity are a function of the distance between the shooter and the victim, ballistic features of the gun and its projectile, and the site of impact on the body [48]. Penetration of the thorax or abdomen has occurred and can cause death [49], but most fatalities arise from cranial injuries that can cause skull fractures, subdural and epidural hematomas, and even penetrating injuries [50]. Facial and eye injuries are not uncommon but usually are not fatal. Even the relatively low level of fatal injuries from these weapons has prompted many of the forces using them to seek other means of crowd control [50].

Air Guns

The Consumer Product Safety Commission, from its emergency room information network, identified 52,499 injuries from air-propelled toys and weapons during the 2-year period of 1980 to 1981 [51]. In the year 2000, 21,840 injuries from gas or air-powered weapons were reported in the United States but apparently with only four deaths [52]. In the United Kingdom, Milroy et al. reported five deaths under various circumstances [53]. Other series often report no fatalities, but the spectrum of injuries primarily in children includes head, facial, eye, and trunk injuries with varying degrees of severity and complications [54,55].

Fatalities tend to result from the more sophisticated pump or compressed gas cylinder devices rather than from the single-compression-stroke toy rifles [56]. Air rifles, depending on the design, can generate 150–1200 ft/s muzzle velocities for the typical .177 caliber B-B or lead-alloy pellet [52]. This places these weapons within the range of muzzle velocities of many powder-powered pistols. Muzzle velocities of a range of about 800 ft/s or less are sufficient to penetrate skin and bone. Sometimes the shot penetrates the thin orbital plate, but we have also seen it perforate the frontal bone, usually in a child. Then it carves out a uniform permanent track until coming to rest against some obstruction, usually the bone of the opposite wall of the cranial vault. The attendant hemorrhage may prove fatal. Embolism of a B-B shot from a wound of the neck to the brain via the internal carotid artery and other intravascular courses has been observed [57,58]. Most air gun injuries are accidental and occur mostly in children who, out of inexperience or youthful exuberance, injure themselves or others, but suicides have been reported with these relatively benign weapons [59].

Gunshot Wounds in the Civilian Population

Because the great majority of fatal head wounds observed by forensic pathologists in the United States are those from handguns, this section will present a detailed analysis of those injuries. These details need to be known not only to forensic pathologists but also to emergency medical personnel, emergency room physicians and neurosurgeons, policemen and field investigators, and attorneys.

The continuing epidemic in this country of firearms injuries and deaths [60] produced 359 fatalities from gunshot wounds to the head in Harris County (Houston, Texas) in 1980. The incidence in the general population from this figure was 15 per 100,000, but it was actually much higher in certain subgroups (young, male, black). Comparisons between rural and metropolitan firearms show important differences [61]. In rural communities, deaths more often result from rifles or shotguns and tend to more likely be suicides and homicides. In urban populations, the handgun predominates and homicide tends to occur more frequently than suicides. A study of the mortality among recent purchasers of handguns in California [62] found that among 238,292 persons who purchased handguns in the state in 1991, in the first year after purchase, suicide was the most common cause of death among purchasers, accounting for nearly 25% of deaths overall and nearly 52% of deaths among women in the 21–44-year age group.

The fatalities reaching the forensic pathologist in the acute period after wounding are, of course, the most severe wounds, typically through the geographic center of the brain and involving both hemispheres and the deep nuclei [63,64]. A study from New York City [65] provides an example of the usefulness of clinical criteria, on receiving first medical attention, for prognosis. For that study, four clinical grades were described:

- Grade 1: Alert with normal neurological examination; had 14 patients, all with functional survival
- Grade 2: Obtunded; had 3 deaths and 2 nonfunctional survivals among 21 patients
- Grade 3: Unresponsive except to pain; had 4 deaths and 2 nonfunctional survivals among 8 patients
- Grade 4: Deep coma; had 39 patients, all of whom died

The grave implications of increased intracranial pressure are recognized by experienced clinicians [60]. The problem of increased intracranial pressure is especially significant in wounds with small-caliber projectiles like that of a .22 caliber bullet, perhaps a .22

"short" that might be fired from a cheap "Saturday night special." These wounds at first may appear not terribly serious because the victim may be conscious and communicating. Later, deterioration may occur, with massive cerebral edema resulting in death. In such cases, quite often the projectile did not exit the head. Controversies have arisen when precipitous declarations of brain death have occurred with organ harvest in these cases, the issue being the legal principle of intervening cause of death where the assailant admitted to shooting the victim but the death of the victim was the result of the actions of the organ salvage team.

The labile condition of survivors has been emphasized, with some being conscious despite severe wounds. Crockard [66] found it "not uncommon" for survivors to be relatively lucid and then to die. Copeland [67] has analyzed the factors that might correlate with survival from handgun wounds and found critical organ systems (brain, heart), larger-caliber bullets (above .38), and populous locations to be more likely to be associated with rapid death. He concludes "that the best evidence for survivability in a specific case is what was documented to have happened." This is an admonition for continued attention to detailed observation and recording of evidence. Obviously, there are still important facts to be discovered about the specific cause of a death, and correlation of symptoms and course with the postmortem findings will remain a challenging and rewarding task.

The more immediate job of the forensic pathologist is to establish the manner and circumstances of death. As Moritz [25] puts it, "make every effort to determine the probable range and direction of fire regardless of the supposed circumstances." For this purpose, certain specific observations need to be sought and recorded in each tissue penetrated by the missile.

Skin Wounds

The missile penetrating the skin will make a depressed collar called the margin of abrasion, surrounding the actual perforation (Figure 8.8). The perforation will usually be just larger than the cross section that the missile presented upon striking the skin. An angled track can

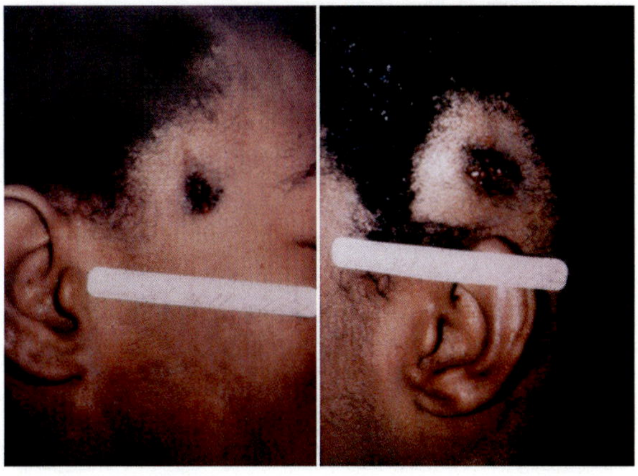

Figure 8.8 Composite photograph of the right side of the face (left panel) where a suicidal contact wound from a small-caliber pistol occurred. Note the faint imprint of the front sight of the weapon above the wound and also a faint stellate pattern of sooting below the wound, probably caused by concentration of gases of firing by the rifling grooves. In the right panel (left side of the head) is the somewhat larger exit wound with slightly everted edges. (Courtesy of the Office of the Medical Examiner, Cook County, IL.)

be observed in some cases, just as occurs from blows that abrade and corrugate the skin in the direction of the blow [8,25]. If the wound is made while the muzzle of the gun is in contact with the skin, the muzzle may imprint its outline as a contusion or create a burn surrounding the missile entry site. Many such illustrations of these phenomena are found in classic texts on gunshot injuries [5,8]. These markings hold great significance for identification of the weapon and should be sought and recorded photographically in every case. Contact wounds often conduct muzzle gases to enter the wound and to create stellate tears in the skin and scalp with sooting, as has already been mentioned. In our experience, these gases usually do not penetrate the brain to any great extent [23], but they can dissect underneath the skin or scalp, elevating and tearing it in patterns that enlarge and distort the entry wound. Note that much of the muzzle gas discharge actually precedes the missile. Gases following the missile can enter the wound, even penetrating the brain, as in the case of an attempted suicide by contact wound from an air rifle [68]. Wadding from blank shells can also penetrate the skin or the brain, as can fragments of fabric, hair, and other foreign materials in some cases.

Powder Markings

Also referred to as burns or tattoos, these deposits of unburned powder and other fouling from the muzzle of the weapon represent significant evidence. To recognize the patterns accurately, it may be required to shave the hair or beard that overlies or is near the wound. Failure to do so may deprive the pathologist or those who may be called upon to evaluate the case in greater detail of valuable evidence. The deposits, which appear as stippled black spots a millimeter or less in diameter around the entry wound (Figure 8.9), should

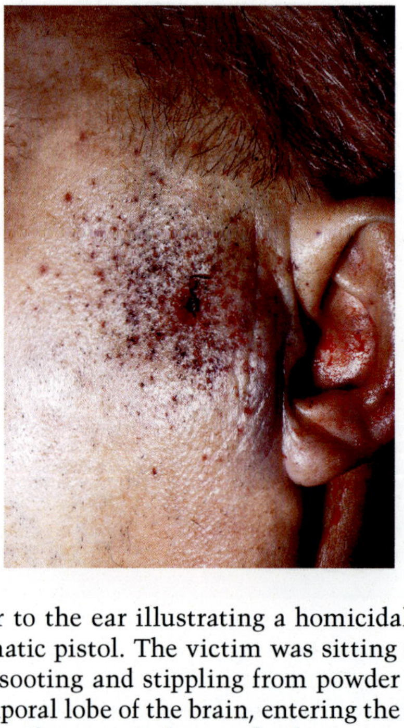

Figure 8.9 Left face anterior to the ear illustrating a homicidal close-range gunshot wound caused by a .25 caliber automatic pistol. The victim was sitting in the driver's seat of his car when he was shot. Note the sooting and stippling from powder fragments about the wound. The bullet penetrated the temporal lobe of the brain, entering the ventricle, but did not exit the cranium. If the weapon or a similar one can be test fired, a reasonably accurate estimate of the distance from weapon to victim can be made. (Courtesy of the Office of the Medical Examiner, Cook County, IL.)

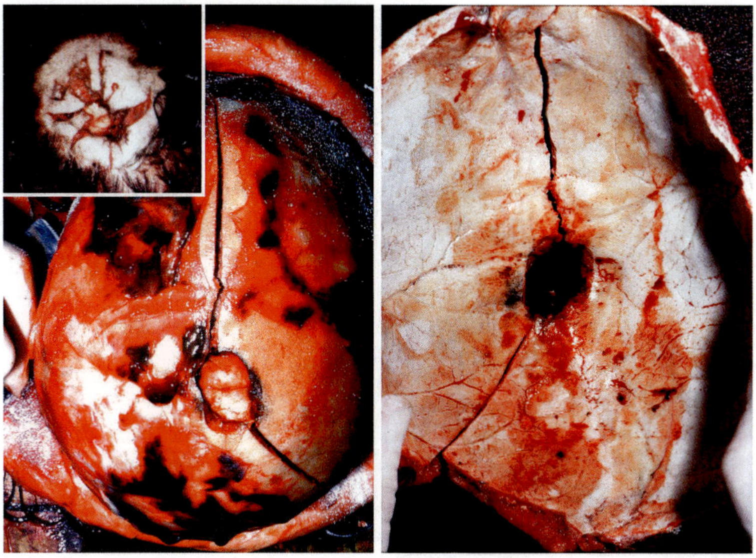

Figure 8.10 Composite photograph illustrating (top left) the contact entrance wound caused by a .357 Magnum service revolver suicidally positioned at the top of the head. Note the stellate tearing of the scalp. In the panel immediately below is the appearance of the vertex of the skull with scalp reflected, showing extensive subgaleal hemorrhage, and a large skull fracture that emanated from the entrance wound. There is a slight amount of outward chip beveling present. In the right panel, showing the undersurface of the vertex skull cap, inward beveling and sooting are obvious in the skull wound. The projectile was found in the third ventricle, curiously not exiting the cranium. (Courtesy of the Office of the Medical Examiner, Cook County, IL.)

be photographed and can be subjected to other tests, which can include swabbing or lifting of the residues for later analysis, perhaps employing modern elemental analysis methods such as energy dispersant x-ray analysis (EDAX), Raman spectroscopy, or other methods as well as scanning electron microscopy [69,70]. Because a surfeit of evidence is always desirable, microscopic sections are also taken from the edge of the entry wound after it has been properly photographed. Metal from the passage of the bullet may be deposited in the margin of abrasion around the entry wound. Other samples frozen and held for possible chromatographic analysis may be indicated.

When the muzzle of a weapon is directly approximated to the skin or scalp, as is often seen in suicidal gunshot wounds, the released gases may split the skin, sometimes in a stellate fashion, and the products of combustion are blown into the tissues, leaving sooting in the deeper tissues (Figure 8.10).

Gunshot Wound—Associated Skull Fractures

Probably the most reliable evidence regarding the entry wound can be obtained from the hole made by the missile as it penetrates the cranial vault. Owing to the architecture of the bone, with the outer and inner tables joined by thin, irregular, diploic struts, a penetration really represents two fractures, one of the outer table and one of the inner table. These are joined by diploë in such a manner that the defect in the outer table in an entry wound is almost always smaller than the defect of the inner table. This is referred to as internal beveling, and the missile can be said to penetrate the skull in a broadening cone (Figure 8.11). If the missile crosses the cranial vault with enough remaining energy to perforate the skull a second time, the principle of the broadening cone along the axis of the missile track will again be observed; that is, the exit fracture will have a smaller hole in the inner table and a larger defect in the outer table (external beveling). Generally, both holes of the exit wound will be larger than the initial entry wound of the outer table, although there are exceptions [71]. Each fracture should be examined carefully and described. It is not sufficient merely to adopt perhaps a police opinion that the wound represents entry or exit. Accurate diagrams may be better than photographs, but at least one of these pictorial methods should be used to preserve the information. Scale markers should be included along with identification numbers in the photograph and written on the diagram with the same pen.

There are several variations that may obscure this important evidence. The entry wound may be so placed that it penetrates very thin bone (orbital plate, temporal squama), and the beveling will not be obvious. In decomposed bodies, the gnawing of rodents can efface the original edges of the fracture. Probably more commonly, the neurosurgeon may have accomplished the same destruction of evidence by his or her placement of burr holes or other operative manipulations. Sadly, many clinicians seem to be unaware of the significance of the fracture patterns and fail to make critical observations and record the essential details. Sometimes neurosurgical burr holes in the skull can be mistaken for gunshot wounds [72]. Missiles striking the very dense petrous portion of the temporal bone cause shattering, which lacks any obvious cone shape [73]. External beveling of entrance wounds can occur from both contact and distant wounds if the missile strikes in an angle very near the perpendicular [74]. Keyhole fractures from tangential shots are created when the entry and exit holes overlap (Figure 8.11), and mixtures of internal and external beveling

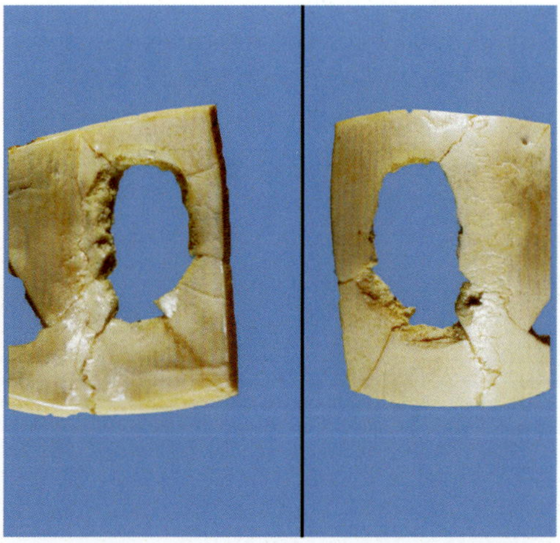

Figure 8.11 Composite photograph of the internal surface of the skull (left) and external surface of the skull (right), which were sawed out of the skull and cleansed, illustrating the uncommon circumstance in which more than one gunshot involved the same wound. In this case of a homicidal shooting in which there were bitemporal wounds, there is an overlapping pattern where both entrance and exit wounds occurred at the same spot. This produced both internal and external beveling on the same hole. (Courtesy of Dr. Lee F. Beamer, Little Rock, AR, and the Office of the Medical Examiner, Cook County, IL.)

are encountered in these wounds. Despite possible confusion of evidence from beveling patterns, there is another possible clue in the pattern of intersecting fracture lines [75]. Because a linear fracture in the skull, originating in the first bullet hole, actually travels faster than the missile, any subsequent fractures, as would arise from the second bullet hole, will meet but not cross the first fracture. This line of observation and reasoning can also be applied to multiple gunshots and confounding fire from multiple directions.

Suicidal Gunshot Wounds

The placement of the entry wound has meaning if suicide is suspected. The majority of right-handed suicides place the muzzle of the gun to the right temple, and left-handers act conversely. Self-inflicted wounds can be posteriorly placed [76]. One study [77] of 23 suicidal wounds found 2 placed in the right occiput, 1 in the mouth, 4 to the right forehead, and the remainder all to the right temple. Sometimes unusual sites of self-inflicted gunshot wounds might suggest homicide. An unusual self-inflicted shot with a .357 Magnum service revolver to the top of the head is illustrated in Figure 8.10. When self-inflicted gunshots via the mouth occur, the injuries may vary, depending on the type of weapon used (handgun, rifle, or shotgun), the caliber of the cartridge, the angle within the mouth, whether the mouth is closed over the gun barrel, and sometimes other factors. Obviously, if the weapon is a high-power one such as a Magnum handgun, high-power rifle (e.g., 30.06), or a shotgun, the destruction may be massive and may essentially destroy the head and expel significant amounts of tissue and brain from the body. With smaller handguns and the lips more or less enclosing the barrel, which is inside the mouth, the gas plume will generally produce tearing or bruising of the lips and cheeks and injure other tissues in the pharynx, larynx, and even esophagus. These tissues will generally be sooted as well. All these types of injuries should be searched for and documented at autopsy.

The recoil of the gun may produce its own injuries, such as fragmenting teeth or lacerating the palate or lips. In the milliseconds after such an intraoral wound, the high-pressure gases from the cartridge will blow back away from the victim and spray blood, tissue, and possibly tooth fragments in patterns that are difficult to predict, sometimes showering other persons who may be present and in front of the victim when the shot occurred. The wounds from handguns will penetrate the back of the mouth, depending on the angle of the shot, and may enter and destroy portions of the cervical spinal column or the skull base, along with whatever neural tissues are nearby. An example of a .38 caliber short barrel intraoral shot is illustrated in Figure 8.12.

Some suicides, and attempted suicides, appear poorly versed in anatomy and miss the vital structures they seek to destroy (Figures 8.13 and 8.14), leaving the victim alive but severely injured. This will account for some cases of suicide with two or more gunshots, which usually involve penetration of the frontal portions of the brain. Multiple self-inflicted gunshot wounds are uncommon but not rare, with many examples having been reported in the literature over the years [78,79]. Quite often such cases involved angled shots to the side of the head, defective ammunition, or just plain bad luck. Occasionally, more than two or three bullets have been fired in a suicide, especially if an automatic weapon was employed [80]. There have been self-filmed or videotaped instances of self-inflicted gunshot wound, sometimes involving more than one shot. These gruesome scenes serve forensic science because it is possible for experts to see what happens following the shot(s), helping them gain insights into future scene inspections and what might or might

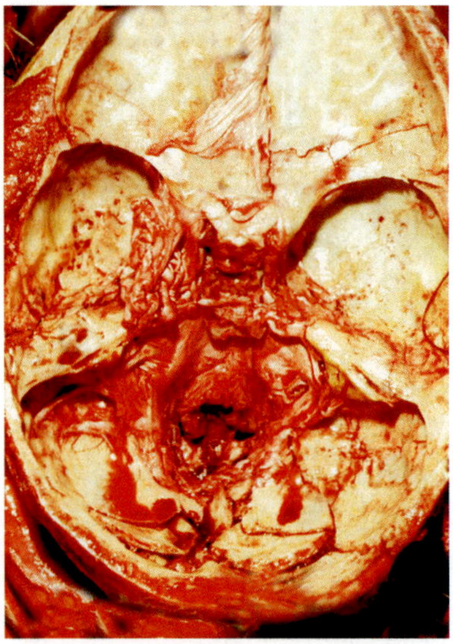

Figure 8.12 Open cranium illustrating a gunshot wound by a .38 caliber short-barrel pistol that had been placed in the mouth. The shot occurred almost exactly in the midline, penetrating just to the left of the midline in the region of the clivus, transecting the cervical–medullary junction, crossing the cerebellum, and finally coming to rest in the subcutaneous tissues of the occiput after shattering the occipital bone. There is an accompanying basilar skull fracture across the anterior fossa.

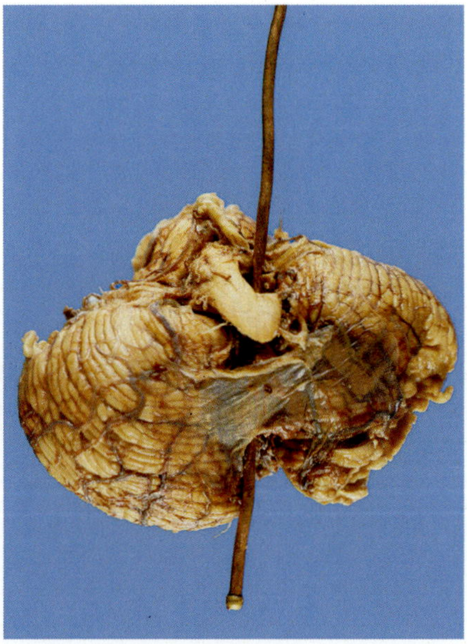

Figure 8.13 Cerebellum and brain stem of a 71-year-old man who had shot himself via the mouth, illustrating the path of bullet. The bullet passed closely to the medulla but did not transect it and lodged in the posterior skull. The victim survived for a month. At autopsy he had hydrocephalus, a chronic subdural hematoma consistent with the survival interval. (Courtesy of Dr. Shaku Teas, Office of the Medical Examiner, Cook County, IL.)

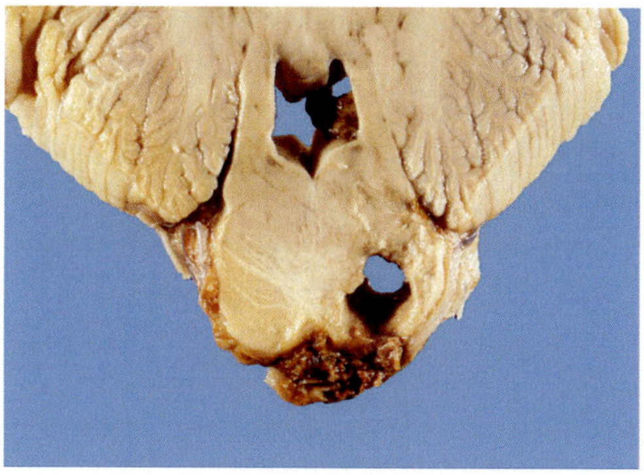

Figure 8.14 Section through the upper pons and cerebellum illustrating a small-caliber gunshot wound involving the pontine tegmentum in a victim who survived several weeks after being wounded. It was reported that the victim was comatose, not always deeply so, but was hemiplegic. (Courtesy of Dr. Carol Haller, Office of the Medical Examiner, Cook County, IL.)

not have occurred. Sometimes the position of the body and the weapon confuse the investigating officials and lead to interpretations that do not reflect the realities of the case. Each case should therefore be documented fully before any movement of the body occurs and any trace evidence collected.

Brain Wounds

The missile, if it does not perforate and pass completely through the head, will almost always travel entirely through the brain tissue in its path and then come to rest against the resistant structure of the skull and dura opposite. The high incidence of ricochet has been noted. Besides "banked shot" ricochets (Figure 8.3), the missile may skitter along the concavity of the inner cranial surface, creating a shallow gutter wound in the adjacent brain. Bone chips that flake off the entry wound may produce significant secondary missiles, which cause additional damage. The paths of the bone chips provide strong evidence of the direction of the missile, and appropriate diagrams or photographs should be added to the record. The tumbling motion of the bullet, which may be deformed from its first encounter with the skull, contributes to irregularity of the permanent track [8,23]. The size and configuration of the track are poor predictors of the caliber and direction of the bullet. The missile track is always hemorrhagic, and the hemorrhages may be large. Sometimes a pattern of perpendicularly oriented small linear hemorrhages alongside the permanent track serves to demarcate the temporary cavity. These are the *in vivo* signs of the fractures observed in gelatin blocks, which Fackler and Malinowski [24] recognize as demonstrating the temporary cavity. The phenomenon of the temporary cavity does occur in many handgun wounds, although it is reduced in size compared with the temporary cavity from a high-velocity missile.

We strongly advocate slicing the gunshot-wounded brain after it has been fixed in formalin for several days, rather than cutting the brain fresh at autopsy. Slicing the fresh brain may be justifiable in some extremely busy services or when time is critical for location of the missile, but the observations that are possible in the jelly-like fresh brain are not as accurate as those in the fixed brain. If cutting the fresh brain is deemed essential, better results can be obtained by making thick (2 cm) sections with a very sharp knife (wet with water before each cut). Another trick for cutting fresh brains is to use a two-bladed oscillating electric knife (turkey knife, available at any hardware store). We prefer to section the brain along the longitudinal axis of the missile track as well as it can be predicted from external examination. This will often make an oblique section necessary, with some corresponding difficulty in anatomical interpretation, but the dramatic demonstration of the path of the missile and bone chips is worth the extra trouble. The missile track should be photographed, with a scale and identification numbers in the picture. Upon location of the missile (perhaps using fluoroscopy or an x-ray plate), it should be carefully removed without abrasion, accurately described, with the prosector's initials inscribed on the base, taking care to preserve any rifling marks for possible later ballistics comparison, some projectiles have no rifling marks (Figure 8.15). The missile, preserved in a plastic bag or container, is an important piece of evidence, and the integrity of the chain of evidence (see Chapter 1) must be maintained. The remaining mass of the missile compared to its original mass (if known) provides a measure of how much fragmentation has occurred. This is an important aspect of the wound profile [24].

The immediate secondary effects of the missile are hemorrhages, disruptions of fiber tracks, and contusions. These may occur at some distance from the missile track due to the temporary cavity and possibly also as a result of damage from the initial shock wave [36,81,82]. An example of massive destruction and hemorrhage along the missile track is illustrated in Figure 8.16. Hemorrhages result from torn blood vessels and may occur in the brain stem acutely due to the forcible downward herniation caused by the volume of the temporary cavity. Intracranial subarachnoid hemorrhage, unaccompanied by other brain injury, has been observed in cases of gunshot wounds to the spine. Apparently, the forceful pressure wave set up in the cerebrospinal fluid can rupture small vessels at some distance from the missile track itself [83]. Brain stem hemorrhages can also occur later, as typical secondary hemorrhages, if the victim survives long enough for hemorrhage and edema to form major supratentorial masses (Figure 8.17). Torn fiber tracks, again especially in the

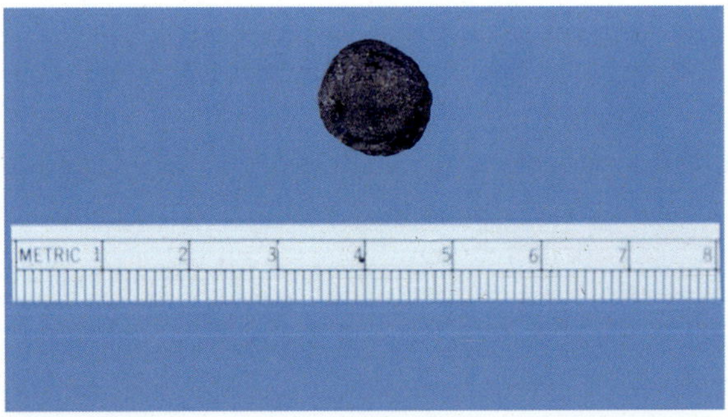

Figure 8.15 This historic specimen is the projectile recovered from the brain of President Abraham Lincoln at his autopsy on or about April 15, 1865. The Army pathologist who performed the autopsy had inscribed on the pellet the initials "AL", which was observed on this specimen by the author when it was examined in 1969. The lead ball was fired from a reported .44 caliber smooth-bore short-barreled derringer by John Wilkes Booth into the back of Lincoln's head at short range on the night of April 14, 1865. Note the deformation of the projectile to a flattened pill-like form. (Courtesy of Dr. Kenneth M. Earle, Armed Forces Institute of Pathology, and the National Archives, Washington, DC.)

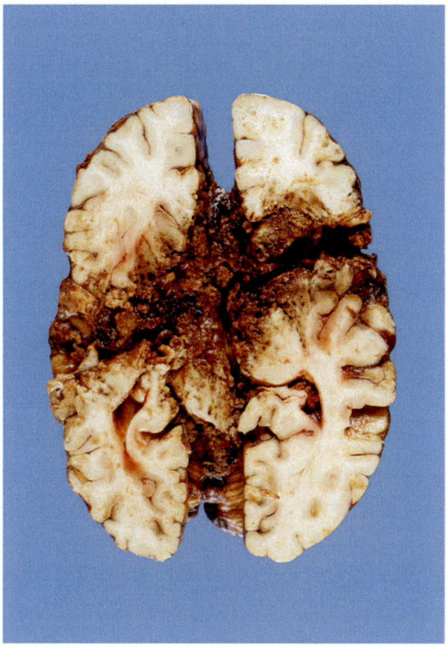

Figure 8.16 Tangential section of the brain of a victim of a homicidal high-power rifle shot to the head illustrating the massive damage that can result from such wounds, with a huge hemorrhagic cavity and many bone and bullet fragments along the track. (Courtesy of the Office of the Medical Examiner, Cook County, IL.)

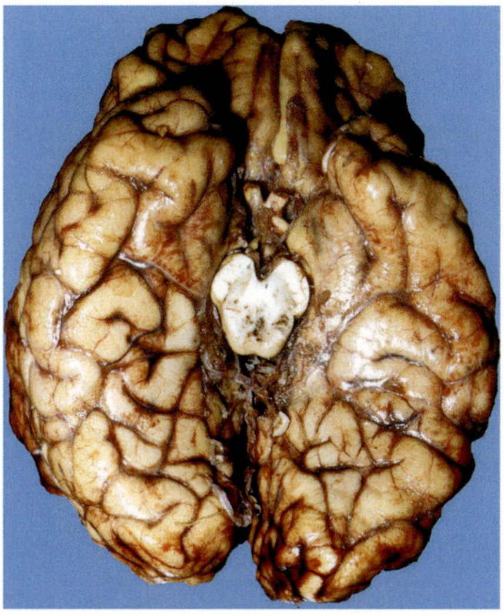

Figure 8.17 Base of the brain with cerebellum and lower brain stem removed from the case shown in Figure 8.10 (suicidal head vertex shot with .357 Magnum pistol), illustrating punctate contusional hemorrhages in the midbrain from the forces of the gunshot. Frequently, contusions of the basal cortex are also seen in such cases.

brain stem, may be present. If the victim survives for a few hours or longer, these will be marked by eosinophilic axonal torpedoes, which can be identified in routine stains or by immunochemical demonstration of β-app accumulation in injured axons [36]. These are caused by continuous movement of axoplasm by axoplasmic flow from the still-intact cell body and proximal axon. As mentioned above, recent experimental evidence suggests that the torn fibers result from shock waves. Obviously, this can be responsible in part for loss of consciousness or focal neurological signs remote from the missile track. Laceration at the corners of the ventricles, caused by bursting of the ventricular walls, has been recognized as a particularly ominous event for survival [48].

Contusions develop on the inferior surfaces of the frontal lobes, on the uncal gyri, and on the cerebellar tonsils. These structures are smashed forcibly against the orbital plates, the tentorial edges, and the foramen magnum, respectively, by the violent expansion of the temporary cavity and also by any subsequent mass effect in victims surviving for any length of time (hours). Contusions to the occipital lobes from glancing or tangential high-velocity missiles can be the cause of pure cortical blindness [84]. The subacute mass effects during the early hours of survival after a gunshot wound to the brain are from hemorrhage and swelling. The closed-box configuration of the cranial vault is altered substantially by open wounds. Swollen brain parenchyma may herniate from the defect, producing the "cerebral fungus," as noted from World War I and earlier battlefields, before rapid evacuation of casualties became possible [41]. Brain swelling can result from the accumulation of water, either intracellularly or in the extracellular space. Ischemia, frequent in survivors of head injury, causes early expansion of the intracellular compartment, especially in glial cell cytoplasm. Hours later, leaks from the vascular endothelium will contribute an additional protein-rich extracellular component. The exact timing of these events is still uncertain, although we have reported very early evidence of brain edema in gunshot wound victims [23]. In our series of 42 fatal cerebral gunshot wounds, 15 had gross evidence of edema on the cut section. This consisted of moist softening and narrowed sulci with flattened gyri. Of these victims, eight survived only 1 hour or less, and six for only a few minutes. This evidence that edema can develop with astonishing rapidity is also suggested from experimental studies [85]. Another early contributor to increasing brain mass is vascular congestion. This has been demonstrated by computerized scanning techniques and is especially likely to occur in children [86]. The cerebral vessels may lose autoregulation, which contributes additional congestion and swelling.

Acute systemic complications from gunshot wounds to the brain may also play a role in the fatal outcome. These can include embolization of brain tissue [87] or the missile [88] to the lungs, consumption coagulopathy from liberation of brain thromboplastin into the systemic circulation, neurogenic pulmonary edema, or gastric erosions. Crockard [89] recorded two patients with gastric erosions severe enough to require gastrectomy among 140 patients with penetrating brain injuries. Neurogenic pulmonary edema has also been observed to follow embolization of a missile (shotgun pellet) from a cervical wound to the brain, causing infarction [90]. Vascular alterations observed experimentally from cerebral missile injuries were caused by defective cardiac muscle contractility and loss of cerebral autoregulation with increase of cerebrovascular resistance [91]. These phenomena probably account for some of the brain ischemia that complicates many head wounds, but the most frequent cause is an inadequate airway initially and later adult respiratory distress syndrome (shock lung).

Long-Term Consequences of Missile Wounds of the Brain and Cord

Delayed Traumatic Intracranial Hemorrhage

Delayed traumatic intracranial hemorrhage is rare, but there are clearly documented examples in the literature. Three large series from a literature review identified three cases among 3731 craniocerebral missile wounds sustained in wartime. The etiology was damage to the wall of an artery, which causes it to balloon outward because of the pressure in the lumen [92]. These traumatic aneurysms or pseudo-aneurysms are prone to rupture 2 weeks or more after the injury [93,94].

Hydrocephalus and Intraventricular Projectiles

Missiles that come to rest alongside one of the cerebral ventricles may become free within the lumen of the ventricle. The changes with position of the head [95] can cause acute decompensation by precipitating acute hydrocephalus [96]. Voracious appetite and thirst may occur after some cerebral gunshot wounds, suggesting hypothalamic or psychogenic involvement, or both [97]. Besides migrating within the ventricular lumen, missiles can migrate in the subarachnoid space [98] or through the substance of the brain itself [99].

Infections and Other Effects of Retained Missiles

A missile left in the brain because of inaccessibility or the proximity of vital structures will become surrounded by a wall of glial scar and sometimes collagen over a period of several months. Foreign-body giant cells and macrophages may form granulomas around the missile [100]. If the missile is steel or steel jacketed, it appears to be relatively innocuous, for as long as 34 years in one case [101]. Lead ions can be released from lead missiles in various body organs, especially if they are within joints, and can cause plumbism (Figure 8.18) [102].

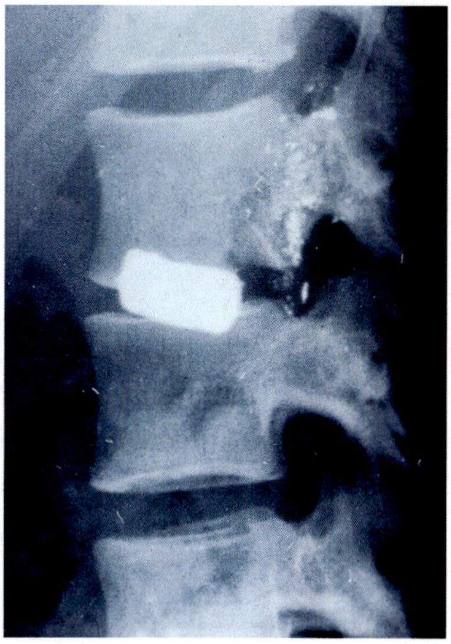

Figure 8.18 Lateral plain spine radiograph illustrating a bullet and bone and lead fragments lodged in the upper lumbar/lower thoracic spine.

If plumbism was observed in association with a cerebral retained lead bullet, it should be reported, because it is theoretically possible. Some authors consider lead bullets less dangerous than copper bullets, because the latter seem more prone to migrate and evoke a more vigorous glial reaction than pure lead alloy bullets [103,104]. The reactive tissue may form a vascular bed receptive to hematogenous abscess formation. This apparently accounted for two of the seven cases of delayed posttraumatic abscesses reported by Arseni and Ghitescu [105]. These two patients had osteomyelitis and purulent tonsillitis before developing a brain abscess around an old retained missile. Although the incidence of bacterial contamination is very high in penetrating wounds, perhaps due to penetration by a fracture through a sinus, it is probably unrealistic to postulate indefinite latent microbism to account for cases that may occur many years after the missile wound. However, studies during World War II did show viable *Staphylococcus aureus* and *Streptococcus* species of bacteria still present in tissue surrounding the wound as long as 86 days following the wounding [106]. Other long-delayed effects of intracranial missile fragments include possible tumor formation [107], which has been discussed in Chapter 3. Such cases are very few and far between [108].

Postwound Complications

The Vietnam Head Injury Study has provided a definitive analysis of epilepsy following penetrating wounds [109]. More than half (53%) of 421 head-injured veterans had posttraumatic epilepsy, and one-fourth of the group still had persistent seizures 15 years after injury. The relative risk of developing epilepsy 10 years after injury was 25 times that of the general population. Larger injuries, large hematomas, and retained metal were significantly correlated with the development of seizures. Injuries in the temporal and frontal lobes were more likely to be associated with seizures. The epileptic group as a whole had decreased life expectancy compared with head-injured veterans without epilepsy or the non-head-injured [110].

Behavioral changes are perhaps even more tragic consequences of penetrating head wounds; only about one in six patients achieves a good recovery [111]. Of course, there are cognitive and other functional residua of cranial wounds, which in time may gradually be overcome; however, the morbidity related to these wounds, especially highlighted from the Iraq War experience, well publicized by the media, illustrates the problems. Such cases may occasionally come to the forensic service in the form of suicides, accidents, and apparently natural deaths; in these kinds of cases, it may fall to the neuropathologist to determine if there is a connection between the death and the injury sustained often long ago. Various aspects of this issue are discussed in Chapter 9.

Blast Injuries and the Nervous System

In recent years, largely in connection with the wars in Afghanistan and Iraq, but most recently in many areas of the world where terrorist activity has proliferated significantly, the number of military personnel and others killed or injured by IEDs and roadside bombs has risen to unprecedented levels. It has been reported that more than 73% of all U.S. military casualties in the Middle East conflicts were due to explosive weaponry [112,113] a significant departure from prior wars. These devices may involve the use of artillery shells, mines, or fabricated devices that are deceptively simple and inexpensive to produce, yet wreak horrible havoc [114]. Most of these devices, however detonated, are constructed from various high explosives such as trinitrotoluene (TNT), C4, Semtex or similar "plastic" explosive formulations, pentaerythritol tetranitrate (PETN), cyclotrimethylene trinitramine (RDX, T4, hexogen), acetone peroxide, and others. Most of these have a very high rate of combustion often exceeding 26,000 ft/s when exploding, yet ironically many will burn peacefully when ignited in small amounts without confinement. It is only when subjected to a shock wave of an initiator (blasting cap) or high heat that explosion occurs. The explosives may be contained in a metal tube capped with a concave copper disk that acts to shape the charge directionally and create very high-velocity, high-temperature fragments that can penetrate vehicular armor, gaining entrance to the vehicle and subjecting its occupants not only to physical components of the device but injurious blast wave and subsequent pressure wave phenomena. Other fabrications can include various containments or combinations of components such as ammonium nitrate, fuel oil and other explosives, which have resulted in terrible destruction and loss of life as in the 1995 bombing of the Murrah Federal Building in Oklahoma City [115].

The chemistry and physics of explosive devices has an extensive literature going back more than 100 years, yet there is still much to be learned. In the past, most damage caused by these devices involved destruction and damage to buildings and facilities and vehicles and inevitably to people, but in recent years the complexion of the use of these devices has changed as has war itself from a former goal to destroy buildings and materiel to inflict serious damage to people in ways not previously appreciated [114,116]. To be sure, injury to extremities of persons in vehicles affected by mostly improvised devices (IEDs) is sometimes devastating, but perhaps more widespread and insidious are the effect on the brain [117]. A great deal of research has gone into understanding this problem involving clinical, radiological, and pathological study of human victims, as well as employing large and small animal experiments and various computer models [118,119].

Explosions, aside from the airborne fragments already mentioned, produce two other phenomena with wounding potential: the blast pressure (shock wave) and the dynamic pressure or blast wind that follows the shock wave [118,120]. There may also be significant thermal injuries if a large flash or conflagration is produced and the victim is close enough to be exposed to it.

Measurements of explosive devices like the typical IED result in a very rapidly traveling shock wave that causes a precipitous rise in ambient pressure in vicinity of the explosion within microseconds of detonation in the range of 10–200 kPa or more in experimental situations to more than 1700 kPa (about 250 psi) in actual IED incidents.* It has been estimated that overpressures of 690–1700 kPa (100–250 psi) are not survivable. After the initial shock wave passes, the ambient pressure falls over the succeeding 4–10 ms then becomes a negative pressure for many more milliseconds until ambient pressure levels are reached only to be replaced by the blast wind, which itself is destructive. This pressure curve has been referred to as the Friedländer curve [118,121,122], which is diagrammatically represented in Figure 8.19. Thereafter, depending on the distance from the explosion, debris and bomb fragments are propelled outward, followed by a thermal wave.

During the high spike in ambient pressure from the shock wave of the explosion, important shock wave–body interactions occur. These interactions especially with the head–brain have been referred to as fluid–structure interactions and have been extensively studied using sophisticated and complex mathematical and computer models and

* kPa refers to kilo-Pascals: measures in metric system for pressure. 1 kPa = 0.145 psi.

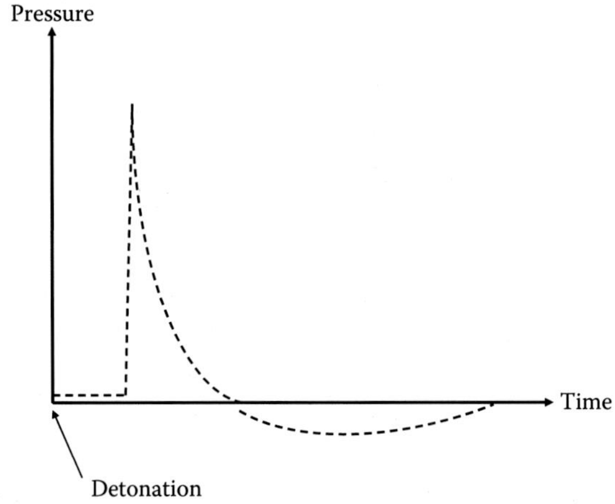

Figure 8.19 This graph depicts time/pressure relationships in close proximity to a high explosive blast event. The time curve after detonation is a function of the distance between the measuring device or victim and the blast. When the blast wave reaches the victim, ambient pressure dramatically rises extremely rapidly to its maximum, then decays into a phase of negative ambient pressure until finally the primary wave dissipates. This curve, often referred to as the Friedländer curve, depicts these events. The negative component of the wave may be sufficient to produce cavitation in tissues and at tissue–fluid interfaces in much the same manner as has been visualized in studies of the contrecoup phenomenon [118]. (From J.M. Varas et al. *Front Neurol*, 2011;2:58–65.)

in animals [118,120,123]. Many complex events occur during the microseconds of the impingement of the detonation shock wave on the human body and its decay. Each body component and tissue offers a different shock wave reaction [121] Those body parts that have air–fluid or air–tissue interfaces, such as the lung, sinuses, gut, and ear, can rupture or suffer profound injury to tissue elements and vessels by a process known as *spallation*, which is defined as the "… disruption that occurs at the boundary between two media of different densities." [118]. This may involve microcavitations. More solid organs have their own tolerance levels and responses. With respect to the brain, the shock wave front interacts with the environmental surface near the head, with whatever head covering might be present, with the skull, brain coverings, cerebrospinal fluid and ventricles, vessels, and the brain itself with reflective phenomena, interference effects, and others to damage tissues in mostly subtle ways. The orientation of the victim's body with respect to the advancing shock wave front as well as the distance from the explosion also affect what ill effects might be suffered.

The interactions with the victim's body occur at a number of levels illustrated in Figure 8.20. Noncranial tissues, as noted above, have individual characteristics and interfaces that interact with the blast wave front causing potentially stress and strain upon vessels, injury to air-filled passages, or fluid-filled passages. The injuries may result in early or later hemorrhages, instigation of the inflammatory cascade (endothelial damage, release of inflammatory mediators), and edema. These in turn can evolve into a host of secondary and tertiary phenomena that evolve over time to lead to air and fat embolism, pulmonary dysfunction, multiorgan failure, sepsis, coagulopathy, fluid and electrolyte imbalances, all of which can complicate any neurological injury that may be present. Direct effects on

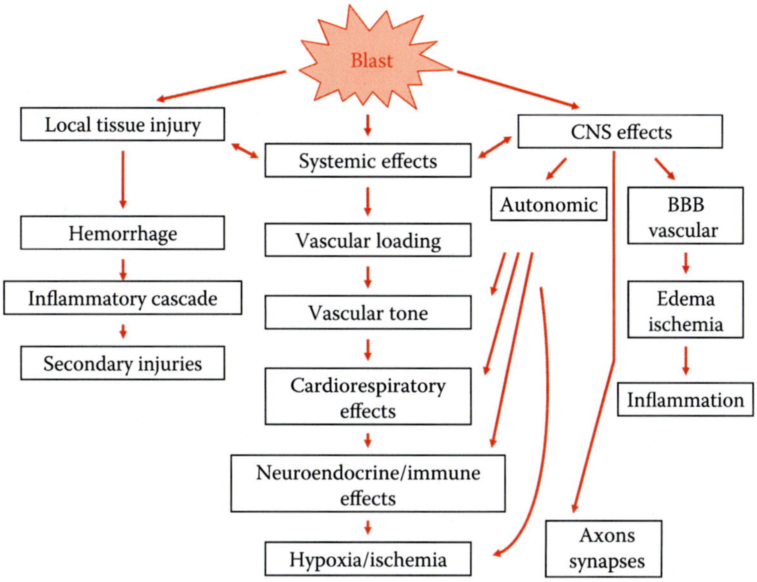

Figure 8.20 This diagram based on the work of Cernak and Nobel-Haeusslein [112] illustrates some of the event cascade in tissues resulting from proximity to a high explosive blast. (From I. Cernak, L.J. Noble-Haeusslein, *J Cereb Blood Flow Metab*, 2010;30:255–66.)

the nervous system involve disruption of the blood–brain barrier, pressure/volume equilibrium, vascular autoregulation, axonal and synaptic membrane functions diffusely or focally at gray–white matter junctions. At the molecular–cellular level, glucose metabolism, energy metabolism, and membrane ionic channel function have been shown to be adversely affected by shock waves [112] in experimental animals. By the same token, alterations in axonal function and microanatomy may also occur [124,125].

In those that have been exposed, often many times, to forceful detonations yet have not suffered apparent physical injury, the incidence of behavioral and cognitional consequences is now appreciated. These problems often involved posttraumatic stress disorder (PTSD), depression, cognitive impairments, and less subtle neurological deficits. In an effort to comprehend what has happened and what the structural lesions that might be associated, a number of studies on human victims as well as large animals (swine, and nonhuman primates) and rodents have modeled the circumstances of IED blasts and attempted to discover their effects. At varying times after blast exposure, imaging studies using advanced MRI technologies (diffusion tensor imaging) have found that blast concussions appear to mimic coup–contrecoup phenomena involving the orbitofrontal and posterior fossa (cerebellum, peduncles, brain stem) [117]. Axonal pathology in these and periventricular regions of the brain (corpus callosum, cingulum, internal capsule, cerebral peduncles) has been found [126].

Injuries to the nervous system aside, blast events have profound effects alluded to above on other organ systems, chiefly the lungs where overpressures may produce devastating injury that with or without the nervous system injury may produce death [127–131], sometimes by mechanisms that are poorly defined. An example of a lethality curve is illustrated in Figure 8.21.

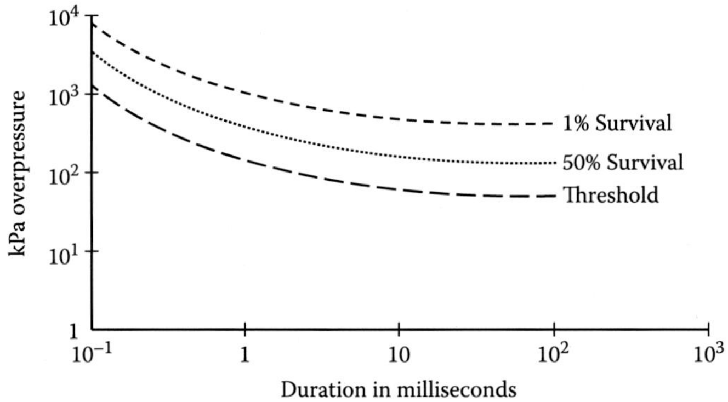

Figure 8.21 This graph depicts lethality curves in large experimental animals exposed to blasts typical for an improvised explosive device (IED) with respect to overpressures and duration of the exposure primarily affecting the lungs. (Modified from Varas JM, Philippens PM, Meijer SR, van den Berg AC, Sibma PC, van Bres JLMJ, de Vries DVWM, *Front Neurol*, 2, 58, 2011.)

Wounds of the Spinal Cord and Canal

As with penetrating wounds to the brain, missile injuries to the spinal cord are caused by three main categories of projectiles: shell fragments and high-velocity bullets, mainly during wartime [132]; low-velocity (handgun) bullets during peacetime; and shotgun pellets [133–135]. In recent years, the explosion of gang violence in American urban areas has left countless victims with spinal cord injuries due to firearms and provided an additional load on forensic pathology services. The particular implication of high-velocity injuries is that they can cause paralysis without grossly obvious damage to the cord. This is probably an example of the effect of shock waves and may also be related to the large temporary cavity that accompanies the high-velocity missile, even if it does not make a direct hit on the cord itself.

Clinicians usually divide the effects of spinal cord missile wounds into four groups [136], depending on the level and extent of injury. The most common injury to the cord itself is complete and permanent paralysis at the level of the wound. Also frequent are conus medullaris and cauda equina injuries [135]. Incomplete paralysis or progressive symptoms are less common, the latter implying a major component of vascular or ischemic injury, which complicates the primary wound.

A major difficulty in studying or treating spinal cord wounds is that the level of cord injury may not correlate well with the level of external wound [137]. This is due to several factors in addition to the shock wave and temporary cavity effects of high-velocity missiles already mentioned. First, the mature spinal cord is anatomically shorter than the axial skeleton, and the disparity increases at the lower levels of the cord (e.g., conus medullaris injuries correspond to a level of about the first lumbar vertebra). Second, there appears to be significant individual variation in relative cord position, some being anatomically prefixed and others postfixed, compared to the norm. Third, the position of the cord within the spinal canal changes with body posture and movement; hence, the exact stance of the victim at the moment of injury is relevant (and difficult to know). Finally, clinicians have observed a condition of spinal shock that causes acute symptoms several segments above the actual wound. These symptoms may improve over several days so that the apparent level of injury descends to that of the permanent wound. The cause of this phenomenon is poorly understood and is discussed in Chapter 6. The problem is significant for the forensic pathologist if the patient has died during the acute period before stabilization of the permanent injury level.

Blast and fragmentation injuries to the spine are common in suicide bombings, in other terrorist bombings of buildings, and in public places. Injuries to the spine are predicated upon proximity to the blast and its character. In recent years, many such incidents have occurred outside the normal combat scenario, but grievous injuries may be caused by mines and booby traps. Although cervical injuries are common, thoracic and lumbar spinal injury is more common and produced by not only huge concussive forces in blasts but also fragmentation of the bomb and its components, as well as secondary fragments from destroyed vehicles or building components [138–141]. The spectrum of injuries is broad and usually involves orthopedic as well as visceral injuries. The legacy of many such injuries include, in addition to neurological damage, damage to vessels and to the integrity of the spinal column and the spinal sac, which may become breached and lead to cerebrospinal fluid fistulas, infection, and major management issues.

The pathological examination may require special adjustments to secure needed forensic information and evidence. We recommend examination of the spinal cord *in situ* in missile wounds to the back and neck. Posterior laminectomy is the most accurate way to correlate nervous tissue injury with bony skeleton injury and to establish trajectory. Prior x-rays are often helpful in identifying fractures and missiles (Figure 8.18) but do not constitute final evidence, because the surgeon's or pathologist's direct visual and tactile observations are conceded to be more accurate. We find complete removal of skeletal muscle attachments to the vertebral laminae to be essential and efficient. After making the laminectomy (with Stryker saw, chisel, or bone rongeurs), the missile or bone fragments are sought while cleaning the spinal canal for photographing of the cord *in situ*. Instability of the spine should be evaluated by careful manual manipulation. As in head injuries, diagrams are useful, and identification numbers and scale markers must be in the photograph. Photographs before and after opening the dural sack are usually justified. The trajectory of the missile can be illustrated in the photograph by placing a probe along the missile track. It should also be remembered that manipulation with instruments of projectiles by the pathologist or diener should be avoided because factitious marks may be introduced that may later confound forensic examination of the projectiles.

The pathologist should seek evidence of gross cord disruption or hematoma, and gentle palpation of the cord is often useful. The cord may be formalin fixed *in situ* by removing the vertebral column, or, after adequate documentation and labeling of at least one specific segment with a tag, it can be elevated gently from the dural sac. A long, slender instrument tray with lid is useful for immersion fixation. It is not necessary to pin the cord to cork board. After fixation, cross sections should be made above and below the injury level. These are especially helpful in chronic injuries, because they assist in documenting the level of injury. Cross- or longitudinal sections may be used at the actual site of the wound.

Microscopic changes may be very subtle [142] and deserve careful study. Petechiae may be truly pathological or may be caused by rough handling of the cord postmortem. Most pathologists are gentler than their dieners, and difficult cases deserve direct personal attention. Whereas small hemorrhages may be somewhat equivocal, margination and early immigration of polymorphonuclear cells are not. This specific pathological change begins within a few minutes near the injury and is usually easy to find within 6 hours postinjury. Swollen axons, as in brain injuries, begin within a few hours and increase in prominence over several days [36].

Wallerian degeneration is a more leisurely process, first becoming evident grossly several weeks after the injury as a chalky white, opaque, slight swelling of the involved tracts. This appearance is due to the degenerating lipids and macrophage activity, which is evident sooner at the microscopic level. Over several months, the removal of cut axons and their myelin continues, and a shrunken glial scar replaces the tract. This will be evident grossly as well as microscopically. A cervical cross section should always be taken. Cauda equina injuries may be recognized accurately by Wallerian degeneration at the cervical level, owing to the medial-to-lateral layering of ascending fibers in the dorsal columns.

Spinal cord injury to the high cervical levels that supply the phrenic nerves may be acutely fatal, but lower levels of injury usually require simultaneous injury to other organ systems to be fatal [133]. Because abdominal or thoracic injuries frequently accompany gunshot wounds to the spine, a complete autopsy is essential. Vascular injuries in particular deserve careful evaluation and description. Any hematomas should be gently washed and probed while still fresh for identification of the torn vessel. This tedious effort does not always succeed at the time of autopsy, but it is almost always doomed to fail if the search is delayed until after the hematoma is fixed. Look first, and then fix!

Stab Wounds

Penetration of the brain by a knife or other sharp object does occur and represents an example of an extremely low-velocity missile (Figure 8.22). There are several reports of pencil wounds in the literature [143], as well as penetrations by a host of objects, including chopsticks and umbrella stems, often via the orbit [144,145]. There is no temporary cavity, as seen in missile injuries, and the damage is inflicted solely by the direct effect of the moving blade or instrument, which may or may not remain in the wound. The clinical findings and the possibility of a fatal issue will be determined by the exact placement of the wound and associated injuries to other organ systems. As with very low-velocity missiles,

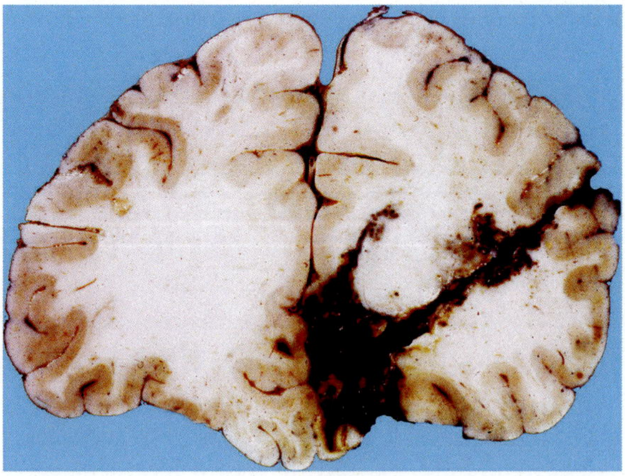

Figure 8.22 This coronal brain section illustrates a knife stab wound to the brain that passed into the brain from the face via the orbital roof. This wound is depicted in Figure 8.23. (Courtesy of Department of Pathology, DC General Hospital, Washington, DC.)

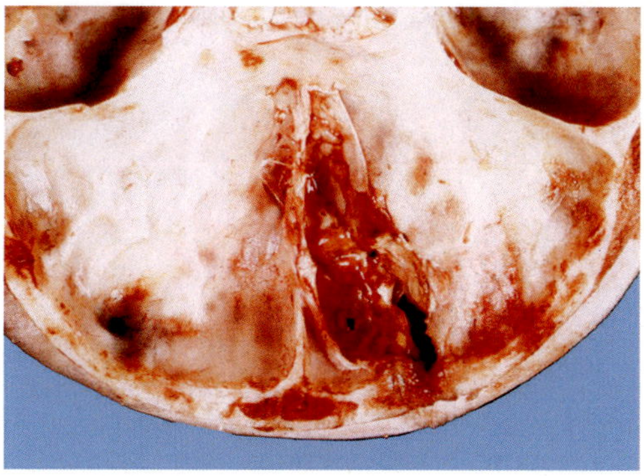

Figure 8.23 Skull base and orbital plates from Figure 8.22 illustrating the entrance wound from a knife stab wound to the face. (Courtesy of Department of Pathology, DC General Hospital, Washington, DC.)

penetration of the bony skull by a knife is more likely at the sites of very thin bone—the orbits and the temporal squama (Figure 8.23). It may occur in penetrating skull wounds that a fragment of bone may be driven into the brain by the instrument. Such bone fragments may or may not ever be discovered but may produce neurological or behavioral abnormalities and may produce a reactive focus for epilepsy.

Whereas ice picks were once, in some parts of the country, a favored weapon, they are now rare, and brain wounds from them are similarly rare. Some "specialists" with this weapon, such as the infamous 1950s-era gangster Israel "Ice Pick Willie" Alderman of Las Vegas [146], were said to be able to murder victims in public places by driving a concealed ice pick via the ear into the brain stem, leaving little or no trace that even a pathologist might miss at autopsy. An example of a thin blade/ice pick homicide is illustrated in Figures 8.24 and 8.25.

Spinal cord stab wounds are more frequent than cranial ones. Incomplete stab wound injuries to the cord account for the classic Brown–Sequard syndrome of paralysis of the same side below a unilateral spinal cord transection, with associated loss of light touch and

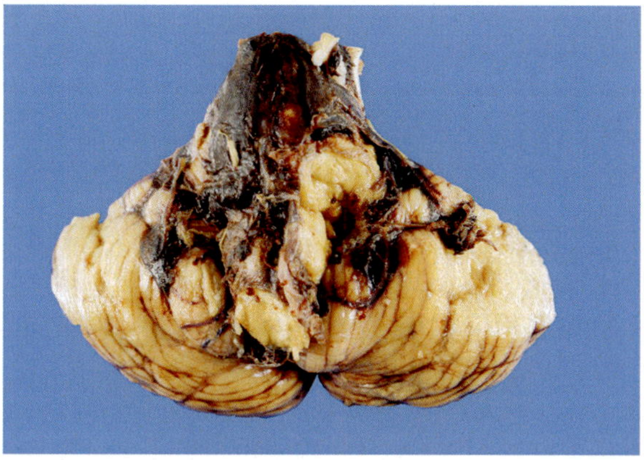

Figure 8.24 View of the brain stem and cerebellum (anterior surface) showing extensive subarachnoid hemorrhage. The weapon apparently was a small kitchen knife driven into the back of the head in this 7-year-old female by the assailant. (Courtesy of Dr. Mitra Kalelkar, Office of the Medical Examiner, Cook County, IL.)

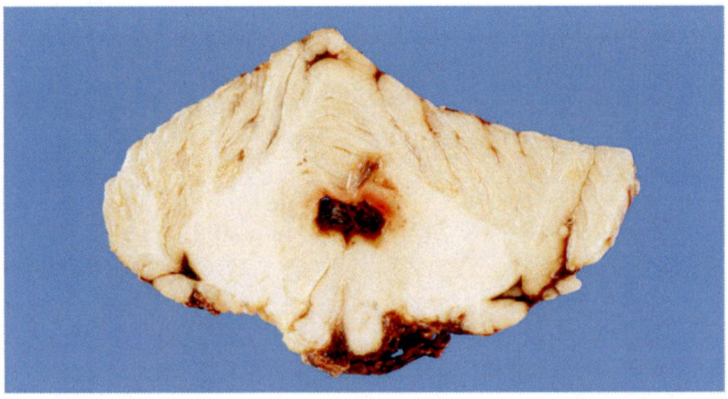

Figure 8.25 This horizontal section of the brain stem and cerebellum from Figure 8.24 shows subarachnoid and intraventricular hemorrhage. (Courtesy of Dr. Mitra Kalelkar, Office of the Medical Examiner, Cook County, IL.)

proprioception on the same side, and loss of pain and temperature sense, a few segments lower, on the opposite side. The pure syndrome is rare because it requires the surgical precision of an exact hemisection of the cord, but incomplete variants are commonly observed. Indeed, Lipschitz [147] observed that almost any combination of symptoms may be encountered.

Stab wounds show the same anatomic and coincidental vagaries of the relationship of the level of neurological damage to the wound of the vertebral column as do gunshot wounds, with an important additional consideration, that is, how the blade must pass if it is to penetrate the almost-complete bony encasement of the spinal cord. Only very heavy blades will fracture and depress the laminae, so to penetrate without fracture, the blade must enter between the laminae. In the thoracic region, this implies that either the laminae must be spread apart, as when the victim is bending over when struck, or the blade must be directed upward from below, to penetrate between the overlapping laminae. In the cervical region, the laminae are narrower, and a horizontal thrust can penetrate, or especially in the high cervical region, the thrust can be downward. Also noteworthy is the ice pick wound of a small narrow blade, which can penetrate dorsolaterally at the intervertebral foramina. Note also that several thrusts may be required to penetrate and that the force needed to achieve penetration may result in the blade's being broken off. After the blade enters the spinal canal, it may penetrate the cord or push the cord aside. The latter circumstance is attributed to the relatively tough fibrous capsule that accompanies the pia mater of the spinal cord. If pushed aside by a dull blade, the cord may be contused by pressure of its opposite side against the bony limit of the canal. This has been called a contrecoup injury and will explain unexpected clinical symptoms, as compared with the anatomical injury. The effect of compression against bone spurs of degenerative osteoarthritis may be a further complicating factor.

There are often a number of associated injuries common with stab wounds. These may be vascular, owing to the vasculature of the spinal cord and other major vessels; or major organs of the pleural sac may be penetrated. Wounds to the brachial plexus, in addition to spinal cord wounds, are not uncommon and present to both clinician and pathologist the difficult problem of central nervous system injury complicated by peripheral nerve injury. Finally, attention is called to the theoretically possible, but rarely seen [147], syndrome of false paraplegia. This results from contusion to the medial motor strips of both cerebral hemispheres from a direct, powerful blow to the vertex. The result is paralysis of both legs, which calls attention first to the spinal cord, which is not the cause. This puzzle can be solved by painstaking, informed examination of the history and the entire body.

Summary and Conclusions

1. The primary aim of the forensic pathologist must be to establish beyond reasonable doubt the facts in each individual case.
2. Accurate observation and recording of evidence are essential and cannot be replaced by terse opinionated diagnoses such as "exit wound" or other imprecise or ambiguous terms.
3. Ballistic principles can be applied to the wounding potential of missiles. The most important variables are velocity, tumbling, and fragmentation of the missile.
4. There is an important practical distinction between military or high-velocity and civilian or low-velocity wounds—the size of the temporary cavity and the tissue injury that occurs.
5. Important details are still lacking in our understanding of the mechanisms of death and morbidity from penetrating head injuries. The forensic pathologist and clinician can help to fill this void by making and publishing informed observations from the abundant material.
6. Blast injuries are dependent on the quantity and type of explosive involved and its rate of combustion, and the proximity and environment of the victim to the device. There are a spectrum of injuries assignable to the blast shock wave (positive and negative—Friedländer curve), to the blast wind, and to the thermal wave. It appears that blast shock wave is responsible for delayed, chronic problems in victims such as PTSD and cognitional deficits.
7. Gunshot wounds of the spine share many aspects of gunshot wounds to the brain; the correlation of the level of neurological damage with the anatomical injury may be a difficult challenge.
8. Stab wounds are like very low-velocity missiles and create damage only in the permanent track. The assailant must use anatomical knowledge, blind chance, or brute force to incise the brain or spinal cord, which are well protected by bony encasements.

References

1. Camps FE, Robinson AE, Lucas BG, eds. *Gradwohl's Legal Medicine*. Bristol: A. John Wright, 1976.
2. DiMaio VJ, DiMaio D. *Forensic Pathology*. Boca Raton, FL: CRC Press, 2001.
3. Gonzales TA, Vance M, Helpern M, Umberger CJ. *Legal Medicine: Pathology and Toxicology*. New York: Appleton-Century-Crofts, 1954.
4. Knight B. *Forensic Pathology*. London: Arnold, 1996.
5. Spitz WU, Spitz DJ, Fisher RS, eds. *Spitz and Fisher's Medicolegal Investigation of Death: Guidelines for the Application of Pathology to Crime Investigation*. Springfield, IL: Charles C. Thomas, 2006.
6. Meirowsky AM. *Penetrating Craniocerebral Trauma*. Springfield, IL: Charles C. Thomas, 1984.
7. Fatteh A. *Medicolegal Investigation of Gunshot Wounds*. Philadelphia: J.B. Lippincott, 1976.
8. Di Maio VJM. *Gunshot Wounds: Practical Aspects of Firearms, Ballistics, and Forensic Techniques*. New York: Elsevier Science, 1985.
9. Dodd M, Byrne K. *Terminal Ballistics: A Text and Atlas of Gunshot Wounds*. Boca Raton, FL: Taylor & Francis, 2006.
10. Sellier KG, Kneubuehl BP. *Wound Ballistics and the Scientific Background*. Amsterdam: Elsevier, 1994.

11. Speer/Omark Industries. *Speer Reloading Manual*, Number 13. Lewiston, ID: Speer/Omark Industries, 2007.
12. Fackler ML, Surinchak JS, Malinowski JA, Bowen RE. Wounding potential of the Russian AK-47 assault rifle. *J Trauma* 1984;24:263–6.
13. Haag LC. The forensic aspects of contemporary disintegrating rifle bullets. *Am J Foren Med Pathol* 2013;34:50–5.
14. Martrille L, Artuso A, Cattaneo C, Baccino E. A deceptive case of gunshot entry wounds—Beware of frangible bullets. *J Foren Leg Med* 2007;14:161–4.
15. Harvey EN, Butler EG, McMillen JH, Puckett WO. Mechanism of wounding. *War Med* 1945;8:91–104.
16. Kirkpatrick JB, Higgins ML, Lucas JH, Gross GW. *In vitro* simulation of neural trauma by laser. *J Neuropathol Exp Neurol* 1985;44:268–84.
17. Povlishock JT, Becker DP, Cheng CL, Vaughan GW. Axonal change in minor head injury. *J Neuropathol Exp Neurol* 1983;42:225–42.
18. Lioubashevski O, Fineberg J. Shock wave criterion for propagating solitary states in driven surface waves. *Phys Rev E Stat Nonlin Soft Matter Phys* 2001;63:035302.
19. Sharon E, Cohen G, Fineberg J. Propagating solitary waves along a rapidly moving crack front. *Nature* 2001;410:68–71.
20. Berloff NG. Solitary wave complexes in two-component condensates. *Phys Rev Lett* 2005; 94: 120401.
21. Oehmichen M, Meissner C, König HG. Brain injury after gunshot wounding: Morphometric analysis of cell destruction caused by temporary cavitation. *J Neurotrauma* 2000;17:155–62.
22. Oehmichen M, Meissner C, König HG, Gehl HB. Gunshot injuries to the head and brain caused by low-velocity handguns and rifles: A review. *Foren Sci Int* 2004;146:111–20.
23. Kirkpatrick JB, Di Maio V. Civilian gunshot wounds of the brain. *J Neurosurg* 1978;49:185–98.
24. Fackler ML, Malinowski JA. The wound profile: A visual method for quantifying gunshot wound components. *J Trauma* 1985;25:522–9.
25. Fatteh A. Gunshot wounds. In Fatteh A. ed., *Handbook of Forensic Pathology*. Philadelphia, Lippincott, 1973, pp. 97–130.
26. Moritz AR. *The Pathology of Trauma*. Philadelphia: Lea & Febiger, 1954.
27. Freytag E. Autopsy findings in head injuries from firearms. *Arch Pathol* 1963;76:215–25.
28. DeMuth WE. Bullet velocity and design as determinants of wounding capacity: An experimental study. *J Trauma* 1966;6:222–32.
29. Bolliger SA, Thali MJ, Ross S, Buck U, Naether S, Vock P. Virtual autopsy using imaging: Bridging radiologic and forensic sciences. A review of the virtopsy and similar projects. *Eur Radiol* 2007;28:44–7.
30. Thali MJ, Yen K, Vock P, Ozdoba C, Kneubuehl BP, Sonnenschein M, Dirnhofer R. Image-guided virtual autopsy findings of gunshot victims performed with multi-slice computed tomography and magnetic resonance imaging and subsequent correlation between radiology and autopsy findings. *Foren Sci Int* 2003;138:8–16.
31. Dimond FC Jr, Rich NM. M-16 rifle wounds in Vietnam. *J Trauma* 1967;7:619–25.
32. Clark MA, Micik W. Confusing wounds of entrance and exit with an unusual weapon. *Am J Foren Med Pathol* 1984;5:75–8.
33. Grey TC. The incredible bouncing bullet: Projectile exit through the entrance wound. *J Foren Sci* 1993;38:1222–6.
34. Byrnes DP, Crockard HA, Gordon DS, Gleadhill CA. Penetrating craniocerebral missile injuries in the civil disturbances in Northern Ireland. *Br J Surg* 1974;61:169–76.
35. Butler EG, Puckett WO, Harvey EN, McMillen JH. Experiments on head wounding by high velocity missiles. *J Neurosurg* 1945;2:358–63.
36. Oehmichen M, Meissner C, Schmidt V, Pedal I, König HG. Pontine axonal injury after brain trauma and nontraumatic hypoxic-ischemic brain damage. *Int J Legal Med* 1999;112:261–7.

37. Lindenberg R, Freytag E. The mechanism of cerebral contusions: A pathological anatomic study. *Arch Pathol* 1960;69:440–69.
38. Carey ME, Sacco W, Merkler J. An analysis of fatal and non-fatal head wounds incurred during combat in Vietnam by U.S. forces. *Acta Chir Scand Suppl* 1982;508:351–6.
39. Bird SM, Fairweather CB. Military fatality rates (by cause) in Afghanistan and Iraq: A measure of hostilities. *Int J Epidemiol* 2007;36:841–6.
40. Roberts L, Lafta R, Garfield R, Khudhairi J, Burnham G. Mortality before and after the 2003 invasion of Iraq: Cluster sample survey. *Lancet* 2004;364:1857–64.
41. Cushing H. *From a Surgeon's Journal*. Boston: Little Brown, 1936.
42. Haag LC. Range of fire determination from the pseudostippling of skin by shotshell buffer material. *Am J Foren Med Pathol* 2013;34:56–62.
43. Fieguth A, Gunther D, Schroeder G, Troger HD. Fatal stun gun injury using a modified animal sedation gun. *Arch Kriminol* 2002;210:39–44.
44. Mosdal C. Cranio-cerebral injuries from Slaughterer's gun. *Acta Neurochir* (Wien) 1985;74:31–4.
45. Spitz WU, Wilhelm RM. Stud gun injuries. *J Foren Med* 1970;17:5–11.
46. Weedn VW, Mittleman RE. Stud guns revisited: Report of a suicide and literature review. *J Foren Sci* 1984;29:670–8.
47. Metress EK, Metress SP. The anatomy of plastic bullet damage and crowd control. *Int J Health Serv* 1987;17:333–42.
48. Mahajna A, Aboud N, Harbaji I, Agbaria A, Lankovsky Z, Michaelson M, Fisher D, Krausz MM. Blunt and penetrating injuries caused by rubber bullets during the Israeli–Arab conflict in October, 2000: A retrospective study. *Lancet* 2002;359:1795–800.
49. Kalebi A, Olumbe AK. Death following rubber bullet wounds to the chest: Case report. *East Afr Med J* 2005;82:382–4.
50. Hiss J, Hellman FN, Kahana T. Rubber and plastic ammunition lethal injuries: The Israeli experience. *Med Sci Law* 1997;37:139–44.
51. Christoffel KK, Tanz R, Sagerman S, Hahn Y. Childhood injuries caused by nonpowder firearms. *Am J Dis Child* 1984;138:557–61.
52. Laraque D. Injury risk of nonpowder guns. *Pediatrics* 2004;114:1357–61.
53. Milroy CM, Clark JC, Carter N, Rutty G, Rooney N. Air weapon fatalities. *J Clin Pathol* 1998;51:525–9.
54. Bhattacharyya N, Bethel CA, Caniano DA, Pillai SB, Deppe S, Cooney DR. The childhood air gun: Serious injuries and surgical interventions. *Pediatr Emerg Care* 1998;14:188–90.
55. Bratton SL, Dowd MD, Brogan TV, Hegenbarth MA. Serious and fatal air gun injuries: More than meets the eye. *Pediatrics* 1997;100:609–12.
56. DiMaio VJ. Homicidal death by air rifle. *J Trauma* 1975;15:1034–7.
57. Padar SC. Air gun pellet embolizing the intracranial internal carotid artery. *J Neurosurg* 1975;43:222–4.
58. Taggart DP, Mackenzie I. Air gun pellet embolism. *Scott Med J* 1988;33:340.
59. Pottker TI, Dowd MD, Howard J, DiGiulio G. Suicide with an air rifle. *Ann Emerg Med* 1997;29:818–20.
60. Lillard PL. Five years experience with penetrating craniocerebral gunshot wounds. *Surg Neurol* 1978;9:79–83.
61. Dresang LT. Gun deaths in rural and urban settings: Recommendations for prevention. *J Am Board Fam Pract* 2001;14:107–15.
62. Wintemute GJ, Parham CA, Beaumont JJ, Wright M, Drake C. Mortality among recent purchasers of handguns. *N Engl J Med* 1999;341:1583–9.
63. Kaufman HH, Loyola WP, Makela ME, Frankowski RF, Wagner KA, Bernstein DP, Gildenberg PL. Civilian gunshot wounds: The limits of salvageability. *Acta Neurochir* (Wien) 1983;67:115–25.
64. Blumenthal R. Suicidal gunshot wounds to the head: A retrospective review of 406 cases. *Am J Foren Med Pathol* 2007;28:288–91.

65. Hubschmann O, Shapiro K, Baden M, Shulman K. Craniocerebral gunshot injuries in civilian practice—Prognostic criteria and surgical management. Experience 82 cases. *J Trauma* 1979;19:6–12.
66. Crockard HA. Penetrating craniocerebral injuries. *Int Anesth Clin* 1979;17:307–26.
67. Copeland AR. Concepts in survival from lethal handgun wounds. *Am J Foren Med Pathol* 1985;6:175–9.
68. Vaquero J, Martinez R, Areitio E, Leunda G. Pneumocephalus after air rifle wound of the brain. *Neuroradiology* 1982;23:161–2.
69. Molina DK, Martinez M, Garcia J. Gunshot residue testing in suicides: Part I, Analysis by scanning electron microscopy with energy-dispersive x-ray. *Am J Foren Med Pathol* 2007;28:187–90.
70. Molina DK, Martinez M, Garcia J. Gunshot residue testing in suicides: Part II. Analysis by inductive coupled plasma-atomic emission spectrometry. *Am J Foren Med Pathol* 2007;28:191–4.
71. Baik SO, Uku JM, Sikirica M. A case of external beveling with an entrance gunshot wound to the skull made by a small caliber rifle bullet. *Am J Foren Med Pathol* 1991;12:334–6.
72. Sauer N, Dunlap SS. The asymmetrical remodelling of two neurosurgical burr holes: A case study. *J Foren Sci* 1985;30:953–7.
73. Hooper RE, Ruben RJ, Mahmood K. Gunshot injuries of the temporal bone. *Arch Otolaryngol* 1972;96:433–40.
74. Coe JJ. External beveling of entrance wounds by handguns. *Am J Foren Med Pathol* 1982;3:215–19.
75. Dixon DS. Pattern of intersection fractures and direction of fire. *J Foren Sci* 1984;29:651–4.
76. Garavaglia JC, Talkington B. Weapon location following suicidal gunshot wounds. *Am J Foren Med Pathol* 1999;20:1–5.
77. Kutscha-Lissberg E, Thetter O. Die Prognose selbstmoerderischer Schädelschussverletzungen. *Wien Med* 1985;120:871–2.
78. Hudson P. Multishot firearm suicide: Examination of 58 cases. *Am J Foren Med Pathol* 1981; 2:239–42.
79. Kury G, Weiner J, Duval JV. Multiple self-inflicted gunshot wounds to the head: Report of a case and review of the literature. *Am J Foren Med Pathol* 2000;21:32–5.
80. al-Alousi LM. Automatic rifle injuries: Suicide by eight bullets. Report of an unusual case and a literature review. *Am J Foren Med Pathol* 1990;11:275–81.
81. Oehmichen M, Meissner C, König HG. Brain injury after survived gunshot to the head: Reactive alterations at sites remote from the missile track. *Foren Sci Int* 2001;115:189–97.
82. Oehmichen M, Gehl HB, Meissner C, Petersen D, Hoche W, Gerling I, König HG. Forensic pathological aspects of postmortem imaging of gunshot injury to the head: Documentation and biometric data. *Acta Neuropathol* (Berl) 2003;105:570–80.
83. Smialek JE, Chason J, Kshirsagar V, Spitz WU. Secondary intracranial subarachnoid hemorrhage due to spinal missile injury. *J Foren Sci* 1981;26:431–4.
84. Adeloye A. Visual disturbances after missile head injuries. *Br J Ophthalmol* 1972;56:905–10.
85. Crockard HA, Brown FD, Calica AB, Johns LM, Mullan S. Physiological consequences of experimental cerebral missile injury and use of data analysis to predict survival. *J Neurosurg* 1977;46:784–94.
86. Zimmerman RA, Bilaniuk L, Bruce DA, Dolinskas C, Obrist W, Kuhl D. Computed tomography of pediatric head trauma: Acute general cerebral swellling. *Radiology* 1978;126:403–8.
87. Hatfield S, Challa VR. Embolism of cerebral tissue to lungs following gunshot wound to head. *J Trauma* 1980;20:353–5.
88. Neheme AE. Intracranial bullet migrating to pulmonary artery. *J Trauma* 1980;20:344–6.
89. Crockard HA. Early intracranial pressure studies in gunshot wounds of the brain. *J Trauma* 1975;15:339–47.
90. Refines HD, Dill L, Saad S, Hungerford GD. Neurogenic pulmonary edema and missile emboli. *J Trauma* 1980;20:698–701.
91. Levett JM, Johns LM, Replogle RL, Mullan S. Cardiovascular effects of experimental cerebral missile injury in primates. *Surg Neurol* 1980;13:59–64.

92. Salar G, Mingrino S. Traumatic intracranial internal carotid aneurysm due to gunshot wound: Case report. *J Neurosurg* 1978;49:100–2.
93. Kaufman HH, Sadhu VK, Clifton GL, Handel SF. Delayed intracerebral hematoma due to traumatic aneurysm caused by a shotgun wound: A problem in prophylaxis. *Neurosurgery* 1980;6:181–4.
94. Sadar ES, Jane JA, Lewis LW, Adelman LS. Traumatic aneurysms of the intracranial circulation. *Surg Gynecol Obstet* 1973;137:59–67.
95. Sternbergh WC Jr, Watts C, Clark K. Bullet within the fourth ventricle: Case report. *J Neurosurg* 1971;34:805–7.
96. Jackson FE, Back J, Pratt R, Fleming P. Artillery fragment in 3rd ventricle of brain producing delayed block of Iter of acqueduct of Sylvius: Case report. *Mil Med* 1971;136:900–3.
97. Greenwood JJ Jr. Removal of foreign body (bullet) from the third ventricle. *J Neurosurg* 1950;7:169–72.
98. Arasil E, Tascioglu AO. Spontaneous migration of an intracranial bullet to the cervical spinal canal causing Lhermitte's sign: Case report. *J Neurosurg* 1982;56:158–9.
99. Liebeskind AL, Anderson RD, Schechter MM. Spontaneous movement of an intracranial missile. *Neuroradiology* 1973;5:129–32.
100. Courville CB. Old missile wounds of the brain. *Bull LA Neurol Soc* 1956;21:49–74.
101. Dillman RO, Crumb CK, Lidsky MJ. Lead poisoning from a gunshot wound: Report of a case and review of the literature. *Am J Med* 1979;66:509–14.
102. DiMaio VJ, DiMaio SM, Garriott JC, Simpson P. A fatal case of lead poisoning due to a retained bullet. *Am J Foren Med Pathol* 1983;4:165–9.
103. Messer HD, Cerza PF. Copper jacketed bullets in the central nervous system. *Neuroradiology* 1976;12:121–9.
104. Ott K, Tarlov E, Crowell R, Papadakis N. Retained intracranial metallic foreign bodies: Report of two cases. *J Neurosurg* 1976;44:80–3.
105. Arseni C, Ghitescu M. Delayed post-traumatic cerebral abscesses due to retained intracerebral foreign bodies. *Acta Neurochir* (Wien) 1967;16:201–17.
106. Ecker AD. Bacteriological study of penetrating wounds of the brain from the surgical point of view. *J Neurosurg* 1946;3:1–6.
107. Cushing H, Eisenhardt L. *Meningiomas: Their Classification, Regional Behavior, Life History and Surgical End Results*. New York: Hafner, 1962.
108. Witzmann A, Jellinger K, Weiss R. Glioblastoma multiforme developing after a gunshot injury of the brain [Author's translation]. *Neurochirurgia* (Stuttg) 1981;24:202–6.
109. Salazar AM, Jabbari B, Vance SC, Grafman J, Amin D, Dillon JD. Epilepsy after penetrating head injury. I. Clinical correlates: A report of the Vietnam Head Injury Study. *Neurology* 1985;35:1406–14.
110. Leestma JE. Sudden unexpected death associated with seizures: A pathological review. In Lathers CM, Schraeder PL, eds., *Epilepsy and Sudden Death*. New York: Marcel Dekker, 1990, pp. 61–88.
111. Kaufman HH, Levin HS, High WM Jr, Childs TL, Wagner KA, Gildenberg PL. Neurobehavioral outcome after gunshot wounds to the head in adult civilians and children. *Neurosurgery* 1985;16:754–8.
112. Cernak I, Noble-Haeusslein LJ. Traumatic brain injury: An overview of pathobiology with emphasis on military populations. *J Cereb Blood Flow Metab* 2010;30(2):255–66.
113. Progressive Management. *2011 Complete Guide to IEDs-Improvised Explosive Devices: Enemy Tactics, Roadside Bombs, Counter-IED Targeting, Defeat the Device, Programs, Technologies, Afghanistan, Iraq, JIEDDO.* Version 1.1: Progressive Management Publications, 2011.
114. Ramasamy A, Harrisson SE, Clasper JC, Stewart MP. Injuries from roadside improvised explosive devices. *J Trauma* 2008;65(4):910–4.
115. Jones S, Israel P. *Others Unknown: Timothy Mc Veigh and the Oklahoma City Bombing Conspiracy*. New York: Public Affairs Books, 1998.

other syndromes [5], some of which have a genetic basis that may or may not have been precisely defined.

Seizure Etiology

An added form of classification and nomenclature takes into consideration the probable etiology of the seizure.

Genetic

While in the prior classification the term "idiopathic" epilepsy was employed and is still applicable, genetic defects have been identified that appear to be the cause of the seizure process and when known and supported by rigorous science, have a place in the classification of the epilepsies. It is here that the recently discovered "ion-channel-opathies" would appear.

Structural/Metabolic

It is now appreciated that many epilepsies have their basis in specific structural abnormalities in neural networks of the brain where anatomic/physiological organization of neurons is responsible for the seizure activity. An example would be congenital malformations, neoplasms and hamartomas, and destructive lesions that destabilize normal function. Some of these structural abnormalities are caused by genetic defects such as in the lipid storage diseases. Disturbances of metabolic processes such as hypoglycemia, hypoxia, and various toxic states would be examples of this etiology.

Unknown

The term *unknown* incorporates the prior "idiopathic" category in which the defect or defects that cause the seizure(s) is unknown.

Characteristics of Epileptic Seizures

The clinical features of epileptic seizures are highly variable, but certain generalizations can be made [3,5]. Many persons with epilepsy experience warning signals of an impending attack, often referred to as a prodrome or aura. The aura is actually an electrical event and can be observed in the EEG [6]. The aura may take the form of a change of mood, headache, minor twitching, nausea or a hollow feeling in the stomach, sweating or other autonomic events, visual or olfactory sensations, thirst or hunger, other sensory phenomena, or unusual behavior [7]. These symptoms may precede the clinical seizure by a few seconds, minutes, hours, or even days. In the case of GTCs (grand mal seizure), there may be no aura or warning of an attack. The classic GTC attack often begins with a loud cry, loss of consciousness, and tonic contraction of muscles leading to collapse, during which bladder and bowel control may be lost. Breathing may be suspended and cyanosis may occur. The pulse may be slow or rapid and bounding, and the blood pressure may be elevated. There may be profuse salivation and frothing at the mouth, and the lips and tongue may be severely bitten during the attack. The tonic phase lasts for a few seconds to a minute and gives way to a cyclical twitching of the body, the clonic phase, which may last for only a few seconds or many minutes. As the seizure ends, the patient may be drenched in sweat, be flaccid or atonic, and show Babinski signs. During the seizure, the individual is unresponsive to external events, and during the postictal phase he or she is usually stuporous and lethargic, may show transitory paralysis (Todd's paralysis), and may sleep for some minutes or longer. Because, during the attack, individuals are unconscious and unable to perform any meaningful or integrated function, they are very vulnerable to accidents. They may fall and injure themselves, drop smoking materials and ignite a fire, or injure others by falling or violent movements. If the seizure occurs in the workplace, the victim may injure himself or herself or others [8–10], and complex medical–legal issues may be raised. If the epileptic is driving an automobile, there may be a collision, and if he or she is bathing, swimming, or diving, he or she may drown [11–13]. GTC seizures may occur infrequently or scores of times each day. GTC is certainly one of the most obvious forms of epilepsy and is probably the most common clinically recognized form of epileptic seizure, accounting for at least 50% of adult cases [14].

Partial or focal fits are typified by the classic Jacksonian seizure, which usually begins with involuntary spasm of a body part, usually an extremity (fingers, hand, toes), but it may include the mouth. This leads to twitching of the affected part, which then spreads up the extremity or across the face (march of symptoms). The seizure may cease or may evolve into a generalized convulsive seizure. Consciousness may be preserved as long as the seizure is localized but is usually lost during the generalized phase. The progression of the seizure often appears to follow the cortical anatomy of the motor strip in ever-widening circles [3].

Other forms of focal fits may affect specific functional regions of the brain, such as the temporal and limbic regions, speech centers, and visual or auditory centers. These seizures may include complex visual or auditory hallucinations, which may be highly organized and stereotyped. There may be perceptions of odors or tastes, which are often unpleasant (burning rubber or flesh, fecal, or putrescent). Some seizures take the form of apparently aversive movements in which the head, an extremity, and the eyes are turned away from one position as if to avoid something. There may be stereotypic complex movements of hands, face, or head resembling a tic. These may include washing or wringing movements of the hands; grimacing or chewing movements; grasping or grabbing movements; flailing or flinging actions; and aimless walking, wandering, or apparent searching motions. Occasionally, verbal automatisms occur, in which nonsensical words are spoken or profanities or abusive words or phrases are yelled. Sometimes these focal events include spitting, involuntary urination, or defecation. Many of these types of seizure symptoms are typical for so-called temporal lobe epilepsy or psychomotor epilepsy. It is in these forms of epilepsy that apparently aggressive or threatening behavior may occur (discussed more fully below) [7–15].

One of the most common forms of epilepsy seen in children, and classified as a form of generalized seizure, is the so-called petit mal or *absence* attack [7]. The appearance of this form of seizure is usually as a staring episode, lasting 5–10 seconds. During this attack, the individual is not conscious of events around him/her and has total amnesia of what occurred during the attack. The individual does not fall but simply becomes immobile and resumes normal activity when the seizure ceases. Sometimes lip movements, grimacing, or small myoclonic jerks may accompany the fit. There is no residue to the seizure, and they may occur hundreds of times each day. Such seizures are often not recognized as such by the affected individual, members of the family, teachers, or friends, and affected individuals may often do poorly in school, apparently for lack of attention or "dreaming." Absence attacks usually affect only children and may begin without prodrome before age 15 years and usually stop by age 20; however, in about 50% of cases, they evolve into GTC seizures in later life. The causes of absence seizures are variable (about 50% are unexplained, 25% have a family history of seizures, and about 25% have some known or suspected underlying disease history, such as birth trauma, meningitis or encephalitis, head injury, or recent immunization) [12,16,17]. Diagnosis rests with a clinical examination and EEG studies, which are needed to demonstrate the typical pattern of abnormal electrical discharges in the brain.

When seizures occur with such frequency that no clear-cut separation between ictal and interictal periods is obvious, the individual is said to be in status epilepticus or continuous seizure state [18]. Status may occur in any form of epilepsy but is commonly associated with GTC seizures and carries a significant mortality of probably more than 10%. In other forms of epilepsy, the constant fits may not immediately be recognized or may present a particular clinical picture of sustained localized twitching of an extremity or face (epilepsia partialis continua). Status may be seen as the first manifestation of seizures, especially in brain trauma and birth trauma, but can be caused by fever, withdrawal of medication, alcohol withdrawal, hypertensive encephalopathy, severe metabolic or electrolyte imbalances, toxic states such as liver failure, Reye's syndrome, lead encephalopathy, and drug reactions. Status may be interrupted by administration of typical antiseizure medications, correction of the underlying disease process, and, in emergencies and intractable cases, general anesthesia [7,18]. The pathological consequences of status epilepticus are discussed below.

Causes and Precipitating Factors for Epilepsy

The neurophysiological basis for epilepsy is not known with certainty, but several classic theories have developed that seek to explain the phenomenon of the seizure. The centrencephalic theory of Penfield and Jasper [19] is based on the notion of functional collections of deep subcortical midline gray matter (the center of the encephalon) that project to and act to control the cerebral cortex and which, in a pathological manner, synchronize epileptiform discharges arising deep in the brain to produce generalized seizures in the cortex. An opposing theory, conceived by Gloor [3], is known as the reticulocortical theory, which proposes that a primary locus of unstable electrical irritability lies in the cerebral cortex that responds to normal driving influences from lower centers, specifically the thalamus and reticular formation, in an abnormal or dysfunctional way to produce the seizure. This latter theory is currently the more popular and seems to adequately explain, at least in part, some aspects of epilepsy. A greater understanding of the organization of the cerebral cortex anatomically and physiologically can explain many forms of seizures, especially those in which there is structural damage or malformation of the cortex and subcortex. Recurrent collateral fibers coming from the cortex extend into the subcortex and then arborize upward into the cortex again to inhibit neural activity. If these recurrent fibers are damaged by an infarction, demyelinating plaque, a tumor, or another destructive lesion, "release" of the cortex may occur and produce a seizure focus [5]. The many "mirror" connections of the cerebral cortex to the opposite hemisphere may also give rise to a kindling focus of instability, which in a way is a form of abnormal conditioning or learning, of course not subject to consciousness.

However, there are many aspects to epilepsy that challenge most theories. Among these is the finding that in chronic epileptics, an epileptogenic cortical region in the brain, as localized by EEG studies or electrode studies, seems to be a region of hypometabolism rather than hypermetabolism, as one might expect in the interictal state. Furthermore, there tends to be a mirror focus of hypometabolism in a comparable anatomic area on the opposite side of the brain in many epileptics. This region may not show electrical abnormality normally but may kindle or join in a seizure early, once the pathological complementary region begins to activate. This phenomenon suggests that patterning or abnormal learning may play a role in the evolution of the epilepsy and, if true, reinforces those who feel that clinical management of epileptics to achieve the fewest number of seizures possible, as early as possible, may prevent intractability later on.

The causes of epilepsy are numerous and include congenital malformations, perinatal brain injury, trauma, infection, metabolic abnormalities, vascular disease, hypoxia, electrolyte abnormalities and dehydration (hypernatremia, hyponatremia, hypocalcemia, hypomagnesemia), renal and hepatic failure, tumors, degenerative diseases, demyelinating diseases, alcohol and drug toxicity and withdrawal, hyperpyrexia, and various poisons [7].

On an anatomic or physiological level, information derived from experimental animals and resected portions (for relief of epilepsy) of human brain thought to be epileptogenic foci indicates that focal pathology may destabilize a population of neurons to the extent that they are hyperexcitable or unstable [20]. This instability may be able to propagate and cause other populations of neurons to fire erratically, extending the abnormality and eventually producing a clinical seizure. The inherent instability can be brought about by destruction of inhibitory fibers derived from recurrent collateral neurites from the population of neurons themselves or from a more distant site, as noted above. Other events may destabilize a group of neurons, such as impulses from facilitatory areas, interstitial electrolyte abnormalities that affect membrane channels, degenerative processes in dendritic or synaptic connections, or interference in the microenvironment brought about by inflammation, glial injury, or proliferation. Microenvironmental neurotransmitter excess (acetylcholine) or deficiencies (GABA or glycine) may also play a role in producing a destabilized cortical focus [7]. These mechanistic possibilities probably all play a role in the epileptogenic focus, and it should be obvious from an analysis of the known precursors to epilepsy that one or more of these processes probably operate.

Events That Precipitate Seizures

There are a number of precipitating events that can cause a seizure in an individual who has had a seizure before, and these are sometimes utilized in the clinical EEG laboratory to elicit abnormal discharges for diagnostic purposes. Some of these precipitating factors are important from a forensic standpoint [3,6]. It is well known that hyperventilation, presumably via production of transitory respiratory acidosis, can precipitate a seizure. This may be important in epileptic individuals who respond to stress or anxiety by hyperventilating. Sometimes emotional factors such as anger, excitement, or fright may precipitate a seizure by themselves via an unknown mechanism. It is well known that epileptics tend to have more seizures near times of awakening or going to sleep than at other times, and it is believed that far more seizures occur during sleep than during the waking state [3]. The role of the reticular activating system on seizure threshold, although poorly understood, is widely accepted.

Fever, especially in children, is another precipitating cause of seizures and an important heralding sign for the possibility of later development of a seizure disorder. Febrile convulsions occur mostly in children (males more frequently than females) between the ages of 6 months and 6 years and do not generally appear until body temperature is greater than 39.2°C (102°F) [7]. They are very common and are said to occur in more than 10% of all children [14]. There is often a strong family history of febrile convulsions, if not of symptomatic epilepsy. The febrile convulsion is usually generalized and results in unconsciousness and tonic–clonic twitchings lasting a few seconds or minutes, but occasionally it lasts longer and may even lead to status epilepticus. The potential for the child with a febrile convulsion to develop recurring seizures later on is difficult to measure and is more likely to occur in very young children with very high fevers, many febrile seizures, underlying brain pathology, or a strong family history of seizures. In any case, an incidence of 15%–40% of febrile convulsions is found in children who later develop symptomatic epilepsy [21]. This figure, however, does not provide a true risk measure for the child with a single febrile convulsion, and some workers [22] disclaim any correlation between the febrile convulsion and later epilepsy.

Some individuals experience increased seizure frequency during menstruation and in pregnancy, where some imbalance in fluid and electrolyte metabolism may be responsible but has not been proven. Some evidence exists that estrogen levels may play a role in seizure thresholds, and birth control pills have been the subject of some concern in this regard. The effect of pregnancy on epilepsy is not always predictable, and some women seem to stabilize their seizure frequency when pregnant, yet others do not. The occurrence of seizures in the terminal stages of pregnancy may be troublesome to differentiate from seizures associated with eclampsia. There is risk to the fetus should the mother have seizures when pregnant, with about twice the expected incidence of malformations and neonatal pathology as in the general population (7% vs. 3% incidence) [3]. This difference is probably due to hypoxia in connection with the seizures or possibly anticonvulsant medication. In this particular connection, there have been many suits alleging teratogenic effects of anticonvulsant drugs, in spite of the significant risk to both mother and child should medication be discontinued.

There are a number of persons with epilepsy who develop seizures in response to highly specific stimuli. These seizure disorders are often referred to as reflex epilepsies. Examples include photostimulative epilepsy produced by flickering lights from a television set, motion pictures, or strobe lights in a discotheque [23]. This propensity can cause seizures in automobile passengers and drivers as they pass flashing lights or as sunlight passes through trees or fences and may cause accidents. Other stimuli can be music or other sounds, such as explosions, voices, or a child's crying. These stimuli possess a heavy emotional connection and may evoke seizures via some psychophysiological mechanism. In the case of a child's crying, this may trigger a highly aggressive outburst (rage reaction) in some individuals, which is not a true epileptic seizure, that may result in the death of a child due to beating. When such cases are prosecuted and come to trial, the defense argument is often based on the premise of lack of culpability because of a seizure disorder that was triggered by an auditory stimulus. This argument is largely unfounded in fact (see below for a discussion of this issue).

A long list of normal activities that have been described to instigate or kindle seizures includes reading or writing [24], brushing one's teeth [25], eating (sometimes specific foods) [26], using the telephone [27], urinating [28], and many others. In some individuals, highly specific visual patterns, as in some types of fabric or wallpaper, may trigger a seizure [29]. Tactile sensations may also induce seizures in some persons; again, an emotional connection in many cases is inescapable and highly individualistic. There is very little opportunity for clinical pathological correlations in most cases, and little is known about the functional basis for such unusual forms of epilepsy. There could be forensic importance to such unusual cases in which an accident occurred to an epileptic person in a specific unusual circumstance, or perhaps the individual died suddenly and unexpectedly in an unusual situation.

The phenomenon of seizures in connection with alcohol withdrawal in heavy and chronic drinkers is well known [30]. However, the true incidence of the phenomenon is not known, but it is common enough that most major medical centers have treated hundreds of cases. The phenomenon usually occurs in persons who have abused alcohol for many years or have been drinking heavily for several days (a binge) and then stop. Usually the seizures are of a generalized nature (grand mal, or GTC) and tend to occur in the immediate 4-day period after alcohol withdrawal, but most are likely to occur within the first 24 hours of sobriety [31]. Seizures may be associated with other signs of alcohol withdrawal, such as tremulousness, agitation, hallucinations, or Wernicke–Korsakoff syndrome. Liver failure is not typical but may be present. About 10%–20% of victims of withdrawal seizures have had seizures before, but most have not. Occasionally, focal seizures may be seen that indicate some focal lesions in the brain, usually from prior head trauma. Although seizure associated with withdrawal from alcohol is the most common situation, seizures induced by acute alcohol intoxication, usually in a chronic drinker, may also occur. These are often referred to as rum fits. Regardless of the type of seizure or its circumstances, all the complications and sequelae of any form of seizure disorder may occur, including status epilepticus, sudden death, and subsequent development of chronic epilepsy. Electrocardiographic abnormalities are common in alcohol withdrawal states and in the presence of seizures [31] and may account for some deaths. The pathogenetic or physiological basis for alcohol-induced seizures is not known with certainty.

Trauma and Seizures

Trauma is a common inducer of the epileptic state, both as a primary acute event and later as a secondary chronic event due to cortical contusion. Seizures of any clinical form, but which are usually generalized, that occur early after trauma often connote a more serious head injury with a much higher fatality rate than if seizures occur later [32]. The seizure can be indicative of intracerebral hemorrhage or extracerebral hemorrhage (subdural or epidural hemorrhage) and is usually associated with prolonged loss of consciousness. The number of individuals who suffer early posttraumatic seizures is variable, ranging from about 2% to 10% or more [14,33]; however, children are three times more likely to suffer this complication than are adults (30% vs. 10%) [33]. Most posttraumatic seizures occur within the first day after the injury and are less commonly seen over the succeeding days and weeks. The period between a few weeks after the trauma and 1 year is usually characterized by very few new episodes of seizures. The development of seizures is an unwelcome complication in the acutely head-injured patient and, when status epilepticus occurs, can cause the death of the patient. The mechanism of seizure production is not always clear but may result from deafferentation of cortical tissue or irritation of instability in viable cortical tissue hemorrhage.

Late development of a seizure disorder after head trauma is also a widely recognized event but probably occurs in only 2%–5%, or more, of cases. Most seizures (about 80%) develop within 2 years of the trauma, but epilepsy may appear 5 or more years later in the remainder [32,33]. The development of late seizures is most likely correlated with brain contusions, previous seizures, and prolonged unconsciousness. About 10% of those who develop late seizures will have had only mild concussive symptoms initially, in which the true extent of the trauma was not recognized or did not produce major clinical symptomatology.

Epidemiological Considerations

Epilepsy is a significant public health problem in every country of the world; however, precise and comprehensive figures on incidence are difficult to obtain because definitions of what constitutes epilepsy vary and methods for obtaining data are not uniform. Nevertheless, if epilepsy is narrowly defined to be limited to chronic seizures only, and if unsubstantiated or sporadic cases and those that occur only during an acute illness (including febrile convulsions of childhood) are excluded, epilepsy prevalence in the general population ranges from 11 to 82 per 100,000 persons, with an average of about 30 per 100,000 [3,16,35]. When statistics are limited to children, the prevalence of seizures is much greater and approaches 2% in some series [34]. The often-quoted statistics derived from a comprehensive study of the population of Denmark [14] seem to indicate that about 1.27% of that population suffers from some form of seizure disorder. These figures are probably also realistic measures of prevalence for most Western countries as well.

The impact on society of epilepsy is significant because the benefits of useful skills are denied society because the affected individual is often compromised in regard to employment opportunities, families suffer increased stress and hardship in many cases, medical costs are often high, and there is a significant loss of life due to accidents, suicide, and complications of epilepsy. Surveys of several large series indicate that life expectancy for an epileptic is significantly diminished, and at any given age the death rate may be two to three times that of an age-matched nonepileptic control [36,37]. More striking are the figures of Rodin as noted by of Laidlaw and Richens [3], who reported that the median age at death for epileptics was between 32.5 and 43.5 years, and for nonepileptics in the general population was between 68.3 and 69.5 years of age. Other series report similar findings [10,12,38]. The causes of death in epileptic persons fall essentially into two groups as outlined by Zielinski [36], those due to or connected with the epilepsy itself and those due to other causes. Numbers must be interpreted with caution because epileptics in the general population may differ significantly from those in institutions, but it appears that about 30% of deaths in epileptics are related in some way to the seizure disorder. These causes include the following: about 25% death in status epilepticus, 20%–25% death due to accidents associated with seizure, and about 50% death occurring suddenly and unexpectedly, but the unexpected–unexplained group varies considerably from series to series [39].

Seizure-unrelated causes of death in epileptics include [11,36,38,40] the following: deaths due to cardiovascular disease, about 35%; brain tumor, 33%; stroke, 27%; visceral neoplasms not involving the brain, 19%; pneumonia, 19%; suicide, 16%; accidents not related to seizures, 9%; and a diverse group of causes not otherwise specified, about 30%.

Mechanisms of Death in Status Epilepticus

As mentioned above, status epilepticus (status) is a significant cause of death in chronic epileptics [12,18]. It occurs with varying frequency among the epileptic population and is said to account for between 2% and 4% of admissions for epilepsy to general hospitals, but some series report much higher relative incidences [41]. Status can be convulsive or nonconvulsive and take many clinical and electrical forms. The underlying causes for status are the following: unknown or idiopathic (12%–50%), tumors (3%–25%), head trauma (5%–39%), cerebrovascular disease (4%–15%), infections (2%–15%), and miscellaneous causes, including malformations and congenital diseases (9%–30%) [18,41]. The reasons why an individual with a seizure disorder may develop status are not clear, but generally the disease process is extensive, rendering larger populations of nerve cells unstable or depressing normal inhibitory influences to such a degree that the usual seizure is not damped in a reasonable period of time. Such systemic conditions as acidosis, hypoxia, severe electrolyte disturbances, and toxic states are especially important. The seriousness of status is not fully appreciated by many physicians, and some argue that it is only rarely fatal. Nevertheless, most series report at least a 10% mortality rate overall and much higher fatality rates in generalized convulsive status epilepticus. The prognosis is directly related to the speed with which control of convulsive status is achieved, and mortality rates of 30%–50% may occur in adults within 6 months after an episode, either secondary to the seizure or as a result of the underlying disease process. The complications and pathological consequences of status are significant [42–44] because many neurons, when subjected to constant electrical activity for 60 minutes or more, are likely to be irreversibly damaged and will probably die from excitotoxicity. The vulnerability to status is variable and related to many factors that include the size and biochemistry of the individual neuron, its anatomic location, degree of systemic hypoxia and metabolic abnormalities, degree and adequacy of cerebral circulation, and plasma glucose levels [18].

The most obvious gross pathological change in individuals who have died in status is brain swelling and even respirator brain changes. Microscopically, fields of neurons in the cerebral cortex will show ischemic cell changes and development of eosinophilia (red neurons). These cells, in time, will shrink, darken, and eventually be lost. Similar changes are seen in typical locations known for their vulnerability to hypoxia, such as the Ammon's horn of the hippocampus, cerebellar Purkinje cells, larger neurons of the dentate nucleus, globus pallidus, and putamen, and neurons of the reticular formation. If status was not immediately fatal, those areas of major neuronal loss will show gliosis and sometimes capillary proliferation if survival is prolonged. Occasionally, laminar or pseudolaminar necrosis of the cortex will be seen, as will necrosis of the globus pallidus or striatum. The pathology seen in human status can be duplicated in animals and appears to be due to metabolic exhaustion, acidosis, and ischemia in connection with edema.

Accidental Death Associated with Seizures

A survey of the various series that deal with causes of death in epileptics reveals that accidents are a significant death risk factor in chronic epileptics [12]. As mentioned previously, up to 25% of epileptic deaths presumed connected with the epilepsy are due to some form of accident [11,17]. These accidents include head and other trauma that occurs in the course of a seizure attack. Trauma can occur in the course of an attack when the individual becomes unconscious and flaccid while climbing stairs (hyperventilation) or in some precarious position (climbing a ladder or working in a hazardous environment) or while operating a machine or driving a vehicle (cycle, motorcycle, or automobile). Some epileptic attacks are very sudden and basically involve immediate collapse (Lennox–Gastaut syndrome, which mostly affects children) [45]. Many persons with epilepsy work in occupations that involve machinery or operation of motor vehicles and have concealed the existence of their seizure disorder from their employers, believing, probably erroneously, that they know when they are going to have a seizure so that they can protect themselves. Of considerable social concern in this context is the tremendous problem of the stigma and limitations often imposed on epileptic persons, which influences some sufferers to conceal their disease and often places physicians, employers, and governmental licensing agencies in a difficult position of judgment regarding what limitations can or should be imposed on a given epileptic to protect the individual and society. Suffice to it say that this issue regularly occurs in the analysis of industrial accidents and traffic fatalities with respect to liability and workers' compensation cases and sometimes in liability actions against physicians, using the argument that the physician failed to adequately warn the individual of risk in the operation of vehicles or of hazards in the workplace. In many states, there is a legal requirement that when a diagnosis of epilepsy is made, the physician must report this diagnosis to appropriate state authorities. The legal and ethical ramifications of this issue pose serious problems that have not been resolved.

Some epileptic persons in the course of their seizures may vomit and are at risk for aspiration, especially after eating a large meal. Aspiration and asphyxia and subsequent pneumonia are often reported as complications of seizures only but generally account for a small percentage of accidental epilepsy-related deaths [17]. It becomes very difficult to analyze such cases when the individual is psychotic and taking tranquilizing medication, which may cause suppression of guarding reflexes and allow massive aspiration, leading to sudden death without any obvious seizures having occurred [46]. Asphyxial deaths may also occur when bedclothes become entwined about the neck or when objects within the mouth, such as dental plates and bridgework, are aspirated in the course of the seizure. Usually careful examination at the scene of such a death provides valuable information about the immediate circumstances of death in such cases. The autopsy will also reveal objects within the pharynx or upper airway that caused the respiratory embarrassment.

Drowning is also a common accidental cause of death in epileptics. The circumstances of drowning almost always involve bathtubs but may involve swimming or SCUBA diving. The risk of bathtub drowning is significant enough [40] that some neurologists suggest that epileptics do not bathe on arising in the morning or before retiring in the evening because there is an increased likelihood of seizures at those times. Needless to say, recreational swimming and certainly scuba or free diving are significant hazards to the epileptic and should probably be avoided because hyperventilation, which is commonly employed in free diving and may occur during SCUBA diving when anxiety exists, is a common precipitating event for seizures [7]. When victims are found dead in bathtubs, immersed or not, the issue of drowning death logically arises. Generally, if the head is immersed, the possibility of drowning is high, but sudden reflex death (discussed below) may also have occurred [2]. The pathology of drowning is complex and not always as obvious to demonstrate in the autopsy as one might intuitively think. When water is found in the lungs or stomach or froth is found in the upper airway, these are often reliable stigmata of a drowning death; however, lack of these findings does not rule out a drowning death [47,48]. The standard works on forensic pathology should be consulted for a thorough discussion of this issue.

Sudden Unexpected (Unexplained) Death and Epilepsy

The phenomenon of sudden unexpected death and epilepsy (SUDEP) has attracted the attention of epileptologists, neurologists, and forensic pathologists but has been a subject of inquiry for many years, although for many years not generally appreciated by physicians or discussed in major works on epilepsy [3] or forensic pathology [49] as a significant complication of seizure disorders [17,50,51]. When some of the older statistics on causes of death in epileptics are examined, some 10%–30% apparently have occurred suddenly and unexpectedly and often show no solid anatomic cause of death after autopsy examination [51]. These cases have formed an enigmatic group that has challenged analysis for many years. In some reports, especially in the older literature, epileptics also suffering from mental illness seemed to suffer unexpected death [52]. In recent years, the role of phenothiazine tranquilizer medication in some of these deaths has been suggested [47,53] and further complicates analysis.

The SUDEP situation is not unlike the problem of sudden infant death syndrome (SIDS), in which one is confronted with an unexpected and apparently unexplained death, with few, if any, relevant autopsy or toxicological findings in someone who had a diagnosis of epilepsy. Thus, like SIDS, SUDEP is not a diagnosis but a label for a problematic death, the cause of which is unclear. The problem for a forensic pathologist when confronted with SUDEP cases is how to properly classify them as to cause and manner of death. A recent survey of pathologists and medical examiners by Schraeder et al. [53] revealed that the majority of pathologists recognized the SUDEP problem but did not incorporate it into the death certificate in some manner. Quite frequently, such deaths were signed out as "natural" or "undetermined," and sometimes as "accidental" when the death occurred in a bathtub but might not have been a typical drowning. It was highly variable that even a mention was made of epilepsy in contributing causes of death, an issue that is evident in many countries [54].

The SUDEP problem has been intensively studied over the past 25 years, and by now probably thousands of cases have been described and analyzed in many publications. There have been two multicontributor books (1990 and 2010) on the subject, each with extensive references and in-depth discussions of all aspects of the SUDEP phenomenon to which the interested reader is referred [55,56] From this author's perspective on the SUDEP problem, nearly 300 cases of this type were collected from the case material of the Cook County Medical Examiner's Office in Chicago between 1977 and 1987. The magnitude of the problem can be put into perspective by an analysis of case statistics that are not markedly different from those of other coroner's and medical examiner's facilities across the United States. In Cook County, Illinois, during the decade of 1977–1987, about 64% of the cases coming to the attention of the medical examiner involved deaths of natural causes. Of these, 9%–12% (or 600–800 cases per year) were sudden and unexpected deaths [57]. Of these 600–800 cases, 8%–12% (70 or more cases per year) occurred in persons who had a history of epilepsy and were found dead or seen to collapse and die suddenly and unexpectedly in connection with a seizure. This number, then, represents about 1%–1.5% of all natural deaths and 8%–12% of all sudden unexpected deaths and amounts to an incidence of at least one or two cases each week in Cook County, where the population at the time was about 5.25 million persons. This rate of occurrence has been steady for nearly 8 years. In a study in Dade County (Miami), Florida, Copeland [11] reported that about 2% of their natural or accidental deaths were linked with seizure disorders, including sudden unexpected deaths. To place this and other figures in perspective against the total number of persons with epilepsy, and to establish some measure of risk of sudden death, is difficult because precise figures for the number of epileptics in the United States in any age group are not accurately known, and the exact number of SUDEP cases is not known either. However, if the figures suggested by Juul-Jensen and Foldspang [14] for the Danish population (1.27% are epileptic) are extrapolated to America, then out of some 66,675 epileptic persons in Cook County, Illinois, at about 1 or 2 cases of SUDEP per week over a year, the risk may be 1 in 1282. A number of other studies from various countries have estimated of the frequency of SUDEP but expressed the frequency as 3.5 of 1000 patient-years [54], 1.21 of 1000 patient-years [58], a minimum of 0.54 of 1000 patient-years, and a maximum of 1.35 of 1000 patient-years [59].

If the study populations are stratified according to age range and the type of seizure disorder is considered (selecting for individuals between 20 and 40 years and those with some form of generalized epilepsy, usually GTC), the risk may be much greater, possibly reaching about 1 in 200–300 persons in this age group, taking no other variable into consideration. In view of the characteristics of the typical SUDEP victim, if other considerations, such as the prevalence of posttraumatic epilepsy, were known, the risks in such a group between the ages of 20 and 40 might be even more impressive.

From an analysis of nearly 100 carefully selected cases collected in 1983 by the Cook County Medical Examiner, the following statistics emerge to provide a profile of the typical SUD/epilepsy victim. The mean age was about 30 years. The usual victim was a black male who had had epilepsy for at least 1 year and probably for 10 years or more. The type of epilepsy was usually generalized and typically of the GTC variety and was usually not intractable and not very frequent (one or two seizures per year or less frequently). However, about 25% of cases had been noted to have had a seizure preceding death, which was often observed by someone. Although many of these seizures were typical, some appeared to be tonic only in comparison to the GTC-type seizures the individual usually suffered. The victim was usually found dead indoors (94%) and in bed (60%), with no signs of foul play or entanglement of bedclothes. The general autopsy usually does not reveal significant disease or an anatomic cause of death but, in most cases, shows pulmonary edema and congestion of the liver as well as a statistically significant greater than expected weight of the heart in the absence of obvious vascular disease. Cases in which the heart showed more than 25% narrowing of coronary arteries were excluded from consideration in this study. This, of course, means that probably some valid SUDEP cases were excluded, a problem in virtually all studies of the phenomenon.

More recent studies have shown that sex differences are probably valid (more males than females), ages vary considerably, compliance with anticonvulsant medications is highly variable from series to series, and there may be a greater incidence of SUDEP in persons taking multiple anticonvulsant medications and seizure intractability [60–66]. Some have suggested that certain anticonvulsant drugs may be accompanied by a greater incidence of SUDEP than others [67], but this is far from clear. It is probably a fair statement that regardless of the therapy (drugs or stimulating devices), SUDEP remains an ever-present risk to the person with epilepsy.

Neuropathological findings that could possibly explain the basis for the epilepsy were more common than in an unselected population of epileptics in that traumatic lesions were found in more than 30% of cases [68,69]. Overall, a structural lesion such as a traumatic contusion, tumor, malformation, subdural hemorrhage, or vascular malformation was found in 60%–70% of cases. Some evidence of brain swelling was commonly observed as evidenced by uncal grooving and tonsillar herniation. Cases with intracranial hemorrhages and other obvious intracranial anatomic causes for death were also excluded from consideration.

Postmortem toxicological studies in this same group revealed that 70%–80% of cases had either no detectable levels of anticonvulsants (phenobarbital or phenytoin) or subtherapeutic levels of these agents, whereas the remainder had therapeutic levels of at least one anticonvulsant at the time of death. Other studies have shown a wide variation in degree of compliance in SUDEP victims, calling into question a causal role for undermedication [64]. Blood alcohol levels were only occasionally found, but easily half of the cases had some history (reliable or not) of chronic alcohol use or abuse. Similar figures were reported by Copeland [11], which raises the question of the role of alcohol withdrawal seizures in the death [70]. Only an occasional case showed any level of opiates or other drugs of abuse, although histories of marijuana and other drug use were commonly obtained from friends or family members. There were three or four cases in which the individual was apparently addicted to caffeine (in the form of excessive coffee or cola drinking).

These observations provide a portrait of the typical SUDEP victim, but a considerable range is observed in the cases, to include children (often mentally retarded and severely epileptic), older individuals, and persons who apparently had only occasional seizures as well as those who had, by all definitions, intractable epilepsy. Of interest are the cases in which persons appeared to die in connection with their first or second seizure and those in which the entire seizure–death was observed. In many of these cases, the seizures were not classic GTC but often appeared to be tonic seizures only (as Freytag and Lindenberg [17] have also reported), even when a history of GTC epilepsy was obtained. In such cases, the individual collapsed and could not be revived, even when persons trained in cardiopulmonary resuscitation (CPR) were present [51]. In other cases, CPR was carried out for protracted periods, and when cardiac action could be restored, the individual was usually in a coma and required ventilatory assistance until death was declared within a few days. Such individuals usually had respirator brains. The finding that most of the victims were found dead in bed or in the bedroom may correlate with the tendency for seizures to occur more frequently in connection with going to sleep or awakening. The fact that few victims, who ordinarily were known to be drinkers, had blood alcohol levels at autopsy may speak highly for the possibility of alcohol withdrawal seizures, especially in the face of low or nonexistent anticonvulsant medication.

The mechanisms behind SUDEP are difficult to substantiate because they involve physiological processes that do not declare themselves directly in the autopsy or in the histological slides. Nevertheless, several mechanisms have been postulated based on clinical observations, neuroanatomical and neurophysiological studies in animals, and pathological observations. These mechanisms may involve the following [51,67–69,71–76]:

1. Sympathetic autonomically induced irreversible cardiac arrhythmia
2. Parasympathetic (vagal) induced cardiac bradycardia or standstill
3. Combined sympathetic and parasympathetic discharges reaching the heart
4. Respiratory failure, possibly due to right heart failure and irreversible apnea
5. Combinations of cardiac arrhythmia and apnea with hypoxia and ischemia, which then lead to further cardiac dysfunction and death

6. Sudden and fatal neurogenic pulmonary edema with cardiac failure
7. Inherited defects in brain and/or heart membrane ion channel function

Although some epileptic patients have been shown to have apparent vagal stoppage of the heart during seizure activity, in most such cases heart action returns spontaneously, apparently due to sympathetic or inherent cardiac pacemaker override [2,77,78]; these cases are probably very rare. The more commonly observed event is that some sympathetic component of the seizure induces an arrhythmia. Such an occurrence has been documented many times and is probably the most likely basis for SUDEP. Recent experimental data [67] in cats treated with subictal doses of metrazol show that electrical but not muscular seizures (by EEG examination) are produced and also a disturbance of the normal symmetrical sympathetic discharges to the heart by sympathetic nerves. Furthermore, additional data by Lathers and Schraeder [68] demonstrated "lock-step" synchrony between induced cerebral ictal discharges and both sympathetic and vagal impulses reaching the heart, as well as paradoxical responses in blood pressure in experimental animals treated with metrazol. These experiments illustrate not only that ictal discharges can produce cardiac and cardiovascular effects but also that an overt muscular seizure is not required for this to occur. An additionally captivating notion is that chronic sympathetic stimulation (stress) to the heart may induce structural lesions that could form a nidus for a later fatal arrhythmia [79–82]. It is unfortunate that no detailed study of the hearts of SUDEP victims has been undertaken to determine if there is any structural basis in the conducting system or of the myocardium or endocardium for what is probably a fatal cardiac arrhythmia in such cases. Conduction system abnormalities have been found in many kinds of sudden death that may parallel the SUDEP phenomenon [83]. It may well be that some individuals have unsuspected "ion-channel-opathies" that could respond poorly under an onslaught of impulses reaching the heart from the brain [84]. Recent studies have identified a number of genetic defects affecting membrane ion channels in the heart and brain that may be involved in SUDEP [74,76,85–90].

A difficult question to answer both experimentally and pathologically is the role of possible apnea in SUDEP. The problems here are similar in complexity to those involved in interpretation of SIDS, in which apnea is felt to be the mechanism of death [91–93]. If apnea plays any role at all, it is probably a secondary one as a part of a purely tonic or inhibitory seizure in which myocardial ischemia may lead to a fatal arrhythmia with or without overlying sympathetic stimulation. The pathological substrate for this event is obviously very difficult to determine by ordinary techniques. Furthermore, the role of neurogenic pulmonary edema and possibly acute cor pulmonale in the syndrome has not been determined but could be significant.

The forensic evaluation of sudden deaths associated with seizures or in persons known to have epilepsy is a challenging one and is often met with skepticism by clinicians, but with the greater experience with the syndrome of many forensic pathologists and epileptologists, it is gradually being accepted as a possibility. To aid in the investigation of such deaths, the reader is referred to Figure 9.1, which illustrates a checklist employed by the scene investigators of the Office of the Medical Examiner of Cook County (Chicago) when SUDEP deaths against a backdrop of epilepsy are encountered [84]. This checklist facilitates the interview process and provides valuable information to the forensic pathologist in further investigating the death and determining its cause, and others are encouraged to employ it for their own uses.

EPILEPSY DEATH CHECK-LIST

Case No.: Name:

Investigator: Date/Time:

Location:

Where victim's body found

Information provided by:

How long did victim have seizures?
How often?
When was the last one?
Was a seizure observed before death?
Did victim take medication for seizures? Was a brain wave test (EEG) ever done?
Hospital/Clinic where treated for seizures?

Doctor who had treated victim: Name:
Address/Phone:

Did victim:
( ) Drink heavily? ( ) Use drugs? ( ) Use marijuana
( ) Have prior head injury? ( ) Have a brain operation?
( ) Have a brain disease? ( ) Have meningitis/encephalitis?
( ) Any chronic health problem? Give details
( ) Take insulin (diabetes)

Additional Information:

Did victim take any of the following medications ? (all that apply)
( ) Dilantin ( ) Phenobarbital ( ) Mysoline ( ) Tegretol
( ) Depakene ( ) Zarontin ( ) Celontin ( ) Lamictal ( ) Other:

Additional Information:

Description of seizures: (check or YES or NO to all that apply)
( ) Stiffening ( ) Violent jerking ( ) Mild twitching ( ) Collapse
( ) Loud cry ( ) Unconsciousness ( ) Staring spells ( ) of one side
( ) Loss of bladder/bowel control ( ) Biting of tongue/cheeks
( ) Repeated automatic or senseless movements of hands, arms, legs
( ) Facial movements-grimacing-chewing movements, etc.
( ) Grogginess-sleeping after attacks
( ) Did victim have any warning of attack?
( ) Could anything bring on an attack?
( ) Could anything prevent an attack?

Additional Information:

Information on labels of any medication found at scene: Pharmacy, Rx number, Doctor, etc:

Figure 9.1 "Check sheet" once employed at the Office of the Medical Examiner, Cook County, Chicago, Illinois, by the field investigators when investigating the scene of a death in which it appears that the victim suffered from epilepsy and died suddenly and unexpectedly. This form has proven valuable in securing the most vital information regarding the death so that the forensic pathologist may make a proper determination in the case. (From Leestma JE, Hughes JR, Teas SS, Kalelkar MB, *Am J Foren Med Pathol* 6, 215, 1985. With permission.)

Pathology of Epilepsy

In the majority of cases of persons who are epileptic and who come to autopsy, there is no obvious gross or microscopic pathology that is diagnostic, and it is said that only about 10%–12% of brains from epileptics will show lesions that could reasonably be expected to have produced the seizures [94]. Remote traumatic lesions were most commonly found and have been reported in 25%–36% of chronic epileptics [84]. It appears that the frequency of traumatic lesions as a cause of epilepsy may have decreased in recent years; nevertheless, traumatic contusions, most commonly of the contrecoup type, are still probably the most common obvious lesions found at autopsy in epileptics who died from all causes. When cases are selected in which SUDEP has occurred, the prevalence of traumatic lesions appears to be increased over that normally expected for epileptic persons autopsied after dying under other circumstances [51,65].

To be sure, many other lesions are encountered in the brains of epileptics at autopsy, which can be causative or associated in some fashion with the seizure disorder. These include Ammon's horn sclerosis (Figure 9.2); ectopic gray matter (Figure 9.3) and other congenital malformations; vascular anomalies (Figure 9.4); old infarctions, tumors, or cysts (Figure 9.5); degenerative diseases, the effects of metabolic diseases, infectious and parasitic processes, and old cerebral contusions (Figure 9.6); brain injuries (Figure 9.7); foreign bodies (Figure 9.8), including fragments of weapons or bone or bullets (Figures 9.9 and 9.10); chronic subdural hematomas; and many others. Often when the clinical parameters of the seizure disorder are known, the structural lesions correlate rather well with the epileptogenic foci observed with the EEG or by means of clinical signs of symptoms. Thus, experience in the case material has allowed interpretation of the sorts of lesions that can apparently cause epilepsy and provide a base of information against which subsequent cases can be compared mechanistically and etiologically. Unfortunately, precise physiological correlations are not usually possible unless more involved morphological methods than are usually available are employed to show the pathology of neuronal connections in the presence of any given lesion, and most interpretations are, of necessity, circumstantial.

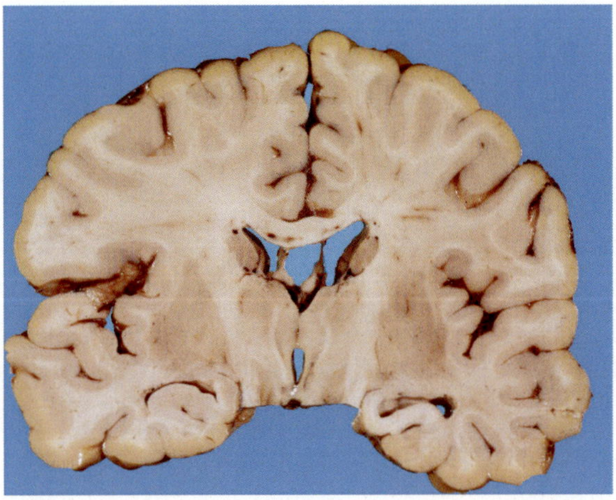

Figure 9.2 This coronal section of the brain from a victim of SUDEP illustrates a right medical temporal lobe (hippocampus) sclerosis. Note comparison with the left hippocampus, which displays the typical Ammon's horn configuration. An incidental finding is a cavum of the septum pellucidum.

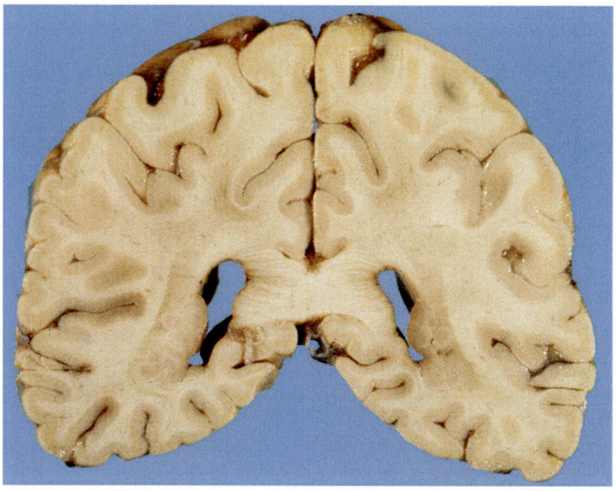

Figure 9.3 This coronal section of the brain from a victim of *absence* epilepsy who died in status epilepticus illustrates bilateral subependymal ectopic gray matter collections. Such collections often extend forward and involve the hippocampus. This individual had had behavioral problems for many years. Deposits of tissue like this are occasionally observed in epileptic persons who die in single-vehicle car crashes, possibly following a seizure.

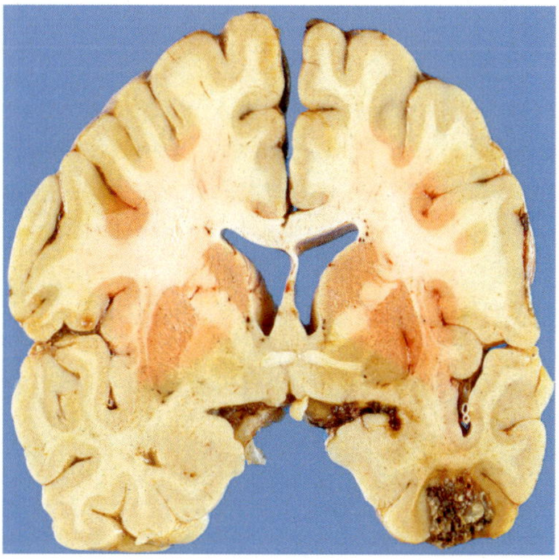

Figure 9.4 This coronal section of the brain of a SUDEP victim, a middle-aged female found dead at home, illustrates a right inferior temporal cryptic arteriovenous malformation that had clearly bled in the past and produced subarachnoid staining at the base of the brain and within the malformation. The proximity of this anomaly to the hippocampal formation likely caused her epilepsy.

Traumatic Lesions in Epilepsy

Traumatic lesions in epileptic persons are usually old contusions that are located most frequently at the base of the brain on the orbital frontal gyri or the temporal lobe tips and inferior surface of the temporal lobe (Figure 9.6). The location of many of these contusions suggests that they arose as contracoup lesions or as gliding contusions as the brain vibrated over bony structures in the base of the skull during head trauma, most usually associated with falls rather than blows. The mechanisms of these contusions are described in

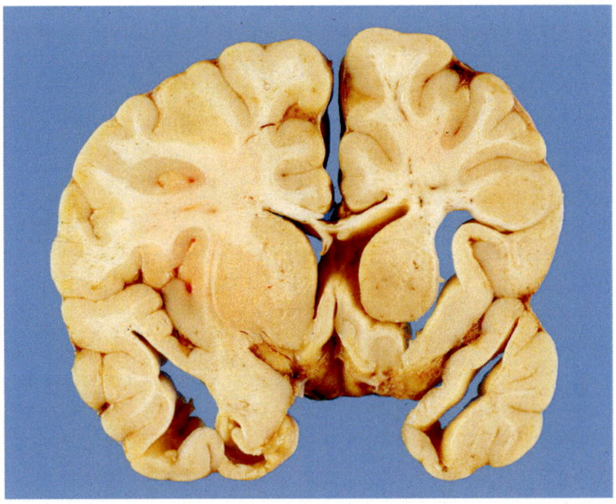

Figure 9.5 This coronal section of the brain of a 6-year-old Hispanic female who was found dead in bed about 90 minutes after having a GTC seizure that lasted for about 20 minutes. The child had been epileptic since she was a baby. There were bilateral chronic subdural hematoma membranes and the ventriculo-peritoneal shunt in place. The original history is not known but abuse was strongly suspected. These clefts, although not hemosiderin stained, suggest old contusional tears from severe deformation of the brain, but may have occurred after severe cerebral edema and electrolyte imbalances. (Courtesy of Dr. Mitra Kalelkar, Office of the Medical Examiner, Cook County, IL.)

Chapter 6. Grossly, these lesions, like any other cortical contusion, are excavated, yellow-brown or orange in color, and tend to reside on the crowns of gyri rather than in the sulci. They do not follow vascular territories and are thus distinguished from infarcts. Sometimes the lesions are subtle but may be extensive and severe. At times contusions may be found over the surface of the brain, especially laterally along the Sylvian triangle or in other locations, where they may be due to contracoup or direct effects of blows (coup lesions).

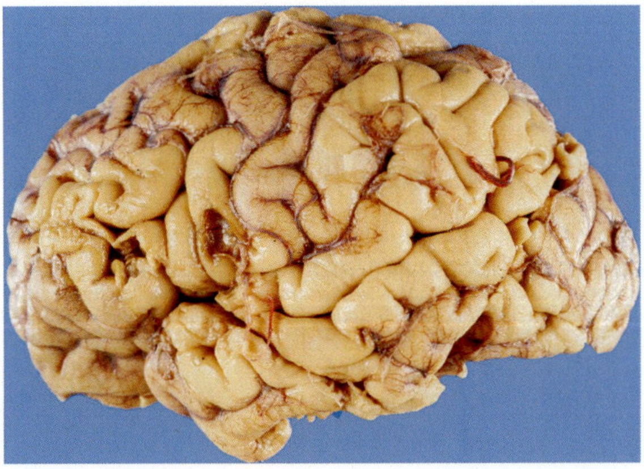

Figure 9.6 This is the brain of a 33-year-old African American man who was found on the floor beside a couch where he had fallen asleep. CPR was administered but he died in hospital the next day without regaining consciousness. He had a history of alcoholism, smoking marijuana, and poor compliance with anticonvulsant medications. Numerous old traumatic brain contusions are illustrated here. There was no anatomic cause of death in the autopsy. (Courtesy of Dr. Yuksel Konacki, Office of the Medical Examiner, Cook County, IL.)

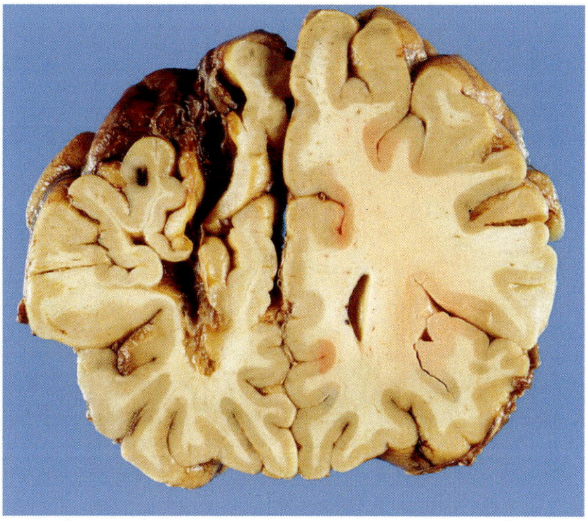

Figure 9.7 This is a coronal section of the brain of a 34-year-old white male who was found dead in bed. He had been an epileptic since age 9 when he was struck by a vehicle while riding his bicycle, suffering an intracerebral hematoma. He had GTC-grand mal epilepsy under poor control. He was apparently addicted to cola soft drinks that would occasionally precipitate seizures. He was very obese and had a 675-g heart but was found to have fresh bites on his tongue. (Courtesy of Dr. Mitra Kalelkar, Office of the Medical Examiner, Cook County, IL.)

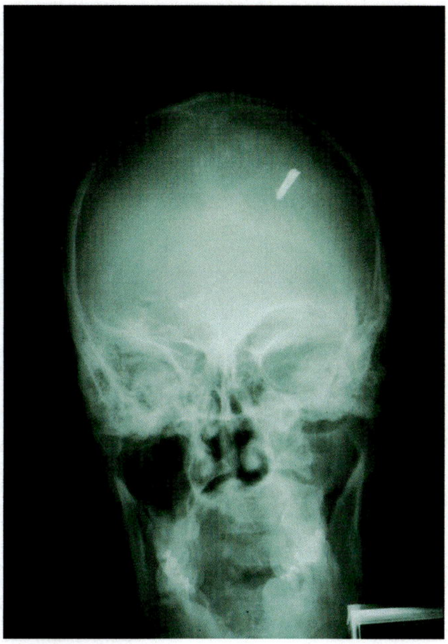

Figure 9.8 This plain radiograph of the head of a 42-year-old chronic epileptic. He had been incarcerated on numerous occasions and was a known epileptic who did not take his anticonvulsant medications. It is not known how this object came to lie in his brain. At autopsy he had bilateral chronic subdural hematomas, and moderate cerebral atrophy. The object resembled a crudely sharpened nail not untypical for a jail house "shiv" or "shank." (Courtesy of Dr. Shaku Teas, Office of the Medical Examiner, Cook County, IL.)

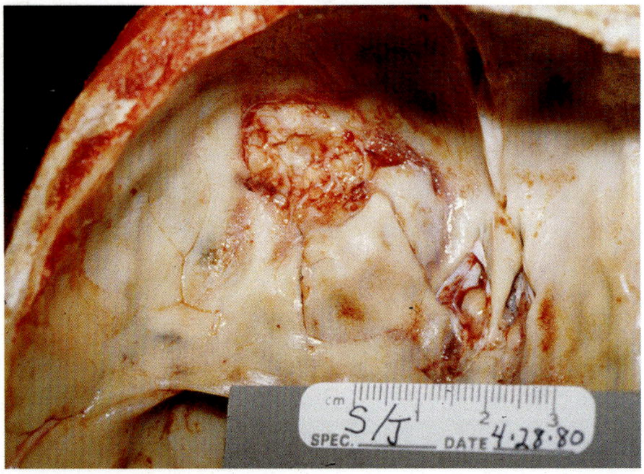

Figure 9.9 This 25-year-old African American female had been the victim of a rape/assault and had been shot several times two months before. One of the gunshot wounds was to the left eye and penetrated the orbital roof and inferior frontal lobe. A dural patch of this wound is illustrated. Her course was complicated by seizures. She was found dead in a bathtub. It was unclear if she had drowned or died from a seizure. (Courtesy of Dr. Robert J. Stein, Office of the Medical Examiner, Cook County, IL.)

The relationship between basal brain lesions and epilepsy is probably related to the inherently lower seizure threshold of these areas as compared with other cortical regions, where lesions are less likely to be associated with seizures. The reasons why basal cortical regions are more epileptogenic than others are not known, but this has been shown in many experimental models [94]. As has been mentioned before, traumatic lesions probably produce irritable or unstable electrical responses by a process of inhibitory influence release or by deafferentation of neuronal populations by a destructive lesion [94,95]. The most likely process is that the cortex or immediate subcortex is damaged, disconnecting recurrent collateral axons that have an inhibitory function on the neighboring cortex rendering populations of neurons unstable. It is possible that the neuronal electrolyte environment,

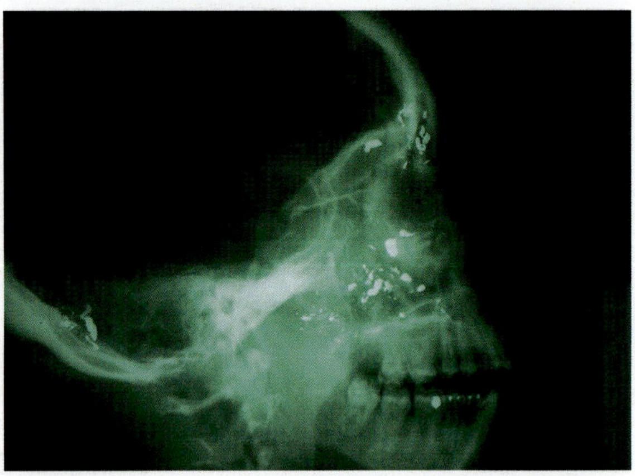

Figure 9.10 This is a lateral plain radiograph of the head of the victim in the case of Figure 9.9, showing many metallic fragments in the facial skeleton as well as intracranially, which is typical of many intracranial gunshot wounds. (Courtesy of Dr. Robert J. Stein, Office of the Medical Examiner, Cook County, IL.)

once injury has occurred, has been altered and that glial reaction may further modify this environment such that instability results. The reason why seizures do not tend to develop until many months or years after trauma may be that glial scars often take months or years to mature, and whatever the effect caused by the scar is only manifested after a long delay.

Ammon's Horn Sclerosis

As illustrated in Figure 9.2, the hippocampal formation contains a region known as Ammon's horn (*cornu ammonis*, CA). It has been recognized for many years that chronic epileptics may show neuronal loss and replacement gliosis in and about this structure [96, 97]. The most common location for neuronal loss is in the CA1 section of the hippocampus (Figure 9.11), also known as Sommer's sector, the region most commonly affected by hypoxia, whereas other portions may or may not be spared. This difference in sensitivity suggests to some workers that the lesion in epileptics may be etiologically separable into the lesion due to hypoxia or uncal herniation in response to anoxia or birth injury (CA1) and the lesion that is caused by the seizure activity itself (CA3) [42,94]. There is some experimental support for this distinction, but it is not universally recognized by all authorities, and much argument still exists concerning the nature of the hippocampal lesion as a cause of epilepsy, an effect of epilepsy, or both [94,96]. In any case, some degree of hippocampal pathology is found in a high percentage of chronic epileptics microscopically. Meldrum and Corsellis [94], for example, have reported that 50%–60% of their cases showed lesions in one or both hippocampi, whereas Spielmeyer [98] indicated that perhaps 80% of cases had lesions. In general, gross evidence of Ammon's horn sclerosis and shrinkage may be found in 5%–10% of cases, and when it is found, it may be bilateral about 2% of the time. When this has occurred, the affected individual is usually neurologically and cognitionally compromised.

The typical gross appearance is illustrated in Figure 9.2, where the Ammon's horn is collapsed and shrunken and may have a firm, white appearance as contrasted with the normal structures. Microscopically, neurons are gone, and there are varying amounts of astroglial scarring present. Neuronal loss may occur elsewhere in the brain, including the parahippocampal regions, amygdala, thalamus, and portions of the cerebral cortex,

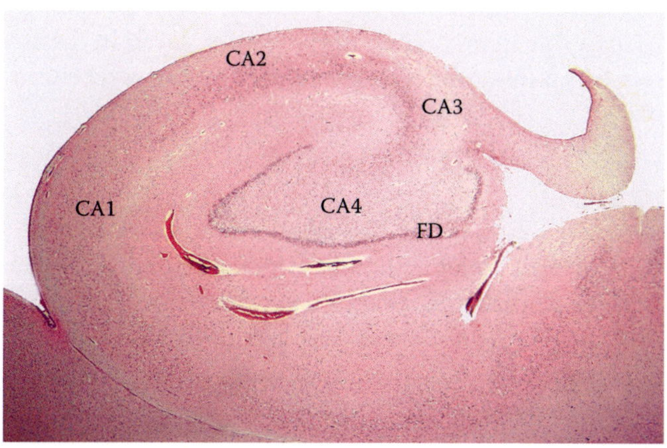

Figure 9.11 This low power photomicrograph illustrates a normal hippocampal formation and the various sectors beginning with the fascia dentata (FD), the CA4 to CA2 sectors, and finally the Sommer's sector, CA1 where the effects of hypoxia are most typically found.

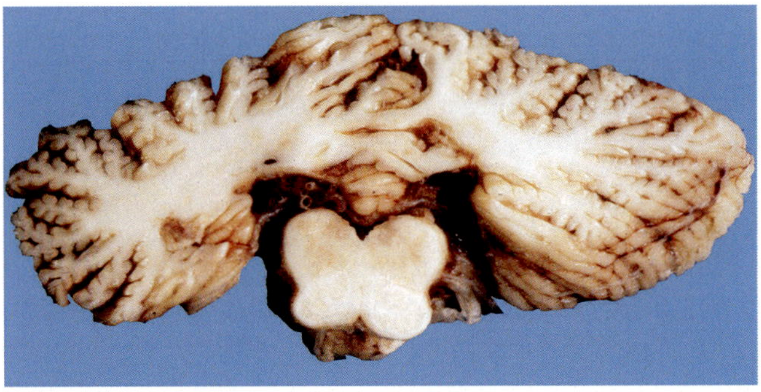

Figure 9.12 This horizontal section of the cerebellum that includes the medulla illustrates profound pan-cerebellar atrophy typical for that found in individuals with chronic and intractable epilepsy. The cerebellum is shrunken to perhaps half its normal mass and is hard and rubbery to the touch. This condition is said to be the effect of prolonged phenytoin administration, but was described in epileptics well before this drug was discovered.

usually with replacement gliosis easily demonstrable with glial fibrillary acidic protein immunostaining. The increasing employment of surgical techniques for epilepsy has provided specimens that show a spectrum of pathology of a chronic nature. The problem of hemiatrophy and intractable seizures is discussed in Chapter 4.

Cerebellar Degeneration with Epilepsy

A common finding in severe chronic epileptics, often those whose seizures have been intractable and resistant to medication, is atrophy of the cerebellum, as illustrated in Figure 9.12. Some degree of cerebellar damage has been reported in up to 45% of cases of chronic epileptics, but its etiology is very much in doubt [94]. To some workers, the often-profound atrophy is thought to be due to an idiosyncratic reaction to chronic treatment with phenytoin anticonvulsants, whereas others interpret the change as being secondary to some effect of the seizure disorders themselves, such as hypoxia or repeated brain swelling with increased intracranial pressure in connection with hypoxia of the seizures. This last assertion is supported by the fact that cerebellar degeneration in epileptics had been reported long before anticonvulsant medications were available; nevertheless, the question has not been resolved. Perhaps a role in exacerbating epilepsy is played in the atrophic cerebellum; however it occurred, it is a loss of inhibitory control by the cerebellum on the brain as a whole.

Chaslin's Gliosis

More than 100 years ago, Chaslin [99] described a process of subpial gliosis of areas of the cerebral cortex in chronic epileptic brains, which he interpreted as being etiologically important in the seizure disorder. Since that time, others, including Spielmeyer [98] and Scholz [20], have debunked this notion and have regarded this reaction as secondary to events in the seizure disorder, such as hypoxia or vascular spasm with ischemia or possibly prior subarachnoid hemorrhage suffered in cranial-trauma-associated falling while having a seizure. In the last 25 years, little attention has been paid by most neuropathologists to this lesion, and most are not familiar with the term. The importance of this reaction remains obscure, but it can regularly be observed in the hippocampal and inferior temporal cortex, usually in severe, chronic epileptics whose disease has incapacitated them.

Systemic Pathology Associated with Epilepsy

Insofar as traumatic injury might be considered a pathological consequence of epilepsy, fractures, contusions, lacerations of the tongue and lips, and other injuries may be seen, as alluded to above, and probably represent the most common form of extra–central nervous system (CNS) lesion encountered. Nevertheless, it is possible that seizure disorders may foster the development of lesions in organs other than the brain. Such an issue has often been raised in connection with the cardiovascular system in the context of sudden unexpected death and seizures. Very little credible work has been done on this issue, but some studies propose that myocardial or subendocardial injury may be caused by seizures or the stress of them [7,71,100]. In a similar vein, the role of seizures in the production of pulmonary edema is also a possible example, although it is poorly understood at present.

One of the most common systemic reactions associated with epilepsy is the reaction to one or more of the medications that were prescribed, not to any obvious effect of seizure disorders. Prominent among these reactions are those caused by phenytoin and include gingival hypertrophy, coarsening of facial features, masculinization and hirsutism, and blood dyscrasia [3,101]. In the case of valproic acid, hepatic toxicity and thrombocytopenia are well known. There are many functional disturbances, usually in the cardiovascular system, produced by other medications, such as carbamazepine, ethosuximide, the benzodiazepines, and phenobarbital-like drugs, which have no obvious pathological stigmata. The role of antiepileptic drugs in pregnant women [60–63] and possible effects on the developing fetus remain an issue for many and have led to discontinuation of medication in some cases, where later the woman died with SUDEP. Litigation has occurred in these cases, usually against the neurologist or family practitioner, but in several cases with which the author is familiar, the plaintiffs were unsuccessful in proving their case that SUDEP was caused by discontinuation of the anticonvulsant medication.

Epilepsy in Relation to Criminal Acts

Epilepsy as a basis for criminal behavior is frequently invoked as a legal defense, and in some sensational cases where an assailant has been killed or committed suicide after commission of a violent crime, legal authorities may look to the forensic pathologist (and by extension to the neuropathologist) to provide clinical–pathological and morphological explanations for the criminal acts performed. Sometimes the pathologist is asked to determine if a seizure disorder was involved in the violent acts of a criminal, dead or alive [102,103]. These issues are almost always beyond the ken of even the most informed forensic pathologists and will probably also confound most neuropathologists. In any case that might occur, there is no possibility of reliable clinical pathological correlation because the relation between structure and function in the nervous system at the level at which most pathological examinations can be carried out is circumstantial at best. That is not to say that no interpretations are possible, but when such an attempt is made, one must carefully take into consideration all available information and probably consult with experts before formulating a conclusion.

In an effort to clarify the question of epilepsy as a cause of criminal acts, specifically of homicide, in 1981 a panel of epileptologists [104] undertook to examine what evidence could be marshaled to support the contention that individuals may be caused to commit homicide while having a seizure. The conclusion of this panel was that true aggressional seizures are very rare, if they occur at all, and that when an individual is truly having an epileptic attack, little highly organized activity is possible. In support of this conclusion, several cases were presented in which the manifestations of the seizures involved rather complex behavior, which in most cases was rather stereotyped and was probably some form of complex partial seizure (temporal lobe in nature). The ictal behavior often involved an attempt by the seizure victim to grasp, hold, or clutch another individual. Sometimes an attempt may be made to reach out and scratch the face, grasp eyeglasses, or reach for the eyes of another during the attack. Why there is a proclivity to reach out and seek the eyes of another individual during such seizures is a very curious issue, perhaps underscoring the strong emotional overlay that occurs in some epileptics. At times some individuals in the seizure state shout obscenities, spit, assume threatening postures, flail about, upset furniture and pull down drapes, or kick at objects or persons near them. Biting behavior in the postictal state in temporal lobe epilepsy is another aspect of the problem [105]. In most instances, these forms of behavior are considered involuntary automatisms, and it can be argued how purposeful they are. In general, such behaviors are short-lived, usually less than 60 seconds, and always accompanied by electrical evidence of seizure activity, which often preceded and followed the overt activity. It is obvious that individuals who had such attacks might be interpreted by uninformed witnesses as dangerous if not homicidal, and it is acknowledged that under some circumstances bodily injury to another could result, but that willful homicide could be accomplished is highly doubtful.

More problematic are the cases in which an individual known to have temporal lobe/partial/complex seizures becomes aggressive and violent when postictal and can attack or appear to attack persons near him or her, including family members and individuals who are called on to render assistance [106], including police, emergency personnel, and firemen. In these circumstances, efforts at restraint may be met with escalating violence on the part of the seizure victim and may result in his or her injury or death [107]. Persons who have exhibited this type of behavior have been studied and reported under various labels, such as dyscontrol syndrome, limbic or frontal lobe seizures, and rage or panic attacks [108–111]. It is curious that in some cases, medication with various anticonvulsants, including carbamazepine, has diminished aggressional attacks and postictal behavior [101].

Some very unusual cases have been reported in the literature in which alleged epileptic attacks have culminated in stabbings of individuals, but it is highly doubtful that such sustained, goal-directed, and purposeful acts occurred in the seizure state; instead, they were likely conscious acts performed by a disturbed individual who may also have had epilepsy [102–105,107–112]. There also remain the cases reported by Gunn and Fenton [102], where automatic criminal acts [15,113] were alleged to have occurred during seizures; however, most current analyses of such cases run counter to the notion that whereas complex automatisms may be acted out during temporal lobe seizures [114,115], goal-directed, complex, and sequential acts are probably not possible under such circumstances and that a functional, much less a structural, basis for such behavior is unlikely [116–118]. When the rare case has been studied with imaging methods, generally structural lesions are rarely found [119] apart from the occasional lesion in the cortex or elsewhere that has a known history. One interesting case is that of a man who had postictal rage and aggressive behavior and was shown to have neuronal ectopias in the ventricle [120]. Another curious but interesting report is that of Caldwell and Little [120], who reported lesions in the limbic systems of eight aggressive and unmanageable dogs. More sophisticated imaging studies have been used as a basis for homicide defense, but there are many controversial aspects to these cases [121]. In cases of Asperger's syndrome and in cases of autism, violence and homicides have occurred, but these are uncommon [122,123]. In cases of mental subnormality with or without severe behavioral symptoms, violent acts against others can occur, as can violence in individuals who apparently have experienced a dissociative reaction, perhaps in connection with posttraumatic stress disorder, which always raises the issue of responsibility for the assailant [124–127].

That behavioral disease may be present along with epilepsy is well known, and the two conditions may have considerable interaction in the dynamics of both illnesses, which often makes interpretation and diagnosis difficult. Pathological correlations in such cases are usually conjectural at best and should be avoided in most instances, although the limbic system is well known to have profound influences on mood and rage reactions [128,129]. When lesions are found in persons who have committed violent crimes, the issue of pathological/clinical correlation becomes important forensically. This issue is discussed below.

Cognitional Disorders

There are many aspects to human mentation that may become disturbed in the course of illnesses, some of which may have an observable pathological and reasonably well-understood pathophysiological basis [130–132]. The forms of higher-order neural dysfunction that are commonly recognized and, to some degree, have morphological or known physiological substrates are the following:

- Observed deficits in recent memory acquisition and retrieval associated with bilateral hippocampal lesions in the Klüver–Bucy syndrome [133], which may occur in herpes simplex encephalitis and occasionally other circumstances
- Cognitive deficits due to deficient cholinergic activity in the cortex, perhaps mediated by lesions of the basal nucleus of Meynert as seen in Alzheimer's disease [134]
- Alterations in the ability to think abstractly and analytically, associated with extensive lesions of the frontal lobe (as in severe cranial trauma or gunshot wounds) or extensive lesions of the dominant cerebral hemisphere due to tumor, infarction, trauma, or hemorrhage [135]
- The loss of ability to use and manipulate language, which may occur when portions of the dominant parietal and para-Sylvian regions are damaged for any reason [136]
- The loss of ability to perceive the environment by means of the senses and to utilize this information appropriately when the relevant visual and auditory cortical association areas, mostly in the parietal lobe, are damaged [137]
- The lack of ability to experience and utilize emotion appropriately and engage in normal interpersonal and social interaction when frontal cortex or limbic structures are damaged [131]

In many circumstances, exact anatomic or physiological associations or correlations with observed clinical symptoms are not possible and will have to await a deeper understanding of the functional anatomy of the nervous system.

Any or all of the complex neural functions alluded to above may be described in what, rather imperfectly, has become known as mental illness, as if this designation implied the lack of a physiological substrate, as opposed to so-called organic brain disease where a known lesion results in the same dysfunctions. Many such disturbances have a neurochemical basis and may not be manifested in a manner that can be detected using the usual morphological methods employed by the neuropathologist [137]. Suffice it to say that only sometimes are clinical correlations possible [136,137], and then only within the context of well-known disease entities such as Alzheimer's disease, Wernicke's disease, traumatic brain injury, metabolic encephalopathies, and neoplasms. The pathophysiology of behavioral or mental illness is only vaguely understood, and there is little that the neuropathologist at present can offer by way of reliable clinical–pathological correlation.

Disturbances of Memory and Dementia

Memory disturbances are one of the more commonly encountered symptoms in neurological degenerative disease and traumatic encephalopathy and may be subdivided into several categories for convenience. Memory loss or impairment that is usually temporary or circumscribed (amnesia) may occur in connection with head trauma, metabolic insult, hypoxia, epileptic attacks, migraine, toxic states as in septic shock or alcoholism, infectious processes, and ischemic vascular disease of the brain. The loss of memory for events may extend to a time before the pathological event (retrograde amnesia) or may include the traumatic event(s) subsequent to the injury (anterograde amnesia). Sometimes amnesia may be long lasting or global [138,139]. In such cases, brain lesions may be found in the following: some part of the limbic system, such as the frontal lobes, medial temporal lobes, and amygdaloid nuclei, and the hippocampal formation; the anterior thalamus; mammillary bodies; cingulate gyri; the hypothalamus; the corpus callosum and anterior commissure; or the fornix [129,131,136–145]. Often only ventricular enlargement, possibly with some element of cerebral atrophy, may be found [144]. Clinical–pathological correlation for specific syndromes is sometimes possible, but in a general sense only [146].

At times memory disturbances seem to be associated with a complex compensatory mechanism that acts to supply missing information, often in a highly inventive manner, as in the case of the confabulation sometimes observed in Wernicke–Korsakoff syndrome. The basis for this mechanism is poorly understood in relation to the structural lesions observed in this condition [141,147].

Longer-lasting disorders of memory due to structural lesions generally apply to the loss of ability to acquire new information and store it for long-term retrieval rather than to the ability to retrieve old information. This situation is most commonly illustrated by conditions in which there are bilateral lesions of the mesial temporal lobe structures, such as the hippocampus, amygdala, and pyriform cortex, as in herpes simplex encephalitis, some cases of severe brain trauma, and embolic vascular disease. Individuals who suffer lesions of this sort may show various attributes of the Klüver–Bucy syndrome [133], which include lack of ability to retain new information, hyperoralism (use of the mouth almost as a substitute for the hands as a source of sensory information), hypersexuality, docility and distractibility, and visual agnosia. These symptoms may so incapacitate affected individuals that they cannot reasonably exist outside an institution because their unconstrained sexual behavior, memory deficits, and tendency to mouth everything would constitute a threat to themselves and possibly to the public if they were not carefully supervised. At times this syndrome may lead to accidental death and homicide, in which case clinical–pathological correlations are important and possible. The anatomic substrate for short-term memory, as implied above, involves mostly mesial temporal lobe structures of the limbic system, and any process that compromises this region by destruction, pressure, irritation, or toxicity can lead to temporary or permanent memory deficits. The precise physiological basis for memory is still subject to theoretical conflict and forms a part of the perennial mind–brain conundrum [131,140].

Broadly defined, dementia is the failure of higher-order neural associational function and involves not only deficits in memory but also integration, sensory processing, and behavior. Classically, the demented patient cannot perform calculations, has disordered perception of time and place, may have difficulty in naming and using objects, is unable to manipulate concepts or achieve understanding of abstractions, and cannot remember recent or remote events or recognize a spouse or children. To be sure, these deficits may be graded and may change with time. Many of the causes of dementia have already been enumerated and include Alzheimer's disease in its many forms, Creutzfeldt–Jakob disease (and its many variants or related conditions), subacute sclerosing panencephalitis (SSPE), the white matter diseases, the lacunar state and multi-infarct state, various toxic and metabolic diseases, and other degenerative diseases that are discussed in Chapters 3 and 4. Many of these conditions are irreversible and untreatable, but there are a number of conditions that produce profound dementia that are treatable or reversible. These include the following: normal-pressure hydrocephalus; chronic subdural hematoma; benign neoplasms and mass lesions; various forms of treatable epilepsy and mental illness; various forms of meningitis, including tuberculosis and fungal disease; syphilis; hypothyroidism; vitamin deficiencies such as hypovitaminosis, folic acid deficiency, and pellagra; encephalopathy in hepatic or renal failure; toxic states due to drugs and hallucinogens; and remote effects of cancer (limbic encephalitis) [148].

Pathology of Dementia

The pathological substrates to dementia can be conceptually divided into the following: those processes that act primarily on the cerebral cortex in a diffuse manner; those acting subcortically in the white matter; those acting on specific critical populations of neurons that control, drive, or pace the cerebral cortex; and complex processes, including diffuse metabolic dysfunctions or toxic states, affecting all elements. Examples of diffuse cortical pathology that produces dementia would be any process producing massive death or disconnection of neurons such as SSPE, Creutzfeldt–Jakob disease and related prion diseases, and terminal Alzheimer's or Pick's disease—all discussed in Chapters 3 and 4. Another rather unique diffuse cortical mechanism is seen in the lipid storage diseases, such as Niemann–Pick disease and Tay–Sachs disease, where, in addition to neuronal distortion by the stored product, abnormal synaptic membranes (meganeurites) are formed on the initial segment of the axon, which probably blocks all meaningful neural transmission from affected neurons [149]. The same individual neuronal dysfunction might apply to neurofibrillary tangle-bearing neurons in Alzheimer's disease, where neuronal associations are interfered with, and in certain cases of apparently congenital mental retardation [150]. The mechanism of disease in these cases is massive destruction or disconnection of enough cortical neurons that effective and accurate association processing is impossible. It is only when substantial populations of neurons are lost that intellectual function markedly deteriorates. For this reason, to produce a demented state, cortical pathology must be extensive and diffuse. Protocols for assessing probable functional impairment in Alzheimer's disease exist and continue to be refined [151].

In diseases where diffuse white matter pathology is present, the effect of this process is to sever axons of passage from gyrus to gyrus and from region to region, thus effectively inhibiting association as effectively as if large areas of the cerebral cortex were isolated from each other and the rest of the brain. This situation is seen in the dementias associated with the following: the leukodystrophies (Krabbe's disease, metachromatic leukodystrophy, adrenal leukodystrophy); chronic carbon monoxide poisoning with white matter degeneration; progressive multifocal leukoencephalopathy; occasional cases of multiple sclerosis; postinfectious or postvaccinial encephalomyelitis; viral leukoencephalitis; Binswanger's disease and extensive *etat crible* (small-vessel disease associated with hypertension); post-traumatic degeneration of white matter; and extensive "inner brain" trauma. Many of these conditions may produce a demented state but may also produce various other disconnection syndromes, such as the apraxias, aphasias, and cortical blindness, which are discussed below. Details of many of these conditions are discussed in Chapters 3 and 4.

Subcortical lesions, other than those in the white matter, that can produce a demented state include lesions of the limbic system, in large part discussed above in association with short-term memory loss, and lesions of diencephalic, thalamic, or other basal nuclei. Diseases in which dementia may be produced in this context are sometimes controversial, for some deny the existence of syndromes such as thalamic dementia. Nevertheless, as diseases such as progressive supranuclear palsy (Steele–Richardson–Olszewski syndrome), multi-infarct dementia and lacunar state, Alzheimer's disease, Parkinson's disease, and Huntington's chorea are understood in light of the new neuropharmacology, a solid basis for the dementing processes seen in these diseases is emerging. It appears that many noncortical neuronal groups have widespread projections to the cerebral cortex and may have a profound influence on it, perhaps providing regulatory, multiplexing, encoding and decoding, as well as clocking, functions. The functional significance of these findings is that lesions in these important nuclei may have wide-ranging effects on cortical function that, alone or in combination with cortical or white matter pathology, can produce defects in higher nervous activity that might be differentiable clinically. By means of an appreciation of the multiple factors that can lead to illnesses such as dementia, it may soon be possible to explain why an individual with minimal cortical neurofibrillary tangles or senile plaques is nevertheless demented (possibly due to subcortical pathology) and why subcortical diseases produce dementing illness. In practice, such clinical–pathological correlations require considerable care and are not always possible with the degree of accuracy one would like; nevertheless, the conceptual basis for interpretations exists [136]. This is especially true in will contests in which the mental competence at the time of the drafting of a will by a now-deceased individual may be at issue. The neuropathologist may be able to determine by a postmortem examination, possibly involving exhumation, that the individual showed the pathological stigmata of Alzheimer's disease and may have suffered impairment as a result.

Pathological Processes Associated with Behavioral Symptoms

Since the dawn of the neurosciences in the late nineteenth century, considerable effort has been expended to understand the neuropathology of behavioral abnormalities and mental disease [131,137,142]. To a large extent, the contributions of neuropathology toward understanding the mind have not provided the insights that neuropharmacology has achieved, although some framework for investigation has been provided by careful case studies in individuals who showed behavioral symptoms and who also had demonstrable lesions at autopsy. However, reliable clinical–pathological analysis is not always possible in predicting, on the basis of pathology and location alone, the kind and degree of psychic symptoms observed. This issue is occasionally raised in the forensic arena, where a violent or habitual criminal is suspected of having or discovered to have some form of focal brain pathology [101,129,152]. A recent study of pedophiles noted a statistically significant volume reduction in the right amydala and related structures in these habitual offenders [152].

Charles Whitman Case

One of the most notorious case examples is that of Charles Whitman, a 25-year-old student who, in 1966, after murdering his mother and wife, went to the top of a building on the University of Texas campus at Austin and, over a period of an hour and a half, shot 45 persons, killing 12 of them, before being killed by a police officer [153–156]. The original autopsy was hastily done by a pathologist with questionable credentials to perform a forensic autopsy, who preserved no specimens, apparently took no photographs, did not document the location of wounds or lesions except before the media, and rendered a report that was less than one typed page of narrative. This pathological debacle left open to doubt the reports, first released at a television news conference, that a "vascular" mass was found in the posterior part of the brain, which may have caused Whitman's behavior. A subsequent attempt to reconstruct the evidence by a panel of consulting experts at the behest of the then-governor of Texas, John B. Connally Jr., resulted in exhumation of the remains, documentation of the wounds, and an attempt to localize where the tumor was reported to have been. Sectioning of more than 100 fragments of the brain that had been returned to the body cavity after the original autopsy did not reveal any residual tumor other than that appearing in the paraffin block submitted by the original pathologist. Examination of this specimen by several consultants revealed that rather than being a vascular malformation, it was a highly vascular glioblastoma multiforme, whose size and location could not independently be confirmed. The final conclusion reached by the panel was that a malignant primary brain tumor existed in a paraffin block, which allegedly came from the brain of Charles Whitman; however, no conclusion, one way or the other, could be made about the veracity of this allegation or what role the tumor, if it came from Whitman's brain, played in the violent events reported. It is indeed unfortunate that a complete and well-documented examination of this case did not take place initially, for the case has now become a folk legend, and the notion that brain tumors can catalyze or cause violent antisocial behavior is perhaps erroneously embedded in the minds of millions of people, laypersons and professionals alike [157].

Richard Speck Case

It is curious that on the day that Whitman committed his atrocity, another mass murderer, Richard Speck, was arraigned in Chicago for the murder of eight student nurses committed on July 13–14, 1966. Speck had entered an apartment complex that served as a dormitory for student nurses near a south Chicago hospital, and as the nurses came home, he murdered them, with the exception of one nurse, who concealed herself and escaped death. Speck was eventually captured and convicted on eight counts of murder. He was sentenced to die in the electric chair, but this sentence was appealed, and eventually the U.S. Supreme Court voided the death sentence on the basis that potential jurors who opposed the death penalty were improperly excluded. He was then sentenced to eight consecutive sentences of 50–150 years in prison. Several appeals for parole were denied, and he died in prison on December 5, 1991.

During Speck's trial, a number of issues were raised concerning his responsibility [157] and included a possible genetic defect (XYY), a brain disorder, and an abnormal electroencephalogram, as well as the role of drugs and alcohol with amnesia at the time of the murders. Pursuant to this, several EEG examinations were undertaken. Apparently in connection with one of them, a barbiturate sedative was administered to collect a sleeping record, to which Speck apparently reacted violently, attacking a fellow inmate. One EEG study was reported to show irregularities in theta rhythms in the frontal and parietal areas along with slow transients maximal in the occipital region, but no epileptiform discharges were noted [158–160]. In histories obtained, it was reported that he had been rendered unconscious several times during his life, beginning at the age of 11 years with a fall from a tree and subsequently by altercations with law enforcement officers. Neurological examinations were said to be normal. A number of scans had been performed on Speck, including computerized tomography (CT) and magnetic resonance imaging (MRI) examinations. Analysis of these by a neuroradiologist indicated that Speck had apparently had a small "encephalocele" involving the frontal lobes and some asymmetry of the left temporal lobe. The radiologist also noted that there was very little right/left volume difference, which to him indicated a possible abnormality of cerebral dominance and the possibility of behavioral abnormality.

After Speck's death, an autopsy was performed and the brain was made available to this author for examination. Portions of the brain stem and cerebellum as well as portions of the frontal lobe tips were missing, apparently due to the manner in which the brain was removed. The brain did not appear atrophic and showed no external abnormality other than mild to moderate cerebral atherosclerosis (Figure 9.13). The encephalocele mentioned in imaging studies did not appear to be present but could have been cut away by the method of brain removal, which left portions of the frontal lobes behind. Coronal sections showed mild subcortical lacunes. The ventricles showed slightly greater volume on the left than the right. The left hippocampal formation appeared somewhat unusual in that there may have been a malformation of the Ammon's horn (see Figure 9.14), with a somewhat smaller than expected, possibly firm and gliotic, right hippocampus. The left temporal lobe appeared somewhat larger than the right, and there may have been slight ventricular asymmetry, with the left lateral ventricle slightly larger than the right, an observation noted in the CT and MRI scans in life. Unfortunately, no microscopic examination of the hippocampal formations was possible because the specimens, while being sent to a consulting expert on hippocampal architecture, were lost in shipment. If a demonstrable abnormality in Speck's hippocampus could have been found, it would have added to the body of knowledge in which hippocampal lesions apparently can have behavioral effects; however, in a specific case, such correlations remain elusive [142,160].

The Speck and Whitman cases are often re-reported whenever someone runs amok and kills several innocent persons in an apparently senseless act of rage. Examples are the Colorado Columbine High School shootings in Littleton, Colorado [161]; the Virginia Tech shootings in Blacksburg, Virginia [162]; the mass murder of 69 young people on Utøya, a small Norwegian island, by Anders Breivik [163]; the recent shootings (July 20, 2012) in a

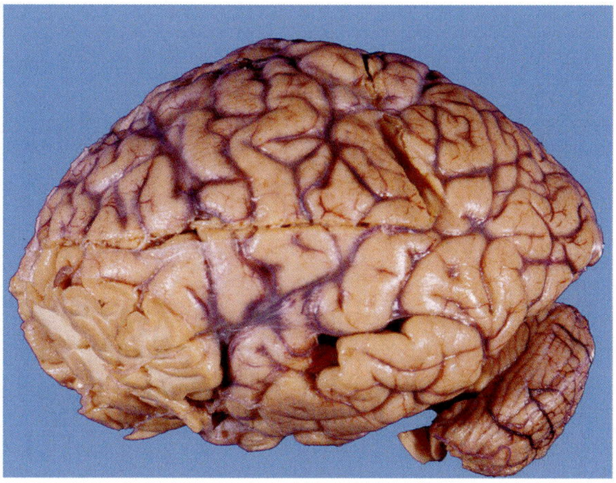

Figure 9.13 This photograph illustrates the left lateral hemisphere of the brain of Richard Speck. Note portions of the frontal lobes are missing. This area was reported to have shown some sort of cortical anomaly, possibly an encephalocele, in imaging studies done in life, but cannot be seen here. No other obvious anomaly is seen.

movie theater in Aurora, Colorado, by James Holmes, a graduate student, that left 12 dead and 59 others wounded. Unfortunately there are, and apparently will be, other such occurrence that scientists will evaluate, perhaps in hopes of making some sense of such blatantly irrational acts. Other, perhaps more horrific cases of the past are those of serial killers whose motives often have a sexual basis. Examples of these kinds of cases are the murders by H.H. Holmes in Chicago during the Columbian Exposition (*Devil in the White City* [164]); the Jeffrey Dahmer case in Wisconsin [165]; the John Wayne Gacy case in Chicago [166]; the Ted Bundy [167] and Gerald Eugene Stano [168] cases in Florida. These are only a few of the hundreds, perhaps thousands, of cases like them worldwide. The fact is that

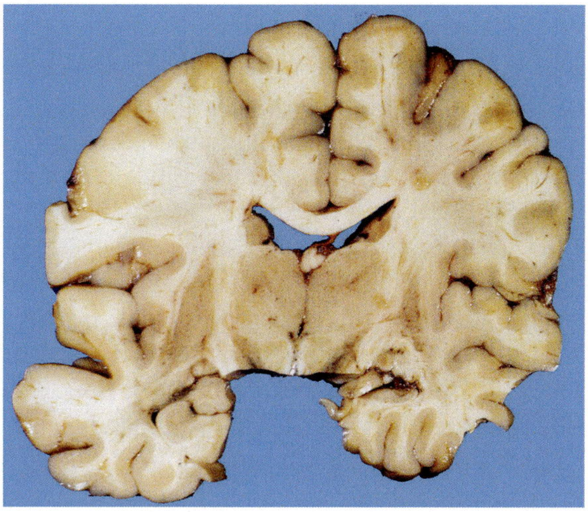

Figure 9.14 This coronal section of the brain of Richard Speck shows a somewhat larger left temporal lobe than usual and also when compared with the right side which has some brain missing owing to the brain removal. The Ammon's horn region shows what appear to be two structures instead of one, and the left hippocampus appears somewhat shrunken. The left lateral ventricle appears slightly larger than the right.

in spite of efforts by the media, the legal profession, and the medical community to connect lesions in the brain with the performance of violent acts, no conclusive evidence has ever been gathered to support what superficially appears to be a reasonable assumption. Unfortunately, no systematic effort has been made to examine the brains of these criminals in a careful manner.

Behavioral Symptoms and Brain Tumors

Mentational, motivational, and behavioral difficulties are, however, common symptoms of brain tumors and it is said that the majority of persons who have frontal, temporal, or parietal lobe tumors have some symptomatology of disturbed mental function; however, this disturbance usually involves memory, cognition, perceptions, or judgment but probably never involves the sort of dysfunction that would lead to highly ordered, goal-directed violent or antisocial acts as described above. Tumors and other lesions of the limbic system, hypothalamus, basal ganglia, and third ventricle may produce psychotic or other severe mental symptoms, including depression and suicidal tendencies, which may abate when the lesion is removed [158]. Such cases indicate that the involved structures were functionally related to clinical symptoms but were not necessarily the seat of mentational or cognitive functions. When cases occur in which such lesions are found and the history is reliable, it is inevitable that conclusions of causality by the lesions will be made. However, it is important to remember that not every lesion in a critical location produces the same symptoms or can be depended on to explain any observed behavior.

Perceptual Disorders

A great deal of clinical, anatomical, and pathological literature exists on the subject of visual perception, auditory perception, speech, and various aspects of the use of language. Defects in these spheres of higher brain function may occasionally confront the forensic pathologist or the neuropathologist acting in the forensic setting. Typical examples are individuals who are aphasic and are involved in traffic or other accidents, or other violence arising out of their perceptual disability, or individuals who have profound visual perceptive deficits or may even be cortically blind yet do not appreciate or deny the degree of their illness and may suffer injuries as a result (Anton's syndrome) [169,170]. Often in litigation, the extent of disability, degree of permanence of such disabilities, and the relationship of the neurological deficit to an injury or illness are the subjects of legal action. In the latter case, the pathologist may be called on to render judgment. It is important that there be some understanding of the nature and anatomic basis for such neurological deficits, but complex and detailed testimony or analysis must usually be obtained from neurologists or other specialists who are very familiar with these syndromes. Nevertheless, a short outline of some of the more common or classic conditions follows.

Aphasia

Aphasias [170–173] may be classified according to the clinical form of the deficit, which often correlates quite well with specific lesions in the brain, usually in the cortex of the dominant hemisphere, but occasionally deep thalamic lesions may also be responsible.

There are three main cortical areas that are important in this class of diseases: Wernicke's area (area 22), Broca's area (areas 44 and 45), and a general region in the posterior–lateral part of the parietal–occipital region, as illustrated in Figure 9.15. Wernicke's area is located near the end of the Sylvian fissure along the superior temporal convolution. Broca's area is located near the posterior end of the inferior temporal convolution just above the Sylvian fissure and in front of the lower end of the motor strip. When there are lesions (such as tumors, infarcts, or other destructive processes) in either or both of these areas or in the pathways that connect them, various syndromes may result. In the case of Wernicke's area lesions (not to be confused with Wernicke–Korsakoff syndrome), the individual may experience what are known as fluent or receptive aphasias. Such aphasias mean that the affected individual may be able to speak or write words appropriately but may be unable to understand the meaning of spoken or written words. Such defects are rarely uniform, and varying degrees of disability may occur. In general, lesions must be in the dominant hemisphere, which in right-handed individuals (93% of the population) is the left cerebral hemisphere 99% of the time. In left-handed persons, left cerebral dominance still predominates about 60% of the time, making the vast majority of persons in the population left-brained (more than 95%) [136,173].

When lesions are in or about Broca's area, the symptoms produced are often referred to as nonfluent, motor, or expressive aphasia. Patients with such lesions will have impaired

Anatomic regions related to linguistic functions

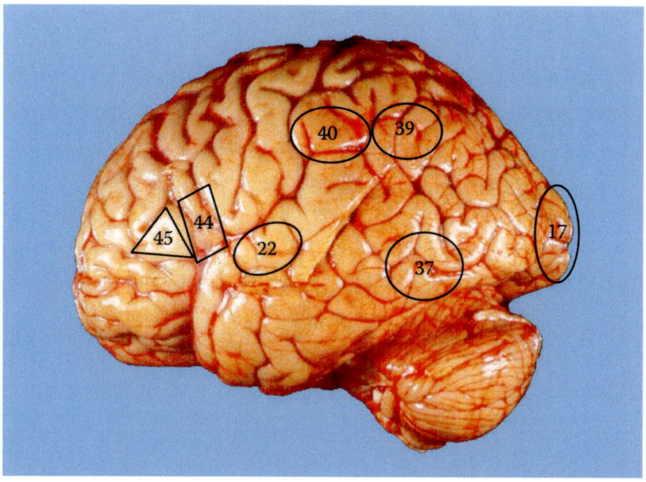

Figure 9.15 The cortical regions of the dominant hemisphere that subserve various linguistic functions are illustrated according to the Brodmann cytoarchitectonic/functional scheme. Areas 44 and 45 constitute Broca's motor speech area. Area 22, at the edge of the Sylvian fissure, and some surrounding areas subserve word meaning and lesions here produce "word" deafness often described as Wernicke's aphasia. Deep to this area within the insula are the primary auditory perception areas (Heschl's gyri), areas 41 and 42 (not shown). Area 40 (supramarginal gyrus) is an important association area involved in perception of the symbolism of language. Lesions of area 39 (angular gyrus) produce receptive aphasia where an affected individual cannot recognize written words (alexia) even when the victim could write them (alexia without agraphia). Area 37 involves visual–auditory association functions and area 17, the most important parts of which are the calcarine gyri on the medial surface of the posterior occipital lobe, are the primary visual perception area [182]. (From Crosby EC, Humphrey T, Lauer EW, eds. *Correlative Anatomy of the Nervous System*. New York: Macmillan, 1962.)

abilities to write and speak. As in the case of Wernicke's area lesions, the disability may be fractional, partial, or complete and may sometimes partially spare one or another function. When both areas are damaged, or the connections between them are disrupted, as in extensive trauma, middle cerebral artery infarction, or tumor involvement, aphasia may be complete or global, with little or no ability to communicate or receive spoken or written words. The cause of the aphasia and the extent of damage may affect the ability to recover, but in general the ability of the nondominant side of the brain to completely compensate is probably limited in most individuals. When faced with the task of clinical–pathological correlation in cases where some form of aphasia is important, a careful anatomical-based dissection approach is advised, along with ample photodocumentation. It is sometimes helpful, if the technology is available, to prepare large paraffin sections to facilitate neuroanatomical analysis.

Apraxia

There are a number of syndromes loosely grouped under the term *apraxia*, in which lesions in the region of the upper end of the dominant Sylvian fissure (temporal–parietal lobe junction) or underlying white matter produce abnormalities of high-order integrative motor function, often overlapping into linguistic dysfunctions. Such abnormalities include the inability to appropriately and correctly perform some movement or movement-linked function, even though the idea is understood and can often be described verbally. For example, an apraxic individual may be unable to appropriately use a key to open a door and may fumble in a confused manner while trying to do so. There may be difficulty in using common objects or performing mundane acts such as shaving, using the lavatory or toilet, or using the telephone. At times the individual may not recognize common objects or what they are used for and may not recognize portions of his or her own body as his or her own, for example, refusing to shave one half of the face "because it's not mine, and belongs to someone else" [174]. These and other similarly interesting and unusual syndromes of disconnection have been extensively described and correlated with structural lesions in the literature [175]. The apraxias have been classified as ideomotor or constructional (inability to perform a mundane physical activity such as brushing one's teeth), ideational (where the executive plan for some action cannot be formulated), kinetic (in which fine motor actions cannot be created), verbal (where the fine movements of tongue and mouth needed for speech cannot be accomplished), and oculomotor (where movements of the eye cannot be coordinated purposefully) [13,176]. Apraxias may often occur in connection with dementing illnesses in which the process may have its initial beginning in the parietal lobe or in the occipital lobe, as in adrenal leukodystrophy, progressive multifocal leukoencephalopathy, Creutzfeldt–Jakob disease, and other degenerative conditions.

Visual Perceptual Disorders

Under some circumstances, individuals who have lesions in the visual system are unable to perceive their lack of visual ability (Anton's syndrome) and may thus drive automobiles or other vehicles and have accidents that are related to their disability [177–179]. In other circumstances, such persons may injure themselves by walking into the path of an oncoming vehicle, suffering falls, or colliding with objects. Although it is not very common, the most classic of these circumstances occur with varying degrees of cortical blindness,

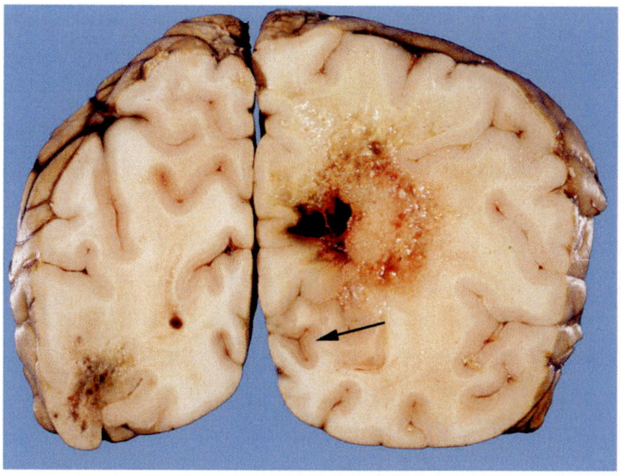

Figure 9.16 This is a coronal section of the brain of a woman who was suffering from advanced ovarian cancer and who died a few days after being involved in a car crash. While driving, she crashed, virtually head on into another automobile coming toward her in the left lane ahead. Given the location of a large metastatic tumor in her right occipital lobe above the calcarine gyrus (Brodmann areas 17 and 18, arrow), it is likely that she had an unperceived left lower visual field defect and never saw the car coming toward her. There are likely two other metastatic lesions in her opposite hemisphere. Her head was traumatized during the accident and she died with cerebral edema and other injuries a few days later. (Courtesy of Department of Pathology, West Suburban Hospital, Oak Park, IL.)

where major areas of the visual cortex (area 17) or its connections to adjacent cerebral cortex (Brodmann areas 18 and 19) may be damaged. Cortically blind persons may deny they have visual difficulty (Anton's syndrome) and appear to compensate by confabulation. It is curious that some persons with this syndrome, in spite of being unaware of visual information, may possess intact visual evoked cortical potentials [169]. There are a number of studies in cortically blind individuals from various causes that appear to have some visual function that is not necessarily privy to consciousness—so-called blind sight [170,178]. Apparently, such individuals can be trained to exploit these evanescent or latent abilities to their advantage.

Usually, visually compromised persons will come fairly promptly to medical attention. Probably a more widespread problem is the individual who has a visual field defect due to a tumor, stroke, or other lesion. In such cases, one half of the visual field in both eyes may be ineffective and such a person faces a real risk of being "blind sided" [180]. An example of a probable visual field defect that likely resulted in a car crash is illustrated in Figure 9.16. Curiously, many victims of homonymous hemianopsia describe only blurriness of vision when, in fact, whole or substantial parts of the visual fields are absent.

Alterations in Consciousness: Stupor and Coma

In a classic work on the neurology of consciousness, Plum and Posner [180] define consciousness as "the state of awareness of the self and the environment and coma as the opposite, i.e., the total absence of awareness of self and environment even when the subject is externally stimulated." This definition captures in perhaps too brief a glimpse the complex nature of consciousness and how it is defined or perceived by not only the medical profession but the public as well. Recent provocative cases of individuals in a state of coma and the decisions to remove life support have energized again the vast differences in perceptions concerning consciousness. Quite often such cases become the province of the forensic pathologist, who must attempt to make judgments that sometimes cannot be made with confidence but which often very vocal segments of the populace demand.

The state of consciousness can be neither black nor white; it is often intermediate, between full consciousness and deep coma, as every physician knows. Determination of the degree of depression of consciousness may be accomplished by the effectiveness of arousal by stimulation, but how reliable and precise are the methods employed? The individual who is unconscious merely because of sleep or mild sedation may be easily arousable to full consciousness by relatively mild stimuli. In deeper states of unconsciousness, arousal may be more difficult, and a fully conscious state may not be achievable even with vigorous stimulation. In addition, stimulation may produce abnormal posturing, which can give some indication of the level and severity of the lesion in the brain stem that is producing unconsciousness. An important contribution to the clinical evaluation and prognosis associated with disturbances of consciousness is the Glasgow Coma Scale, which details various parameters of observation in individuals who have suffered head injury. A numerical score is attached to each parameter, and a summation of them provides a numerical score range that can be correlated with expectations of clinical outcome (based on a large series of past observations). The practical importance of this scale is that some idea of prognosis is achieved and an appropriate therapeutic plan can be made with this in mind [180].

Various descriptives may be employed in characterizing gradations in the spectrum of consciousness, such as lethargy, drowsiness, confusion, obtundation, delirium, stupor, and coma. Special cases of unconsciousness, which have specific meaning, are akinetic mutism, coma vigil or apallic state, and locked-in and locked-out syndromes [130,180]. The type of disturbance is, in large measure, related to the location of the lesion, be it systemic, diffuse, multifocal, or focal.

The anatomical and physiological substrate of consciousness is most importantly vested in the so-called ascending reticular activating system, which, for the most part, resides in the pontine tegmentum, midline midbrain, and medial diencephalon, but also depends on sufficient cerebral cortical association to permit meaningful processing of information [132,180–182]. Insofar as the cerebral cortex is involved, the frontal lobes are especially important, but mostly in a general way. However, the degree of alertness is probably related more to the volume of cortical matter that is preserved than to its location [180]. In the case of lesions of the limbic system, a special form of consciousness disorder may be seen, an akinetic mute state (discussed below). Curiously, the medulla is probably not important in the maintenance of consciousness because transecting lesions will still permit a high order of functioning in spite of severe motor deficits that challenge communication. These insights have been gained over the years empirically by observing human case material and extending the observations by animal experiments.

Lesions that most commonly result in unconsciousness can be divided into those occurring above the tentorium, those occurring below it, and those that involve more than one location or are diffuse processes. When the etiology of coma is not immediately known (coma of unknown cause) and only becomes clear after some study, supratentorial lesions are most commonly due to intracerebral hemorrhages, epidural or subdural hematomas, and massive infarctions; however, tumors, severe hypoxia, and hypoglycemia, as well as diffuse axonal injury (diffuse inner brain trauma) and extensive traumatic contusion, may also be responsible. The subtentorial lesions most commonly also involve vascular diseases, usually infarctions, but may also include hemorrhages, tumors, and subarachnoid hemorrhages [183]. When the cause of unconsciousness or its degree of severity is not an issue, head trauma and some transient disorders of cerebral circulation (due to hypotension, shock, vascular disease) become the most common etiologies. Many systemic or diffuse processes also result in some degree of unconsciousness and most commonly include drug overdoses, metabolic comas (diabetic, hypoglycemic, hepatic, etc.), postictal states and seizure disorders, and toxic states [148,180,184]. Psychogenic disturbances of consciousness are also seen in cases of depression, conversion neurosis, and catatonia, where the cause may be neurochemical.

Apallic State and Related Conditions

The apallic state and related conditions are most curious forms of coma in which there has been massive bilateral loss of functional cortical matter, as in hypoxic encephalopathy, closed- or open-head trauma, viral encephalitis, or extensive white matter lesions resulting in a so-called vegetative state [185,186]. Individuals suffering this form of injury may in some respects appear to be conscious, with their eyes open and apparently scanning about the room or even following objects (coma vigil or apallic state) [187]. There may be spontaneous limb movements that are usually not purposeful, and there may be grasping of objects placed in the hands. There may be moaning or groaning sounds, but no speech occurs. Such movements may erroneously be interpreted as signs of consciousness, yet the individual is in coma and all responses come from subcortical—automatic—reflexes. The vegetative state may persist for long periods until infection, heart failure, or life support termination causes loss of vital signs.

In recent years, there have been many incidents in which a victim after some event remains alive but in coma and maintained on life support but does not fulfill the commonly accepted criteria for brain death [188] and thus life support probably may not be removed. Although the term *persistent vegetative state* (PVS) [189,190] has been employed for some time, it has come into common parlance and to a large degree has replaced other designations, such as apallic state or coma vigil. With advancing technologies, it is becoming possible to penetrate the veil of coma and to determine sometimes if the comatose victim is, in fact, processing information and thus fulfilling at least some aspect of the fundamental definition of consciousness. Numerous cases have now been reported in which, by using functional MRI [191] and other methods such as advanced EEG processing [192], coma victims can be shown to respond to parental or familiar voices and to activate portions of their brains appropriate for certain activities described or elicited by voices of observers, all without any sign of movement or response. These cases and those in which victims of PVS or minimally conscious states have recovered for various periods of time [193,194] have renewed serious questions of termination of life support and the treatment of such victims, even though it appears that they are oblivious to their surroundings.

A special form of coma is akinetic mutism, in which diffuse cortical or white matter lesions have occurred, leaving the victim in a state that resembles sleep, which may be punctuated by periods of apparent wakefulness, but no meaningful vocalization is possible, voluntary control of movements is not possible, and there is usually complete incontinence of bladder and bowel. The EEG may show typical wake–sleep cyclical patterns [181,195]. It is said that akinesia is a prominent feature of extensive frontal lobe damage or limbic destruction. In some cases where neurological improvement occurs, for example, following closed-head injury after prolonged unconsciousness, some aspects of consciousness may eventually emerge, yet the victim remains unable to speak or initiate actions that constitute a meaningful response to external events. On such occasions, the distinction between severe dementia and mutism becomes blurred.

Locked-In Syndrome

This graphic description applies to individuals who have sustained destructive lesions such as infarctions, hemorrhages, tumors, or traumatic lesions of the lower brain stem (lower pons–medulla) that have effectively precluded voluntary motor movements but which have not precluded consciousness and mentation. In this state, the individual is able to hear and see but is unable to communicate except by blinking the eyes in response to questions. Survival is limited, owing to inability to control secretions and the liability to infection, although very long survivals in this state have been reported [180,194].

Locked-Out Syndrome

Although this clinical condition is not specific in the same sense that is seen in the locked-in syndrome and overlaps to a great degree with vegetative states, in that the individual may show electrical evidence of waking and sleeping cycles (so-called alpha coma), the classic lesion that produces this condition is a midbrain or upper-pontine destructive process such as a primary pontine hemorrhage [196]. Such a lesion effectively destroys the vital midbrain–pontine ascending reticular formation so that there is no possibility of consciousness. In effect, the upper brain is prevented from waking up. Individuals with this problem do not usually survive for protracted periods of time and usually require ventilatory assistance, but prolonged survivals do occur. The case of Karen Ann Quinlan from 1977 is an example [188]. Such cases often pose ethical dilemmas because the classic criteria for brain death are not met and life support system withdrawal may not be permissible; however, when it is, sometimes the victim is able to breathe on his or her own against the prognostications of the clinicians. Such cases then pose an additional dilemma, most recently embodied in the case of Terri Schiavo [196–198].

Forensic Aspects of Consciousness

The importance of an understanding of disturbances of consciousness to forensic medicine emerges most commonly in the context of civil litigation, where the issue of conscious pain and suffering after an injury is often paramount. An analysis of the neuropathological and clinical findings is often decisive in adjudicating such cases, and the neuropathologist may be very helpful in resolving what might initially appear to be an impossible situation. A common problem arises out of the observations by family members of a severely injured relative in a hospital and possibly on respiratory assistance who, although not able to communicate, appears to moan and move spontaneously or in response to physical stimuli and to grasp another's hand. The family members may interpret these movements or vocalizations as evidence that the individual is suffering conscious pain, prompting them and their legal advisors to seek punitive damages based on the perceived suffering, when in reality the observations, painful to them as they are, may not reflect consciousness on the part of the victim, although as mentioned above, functional testing of the brain (MRI, evoked potentials, and advanced EEG studies) may appear to confirm what the family members are maintaining. All of this reinforces the need for careful and competent analysis of PVS cases from every perspective, including at autopsy, so that possible correlations of function and structure can be made. The analysis of the Quinlan case provides one of the rare opportunities for such correlation [198,199]. Unfortunately, most recently in the Schiavo case (in which a young woman sustained a cardiac arrest, apparently in connection with an eating disorder and profoundly abnormal serum electrolytes, and suffered global hypoxia/ischemia), an autopsy was done many years after her illness and a neuropathological study by a neuropathologist was undertaken, but there is little likelihood that the case will ever be reported in the professional literature owing to restrictive legislation in the state of Florida, which precludes such an effort because of concerns of patient confidentiality and the possibility of sensationalism and commercial gain. Nevertheless, a CT scan image taken in 2002 of a portion of Ms. Schiavo's brain has appeared on the Internet [197] and shows profound ventricular dilation (hydrocephalus *ex vacuo*) from severe brain tissue volume loss, which was also confirmed at the autopsy after life support and nutritional support were withdrawn after a tortuous legal battle over the right to die and the power of the next of kin [105,198,200]. There are many lessons that can be learned at all levels from the Schiavo case.

When confronted with a case like Schiavo's or Quinlan's, it is likely that a medical examiner or other forensic facility will be involved. It behooves anyone involved with such a case, media attention notwithstanding, to preserve confidentiality and perform a thorough autopsy and preserve the brain for later examination by a competent neuropathologist, or perhaps a group of them, who can plan the examination and do a scholarly job. Such an examination may have to involve expensive and hard-to-obtain technologies such as window-pane, large histological sections of the brain in order to determine the degree of volume loss, where loss has occurred, and in essence what is connected to what. Other advanced morphometric methods might also be needed that are not available generally in coroner's or medical examiner's facilities.

Agitated Delirium

There are circumstances in which an individual in a delirious, agitated state behaves in a threatening or harmful manner to others or whose behavior constitutes a high potential for self-harm. Under such circumstances, it is very common for security personnel, police, firemen, prison guards, emergency medical personnel, or bystanders to become involved in subduing the delirious person. In conjunction with such interventions, at a scene or later, the delirious person may die. The death may occur at the scene where the victim simply becomes quiet and is found apneic and in cardiac arrest, or may occur later under the same circumstances. Often such deaths are referred to as restraint deaths and invariably come to the medical examiner or coroner for investigation. It is common for those involved in the restraint of the individual to be under suspicion for overreacting and causing the death by what many have referred to as positional asphyxia, owing to the fact that often the delirious individual's struggles are violent and very forceful and result in handcuffing or "hog tying," often with a number of individuals on top of the struggling victim, allegedly preventing him or her from breathing. It is no surprise that quite often the media become involved in such cases, especially if the people involved are of different races. Civil and criminal lawsuits are also common in such cases. The forensic issues involved in these cases are complex and often controversial.

The causes of agitated or exciting delirium are many and may involve epilepsy and the postictal state (particularly in individuals with complex or partial seizures that commonly involve the temporal lobe); alcohol intoxication; drugs such as cocaine, phencyclidine (PCP or angel dust), amphetamines, and combinations of these; or individuals with severe psychiatric problems, possibly involving acute psychosis, panic disorders, or fugue states [105,201]. Medication with and without drugs of abuse may precipitate an agitated delirious state and may be mediated by excess dopamine [202]. The agitated state may occur in the home, at school, at work, or in connection with a crime such as shoplifting or a robbery when an arrest attempt may be made by authorities. Other circumstances may involve arrest and incarceration, transfer of a prisoner within a prison or police lockup to another cell or solitary confinement, and many other circumstances.

The forensic analysis of agitated delirium cases is often difficult. A full investigation of the history of the victim must be undertaken, including past medical records of hospitalization, treatments, and medications, including history of substance abuse. Toxicological investigations are paramount and very commonly reveal multidrug patterns of abuse. The circumstances under which the agitated state occurred must be documented and investigated. A thorough forensic autopsy must be conducted with extensive photodocumentation of the body, organs, and nervous system and a similar extensive histological study of all the organs, especially the heart and the brain. Guidelines for autopsy procedures in these cases have been outlined by DiMaio and DiMaio [105]. The forensic challenges lie mostly in processes that are physiological and not morphological.

There are a number of causes and mechanisms that have been established for deaths in agitated delirium and several that are controversial or unproven. The former involve clearly toxic and pharmacological effects of drugs of abuse as mentioned above [46,105], including prescription drugs such as the major tranquilizers [203], all of which are known to cause sudden deaths probably by means of catecholamine release [204]; direct cardiac or CNS effects; or combinations of these. Many cases suffer hyperpyrexia with or without rhabdomyolysis [201]. The interplay of these effects on top of diseases such as asthma, lowered pulmonary function, extreme obesity, cardiovascular disease, and gastroesophageal reflux disease many times can explain the death, whether restraint was involved or not. When there has been restraint, the situation becomes more complicated by the issue of hog tying and so-called positional asphyxia [204–206] and physical pressure on the chest, usually in the prone position by multiple persons, or by positioning the restrained individual in an unnatural position that would allegedly preclude respiration [105,207,208]. Neck holds can cause death by several mechanisms: crushing of the larynx, external compressive pressure on the airway, and carotid artery compression. Some insights into the course of events that may follow strangulation scenarios in the context of autoerotic practices or suicidal hangings have been provided by the studies of Sauvageau and colleagues [209,210]. These studies involved video recordings by the individuals involved and indicated that with ligature compressions of the neck in autoerotic situations, consciousness was lost within 11 seconds and that convulsions occurred within 7–11 seconds. Whereupon, when the ligature was removed, the individual regained consciousness without apparent ill effect. In videotaped lethal ligature hangings, the onset of unconsciousness and convulsions was almost identical, followed in about 40 seconds by decerebrate posturing. Cessation of respiratory effort occurred at about 2 minutes after ligature pressure, and most muscle movements ceased after about 4 minutes. The significance of these observations is that within one circulation time, the consciousness is lost, but if circulation is restored, it will rapidly return. Precisely how long an interval of little or no brain circulation is recoverable, is not addressed specifically by these studies.

When laryngeal fracture and crushing occur, the airway may be sufficiently compromised that even if the compressive force is removed, respiratory embarrassment may occur. Death has been alleged to be due to compressive forces on the chest during restraint; however, this phenomenon has been studied physiologically by Chan and colleagues [84,211,212], who found insufficient interference with ventilation by thorax loading to cause death and that body position, even while hog tied, did not sufficiently compromise respiratory physiology. Rather, there are more likely causes of death, namely, underlying disease states, presence of one or more drugs in the circulation, and possibly idiosyncratic physiological responses to stress in the victim.

Respiratory Control

Historically it has long been recognized that stimulation of or disconnection/destruction of the reticular formation of the pons and medulla can produce profound changes in respiratory control in animals and man [182,213,214]. Modern methods of neural connection tracing using radiolabeling and various tagging methods that employ retrograde axonal transport (horseradish peroxidase, pseudorabies, and herpes viruses), as well as *in vivo* neurophysiological stimulation and recordings, over many years have given precise interconnections of groups of neurons and their physiological actions during respiration; however, a great deal of information remains incomplete. Of necessity, much of the research on the neuroanatomy and neurophysiology of respiratory control has had to be performed in animals (rat, cat, goats, and primates), like much else of neuroanatomy has been. Yet this impediment has not stymied an understanding of human neuroanatomy and neurophysiology due to opportunities to use “nature’s experiments” through disease and injuries to seek comparisons and affirmations about what the animal work has revealed.

Brain Stem Anatomy and Physiology Related to Respiratory Control

The anatomy and physiology of respiration is highly complex with many stimulative, inhibitory, interactive, and feedback control functions that are only partially understood in man. The anatomic locations where most of the control functions occur are in the paramedian and lateral reticular formations of the pons and medulla (see Figures 9.17 and 9.18). These various neuronal groups’ neurochemical profiles and receptors have been the subject of investigation and have been characterized [215].

There are several groups of neurons in the upper pons that receive inputs from the frontal and temporal cerebral cortex, hypothalamus, and probably other supratentorial sites that contribute to both conscious–voluntary and unconscious–involuntary aspects of respiration. These groups of neurons are clustered about the superior cerebellar peduncle (brachium conjunctivum) in the pontine tegmentum (dorsal), and for simplicity’s sake are referred to at

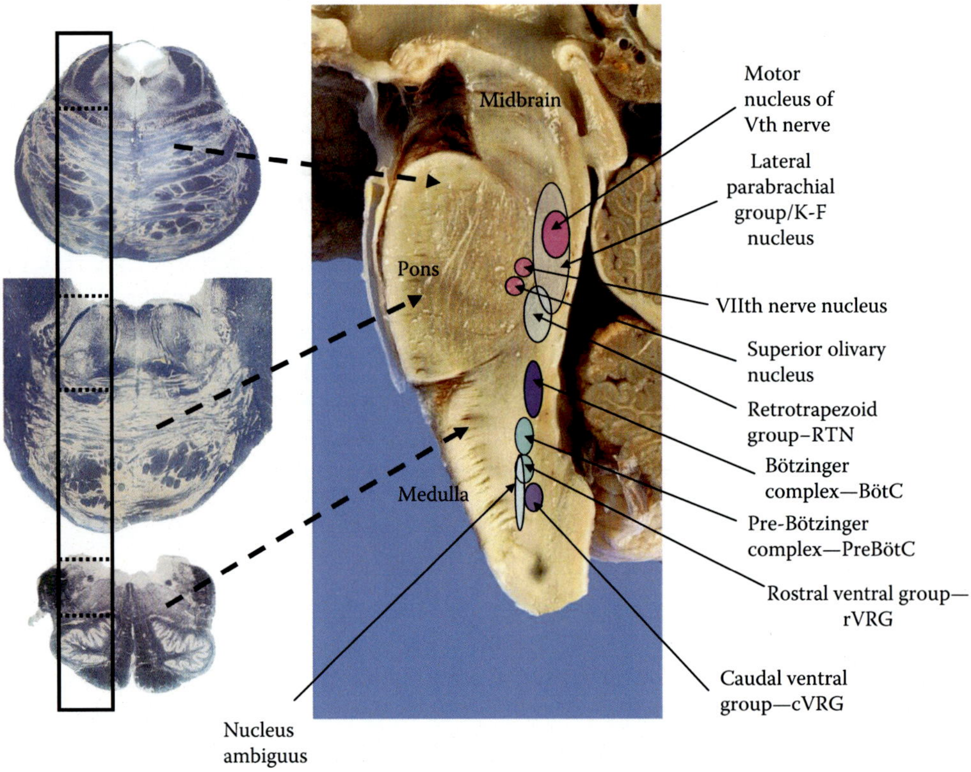

Figure 9.17 This figure illustrates the anatomic locations of major respiratory control–related nuclear groups of the pontine and medullary reticular formation diagrammatically represented in (right) a midline section through the brain stem and cerebellum. The series of myelin-stained section in the left depict the general locations of the major neuronal groups in cross sections. K-F refers to the Kölliker–Fuse nucleus, the existence of which is controversial in man. (From Petrovicky P, *J Hirnforschung*, 30, 551–63, 1989.)

the parabrachial nuclear complex and include the so-called Kölliker–Fuse nucleus [216,217]. The cytology and organization of these nuclei in man have been described by Olszewski and Baxter in their classic atlas [218]. Nomenclature for these and other brain stem neuronal groups is complex and confusing, since other workers have employed different systems than Olszewski and Baxter but generally provide a lexicon in their papers that relates to specific pages or plates in the Olszewski monograph [216] along with diagrams. It is interesting, although not unexpected, that the organization of these nuclear groups is very similar in all of the higher animals (mammals), perhaps because respiration is such an integral part of basic brain function absolutely vital to survival and thus highly conserved in evolution.

The pontine reticular formation neuronal groups with contributions from the fifth and seventh cranial nerve nuclei and from the nucleus solitarius project connections to the medulla where there are thought to be loci of neuronal groups variously referred to at the dorsal respiratory group that contain the so-called pre-Bötzinger complex and the ventral respiratory group. These groups of neurons are essentially stacked one upon the other, rostral-caudally [219]. Collectively they control rhythmicity of respiratory movements and responses to changes in blood carbon dioxide and oxygen levels. It appears that the main CO_2 sensory input in man comes via the carotid body and the ninth cranial nerve [220] via connections with the tractus solitarius [213], while O_2 sensing functions and possibly also some CO_2 and

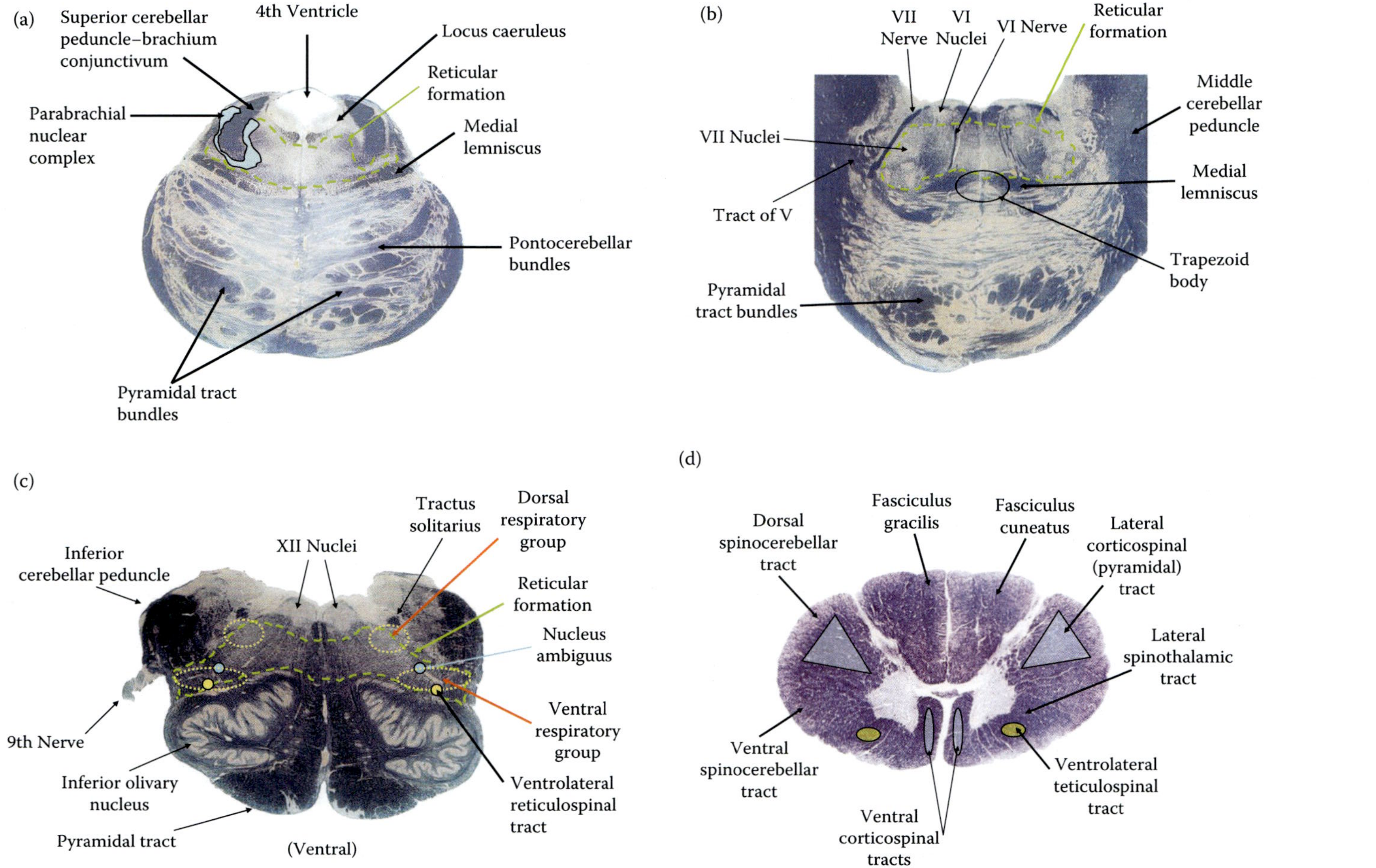

Figure 9.18 This figure illustrates reference anatomic landmarks for the respiratory control apparatus in the pons, medulla, and spinal cord in myelin-stained cross sections of the brain stem. (a) Upper pons, (b) mid pons, (c) mid medulla, and (d) middle cervical spinal cord.

pH sensory inputs are detected more or less locally in the respiratory nuclei or nearby structures [219,221–223]. The mechanism of this sensitivity may or may not be primarily neuronal, since a role for astroglia in detection of pH and adenosine has been suggested [223].

It appears that chemoreception and responses to changes in blood pH, CO_2, and O_2 are more sluggish during sleep. During an awake cycle, CO_2 sensitivity is much more robust and as everyone has experienced, air hunger is the result [222]. The responses to hypoxia are more muted than for CO_2 and is generally not perceived as such with any significant feeling of air hunger, a fact demonstrated graphically and experientially to anyone who has undergone "high altitude" simulation in a chamber where erratic behavior and eventual rather rapid unconsciousness occurs before any particular sensory warning reaches consciousness [224].

Respiratory movements out of necessity require phase control. Inspiration is and must be separate from expiration just as flexion and extension is in the extremities (see Figure 9.19). It appears that the medullary pre-Bötzinger complex neurons control inspiration via interaction with the ventral respiratory group neurons that project to the upper spinal cord and then via the phrenic nerve to the diaphragm. The Bötzinger complex neurons control expiration and inhibit inspiration [219,225].

Management of respiratory phase control requires feedback from peripheral sensory sources. In several mammals, apparently fibers carried by the vagus nerve (10th cranial nerve) project to the respiratory "field" in the medulla [226]. Also impinging on the respiratory "centers" are proprioceptive sensory fibers from the chest wall and diaphragm carried

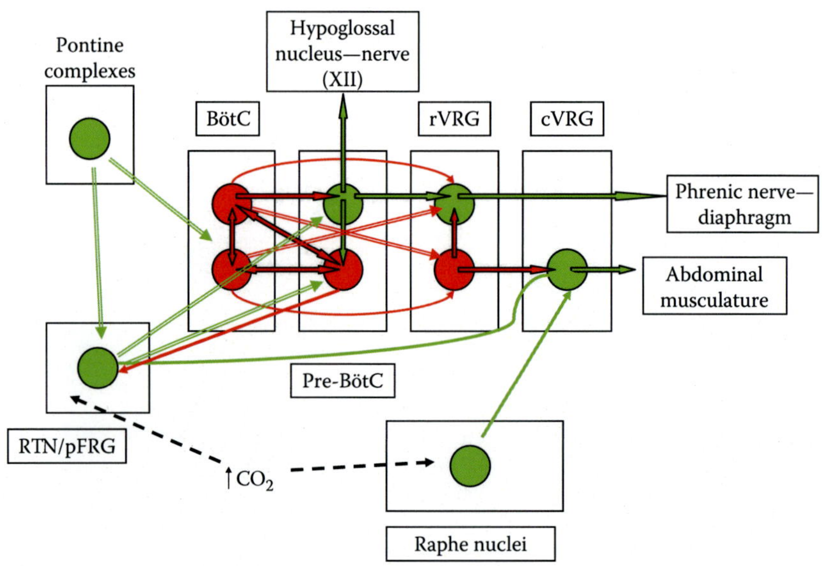

Figure 9.19 This diagram depicts the interconnections and functional contributions to respiratory control by pontine and medullary reticular formation nuclei. Green circles and arrows indicate stimulatory or facilitative functions. Red circles and arrows indicate inhibitory functions. BötC and Pre-BötC refer to the Bötzinger complex and pre-Bötzinger complex in the medulla (see Figure 9.21). RTN/pFRG refer to retrotrapezoid/parafacial respiratory groups of neurons, rostral to the Bötzinger complex in the rostral medulla. rVRG and cVRG refer to the rostral ventral and caudal ventral groups of neurons in the caudal medulla (see Figure 9.17). (From Smith JC et al., *Philos Trans R Soc Lond B Biol Sci*, 364, 2577–87, 2009; Alheid GF et al., *Respir Physiol Neurobiol*, 164, 3–11, 2008; Darnall RA, *Respir Physiol Neurobiol*, 173, 201–12, 2010; Guyenet PG et al., *J Comp Neurol*, 518, 3883–906, 2010.)

rostrally by the fasciculus gracilis and cuneatus. The output from the medullary respiratory centers descends via the medullary ventrolateral and possibly medial reticulospinal tracts to reach the phrenic nerve nuclei in the upper cervical spinal cord, which drives the diaphragm. Other reticulospinal fibers probably innervate muscles of the pharynx and larynx and also communicate with and through the spinal accessory nerve (11th cranial nerve) that controls accessory muscles of respiration in the neck. Other important inputs to the medullary reticular formation come from the pontine reticular formation, which in turn receives inputs from the hypothalamus, basal ganglionic, and also cerebral cortical centers that influence respiration in complex ways, including voluntary respiratory drive [213].

Abnormal Patterns of Breathing

There are a number of well-characterized disorders of breathing observed in man that are caused by lesions that disrupt the interplay between normal inspiration and expiration and respiratory drive. Depending on where the lesions are, various portions of the reflex arcs are affected.

Cheyne–Stokes Respiration

This characteristic pattern of breathing displays periodic rapid breathing alternating with periodic apnea and periods of normal periodicity. The pathophysiology involved probably represents a combination of frontal lobe "release" in the face of responses to increased blood levels of CO_2 after insufficient respiratory effort or the lack of response to respiratory effort from whatever the cause. This type of breathing pattern can be seen in individuals with sleep disorders [180,227], but when sustained it is generally associated with semicomatose or comatose states with intracranial pathology that can be localized or rather diffuse in the cerebrum or deep nuclei generally above the pontine level of the brain stem. Cortical infarcts or hemorrhages, usually multiple or widespread, and/or lesions of the diencephalon are some of the most common causes, but brain hypoxia, heart failure, extensive deep brain trauma, brain tumors, cardiac arrhythmias, hypertensive encepehalopathy, uremia, hypoglycemia, and other metabolic conditions may lead to Cheyne–Stokes respirations [228].

Hyperventilation

Another form of respiratory dysfunction is unremitting and sustained hyperventilation. This pattern of breathing can be seen in man, although apparently rarely, but apparently not in animals [228]. Central hyperventilation syndrome diagnosis requires that arterial PO_2 and pH be elevated, while arterial PCO_2 is lowered even during sleep [228] to differentiate it from other causes of hyperventilation.

Autopsy studies have shown that when hemorrhages, infarcts, and other lesions occur in the upper midline pontine reticular formation and/or above in the midbrain, this pattern of respiration occurs. This is often associated with upper basilar artery thrombosis and infarction. Because of the location of the destructive lesions at upper pontine and midbrain reticular formation, the victim is usually comatose and unarousable. However, hyperventilation may be observed in conscious patients who may be suffering from multiple sclerosis, encephalitis, brain stem gliomas, and other neoplasms [229,230]. The presence of form of abnormal respiration is an ominous sign with very few survivors, although the victim may survive for days or longer if fluid and electrolytes are supported.

Apneustic Respirations

This abnormal form of respiration represents a prolonged inspiratory phase with a delay in initiating an expiratory phase. It results from destruction by infarct or other process of the region around the brachium conjunctivum (superior cerebellar peduncle) in the upper pons (the parabrachial respiratory complex), which projects to the medullary respiratory complexes where rhythmicity and coordination of respiratory phases are regulated [231–233]. While relatively uncommon, it is most often associated with pontine hemorrhages or infarctions [180,228].

Ataxic Breathing

This form of abnormal respiration is characterized by random, disorganized inspiratory and expiratory phases with breaths of varying depth, rhythm, and duration occurring. Periods of apnea are common. The apparent randomness of the respiratory pattern distinguishes ataxic breathing from Cheyne–Stokes respiration, which is rhythmical [180,228]. This form of respiratory pattern results from destruction or dysfunction of the medullary respiratory complexes, which mediate rhythmicity and coordination between the phases of respiration. This disruption can occur with infarctions, hemorrhages, or other lesions of the medulla that can include viral infections such a poliomyelitis [232]. Lesions of the cerebellum can also give rise to ataxic breathing [234].

Hypoventilation Syndromes

There are conditions, often congenital, that result in failure to maintain normal respiratory rates during sleep that may result in fatal apnea. Infants affected with congenital hypoventilation syndrome (CCHS) are not capable of the typical automatisms of respiration, which results in progressive hypercapnia and hypoxemia [180]. This condition has been immortalized in mythology under the name "Ondine's curse." Individuals so affected can respire normally when awake but lose the ability for automatic breathing while sleeping. Even when awake, affected individuals do not respond normally when challenged with hypoxia or hypercarbia [235]. The condition, when congenital, appears to be caused by mutations in the paired-like homeobox 2b (*PHOX2B*) gene, which is located on chromosome 4 [236]. This gene is also associated with Hirschprung's disease. Hypoventilation syndromes may also accompany brain stem injury due to trauma and Leigh's disease, which appears to be caused by defective mitochondrial genes [237]. Affected individuals require ventilatory support while sleeping to avoid fatal apnea. It should be pointed out that CCHS has a different mechanism than the far more common sleep-associated apnea, which is involved in many adult onset sleep disorders.

Respiratory Arrest

The complete failure of respiration has many causes but is a common presenting problem in infancy and later in life. In infancy, respiratory arrest can follow periods of apnea during sleep leading to the so-called sudden infant death syndrome (SIDS), which is covered in Chapter 4. It is a common presenting issue in allegedly abused infants where the infant may experience an acute life-threatening event with difficulty in breathing or frank respiratory failure following an episode of "choking." CPR may or may not occur rapidly enough and/or failed intubation and resuscitation may have profound effects of brain vitality and function regardless of the pathological basis for the respiratory arrest. In infancy, a major causal or mechanistic issue is increased intracranial pressure associated with brain stem herniation. This process is discussed in detail in Chapter 5 and will not be repeated here. The central issue in all of these causes is how long a period of compromise can exist before the respiratory apparatus cannot respond and respiration cannot occur with disastrous consequences for the brain, heart, and other organs.

Non-neurological causes of respiratory failure are well known to every forensic pathologist and include the so-called café coronary where food has been aspirated and blocks the airway, sometimes with fatal results. It can also include aspiration of gastric contents, water as in drowning, blood, or sand or dirt in connection with work site cave-in accidents. Failure of gas transfer in the lungs can follow crushing injuries (flail chest), pneumothoraces from many causes, compression forces on the chest and abdomen, constriction of the airway by smothering, strangulation, hanging, fracture of larynx, or entanglement. Metabolic interference with proper gas transfer or utilization would include carbon monoxide, cyanide, hydrogen sulfide, and other poisonous gas inhalations. Hypotension and related problems with or without blood loss, or sepsis can cause respiratory distress syndromes and "shock lung" often also associated with multiorgan failure with a high mortality rate [238]. Other non-neurological scenarios include overdose of opioids and sedatives; paralytic agents such as curare, succinyl choline, and others; and certain venoms and toxins.

References

1. Schraeder PL, Lathers CM, Charles JB. The spectrum of syncope. *J Clin Pharmacol* 1994;34:454–9.
2. Johnson RH, Lambie DG, Spalding JMK, eds. *Neurocardiology: The Interrelationships between Dysfunction in the Nervous and Cardiovascular Systems*, Vol. 13. Philadelphia: W.B. Saunders, 1984.
3. Laidlaw J, Richens A. *A Textbook of Epilepsy*. Edinburgh: Churchill-Livingstone, 1982.
4. Berg AT, Scheffer IE. New concepts in classification of the epilepsies: Entering the 21st century. *Epilepsia* 2011;52(6):1058–62.
5. Engel J Jr. *Seizures and Epilepsy*. Philadelphia: F.A. Davis, 1989.
6. Hughes JR. *EEG in Clinical Practice*. Boston: Butterworth-Heinemann, 1994.
7. Engel J Jr, Pedley TA, Aicardi J, eds. *Epilepsy: A Comprehensive Textbook*, 2nd ed. Philadelphia: Wolters, Kluwer, Lippincott, Williams & Wilkins, 2008.
8. Cockerell OC, Johnson AL, Sander JW, Shorvon SD. Prognosis of epilepsy: A review and further analysis of the first nine years of the British National General Practice Study of Epilepsy, a prospective population-based study. *Epilepsia* 1997;38:31–46.
9. Day SM, Wu YW, Strauss DJ, Shavelle RM, Reynolds RJ. Causes of death in remote symptomatic epilepsy. *Neurology* 2005;65:216–22.
10. Krohn W. Causes of death among epileptics. *Epilepsia* 1963;74:315–22.
11. Copeland AR. Seizure disorders: The Dade County experience from 1978 to 1982. *Am J Foren Med Pathol* 1984;5:211–5.
12. Leestma JE. Natural history of epilepsy. In Lathers CM, Schraeder PL, eds., *Epilepsy and Sudden Death*. New York: Marcel Dekker, 1990, pp. 1–26.
13. Freytag E, Sacks JG. Abnormalities of the central visual pathways contributing to traffic accidents. *JAMA* 1968;204:871–3.
14. Juul-Jensen P, Foldspang A. Natural history of epileptic seizures. *Epilepsia* 1983;24:297–312.
15. Knox SJ. Epileptic automatism and violence. *Med Sci Law* 1968;8:96–104.
16. Blom S, Heijbel J, Bergfors PG. Incidence of epilepsy in children: A follow-up study three years after the first seizure. *Epilepsia* 1978;19:343–50.
17. Freytag E, Lindenberg R. 294 medicolegal autopsies in epileptics. *Arch Pathol* 1964;78:274–86.

18. Wasterlain CG, Treiman DM, eds. *Status Epilepticus: Mechanisms and Management*. Cambridge, MA: MIT Press, 2006.
19. Penfield W, Jasper H. *Epilepsy and the Functional Anatomy of the Human Brain*. Boston: Little Brown, 1954.
20. Scholz W. The contribution of patho-anatomical research to the problem of epilepsy. *Epilepsia* 1959;12:36–55.
21. Annegers JF, Hauser WA, Elveback LR, Kurland LT. The risk of epilepsy following febrile convulsions. *Neurology* 1979;29:297–303.
22. Nelson KB, Ellenberg JH. Prognosis in children with febrile seizures. *Pediatrics* 1978;61:720–7.
23. Binnie CD, Darby CE, Hindley AT. Electroencephalographic changes in epileptics while viewing television. *Br Med J* 1973;4:378–9.
24. Abreu P, Ribeiro M, Forni A, Pires I, Sousa G. Writing epilepsy: A neurophysiological, neuropsychological and neuroimaging study. *Epilepsy Behav* 2005;6:463–6.
25. Chuang YC, Lin TK, Lui CC, Chen SD, Chang CS. Tooth-brushing epilepsy with ictal orgasms. *Seizure* 2004;13:179–82.
26. Nakazawa C, Fujimoto S, Watanabe M, Tanaka M, Kageyama M, Ishikawa T, Watanabe Y. Eating epilepsy characterized by periodic spasms. *Neuropediatrics* 2002;33:294–7.
27. Michelucci R, Gardella E, de Haan GJ, Bisulli F, Zaniboni A, Cantalupo G, Alberto Tassinari C, Tinuper P, Nobile C, Nichelli P et al. Telephone-induced seizures: A new type of reflex epilepsy. *Epilepsia* 2004;45:280–3.
28. Okumura A, Kondo Y, Tsuji T, Ikuta T, Negoro T, Kato K, Watanabe K. Micturition induced seizures: Ictal EEG and subtraction ictal SPECT findings. *Epilepsy Res* 2007;73:119–21.
29. Radhakrishnan K, St. Louis EK, Johnson JA, McClelland RL, Westmoreland BF, Klass DW. Pattern-sensitive epilepsy: Electroclinical characteristics, natural history, and delineation of the epileptic syndrome. *Epilepsia* 2005;46:48–58.
30. Rathlev NK, Ulrich AS, Delanty N, D'Onofrio G. Alcohol-related seizures. *J Emerg Med* 2006;31:157–63.
31. Cuculi F, Kobza R, Ehmann T, Erne P. ECG changes amongst patients with alcohol withdrawal seizures and delirium tremens. *Swiss Med Wkly* 2006;136:223–7.
32. Jennett B, Teasdale G. *Management of Head Injuries*. Philadelphia: F.A. Davis, 1981.
33. Annegers JF, Grabow JD, Groover RV, Laws ER Jr, Elveback LR, Kurland LT. Seizures after head trauma: A population study. *Neurology* 1980;30:683–9.
34. Rose SW, Penry JK, Markkush RE, Radloff LA, Putnam PL. Prevalence of epilepsy in children. *Epilepsia* 1973;14:133–52.
35. Hauser WA, Kurland LT. The epidemiology of epilepsy in Rochester, Minnesota, 1935 through 1967. *Epilepsia* 1975;16:1–66.
36. Zielinski JJ. Epilepsy and mortality rate and cause of death. *Epilepsia* 1974;15:191–201.
37. Woodbury LA. *Shortening of the Life Span and Mortality of Patients with Epilepsy: Plan for Nationwide Action on Epilepsy*, Vol. 4. Washington, DC: Department of Health Education and Welfare, 1978, pp. 107–14.
38. Spratling WP. The cause and manner of death in epilepsy. *Med News* 1902;80:1225–7.
39. Rafnsson V, Olafsson E, Hauser WA, Gudmundsson G. Cause-specific mortality in adults with unprovoked seizures: A population-based incidence cohort study. *Neuroepidemiology* 2001;20:232–6.
40. Geertinger P, Voigt J. Death in the bath: A survey of bathtub deaths in Copenhagen, Denmark, and Gothenburg Sweden from 1961 to 1969. *J Foren Med* 1970;17:135–47.
41. Lederman RJ. Status epilepticus. *Clev Clin Q* 1984;51:261–6.
42. Dam MA. Hippocampal neuron loss in epilepsy and after experimental seizures. *Acta Neurol Scand* 1982;66:601–42.
43. Corsellis JAN, Bruton CJ. Neuropathology of status epilepticus in humans. In Delgado-Esquela AV, Wasterlain CG, Treiman DM, Porter RJ, eds., *Status Epilepticus: Mechanisms of Brain Damage and Treatment*. New York: Raven Press, 1983, pp. 129–39.

44. Meldrum BS, Brierley JB. Prolonged epileptic seizures in primates. Ischemic cell change and its relations to ictal physiological events. *Arch Neurol* 1973;28:10–7.
45. Crumrine PK. Lennox–Gastaut syndrome. *J Child Neurol* 2002;17(Suppl 1):S70–5.
46. Leestma JE, Koenig KL. Sudden death and phenothiazines: A current controversy. *Arch Gen Psychiatr* 1968;18:137–48.
47. Knight B. *Forensic Pathology*. London: Arnold, 1996.
48. Sptiz WU, Spitz DJ, Fisher RS, eds. *Spitz and Fisher's Medicolegal Investigation of Death: Guidelines for the Application of Pathology to Crime Investigation*. Springfield, IL: Charles Thomas, 2006.
49. Kuller L. Sudden and unexpected non-traumatic death in adults: A review of epidemiological and clinical studies. *J Chron Dis* 1966;19:1192.
50. Hirsch CS, Martin DL. Unexpected death in young epileptics. *Neurology* 1971;21:682–90.
51. Jay GW, Leestma JE. Sudden death in epilepsy: A comprehensive review of the literature and proposed mechanisms. *Acta Neurol Scand* 1981;63(Suppl 82):1–66.
52. Wendkos MH. *Sudden Death and Psychiatric Illness*. New York: SP Medical and Scientific Books, 1979.
53. Schraeder PL, Delin K, McClelland RL, So EL. Coroner and medical examiner documentation of sudden unexplained deaths in epilepsy. *Epilepsy Res* 2006;68(2):137–43.
54. Leestma JE, Annegers JF, Brodie MJ, Brown S, Schraeder P, Siscovick D, Wannamaker BB, Tennis PS, Cierpial MA, Earl NL. Sudden unexplained death in epilepsy: Observations from a large clinical development program. *Epilepsia* 1997;38:47–55.
55. Lathers CM, Schraeder PL, eds. *Epilepsy and Sudden Death*. New York: Marcel Dekker, 1990.
56. Lathers CM, Schrader P, Bungo M, Leestma J, eds. *Sudden Death in Epilepsy: Forensic and Clinical Issues*. New York: Taylor & Francis, 2010.
57. Office of the Medical Examiner, Cook County, Illinois. *Annual Report, 1977–79*. Chicago, IL: Author, 1979.
58. Walczak TS, Leppik IE, D'Amelio M, Rarick J, So E, Ahman P, Ruggles K, Cascino GD, Annegers JF, Hauser WA. Incidence and risk factors in sudden unexpected death in epilepsy: A prospective cohort study. *Neurology* 2001;56:519–25.
59. Tennis P, Cole TB, Annegers JF, Leestma JE, McNutt M, Rajput A. Cohort study of incidence of sudden unexplained death in persons with seizure disorder treated with antiepileptic drugs in Saskatchewan, Canada. *Epilepsia* 1995;36:29–36.
60. Bell GS, Sander JW. Sudden unexpected death in epilepsy. Risk factors, possible mechanisms and prevention: A reappraisal. *Acta Neurol Taiwan* 2006;15:72–83.
61. Walczak T. Do antiepileptic drugs play a role in sudden unexpected death in epilepsy? *Drug Saf* 2003;26:673–83.
62. Tomson T, Walczak T, Sillanpaa M, Sander JW. Sudden unexpected death in epilepsy: A review of incidence and risk factors. *Epilepsia* 2005;46(Suppl 11):54–61.
63. Opeskin K, Berkovic SF. Risk factors for sudden unexpected death in epilepsy: A controlled prospective study based on coroners cases. *Seizure* 2003;12:456–64.
64. Timmings PL. Sudden unexpected death in epilepsy: Is carbamazepine implicated? *Seizure* 1998;7:289–91.
65. Leestma JE, Kalelkar MB, Teas SS, Jay GW, Hughes JR. Sudden unexpected death associated with seizures: Analysis of 66 cases. *Epilepsia* 1984;25:84–8.
66. Leestma J. Sudden unexpected death associated with seizures: A pathological review. In Lathers CM, Schraeder PL, eds., *Epilepsy and Sudden Death*. New York: Marcel Dekker, 1990, pp. 61–88.
67. Kennedy GM, Lhatoo SD. CNS adverse events associated with antiepileptic drugs. *CNS Drugs* 2008;22:739–760.
68. Lathers CM, Schraeder PL. Stress and sudden death. *Epilepsy Behav* 2006;9:236–42.
69. Critchley HD, Taggart P, Sutton PM, Holdright DR, Batchvarov V, Hnatkova K, Malik M, Dolan RJ. Mental stress and sudden cardiac death: Asymmetric midbrain activity as a linking mechanism. *Brain* 2005;128:75–85.
70. Chan AWK, Lathers CM, Leestma JE. Alcohol arrhythmias, seizures, and sudden death. In Lathers CM, Schraeder PL, eds., *Epilepsy and Sudden Death*. New York: Marcel Dekker, 1990, pp. 329–73.

71. Stollberger C, Finsterer J. Cardiorespiratory findings in sudden unexplained/unexpected death in epilepsy (SUDEP). *Epilepsy Res* 2004;59:51–60.
72. Ryvlin P, Montavont A, Kahane P. Sudden unexpected death in epilepsy: From mechanisms to prevention. *Curr Opin Neurol* 2006;19:194–9.
73. Leung H, Kwan P, Elger CE. Finding the missing link between ictal bradyarrhythmia, ictal asystole, and sudden unexpected death in epilepsy. *Epilepsy Behav* 2006;9:19–30.
74. Hedley PL, Jorgensen P, Schlamowitz S, Moolman-Smook J, Kanters JK, Corfield VA, Christiansen M. The genetic basis of Brugada syndrome: A mutation update. *Hum Mutat* 2009;30(9):1256–66.
75. Ptacek LJ. Channelopathies: Ion channel disorders of muscle as a paradigm for paroxysmal disorders of the nervous system. *Neuromuscul Disord* 1997;7(4):250–5.
76. Akalin F, Tirtir A, Yilmaz Y. Increased QT dispersion in epileptic children. *Acta Paediatr* 2003;92(8):916–20.
77. Armour JA, Ardell JL, eds. *Neurocardiology*. New York: Oxford University Press, 1994.
78. Lathers CM, Schraeder PL. Autonomic dysfunction in epilepsy: Characterization of autonomic cardiac neural discharge associated with pentylenetetrazol-induced epileptogenic activity. *Epilepsia* 1982;23:633–47.
79. Falconer B, Rajs J. Post-mortem findings of cardiac lesions in epileptics: A preliminary report. *J Foren Sci* 1976;8:63–71.
80. Bharati S, Lev M. *The Cardiac Conduction System in Unexplained Sudden Death*. Mt. Kisco, NY: Futura, 1990.
81. Bohus B, Korte S. Stress, the hypothalamo–pituitary–adrenal system and the heart, Chapter 6. In Ter Horst G, ed., *The Nervous System and the Heart*. Totowa, NJ: Humana Press, 2000, pp. 241–64.
82. Lathers CM, Schraeder PL. Stress and SUDEP. In Lathers CM, Schrader PL, Bungo MW, Leestma, JE, eds., *Sudden Death in Epilepsy: Forensic and Clinical Issues*. New York: Taylor and Francis/CRC Press, 2010, pp. 253–283.
83. Ackerman MJ. Cardiac causes of sudden unexpected death in children and their relationship to seizures and syncope: Genetic testing for cardiac electropathies. *Semin Pediatr Neurol* 2005;12:52–8.
84. Leestma JE, Hughes JR, Teas SS, Kalelkar MB. Sudden epilepsy deaths and the forensic pathologist. *Am J Foren Med Pathol* 1985;6:215–8.
85. Aurlien D, Leren TP, Tauboll E, Gjerstad L. New SCN5A mutation in a SUDEP victim with idiopathic epilepsy. *Seizure* 2009;18(2):158–60.
86. Brugada R, Hong K, Dumaine R, Cordeiro J, Gaita F, Borggrefe M, Menendez TM, Brugada J, Pollevick GD, Wolpert C et al. Sudden death associated with short-QT syndrome linked to mutations in HERG. *Circulation* 2004;109(1):30–5.
87. Cannon SC. Pathomechanisms in channelopathies of skeletal muscle and brain. *Annu Rev Neurosci* 2006;29:387–415.
88. Lehnart SE, Wehrens XH, Laitinen PJ, Reiken SR, Deng SX, Cheng Z, Landry DW, Kontula K, Swan H, Marks AR. Sudden death in familial polymorphic ventricular tachycardia associated with calcium release channel (ryanodine receptor) leak. *Circulation* 2004;109(25):3208–14.
89. Schimpf R, Veltmann C, Wolpert C, Borggrefe M. Channelopathies: Brugada syndrome, long QT syndrome, short QT syndrome, and CPVT. *Herz* 2009;34(4):281–8.
90. Ghali N, Nashef L. Genetics of sudden death in epilepsy. In: Lathers CM, Schraeder P, Bungo M, Leestma J, eds., *Sudden Death in Epilepsy: Forensic and Clinical Issues*. New York: Taylor & Francis, 2010.
91. Langan Y, Nashef L, Sander JW. Sudden unexpected death in epilepsy: A series of witnessed deaths. *J Neurol Neurosurg Psychiatry* 2000;68(2):211–3.
92. Lhatoo SD, Faulkner HJ, Dembny K, Trippick K, Johnson C, Bird JM. An electroclinical case–control study of sudden unexpected death in epilepsy. *Ann Neurol* 2010;68(6):787–96.

93. Nashef L, Walker F, Allen P, Sander JW, Shorvon SD, Fish DR. Apnoea and bradycardia during epileptic seizures: Relation to sudden death in epilepsy. *J Neurol Neurosurg Psychiatry* 1996;60(3):297–300.
94. Meldrum BS, Corsellis JAN. Epilepsy. In Adams JH, Corsellis JAN, Duchen LW, eds., *Greenfield's Neuropathology*. New York: Wiley, 1984, pp. 921–50.
95. Ward AA. The epileptic neurone: Chronic foci in animals and man. In Jasper HH, Ward AA, Pope A, eds., *Basic Mechanisms of the Epilepsies*. London: Churchill-Livingstone, 1969, pp. 263–77.
96. Sano K, Malamud N. Clinical significance of sclerosis of the cornu ammonis. *Arch Neurol Psychiatr* 1953;70:40–53.
97. Lindenberg R. Patterns of CNS vulnerability in acute hypoxemia, including anaesthesia accidents. In Schade J, McMenemey WH, eds., *Selective Vulnerability of the Brain in Hypoxaemia*. Oxford: Blackwell, 1963, pp. 189–209.
98. Spielmeyer W. Die Pathogenese des epileptischen Krampfes. *Ztr Ges Neurol Psychiatr* 1927;109:501–20.
99. Chaslin P. Note sur l'anatomie pathologique de l'épilepsie dite essentielle—La sclérose nevroliques. *C R Séances Soc Biol* 1889;1:1698–71.
100. Manno EM, Pfeifer EA, Cascino GD, Noe KH, Wijdicks EF. Cardiac pathology in status epilepticus. *Ann Neurol* 2005;58:954–7.
101. Elliott FA. Neurological factors in violent behavior (the dyscontrol syndrome). *Bull Am Acad Psychiatry Law* 1976;4:297–315.
102. Gunn J, Fenton G. Epilepsy, automatism, and crime. *Lancet* 1971;1:1173–6.
103. Delgado-Escueta AV, Mattson RH, King L, Goldensohn ES, Spiegel H, Madsen J, Crandall P, Dreifuss F, Porter RJ. Special report: The nature of aggression during epileptic seizures. *N Engl J Med* 1981;305:711–6.
104. Alberto Tassinari C, Tassi L, Calandra-Buonaura G, Stanzani-Maserati M, Fini N, Pizza F, Sartori I, Michelucci R, Lo Russo G, Meletti S. Biting behavior, aggression, and seizures. *Epilepsia* 2005;46:654–63.
105. DiMaio TG, DiMaio VJM. *Excited Delirium Syndrome: Cause of Death and Prevention*. Boca Raton, FL: CRC Taylor & Francis, 2006.
106. Fazel S, Lichtenstein P, Grann M, Langstrom N. Risk of violent crime in individuals with epilepsy and traumatic brain injury: A 35 year Swedish population study. *PLoS Med* 2011;8(12):e1001150.
107. Monroe RR. Dyscontrol syndrome: Long-term follow-up. *Compr Psychiatry* 1989;30:489–97.
108. Pellegrini A, Lippmann SB, Crump G, Manshadi M. Psychiatric aspects of complex partial seizures: Case report. *J Clin Psychiatry* 1984;45:269–71.
109. Stern TA, Murray GB. Complex partial seizures presenting as a psychiatric illness. *J Nerv Ment Dis* 1984;172:625–7.
110. Yankovsky AE, Veilleux M, Dubeau F, Andermann F. Post-ictal rage and aggression: A video-EEG study. *Epileptic Disord* 2005;7:143–7.
111. Stone JL, McDaniel KD, Hughes JR, Hermann BP. Episodic dyscontrol disorder and paroxysmal EEG abnormalities: Successful treatment with carbamazepine. *Biol Psychiatry* 1986;21:208–12.
112. Elliott FA. Neurological findings in adult minimal brain dysfunction and the dyscontrol syndrome. *J Nerv Ment Dis* 1982;170:680–7.
113. Jang D, Coles EM. The evolution and definition of the concept of "automatism" in Canadian case law. *Med Law* 1995;14:221–38.
114. Mendez MF. Postictal violence and epilepsy. *Psychosomatics* 1998;39(5):478–80.
115. Reuber M, Mackay RD. Epileptic automatisms in the criminal courts: 13 cases tried in England and Wales between 1975 and 2001. *Epilepsia* 2008;49(1):138–45.
116. Chio A, Spreafico R, Avanzini G, Ghiglione P, Vercellino M, Mutani R. Cesare Lombroso, cortical dysplasia, and epilepsy: Keen findings and odd theories. *Neurology* 2003;61(10):1412–6.
117. Granieri E, Fazio P. The Lombrosian prejudice in medicine. The case of epilepsy. Epileptic psychosis. Epilepsy and aggressiveness. *Neurol Sci* 2012;33(1):173–92.

118. Monaco F, Mula M. Cesare Lombroso and epilepsy 100 years later: An unabridged report of his original transactions. *Epilepsia* 2011;52(4):679–88.
119. Hollister LE, Shah NN. Structural brain scanning in psychiatric patients: A further look. *J Clin Psychiatry* 1996;57:241–4.
120. Caldwell DS, Little PB. Aggression in dogs and associated neuropathology. *Can Vet J* 1980; 21:152–4.
121. Rojas-Burke J. PET scans advance as tool in insanity defense. *J Nucl Med* 1993;34:13N–6N, 25N–6N.
122. Schwartz-Watts DM. Asperger's disorder and murder. *J Am Acad Psychiatry Law* 2005;33:390–3.
123. Katz N, Zemishlany Z. Criminal responsibility in Asperger's syndrome. *Isr J Psychiatry Relat Sci* 2006;43:166–73.
124. McSherry B. Criminal responsibility, "fleeting" states of mental impairment, and the power of self-control. *Int J Law Psychiatry* 2004;27:445–57.
125. McSherry B. Getting away with murder? Dissociative states and criminal responsibility. *Int J Law Psychiatry* 1998;21:163–76.
126. Bisson JI. Automatism and post-traumatic stress disorder. *Br J Psychiatry* 1993;163:830–2.
127. Solomon Z, Neria Y, Ohry A, Waysman M, Ginzburg K. PTSD among Israeli former prisoners of war and soldiers with combat stress reaction: A longitudinal study. *Am J Psychiatry* 1994;151:554–9.
128. Doane BK, Livingston KF. *The Limbic System*. New York: Raven Press, 1986.
129. Eichelman B. The limbic system and aggression in humans. *Neurosci Biobehav Rev* 1983;7:391–4.
130. Eccles JC, ed. *Brain and Conscious Experience*. New York: Springer-Verlag, 1966.
131. Charney DS, Nestler EJ, Bunney BS, eds. *Neurobiology of Mental Illness*. New York: Oxford University Press, 1999.
132. Chapman LF, Wolff HG. The cerebral hemispheres and the highest integrative functions of man. *Arch Neurol* 1959;1:357–424.
133. Lilly R, Cummings JL, Benson DF, Frankel M. The human Klüver–Bucy syndrome. *Neurology* 1983;33:1141–5.
134. Davies P, Maloney AJ. Selective loss of central cholinergic neurons in Alzheimer's disease. *Lancet* 1976;2:1403.
135. Levin S. Frontal lobe dysfunctions in schizophrenia: II. Impairments of psychological and brain functions. *J Psychiatr Res* 1984;18:57–72.
136. Watson C, Kirkcaldie M, Paxinos G. *The Brain: An Introduction to Functional Neuroanatomy*. New York: Academic Press, 2010.
137. Parker B, Deibler S, Feldshuh B, Frosch W, Laureano E, Sillen J. Finding medical reasons for psychiatric behavior. *Geriatrics* 1976;31:87–91.
138. Suranyi L. Transient global amnesia and the law. *Arch Neurol* 1983;40:393.
139. Porter S, Birt AR, Yuille JC, Herve HF. Memory for murder. A psychological perspective on dissociative amnesia in legal contexts. *Int J Law Psychiatry* 2001;24:23–42.
140. Heilman KM. Exploring the enigmas of frontal lobe dysfunction. *Geriatrics* 1976;31:81–7.
141. Heilman KM, Sypert GW. Korsakoff's syndrome resulting from bilateral fornix lesions. *Neurology* 1977;27:490–3.
142. Lectenberg R. *The Psychiatrist's Guide to Diseases of the Nervous System*. New York: Wiley, 1982.
143. Squire LR, Moore RY. Dorsal thalamic lesion in a noted case of human memory dysfunction. *Ann Neurol* 1979;6:503–6.
144. Earnest MP, Heaton RK, Wilkinson WE, Manke WF. Cortical atrophy, ventricular enlargement and intellectual impairment in the aged. *Neurology* 1979;29:1138–43.
145. Dusoir H, Kapur N, Byrnes DP, McKinstry S, Hoare RD. The role of diencephalic pathology in human memory disorder: Evidence from a penetrating paranasal brain injury. *Brain* 1990;113:1695–706.
146. Pfefferbaum A, Zipursky RB, Lim KO, Zatz LM, Stahl SM, Jernigan TL. Computed tomographic evidence for generalized sulcal and ventricular enlargement in schizophrenia. *Arch Gen Psychiatry* 1988;45:633–40.

147. Victor M, Adams RD, Collins GH. *The Wernicke-Korsakov Syndrome: A Clinical Pathological Study of 245 Patients, 82 with Post-Mortem Examinations*. Oxford: Blackwell, 1971.
148. Norenberg MD, Gregorios JB. Central nervous system manifestations of systemic disease. In Davis RL, Robertson DM, eds., *Textbook of Neuropathology*. Baltimore: Williams & Wilkins, 1985, pp. 403–67.
149. Purpura D, Baker HJ. Meganeurites and other aberrant processes of neurons in feline GM1-gangliosidosis: A Golgi study. *Brain Res* 1978;143:13–26.
150. Pupura DP. Dendritic spine dysgenesis and mental retardation. *Science* 1974;186:1126–8.
151. Alafuzoff I, Iqbal K, Friden H, Adolfsson R, Winblad B. Histopathological criteria for progressive dementia disorders: Clinical–pathological correlation and classification by multivariate data analysis. *Acta Neuropathol* (Berl) 1987;74:209–25.
152. Schiltz K, Witzel J, Northoff G, Zierhut K, Gubka U, Fellmann H, Kaufmann J, Tempelmann C, Wiebking C, Bogerts B. Brain pathology in pedophilic offenders: Evidence of volume reduction in the right amygdala and related diencephalic structures. *Arch Gen Psychiatry* 2007;64:737–46.
153. Crime. The madman in the tower. *Time Magazine*, August 12, 1996, 88(7), pp. 14–19.
154. The Texas sniper. *Life Magazine*, August 12, 1966, pp. 28a–28c.
155. Charlie Whitman: The Eagle scout who grew up with a tortured mind. *Life Magazine*, Nevin D, August 12, 1996, pp. 28d–29.
156. Lavergne GM. *The Sniper in the Tower: The Charles Whitman Murders*. New York: Bantam (Random House), 1998.
157. Restak RM. See no evil: The neurological defense would blame violence on the damaged brain. *Sciences* 1992;32:16–21.
158. Luchins DJ. A possible role of hippocampal dysfunction in schizophrenic symptomatology. *Biol Psychiatry* 1990;28:87–91.
159. Gibbs FA. Round table discussion: Violent behavior and the electroencephalogram. *Clin Electroencephalogr* 1972;3:180–214.
160. Lorimer FM. Six year studies of growth and development of an electroencephalographic laboratory in prison. *Clin Electroencephalogr* 1973;4:117–25.
161. Cullen D. *Columbine*. New York: Hachette, 2009.
162. Roy L. *No Right to Remain Silent: The Tragedy at Virginia Tech*. New York: Three Rivers Press, 2009.
163. Humphreys P, Rundle G, Tietze T, eds. *On Utøya: Anders Breivik, Right Terror, Racism and Europe*. Elguta Press, 2011.
164. Larson E. *Devil in the White City*. New York: Crowne (Random House), 2003.
165. Davis DA. *The Jeffrey Dahmer Story: An American Nightmare*. New York: Macmillan, 1991.
166. Sullivan T, Maiken P. *Killer Clown: The John Gacy Murders*. New York: Pinnacle Books (Windsor Publishing Co.), 1983.
167. Michaud SG, Aynesworth H. *The Only Living Witness: The True Story of Serial Sex Killer Ted Bundy*. Irving, TX: Authorlink Press, 1999.
168. Kelly AM, Montane D. *I Would Find a Girl Walking*. New York: Berkeley-Penguin, 2011.
169. Stoerig P. Blindsight, conscious vision, and the role of primary visual cortex. *Prog Brain Res* 2006;155:217–34.
170. Goodwin J. Disorders of higher cortical visual function. *Curr Neurol Neurosci Rep* 2002;2:418–22.
171. Geschwind N. Current concepts: Aphasia. *N Engl J Med* 1971;284:654–6.
172. McNeil MR. Current concepts in adult aphasia. *Int Rehabil Med* 1984;6:128–34.
173. Albert ML, Helm-Estabrooks N. Diagnosis and treatment of aphasia. Part I. *JAMA* 1988;259:1043–7.
174. Watson RT, Heilman KM. Thalamic neglect. *Neurology* 1979;29:690–4.
175. Trojano L, Labruna L, Grossi D. An experimental investigation of the automatic/voluntary dissociation in limb apraxia. *Brain Cogn* 2007;65:169–76.
176. McGeoch PD, Brang D, Ramachandran VS. Apraxia, metaphor and mirror neurons. *Med Hypotheses* 2007;69:1165–8.

177. Keane JR. Automobile accidents caused by unsuspected neurological disease. *J Neurosurg* 1973;38:581–3.
178. Lindenberg R, Walsh FB, Sacks JG. *Neuropathology of Vision: An Atlas*. Philadelphia: Lea & Febiger, 1973.
179. Spehlmann R, Gross RA, Ho SU, Leestma JE, Norcross KA. Visual evoked potentials and postmortem findings in a case of cortical blindness. *Ann Neurol* 1977;2:531–4.
180. Plum F, Posner JB. *The Diagnosis of Stupor and Coma*. Philadelphia: F.A. Davis, 1982.
181. Al-Wardi DAM, Adams AH, Hamilton A. Four cases of "locked in" syndrome and review of literature. *Bull LA Neurol Soc* 1975;40:60–70.
182. Crosby EC, Humphrey T, Lauer EW, eds. *Correlative Anatomy of the Nervous System*. New York: Macmillan, 1962.
183. Young GB, Ropper AH, Bolton CF, eds. *Coma and Impaired Consciousness: A Clinical Perspective*. New York: McGraw-Hill, 1998.
184. Hoyumpa AM Jr, Schenker S. Perspectives in hepatic encephalopathy. *J Lab Clin Med* 1982; 100:477–87.
185. Jennett B. Thirty years of the vegetative state: Clinical, ethical and legal problems. *Prog Brain Res* 2005;150:537.
186. Walker AE, Diamond EL, Moseley J. The neuropathological findings in irreversible coma: A critique of the "respirator." *J Neuropathol Exp Neurol* 1975;34:295–323.
187. Wijdicks EFM, ed. *Brain Death*. Philadelphia: Lippincott Williams & Wilkins, 2001.
188. Wijdicks EF. Minimally conscious state vs. persistent vegetative state: The case of Terry (Wallis) vs. the case of Terri (Schiavo). *Mayo Clin Proc* 2006;81:1155–8.
189. Mappes TA. Persistent vegetative state, prospective thinking, and advance directives. *Kennedy Inst Ethics J* 2003;13:119–39.
190. Owen AM, Coleman MR, Boly M, Davis MH, Laureys S, Pickard JD. Using functional magnetic resonance imaging to detect covert awareness in the vegetative state. *Arch Neurol* 2007; 64:1098–102.
191. Machado C, Korein J, Aubert E, Bosch J, Alvarez MA, Rodriguez R, Valdes P, Portela L, Garcia M, Pérez N et al. Recognizing a mother's voice in the persistent vegetative state. *Clin EEG Neurosci* 2007;38:124–6.
192. Sara M, Sacco S, Cipolla F, Onorati P, Scoppetta C, Albertini G, Carolei A. An unexpected recovery from permanent vegetative state. *Brain Inj* 2007;21:101–3.
193. Taylor CM, Aird VH, Tate RL, Lammi MH. Sequence of recovery during the course of emergence from the minimally conscious state. *Arch Phys Med Rehabil* 2007;88:521–5.
194. Hughes J, Cayaffa J, Leestma J, Mizuno Y. Alternating "waking" and "sleep" EEG patterns in a deeply comatose patient. *Clin Electroencephalogr* 1972;3:86–93.
195. Hughes JR. Limitations of the EEG in coma and brain death. *Ann NY Acad Sci* 1978;315:121–36.
196. Kinney HC, Korein J, Panigrahy A, Dikkes P, Goode R. Neuropathological findings in the brain of Karen Ann Quinlan: The role of the thalamus in the persistent vegetative state. *N Engl J Med* 1994;330:1469–75.
197. Marks TC. A dissenting opinion, *Bush v. Schiavo*, 885 So. 2d 321 (Fla. 2004). *Stetson Law Rev* 2005;35:195–205.
198. Kollas CD, Boyer-Kollas B. Closing the Schiavo case: An analysis of legal reasoning. *J Palliat Med* 2006;9:1145–63.
199. Abrams D. *The Abrams Report*. MSNBC, 2005.
200. Cerminara KL. Theresa Marie Schiavo's long road to peace. *Death Stud* 2006;30:101–12.
201. Ruttenber AJ, McAnally HB, Wetli CV. Cocaine-associated rhabdomyolysis and excited delirium: Different stages of the same syndrome. *Am J Forensic Med Pathol* 1999;20(2):120–7.
202. Mack DR, Barbarello-Andrews L, Liu MT. Agitated delirium associated with therapeutic doses of sustained-release bupropion. *Int J Clin Pharm* 2012;34(1):9–12.
203. Dimsdale JE. Emotional causes of sudden death. *Am J Psychiatry* 1977;134:1361–6.

204. Reay DT, Fligner CL, Stilwell AD, Arnold J. Positional asphyxia during law enforcement transport. *Am J Foren Med Pathol* 1992;13:90–7.
205. Stratton SJ, Rogers C, Green K. Sudden death in individuals in hobble restraints during paramedic transport. *Ann Emerg Med* 1995;25:710–2.
206. Stratton SJ, Rogers C, Brickett K, Gruzinski G. Factors associated with sudden death of individuals requiring restraint for excited delirium. *Am J Emerg Med* 2001;19:187–91.
207. O'Halloran RL, Lewman LV. Restraint asphyxiation in excited delirium. *Am J Foren Med Pathol* 1993;14:289–95.
208. Chan TC, Vilke GM, Neuman T, Clausen JL. Restraint position and positional asphyxia. *Ann Emerg Med* 1997;30:578–86.
209. Sauvageau A, Laharpe R, King D, Dowling G, Andrews S, Kelly S, Ambrosi C, Guay JP, Geberth VJ; Working Group on Human Asphyxia. Agonal sequences in 14 filmed hangings with comments on the role of the type of suspension, ischemic habituation, and ethanol intoxication on the timing of agonal responses. *Am J Forensic Med Pathol* 2011;32(2):104–7.
210. Sauvageau A, Ambrosi C, Kelly S. Three nonlethal ligature strangulations filmed by an autoerotic practitioner: Comparison of early agonal responses in strangulation by ligature, hanging, and manual strangulation. *Am J Forensic Med Pathol* 2012;33:339–40.
211. Chan TC, Vilke GM, Neuman T. Reexamination of custody restraint position and positional asphyxia. *Am J Foren Med Pathol* 1998;19:201–5.
212. Chan TC, Neuman T, Clausen J, Eisele J, Vilke GM. Weight force during prone restraint and respiratory function. *Am J Foren Med Pathol* 2004;25:185–9.
213. Ranson SW, Clark SL. *The Anatomy of the Nervous System: Its Development and Function*, 8th ed. Philadelphia: Saunders, 1948, pp. 341–345.
214. Brodal A. The reticular formation and some related nuclei. In Brodal A, ed., *Neurological Anatomy*, 3rd ed. New York: Oxford University Press, 1981, pp. 394–447.
215. Alheid GF, McCrimmon DR. The chemical neuroanatomy of breathing. *Respir Physiol Neurobiol* 2008;164(1–2):3–11.
216. Petrovicky P. The nucleus Kölliker–Fuse (K-F) and parabrachial complex (PNBC) in man: Location, cytoarchitectonics and terminology in embryonic and adult periods, and comparison with other animals. *J Hirnforschung* 1989;30:551–63.
217. Yokota S, Tsumori T, Ono K, Yasui Y. Glutamatergic pathways from the Kölliker–Fuse nucleus to the phrenic nucleus in the rat. *Brain Res* 2004;995(1):118–30.
218. Olszewski J, Baxter D. *Cytoarchitecture of the Human Brain Stem*. Philadelphia: Lippincott, 1954.
219. Smith JC, Abdala AP, Rybak IA, Paton JF. Structural and functional architecture of respiratory networks in the mammalian brainstem. *Philos Trans R Soc Lond B Biol Sci* 2009;364(1529):2577–87.
220. Darnall RA. The role of CO(2) and central chemoreception in the control of breathing in the fetus and the neonate. *Respir Physiol Neurobiol* 2010;173(3):201–12.
221. Guyenet PG, Bayliss DA, Stornetta RL, Fortuna MG, Abbott SB, DePuy SD. Retrotrapezoid nucleus, respiratory chemosensitivity and breathing automaticity. *Respir Physiol Neurobiol* 2009; 168(1–2):59–68.
222. Guyenet PG, Stornetta RL, Bayliss DA. Central respiratory chemoreception. *J Comp Neurol* 2010;518(19):3883–906.
223. Mulkey DK, Wenker IC. Astrocyte chemoreceptors: Mechanisms of H+ sensing by astrocytes in the retrotrapezoid nucleus and their possible contribution to respiratory drive. *Exp Physiol* 2011;96(4):400–6.
224. Nattie E. Julius H. Comroe, Jr., distinguished lecture: Central chemoreception: Then and now. *J Appl Physiol* 2011;110(1):1–8.
225. Beaton L, Magoun H. Localization of the medullary respiratory centers in the monkey. *Am J Physiol* 1941;134(177):185.
226. Baumgarten R, Aranda Coddou L. Distribucion de las aferencias cardiovasculares y respiratorias en las raices bubares del nervio vago. *Acta Neurol Lat Am* 1959;5:267–78.

227. Pinna GD, Robbi E, La Rovere MT, Maestri R. A hybrid approach for continuous detection of sleep-wakefulness fluctuations: Validation in patients with Cheyne–Stokes respiration. *J Sleep Res* 2012;21(3):342–51.
228. Naughton MT. Cheyne–Stokes respiration: Friend or foe? *Thorax* 2012;67(4):357–60.
229. Tarulli AW, Lim C, Bui JD, Saper CB, Alexander MP. Central neurogenic hyperventilation: A case report and discussion of pathophysiology. *Arch Neurol* 2005;62(10):1632–4.
230. Van Wamelen DJ, Hama-Amin AD, Gilhuis HJ, De Bruijn SF. Central neurogenic hyperventilation due to pontine glioma. *Neurol India* 2011;59(5):782–3.
231. St. John WM. Rostral medullary respiratory neuronal activities of decerebrate cats in eupnea, apneusis and gasping. *Respir Physiol* 1999;116(1):47–65.
232. Morrison SF, Cravo SL, Wilfehrt HM. Pontine lesions produce apneusis in the rat. *Brain Res* 1994;652(1):83–6.
233. Saito Y. Reflections on the brainstem dysfunction in neurologically disabled children. *Brain Dev* 2009;31(7):529–36.
234. Ebert D, Hefter H, Dohle C, Freund HJ. Ataxic breathing during alternating forearm movements of various frequencies in cerebellar patients. *Neurosci Lett* 1995;193(3):145–8.
235. Chen ML, Keens TG. Congenital central hypoventilation syndrome: Not just another rare disorder. *Paediatr Respir Rev* 2004;5(3):182–9.
236. Rand CM, Yu M, Jennings LJ, Panesar K, Berry-Kravis EM, Zhou L, Weese-Mayer DE. Germline mosaicism of PHOX2B mutation accounts for familial recurrence of congenital central hypoventilation syndrome (CCHS). *Am J Med Genet* 2012;158A:2297–301.
237. Zinka B, Buettner A, Graw M. Leigh's disease: The acute clinical course of a two-year-old child with subacute necrotizing encephalomyelopathy. *Case Report Med* 2010;2010:986302.
238. Vincent JL. Acute kidney injury, acute lung injury and septic shock: How does mortality compare? *Contrib Nephrol* 2011;174:71–7.

Index

Page numbers followed by f and t indicate figures and tables, respectively.

C

D

F

G

M

O

P

W

Y

Z